Dietary Reference Intakes: Recommended Intakes for Individuals: Minerals

Life Stage Group	Calcium (mg/d)	Chromium (µg/d)	Copper (µg/d)	Fluoride (mg/d)	Iodine (µg/d)	Iron (mg/d)	Magnesium (mg/d)	Manganese (mg/d)	Molybdenum (µg/d)	Phosphorus (mg/d)	Selenium (µg/d)	Zinc (mg/d)
Infants												
0–6 mo	210°	0.2°	200°	0.01°	110°	0.27°	30°	0.003°	2°	100°	15°	2°
7–12 mo	270°	5.5°	220°	0.5°	130°	11	75°	0.6°	3°	275°	20°	3
Children												
1–3 y	500°	11°	340	0.7°	90	7	80	1.2°	17	460	20	3
4–8 y	800°	15°	440	1°	90	10	130	1.5°	22	500	30	5
Males												
9–13 y	1,300°	25°	700	2°	120	8	240	1.9°	34	1,250	40	8
14–18 y	1,300°	35°	890	3°	150	11	410	2.2°	43	1,250	55	11
19–30 y	1,000°	35°	900	4°	150	8	400	2.3°	45	700	55	11
31–50 y	1,000°	35°	900	4°	150	8	420	2.3°	45	700	55	11
51–70 y	1,200°	30°	900	4°	150	8	420	2.3°	45	700	55	11
> 70 y	1,200°	30°	900	4°	150	8	420	2.3°	45	700	55	11
Females												
9–13 y	1,300°	21°	700	2°	120	8	240	1.6°	34	1,250	40	8
14–18 y	1,300°	24°	890	3°	150	15	360	1.6°	43	1,250	55	9
19–30 y	1,000°	25°	900	3°	150	18	310	1.8°	45	700	55	8
31–50 y	1,000°	25°	900	3°	150	18	320	1.8°	45	700	55	8
51–70 y	1,200°	20°	900	3°	150	8	320	1.8°	45	700	55	8
> 70 y	1,200°	20°	900	3°	150	8	320	1.8°	45	700	55	8
Pregnancy												
≤ 18 y	1,300°	29°	1,000	3°	220	27	400	2.0°	50	1,250	60	13
19–30 y	1,000°	30°	1,000	3°	220	27	350	2.0°	50	700	60	11
31–50 y	1,000°	30°	1,000	3°	220	27	360	2.0°	50	700	60	11
Lactation												
≤ 18 y	1,300°	44°	1,300	3°	290	10	360	2.6°	50	1,250	70	14
19–30 y	1,000°	45°	1,300	3°	290	9	310	2.6°	50	700	70	12
31–50 y	1,000°	45°	1,300	3°	290	9	320	2.6°	50	700	70	12

NOTE: This table presents Recommended Dietary Allowances (RDAs) in bold type and Adequate Intakes (AIs) in ordinary type followed by an asterisk (°). RDAs and AIs may both be used as goals for individual intake. RDAs are set to meet the needs of almost all (97 to 98%) individuals in a group. For healthy breast-fed infants, the AI is the mean intake. The AI for other life stage and gender groups is believed to cover needs of all individuals in the group, but lack of data or uncertainty in the data prevent being able to specify with confidence the percentage of individuals covered by this intake.

Source: Trumbo, P., Schlicker, S., and Poos, M. Dietary Reference Intakes: vitamin A, vitamin K, arsenic, boron, chromium, copper, iodine, manganese, molybdenum, nickel, silicon, vanadium, and zinc. *J. Am. Diet. Assoc.* 101:294–301, 2001.

NUTRITION

SCIENCE AND APPLICATIONS

Fourth Edition

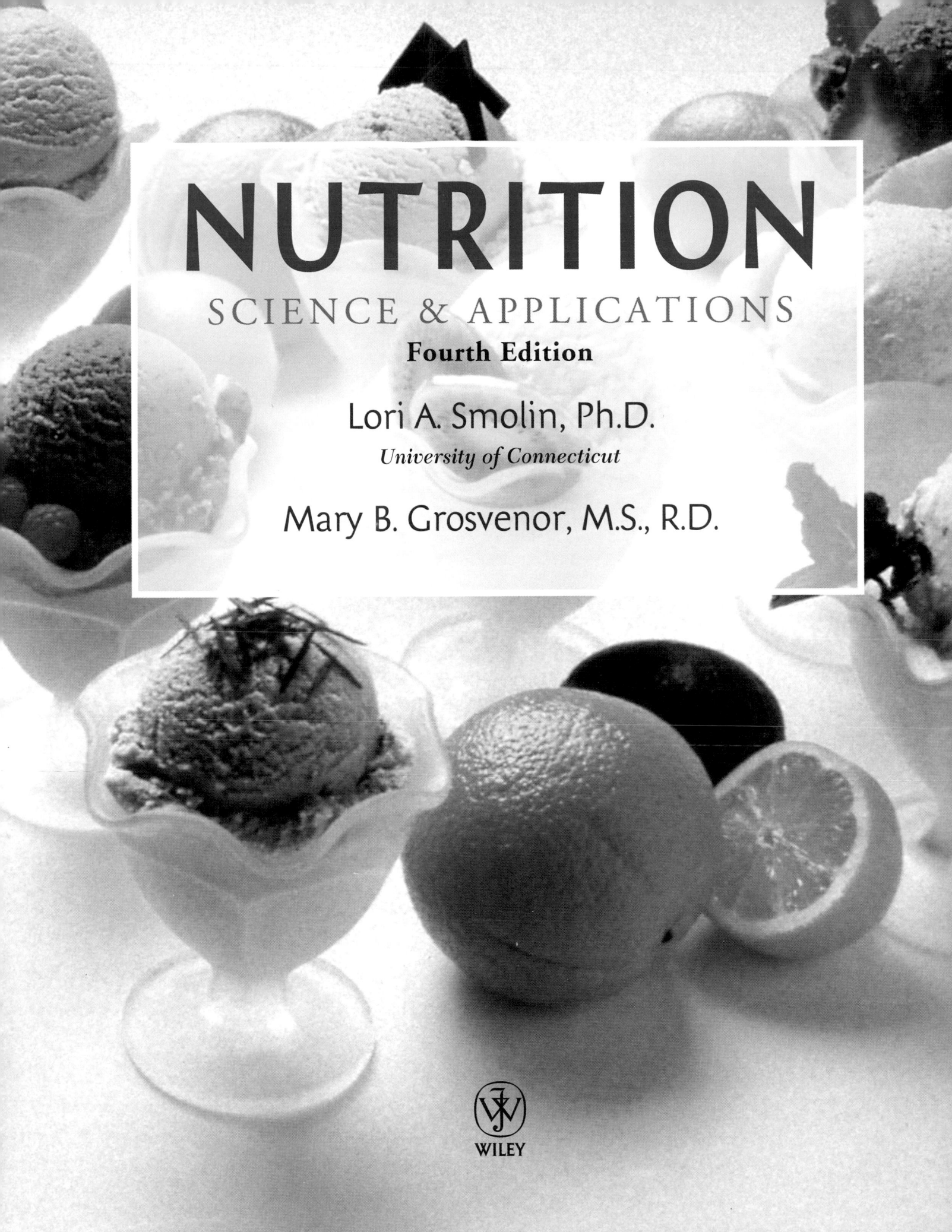

NUTRITION
SCIENCE & APPLICATIONS
Fourth Edition

Lori A. Smolin, Ph.D.
University of Connecticut

Mary B. Grosvenor, M.S., R.D.

WILEY

To our sons, Zachary and Max and David and John.
Their view of the world helps us to keep life in perspective.

To our husbands, David Knecht and Peter Ambrose,
who have given their support, patience, and understanding
over the years as well as their expertise as
computer and literary consultants.

Executive Editor	Bonnie Roesch
Associate Director of Development	Johnna Barto
Marketing Manager	Clay Stone
Production Editor	Barbara Russiello
Senior Designer	Dawn Stanley
Illustration Editor	Anna Melhorn
Photo Editor	Hilary Newman
Photo Researcher	Elyse Rieder
Cover Design	David Levy
Cover Photo	© Tom DeSanto/Stock Food America

This book was set in 10/12 New Caledonia by UG / GGS Information Services, Inc. and printed and bound by Von Hoffman Press, Inc. The cover was printed by Von Hoffman Press.

This book is printed on acid free paper. ∞

To order books or for customer service please, call 1(800)-CALL-WILEY (225-5945).

ISBN 0-471-26879-8

Printed in the United States of America

10 9 8 7 6 5 4 3

About the Authors

Lori A. Smolin, Ph.D.   Lori Smolin received her B.S. degree from Cornell University, where she studied human nutrition and food science. She received her doctorate from the University of Wisconsin at Madison. Her doctoral research focused on B vitamins, homocysteine accumulation, and genetic defects in homocysteine metabolism. She completed postdoctoral training both at the Harbor–UCLA Medical Center, where she studied human obesity, and at the University of California at San Diego, where she studied genetic defects in amino acid metabolism. She has published in these areas in peer-reviewed journals. Dr. Smolin is currently at the University of Connecticut, where she teaches both in the Department of Nutritional Sciences and in the Department of Molecular and Cell Biology. Courses she has taught include introductory nutrition, lifecycle nutrition, food preparation, nutritional biochemistry, general biochemistry, and biology. Dr. Smolin spent the 2001/2002 academic year in England where she was able to experience the food and nutrition culture on the other side of the Atlantic.

Mary B. Grosvenor, M.S., R.D.   Mary Grosvenor received her B.A. degree in English from Georgetown University and her M.S. in Nutrition Science from the University of California at Davis. She is a registered dietitian who worked for many years managing nutrition research studies at the General Clinical Research Center at Harbor–UCLA Medical Center. She has published in peer-reviewed journals in the areas of nutrition and cancer and methods of assessing dietary intake. She has taught introductory nutrition at the community college level and currently lives with her family in a small town in Colorado. She is continuing her teaching and writing career and is still involved in nutrition research via the electronic superhighway.

Preface

Life is full of choices. Whether you choose plain vanilla ice cream, orange sorbet, or a fresh orange depends on many factors, including nutrition. How this choice affects your nutritional health depends on the other choices you make. This text conveys to students that each dietary choice makes up only one part of the total diet. So, no one choice is a bad one as long as the sum of food choices over a period of days or weeks makes up a healthy overall diet. Knowing how to make wise choices is the key to applying nutritional principles. The Fourth Edition of *Nutrition: Science and Applications* continues with and expands upon the theme of choice that was used in the previous editions.

The goal of the authors is to provide a text that teaches students both the basic principles of nutrition science and how to apply them to choices about the foods they eat and the nutrition information they encounter. Students frequently ask: Is this food good for me or bad for me? Should I be eating a lowfat diet? Should I take a protein supplement to improve my athletic performance? Are herbal supplements safe? How can I lose 10 pounds? The answers to all these questions involve choices. And it is these personal concerns that trigger student interest in nutrition. When introductory nutrition classes and textbooks present the basics—What is carbohydrate? Protein? Fat?—but fail to prepare students to make choices about foods and popular nutrition issues, it is difficult for students to apply what they have learned to their daily lives. *Nutrition: Science and Applications* presents a complete introduction to the science of nutrition while at the same time teaching students how to use a scientific approach in making decisions about the nutrition-related choices they face every day.

Approach

A scientific approach is employed throughout the text. The goal is to teach students how to apply the logic of science to their own nutrition concerns. We present the process of scientific inquiry and demonstrate how it is used to evaluate the role of nutrition in health. The text contains all of the information students need to analyze and modify their own diets to promote health and to reduce the risk of deficiencies and chronic diseases related to nutrition.

Several themes are used throughout the book to provide a broad view of both the science of nutrition and its applications. These include

(1) An emphasis on the importance of the total diet, not just individual nutrients or food choices

(2) Attention to health promotion and disease prevention

(3) A focus on the methods of science to provide students with the tools needed to make healthy food and nutrition decisions

(4) An emphasis on critical thinking, which guides students through the thought processes necessary to make nutrition decisions

(5) A broad cultural view of our ethnically diverse population and food supply.

The Fourth Edition continues the integrated approach that was so successful in previous editions. Health and disease, metabolism, cultural diversity, and life-stage topics are incorporated into each chapter. For example, the relationship of dietary fat intake, lipid metabolism and transport, and heart disease is discussed in the lipids chapter. How this information applies to young children, pregnant women, and older adults is also presented. This integration engages students early on because it presents the topics of greatest interest to them, such as the role of nutrition in health and disease, along with basic nutrition principles. Students are then more motivated to learn the basics and are prepared to apply them to their personal health and nutrition.

Continuing and New Features of the Fourth Edition

The Fourth Edition continues with, enhances, and adds to the features of earlier editions. These features help to emphasize the importance of the total dietary pattern as well as individual nutrients in health and disease. They also support the scientific approach used throughout the text, encourage the students to learn and use critical thinking skills, and enhance the educational effectiveness and visual appeal of the book.

The Total Diet The more science discovers about nutrition, the more clear it becomes that it is not a single food or nutrient that determines our nutritional health. Rather it is the total diet, including the overall combination of nutrients, foods, and other health-promoting substances, that determines nutritional status. This concept is highlighted by chapter sections that address the role of a nutrient as one part of the total diet. These sections stress the importance of a diet based on whole grains, fruits, and vegetables and the importance of meeting nutrient needs with a variety of foods. This type of diet provides a variety of nonnutrient substances such as phytochemicals that are also important to health and are lacking when people rely on vitamin and mineral supplements, rather then foods, to meet their nutrient needs. Several of the Critical Thinking exercises help illustrate that each dietary choice we make affects more than one nutrient in the diet. This focus on the importance of the diet as a whole rather than on single foods or nutrients helps students understand that one choice does not make or break a diet.

New: Dietary Reference Intakes (DRIs) for Energy, Carbohydrates, Fiber, Fat, Protein, and Amino Acids This text incorporates the new DRI recommendations for energy and the macronutrients, which were released in September 2002. These new DRIs emphasize that carbohydrate, fat, and protein all serve as energy sources in the diet and must therefore be considered together. Acceptable Macronutrient Distribution Ranges (AMDR) of 45 to 65% of energy from carbohydrate, 20 to 35% from fat, and 10 to 35% from protein have been recommended. Adequate Intakes have been established for fiber and essential fatty acids; RDAs have been set for dietary carbohydrate and protein; Estimated Energy Requirements have been developed for four different activity levels; and new physical activity recommendations have been presented. The DRIs for nutrients involved in bone formation (calcium, phosphorus, magnesium, vitamin D, and flouride), for B vitamins and choline, for antioxidants (vitamin C, vitamin E, selenium, and carotenoids), and for vitamins A and K and the trace elements are also included in this text and updates will be provided throughout the life of this edition for DRI sets that have not yet been completed.

New: A Separate Chapter on Meeting Nutrient Needs with Food, Fortified Foods, and Dietary Supplements The modern food supply offers a variety of ways to meet nutrient needs. For many people, a well-planned diet made up of minimally processed foods can provide all their nutrient needs. For others, supplemental sources (that is, fortified foods and dietary supplements) may be desired or required to meet needs. For the first time, government recommendations on nutrient needs, the Dietary Reference Intakes, have recognized that these products may be the best way for certain life-stage groups to meet their needs. However, the increase in the availability of these products has also opened the door for toxicity. Even those who do not take supplements may consume more than the recommended amounts of certain nutrients in fortified products such as breakfast cereals and beverages. To address these issues, this edition has included a new chapter (12) that discusses the benefits and drawbacks of meeting needs with foods, fortified foods, and supplements as well as the role of many supplements that are not nutrients, including herbal supplements. A text that does not address this topic invites students to seek information from less reliable sources. Discussions of many popular dietary supplements are also integrated throughout the text with information

about individual nutrients and topics such as weight loss, exercise, and aging.

Staying Abreast of New Information The Fourth Edition continues to provide up-to-date coverage of the most recent advances in nutrition science, such as the relationship between genetics and body weight regulation, the ecological impact of genetically modified foods and organic food production, and the nutritional and health impact of phytochemicals and dietary supplements. The text is well referenced with the majority of references from the last five years. The authors would be happy to provide sources for information that is not referenced in the text. Recent public health messages are also included. For example, the Dietary Guidelines for Americans, 2000 are covered thoroughly in Chapter 2 and highlighted throughout the text. When one or more of the recommendations of the Dietary Guidelines applies to the topic being addressed, a graphic depicting these guidelines appears.

Easy-to-Understand Metabolism Information Metabolism is one of the most challenging topics for nutrition students. To prevent students from being overwhelmed, this text integrates coverage of metabolism with discussions of each of the macronutrients rather then concentrating it into one long chapter. This approach allows information on metabolism to build on and reinforce what was learned in the previous chapter. For example, the information on fat metabolism in Chapter 5 builds on the presentation of carbohydrates in Chapter 4. Chapter 7 integrates all of the information on energy production. Chapters 8 through 11 discuss the role of micronutrients in metabolism, and Chapter 13 provides an overview and review by applying this knowledge to a discussion of fitness and the exercising body.

Environmental Issues Discussions of environmental issues are included because they can have an impact on the nutrient composition of foods as well as on food choices. For example, the amounts of certain nutrients in a food, such as iodine and selenium, depend on the environmental conditions where that food is produced. In addition, the foods we choose are often affected by our concern for the environment. This is discussed in depth in Chapters 17 and 18 where the impact of food production on the environment and the benefits and risks of organic food production and genetically modified foods are discussed.

Ethnic Diversity This text uses statistics and examples to reflect the broad cultural base of a diverse student population. Incorporating ethnic foods in text examples and in Critical Thinking exercises throughout make the book more relevant for this audience. In addition, these examples expose students to the foods and eating patterns of other cultures. Differences in the disease risks of various ethnic groups in relation to their genetic makeup and their native diets are also addressed.

Concise, Easy-to-Read Style As the field of nutrition progresses, more and more information becomes available and textbooks get longer and longer. To help instructors and students cover the important and interesting aspects of macronutrients and micronutrients, the length of the Fourth Edition has been kept in check. The writing style is concise, consistent, engaging, and easy to read. The organization from chapter to chapter is uniform, each chapter starting with a "friendly" or familiar topic to capture students' interest. Throughout the book, similar illustration designs—such as those depicting the metabolism of carbohydrate, fat, and protein; the nutrient content of foods; and the recommendations of the Dietary Guidelines—help students identify analogous information and reinforce and build upon knowledge acquired in previous sections. Colors are also used consistently to represent carbohydrate, fat, and protein and to identify certain steps in metabolism.

Critical Thinking Exercises These unique exercises appear in each chapter. They use case histories to introduce a nutritional problem and then guide students through the logical thought processes involved in solving the problem. Some questions are answered to provide a model for students, and others require students to critically think through the answers themselves (solutions are included in the Appendices). The Critical Thinking exercises also provide a guide for students to use when answering Applications questions at the end of the chapter. In the Fourth Edition many Critical Thinking exercises have been revised to improve clarity and reflect changes in the field.

Off the Shelf These boxed features discuss issues that relate to items that can be obtained off the shelves of stores, such as foods, books, and supplements. They focus on consumer issues and choices and on evaluating nutrition information. Off the Shelf discussions are a unique aspect of this text, briefly highlighting topics of special interest that deserve more explanation. They can be read separately or in conjunction with the body of the text. In the Fourth Edition, new boxes have been added and old ones updated to reflect new information relating to the topic being discussed.

Off the Label These features present in-depth information on food labels as they apply to specific nutrients or issues. The most up-to-date information is included. For example, in Chapter 3 the box "Antacids: Getting the Drug Facts" points out that taking medications can add nutrients to the diet and explains how the drug facts label can be used to assess the nutrient contribution made by a medication. Other new Off the Label boxes show how to use labels to get enough calcium in your diet and how to understand the information about micronutrients that is given on the label.

Life Stage Icons In each chapter, life stage icons highlight issues and recommendations that apply to specific stages and circumstances of life. This information helps students understand how nutrient requirements are affected by one's life stage as well as offering information relevant to students in all phases of life. These topics are also covered in depth in separate chapters (14, 15 ,16).

The Fourth Edition, Chapter-by-Chapter

The text includes five parts. The first part, "Nutrition: Sorting Fact from Fantasy," introduces the reader to the basic concepts of nutrition, the scientific method, and the principles of digestion and absorption necessary to understand issues presented throughout the book. The second part, "Energy-Yielding Nutrients," includes chapters on carbohydrates, lipids, and proteins, as well as a chapter that covers energy balance, weight control, and eating disorders. The third part, "Water and the Micronutrients," examines the non-energy-yielding nutrients: water, vitamins, and minerals as well as supplemental sources of nutrients. The fourth part, "Applying Nutrition to Life," applies the basics of nutrition to different lifestyle issues and stages of development. The final part, "Nutrition in Today's World," addresses food safety and discusses issues related to malnutrition in North America and the world. The material is presented in a consistent and logical order, but the chapters and sections can be taught in any order.

Chapter 1, "Nutrition: Everyday Choices," provides an overview of the nutrients and their roles in the body, and introduces the scientific method. Chapter 1 also teaches students how to sort accurate from inaccurate nutrition information. A mock ad featuring a protein supplement for athletes is used to help students learn how to interpret nutrition information from many sources.

Chapter 2, "Applying the Science of Nutrition," shows how the results of scientific studies are used to develop dietary standards and guidelines. The Dietary Reference Intakes (DRIs) are introduced here, and tools for diet planning, including the Food Guide Pyramid, Exchange Lists, and food labels, are presented so that students can begin applying them to their own diets. The Dietary Guidelines for Americans, 2000 are discussed and help tie together other recommendations and guidelines. The final section of this chapter discusses how these and other tools can be used to assess the nutritional health of populations and individuals. Information from the most up-to-date surveys (NHANES IV) and programs (Healthy People 2010) is provided here and throughout the text. The Critical Thinking exercises in this chapter demonstrate how to plan diets using the Food Guide Pyramid and how nutritional assessment can be used to identify nutrition-related health problems.

Chapter 3, "The Human Body: From Meals to Molecules," presents digestion and absorption by showing how a particular meal is digested, its nutrients absorbed into the body and transported to the cells where metabolism occurs, and finally how wastes are removed. A new Off the Label box discusses the potential nutritional impact of over the counter medications.

Chapters 4, 5, and 6 discuss carbohydrates, lipids, and proteins, respectively. Each begins with information about the types of foods that contain these nutrients, followed by a discussion of their basic structures. Key points about the digestion and absorption of these nutrients are followed by a section addressing their role in the body. In each chapter, energy production is summarized using a figure that illustrates how the metabolism of each nutrient interfaces with that of others. A separate section on health and disease is followed by a section that discusses the role of each individual nutrient as one part of the total diet. Nutrient requirements and how they vary through life, as well as how to make dietary choices to meet recommendations, are presented. To teach students how to select a healthy diet, the recommendations of the DRIs and Dietary Guidelines are integrated with the information provided by food labels and the Food Guide Pyramid.

In Chapter 4 information on diabetes has been updated and expanded to provide students with a better understanding of the long-term consequences of this growing public health problem. The DRI recommendations, including the RDA and Acceptable Macronutrient Distribution Range (AMDR) for carbohydrate intake and the AI fiber, are presented and discussed. Chapter 5 has been updated to reflect the new DRI recommendations and the most recent recommendations regarding blood cholesterol levels. Improvements and additions to the art program help students to better understand lipid structure, digestion, absorption, and metabolism. In Chapter 6, the discussion of protein synthesis and gene expression has been strengthened, and intake recommendations have been updated to reflect the new DRIs. A new vegetarian Food Guide Pyramid has been added, and information on the potential health benefits of soy protein has been updated.

Chapter 7, "Energy Balance and Weight Management," presents the concept of energy balance and applies it to weight management. This chapter includes the new DRI Estimated Energy Requirements (EERs), which are based on physical activity levels. The presentation of obesity reflects the newer view that it is a disease that should be treated using an individualized plan that includes diet, exercise, behavior modification, and, when appropriate, medication. Information on assessing body weight using body mass index (BMI) has been updated to include the recommendations of the Dietary Guidelines for Americans, 2000. Updated information is also included on how body weight is regulated and the role of genetic versus environmental factors in determining body fatness. A new Off the Shelf feature discusses the risks of using weight-loss supplements called fat burners. The health risks of too much or too little body fat as well as of eating disorders are addressed.

Chapter 8, "The Water-Soluble Vitamins," begins with a general overview of vitamins—where they are found in the diet, factors affecting bioavailability, and how they function. Each of the B vitamins and vitamin C are discussed individually, but the B vitamins are grouped according to common roles as coenzymes in energy production, amino acid metabolism, and cell division. Discussions of each of the water-soluble vitamins include sources in the diet, func-

tions in the body, impact on health, recommended intakes, supplement use, and potential for toxicity. This chapter also discusses choline, a substance that is not currently classified as a vitamin but one for which DRIs have been established. Improved line art helps identify Food Guide Pyramid Groups that are good sources of these vitamins and point out functional relationships among the B vitamins. The section on vitamin C includes an expanded discussion of the role of antioxidants in protecting the body from damage.

Chapter 9, "The Fat-Soluble Vitamins," presents each of the fat-soluble vitamins and discusses sources in the diet, functions in the body, impact on health, recommended intakes, supplement use, and potential for toxicity. A discussion (with line art) of how vitamins A and D act by affecting gene expression is presented in this chapter.

Chapter 10, "The Internal Sea: Water and the Major Minerals," presents information on where these nutrients are found and discusses their function in the body, their relationship to health and disease, and recommended intakes. Water is discussed first, followed by the electrolytes sodium, potassium, and chloride, which interact closely with water. Some general information about minerals is followed by a discussion of the minerals involved in bone formation—calcium, phosphorus, and magnesium. The impact of diet and lifestyle on hypertension and osteoporosis is also addressed here. Advances in our understanding of the impact of total dietary patterns on hypertension is stressed by an expanded discussion of the DASH diet, a dietary pattern that has been shown to lower blood pressure.

Chapter 11, "The Trace Minerals: Our Elemental Needs," discusses the trace elements in a format similar to that used for other micronutrients. An emphasis is placed on the unique roles of some minerals and on the similarities in function and the interactions that exist among them. Discussions of the health issues related to these nutrients help create interest, as do discussions of the pros and cons of trace element supplements. For example, the discussion of iron has been expanded to place emphasis on the problems of iron overload as well as iron deficiency, and an Off the Shelf feature on the effectiveness of zinc lozenges for treating cold symptoms has been updated.

The new Chapter 12, "Meeting Our Needs: Food, Fortified Food, and Supplements," addresses the fact that Americans today get their nutrients from fortified food and dietary supplements as well as food. This new chapter has been added to address the role that fortified foods and supplements have in the diet and the advantages and disadvantages of using these products. We emphasize the fact that food sources of nutrients also provide other substances, such as phytochemicals, which, although they are not nutrients, may have health benefits. An expanded section on dietary supplements uses a risk-benefit approach to help students evaluate all products defined as dietary supplements. We have added an Off the Shelf feature that discusses foods that have been highly fortified with micronutrients and herbs. A new Critical Thinking exercise helps students learn how to evaluate the safety and efficacy of dietary supplements.

Discussions of dietary supplements are also integrated throughout the book, with applicable topics.

Chapter 13, "Fueling Fitness: Nutrition and Exercise," is designed to emphasize the importance of fitness to nutritional health as well as to provide information on nutrition and athletic performance. This chapter includes the new DRI exercise recommendations and serves as a review of metabolism and energy production. By this point in the text, students have studied all the essential nutrients, so a complete discussion of the macronutrient and micronutrient needs for energy production can be included. An expanded discussion of ergogenic aids for more competitive athletes directs students to use a risk-benefit analysis of these products before deciding whether or not to use them. A new Off the Shelf feature discusses anabolic steroids, androstenedione, and other ergogenic hormones.

Chapter 14, "In the Beginning: Nutrition for Mothers and Infants," addresses the role of nutrition in development by discussing the nutritional needs of the mother during pregnancy and lactation as well as the nutritional needs of the infant. Current recommendations and practical information about breast and formula feeding of infants are given. The DRI recommendations for pregnancy and lactation are included.

Chapter 15, "The Growing Years: Infancy to Adolescence," begins by discussing the importance of learning healthy eating habits early in life. The chapter discusses nutrient needs from the first solid foods offered to infants to the independent choices of adolescents. Exercise recommendations and an activity pyramid for children are included. A discussion of nutrition and alcohol consumption is included in this chapter because adolescents are often faced with the important choice of whether or not to use alcohol.

Chapter 16, "Nutrition and Aging: The Adult Years," addresses how nutrition affects aging and how aging affects nutrition. It includes updated information on the interrelationships between aging and nutritional status. It discusses nutrient-drug interactions, including an expanded discussion of the risks and benefits of alcohol consumption. Also presented are nutrition programs such as the Older Americans Act and the Nutrition Screening Initiative. The chapter includes a new Critical Thinking exercise that shows how the DETERMINE checklist can be used to identify and prevent malnutrition in the elderly.

Chapter 17, "How Safe Is Our Food Supply?" discusses the risks and benefits associated with the U.S. food supply and includes information on the impact of microbial hazards, chemical toxins, food additives, irradiation, and genetically modified foods. The directives of the Food Safety Initiative are addressed, including the use of HACCP (Hazard Analysis Critical Control Point) to ensure safe food and advances in technology that help identify the sources of food-borne illness. Information on genetically modified food production and the debate surrounding its benefits and risks has been expanded. A new Off the Shelf box has been added discussing Mad Cow disease and the potential risk associated with consuming meat from affected animals.

Chapter 18, "The Global View: Feeding the World," deals with the problems of hunger and malnutrition both at home and globally. It discusses the issue of providing enough of the right kinds of food and distributing it equitably. It examines the causes of world hunger, along with potential solutions. Updated information on the status of world hunger and micronutrient deficiencies is presented. The health impact of the "Westernization" of the diet in many developing countries is discussed.

Ancillaries

This Fourth Edition of *Nutrition: Science and Applications* is accompanied by a complete set of supplementary teaching and learning materials. The materials available for *students* are as follows:

Diet Analysis Software The diet analysis software package includes values for energy and 25 nutrients for about 4000 foods. It includes a feature that allows users to add 30 foods to the database to keep pace with the ever-growing market of available products. The database has been designed to incorporate the foods mentioned throughout the text, including foods from a variety of cultures. The database includes updated folate values for all non-brand-name foods and for many brand-name items. The software includes an analysis of the diet based on the number of servings recommended by the Food Guide Pyramid.

Study Guide This guide, written by Melanie Burns of Eastern Illinois University, includes chapter outlines, multiple-choice questions, matching exercises, short-answer review questions, and a variety of learning activities designed for use by individual students and by groups in the classroom.

The teaching materials available to *instructors* include the following:

Instructor's Manual The Instructor's Manual, available online from the text Web site, is written by the authors and includes key concepts, complete chapter outlines, new Critical Thinking exercises, diet assessment forms, key terms, student self-assessment forms, and sources of other materials, including useful Web sites.

Test Bank The Test Bank, written by Kathy Beerman and Lois Jensen, both of Washington State University, includes multiple-choice and short-answer questions as well as short case studies with attendant questions that encourage students to apply what they have learned.

Overhead Transparencies This set of 100 full-color overheads helps instructors illustrate the book's more complicated concepts in the classroom.

Instructor's Resource CD-ROM for Nutrition This dual-platform presentation CD-ROM (for Macintosh and

Windows) features all of the illustrations and tables from the text in both jpeg and PowerPoint formats.

Both students and instructors will find additional resources on the text's companion Web site: www.wiley.com/college/smolin.

Acknowledgments

The authors wish to thank the many professors and students who helped in the development of this text. Their endless hours of careful reading and their many thoughtful suggestions from diverse viewpoints have helped to make this text the best available on today's market. The reviewers, who offered comments and suggestions on both the presentation and the accuracy of this information, include the following:

Beverly Benes, *University of Nebraska, Lincoln*

Debra Boardley, *University of Toledo*

Tammy Collum, *University of Northern Iowa*

Eileen L. Daniel, *SUNY, Brockport*

Roberta Durschlag, *Boston University*

Marjorie Fitch-Helgenberg, *University of Arkansas*

David Holben, *Ohio University*

Laura Kruskall, *University of Nevada, Las Vegas*

Heather Lynne, *West Valley Mission Community College*

Jennifer Ricketts, *University of Arizona*

Karen Schuster, *University of North Florida*

Paul S. Weiss, *Queensborough Community College*

Fred Wolfe, *University of Arizona*

We are grateful to the editorial and production staff at John Wiley & Sons for their help and support. We are new authors in this company, and everyone has welcomed us warmly and put forth an exceptional effort to produce this edition in a timely fashion. We thank our Acquisitions Editor Bonnie Roesch for her enthusiasm and excitement about publishing in the field of nutrition, our Development Editor Johnna Barto for managing the day-to-day and minute-to-minute problems that occur during the course of writing a book, our Associate Editor Mary O'Sullivan who carefully developed all the ancillaries, and our Marketing Manager, Clay Stone, for coordinating the advertising, marketing, and sales efforts for the book and its supplements. We also thank our Photo Editor Hilary Newman for ensuring the outstanding quality of the photos in this text, our Illustration Editor Anna Melhorn for assuring high-quality artwork, even when last minute corrections were needed, our studio, Senior Designer Dawn Stanley for delivering an attractively designed text, and our Production Editor, Barbara Russiello, for her patience and efficiency in guiding this project through production, especially considering the fact that the authors lived on different continents during the writing of this edition.

To the Student

Ice cream on the cover of a nutrition text, what were they thinking? Most nutrition texts choose to put a photo of fruits, vegetables, or grain products on the cover. These foods make up the basis of a healthy diet. We choose to put ice cream on our cover to emphasize the concept of choice—any food can be part of a healthy diet. Your diet is made up of all the food choices you make throughout the course of a day. And no one food makes or breaks a diet. If you choose ice cream, the nutrients you get are different than if you choose to eat an orange. Even the choice of fruit sorbet instead of mocha almond fudge makes a different nutrient contribution. Fresh fruit may provide more nutrients with fewer kcalories than ice cream, but ice cream can be part of a healthy diet as long as all of your choices put together provide an overall diet that promotes health, protects you from disease, and provides enjoyment. Each food and lifestyle choice you make must be balanced with other choices you have made or intend to make. Good nutrition does not mean giving up all the foods you like; it means making wise choices. To help you with nutrition choices, we have provided a text that bridges the gap between popular nutrition and nutrition science. Our goal is not to tell you, for instance, that you should or should not eat ice cream or potato chips. Instead, we have provided you with the information you need to make your own informed decisions. This text takes nutrition science out of the classroom and allows you to apply it to the choices you make about foods, dietary supplements, and other lifestyle factors important to your health.

How to Use This Book to Make Informed Choices

In order to help you understand and apply the principles of nutrition, we have designed and incorporated some very useful learning aids. From the menu of features below, you can choose which will be most helpful to you in learning, retaining, and applying the information presented in this text.

Just a Taste What do you know, or think you know? Find out by answering these questions at the beginning of each chapter. They offer a simple self-test that targets common nutrition misconceptions.

Chapter Outline What's in store? This outline of the chapter's content provides you with an overview of all the material presented in this chapter.

Chapter Concepts Need a concept check? Each chapter opens with a checklist of the concepts to be explored. These help you preview how the material will be covered. You can go back and review them once you have completed the chapter to see how well you have digested the material in the chapter.

Boldfaced Terms and Margin Definitions See an unfamiliar term? Important terms are shown in boldfaced type throughout the text. These help point out words that may be new to you. Each boldfaced term is defined in the margin for easy reference. These terms and many others are also included in the main glossary at the back of the book.

Off the Shelf Intrigued by an idea in the chapter? We have chosen some of the most common consumer choices related to products available off the shelves of stores and presented the pros and cons of selecting them. These Off the Shelf discussions will help you think more logically and scientifically about nutrition decisions in your life. They can be read separately or in conjunction with the body of the text.

Off the Label Trying to figure out which breakfast cereal is better for you? Try reading the Nutrition Facts label. Food labels provide a wealth of information on dietary recommendations and the nutritional contributions made by specific foods. Off the Label features will teach you how to choose low-kcalorie items, how to figure out how much vitamin C is in a food, and how to tell if a food is low in fat. This practical knowledge about food labels will help you choose foods wisely and know what you are choosing.

Critical Thinking You think you understand the concept? Now, try applying it. Use the Critical Thinking exercises in each chapter to see if you can apply the concepts covered. Following the thought processes outlined in these exercises can help you to better address your own nutrition concerns.

Applications Try again. These exercises at the end of each chapter give you an opportunity to apply the critical thinking skills developed in Critical Thinking exercises and the knowledge gained throughout the chapter to your own diet and lifestyle.

Art and Photography Are you a visual learner? The art was carefully developed and the photography chosen to enhance your understanding of and interest in the material discussed in the text. Use these to complement and enhance the information in the text.

On the Web Need more information? The On the Web feature offers the names and web addresses of sites where you can find additional information about topics discussed in the chapter.

Chapter Summary Have you remembered the most important concepts? A summary at the end of each chapter parallels but provides more detail about the concepts used to introduce each chapter. Use this summary of important information to review the chapter topics.

Review Questions Check your knowledge. If you can answer the review questions at the end of each chapter, you have grasped the most important concepts covered in the chapter. They are designed to review in a simple manner the key points of each chapter and to serve as a study guide.

Inside the Covers Need a quick reference? Opening the front and back covers will give you instant access to the DRI values. Tables that include the RDAs and AI values for vitamins and minerals as well as those that list the recommendations for carbohydrate, fat, protein, and energy can be found here.

Appendices We tried, but we couldn't fit everything in the text. Additional information has been put in appendices at the end of the text. These include a comprehensive food composition table containing information on energy and 25 nutrients in about 4000 foods, including fast foods and convenience foods. Other appendices include standards for nutritional indices, such as height and weight charts for infants through the elderly; normal blood values used in nutrition assessment; reliable sources of nutrition information; dietary recommendations from the United States, Canada, and the World Health Organization; recommendations for risk reduction from various special interest groups, such as the American Heart Association; the Exchange Lists; versions of the Food Guide Pyramid that reflect ethnically diverse food choices; an extensive review of food labeling guidelines; energy expenditure values; and answers to Critical Thinking exercises.

Glossary Forgot what the term means? An extensive glossary of terms is included at the end of the text to provide a quick reference for terminology with which you may be unfamiliar or for which you may need review.

Index Want to review a specific concept? The text is well indexed to allow easy cross-reference to material of interest.

We have offered plenty of choices on how to absorb and apply this material. We hope that you benefit from the variety of options while learning to apply your knowledge and enjoy a healthy diet chosen from the diversity of flavors, textures, and tastes that are available in today's food supply.

Lori Smolin
Storrs, Connecticut
Mary Grosvenor
Delta, Colorado
October 2002

Brief Contents

Contents

WATER AND THE MICRONUTRIENTS

Nutrition: Everyday Choices   Chapter 1

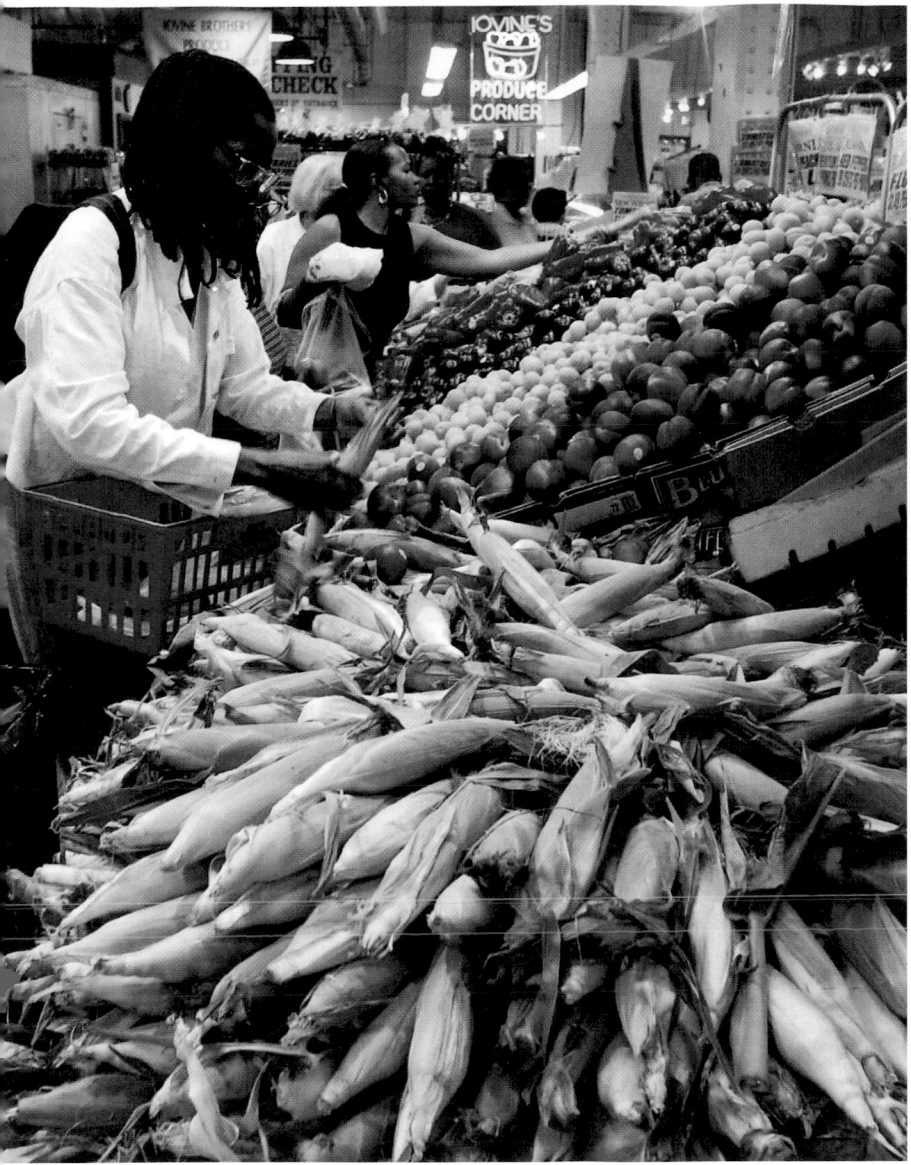

(© AP/Wide World Photos)

Chapter Outline

WHAT IS NUTRITION?
What Are Nutrients?
What Do Nutrients Do?
How Much of Each Nutrient Do We
  Need?
Effects of Poor Nutrient Intake

WHAT ARE WE CHOOSING?
How Healthy Is the American Diet?
How Do We Make Food Choices?

WHAT IS RELIABLE NUTRITION INFORMATION?
Sources of Nutrition Information
Understanding the Process of Science:
  The Scientific Method
Types of Nutrition Research Studies
Judging Nutrition Information

Chapter Concepts

✔ Nutrition studies all of the interactions of living organisms with food.

✔ Nutrients are substances found in food that provide energy, structure, and regulation for the body processes of maintenance and repair, growth, and reproduction.

✔ Nutrients must be consumed in the proper amounts and proportions to meet nutritional needs and maintain health.

✔ Any food can be part of a healthy diet as long as the overall pattern of food choices is consistent with recommendations for a healthy diet.

✔ Our food choices are based on what is available, what we like and are culturally conditioned to eat, as well as what we think we should be eating.

✔ Advances in our understanding of nutrition are made by using the scientific method.

✔ Well-conducted experiments must use quantifiable measurements, proper experimental controls, and the right experimental population and must be interpreted carefully.

✔ Many types of research are used to study relationships among diet, health, and disease.

✔ Consumers must be skeptical when evaluating nutrition information.

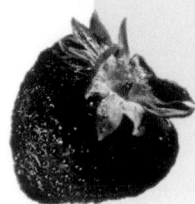

Just a Taste

Can ice cream be part of a healthy diet?

Can your food choices today affect your future health?

Which nutrition headlines should you believe?

Ice cream—cold, creamy, delicious—but is it nutritious? Should it be a part of your diet? The answer depends on the choices you make. Ice cream and other frozen desserts come in many colors, flavors, and varieties: Neapolitan, rainbow sherbet, heavenly hash, fudge swirl, frozen yogurt, sorbet, fat-free, sugar-free . . . . Each tastes different, looks different, and makes a different contribution to your total diet. None of these choices is bad, nor is the decision to include ice cream in your diet, as long as it constitutes one part of an overall healthy diet.

Whether you are deciding to have a bowl of ice cream or wondering if you should believe a news headline—the choices you make depend on who you are, what your individual goals are, and what your genetic and cultural background is. Are you an athlete? Are you planning a pregnancy, breast feeding an infant, or trying to prevent the physical decline that occurs with aging? Did your mother die of a heart attack? Does cancer run in your family? Are you trying to keep kosher, lose weight, or eat a vegetarian diet? Is your heritage Asian, African, European, Central or South American? In order to choose foods that satisfy your personal and cultural preferences but also contribute to a healthy diet and prevent chronic diseases, you must have information about what nutrients you require, what role they play in health and disease, and what foods contain them. You must also be able to judge the validity of the nutrition information you encounter. Should you be taking antioxidant supplements, eating fat-free foods, or drinking calcium-fortified orange juice? Should you believe the story you saw on the news about vitamin E and heart disease? Filtering out the worthless and understanding the worthwhile can be a mind-boggling task. It requires an understanding of the principles of nutrition; the nutrient content of foods; the interactions of nutrition, health, and disease; and how scientists study nutrition.

• WHAT IS NUTRITION?

Nutrition is a science that studies all the interactions that occur between living organisms and food. It studies the psychological, social, cultural, economic, and technological factors that influence which foods we choose to eat. The science of nutrition also studies the biological processes by which we consume food and utilize the nutrients it contains.

What Are Nutrients?

Nutrients are substances contained in food that are necessary to maintain life and allow growth and reproduction. Nutrients provide energy, contribute to structure, and regulate biological processes. To date, approximately 45 nutrients are considered essential to human life. **Essential nutrients** are those substances necessary to support life that must be supplied in the diet because they either cannot be made by the body or cannot be made in large enough quantities to meet needs. Protein, for example, is an essential nutrient needed for the growth and maintenance of body tis-

Nutrition A science that studies the interactions that occur between living organisms and food.

Nutrients Chemical substances in foods that provide energy, structure, and regulation of body processes.

Essential nutrients Nutrients that must be provided in the diet because the body either cannot make them or cannot make them in sufficient quantities to satisfy its needs.

2

sues and the synthesis of regulatory molecules. Food also contains substances classi-fied as nonessential. Some of these are not essential to sustain life but have health-promoting properties. For example, a **phytochemical** found in broccoli, called sulforaphane, is not essential but may reduce the risk of cancer. Others are required by the body but can be produced in sufficient amounts to meet needs. For example, lecithin, which is needed for nerve function, is not an essential nutrient because it can be manufactured in the body.

Chemically, there are six classes of nutrients: carbohydrates, lipids, proteins, water, vitamins, and minerals. Carbohydrates, lipids, and proteins provide energy to the body and thus are referred to as energy-yielding nutrients. Along with water, they constitute the major portion of most foods. They are referred to as **macronu-trients** because they are required in relatively large amounts ("macro" means large). Their requirements are measured in kilograms (kg) or grams (g) (see Appendix L). Alcohol also provides energy but is not considered a nutrient because it is not needed to support life.

Carbohydrates include sugars such as those in table sugar, fruit, and milk, and starches such as those in vegetables and grains. Sugars are the simplest form of car-bohydrate, and starches are more complex carbohydrates made of many sugars linked together (Figure 1.1). Carbohydrates provide a readily available source of en-ergy to the body. Most fiber is also carbohydrate. It cannot be completely broken down by the body, so it provides little energy. However, it is important for gastroin-testinal health. Fiber is found in vegetables, fruits, legumes, and whole grains.

Lipids, commonly referred to as fats and oils, provide a storage form of energy. Lipids in our diets come from foods that naturally contain fats, such as meat and whole milk, and from processed fats, such as vegetable oils and butter, that we add

Phytochemical A substance found in plant foods that is not an essential nutrient but may have health-promoting properties.

Macronutrients Nutrients needed by the body in large amounts. These include water and the energy-yielding nutrients carbohydrates, lipids, and proteins.

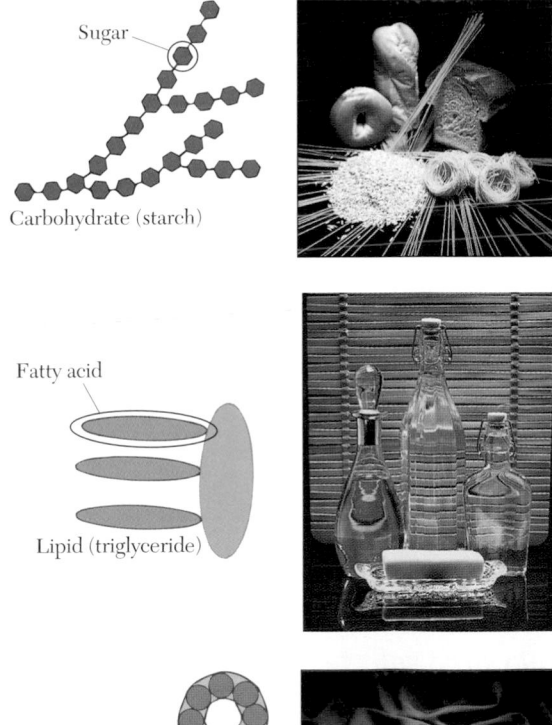

Figure 1.1
Starches are made of sugars linked together; most lipids such as the triglyceride shown here contain fatty acids; and proteins are made of folded chains of amino acids.
(Photographs, Charles D. Winters)

to food. Most lipids contain fatty acids, some of which are essential in the diet. The amount and type of lipid in the diet affects the risk of cardiovascular disease and certain types of cancer.

Protein, such as that in meat, fish, poultry, milk, grains, and legumes, is needed for growth and maintenance of body structures and regulation of body processes. Protein is made up of units called amino acids. Some amino acids can be made by the body, and others are essential in the diet. Dietary protein must meet the need for the essential amino acids.

Water is a nutrient in a class by itself. Water makes up about 60% of the human body and is required in kilogram amounts in the daily diet. It is a macronutrient that doesn't provide energy. Water serves many functions in the body, including acting as a lubricant, a transport fluid, and a regulator of body temperature.

Vitamins and minerals are classified as **micronutrients** because they are needed in small amounts in the diet ("micro" means small). The amounts required are expressed in milligrams (1 mg = 1/1000 g) or micrograms (1 μg = 1/1,000,000 g). They do not provide energy, but many help regulate the production of energy from carbohydrates, lipids, and proteins. They also have unique roles in processes such as bone growth, oxygen transport, and tissue growth and development. Vitamins and minerals are found in most of the foods we eat. Fresh foods are a good natural source of vitamins and minerals, and many processed foods have micronutrients added to them during manufacture. For example, breakfast cereals are a good source of iron and B vitamins because these are added during processing. Processing can also cause nutrient losses. Light, heat, and exposure to oxygen destroy some micronutrients, and others are lost in the water used in cooking and processing. Nevertheless, frozen, canned, and otherwise processed foods can still be good sources of vitamins and minerals. Vitamin and mineral supplements are also a common source of micronutrients in today's diet.

Micronutrients Nutrients needed by the body in small amounts. These include vitamins and minerals.

What Do Nutrients Do?

Together, the macronutrients and micronutrients provide energy, structure, and regulation, which are needed for growth, maintenance and repair, and reproduction. Each nutrient provides one or more of these functions, but all nutrients together are needed to maintain health.

Carbohydrates, lipids, and proteins provide the fuel or energy that is required to maintain life. If less energy is consumed than is needed, the body will burn its own fat as well as carbohydrate and protein to meet its energy needs. If more energy is consumed than is needed, the extra is stored as body fat. The energy needed for all body processes and activities is measured in **kilocalories** (abbreviated as *kcalories* or *kcals*) or in **kilojoules** (abbreviated as *kjoules* or *kJs*). The more common term "calorie" is technically 1/1000 of a kilocalorie, but when spelled with a capital "C" it indicates kilocalories. For instance, the term "Calories" on food labels actually refers to kilocalories. One gram of carbohydrate or protein provides 4 kcalories. One gram of fat provides 9 kcalories. Alcohol contributes about 7 kcalories per gram (Table 1.1).

Kilocalorie A unit of heat that is used to express the amount of energy provided by foods.

Kilojoule A measure of work that can be used to express energy intake and energy output; 4.18 kjoules = 1 kcalorie.

Table 1.1 *Energy Content of Carbohydrate, Protein, Lipid, and Alcohol*

	Kcalories/gram	Kjoules/gram
Carbohydrate	4	16.7
Protein	4	16.7
Lipid	9	37.6
Alcohol	7	29.3

Table 1.2 *Examples of How Nutrients Function in the Body*

Function	Nutrient	Example
Energy	Carbohydrate	Blood glucose is a carbohydrate that fuels body cells.
	Lipid	Fat is the most plentiful source of stored fuel in the body.
	Protein	Protein consumed in excess of protein needs will be used for energy.
Structure	Lipid	The membranes that surround each cell are primarily lipid.
	Protein	Connective tissue protein holds bones together and holds muscles to bones.
	Minerals	The minerals calcium and phosphorus make teeth and bones hard.
Regulation	Lipid	Estrogen is a lipid hormone that helps regulate the reproductive cycle in women.
	Protein	Leptin is a protein that helps regulate body fat.
	Water	Water lost as sweat helps cool the body to regulate body temperature.
	Vitamins	B vitamins regulate the use of macronutrients for energy.
	Minerals	Sodium helps regulate blood volume.

Nutrients are also needed to form and maintain body structures. Water, proteins, lipids, and minerals are important structural nutrients. For example, muscle is made up primarily of protein and water, and bone is composed of a protein framework embedded with minerals. Nutrients also regulate biochemical reactions in the living body. Together all of the reactions that occur in the body are referred to as **metabolism**. Metabolic processes must be regulated to maintain a constant environment inside the body, referred to as **homeostasis**. Vitamins, minerals, water, and proteins are important regulatory nutrients. For example, water helps to regulate body temperature. When body temperature increases, water lost through sweat helps to cool the body. Proteins, vitamins, and minerals help to speed up or slow down the reactions of metabolism as needed to maintain homeostasis (Table 1.2).

Metabolism The sum of all the chemical reactions that take place in a living organism.

Homeostasis A physiological state in which a stable internal body environment is maintained.

How Much of Each Nutrient Do We Need?

In order to support life, an adequate amount of each essential nutrient must be consumed in the diet. The amount of a nutrient that is optimal will avoid deficiencies and excesses and promote short-term and long-term health. The exact amount that is optimal is different for each individual. It depends on genetic makeup, lifestyle, and overall diet. A person with a genetic predisposition to heart disease needs to consume different amounts of certain nutrients to maintain long-term heart health than does a person with no genetic risk of heart disease. Individuals who smoke cigarettes need more vitamin C than nonsmokers, and athletes need more energy than their less active counterparts. The amount of each nutrient required is also dependent on the other nutrients and non-nutrient substances present in the diet. For example, adequate fat is essential for the absorption of vitamin A. The amount of vitamin E that is optimal may be affected by the amount of selenium, vitamin C, and beta-carotene (β-carotene) available; the amount of iron absorbed is affected by the presence of vitamin C and calcium. Therefore, it is difficult to make generalizations about how much is enough or too much without considering both individual needs and overall diet.

Effects of Poor Nutrient Intake

Consuming either too much or too little of one or more nutrients or energy can cause **malnutrition** (Figure 1.2). We usually think of malnutrition as **undernutrition**, a deficiency of energy or nutrients. Undernutrition may occur due to a deficient intake of energy or nutrients, increased requirements, or an inability to absorb or use nutrients. Starvation, the most severe form of undernutrition, is a deficiency of energy that causes weight loss, poor growth, the inability to reproduce, and if

Malnutrition Any condition resulting from an energy or nutrient intake either above or below that which is optimal.

Undernutrition Any condition resulting from an energy or nutrient intake below that which meets nutritional needs.

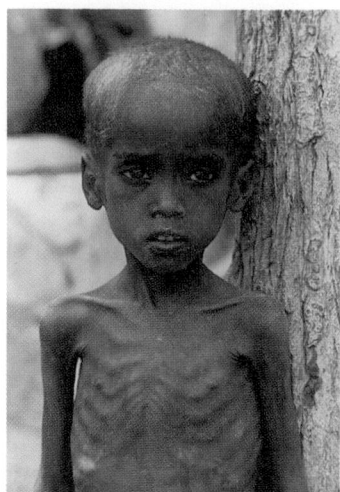 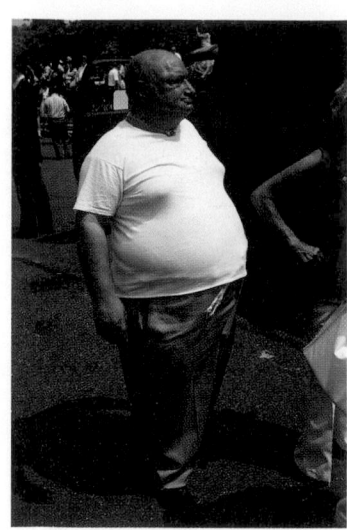

Figure 1.2
Malnutrition includes both undernutrition and overnutrition. (*Left*, Gamma Liaison/Camera Pix. Right, © Van Bucher/Photo Researchers, Inc.)

Overnutrition Poor nutritional status resulting from a dietary intake in excess of that which is optimal for health.

Toxic The capacity to produce injury at some level of intake.

Risk factor A characteristic or circumstance that is associated with the occurrence of a particular disease.

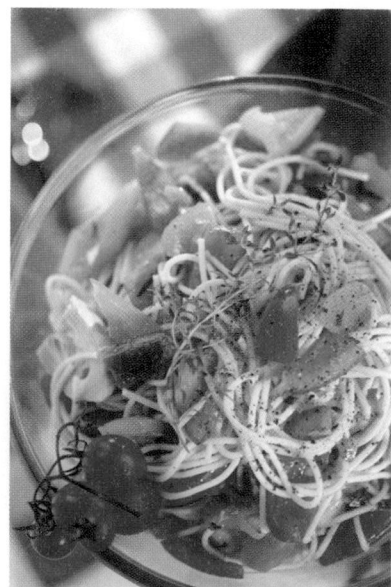

Figure 1.3
We don't eat nutrients; we eat foods that we choose for a variety of reasons including taste, color, and texture. (© Image State)

severe enough, death. Iron deficiency is a form of undernutrition that is common in young children and adolescents because their rapid growth increases the need for iron. Vitamin B$_{12}$ deficiency is a risk for older adults because changes in the stomach that often occur with age decrease vitamin B$_{12}$ absorption. When undernutrition is caused by a specific nutrient deficiency, the symptoms often reflect the body functions that rely on the deficient nutrient. For example, vitamin A is necessary for vision; a deficiency of vitamin A can result in blindness.

Overnutrition, an excess of nutrients, is also a form of malnutrition. When food is consumed in excess of energy need, the extra is stored as body fat. Some fat is necessary as insulation and an energy store, but an excess of body fat, called obesity, increases the risk for high blood pressure, heart disease, diabetes, and other chronic health problems. When excesses of specific nutrients are consumed, an adverse or **toxic** reaction may occur. Because foods generally do not contain high enough concentrations of nutrients to be toxic, most nutrient toxicities result from the overconsumption of vitamin and mineral supplements.

The symptoms of a nutritional deficiency or excess may appear rapidly or take a lifetime to develop. For example, an athlete exercising in hot weather may become dehydrated in a matter of hours, developing symptoms such as headache and dizziness. Drinking water relieves the symptoms as rapidly as they appeared. Nutritional imbalances that take weeks or months to manifest themselves are no less important. For example, if excess energy is consumed, body fat is deposited, but it may take months before a significant amount of weight is gained. Likewise, as anyone who has tried to lose weight knows, it can take months of reduced energy consumption to use up the excess fat.

Nutritional effects that occur over a much longer time are also an important health concern. An individual's nutrient intake today may affect the development of osteoporosis, cancer, or heart disease 20, 30, or 40 years from now. However, the effects of nutrition on the development of chronic disease are difficult to determine because other variables or **risk factors**, such as age, genetics, and gender, are also often involved. These risk factors cannot be changed, but diet is a lifestyle variable that can be changed because it is determined by individual choices.

• WHAT ARE WE CHOOSING?

We need nutrients to survive—but we eat food, not nutrients (Figure 1.3). There are hundreds of food choices to make and hundreds of reasons for making them. Each of these choices contributes to our total nutrient intake. Some foods are rich in protein and minerals, others in vitamins and phytochemicals. Choosing a healthy

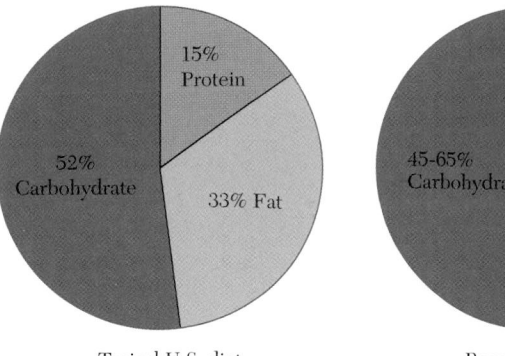

Typical U.S. diet   Recommended diet

Figure 1.4
Americans are now eating a diet that is within the recommended ranges of intake for carbohydrate, fat, and protein.

diet does not mean you have to give up favorite foods. None of the foods we choose are good or bad in and of themselves, but together they make up a healthy or a not-so-healthy diet.

How Healthy Is the American Diet?

Recommendations for a healthy diet suggest that we consume a diet that provides about 45 to 65% of energy from carbohydrate, 10 to 35% from protein, and 20 to 35% from fat. The typical diet in the United States is within these recommendations. As a nation we eat about 52% carbohydrate, 15% protein, and 33% fat (Figure 1.4).[1] The percentages of energy from macronutrients in the American diet have improved over the last 20 years. For example, the typical fat intake has decreased by 3% since 1980.[2] Despite this, the American diet is not as healthy as it could be. The diet should be based on whole grains, vegetables, and fruits, with smaller amounts of dairy products and high protein foods and limited amounts of fats and sweets. But few Americans follow these recommendations (Table 1.3). As a population, we don't eat enough grains, legumes, fruits, dairy products, or lean meats, and we eat too much fat and added sugar. This dietary pattern along with a lack of physical activity increases the risk of developing chronic diseases, such as diabetes, obesity, heart disease, and cancer, which are the major causes of illness and death in our population.[3] Recommendations for reducing disease risk focus on changes in the foods we choose and the amount of exercise we get (see *Off the Shelf*: Can "Bad" Foods Be Part of a Healthy Diet?).

ON THE WEB
For more information on food intake patterns in the United States, go to the USDA Economic Research Service at www.ers.usda.gov

Table 1.3 *Typical American Diet*

	Daily Recommendation	Typical Diet
Grains	6–11 servings—several should be whole grains	50% do not eat even 6 servings. Most people only eat one serving of whole grains
Vegetables	3–5 servings—include legumes and leafy greens	59% do not meet recommendations— 33% of vegetable servings are white potatoes, only 3% are leafy greens, and 6% are legumes
Fruits	2–4 servings daily	76% do not meet recommendations—48% do not eat any at all
Dairy	2–3 servings	77% of people do not meet recommendations—over 80% of women do not meet recommendations
Meats	2–3 servings or a total of 5–7 ounces	48% of men and 75% of women meet this recommendation
Fats and sweets	20 to 30% fat and limit added sugars to less than 18 teaspoons per day	The typical diet contains 33% fat and includes 19 teaspoons of added sugars per day

Source: Cleveland, L. E., Cook, A. J., Wilson, J. E., et al., Pyramid Servings Data, ARS Food Survey Research Group. Available online at *www.barc.usda.gov/bhnrc/foodsurvey/home.htm*

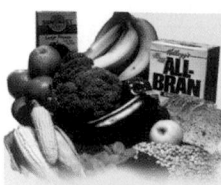

Off the Shelf

Can "Bad" Foods Be Part of a Healthy Diet?

Collard greens are rich in vitamin A. Potato chips are high in fat. Does that mean you should eat collard greens every day and swear off potato chips? What if the collard greens are swimming in pork fat? What if the potato chips are fat free? Are they healthy choices then? Can they be part of a healthy diet?

The first step toward making healthy choices is understanding that there is no such thing as a good food or a bad food—any food can be part of a healthy diet. A healthy diet does not need to exclude the foods you love. Whether your cravings are for ice cream or potato chips, you can fit favorite foods into your diet. High-fat foods must be balanced with lower fat choices and sweet treats offset by foods naturally low in sugar. Choosing special foods like fat-free chips, sugar-free candy, or lowfat cookies doesn't guarantee a healthy diet. These foods are lower in fat and/or sugar, but they still add kcalories to the diet and contribute few other nutrients.

A healthy diet is based on grains, fruits, vegetables, milk, and meats or meat substitutes. It includes a wide variety of foods we enjoy. But selecting a diet based on these is not necessarily easy. The multitude of choices that modern food production and processing provides makes choosing difficult. Chicken, rice, and vegetables sounds like a healthy meal. But even purchasing the foods for such a simple meal involves hundreds of decisions that can impact on the overall healthiness and appeal of the diet. Is it lower in fat if you purchase a whole raw chicken, boneless, skinless chicken breasts, or frozen breaded nuggets of chicken? Is brown rice healthier than white because it adds more fiber to the diet? Instant rice is convenient, but is it as nutritious and does it taste good? Is the packaged rice with added flavorings too high in fat and salt? The healthiness of the diet is also a concern when choosing produce. You need to decide not only which vegetable to eat, but whether you want it grown organically and whether to buy it fresh, frozen, or in a can. And variety is important too. Carrots every day is not bad, but a variety of vegetables is even better. Including legumes and leafy green vegetables and eating some vegetables raw and others cooked can add variety to your plate, your palate, and the nutrients supplied by your diet.

A healthy choice can be any choice that is part of an overall healthy diet. For example, fat-free ice cream does not make a diet healthy if the diet's overall fat content is too high and it is low in whole grains, fruits, and vegetables; but a diet rich in whole grains, fruits, and vegetables can still be healthy even if you have regular ice cream for dessert. Subsequent chapters and *Off the Shelf* boxes throughout this text provide information that will help you understand what makes a healthy diet and how to make wise decisions about individual foods and supplements you buy off the shelf.

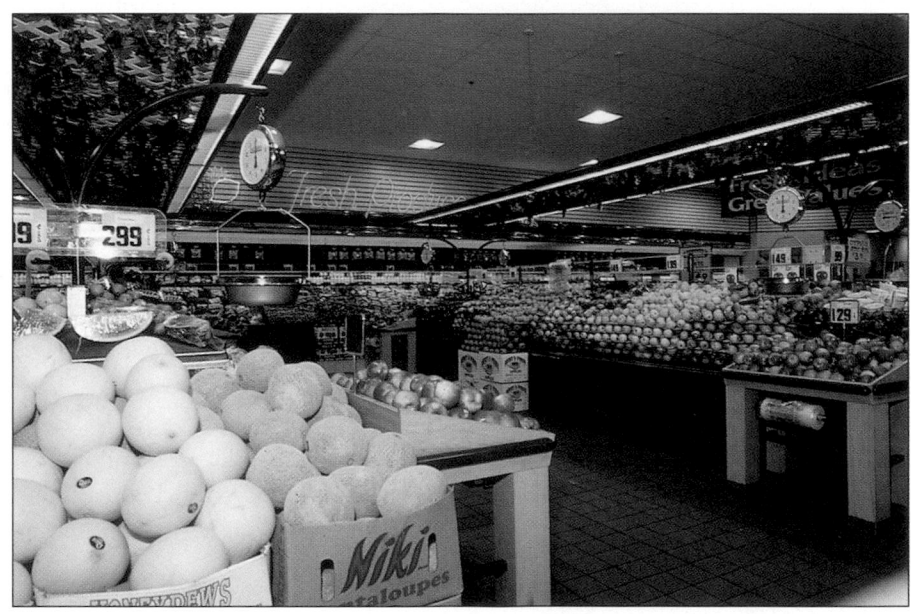

(George Semple)

How Do We Make Food Choices?

Why do we choose the foods we do? Most Americans understand that nutrition is important to their health, yet people don't want to give up their favorite foods and they don't want to eat foods they don't like.[4] Our food choices and food intake are affected not only by nutrient needs but also by what is available to us, where we live, what is within our budget and compatible with our lifestyle, what we like, what is culturally acceptable, what mood we are in, and what we think we should eat.

Availability The food available to an individual or a population is affected by geography, socioeconomics, and health status. In many parts of the world, food choices are limited to foods produced locally. Nutrients that are lacking in local foods will be

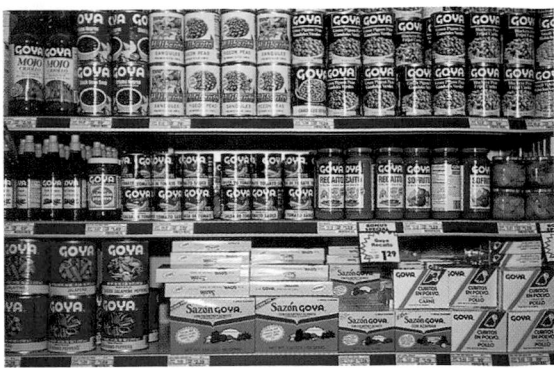

Figure 1.5
Modern processing and transportation make foods from around the world available in local grocery stores. (George Semple)

lacking in the population's diet. In more developed parts of the world, the ability to store, transport, and process food allows year-round access to seasonal foods and foods grown and produced at distant locations. (Figure 1.5).

Even if foods are available in the store, it doesn't mean that they are available to all individuals. Socioeconomic factors such as income level, living conditions, and lifestyle as well as education affect the types and amounts of foods that are available. Individuals with limited incomes can choose only the types and amounts of foods that they can afford. Individuals who don't own cars can only purchase what they can carry home. Those without refrigerators or stoves are limited in what foods can be prepared at home. And those who can't or don't have time to cook are limited to prepared foods and restaurant meals.

Health status also affects the availability of food. People who cannot carry heavy packages are limited in what they can purchase. People with food allergies, digestive problems, and dental disease are limited in the foods they can consider for consumption. People consuming special diets for disease conditions are limited to foods that meet their dietary prescriptions.

Personal and Cultural Preferences Availability affects the foods we have to choose from; but individual palates and convictions determine what we actually consume, and tradition, religion, and social values may dictate what foods we consider appropriate. Personal preferences for taste, smell, appearance, and texture affect which foods we select. Not wanting to give up the foods they like is the number one reason people give for not choosing a healthier diet.[4] Personal convictions also affect food choices; a vegan will not choose a meal that contains meat, and an environmentalist may not buy food packaged in nonrecyclable containers.

Food preferences and eating habits are learned as part of each individual's family, cultural, national, and social background. They are among the oldest and most entrenched features of every culture. An individual of Asian descent may consider rice the focus of the meal, whereas Italians may include pasta with every meal. The foods we are exposed to as children influence what foods we buy and cook as adults. If your mother never served artichokes or Swiss chard you may not consider eating them as an adult. If you grow up eating turkey on Thanksgiving and tamales at Christmastime you will likely continue these traditions. Religious background also affects food intake: Seventh-Day Adventists are vegetarians; Jews and Muslims do not eat pork. Even for those who choose not to observe religious dietary rules, habit may dictate many mealtime decisions. Jewish kosher laws prohibit the consumption of meat and milk in the same meal. Even Jews who do not follow kosher law may choose not to serve milk at dinner because they never had it as children.

Food is a focus for social interaction and may be a determinant of social acceptance. Peer pressure exerts a tremendous influence on what foods we choose. For an adolescent, stopping for a cheeseburger or taco after school can be the basis for acceptance by one's peers. Food may also be an expression and a moderator of mood and emotional states. Some of us eat more when we are upset, while others eat less. Food and certain specific foods are associated with comfort, love, and security.

Our attitudes about what foods we think are good for us also affect what we choose. We may choose a lowfat diet because we think it is good for our heart, organic produce because we are concerned about exposure to pesticides, or green tea to increase our intake of cancer-fighting antioxidants.

• What Is Reliable Nutrition Information?

We are bombarded with nutrition information. Some of what we hear is accurate and some of it is incorrect or exaggerated to sell products or make news headlines more enticing: oat bran lowers cholesterol, β-carotene prevents cancer, obesity is genetic, vitamin C cures the common cold, vitamin E slows aging. Sifting through this information and distinguishing the useful from the useless may seem overwhelming. An understanding of the process of science and how it is used to study the relationship between nutrition and health will allow you to develop the nutrition sense needed to judge the validity of nutrition headlines.

Sources of Nutrition Information

Some nutrition information comes from individual contact with physicians and dietitians; some is printed on food labels and in educational pamphlets; but much of it reaches us through television, radio, newspapers, and magazines (Figure 1.6). Although dietitians and physicians are viewed as the most valuable source of nutrition information, Americans today get most of their food and nutrition information from the mass media.[4] Mass media are very powerful tools in promoting health and nutrition messages. Information that would take individual health-care workers years to disseminate can reach millions of individuals in a matter of hours or days. Much of this information is reliable, but some can be misleading. The motivation for news stories is often to sell subscriptions or improve ratings, not to promote the nutritional health of the population. Some nutrition and health information originates from food manufacturers. It is usually in the form of marketing and advertising designed to sell existing products or target new ones. This promotional information can be confusing to the consumer, who may not know how to interpret it. For instance, the scientific evidence that reducing dietary fat intake can protect you from heart disease and help maintain a healthy weight has created a vast market for products low in fat. Food manufacturers responded by creating fat-free, lowfat, and reduced-fat products at an astonishing rate. Weight- and health-conscious consumers responded by increasing their consumption of fat-free foods, but the girth of American waists continued to increase. The message that reducing fat intake promotes health was received, but consumers did not understand that fat-free foods are not kcalorie free and simply adding lowfat foods to the diet was not a prescription for good health. Knowing what information to believe and how to use this information to choose a diet can be difficult (see *Off the Label*: Read the Whole Label to Know What You Are Choosing).

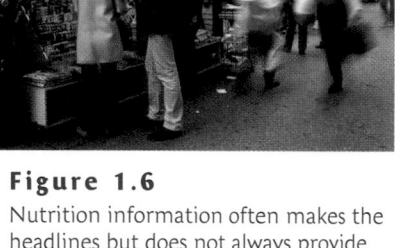

Figure 1.6
Nutrition information often makes the headlines but does not always provide an accurate presentation of new discoveries.(© Hugh Sitton/Stone)

Scientific method The general approach of science that is used to explain observations about the world around us.

Hypothesis An educated guess made to explain an observation or to answer a question.

Theory An explanation based on scientific study and reasoning.

Understanding the Process of Science: The Scientific Method

Advances in nutrition are made using the **scientific method**. The scientific method offers a systematic, unbiased approach to evaluating the relationships between food and health. The first step of the scientific method is to make an observation and ask questions about the observation. The next step is to propose an explanation for the observation. This explanation is called a **hypothesis**. Once a hypothesis has been proposed, experiments can be designed to test it. The experiments must provide objective results that can be measured and repeated. If the experimental results do not prove the hypothesis to be wrong, a **theory**, or a scientific explanation based on experimentation, can be established (Figure 1.7). Scientific theories are accepted only as long as they cannot be disproved and con-

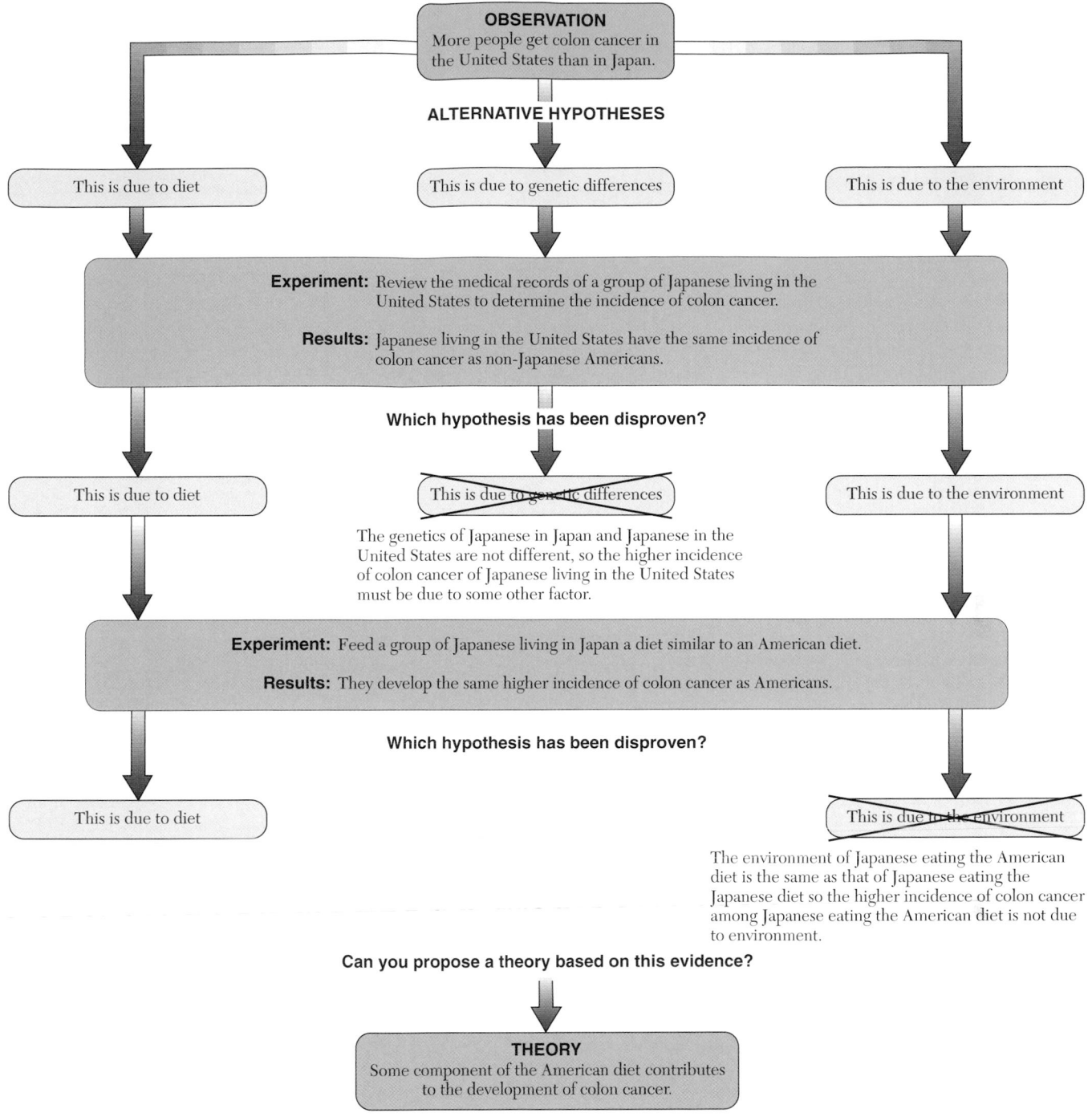

Figure 1.7
This example illustrates how the scientific method can be used to formulate hypotheses based on observations, design experiments to test these hypotheses, and interpret the results to support or disprove the hypotheses, helping establish a theory.

tinue to be supported by all new evidence that accumulates. Even a theory that has been accepted by the scientific community for years can be proved wrong. This flux allows the body of knowledge to increase, but it can be confusing as old theories give way to new ones.

The discovery of the relationship between nutrition and pellagra, a disease now known to be caused by a deficiency of the vitamin niacin, is an example of how the scientific method has been used in nutrition research. The events leading to this discovery began with the observation in 1914 that individuals in institu-

Off the Label
Read the Whole Label to Know What You Are Choosing

Healthy! Fresh! Light! The first thing that may catch your eye when shopping is a large-print banner describing some nutritious feature of a product. Food labels with eye-catching banners and names sell better. Although food labels must conform to federal guidelines and use standard definitions for most terms, they can still be misleading. Understanding what these terms mean on food labels will help you know what you are choosing and how it fits into your diet.

Many of these descriptors highlight individual nutrients, and just as no single food determines the healthiness of a diet, no single nutrient makes a food good or bad for you. Look beyond the banner and see what other contribution the food makes to your diet. For example, chocolate cookies labeled "fat free" may not be your best choice if you are trying to reduce your sugar intake or increase the amount of fiber in your diet. A food labeled "fresh" may sound appealing. Any raw food that has not been frozen, heat processed, or otherwise preserved can be labeled fresh. The term "fresh" however, doesn't provide any information about the nutrient content of the product or how long it took for this food to travel from the farm to the grocery store shelf. "Healthy" is another attractive

byline that applies to more than a single nutrient. It implies that the product is wholesome and nutritious. In fact, to use the term "healthy" a food must be low in fat and saturated fat, contain no more than 360 mg of sodium and 60 mg of cholesterol per serving, and be a good source of one or more important nutrients. Since vegetables, fruits, and grain products are an important part of a healthy diet, fresh fruits and vegetables and some canned and frozen ones as well as enriched grain products may be labeled healthy even if they are not a good source of one or more of the specified nutrients.[1] While all of the qualities specified by the term "healthy" are part of a healthy diet, foods that fit this definition are not necessarily the basis for a healthy diet. For instance, some fat-free brownies fit the labeling definition of healthy. They are low in fat, saturated fat, cholesterol, and sodium, and supply 10% of the recommended intake for iron. But they are a good choice only in limited quantities because they are high in sugar and contain few other nutrients. Likewise, a food that doesn't meet the labeling definition of healthy is not necessarily a poor choice. Vegetable soup, for example, contains more sodium than the definition of healthy will allow, but if the rest of the diet

is not high in sodium, the soup can be a healthy choice.

Enticing product names can also be misleading. However, unless you have memorized the U.S. Department of Agriculture (USDA) and Food and Drug Administration (FDA) labeling regulations you can't tell exactly what you are buying. These standards determine how much beef is in a beef enchilada, how much chicken is in chicken soup, and how much fruit is in a Fruit Roll-Up. Product names must comply with legal definitions, but they don't have to make sense to consumers. For example, "lasagna with meat sauce" must be 6% meat, but "lasagna with meat and sauce" must be 12% meat.

To get the whole picture, you need to look beyond the healthy sounding banner and the name of the product. Since the nutrient content of foods must be listed, as well as information on how a food fits into the diet as a whole, reading the label thoroughly will provide you with the information you need to make wise choices. Chapter 2 and *Off the Label* boxes throughout this book provide more information on how to read food labels.

[1]More foods can carry "healthy" label. *FDA Consumer* 32:2, July/August, 1998.

---

tions such as hospitals, orphanages, and prisons suffered from pellagra, but the staff there did not. If pellagra was an infectious disease, both populations would be equally affected. The hypothesis proposed was that pellagra was due to a dietary deficiency. To test this hypothesis, nutritious foods such as fresh meats and vegetables were added to the diet. The symptoms of pellagra disappeared, supporting the hypothesis that pellagra is due to a deficiency of something in the diet. This experiment and others led to the theory that pellagra is caused by a dietary deficiency. This theory, further developed by the discovery of the vitamin niacin, still holds today.

For the scientific method to generate reliable theories, the experiments done to test hypotheses must generate reliable results and be interpreted accurately. The public hears about nutrition-related experiments in the news, and reads about them in magazines or in advertisements and promotional material for nutritional products. For example, the hypothetical advertisement for Power Boost illustrated in Figure 1.8 discusses one study that supports its claim to increase muscle mass and decrease body fat. Was this experiment conducted properly? Do the results mean that Power Boost will increase your muscle mass?

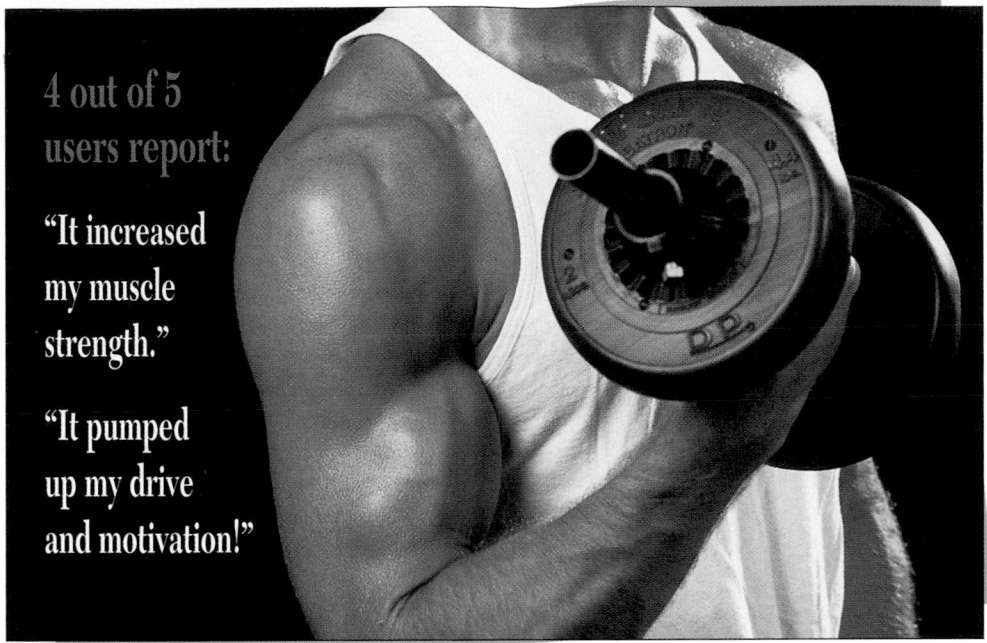

POWER BOOST

BOOST your STRENGTH • POWER up your DRIVE • MAXIMIZE your MASS

4 out of 5
users report:

"It increased
my muscle
strength."

"It pumped
up my drive
and motivation!"

Years of research have developed this special nutritional formulation. Just mix with water and stack one shake with every meal or snack.

University Study Shows: 25 experienced weight lifters added one POWER BOOST shake at meals and snacks 5 times a day for 4 weeks.
Body muscle mass and fat mass were measured by underwater weighing before POWER BOOST was added and after 4 weeks of training with POWER BOOST.

RESULTS
The weight lifters gained an average of 5.2 pounds of lean muscle and lost 4.5 pounds of unwanted fat.

Figure 1.8
This hypothetical advertisement illustrates the types of nutrition claims that consumers must be prepared to evaluate. (Lawrence Migdale/Photo Researchers, Inc.)

What Makes a Good Experiment? A well-conducted experiment must collect quantifiable data using proper experimental controls and the right experimental population.

Quantifiable Data Scientific experiments are designed to provide measurable data that can be quantified and repeated. For instance, body weight and blood pressure are parameters that can be measured reliably. Feelings are more difficult to assess. They can be quantified with standardized questionnaires, but individual testimonies or opinions, referred to as **anecdotal**, have not been measured objectively. In the Power Boost ad, the quotes from users who report increased muscle strength and pumped-up motivation are anecdotal and are not quantifiable. The increase in muscle mass and loss of fat determined by underwater weighing are objective measurements that can be quantified and repeated.

Proper Controls **Experimental controls** ensure that each factor or **variable** studied can be compared with a known situation. A **control group** acts as a standard of comparison for the treatment being tested. A control group is treated in the same way as the **experimental groups** except no experimental treatment is implemented. For example, in the experiment described in the Power Boost ad the experimental group consists of athletes consuming the Power Boost drink for four weeks. An appropriate

Anecdotal Information based on a story of personal experience.

Experimental controls Factors included in an experimental design that limit the number of variables, allowing an investigator to examine the effect of only the parameters of interest.

Variable A factor or condition that is changed in an experimental setting.

Control group A group of participants in an experiment that are identical to the experimental group except that no experimental treatment is used. They are used as a basis of comparison.

Experimental groups Groups of participants in an experiment who are subjected to an experimental treatment.

control group would consist of athletes of similar age, gender, and ability eating similar diets and following similar workout regimens, but not consuming Power Boost. Both groups would have their body fat measured before and after the four-week period.

In order to make the control and experimental groups indistinguishable, a **placebo** is sometimes used. The placebo, often a sugar pill, is identical in appearance to the actual treatment but has no therapeutic value. In the Power Boost example the experimental group is consuming a protein drink. An appropriate placebo for the control group would be a drink that looks and tastes just like Power Boost but doesn't contribute any nutrients. By using a placebo, participants in the experiment would not know if they were receiving the actual supplement. When the subjects do not know which treatment they are receiving, the study is called a **single-blind study**. Using a placebo in a single-blind study helps to prevent the expectations of subjects from biasing the results. For example, if the athletes think they are taking Power Boost, they may be convinced that they are getting stronger and as a result they work harder in their training and develop bigger muscles even without the supplement. Errors can also occur if investigators allow their own desire for a specific result to affect the interpretation of the data. This type of error can be avoided by designing a **double-blind study** in which neither the subjects nor the investigators know who is in which group until after the results have been analyzed.

The Appropriate Experimental Population In order for an experiment to produce reliable results, it must be conducted in the right population. Therefore, if Power Boost claims to improve performance in trained athletes, it should be tested on trained athletes.

The number of subjects included in a study is also important. To be successful, an experiment must show that the treatment being tested causes a result to occur more frequently than it would occur by chance. Fewer subjects are needed to demonstrate an effect that rarely occurs by chance. For example, if only one person in a million can increase muscle mass by weight training for four weeks, then the experiment to see if Power Boost increases muscle mass in athletes weight training for four weeks would require only a few subjects to demonstrate an effect. If one in four athletes can improve his muscle mass by weight training for four weeks, then many more subjects are needed. Statistical methods should be applied before a study is conducted to determine how many subjects are needed to show the effect of the experimental treatment. The number of subjects will depend on the type of study and the effect being tested. The fewer variables included in a study, the fewer experimental subjects needed to demonstrate an effect.

Interpretation of Experimental Results In science, the interpretation of results is as important as the way studies are done. If Power Boost is tested in experienced weight lifters, the product cannot claim that it will help novices in the gym. One way to ensure that experiments are correctly interpreted is to use a **peer-review** system. Most scientific journals require that reports of studies be reviewed by two or three experts in the field who did not take part in the research that is being evaluated. Before an article can be published in the journal, these scientists must agree that the experiments were well conducted and that the results were interpreted fairly. Nutrition articles can be found in peer-reviewed journals such as *The American Journal of Clinical Nutrition, The Journal of Nutrition, The Journal of the American Dietetic Association, The New England Journal of Medicine,* and *The International Journal of Sport Nutrition.*

Types of Nutrition Research Studies

Nutrition research studies are done to determine nutrient requirements, to learn more about the metabolism of nutrients, and to understand the role of nutrition in health and disease. Perfect tools do not exist for addressing all these questions. However, many types of research can be useful, including epidemiological observations and studies, human intervention studies, and a variety of types of laboratory studies.

Placebo A fake medicine or supplement that is indistinguishable in appearance from the real thing. It is used to disguise the control and experimental groups in an experiment.

Single-blind study An experiment in which either the study participants or the researchers are unaware of who is in a control or an experimental group.

Double-blind study An experiment in which neither the study participants nor the researchers know who is in a control or an experimental group.

Peer review Review of the design and validity of a research experiment by experts in the field of study who did not participate in the research.

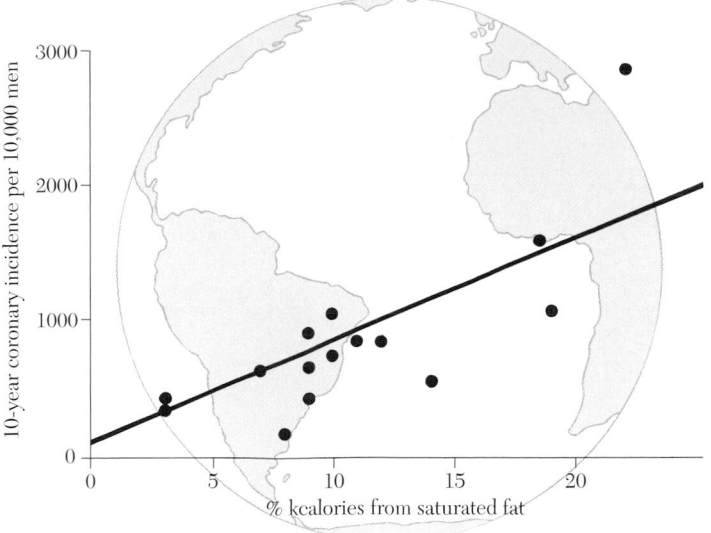

Figure 1.9
This graph shows the incidence of coronary heart disease versus the amount of saturated fat in the diet of different populations. As the amount of saturated fat in the diet increases, so does the incidence of coronary heart disease. (Keys, A. *Seven Countries: A Multivariate Analysis of Deaths and Coronary Heart Disease.* Cambridge, MA: Harvard University Press, 1980)

Epidemiology **Epidemiology** is the study of patterns that occur within populations. In nutrition, epidemiological studies are used to suggest relationships between diet and health. For instance, epidemiology can be used to identify the typical intake of a nutrient in a healthy population. **Cross-sectional data** can be collected from a cross section of the population at one point in time, or **longitudinal data** can be collected from the same group of individuals over a period of time.

Epidemiology does not determine cause and effect relationships—it just identifies patterns. For instance, epidemiology was used to identify the association, or **correlation**, between high-fat diets and heart disease. This was done by looking at the incidence of heart disease in different countries and then finding dietary factors that follow the same pattern (Figure 1.9). From the observation that populations with high dietary fat intakes also have high incidences of heart disease, one possible hypothesis is that a high intake of fat in the diet predisposes to cardiovascular disease. This hypothesis must then be tested by controlled intervention and laboratory studies.

Human Intervention Studies The observations and hypotheses that come from epidemiology can be tested in human **intervention studies**. This type of experiment actively intervenes in the lives of individuals in a population and examines the effect of this intervention. Nutrition intervention studies generally explore the effects of altering people's diets. For example, if it is determined by epidemiology that populations who eat a lowfat diet have a lower incidence of heart disease, an intervention trial may be designed with an experimental group that consumes a diet lower in fat than is typical in the population and a control group that consumes the typical higher fat diet. The groups can be monitored to see if the dietary intervention affects the incidence of heart disease over the long term.

Laboratory Studies Laboratory studies are conducted in research facilities such as hospitals and universities. They are used to test hypotheses; to learn more about how nutrients function; and to evaluate the relationships among nutrient intake, levels of nutrients in the body, and health. They may study nutrient requirements and functions in the human or animal body, or they may use specific types of cells or molecules.

Studies Using Whole Organisms Many nutrition studies are done by feeding a specific diet to a person or animal and monitoring the physiological effects of that diet. **Depletion-repletion studies** are a classic method for studying the functions of nutrients and estimating the requirement for a particular nutrient. They involve deplet-

Epidemiology The study of the interrelationships between health and disease and other factors in the environment or lifestyle of different populations.

Cross-sectional data Information obtained by a single broad sampling of many different individuals in a population.

Longitudinal data Information obtained by repeatedly sampling the same individuals in a population over time.

Correlation Two or more factors occurring together.

Intervention study A study of a population in which there is an experimental manipulation of some members of the population; observations and measurements are made to determine the effects of this manipulation.

Depletion-repletion study A study that feeds a diet devoid of a nutrient until signs of deficiency appear, and then adds the nutrient back to the diet to a level at which symptoms disappear.

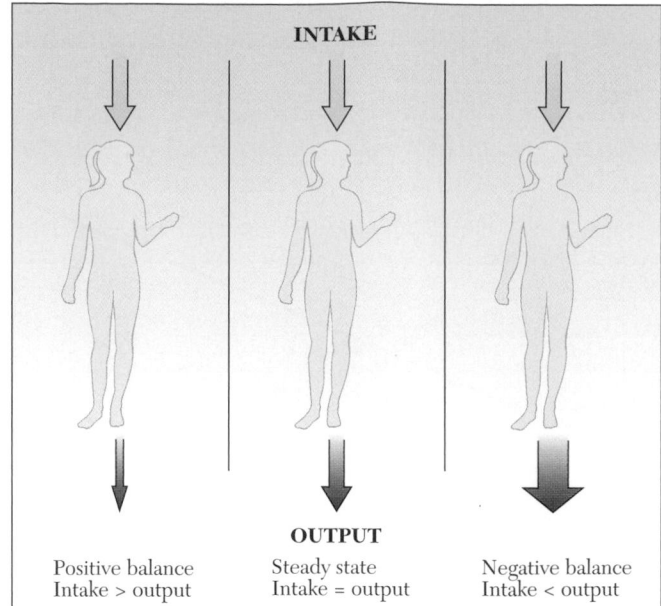

Figure 1.10
The concept of nutrient balance is illustrated here. If more of a nutrient is consumed than excreted, balance is positive; if the same amount is consumed and excreted, balance or a steady state exists; and if less is consumed than excreted, balance is negative.

Balance study A study that compares the total amount of a nutrient that enters the body with the total amount that leaves the body.

ing a nutrient by feeding a subject a diet devoid of that nutrient. After a period of time, if the nutrient is essential, symptoms of a deficiency will develop. The symptoms provide information on how the nutrient is functioning in the body. The nutrient is then added back to the diet, or repleted, until the symptoms are reversed. The requirement for that nutrient is the amount needed to reverse the deficiency symptoms.

Another method for determining nutrient functions and requirements is to compare the intake of a nutrient with its excretion. This type of study is known as a **balance study**. If more of a nutrient is consumed than is excreted, it is assumed that the nutrient is being used or stored by the body. If more of the nutrient is excreted than is consumed, some is being lost from body stores. When the amount consumed equals the amount lost, the body is neither gaining nor losing that nutrient and is said to be in balance (Figure 1.10). By varying the amount of a nutrient consumed and then measuring the amount excreted, it is possible to determine the minimum amount of that nutrient needed to replace the body losses. This type of study can be used to determine requirements for nutrients such as protein that are not stored in the body but not for nutrients such as fat that are stored when an excess is consumed.

Why Use Animals to Study Human Nutrition? Ideally, studies of human nutrition should be done in humans. However, because studying humans is costly, time consuming, inconvenient for subjects, and in some cases impossible for ethical reasons, many studies are done in animals.

An ideal animal model is one with metabolic and digestive processes similar to those in humans. For example, cows are rarely used in human nutrition research because they digest their food in four stomach-like chambers as opposed to a single stomach. Pigs, on the other hand, are a good model because they digest food in a manner similar to that of humans. However, in addition to digestion and metabolism, factors such as cost and time must be considered. Pigs and other large animals are expensive to use, and they take a long time to develop nutrient deficiencies. Smaller laboratory animals, such as rats and mice, are therefore the most common experimental animals. They are inexpensive, have short life spans, reproduce quickly, and the effects of nutritional changes develop rapidly. Their food intake can be easily controlled, and their excretions can be measured accurately using special cages. Even when using small animals, the species of animal must be carefully cho-

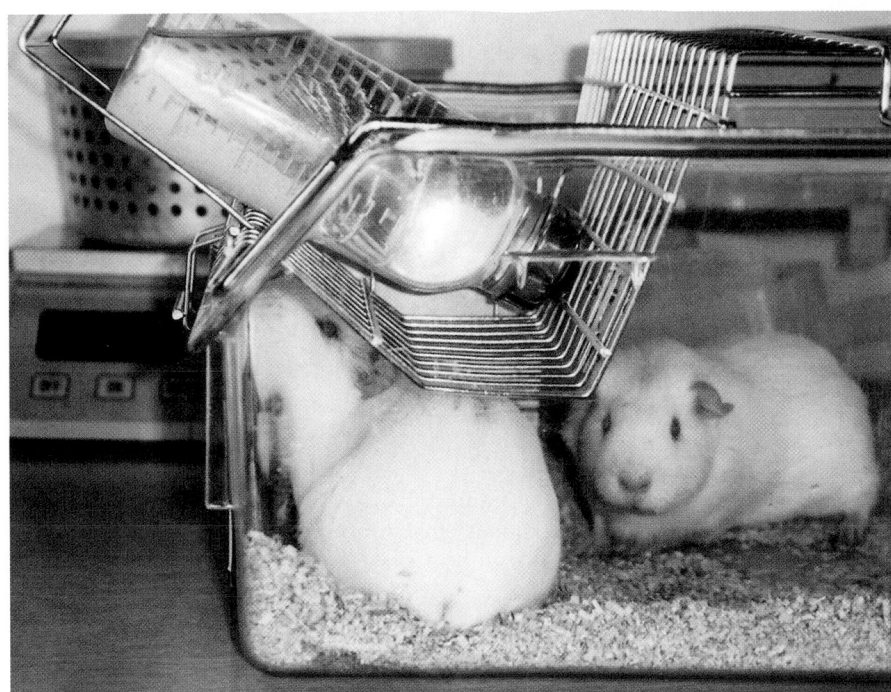

Figure 1.11
Laboratory animals, such as these guinea pigs, are used to study human nutrition. (Lori Smolin)

Molecular biology The study of cellular function at the molecular level.

DNA (deoxyribonucleic acid) The genetic material that codes for the synthesis of proteins.

Genes Lengths of DNA that provide instructions for heritable traits.

sen. For example, rats are more resistant to heart disease than are humans, so they are not a good model for studying the effect of diet on heart disease. Rabbits, on the other hand, do develop heart disease and can be used to study diet-heart disease relationships. Both rabbits and rats, however, are poor choices for a study of vitamin C requirements because they can synthesize this vitamin. Guinea pigs would be a better choice because the guinea pig is one of the few animals, other than humans, that cannot make vitamin C in its body (Figure 1.11). Even the best animal model is not the same as a human, and care must be taken when extrapolating the results to the human population. For example, a study that uses rats to show that a calcium supplement increases bone density can hypothesize, but not conclude, that the supplement will have the same effect in humans.

Studies Using Cells Another alternative to conducting studies in humans is to study cells either extracted from humans or animals or grown in the laboratory (Figure 1.12). Biochemistry can be used to study how nutrients are used for energy and how they regulate chemical reactions in cells. **Molecular biology** can be used to study how segments of **DNA (deoxyribonucleic acid)**, called **genes**, regulate functions of body cells. The types and amounts of nutrients available to cells can affect the action of genes. For example, vitamin A can directly activate or inactivate certain genes.

Knowledge gained from biochemical and molecular biology research can be used to study nutrition-related conditions that affect the entire organism. These methods help us understand the hereditary basis of diseases like heart disease, cancer, and obesity. These advances may enable us to identify individuals who are susceptible to specific diseases so that intervention can begin early. For example, it may someday be possible to identify individuals at high risk of developing heart disease by analyzing their DNA. These individuals could then modify their diet and lifestyle to delay or prevent disease onset.

Ethical Concerns Ethical issues are often raised in the process of conducting nutrition research. To avoid harm to study subjects or experimental animals, researchers use alternatives whenever possible. For example, extracted fluids, cells grown in the laboratory, and even computer models are used to predict how changes in nutrient

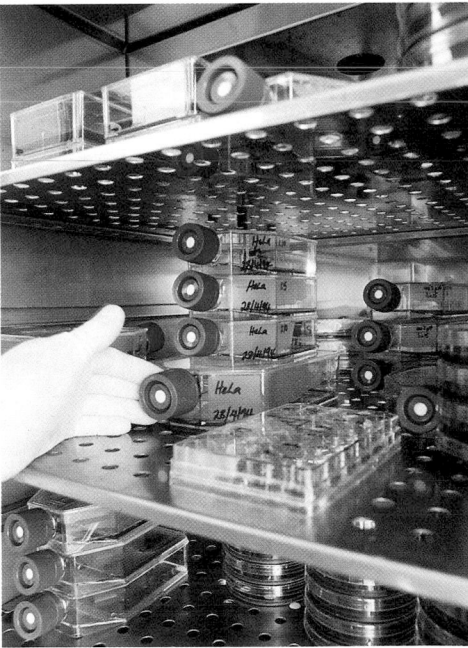

Figure 1.12
With technological advances, more and more research is being done using cells grown in the laboratory. (James King-Holmes/Science Photo Library/Photo Researchers, Inc.)

intake affect body processes. Such alternatives cannot always be used; therefore, human and animal experimentation is still necessary to answer many questions. To protect the rights of humans and animals used in experimental research, government guidelines have been developed.

Before an experiment involving human subjects can be conducted, the study must first be reviewed by a committee of scientists and nonscientists to ensure that the rights of the subjects are respected and that the risk of physical, social, and psychological injury is balanced against the potential benefit of the research. This was not always the case. Much of what we know today about the effects of starvation in humans was determined during World War II by conducting depletion-repletion studies using conscientious objectors as experimental subjects. These subjects were monitored physically and psychologically while they were starved and then refed. Because starvation causes physical discomfort, these individuals experienced some level of suffering during the trials and risked longer lasting physical and psychological harm.

As with experiments involving humans, the federal government mandates that panels of scientists review experiments that propose to use animals. These panels consider whether the need for animals is justified and whether all precautions will be taken to avoid pain and suffering. Animal housing and handling are strictly regulated, and a violation of these guidelines can close a research facility.

The development of the techniques of molecular biology has given rise to ethical issues regarding the manipulation of genes. Guidelines for manipulating genes have been developed and are constantly being revised to stay abreast of advances in this field.

Judging Nutrition Information

Nutrition, like all science, continues to develop as new discoveries provide clues to the right combination of nutrients needed for optimal health. As knowledge and technology advance, new nutrition principles are developed. Sometimes, established beliefs and concepts must give way to new ideas. As knowledge increases, recommendations change. Consumers may find this frustrating because the experts seem to change their minds so often. One day you are told margarine is better for you than butter; the next day a report says that it is just as bad. Which should you believe? Who are the experts?

Just as scientists use the scientific method to expand their understanding of the world around us, each of us can use an understanding of how science is done to evaluate nutrition claims. For example, the advertisement for Power Boost illustrated in Figure 1.8 states that this product contains a special nutritional information. It claims to increase your muscle mass, decrease body fat, improve strength, and increase your drive. These claims are certainly appealing, but must be evaluated before they can be accepted.

Does the Information Make Sense? The first question to ask yourself when evaluating a nutrition claim is, Does the information make sense? (See Table 1.4.) Some claims are too outrageous to be true. If, for example, Power Boost had claimed to increase muscle mass and decrease body fat in only one week with no exercise or change in diet, common sense should tell you it is too good to be true. The claim that it will increase muscle mass over a four-week period with a strict training regimen is not so outrageous.

Where Did the Information Come From? If the claim seems reasonable, look to see where it came from. Was it a personal testimony, a government recommendation, or advice from a health professional? Was it the result of a research study? Is it in a news story or an advertising promotion?

Claims that come from individual testimonies have not been tested by experimentation. For example, the claim that Power Boost improves drive and motivation

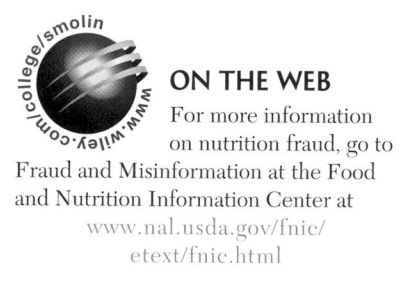

ON THE WEB
For more information on nutrition fraud, go to Fraud and Misinformation at the Food and Nutrition Information Center at www.nal.usda.gov/fnic/etext/fnic.html

Table 1.4 *Evaluating Nutrition Information*

1. Does the information make sense?

   Is it too outrageous to believe?

   Is it based on a cultural or religious belief?

2. Where did the information come from?

   Is it based on a government recommendation?

   Is it based on a study in a peer-reviewed journal?

   Have other studies confirmed the results?

   Is it based on someone's personal experience?

   Is it in a news story or an advertising promotion?

3. Were the experiments well designed?

   Were proper controls used?

   Were enough study subjects used to get reliable results?

   Were quantifiable data evaluated?

4. Is the information interpreted accurately?

   Were the results or importance of the study exaggerated?

   If the study was done in animals, can it be applied to humans?

   Was the level of food or nutrient used compatible with amounts in a human diet?

5. Who is making the recommendation and who stands to benefit?

   Is it helping to sell a product?

   Does the reporter stand to benefit from your believing the information?

   Is it making a magazine cover or newspaper headline more appealing?

   Is it designed to improve public health?

is anecdotal—it has not been studied using controlled experiments. Therefore, it cannot be assumed that similar results will occur in other people.

Government recommendations regarding healthy dietary practices are developed by committees of scientists who interpret the latest well-conducted research studies and use their conclusions to develop recommendations for the population as a whole. The government provides information about food safety and recommendations on food choices and the amounts of specific nutrients needed to avoid nutrient deficiencies and excesses and to prevent chronic diseases. These recommendations are used to develop food-labeling regulations and are the basis for public health policies and programs. They are published in pamphlets and brochures designed for consumers.

Research studies published in peer-reviewed journals are well scrutinized. But results presented at conferences or published in popular magazines, although they may be legitimate, have not been scrutinized by the scientific community to determine their quality and validity. The Power Boost ad states that the study was a university research study. They do not indicate if it was published, and if so, if it was published in a peer-reviewed journal.

Was the Study Well Designed and Accurately Interpreted? If the source of the information seems reliable, ask if the study was well designed and if the results were interpreted accurately. Even well-designed, carefully executed, peer-reviewed experiments can be a source of misinformation if the experimental results are interpreted incorrectly or if the implications of the results are exaggerated. For example, a study that shows that rats fed a diet high in vitamin E live longer than those consuming less vitamin E could be the basis of the headline, "Vitamin E Supplements Increase Longevity." The fact that a diet high in vitamin E increased longevity does not mean that supplements will have the same effect. In addition, this study was done in rats. Can the result be extrapolated to human health? Just because rats consuming diets high in vitamin E live longer does not mean that the same is true for humans.

Some sources provide the details of how a study was done. For others it is not possible to evaluate how studies were done. For example, the Power Boost ad (Figure 1.8) gives some information on how the study was done. We know that 25 experienced weight lifters were studied and that underwater weighing was used to assess muscle mass and body fat at the beginning and end of the study. However, we don't know if there was a control group not taking Power Boost, or whether there was any control over what the subjects ate or how much they worked out. There is no mention of a placebo that would have made control and experimental groups indistinguishable. Without a placebo to eliminate bias, the athletes taking a supplement they believed would increase strength and muscle mass could have been motivated to eat better and work out more strenuously. We know that athletes taking Power Boost gained an average of 5.2 pounds of lean tissue, but we don't know if controls not taking Power Boost would have gained more, less, or the same amount of lean tissue.

Who Stands to Benefit? The final question in judging nutrition claims is, Who is presenting the information or who stands to benefit from the information? Is the claim making a magazine cover or newspaper headline more appealing? If a claim is part of a news headline, it may be true but exaggerated to sell newspapers or magazines. Is it helping to sell a product? The claims for Power Boost are part of an advertisement to increase sales. The company stands to profit from your believing the claim.

Information in public health bulletins is designed to improve the health of the population. Information presented to individuals by nutritionists is designed to improve personal nutritional health. However, care must be taken even when obtaining information from nutritionists. Although "nutritionists" and "nutrition counselors" may provide accurate information, it is important to determine the credentials of these individuals. The term *nutritionist* is not legally defined and is used by a wide range of individuals from college professors with doctoral degrees from reputable universities to health food store clerks with no formal training. One reliable source of nutrition information is the registered dietitian. Registered dietitians (RDs) are nutrition professionals who have completed a four-year college degree in a nutrition-related field and who have met established criteria to certify them in providing nutrition counseling (see *Critical Thinking*: What Is Wrong with This Experiment?).

CRITICAL THINKING

What Is Wrong with This Experiment?

After seeing the advertisement for Power Boost in Figure 1.8, Jake wrote the company and asked about the "years of research" that were done to develop this product. He received the company's newsletter, which discussed these three experiments.

Experiment 1

Eight healthy male college students who regularly weight train were studied in two groups. They were asked to follow their regular weight-training regimens, but one group took Power Boost at every meal while the other group received a placebo. The study was double blind. After three weeks, the subjects were asked how energetic and motivated they felt during workouts. The individuals in the experimental group reported higher energy and motivation levels than those in the control group.

Was the study well controlled?
▼

The study used a placebo control and was double blind; however, individuals were not asked to evaluate their motivation and energy level before the study started, so it cannot be concluded that the Power Boost improved their energy or motivation. The experimental group may have been more energetic and motivated even without taking Power Boost. In addition, the study did not control for differences in diet or training level among the subjects. A better controlled study would have evaluated the subjects both before and after Power Boost and would have standardized dietary intake and workout regimens.

Was the proper number of experimental subjects used?
▼

No mention was made of a statistical analysis. It is unlikely that the small number of people in the experimental group could have conclusively demonstrated the advertised benefits of Power Boost.

Was quantifiable data evaluated?
▼

No. The data collected consisted of the opinions of the study subjects regarding their motivation or energy level.

Is the conclusion valid?
▼

No. Because no data were collected prior to giving Power Boost or the placebo, it cannot be concluded that the effect seen was due to Power Boost.

Experiment 2

Five groups of rats were used to test the absorption and muscle-building properties of the nutrients contained in Power Boost. Each group of four rats was fed rat chow plus a different formulation of nutrients. Rat feces were collected and analyzed to see which nutrients were absorbed and which were excreted. To measure muscle mass, body composition was determined by carcass analysis at the end of the study. The average amount of muscle mass in one group was 1.2 grams greater than any other group. This same group of rats excreted smaller amounts of the supplemental nutrients in their feces. It was concluded that the formulation given to this group of rats was best absorbed and resulted in an increase in muscle mass.

Was the study well controlled?
▼

No. There was no control group. All groups were taking some formulation of the supplement. No measurements of nutrient excretion or muscle mass were made at the beginning of the study before the supplement was given. Therefore, the change in nutrient excretion and muscle mass caused by adding these supplement formulations cannot be determined, only the differences between groups receiving the various formulations. There was also no control of activity, a variable that affects muscle development.

Was the proper number of experimental subjects used?

▼

The use of four rats per group may have been sufficient, but no statistical analysis was reported to verify that one group was truly different from the others. An increase in average muscle mass of 1.2 grams may simply be due to one large rat in that group and may not reflect an increase in the muscle mass of all rats in the group.

Was quantifiable data evaluated?

▼

Yes. Measures of muscle mass and nutrients in the feces are both quantifiable.

Given that this study was done using an experimental animal, is the conclusion valid?

▼

Rats may have been an adequate experimental model for nutrient absorption, but showing that rats absorb the supplement does not necessarily mean that humans will. Further, a study that demonstrates increased muscle mass in rats cannot conclude that the same supplement will improve muscle mass in humans.

Experiment 3

Two groups of 25 nutrition majors were studied over a four-week period. At the beginning of the study, leg and arm muscle strength was measured in all participants. One group then added the Power Boost supplement at every meal and snack. The other group received no supplement. Both groups were instructed to consume their typical diet. After four weeks, arm and leg muscle strength was again measured. The group taking Power Boost increased leg muscle strength by 5 pounds. There was no difference in leg strength in the group not taking Power Boost or in arm strength in any group. It was concluded that Power Boost helps improve muscle strength.

Was the experiment subjected to the peer-review process?

▼

No. This study, like the other two, was done and published by the company that makes the formula. There was no mention of a peer-review process by scientists who did not participate in the study.

Was the study well controlled? Was the proper number of experimental subjects used? Was quantifiable data evaluated? Is the conclusion valid?

▼

Answer:

• APPLICATIONS •

1. List four food items you ate today or yesterday.
   a. For each, indicate the factor or factors that influenced your selection of that particular food. For example, if you ate a candy bar before your noon class, did you choose it because the machine was available outside the lecture hall, because you didn't have enough money for anything else, because you just like candy bars, because you were depressed, because all of your friends were eating them, because it is good for you, or for some other reason?
   b. For each food, indicate what information you used in making the selection. For example, did you read the label on the product, or consider something you read or heard recently in the news media, or simply choose it because you like the taste?
   c. List three factors that commonly influence your food choices.
   d. List three types of information you regularly use to make your food choices.

2. Examine a nutritional supplement ad provided by your instructor or select one from a health or fitness-related magazine.
   a. Is the claim made about this product believable?
   b. Does the ad refer to any research studies? If so, do they seem well controlled? Were the results based on quantifiable measurements? Were the conclusions consistent with the results obtained? Were they published in peer-reviewed journals?
   c. Were claims based on anecdotal reports of individual users?
   d. Who stands to benefit if you spend money on this product?
   e. Based on this ad, would you choose to take this supplement?

3. Use an Internet search program to explore the types of nutrition information available on the Web. Search for the word nutrition. Make a list of four organizations that you find. Why do these organizations have Web sites? For example, one might be listed to sell products directly to the consumer, whereas another might provide public health messages.

SUMMARY

1. Nutrition is a science that encompasses all the interactions that occur between living organisms and food. These include the physiological processes by which an organism ingests and uses food; the biological actions and interactions of food with the body and their consequences for health and disease; and the psychological and sociocultural factors that influence what foods we eat.

2. Food contains nutrients that are needed by the body for growth, maintenance and repair, and reproduction. Nutrients are grouped into six classes: carbohydrates, lipids, proteins, water, vitamins, and minerals.

3. Nutrients provide energy, which is measured in kcalories or kjoules. They provide structure to the body and regulate the biochemical reactions of metabolism to maintain homeostasis. When energy or one or more nutrients are deficient or excessive in the diet, malnutrition may result.

4. Malnutrition includes both undernutrition and overnutrition. Its effects can occur in the short term or over the course of many weeks, months, or even years.

5. Consumers make many food choices every day. No one food choice is good or bad and no one choice can make a diet healthy or unhealthy—each choice contributes to the diet as a whole. The typical diet in North America does not meet the recommendations for a healthy diet and contributes to the incidence of chronic diseases such as diabetes, obesity, and heart disease.

6. Our food choices are affected by food availability, personal tastes, sociocultural influences, and what we think we should eat. What we think we should eat is affected by information received via media reports and advertising.

7. The science of nutrition uses the scientific method to determine the relationships between food and the nutrient needs of the body. The scientific method involves making observations of natural events, formulating hypotheses to explain these events, designing and performing experiments to test the hypotheses, and developing theories that explain the observed phenomenon based on the experimental results.

8. To be valid, a nutrition experiment must use quantifiable measurements, appropriate controls, the right type and number of experimental subjects, and a careful interpretation of experimental results.

9. The science of nutrition uses many different types of experimental approaches to determine nutrient functions and requirements. Epidemiology identifies relationships in populations. Intervention trials can test hypotheses developed from epidemiology. Laboratory studies, including those that study the whole organism such as depletion-repletion and balance studies, and those that study cells such as biochemical and molecular biological studies, are used to evaluate the relationships among nutrient intake, levels of nutrients in the body, and other parameters of metabolism or health.

10. When judging nutrition claims you need to consider whether the information makes sense, whether it came from a reliable source, whether the study was well done and accurately interpreted, and who stands to benefit from making the claim.

REVIEW QUESTIONS

1. What is nutrition?
2. What is an essential nutrient?
3. List the energy-yielding nutrients.
4. List three functions provided by nutrients.
5. What is malnutrition?
6. What is a toxicity?
7. How does the typical North American diet compare to recommendations for a healthy diet?

8. List three factors other than biological need that influence what we eat.

9. List the steps of the scientific method.

10. What is a control group?

11. What is a placebo?

12. What is a double-blind study?

13. What type of information can be obtained using epidemiology?

14. Why are animals used to study human nutrition?

15. What factors should be considered when judging nutrition claims?

REFERENCES

1. Institute of Medicine, Food and Nutrition Board. *Dietary Reference Intakes for Energy, Carbohydrates, Fiber, Fat, Protein and Amino Acids.* Washington, D.C.: National Academy Press, 2002.

2. Healthy People 2000 Progress Report for Nutrition. July 5, 1994. Available online at dphp.osophs.dhhs.gov/pubs/hp2000/ Accessed March 6, 2002.

3. Frazao, E. *America's Eating Habits: Changes and Consequences.* Agriculture Information Bulletin No. 750. ERS, USDA, 1999 Beltsville, MD. Available online at www.ers.usda.gov/publications/aib750/ Accessed March 7, 2002.

4. American Dietetic Association *Nutrition and You: Trends 2002.* Available online at www.eatright.org/ Accessed June 18, 2002.

Applying the Science of Nutrition   Chapter 2

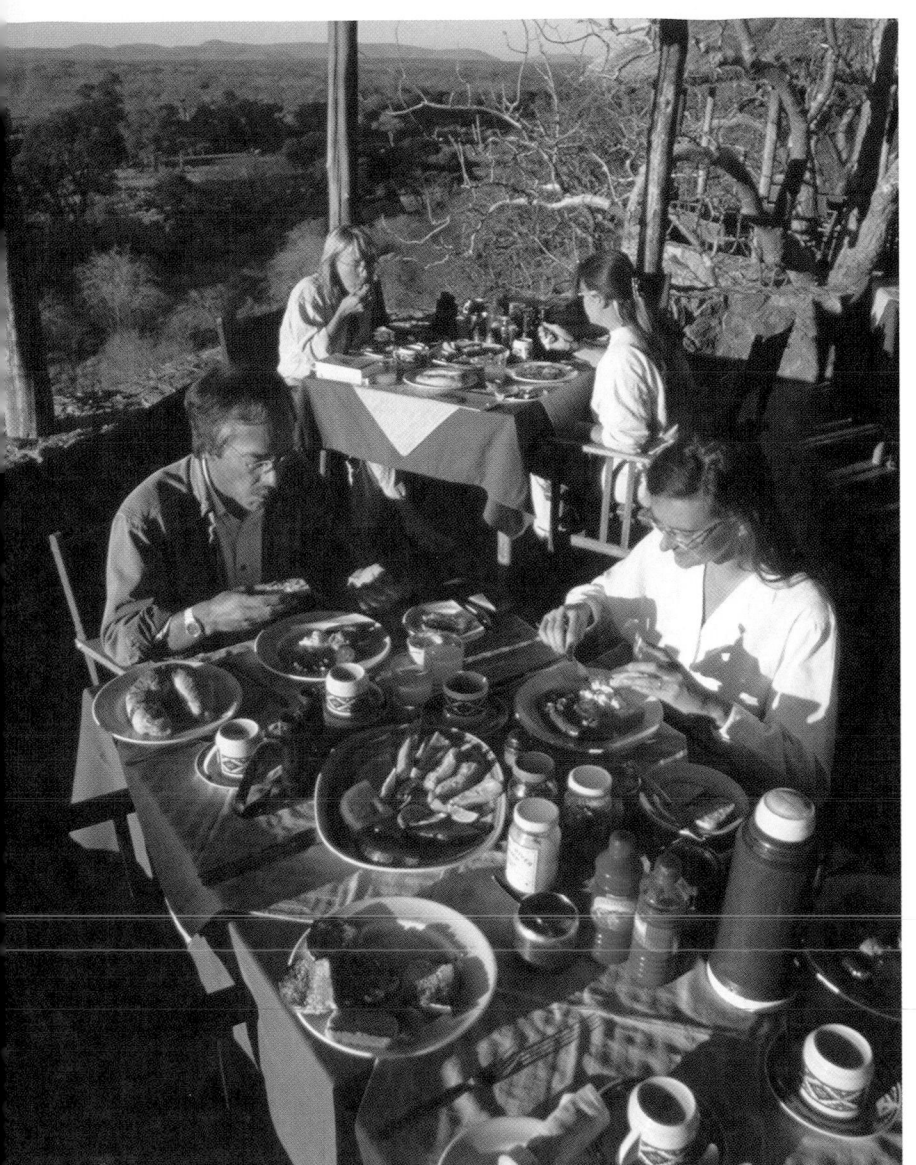

(© Tim Wright/Corbis)

Chapter Concepts

✔ Knowledge gained from nutrition research is used to develop standards and guidelines for dietary intake.

✔ The Dietary Reference Intakes are a set of reference values for the amounts of nutrients and food components needed in the diets of healthy individuals.

✔ The Food Guide Pyramid is a tool that can be used by individual consumers to plan diets that meet nutrition recommendations.

✔ Food labels provide information about the nutrient content of individual foods and help consumers determine how specific food products fit into their overall diet.

✔ The Dietary Guidelines for Americans are a set of nutrition and lifestyle recommendations that help consumers reduce the risks of chronic disease.

✔ The Exchange Lists is a food group system that can be used in planning diets with specific energy and macronutrient goals.

✔ The nutritional status of the population is monitored by identifying and comparing trends in food intake, health, and disease in the population.

✔ An individual's nutritional status can be assessed by evaluating dietary intake along with medical history and anthropometric and laboratory measures.

25

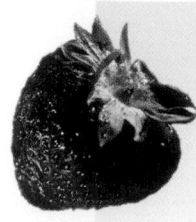

Just a Taste

How do you know if you are eating a healthy diet?

If your diet does not meet the RDAs, will you develop a nutrient deficiency?

Does what you eat for lunch affect what you should have for dinner?

People need to eat to survive, but health-conscious individuals want to do more than survive. They want to choose diets that will optimize their health. How do we know what an optimal diet is? We know it should contain just the right amount of each nutrient. But what is the right amount? Is it the amount needed to prevent a deficiency, the amount needed to maintain a certain nutrient level in the blood, the amount that minimizes cancer risk, maximizes immune function, or extends life span? For each nutrient, the optimal amount may vary depending on what parameter is being measured. The optimum is also different for each individual and depends on the amounts of other nutrients in the diet. Men have different needs from women, growing children have different needs from adults, athletes have different needs from sedentary individuals, and each of us has a unique genetic makeup that affects our nutrient requirements.

The science of nutrition has determined which nutrients are necessary for the survival of the species and how these needs vary at different stages of life, such as pregnancy or infancy. But it is not currently possible to determine the optimal amount of each nutrient that should be included in the diet of each individual. Instead, the methods of science have been used to establish general recommendations for the types and amounts of nutrients that will maintain the health of individuals and populations. To be useful to health-conscious consumers, these amounts have been translated into recommendations about food choices. These recommendations are also used as a standard of comparison to assess whether populations and individuals are consuming diets that promote health.

• NUTRITION RECOMMENDATIONS

Some of the first nutrition recommendations were made in England in the 1860s when the Industrial Revolution caused a rise in urban populations with large numbers of homeless and hungry people. The government wanted to know the least expensive way to keep these people alive and maintain the work force. As a result, a dietary standard was established based on what the average working person ate in a typical day. This method of estimating nutrient needs was used until World War I, when the British Royal Society made specific recommendations about foods that not only would sustain life but also would be protective of health. They recommended that fruits and green vegetables be included in a healthy diet and that milk be included in the diets of all children. Since then, the governments of many countries have established their own sets of dietary standards based on the nutritional problems and dietary patterns specific to their populations and the interpretations of their scientists. Most of the differences between guidelines from country to country are small. The World Health Organization and the Food and Agriculture Organization of the United Nations, organizations concerned with international health, publish a set of dietary standards to apply worldwide[1] (see Appendix F).

Because nutrition recommendations must satisfy a variety of needs, a number of different types of recommendations have been developed in the United States. Some describe the amounts of individual nutrients that are needed and some recommend patterns of food intake that promote health and prevent disease. The nature of each set of recommendations depends on the population it is targeting, who is developing it, what their goals are, and how it will be used. These recommendations are updated periodically as our understanding of nutrition evolves and new discoveries are made.

• DIETARY REFERENCE INTAKES: DEFINING NUTRIENT NEEDS

The current standard for recommended intakes of nutrients and other food components in the United States is a set of standards called the **Dietary Reference Intakes (DRIs)**. The DRIs are designed to be used for planning and assessing the diets of healthy people. They provide recommendations for the amounts of nutrients and other food components that should be consumed on an average daily basis—they are not requirements that must be consumed each day. The United States and Canada are collaborating to develop the DRIs, which are replacing both the 1989 RDAs in the United States and the Recommended Nutrient Intakes (RNIs) in Canada. This joint United States–Canadian effort will help to standardize recommendations for North America.

Development of the Dietary Reference Intakes

The original dietary standard in the United States was the Recommended Dietary Allowances (RDAs). They were developed in response to the widespread food limitations created by World War II (Figure 2.1). They were first published in 1943 and were revised every few years by the Food and Nutrition Board of the National Research Council until 1989.[2] The RDAs were set at levels that would prevent nutrient deficiencies. Recommendations were made for energy and nutrients at risk for deficiency—protein, vitamins, and minerals. Over the years since these first standards were developed, our knowledge of nutrient needs has increased and patterns of dietary intake and disease have changed. Overt nutrient deficiencies are now rare in most developed countries, but the incidence of chronic diseases whose risk is affected

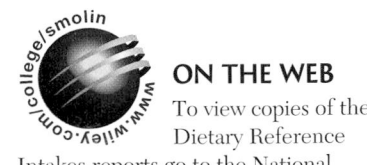

ON THE WEB
To view copies of the Dietary Reference Intakes reports go to the National Academy Press at
www.nap.edu/

Dietary Reference Intakes (DRIs) A set of four reference values for the intake of nutrients and food components that can be used for planning and assessing the diets of healthy people in the United States and Canada.

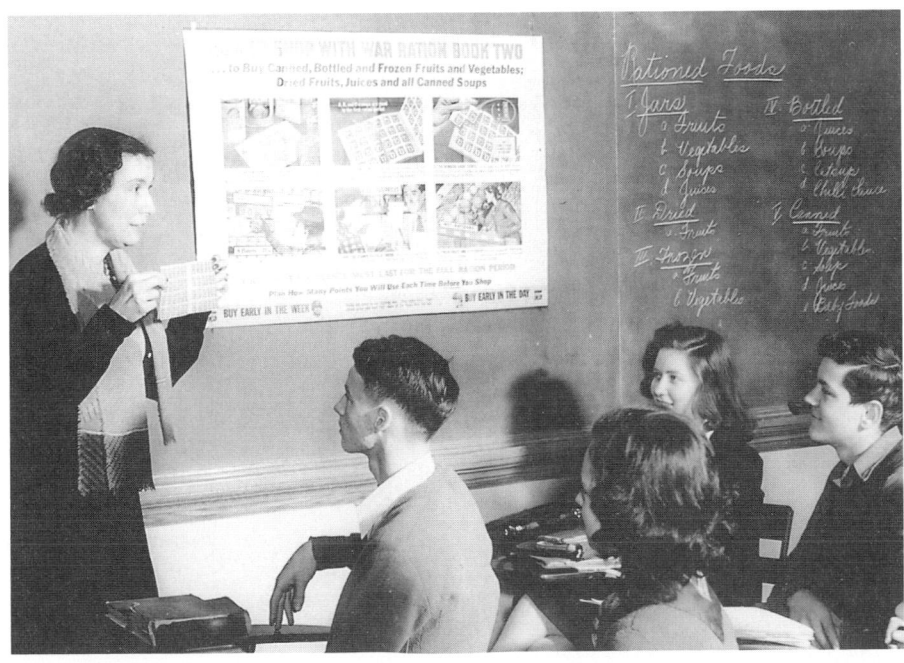

Figure 2.1
Food shortages during World War II prompted the U.S. government to establish dietary standards. (Office of War Information)

by diet such as heart disease, cancer, and obesity has increased. In response to these changes in our diet and health, the original RDAs are being replaced by the DRIs.

The DRIs are an expansion of the concept originally developed in the RDAs. They include values not only for energy, protein, and micronutrients but also for macronutrients (carbohydrate, fat, and protein) and food components that affect health, such as phytochemicals. The recommendations of the DRIs aim to promote health and reduce the incidence of chronic disease as well as prevent deficiencies.

The DRIs are being developed for seven nutrient groups: (1) calcium, phosphorus, magnesium, vitamin D, and fluoride; (2) B vitamins and choline; (3) antioxidants (vitamin C, vitamin E, selenium, and β-carotene) (4) vitamins A and K and the trace elements (e.g., iron, zinc, copper); (5) energy and macronutrients; (6) electrolytes and water; and (7) other food components (e.g., phytochemicals). Values for some groups have been established, others are in the process of being finalized. At the time this book was published values had been established for nutrients involved in bone formation (calcium, phosphorus, magnesium, vitamin D, and fluoride), for B vitamins and choline, for antioxidants, for vitamins A and K and the trace elements, and for energy and macronutrients (see inside cover).

Dietary Reference Intake Values

The DRIs include four different sets of values.[3] The **Estimated Average Requirement (EAR)** is the amount of a nutrient that is estimated to meet the needs of 50% of people in the same gender and life-stage group. The Estimated Average Requirement is a value that is useful for evaluating the adequacy of, and planning for, the nutrient intake of population groups. The prevalence of inadequate nutrient intakes can be estimated by looking at the proportion of the population with intakes below the EAR.

The **Recommended Dietary Allowances (RDAs)** are recommendations calculated to meet the needs of nearly all healthy individuals in each gender and life-stage group. The RDAs are determined by starting with the EAR value and using the variability in the requirements among individuals to increase it to an amount that meets the needs of 97 to 98% of healthy individuals. The RDA is the value that can be used by individuals as a guide to achieve adequate nutrient intake. Because the RDA is only a target, an intake less than the RDA does not necessarily indicate that the needs of that particular individual have not been met.[4] However, the risk of a deficiency is low if intake meets the RDA and increases as intake falls below the RDA.

The **Adequate Intakes (AIs)** are estimates used when there is insufficient scientific evidence to set an EAR and calculate an RDA. The AIs are based on observed or experimentally determined approximations of the average nutrient intake by a healthy population. When an AI value rather than an RDA is set, it targets the need for more research on the requirement of that nutrient. The AI values, like the RDAs, can be used as a goal for individual intake. A healthy individual whose intake of a specific nutrient is at or above the AI is unlikely to be deficient in that nutrient.

The fourth set of values, the **Tolerable Upper Intake Levels (ULs)**, represent the maximum level of daily intake of a nutrient that is unlikely to pose a risk of adverse health effects to almost all individuals in the specified group. It is not a recommended level, but it is a level of intake that can probably be tolerated. Tolerable Upper Intake Levels are used as a guide for limiting intake when planning diets and evaluating the possibility of over-consumption. The exact level of intake that will cause an adverse effect cannot be known with certainty for each individual, but if an individual's intake is below the UL, there is good assurance that an adverse effect will not occur.

Life-Stage Groups

The DRIs include values that apply to different **life-stage groups**. These have been established to account for the physiological differences among infants, children, adolescents, adults, older adults, and pregnant and lactating women. The

Estimated Average Requirements (EARs) Intakes that meet the estimated nutrient needs of 50% of individuals in a gender and life-stage group.

Recommended Dietary Allowances (RDAs) Intakes that are sufficient to meet the nutrient needs of almost all healthy people in a specific life-stage and gender group.

Adequate Intakes (AIs) Intakes that should be used as a goal when no RDA exists. These values are an approximation of the average nutrient intake that appears to sustain a desired indicator of health.

Tolerable Upper Intake Levels (UL) Maximum daily intakes that are unlikely to pose risks of adverse health effects to almost all individuals in the specified life-stage and gender group.

Life-stage groups Groupings of individuals based on stages of growth and development, pregnancy, and lactation that have similar nutrient needs.

pregnancy and lactation life stages also include age categories to distinguish the unique nutritional needs of pregnancy and lactation in teenagers and older mothers (see inside front cover).

How the Dietary Reference Intakes Are Determined

Determining levels of intake to reduce the risk of chronic disease, developmental disorders, and other health problems—as well as prevent deficiency diseases—is challenging. In order to meet this goal, appropriate criteria of adequate intake must be established for each nutrient in each life-stage and gender group. This **criterion of adequacy** is an indicator, such as the amount of a nutrient in the blood, that can be evaluated to determine the biological effect of a level of nutrient intake. The criteria may not be the same for different life-stage groups (Figure 2.2). For example, the AI for calcium for infants is based on the amount consumed in human milk. For children the AI is based on the amount needed for maximal calcium accumulation to support bone growth. For older adults the AI is set to support maximal calcium retention, which may decrease the risk of bone fractures. One or more criteria may be used to establish each EAR or AI. For all DRI values, the recommendations consider how much of a nutrient in food is available to the body for use.

To establish a UL, a specific adverse effect or indicator of excess is used. The lowest level of intake that causes the adverse effect is determined, and the UL is set far enough below this level that even the most sensitive people in the population are unlikely to be affected. If adverse effects have been associated only with intake from supplements, the UL is based only on this source. Therefore, for some nutrients these values represent intake from supplements alone; for some, intake from supplements and fortified foods; and for others, total intake from food, fortified food, water, nonfood sources, and supplements. For many nutrients, data are insufficient to establish a UL value.

Applications of the Dietary Reference Intakes

The DRIs have many uses. They provide a set of standards that can be used to plan diets, to assess the adequacy of diets, and to make judgments about excessive intakes for individuals and populations.[3] For example, they can be used as a standard for meals prepared for schools, for hospitals and for other health-care facilities, for government feeding programs for the elderly, and even for meals for space-shuttle astronauts. They can be used to determine standards for food labeling and to develop practical tools for diet planning, such as the Food Guide Pyramid.[5] They can also be used to interpret information gathered about the food consumed by a population to help identify potential nutritional inadequacies that may be of public health concern.

Despite their many uses, dietary standards cannot be used to identify with certainty whether a specific person has a nutritional deficiency or excess. To ascertain this, an evaluation of an individual's nutritional status using dietary, clinical, biochemical, and body-size measurements is needed, as discussed later in this chapter.

• THE FOOD GUIDE PYRAMID: A TOOL FOR DIET PLANNING

The DRIs recommend amounts of specific nutrients and food components, but they do not tell you how much of which foods you should choose to meet these. To help individuals follow the recommendations for a healthy diet, a number of systems have been developed to translate the recommendations for nutrient intake into food choices. The most commonly used tools are food groups. These divide foods into groups based on the nutrients they supply most abundantly and then recommend the number of servings from each group needed to provide a healthy diet. The most recent version of a food group system used in the United States is the Food Guide Pyramid (Figure 2.3). In Canada, the Food Guide to Healthy Eating is used (Appendix E).

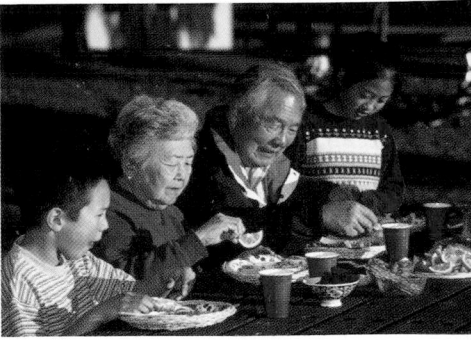

Figure 2.2
The nutrient requirements of growing children differ from those of older adults. The criteria used to determine the DRI values for a particular nutrient as well as the recommendations themselves may be different for different life-stage groups. (David Young-Wolff/PhotoEdit)

Criterion of adequacy An indicator such as the level of a nutrient in the blood or the appearance of a deficiency symptoms that can be evaluated to determine the biological effect of a level of nutrient intake.

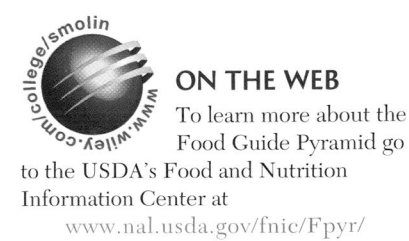

ON THE WEB
To learn more about the Food Guide Pyramid go to the USDA's Food and Nutrition Information Center at
www.nal.usda.gov/fnic/Fpyr/pyramid.html

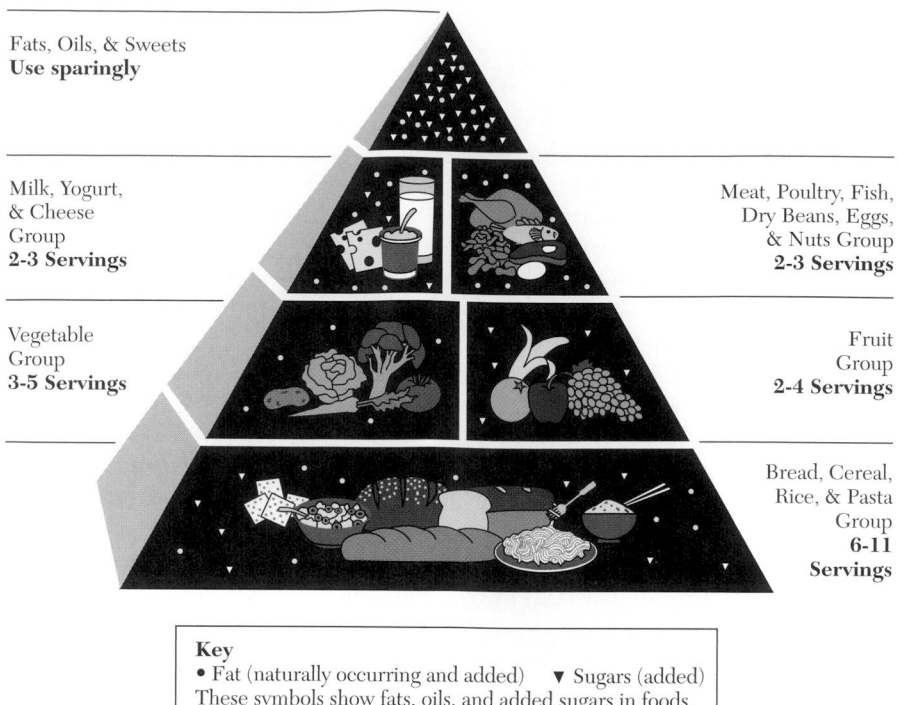

Figure 2.3
The Food Guide Pyramid. (USDA, 1992)

Food Guide Pyramid A guide for diet planning that is based on five major food groups. Following serving and selection recommendations helps individuals select diets that meet nutrient requirements and the recommendations for health promotion and disease prevention.

The **Food Guide Pyramid** is a guide for planning diets that meet nutrient requirements and the recommendations for health promotion and disease prevention. It proposes a diet plan based on servings from five food groups: Bread, Cereal, Rice, & Pasta; Vegetable; Fruit; Milk, Yogurt, & Cheese; and Meat, Poultry, Fish, Dry Beans, Eggs, & Nuts. The Pyramid also includes a recommendation to use Fats, Oils, & Sweets sparingly in the diet. The serving sizes within each group of the Pyramid are fairly constant. For instance, 1 serving from the Bread, Cereal, Rice, & Pasta Group is 1 slice of bread; 1 ounce of dry cereal; or 1/2 cup of cooked cereal, rice, or pasta (Table 2.1). Foods within each food group supply similar nutrients. For example, foods in the Milk, Yogurt, & Cheese Group are good sources of protein, calcium, and riboflavin.

Why Use a Pyramid Shape?

The shape of the Pyramid helps emphasize the relative contribution each food group should make to the diet. The large base of the Pyramid is made up of foods that come from grains: bread, cereal, rice, and pasta. These high-carbohydrate foods are the foundation of a healthy diet; between 6 and 11 servings per day are recommended. In the next level of the Pyramid are two groups of foods that also come from plant sources: the Vegetable Group, of which three to five servings per day are recommended, and the Fruit Group, of which two to four servings per day are recommended. The next level, where the decreasing size of the Pyramid boxes reflects the smaller number of recommended servings, comprises two groups of foods that come primarily from animals: the Milk, Yogurt, & Cheese Group, of which two to three servings are recommended, and the Meat, Poultry, Fish, Dry Beans, Eggs, & Nuts Group, of which two to three servings a day are recommended. At the narrow tip of the Pyramid are Fats, Oils, & Sweets. These should be used sparingly after other nutrient needs have been met.

Table 2.1 *Servings and Selections from the Food Guide Pyramid*

Food Group/Serving Size	Nutrients Provided	Selection Tips
Bread, Cereal, Rice, & Pasta (6 to 11 servings) 1/2 cup cooked cereal, rice, or pasta 1 ounce dry cereal 1 slice bread, 1 tortilla 2 cookies 1/2 medium doughnut	B vitamins, fiber, iron, magnesium, zinc, complex carbohydrates	Choose whole-grain breads, cereals, and grains such as whole wheat or rye, oatmeal, and brown rice. Use high-fat, high-sugar baked goods such as cakes, cookies, and pastries in moderation. Limit fats and sugars added as spreads, sauces, or toppings.
Vegetable (3 to 5 servings) 1/2 cup cooked or raw chopped vegetables 1 cup raw leafy vegetables 3/4 cup vegetable juice 10 french fries	Vitamin A, vitamin C, folate, magnesium, iron, fiber	Eat a variety of vegetables, including dark-green leafy vegetables like spinach and broccoli, deep-yellow vegetables like carrots and sweet potatoes, starchy vegetables such as potatoes and corn, and other vegetables such as green beans and tomatoes. Cook by steaming or baking. Avoid frying, and limit high-fat spreads or dressings.
Fruit (2 to 4 servings) 1 medium apple, banana, or orange 1/2 cup chopped, cooked, or canned fruit 3/4 cup fruit juice 1/4 cup dried fruit	Vitamin A, vitamin C, potassium, fiber	Choose fresh fruit, frozen without sugar, dried, or fruit canned in water or juice. If canned in heavy syrup, rinse with water before eating. Eat whole fruits more often than juices; they are higher in fiber. Regularly eat citrus fruits, melons, or berries rich in vitamin C. Only 100% fruit juice should be counted as fruit.
Milk, Yogurt, & Cheese (2 to 3 servings) 1 cup milk or yogurt 1 1/2 ounces natural cheese 2 ounces process cheese 2 cups cottage cheese 1 1/2 cups ice cream 1 cup frozen yogurt	Protein, calcium, riboflavin, vitamin D	Use lowfat or skim milk for healthy people over 2 years of age. Choose lowfat and nonfat yogurt, "part skim" and lowfat cheeses, and lower-fat frozen desserts like ice milk and frozen yogurt. Limit high-fat cheeses and ice cream.
Meat, Poultry, Fish, Dry Beans, Eggs, & Nuts (2 to 3 servings) 2–3 ounces cooked lean meat, fish, or poultry 2–3 eggs 4–6 tablespoons peanut butter 1 to 1 1/2 cups cooked dry beans 2/3 to 1 cup nuts	Protein, niacin, vitamin B_6, vitamin B_{12}, iron, zinc	Select lean meat, poultry without skin, and dry beans often. Trim fat, and cook by broiling, roasting, grilling, or boiling rather than frying. Limit egg yolks, which are high in cholesterol, and nuts and seeds, which are high in fat. Be aware of serving size; 3 ounces of meat is the size of an average hamburger.
Fats, Oils, & Sweets (use sparingly) Butter, mayonnaise, salad dressing, cream cheese, sour cream, jam, jelly		These are high in energy and low in micronutrients. Substitute lowfat dressings and spreads.

Human Nutrition Information Service. *The Food Guide Pyramid*. Home and Garden Bulletin No. 252. Hyattsville, Md.: U.S. Department of Agriculture, 1992, 1996, revised.

Planning Diets Using the Food Guide Pyramid

To plan a diet that satisfies the recommendations of the Food Guide Pyramid, several servings of breads and grains and fruits or vegetables should be included at each meal. From this base, servings from the milk and meat groups can be added. Mixed dishes can be planned with the Pyramid by considering the component parts. For example, a chicken taco consists of a tortilla (a bread), chicken (a meat), and lettuce and tomatoes (vegetables). A beef with broccoli stir-fry consists of beef (a meat) and broccoli (a vegetable), served over rice (a grain). However, just choosing the specified number of servings from each group of the Food Guide Pyramid will not assure an optimal diet. Wise choices must be made from each food group.

Nutrient density A measure of the nutrients provided by a food relative to the energy it contains.

Choosing for Balance and Variety Planning a diet to meet nutrient needs must consider the **nutrient density** of foods as well as the variety and balance of the foods chosen. Nutrient density refers to the amount of essential nutrients in a food relative to the energy provided. For example, both skim milk and ice cream are in the Milk, Yogurt, & Cheese Group. However, a 1-cup serving of skim milk provides 300 mg of calcium in 90 kcalories, whereas a cup of ice cream provides 168 mg of calcium in 265 kcalories. The skim milk is considered to have a higher nutrient density because it provides more nutrients per kcalorie than the ice cream. The Food Guide Pyramid offers selection tips for choosing a nutrient-dense diet, which are listed in Table 2.1.

Choosing a variety of foods is also essential to meeting nutrient needs. There are similarities in the nutrients provided by different foods from within each food group, but there are also important differences in the amounts and types of nutrients. For example, white potatoes and carrots are both in the vegetable group of the Food Guide Pyramid. White potatoes are a good source of vitamin C but contain almost no vitamin A; carrots provide vitamin A , but have little vitamin C. A diet that meets the recommended 3 servings of vegetables each day but includes 3 servings of potatoes will be missing out on vitamin A and other nutrients that you would have consumed in a more varied diet. Choosing a varied diet is also important because there are interactions between different foods and nutrients. These interactions may be positive, enhancing nutrient utilization, or negative, inhibiting nutrient use. For example, consuming iron with orange juice enhances its absorption, while consuming iron with milk may reduce its absorption. In a varied diet these interactions balance out. In addition, some foods may contain toxic substances such as pesticides, fertilizers, and natural toxins. Choosing a variety of foods avoids an excess of any one of these substances (see *Critical Thinking*: Using the Food Guide Pyramid).

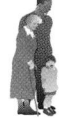

Meeting Individual Needs and Preferences The Food Guide Pyramid is designed to meet a variety of energy needs as well as to be flexible enough to suit the preferences of people from diverse cultures and lifestyles. By choosing within the

Table 2.2 *Number of Food Guide Pyramid Servings for Three Daily Energy Levels**			
	1600 kcalories (sedentary women and some older adults)	2200 kcalories (children, teenage girls, active women, and many sedentary men)	2800 kcalories (teenage boys, many active men, and some very active women)
Bread, Cereal, Rice, & Pasta Group	6	9	11
Vegetable Group	3	4	5
Fruit Group	2	3	4
Milk, Yogurt, & Cheese Group	2–3†	2–3†	2–3†
Meat, Poultry, Fish, Dry Beans, Eggs, & Nuts Group	2 (5 oz total)	2 (6 oz total)	3 (7 oz total)

*Assumes that food choices are mostly lowfat and low kcalorie.

†Women who are pregnant or breastfeeding, teenagers, and young adults to age 24 need three servings.

U.S. Department of Agriculture. *The Food Guide Pyramid*. Home and Garden Bulletin 252, 1992, revised 1996.

range of recommended servings, individuals can satisfy a variety of energy needs. For example, those who need 1600 kcalories per day could meet their needs by using the low end of the range of servings, for instance, 6 bread servings per day. Someone who needs 2800 kcalories per day should choose from the high end of the range for each food group, for instance, 11 breads, 5 vegetables, 4 fruits, and so on (Table 2.2).

The Pyramid can also be used for groups with special needs. Pregnant and lactating women, children, adolescents, and adults under 25 years of age should consume three servings from the milk group. Modified Food Guide Pyramids have been developed for vegetarians, young children, and older adults (see Chapters 6, 15, and 16). In addition, pyramids designed around various ethnic diets have been developed to provide food choices that meet the needs of different cultures (see Appendix H).

CRITICAL THINKING

Using the Food Guide Pyramid

For the first time in his life, Jarad is living on his own. He has gained a few pounds and is beginning to realize that he needs to pay more attention to the kinds of foods he eats. To evaluate his nutrient intake, he records everything he consumes for one day and compares it with the number of servings recommended by the Food Guide Pyramid.

▼

Food	Serving Size	Number of Servings	Food Group
Breakfast			
Cornflakes	3/4 cup	1	Grain
Whole milk	3/4 cup	3/4	Milk
Orange juice	3/4 cup	1	Fruit
Coffee	1 cup		
with cream	1 Tbsp		Fats and sweets
and sugar	1 tsp		Fats and sweets
Snack			
Doughnut	1	2	Grain
Lunch			
Hamburger			
roll	1 whole	2	Grain
patty	2 oz	1	Meat
onions	1 Tbsp	1/8	Vegetable
sauce	1 Tbsp		Fats and sweets
French fries	25 pieces	2 1/2	Vegetable
Milk shake	12 fluid oz	1 1/2	Milk
Snack			
Soda	1 can		Fats and sweets
Dinner			
Frozen lasagna			
noodles	1 cup	2	Grain
tomato sauce	1/2 cup	1	Vegetable
ground beef	4 oz	2	Meat
cheese	1 oz	2/3	Milk
Soda	1 can		Fats and sweets
Ice cream	1 cup	2/3	Milk

Does Jarad's diet meet the minimum number of servings recommended by the Food Guide Pyramid?

▼

Recommended Servings	Total Number of Servings in the Diet
Bread, Cereal, Rice, & Pasta (6–11 servings)	_____
Vegetable (3–5 servings)	_____
Fruit (2–4 servings)	_____
Milk, Yogurt, & Cheese (2–3 servings)	_____
Meat, Poultry, Fish, Dry Beans, Eggs, & Nuts (2–3 servings)	_____

Jarad consumes adequate numbers of servings from all the food groups except the fruit group. He can easily increase his fruit consumption by taking a piece of fruit as a snack or adding fruit to his cereal in the morning.

How many foods did he have during the day that contribute primarily sugar and/or fat?

▼

Fats, oils, and sweets (sparingly)_____

How would you rate Jarad's food selections in terms of their nutrient density and variety?

▼

He does not choose many nutrient-dense foods. Many of Jarad's choices, such as doughnuts, soda, ice cream, and french fries, are of low nutrient density. Lack of variety is also a problem in his diet. His selections from the base of the Pyramid include no whole grains, and almost all his vegetable servings are from french fries. An occasional serving of french fries is fine, but it is important to also include green and yellow-orange vegetables in the diet because they contain nutrients that may be missing from potatoes.

How would more nutrient-dense choices affect the energy content of his diet?

▼

More nutrient-dense choices, such as fruit instead of a doughnut for a morning snack and lowfat milk and frozen desserts, will reduce the energy and fat content of his diet. This will allow him to add more whole grains and vegetables without exceeding his energy needs.

To increase the variety and nutrient density of his diet, Jarad decides to try having lunch at a local sandwich shop that assembles sandwiches to order.

Suggest a nutrient-dense sandwich order that includes selections from at least three Food Guide Pyramid food groups.

▼

Answer:

• FOOD LABELS: KNOWING WHAT YOU CHOOSE

Food labels are another tool that can be used in diet planning. They are designed to help consumers make healthy food choices by providing information about the nutrient composition of foods and about how a food fits into the overall diet. To make this information uniform and easy to use, food labeling standards are specified by the Nutrition Labeling and Education Act of 1990.[6]

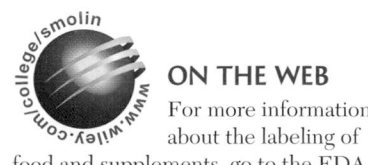

ON THE WEB
For more information about the labeling of food and supplements, go to the FDA Center for Food Safety and Applied Nutrition at

www.cfsan.fda.gov/

What Must Be Labeled

Food labeling laws regulate about 75% of all food consumed in the United States.[7] The Food and Drug Administration (FDA) regulates the labeling of all foods except meat and poultry products, which are regulated by the U.S. Department of Agriculture (USDA). All packaged foods except those produced by small businesses and those in packages too small to fit the labeling information must be labeled. Some restaurant food and ready-to-eat food, such as that served in bakeries and delicatessens, is also exempt, but if a claim about a food's nutritional content or health benefits such as "lowfat" or "heart healthy" is included on a menu, the eating establishment must provide nutritional information about this food when requested[8] (see *Off the Shelf*: Choosing Off the Menu). Raw fruits, vegetables, fish, meat, and poultry are not required to carry individual labels. The FDA has asked grocery stores to voluntarily provide nutrition information for the raw fruits, vegetables, and fish most frequently eaten in the United States, and the USDA encourages voluntary nutrition labeling of raw meat and poultry. About 75% of stores comply with the request to provide nutrient information for raw produce and fish.[7] The information can appear on large placards or in consumer pamphlets or brochures (Figure 2.4).

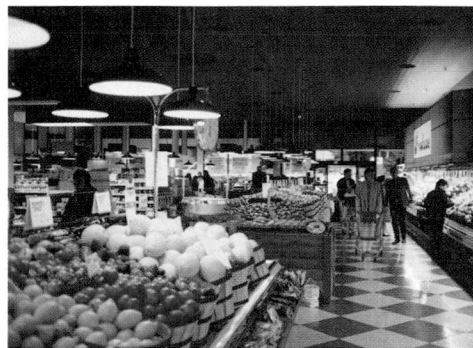

Figure 2.4
Fresh produce is not required to carry individual labels, but the information is usually displayed in the produce section of the store. (PhotoDisc, Inc.)

What Must Be Listed

All labels contain basic product information such as the name of the product; the net contents or weight; the date by which the product should be sold; and the name and place of business of the manufacturer, packager, or distributor. In addition, most food labels contain a list of the food's ingredients and a "Nutrition Facts" panel that provides information about the nutrient content of the product and its contribution to a healthy diet.

List of Ingredients   The ingredients section of the label lists the contents of the product in order of their prominence by weight. An ingredient list is required on all products containing more than one ingredient. Food additives, including food colors and flavorings, must be listed among the ingredients.

Nutrition Facts   The nutrition information section of the label is entitled "Nutrition Facts" (Figure 2.5). In this section, the serving size is listed in common household and metric measures, and is based on a standard list of serving sizes designed to be representative of the serving sizes people choose. The use of standard serving sizes allows comparisons to be made easily between products. For example, comparing the energy content of different types of crackers is simplified because all packages list energy values for a standard serving size of about 30 grams and tell you the number of crackers per serving. These serving sizes are not always the same as the serving sizes in the Food Guide Pyramid.

The serving size on the label is followed by the number of servings per container. The label must then list the total kcalories (on food labels the term "Calorie" is used to represent kcalories), kcalories from fat, total fat, saturated fat, cholesterol, sodium, total carbohydrate, dietary fiber, sugars, and protein. The amounts of these nutrients are given per serving, and most are also listed as a percentage of a standard called the **Daily Value**. Daily Values help consumers determine how a food fits into

Daily Value A nutrient reference value used on food labels to help consumers see how foods fit into their overall diets.

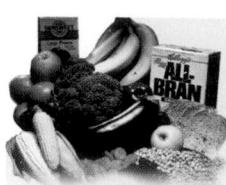

Off the Shelf

Choosing Off the Menu

Treating yourself to an occasional dinner out has little long-term impact on your total diet, but for many Americans eating out is more than an occasional treat. Today, more Americans than ever are eating away from home, and the restaurant meals they consume are usually higher in fat and cholesterol than meals eaten at home.[1] The change in our lifestyle to include more restaurant and fast-food meals has made choosing healthy foods from restaurant menus an important skill—but it can be a challenge.

Some healthy choices are easy, even at restaurants. If you are looking for a low-fat meal, skip the fried fish and have it broiled instead. Minimize sauces and spreads (like the honey butter on your corn bread) that add fat, sugar, and kcalories. Use less salad dressing by asking that it be served on the side. Be conscious of portion sizes. Those served in restaurants are often much larger than what we prepare at home. You don't have to finish everything—take it home for tomorrow's lunch.

Other restaurant choices are more difficult to make. Items that sound like part of a healthy diet are not always what they seem. What's in that house special turkey tetrazzini, beef lo mein, or a fajita wrap? Without the chef's recipe it is impossible to know. The amounts of specific nutrients are usually not given on menus and the ingredients can be a mystery. Even when you know what ingredients are usually in a dish like eggplant parmesan, you can never be sure how much oil or salt was used. Even an order of plain old green beans might come floating in butter.

Many restaurants and fast-food establishments have responded to consumer concern about healthy diets with healthier choices. Menus often highlight healthy items by making claims about nutrient content, such as lowfat tostados, low-salt lo mein, or reduced kcalorie lasagna. The food labeling laws that regulate packaged foods also apply to menus so the definition of these terms must match those used on food labels. For example, if you order low-fat tostados, the term "lowfat" should mean the same as it does on labeled packaged foods—that it contains 3 grams or less of fat per serving.

Menus may also include statements that give general dietary guidance or make specific claims about the relationship between a nutrient and a disease or health condition. For example, the salad section may start with the statement that "eating five fruits and vegetables a day is an important part of a healthy diet."[2] A dish that is low in fat, saturated fat, and cholesterol might carry a claim that diets low in saturated fat and cholesterol may reduce the risk of heart disease. To carry a health claim, menu items must contain a signifi-

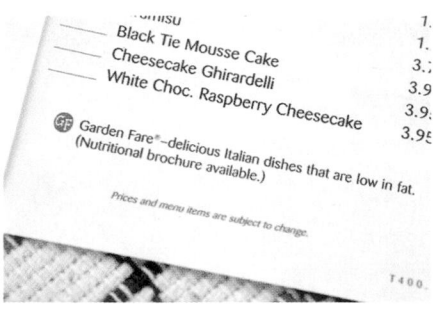

George Semple

cant amount of at least one of six key nutrients (vitamin A, vitamin C, iron, calcium, protein, or fiber) and cannot contain a food substance at a level that increases the risk of a disease or health condition.

Nutrient content claims and health claims about items on the menu must be backed up with appropriate material when requested. This information can be on the menu or in accompanying nutrition information available upon request. It can be presented in any format, such as printed in a notebook or recited by the staff, and only needs to provide information about the nutrient or nutrients to which the claim is referring. Restaurants do not have to provide nutrition information about items that do not carry nutrient content or health claims or that are referred to in general dietary messages.

When choosing from a menu, look for items that fit into an overall healthy diet—and are also things you enjoy. Choose foods you like and remember that a high-fat or high-kcalorie meal now and then doesn't make your overall diet unhealthy. But, if you eat out frequently, these meals make up a greater part of your overall diet and should be chosen carefully. Use nutrient content claims and health claims to choose items that meet your dietary needs.

[1] USDA, Agricultural Service, 1997, Results from USDA's 1994–1996 Continuing Survey of Food Intakes by Individuals and 1994–1996 Health Knowledge Survey. ARS Food Surveys Research Group. Available online at www.barc.usda.gov/bhnrc/foodsurvey/home/htm/ Accessed February 28, 2002.

[2] Kurtzweil, P. Today's special nutrition information. *FDA Consumer* 31:21–25, May–June, 1997.

Reference Daily Intakes (RDIs)
Reference values established for vitamins and minerals that are based on the highest amount of each nutrient recommended for any adult age group by the 1968 RDAs.

Daily Reference Values (DRVs)
Reference values established for protein and seven nutrients for which no original RDAs were established. The values are based on dietary recommendations for reducing the risk of chronic disease.

their overall diet. The percent Daily Value is the amount of a nutrient in a food as a percentage of the recommendation for a 2000-kcalorie diet. For example, if a food provides 10% of the Daily Value for dietary fiber, then the food provides 10% of the recommended daily intake for dietary fiber in a 2000-kcalorie diet. Daily Values are based on two sets of standards, the **Reference Daily Intakes (RDIs)** and the **Daily Reference Values (DRVs)**. To avoid confusion, only the term "Daily Value" appears on food labels.

The Reference Daily Intakes (Table 2.3) are used to determine Daily Values for vitamins and minerals for which original RDAs were established. Although the name has changed, most of the current RDI values are the same as the old U.S. RDAs (U.S. Recommended Daily Allowances). They are based on the highest amount of

Standardized serving sizes simplify comparison of the nutrient content of similar products

The list of nutrients includes those most important to the health of today's consumer

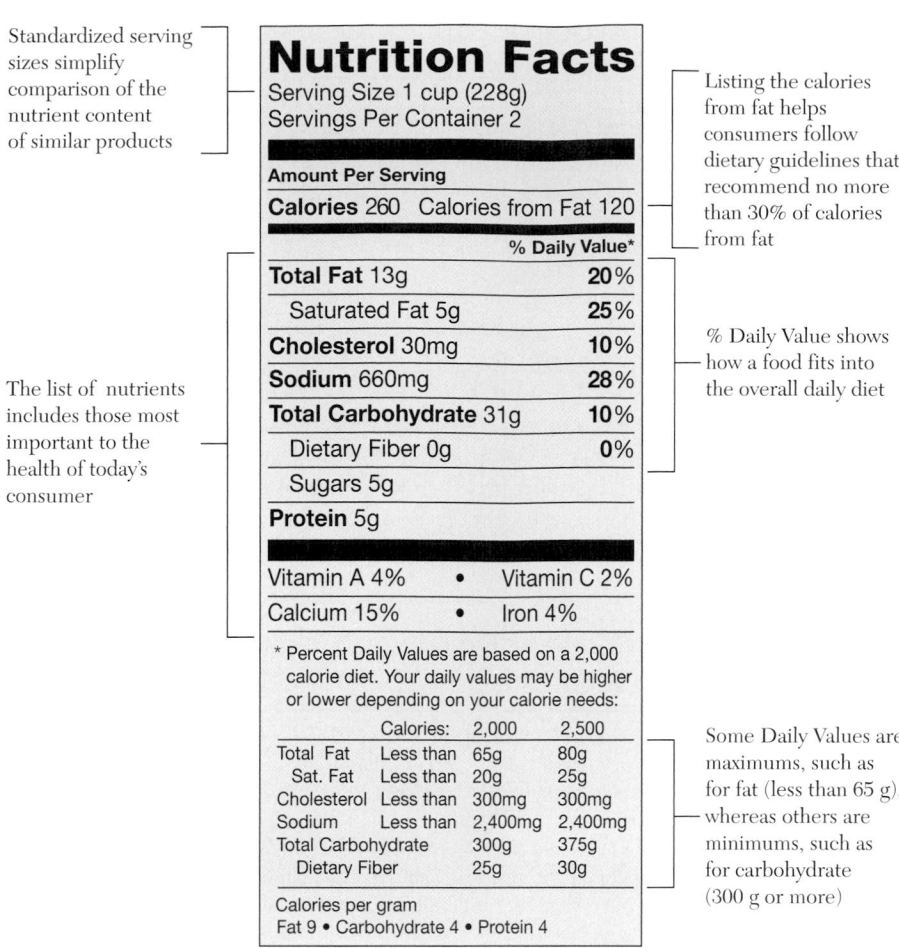

Listing the calories from fat helps consumers follow dietary guidelines that recommend no more than 30% of calories from fat

% Daily Value shows how a food fits into the overall daily diet

Some Daily Values are maximums, such as for fat (less than 65 g), whereas others are minimums, such as for carbohydrate (300 g or more)

Figure 2.5
The Nutrition Labeling and Education Act of 1990 required standardization of the information on food labels. (*FDA Consumer* 27:23, May 1993)

each nutrient recommended for any adult age group by the 1968 RDAs. These may overestimate the amount of a nutrient needed for some groups, but they do not underestimate the requirement for any group (except pregnant and lactating women). Label regulations require that percent Daily Values, based on RDIs, be listed for vitamin A, vitamin C, calcium, and iron. A manufacturer may voluntarily include information about other vitamins and minerals.

Daily Reference Values are guidelines for the amounts of total fat, saturated fat, carbohydrate, fiber, cholesterol, sodium, potassium, and protein that should be included in

Table 2.3 *Reference Daily Intakes**

Nutrient	Amount	Nutrient	Amount	Nutrient	Amount
Vitamin A	5000 IU†	Vitamin E	30 IU†	Biotin	300 μg
Vitamin C	60 mg	Vitamin B$_6$	2.0 mg	Pantothenic acid	10 mg
Thiamin	1.5 mg	Folic acid	400 μg	Vitamin K	80 μg
Riboflavin	1.7 mg	Vitamin B$_{12}$	6 μg	Chromium	120 μg
Niacin	20 mg	Phosphorus	1000 mg	Selenium	70 μg
Calcium	1000 mg	Iodine	150 μg	Molybdenum	75 μg
Iron	18 mg	Magnesium	400 mg	Manganese	2 mg
Vitamin D	400 IU†	Zinc	15 mg	Chloride	3400 mg
		Copper	2 mg		

*Based on National Academy of Sciences' 1968 Recommended Dietary Allowances.

†The RDIs for some fat-soluble vitamins are expressed in International Units (IU). The DRIs use a newer system of measurement.

Table 2.4
Daily Reference Values

Food Component	Daily Reference Value (2000 kcal)
Total fat	Less than 65 g (30% of energy)
Saturated fat	Less than 20 g (10% of energy)
Cholesterol	Less than 300 mg
Total carbohydrate	300 g (60% of energy)
Dietary fiber	25 g (11.5 g/1000 kcal)
Sodium	Less than 2400 mg
Potassium	3500 mg
Protein	50 g (10% of energy)

a healthy diet (Table 2.4). The DRV for fat, for example, is based on the recommendation that dietary fat should account for less than 30% of energy, or less than 65 grams for a 2000-kcalorie diet. The DRVs are used on food labels to calculate the percent Daily Values for nutrients based on a diet containing 2000 kcalories. To illustrate that the recommended intake of some nutrients depends on energy needs, Daily Values based on DRVs are listed on food labels for both a 2000- and a 2500-kcalorie diet.

Nutrient Content Claims

In addition to the required nutrition information, food labels often highlight specific characteristics of a product that might be of interest to the consumer, such as "low in Calories" or "high in fiber." Definitions for nutrient content descriptors such as "free," "low," and "light" have been established by the FDA and are based on how these terms relate to nutrient content. In selecting a product labeled with a descriptor such as "fat free," consumers can be assured that the food meets the defined criteria, in this case that the product contains less than 0.5 gram of fat per serving. The specific definition of each of these descriptors is given in Table 2.5 and their use in relation to specific nutrients is discussed in *Off the Label* features throughout this text.

Table 2.5 *Nutrient Content Descriptors Commonly Used on Food Labels*

Free	Product contains no amount of, or a trivial amount of, fat, saturated fat, cholesterol, sodium, sugars, or kcalories. For example, "sugar free" and "fat free" both mean less than 0.5 g per serving. Synonyms for "free" include "without," "no," and "zero."
Low	Used for foods that can be eaten frequently without exceeding the Daily Value for fat, saturated fat, cholesterol, sodium, or kcalories. Specific definitions have been established for each of these nutrients. For example, "lowfat" means that the food contains 3 g or less per serving, and "low cholesterol" means that the food contains less than 20 mg of cholesterol per serving. Synonyms for "low" include "little", "few", and "low source of."
Lean and extra lean	Used to describe the fat content of meat, poultry, seafood, and game meats. "Lean" means that the food contains less than 10 g fat, less than 4.5 g saturated fat, and less than 95 mg of cholesterol per serving and per 100 g. "Extra lean" means that the food contains less than 5 g fat, less than 2 g saturated fat, and less than 95 mg of cholesterol per serving and per 100 g.
High	Used for foods that contain 20% or more of the Daily Value for a particular nutrient. Synonyms for "high" include "rich in" and "excellent source of."
Good source	Food contains 10 to 19% of the Daily Value for a particular nutrient per serving.
Reduced	Nutritionally altered product contains 25% less of a nutrient or of energy than the regular or reference product.
Less	Food, whether altered or not, contains 25% less of a nutrient or of energy than the reference food. For example, pretzels may claim to have "less fat" than potato chips. "Fewer" may be used as a synonym for "less."
Light	Used in different ways. First, it can be used on a nutritionally altered product that contains one-third fewer kcalories or half the fat of a reference food. Second, it can be used when the sodium content of a low-calorie, lowfat food has been reduced by 50%. The term "light" can be used to describe properties such as texture and color as long as the label explains the intent—for example, "light and fluffy".
More	Serving of food, whether altered or not, contains a nutrient that is at least 10% of the Daily Value more than the reference food. This definition also applies to foods using the terms "fortified", "enriched", or "added."
Healthy	Used to describe foods that are low in fat and saturated fat and contain no more than 360 mg of sodium and no more than 60 mg of cholesterol per serving and provide at least 10% of the Daily Value for vitamins A or C, or iron, calcium, protein, or fiber.
Fresh	Used on foods that are raw and have never been frozen or heated and contain no preservatives.

Federal Register 58, Jan. 6, 1993. U.S. Government Printing Office, Superintendent of Documents, Washington, D.C.

Health Claims

Food labels are also permitted to include a number of health claims if they are relevant to the product. Health claims refer to a relationship between a nutrient or a food and the risk of a disease or health-related condition. They can be used on conventional foods or dietary supplements and can help consumers choose products that will meet their dietary needs or health goals. For example, lowfat milk, a good source of calcium, might include on the package label a statement indicating that a diet high in calcium will reduce the risk of developing osteoporosis. Health claims are permitted only after the scientific evidence is reviewed and found to be factual and truthful. The claims listed in Table 2.6 are currently approved by the FDA for use on food labels.[9]

Despite the wealth of information available on food labels, today's consumer must be educated about the benefits and pitfalls of foods that are not labeled and about food and nutrition issues that are not addressed by food labels. Such issues include the advantages and disadvantages of fresh, frozen, and canned produce, and the safe selection, storage, and preparation of food. Food labels cannot tell you what you should eat, or how you should prepare it, but they are an important source of information about what you are eating (see *Off the Label*: Using Food Labels to Choose a Diet That Meets Recommendations).

Table 2.6 *FDA-Approved Health Claims**

Calcium and osteoporosis	Adequate calcium intake throughout life helps maintain bone health and reduce the risk of osteoporosis.
Sodium and hypertension (high blood pressure)	Diets low in sodium may reduce the risk of high blood pressure in some people.
Dietary fat and cancer	Diets low in fat may reduce the risk of some types of cancer.
Saturated fat and cholesterol and risk of coronary heart disease	Diets low in saturated fat and cholesterol help reduce blood cholesterol and, thus, the risk of heart disease.
Fiber-containing grain products, fruits, and vegetables, and cancer risk	Diets low in fat and rich in fiber-containing grain products, fruits, and vegetables may reduce the risk of some types of cancer.
Fruits, vegetables, and grain products that contain fiber, particularly soluble fiber, and risk of coronary heart disease	Diets low in saturated fat and cholesterol and rich in fruits, vegetables, and grain products that contain fiber, particularly soluble fiber, may reduce the risk of coronary heart disease.
Fruits and vegetables and cancer	Diets low in fat and rich in fruits and vegetables may reduce the risk of some types of cancer.
Folic acid and neural tube birth defects	Adequate folic acid intake by the mother reduces the risk of birth defects of the brain or spinal cord in her baby.
Soluble fiber from certain foods and risk of coronary heart disease	Diets low in fat, saturated fat, and cholesterol that include soluble fiber from whole oats or psyllium seed husk may reduce the risk of heart disease.
Dietary sugar alcohol and dental caries (cavities)	Sugar-free foods that are sweetened with sugar alcohols do not promote tooth decay and may reduce the risk of dental caries.
Soy protein and risk of coronary heart disease	Soy protein included in a diet that is low in saturated fat and cholesterol may reduce the risk of coronary heart disease by lowering blood cholesterol levels.
Plant sterol/stanol esters and risk of coronary heart disease	Plant sterols and plant stanols included in a diet that is low in saturated fat and cholesterol may reduce the risk of coronary heart disease by lowering blood cholesterol levels.

*A food carrying a health claim must be a naturally good source (10% or more of the Daily Value) for one of six nutrients (vitamin A, vitamin C, protein, calcium, iron, or fiber) and must not contain more than 20% of the Daily Value for fat, saturated fat, cholesterol, or sodium. These claims have been approved for use on food labels. The FDA continues to evaluate new claims, many of which are in various stages of approval.

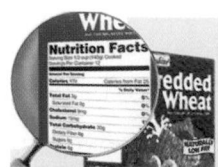

Off the Label

Using Food Labels to Choose a Diet That Meets Recommendations

ood labels can't help you include three to five servings of vegetables and two to four servings of fruit in your diet each day, or ensure that you select a varied diet, but they can help you choose foods that meet the recommendations of the Dietary Guidelines and the Food Guide Pyramid.

Food labels are a readily available source of nutrition information. Yet 36% of Americans say they pay only slight or no attention to these valuable tools.[1] Reviewing

labels while in the grocery store can have a big impact on your nutrient intake for the day. For example, if you are selecting foods for breakfast, your choice could be granola with whole milk or oatmeal made with skim milk. The labels on the milk and the cereal boxes can help you choose which fits best into a diet that is low in fat, moderate in sugar, and high in nutrient density. Whole milk provides 150 kcalories and 8 grams of fat in a cup. This 8 grams of fat represents 12% of the Daily Value—that is, 12% of

the total amount of fat recommended per day for a 2000-kcalorie diet. The fat-free milk contains no fat and only 90 kcalories per cup. Both are sources of calcium and vitamins A and D, and both count as a serving from the milk group of the Food Guide Pyramid. In terms of meeting the Dietary Guideline to choose a diet low in fat, saturated fat, and cholesterol, fat-free milk is a better choice. And, if you don't like the taste of fat-free milk, there are reduced-fat and lowfat choices.

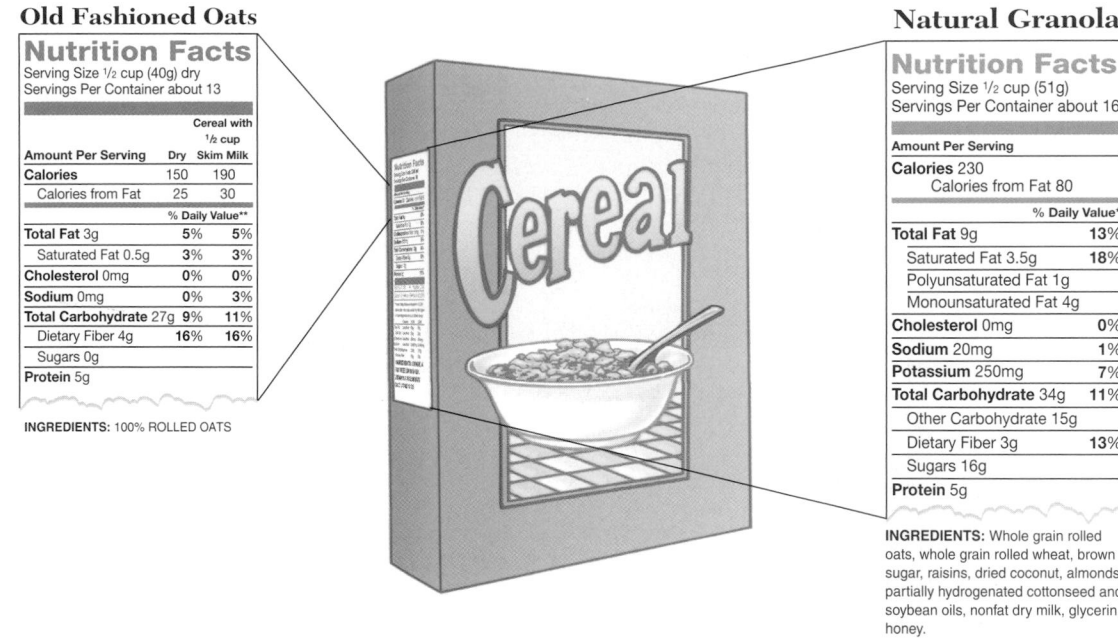

Old Fashioned Oats

Nutrition Facts
Serving Size 1/2 cup (40g) dry
Servings Per Container about 13

Amount Per Serving	Dry	Cereal with 1/2 cup Skim Milk
Calories	150	190
Calories from Fat	25	30

	% Daily Value**	
Total Fat 3g	5%	5%
Saturated Fat 0.5g	3%	3%
Cholesterol 0mg	0%	0%
Sodium 0mg	0%	3%
Total Carbohydrate 27g	9%	11%
Dietary Fiber 4g	16%	16%
Sugars 0g		
Protein 5g		

INGREDIENTS: 100% ROLLED OATS

Natural Granola

Nutrition Facts
Serving Size 1/2 cup (51g)
Servings Per Container about 16

Amount Per Serving	
Calories 230	
Calories from Fat 80	

	% Daily Value*
Total Fat 9g	13%
Saturated Fat 3.5g	18%
Polyunsaturated Fat 1g	
Monounsaturated Fat 4g	
Cholesterol 0mg	0%
Sodium 20mg	1%
Potassium 250mg	7%
Total Carbohydrate 34g	11%
Other Carbohydrate 15g	
Dietary Fiber 3g	13%
Sugars 16g	
Protein 5g	

INGREDIENTS: Whole grain rolled oats, whole grain rolled wheat, brown sugar, raisins, dried coconut, almonds, partially hydrogenated cottonseed and soybean oils, nonfat dry milk, glycerin, honey.

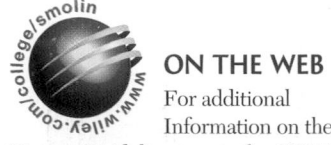

ON THE WEB

For additional Information on the Dietary Guidelines, go to the USDA's Food and Nutrition Information Center at www.nal.usda.gov/fnic/dga/index.html

Dietary Guidelines for Americans A set of nutrition and lifestyle recommendations designed to promote population-wide dietary changes to reduce the incidence of nutrition-related chronic disease.

• THE DIETARY GUIDELINES FOR AMERICANS: TYING IT ALL TOGETHER

The **Dietary Guidelines for Americans** is a set of recommendations on diet and lifestyle designed to promote health, support active lives, and reduce chronic disease risks in the general population (Figure 2.6 and Appendix G).

Development of the Dietary Guidelines

The first broad-based recommendation for health promotion—rather than just deficiency prevention—was the Dietary Goals for the United States, established in 1977 by the Senate Select Committee on Human Needs.[10] The Dietary Goals were subsequently modified and published as the Dietary Guidelines for Americans in 1980 by the U.S. Department of Agriculture and the U.S. Department of Health and Human

The granola and the oatmeal both provide a serving from the grain group, but the amounts of fat and sugars differ. According to the labels, a serving of granola provides 230 kcalories and 9 grams of fat, whereas oatmeal provides only 150 kcalories and 3 grams of fat. A review of the ingredient list reveals that oatmeal contains only rolled oats, whereas granola contains rolled oats plus added sugars in the form of brown sugar and honey. The oatmeal is a choice that is lower in both fat and refined sugars and is higher in nutrient density.

Knowing how to interpret the information on food labels can help you choose a diet that meets the recommendations of the Dietary Guidelines and follows the selection tips of the Food Guide Pyramid. This doesn't mean you can never have a doughnut for breakfast because the label identifies it as high in fat and kcalories.

Even a high-fat food choice can be part of a healthy diet as long as it is balanced with healthy lowfat choices throughout the day. Remember, it is your total diet—not each choice—that counts.

[1]American Dietetic Association, Americans Food and Nutrition Attitudes and Behavior: Trends 2000. Available online at www.eatright.org/pr/2000/01300a.html/ Accessed February 28, 2002.

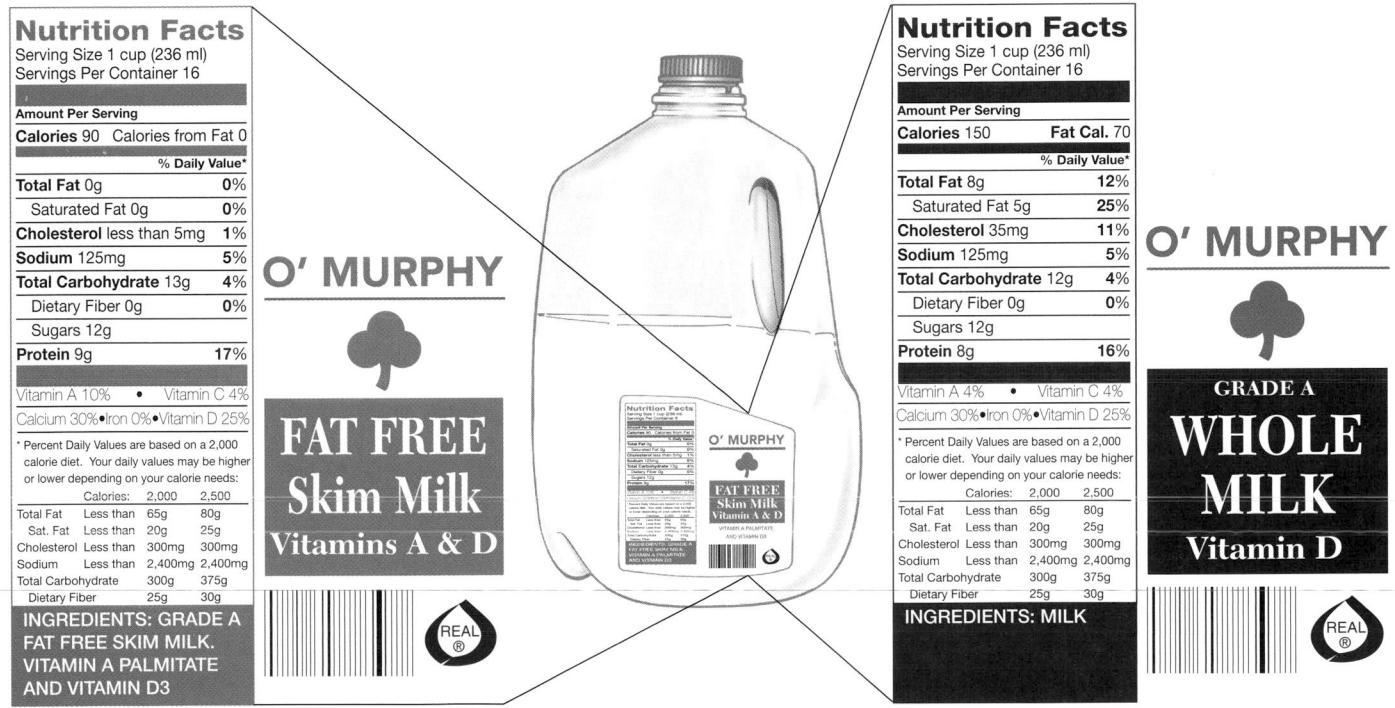

Services. Since then, they have been revised every five years to reflect advances in our scientific understanding of what constitutes a diet that promotes health. The most recent (fifth) edition was released in February 2000.

The Dietary Guidelines for Americans, 2000 takes advantage of many of the other tools developed for selecting a healthy diet; for example, consumers are encouraged to use the Food Guide Pyramid and food labels to select a diet that meets the recommendations of the Dietary Guidelines.[11] In this way, the Dietary Guidelines ties together other recommendations to present a consumer-friendly package of information on choosing a healthy diet and lifestyle.

ABCs for Good Health

The Guidelines are organized using a three-tier system called the ABCs for Good Health. The first tier of the Dietary Guidelines, **Aim for Fitness**, contains two guide-

Nutrition and Your Health:
DIETARY GUIDELINES FOR AMERICANS

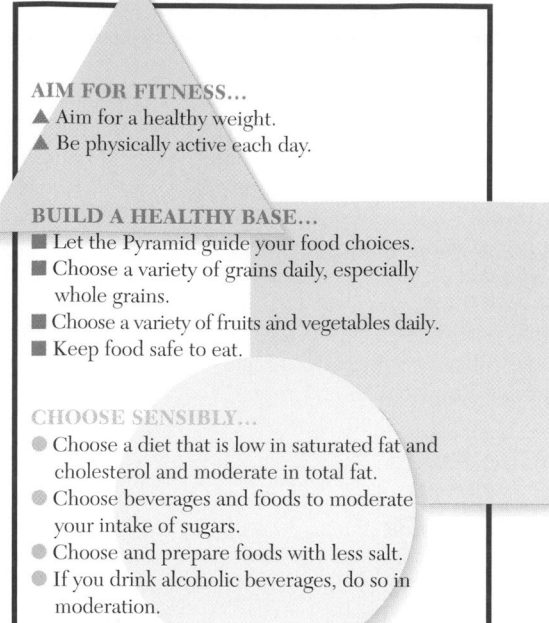

AIM FOR FITNESS...
▲ Aim for a healthy weight.
▲ Be physically active each day.

BUILD A HEALTHY BASE...
■ Let the Pyramid guide your food choices.
■ Choose a variety of grains daily, especially whole grains.
■ Choose a variety of fruits and vegetables daily.
■ Keep food safe to eat.

CHOOSE SENSIBLY...
● Choose a diet that is low in saturated fat and cholesterol and moderate in total fat.
● Choose beverages and foods to moderate your intake of sugars.
● Choose and prepare foods with less salt.
● If you drink alcoholic beverages, do so in moderation.

...for good health

Figure 2.6
The Dietary Guidelines for Americans promotes healthy diets and lifestyles. (USDA, DHHS, 2000)

lines that focus on the importance of maintaining a healthy weight and being physically active. The second tier, **Build a Healthy Base**, contains four guidelines that focus on encouraging healthy food practices, and the third tier, **Choose Sensibly**, contains four guidelines that focus on dietary components that should be limited.

Aim for Fitness Concerns about the rising incidence of obesity in the United States and the sedentary lifestyles of most Americans have prompted an emphasis in the Dietary Guidelines on a healthy body weight and active lifestyle. The tier called Aim for Fitness recommends that we "Aim for a healthy weight." Specific guidelines for evaluating body weight are given (see Chapter 7). Emphasis is placed on encouraging healthy weight in children. This tier also encourages us to "Be physically active each day." This guideline is backed up by specific recommendations about the intensity, amount, and variety of activity that will benefit health (see Chapter 13).

Build a Healthy Base This tier offers four guidelines on choosing a variety of foods and handling these foods safely. It emphasizes that no one food or food group provides all the nutrients and other healthful substances in the amounts needed. The first guideline recommends a diet based on the Food Guide Pyramid and emphasizes variety among food groups by advising "Let the Pyramid guide your food choices." The next guideline emphasizes variety in the choices from the base of the Pyramid by stating "Eat a variety of grains daily, especially whole grains." Whole grains are emphasized because of increasing evidence that these foods may reduce the risk of coronary heart disease, bowel diseases, diabetes, and certain types of cancer (see Chapter 4). Variety is also encouraged in the guideline that suggests "Eat a variety of fruits and vegetables daily." Fruits and vegetables are high in nutrients and health-promoting phytochemicals. Most Americans do not consume the recommended minimum of five servings of fruits and vegetables each day.

The fourth recommendation in this tier cautions Americans to "Keep food safe to eat." This is the first edition of the Dietary Guidelines to include a food safety guideline. The topic has become a focus of public health education because most of the foodborne illness in the United States is caused by food prepared at home (Table 2.7).

Choose Sensibly The third tier focuses on choices designed to limit certain dietary components. The first guideline in this tier states that Americans should "Choose a diet low in saturated fat and cholesterol and moderate in fat." This wording reflects the understanding that diets low in saturated fat and cholesterol can improve blood cholesterol levels, even if the total diet is moderate rather than low in total fat. The guideline suggests that if your total fat intake is more than 30% of kcalories, it should be reduced by decreasing saturated and *trans* fats (see Chapter 5).

The guideline to "Choose beverages and foods that limit your intake of sugars" is in response to the rising intake of sugars in the United States, particularly from soft drinks. The Dietary Guidelines points out that the Nutrition Facts label will indicate total grams of sugars in a food product, but to distinguish how much is from added sugars consumers must be able to identify sources of added sugar listed in the ingredient list (see Chapter 4).

The guideline to "Choose and prepare foods with less salt" is based on research that indicates that a diet high in salt increases blood pressure in some individuals. This recommendation is included because there is no way to identify who might benefit from reduced salt intake and reducing salt intake is not harmful for healthy individuals. In addition there is evidence that lower salt intakes might reduce the loss of calcium from bone (see Chapter 10).

The final guideline states that "If you drink alcoholic beverages, do so in moderation." It emphasizes the dangers of excess alcohol consumption but includes the fact that in men over 45 and women over 55 moderate drinking can lower the risk of heart disease.

• EXCHANGE LISTS

The **Exchange Lists** is a food group system that is useful in planning diets to meet specific energy and macronutrient goals. It was first developed in 1950 by the American Dietetic Association and the American Diabetes Association as a meal-planning tool for individuals with diabetes. Since then, its use has been expanded to planning weight-loss diets and diets in general. The latest revision of the Exchange Lists divides foods into three main groups based on their macronutrient content: the carbohydrate group, the meat and meat-substitute group, and the fat group. The carbohydrate group includes exchange lists for foods that are sources of carbohydrates: starches, fruits, milk, and vegetables. It also defines a list of other high-carbohydrate foods and indicates how to fit these foods into a diet based on exchanges. The meat and meat- substitute group includes an exchange list with four subgroups: very lean, lean, medium-fat, and high-fat meat. The fat group includes an exchange list with subgroups of monounsaturated, polyunsaturated, and saturated fats (Table 2.8)[12] (see Appendix I).

The serving sizes for foods within each exchange list are different from those in the Food Guide Pyramid. The exchanges are set so that each food within a list contains approximately the same amount of energy, carbohydrate, protein, and fat. For instance, each fruit in the fruit exchange list provides about 60 kcalories, 15 grams of carbohydrate, no protein, and no fat, whereas foods in the starch list provide about 80 kcalories, 15 grams of carbohydrate, 3 grams of protein, and 0 to 1 gram of fat. The food groupings of the Exchange Lists differ from the Food Guide Pyramid groups because the lists are designed to meet energy and macronutrient criteria, whereas the Pyramid groups are designed to be good sources of certain nutrients regardless of their energy content. For example, a potato is included in the starch exchange list because it contains about the same amount of energy, carbohydrate, protein, and fat as breads and grains, but in the Food Guide Pyramid a potato is in the Vegetable Group because it is a good source of vitamins, minerals, and fiber.

Table 2.7
Steps to Keeping Food Safe

1. Clean—Wash hands and surfaces often.
2. Separate—Separate raw, cooked, and ready-to-eat foods while shopping, preparing, and storing.
3. Cook—Cook food to a safe temperature.
4. Chill—Refrigerate perishable foods promptly.
5. Follow the label.
6. Serve safely.
7. If in doubt, throw it out.

The Dietary Guidelines for Americans, 2000, USDA, DHHS, 2000.

Exchange Lists A food group system that groups foods according to energy and macronutrient content. It is used extensively in planning diabetic and weight loss diets.

Table 2.8 *Energy and Macronutrient Values of the Exchange Lists*

Exchange Group/Lists	Serving Size	Energy (kcals)	Carbohydrate (g)	Protein (g)	Fat (g)
Carbohydrate Group					
Starch	1/2 cup pasta, cereal, rice; 1 slice bread	80	15	3	0–1
Fruit	1 small apple, peach, or pear; 1/2 banana; 1/2 cup canned fruit (in juice)	60	15	0	0
Milk					
Nonfat	1 cup milk or yogurt	90	12	8	0
Lowfat		110	12	8	3
Reduced fat		120	12	8	5
Whole		150	12	8	8
Other carbohydrates	Serving sizes vary	Varies	15	Varies	Varies
Vegetables	1/2 cup cooked vegetables, 1 cup raw	25	5	2	0
Meat/Meat Substitute Group	1 oz meat or cheese				
Very lean		35	0	7	0–1
Lean		55	0	7	3
Medium fat		75	0	7	5
High fat		100	0	7	8
Fat Group	1 tsp butter, margarine, or oil; 1 Tbsp salad dressing	45	0	0	5

The exchange system can be used to design diets to meet individual tastes and preferences at specific energy and macronutrient levels. For instance, a diet could be calculated to provide 1600 kcalories with 75 grams of protein, 200 grams of carbohydrate, and 50 grams of fat. The consumer would meet these nutrient criteria by consuming a prescribed number of servings from each of the exchanges. For example, he would be instructed to choose 6 starch exchanges, 2 milk exchanges, 3 vegetable exchanges, and so on.

• OTHER GUIDELINES FOR HEALTH PROMOTION AND DISEASE PREVENTION

In addition to the recommendations and guidelines discussed in the previous section, there are a number of other types of recommendations made to promote a healthy diet and lifestyle. The Healthy People Initiative is a health promotion program that includes nutrition in its recommendations. Special interest groups also make nutrition recommendations for reducing the risks of specific diseases such as heart disease and cancer.

The Healthy People Initiative

Healthy People A set of national health promotion and disease prevention objectives for the U.S. population.

The U.S. Public Health Service along with 300 private and public organizations has developed a set of public health objectives called **Healthy People**. The first set, Healthy People 2000, developed in 1990, was directed toward the year 2000. The most recent objectives, Healthy People 2010, target the current decade. Healthy People 2010 is committed to a single, overarching purpose: promoting health and preventing illness, disability, and premature death. From this broad view it defines goals and objectives for health promotion. The goals for the Healthy People initiative include increasing the span of healthy life for Americans and eliminating health disparities among Americans. These goals are to be met through the broad approaches of promoting healthy behaviors, protecting health, assuring access to quality health care, and strengthening community prevention.[13] Many of these objectives are directed toward improving the nutritional status of the population (see Appendix G). For instance, Healthy People is working toward reducing the number of cancer and heart disease deaths and the prevalence of obesity in adults by promoting active lifestyles and diets low in fat and sodium and high in fiber. It promotes a reduction in growth retardation in children by encouraging healthy feeding practices, including breast feeding for infants. Other nutrition-related objectives are designed to improve the delivery of nutrition information and services.

Recommendations for Reducing Risks for Specific Diseases

In addition to guidelines for a healthy diet for the general population, recommendations to populations at risk for certain diseases have been published by groups such as the American Heart Association and the American Institute for Cancer Research (see Appendix G). These groups base their recommendations on sound scientific literature, but because of their special interest in preventing a specific disease, their recommendations may differ slightly from one another in emphasis and focus. For example, to reduce the risk of heart disease, the guidelines developed by the American Heart Association include a recommendation to restrict dietary cholesterol to less than 300 mg per day, whereas the recommendations of the American Institute for Cancer Research, which are designed to reduce the incidence of cancer, do not comment on cholesterol intake, because a correlation has not been established between cholesterol intake and cancer incidence. On the other hand, the American Institute for Cancer Research recommends a reduction in the consumption of cured and smoked meats because of a correlation with cancer, but these foods are not mentioned in the American Heart Association guidelines.

• ASSESSING NUTRITIONAL HEALTH

To be healthy, populations and individuals need to consume combinations of foods that provide appropriate amounts of nutrients. Scientists have developed standards for the amounts of nutrients we need and tools for planning diets to meet these needs. But how do we know if the nutritional needs of a population or an individual are being met? Evaluating the **nutritional status** of populations and individuals can identify nutritional needs and be used to plan diets to meet these needs.

Nutritional status State of health as it is influenced by the intake and utilization of nutrients.

Nutritional Health of the Population

We know that there is enough food available in the United States to meet the needs of the population. We also know that poor nutritional choices from this food supply result in diets high in some nutrients and low in others. This kind of information is obtained by monitoring what foods are available (the supply) and what is consumed. In the United States, the National Nutrition Monitoring and Related Research Program is responsible for providing an ongoing description of nutrition conditions in the population by collecting information about food availability and consumption; food composition; and the eating behaviors, health, and nutritional status of the population.[14] These epidemiological data are used for the purpose of planning nutrition-related policies and programs and predicting future trends of public health importance. The information gathered from population surveys can be used to identify the need for nutrition education, food assistance programs, or addition of a specific nutrient to the food supply. These surveys are key in establishing relationships among diet, nutritional status, and the health of the U.S. population.

Monitoring the Food Supply The food available to a population is estimated using **food disappearance surveys**. The food supply includes all that is grown, manufactured, or imported for sale in the country. Food use or "disappearance" is estimated by

Food disappearance surveys A method that estimates the food use of a population by monitoring the amount of food that leaves the marketplace.

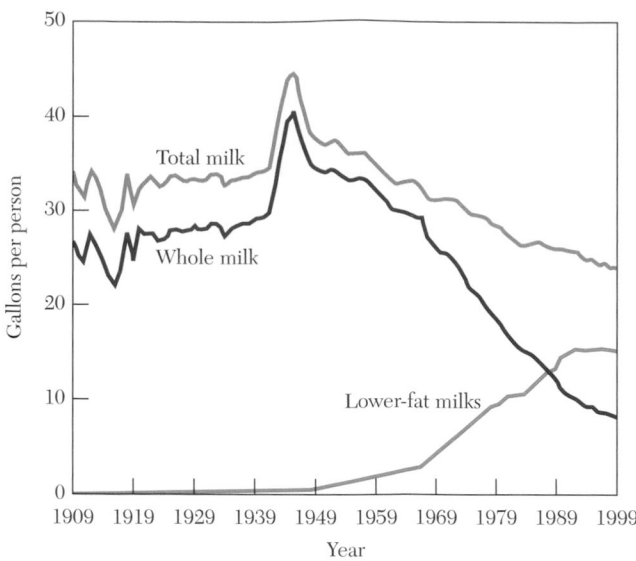

Figure 2.7
Food disappearance data can identify population trends in food intake such as the increase in the consumption of lower-fat milks and the decrease in whole milk consumption that has occurred over the last 50 years. (Source: USDA Economic Research Service, Major trends in the U.S. food supply, 1909–1999, *Food Review* 23:12, 2000, Available online at www.ers.usda. gov/epubs/pdf/foodrevw/jan2000/)

measuring what food is sold. These types of surveys are used to estimate what is available to the population, provide year-to-year comparisons, and identify trends in the diet; but they tend to overestimate actual intake because they do not consider losses that occur during processing, marketing, and home use. Also, the surveys do not assess the distribution of food throughout the population. For example, Figure 2.7 illustrates the food disappearance data on milk consumption over the past 90 years. It shows that the consumption of whole milk, which is high in fat, has declined since the 1950s and the consumption of lower-fat milks has increased. From this it can be concluded that fat intake from milk has declined. But the graph also indicates that total milk consumption has been declining. This may alert the government that calcium intake from milk has decreased and that there may be a risk for calcium deficiency in the population. The numbers in this graph do not give any information about how much milk each person is drinking or who is at risk of inadequate calcium intake.

Monitoring Nutritional Status The nutritional status of the population is monitored by examining and comparing trends in food intake and health. This is done by interviewing individuals within the population to determine what food is actually consumed, and collecting information on health and nutritional status. The Department of Health and Human Services conducts the **National Health and Nutrition Examination Survey (NHANES)**, which combines information on food consumption with medical histories, physical examinations, and laboratory measurements to monitor both nutritional and health information. Data on food, energy, and nutrient intake can be assessed by comparing population intakes with reference values such as the DRIs or with other guidelines such as the recommendations of the Dietary Guidelines or the Food Guide Pyramid. For example, we know that few people eat the five or more servings of fruits and vegetables per day recommended by the Food Guide Pyramid, that there has been a slight drop in dietary fat intake, and that the number of people who are overweight has increased in all adult age groups in the past decade.

A system that has been developed to evaluate the adequacy of the diet of Americans is the Healthy Eating Index.[15] This provides a measure that summarizes overall diet quality by scoring 10 components of the diet, each representing different aspects of a healthy diet. Five of these components measure how well a person's diet complies with the serving recommendations for the five food groups of the Food Guide Pyramid. The other five components score the diet based on how well it complies with the recommendations of the Dietary Guidelines regarding total fat, saturated fat, cholesterol, sodium, and variety. Each component has a maximum score of

National Health and Nutrition Examination Survey (NHANES) A survey that collects information about the health and nutritional status of individuals in the population.

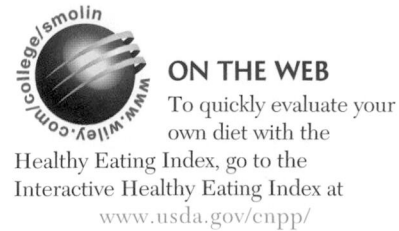

ON THE WEB
To quickly evaluate your own diet with the Healthy Eating Index, go to the Interactive Healthy Eating Index at www.usda.gov/cnpp/

10, so an individual who follows all of these guidelines would have a Healthy Eating Index score of 100. Since the index was first computerized in 1989, the typical American diet has improved slightly from a score of 61.5 in 1989 to 63.8 in 1996.

Individual Nutritional Health

What about your own nutritional status? Are you losing weight? Gaining weight? Do you have a history of heart disease in your family? Are you at risk for a nutrient deficiency because you can't get to the store, can't afford to buy healthy foods, or you don't know what to eat or how to cook? An individual **nutritional assessment** requires a review of past and present dietary intake, an assessment of body size, a medical history and physical exam, and laboratory measurements. Even with all these tools, diagnosing a nutritional deficiency or excess is not trivial. Estimates of dietary intake are not always accurate, and symptoms may be indistinguishable from other medical conditions.

Estimating Dietary Intake A good place to start when evaluating people's nutritional status is to determine what they typically eat. This can be done by observing all the food and drink consumed by the individual for a specified period of time or by asking the individual to record or recall their intake. Neither option is ideal because being observed can affect an individual's intake. Similarly recording and recalling intake are imprecise measures because these methods rely on the memory and reliability of the consumer. For instance, a person who is attempting to lose weight may tend to report smaller portions than were actually eaten.[16] Despite this problem, the commonly used methods described below are the best tools available for evaluating dietary intake to predict nutrient deficiencies or excesses. Once this information on intake has been collected, the nutrient content of the foods consumed can be estimated using food composition tables or computer software.

24-Hour Recall The most common method of assessing dietary intake is a **24-hour recall** in which a trained interviewer asks people to recall exactly what they ate during the preceding 24-hour period. A detailed description of all food and drink, including descriptions of cooking methods and brand names of products, is recorded. Since food intake varies from day to day, repeated 24-hour recalls on the same individuals provides a more accurate estimate of typical intake.

Food Diary or Food Intake Record Food intake information can also be gathered by having a consumer keep a **food diary**, or record, of all the food and drink consumed for a set period of time. Typically, this is done for two to seven days including at least one weekend day, since most people eat differently on weekends than during the school or work week. Foods may be weighed or portion sizes just estimated (Figure 2.8). The record should be as complete as possible, including all beverages, condiments, and the brand names and preparation methods. The tedious nature of this type of record can be a disadvantage because in some cases it may cause the consumer to change her intake rather than record certain items.

Food Frequency A **food frequency questionnaire** lists a variety of foods, and the consumer is asked to estimate the frequency with which they consume each item or food group. For example, "How often do you drink milk?" or "How many times a week do you eat red meat?" This method cannot be used to itemize a specific day's intake, but it can give a general picture of one's typical pattern of food intake (Figure 2.9).

Diet History A **diet history** is a general term for collecting information about dietary patterns. It may review eating habits: Do you cook your own meals? Do you skip lunch? It may also include a combination of other methods such as a 24-hour recall along with a food frequency questionnaire. The combination of two or more methods often provides more complete information than one method alone. For in-

Nutritional assessment The process of determining the nutritional status of individuals or groups for the purpose of identifying nutritional needs and planning personal health-care or community programs to meet these needs.

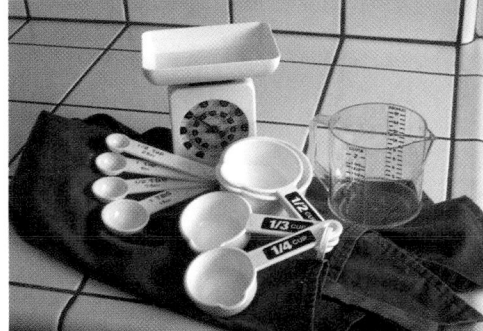

Figure 2.8
Accurate food diaries require recording the correct amounts of all food and drink consumed. (Tony Freeman/PhotoEdit)

24-hour recall A method of assessing dietary intake in which a trained interviewer helps an individual remember what he ate during the previous day.

Food diary A method of assessing nutrient intake that involves an individual keeping a written record of all food and drink consumed during a defined period.

Food frequency questionnaire A method of assessing nutrient intake that gathers information about how often certain categories of food are consumed.

Diet history Information about dietary habits and patterns. It may include a 24-hour recall, a food record, or a food frequency questionnaire to provide information about current intake patterns.

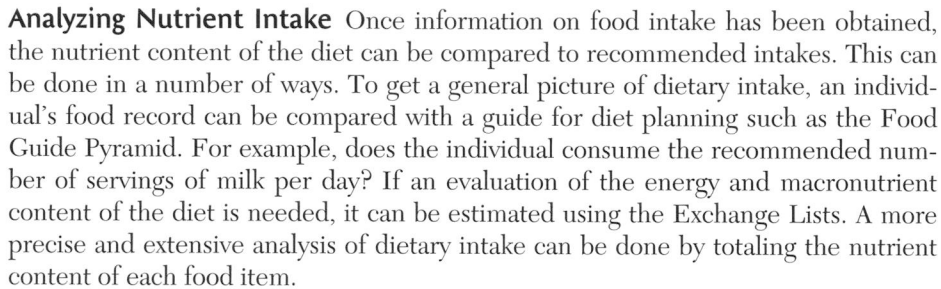

Food Frequency Questionnaire

On the following pages, please check the appropriate column indicating how often you consume each food.

	Once a day	Twice or more a day	Once a week	Twice or more a week	Once a month	Twice or more a month
Milk						
Whole						
Reduced fat						✔
Nonfat	✔					
Yogurt						
Whole						
Reduced fat			✔			
Nonfat						
Cheese						
Hard					✔	
Soft						✔
Reduced fat						
Ice cream						
Regular						
Reduced fat	✔					

Figure 2.9
This section of a sample food frequency questionnaire obtains information about dairy product consumption patterns.

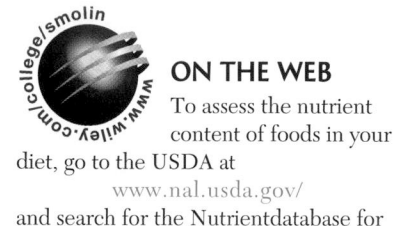

ON THE WEB
To assess the nutrient content of foods in your diet, go to the USDA at
www.nal.usda.gov/
and search for the Nutrientdatabase for Standard Reference.

stance, if an individual's 24-hour recall does not include milk, but a food frequency questionnaire suggests that the individual usually drinks milk once a day, the two can be combined to provide a more accurate picture of this individual's typical intake.

Analyzing Nutrient Intake Once information on food intake has been obtained, the nutrient content of the diet can be compared to recommended intakes. This can be done in a number of ways. To get a general picture of dietary intake, an individual's food record can be compared with a guide for diet planning such as the Food Guide Pyramid. For example, does the individual consume the recommended number of servings of milk per day? If an evaluation of the energy and macronutrient content of the diet is needed, it can be estimated using the Exchange Lists. A more precise and extensive analysis of dietary intake can be done by totaling the nutrient content of each food item.

Information on the nutrient composition of foods is available on food labels, in published food composition tables, and in computer databases. Food labels provide information only for some nutrients, and they are not available for all foods. Food composition tables generated by government and industry laboratories can provide more extensive information on food composition (see Appendix A for an abbreviated list). The major source of food composition data in the United States is *USDA Nutrient Database for Standard Reference,* which is available online.[17] Computer programs with food composition databases are now readily available for professionals and for home use.

To analyze nutrient intake using a computer program, one must enter each food and the exact portion consumed into the program. If a food is not found in the computer database, an appropriate substitute can be used or the food can be broken down into its individual ingredients. For example, homemade vegetable soup could be entered as generic vegetable soup, or as vegetable broth, carrots, green beans, rice, and so on. If a new product has come on the market, the information from the food label can be added to the database. The advantage of computer diet analysis is that it is fast and accurate. A program can calculate the nutrients for each day or average them over several days. It can also compare nutrient intake to recommended amounts. However, the information generated by computer diet analysis is only useful if it is entered correctly and interpreted appropriately. Also, a nutrient intake that is below the recommended amount does not always indicate a deficiency, and intake that meets recommendations does not ensure adequate nutritional status. Figure 2.10 shows a typical printout for a computerized diet analysis.

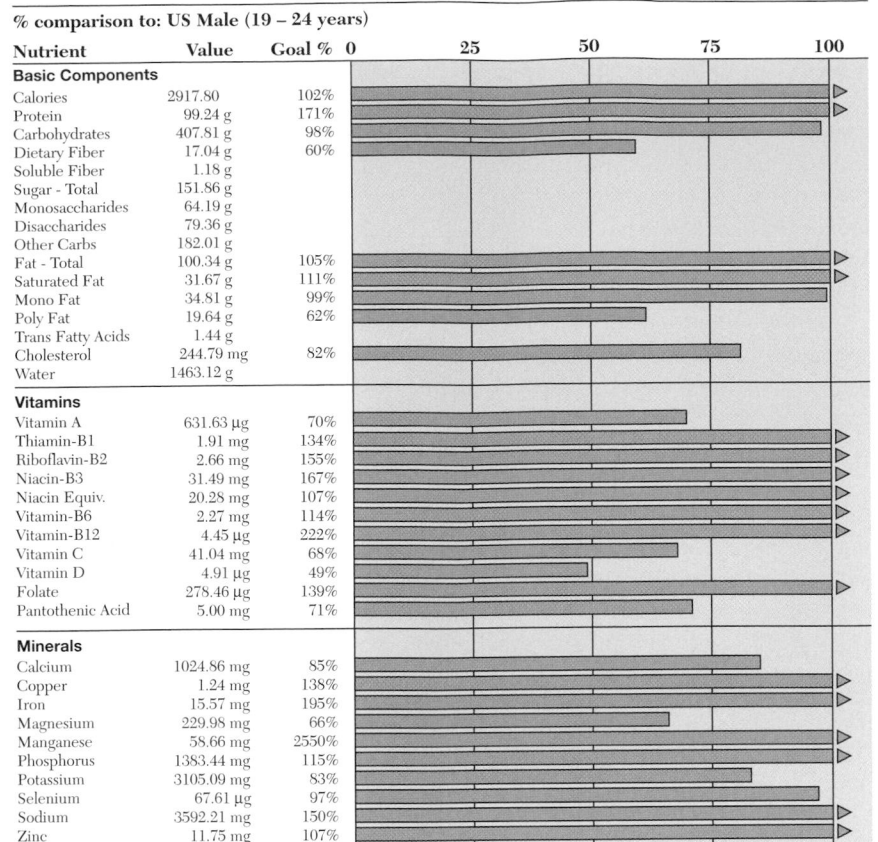

% comparison to: US Male (19 – 24 years)							
Nutrient	Value	Goal %	0	25	50	75	100
Basic Components							
Calories	2917.80	102%					
Protein	99.24 g	171%					
Carbohydrates	407.81 g	98%					
Dietary Fiber	17.04 g	60%					
Soluble Fiber	1.18 g						
Sugar - Total	151.86 g						
Monosaccharides	64.19 g						
Disaccharides	79.36 g						
Other Carbs	182.01 g						
Fat - Total	100.34 g	105%					
Saturated Fat	31.67 g	111%					
Mono Fat	34.81 g	99%					
Poly Fat	19.64 g	62%					
Trans Fatty Acids	1.44 g						
Cholesterol	244.79 mg	82%					
Water	1463.12 g						
Vitamins							
Vitamin A	631.63 µg	70%					
Thiamin-B1	1.91 mg	134%					
Riboflavin-B2	2.66 mg	155%					
Niacin-B3	31.49 mg	167%					
Niacin Equiv.	20.28 mg	107%					
Vitamin-B6	2.27 mg	114%					
Vitamin-B12	4.45 µg	222%					
Vitamin C	41.04 mg	68%					
Vitamin D	4.91 µg	49%					
Folate	278.46 µg	139%					
Pantothenic Acid	5.00 mg	71%					
Minerals							
Calcium	1024.86 mg	85%					
Copper	1.24 mg	138%					
Iron	15.57 mg	195%					
Magnesium	229.98 mg	66%					
Manganese	58.66 mg	2550%					
Phosphorus	1383.44 mg	115%					
Potassium	3105.09 mg	83%					
Selenium	67.61 µg	97%					
Sodium	3592.21 mg	150%					
Zinc	11.75 mg	107%					

Figure 2.10

To be meaningful, the information on computer printouts from diet analysis must be accurately interpreted. This printout shows one day's intake for a 19- to 24-year-old male. The "Value" column gives the total amount of a nutrient consumed that day and the "Goal %" column compares this amount to dietary standards. For example, this individual's vitamin C intake on this day is only 68% of the recommended goal. For some nutrients, such as vitamin C, the goal is a target for average daily intake. A goal % that is consistently below 100% indicates an increased risk of inadequate intake.

Height, Weight, and Body Size Evaluating nutritional health also involves an assessment of an individual's **anthropometric measurements**—that is, height, weight, and body size. These measurements can be compared with population standards (see Appendix B) or used to monitor changes in an individual over time (Figure 2.11). If an individual's measurements differ significantly from standards, it could indicate a nutritional deficiency or excess; however, this information should be evaluated only within the context of that person's personal and family history. For example, children who are small for their age may have a nutritional deficiency or may simply have inherited their small body size. Individuals who weigh less than the standard may be adequately nourished if they have never weighed more than their current weight and are otherwise healthy.

Anthropometric measurements External measurements of the body, such as height, weight, limb circumference, and skinfold thickness.

Medical History and Physical Exam A medical history can also be used to assess symptoms of, or risk factors for, nutrition-related diseases. This should include information about family medical history and individual health and socioeconomic status. For instance, a medical history could reveal that an individual's mother died of a heart attack at age 50. This individual has a higher than average risk of developing heart disease and therefore would want to select a diet that reduces the risk of developing this disease (see Chapter 5). Someone who has a family history of diabetes has an increased risk of developing this disease, especially if the individual carries excess body fat.

In a physical exam all areas of the body including the mouth, skin, hair, eyes, and fingernails are examined for indications of poor nutritional status. Symptoms, such as dry skin, cracked lips, or lethargy, may indicate a nutritional deficiency, but these types of symptoms are nonspecific and may be due to factors unrelated to nutritional status. Determining whether the symptoms noted in a physical exam are due to malnutrition or another disease requires that they be evaluated in conjunction with the results of laboratory measurements and within the context of each individual's medical history (see *Critical Thinking*: Nutritional Assessment).

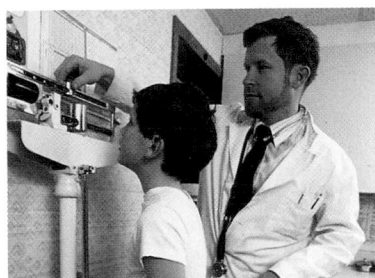

Figure 2.11

Measures of height, weight, and body circumference are examples of anthropometric measurements. (Andy Levin/Photo Researchers)

Laboratory Measurements Measures of nutrients or their by-products in body cells or fluids such as the blood and urine can be used to detect nutrient deficiencies and excesses (see Appendix C). For instance, levels of the blood protein albumin are often used to assess protein status. Because blood carries newly absorbed nutrients to the cells of the body, the amounts of some nutrients in the blood may reflect the amount in the current diet rather than the total body status of the nutrient. To assess the status of these nutrients, it may therefore be necessary to analyze the cells in the blood or other tissues for indications of abnormal function such as altered rates of chemical reactions. For example, vitamin B_6 is needed for chemical reactions involved in amino acid metabolism. When vitamin B_6 is deficient the rate of these reactions is slower than normal.

If the measure does not reflect body status, then it is not useful in nutritional assessment. For instance, hair analysis has been suggested as a means of assessing body mineral levels. However, because many factors, including exposure to environmental contaminants, shampoos, and hair treatments, affect the mineral content of hair, this analysis may not provide much useful information about mineral status in the body.

Laboratory data can also be used to evaluate risk for nutrition-related chronic diseases. For instance, heart disease risk can be assessed by measuring levels of cholesterol in the blood. Measuring the amount of glucose in the blood can be used to diagnose diabetes. More sophisticated medical tests can be used to obtain additional information about the risk and progression of nutrition-related diseases. For example, procedures are available to determine the extent of coronary artery blockage in an individual with heart disease or to assess bone density in someone at risk for osteoporosis.

CRITICAL THINKING

Nutritional Assessment

Alison is 23 years old and has just started college. Recently she has been feeling tired and has had difficulty concentrating in class. She goes to the health clinic where she is weighed and measured. A physician does a physical exam and asks about her medical history. Blood and urine samples are collected for laboratory analysis, and she is referred to a dietitian to assess her dietary intake.

▼

Clinical assessment

The physician notes that she appears thin and pale. Anthropometric measurements of height and weight tell us that she is 5 feet 4 inches tall and weighs 114 pounds. She recalls that a year ago she weighed 120 pounds and hasn't been trying to lose weight. Although her body weight is in the normal range, her unintentional weight loss is a concern.

Dietary assessment

Alison tells the dietitian that she stopped eating red meat last year. Using information from a 24-hour recall, the dietitian enters her diet into a computer program. A portion of the analysis is shown below.

Nutrient	Value	Goal %
Kcalories	1500	68%
Protein	46 g	100%
Vitamin C	110 mg	146%
Vitamin A	1028 μg	147%
Iron	6 mg	33%
Calcium	1300 mg	130%

Use the values given on this computer printout to identify nutrients that do not meet recommendations.

▼

Alison consumes more than the recommended amounts of vitamin A, vitamin C, and calcium. Her energy intake is less than the recommended amount and, since she is losing weight, is not enough to maintain her body weight. Her iron intake is well below the recommendation for young women.

Laboratory assessment

The results of her blood test indicate that blood hemoglobin level is 11.2 g per 100 ml of blood and that her hematocrit, which measures the total volume of blood cells, is 35 ml per 100 ml of blood.

Look up the normal values for hemoglobin and hematocrit in Appendix C. Are her values in the normal range?

▼

Her values for both hemoglobin and hematocrit are below normal. This along with her diet history suggests that she hasn't been consuming enough iron to produce adequate hemoglobin, the oxygen-carrying protein in red blood cells. This reduces her ability to deliver oxygen to her cells, which could be the cause of her tiredness and difficulty in concentrating. The dietitian recommends that she take an iron supplement for a few months and increase plant sources of iron in her diet.

Should she be concerned about the nutrients she is consuming in excess of her goal? Use the DRI tables to determine if they are likely to pose a risk.

▼

Answer:

• APPLICATIONS •

1. Make a form similar to the sample shown here or use one provided by your instructor to keep a food diary of everything you eat for three days. Since you may eat differently on weekends, record for two weekdays and one weekend day. To make sure you don't forget anything, carry your record with you and record food as it is consumed. This record will be used in Applications throughout this book to focus on particular nutrients. Make the record as complete as possible by using the following tips:
   a. Include all food and drink, and be as specific as possible. For example, did you eat a chicken breast or thigh?
   b. Estimate as carefully as possible the portion size that you ate; for example, 1/2 cup of rice, 10 potato chips, 2 ounces of tofu, and 6 ounces of milk.
   c. Record the preparation or cooking method. For example, was your potato peeled? Was your chicken skinless? Was it baked or fried?
   d. Include anything added to your food, for instance, butter, ketchup, or salad dressing.
   e. Don't forget snacks, beverages, and desserts.
   f. If the food is from a fast-food chain, list the name.

   g. You may have to break down mixed dishes into their ingredients. For example, a tuna sandwich can be listed as 2 slices of whole wheat bread, 1 tablespoon of mayonnaise, and 3 ounces of tuna packed in water.

Sample Food Record

Food or Beverage	Kind/How Prepared	Amount
Chicken salad sandwich:		
wheat bread		2 slices
chicken	skinless breast	1/2 cup
mayonnaise	lowfat	1 tablespoon
Diet cola		1 can

2. Make a form similar to the sample shown here or use one provided by your instructor to list the foods from one day of your food record. Next to each food list the Food Guide Pyramid food group to which it belongs. In the next column list the number of Food Guide Pyramid servings or fractions of servings it provides. For mixed foods, list all ingredients separately and identify the food groups and serving sizes that apply.

Sample Food Guide Pyramid Serving Record

Food	Amount	Pyramid Group	Number of Servings
2 Egg rolls:			
wrappers	2	Grain	1
carrots	1/2 cup	Vegetable	1
pork	1 oz	Meat	1/2
peanut oil	1 Tbsp	Fats and sweets	
Rice	1/2 cup	Grain	1

   a. How many servings from each food group did you consume?

   b. Does your diet meet the guidelines of the Food Guide Pyramid? If not, what types of food(s) do you need to add to or eliminate from your diet?

   c. Are your food choices consistent with the selection tips described in Table 2.1? How might you modify your food choices to more closely follow these suggestions?

3. From your kitchen cupboard or the grocery store, select three packaged foods with food labels.

   a. What is the percent of kcalories from fat in each of these foods?

   b. How much carbohydrate, fat, and fiber are in a serving of each?

   c. How does each of these foods fit into your overall daily diet with regard to total carbohydrate? total fat? dietary fiber?

   d. If you consumed a serving of each of these three foods, how much more fat could you consume during the day without exceeding the recommendations? How much more total carbohydrate and fiber should you consume that day to meet recommendations for a 2000-kcalorie diet?

SUMMARY

1. Nutrition recommendations made to the public for health promotion and disease prevention are based on available scientific knowledge. Dietary standards such as the Dietary Reference Intakes (DRIs) provide recommendations for intakes of nutrients and other food components that can be used to plan and assess the diets of individuals and populations. Intakes at these levels will avoid deficiencies and excesses and prevent chronic diseases in the majority of healthy persons.

2. The DRIs include four sets of standards. The Estimated Average Requirement (EAR) is the amount of a nutrient that is estimated to meet the needs of half of the people in a particular gender and life-stage group. The EARs can be used to evaluate and plan nutrient intakes for population groups and are the basis for the Recommended Dietary Allowances (RDAs). The RDAs are recommendations calculated to meet the needs of nearly all healthy individuals (97 to 98%) in a specific group and can be used by individuals as a guide to achieve an adequate intake. Adequate Intakes (AIs) serve the same purpose as the RDAs but are estimated from average intakes by healthy populations when there is insufficient scientific evidence to calculate an EAR and RDA. Tolerable Upper Intake Levels (ULs) provide a guide for a safe upper limit of intake.

3. The Food Guide Pyramid is a tool for planning diets that meet recommendations. It emphasizes variety and recommends servings from each of five major food groups. The pyramid shape reflects the relative proportions of each food group that should be included in the diet. The number of servings is given as a range so it can be used by individuals with different energy needs.

4. Food labels follow a standard format and are designed to provide consumers with information they need to make wise food choices. The percent Daily Values show how foods fit into the recommendations for a healthy diet.

5. The Dietary Guidelines for Americans, 2000 makes dietary and lifestyle recommendations that help Americans "Aim for Fitness" by targeting body weight and physical activity, "Build a Healthy Base" by encouraging healthy food choices and food safety, and "Choose Sensibly" by limiting certain dietary components. These recommendations promote good health and help reduce the risk of chronic diseases that are common in developed countries today. It instructs consumers on how to use the Food Guide Pyramid and food labels as tools to meet these guidelines.

6. The Exchange Lists are used to plan individual diets that provide specific amounts of energy, carbohydrate, protein, and fat.

7. The nutritional status of populations is monitored by measuring what foods are available, what foods are consumed, and how nutrient intake is related to overall health.

8. Individual nutritional status is assessed by evaluating dietary intake, examining clinical parameters such as body size, and interpreting laboratory values within the context of an individual's medical history.

REVIEW QUESTIONS

1. Describe the four types of standards that make up the DRIs.

2. What is the basis for the shape of the Food Guide Pyramid?

3. List the food groups of the Food Guide Pyramid.

4. What is meant by nutrient density? Give an example.

5. Why is variety important to a healthy diet?

6. Why are the serving sizes standardized on food labels?

7. What determines the order in which food ingredients are listed on a label?

8. How do the Daily Values help consumers determine how foods fit into their overall diets?

9. What are the three tiers of the Dietary Guidelines?

10. How are the Exchange Lists used in planning diets?

11. What is nutritional status?

12. List the components of individual nutritional assessment.

REFERENCES

1. FAO/WHO/UNU. *Energy and Protein Requirements*. WHO Technical Report Series No. 724. Geneva: World Health Organization, 1985.

2. National Research Council, Food and Nutrition Board, *Recommended Dietary Allowances*, 10th ed. Washington, D.C.: National Academy Press, 1989.

3. Institute of Medicine, Food and Nutrition Board. *Dietary Reference Intakes for Calcium, Phosphorus, Magnesium, Vitamin D, and Fluoride*. Washington, D.C.: National Academy Press, 1997.

4. Institute of Medicine, Food and Nutrition Board. *Dietary Reference Intakes for Thiamin, Riboflavin, Niacin, Vitamin B-6, Folate, Vitamin B-12, Pantothenic Acid, Biotin, and Choline*. Washington, D.C.: National Academy Press, 1998.

5. U.S. Department of Agriculture. The Food Guide Pyramid, revised 2000. Available online at www.pueblo.gas.gov/cic_text/food/food-pyramid/main.htm/ Accessed February 28, 2002.

6. Federal Register 58, 1993, January 6. Washington, D.C.: U.S. Government Printing Office, Superintendent of Documents.

7. Food and Drug Administration, Center for Food Safety and Applied Nutrition: *Food Labeling and Nutrition: A Food Labeling Guide*. Available online at www.cfsan.fda.gov/~dms/lab-ind.html/ Accessed February 28, 2002.

8. U.S. Food and Drug Administration Center for Food Safety and Applied Nutrition. *Food Labeling: A Guide for Restaurants and Other Retail Establishments, Questions*, August, 1995; Revised February 1996. Available online at www.cfsan.fda.gov/~frf/qaintro.html/ Accessed February 28, 2002.

9. Food and Drug Aministration, Center for Food Safety and Applied Nutrition. *A Food Labeling Guide*. Appendix C, Health Claims, August 12, 1997. Available online at www.cfsan.fda.gov/~frf/qaintro.html/ Accessed February 28, 2002.

10. Report of the Select Committee on Nutrition and Human Needs, U.S. Senate. *Eating in America: Dietary Goals for the United States*. Cambridge, Mass.: MIT Press, 1977.

11. U.S. Department of Agriculture, U.S. Department of Health and Human Services. *Nutrition and Your Health: Dietary Guidelines for Americans*, 5th ed., 2000. Item Number 147-G. Hyattsville, Md.: U.S. Government Printing Office, 2000.

12. The American Diabetes Association, Inc., and the American Dietetic Association. Exchange Lists for Meal Planning, 1995.

13. Maiese, D. R., and Fox, C. E. *Laying the Foundation for Healthy People 2010—The First Year of Consultation* Available online at web.health.gov/healthypeople/ Accessed November 13, 2000.

14. CDC Nutrition Monitoring in the United States: The Directory of Federal and State Nutrition Monitoring and Related Research Activities, March 21, 2000. Available online at www.cdc.gov/nchs/about/otheract/nutrishn/nutrishn.htm/ Accessed February 28, 2002.

15. Bowman, S. A., Lino, M., Gerrior, S. A., and Bastiotis, P. P. *The Healthy Eating Index: 1994–96*. U.S. Department of Agriculture, Center for Nutrition Policy and Promotion, 1998. CNPP-5. Available online at www.usda.gov/cnpp/hei94-96.PDF/ Accessed June 22, 2002.

16. Johansson, L., Solvoll, K., Bjørneboe, G-E. A., and Drevon, C. A. Under- and overreporting of energy intake related to weight status and lifestyle in a nationwide sample. *Am. J. Clin. Nutr.* 68:226–274, 1998.

17. USDA, *USDA Nutrientdatabase for Standard Reference*. Available online at www.nal.usda.gov/fnic/foodcomp/ Accessed February 28, 2002.

The Human Body: From Meals to Molecules

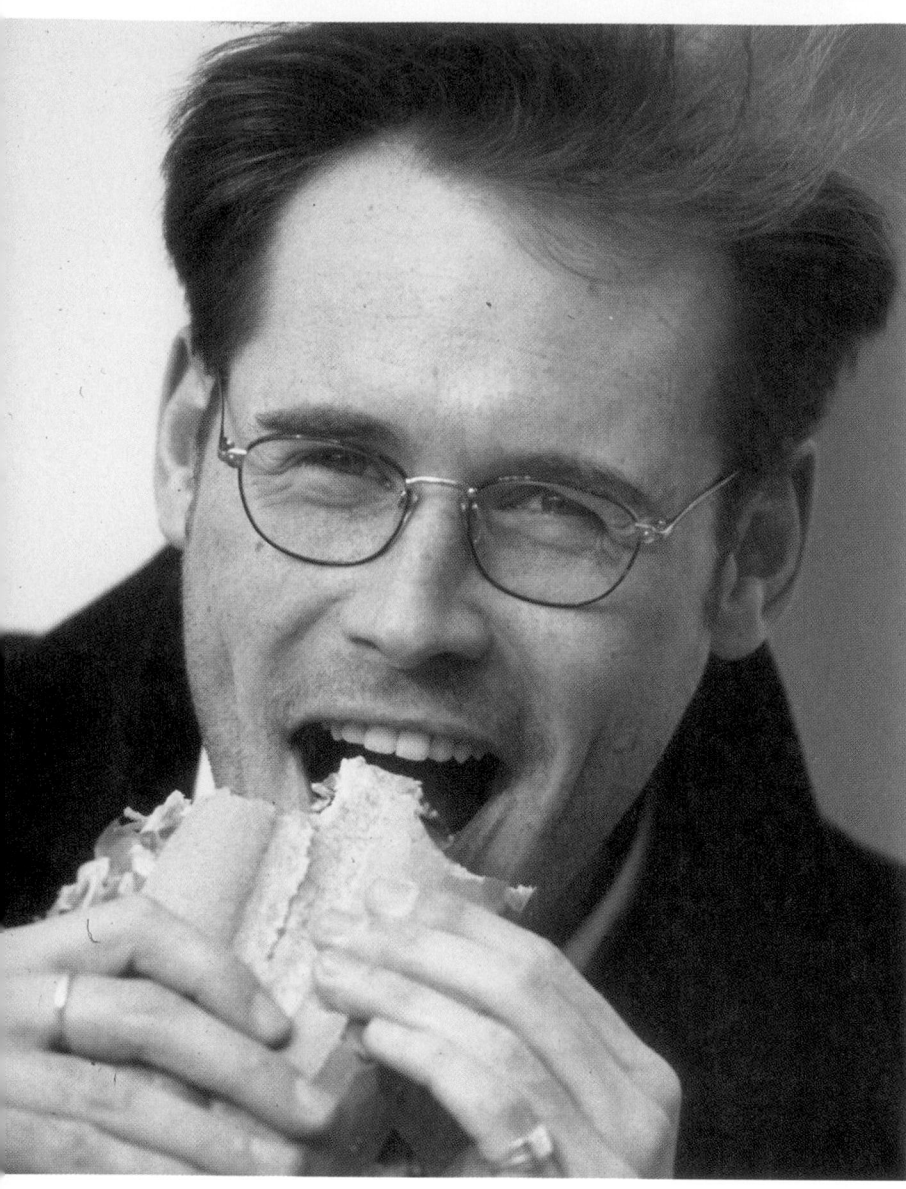

(© Carol Kohen/The Image Bank)

Chapter Concepts

✔ All plant and animal life is made up of atoms bound together to form molecules that are organized into cells. Cells form tissues that compose the organs and organ systems of a living organism.

✔ The food we eat is digested in the gastrointestinal tract, and nutrients are absorbed into the body.

✔ Hormones released into the blood and enzymes released into the gastrointestinal tract facilitate the digestion of food and the absorption of nutrients.

✔ The small intestine is the primary site of digestion and absorption.

✔ Water-soluble materials are absorbed into the blood. Most fat-soluble materials are absorbed into the lymph.

✔ Nutrients delivered to the cells can be used to produce energy in the form of ATP and to synthesize molecules for immediate use or for storage.

✔ Materials that are consumed but not absorbed are excreted in feces. The waste products generated inside the body by metabolism are eliminated via the lungs, skin, and kidneys.

Just a Taste

Can simply seeing or smelling food activate digestion?

Why are you hungry very soon after eating some meals while others stick with you longer?

Is it healthy to have bacteria living in your gastrointestinal tract?

No matter what food choices you make, the processes by which your body uses the nutrients in food are the same. After being consumed, food must be broken into smaller components, absorbed into the body, and then converted into forms that the body can use. Converting the meals we eat into energy or molecules that are a part of our body involves the integration of a number of processes and interaction among almost all the systems of the body. Digestion breaks food into its component parts; absorption brings these components into the body; and metabolism uses the nutrients for energy production, building new tissues, maintaining and repairing existing tissues, and regulating these processes. Whether you choose to eat a burrito, a mango, and arroz con leche (rice with milk), or a turkey sandwich, an apple, and a glass of milk—if the food cannot be properly digested, absorbed, and metabolized by the body, it will be of little benefit.

An understanding of nutrition requires comprehending the processes by which food provides fuel and function to the human body. The unique features of the digestion, absorption, and metabolism of specific nutrients will be more thoroughly discussed in subsequent chapters.

• THE CHEMISTRY OF LIFE

The organization of life, as of all matter, begins with **atoms**. Atoms are units of matter that cannot be further broken down by chemical means. Atoms of different **elements** have different characteristics. Carbon, hydrogen, oxygen, and nitrogen are the most abundant elements in our bodies and in the foods we eat. These atoms can be linked by forces called **chemical bonds** to form **molecules**. The chemistry of all life on earth is based on **organic molecules**, which are those that contain carbon. Carbohydrates, lipids, proteins, and vitamins are nutrient classes that are made up of organic molecules. Substances that do not contain carbon, such as water and minerals, are referred to as **inorganic**.

In any living system, whether a broccoli plant, a cow, or a human being, molecules are organized into structures that form cells, the smallest unit of life (Figure 3.1). **Cells** of similar structure and function are organized into tissues. The human

Atoms The smallest units of an element that still retain the properties of that element.

Elements Substances that cannot be broken down into products with different properties.

Chemical bonds Forces that hold atoms together.

Molecules Units of two or more atoms of the same or different elements bonded together.

Organic molecules Molecules that contain carbon atoms.

Inorganic Substances that contain no carbon atoms.

Cells The basic structural and functional units of plant and animal life.

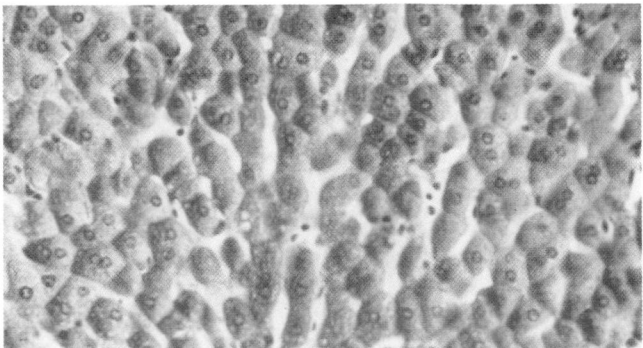

Figure 3.1
Living things are made up of cells such as these human liver cells. (Courtesy Dr. Roger Wagner)

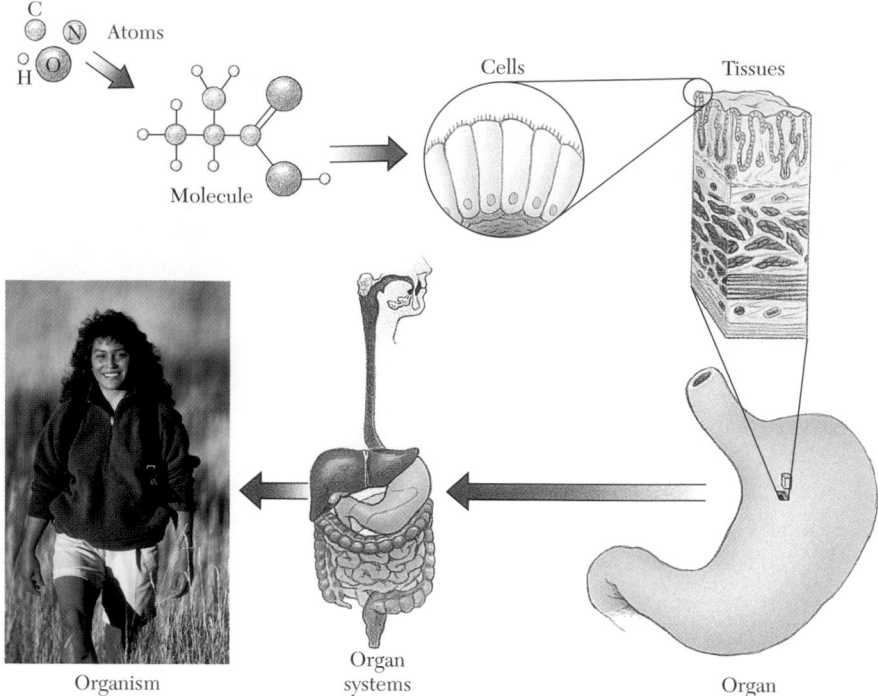

Figure 3.2
The organization of life begins with atoms that form molecules, which are then organized into cells to form tissues, organs, and organisms. (Photo, © Brian Bailey/Stone)

Table 3.1   *The Role of Body Organ Systems*

Organ System	Components	Functions
Nervous	Nerves, sense organs, brain, and spinal cord	Responds to stimuli from the external and internal environments; conducts impulses to activate muscles and glands; integrates activities of other systems.
Respiratory	Lungs, trachea, and air passageways	Supplies the blood with oxygen and removes carbon dioxide.
Urinary	Kidneys and associated structures	Eliminates wastes and regulates the balance of water, electrolytes, and acid in the blood.
Reproductive	Testes, ovaries, and associated structures	Produces offspring.
Cardiovascular	Heart and blood vessels	Transports blood, which carries oxygen, nutrients, and wastes.
Lymphatic/ Immune	Lymph and lymph structures, leukocytes	Defends against foreign invaders; picks up fluid leaked from blood vessels; transports fat-soluble nutrients.
Muscular	Skeletal muscles	Provides movement and structure.
Skeletal	Bones and joints	Protects and supports the body, provides a framework for the muscles to use for movement.
Endocrine	Pituitary, adrenal, thyroid, and other ductless glands	Secretes hormones that regulate processes such as growth, reproduction, and nutrient use.
Integumentary	Skin, hair, nails, and sweat glands	Covers and protects the body; helps control body temperature.
Digestive	Mouth, esophagus, stomach, intestines, pancreas, liver, and gallbladder	Ingests and digests food; absorbs nutrients into the blood; eliminates nonabsorbed food residues.

Adapted from E. N. Marieb, *Human Anatomy and Physiology*, 5th ed. Redwood City, Calif.: Benjamin/Cummings Publishing Co., 2000.

body contains four types of tissues: muscle, nerve, epithelial, and connective. These tissues are organized in varying combinations into **organs**, which are discrete structures that perform specialized functions in the body (Figure 3.2).

Most organs do not function alone but are part of a group of cooperative organs called an organ system. The organ systems in humans include the nervous system, respiratory system (lungs), urinary system (kidneys and bladder), reproductive system, cardiovascular system (heart and blood vessels), lymphatic/immune system, muscular system, skeletal system, endocrine system (hormones), integumentary system (skin and body linings), and digestive system (Table 3.1). An organ may be part of more than one organ system. For example, the pancreas is part of the endocrine system as well as the digestive system.

The digestive system is the organ system primarily responsible for the movement of nutrients into the body; however, several other organ systems are also important in the process of using these nutrients. The endocrine system secretes chemical messengers that help regulate food intake and absorption. The nervous system aids in digestion by sending nerve signals that help control the passage of food through the digestive tract. Once absorbed, nutrients are transported to individual cells by the cardiovascular system. The body's urinary, respiratory, and integumentary systems allow for the elimination of metabolic waste products.

Organ A discrete structure composed of more than one tissue that performs a specialized function.

• THE DIGESTIVE SYSTEM: AN OVERVIEW

The digestive system provides two major functions: **digestion** and **absorption**. Carbohydrate, fat, and protein are digested and absorbed as sugars, fatty acids, and amino acids, respectively. Some substances, such as water, can be absorbed without digestion, and others, such as dietary fiber, cannot be digested by humans and therefore cannot be absorbed. These unabsorbed substances pass through the digestive tract and are excreted in the **feces**.

The main part of the digestive system is the **gastrointestinal tract**. It is also referred to as the GI tract, gut, digestive tract, intestinal tract, or alimentary canal. It can be thought of as a hollow tube that runs from the mouth to the anus. The organs of the gastrointestinal tract include the mouth, pharynx, esophagus, stomach, small intestine, large intestine, and anus (Figure 3.3). The inside of the tube that these organs form is called the **lumen**. Food within the lumen of the gastrointestinal tract has not been absorbed and is therefore technically still outside the body. Only after food is transferred into the cells of the intestine by the process of absorption is it actually "inside" the body.

The amount of time it takes for food to pass from mouth to anus is referred to as **transit time**. In a healthy adult, transit time is about 24 to 72 hours. It is affected by the composition of the diet, physical activity, emotions, medications, and illnesses. To measure transit time, researchers add a nonabsorbable dye to a meal and measure the time between consumption of the dye and its appearance in the feces. The shorter the transit time, the more rapid the passage through the digestive tract.

The digestive process is aided by substances that are secreted into the digestive tract both by cells lining the digestive tract and by a number of accessory organs. One of these substances is **mucus**, a viscous material produced by mucosal cells that line the gut. Mucus moistens, lubricates, and protects the digestive tract. **Enzymes**, protein molecules that speed up chemical reactions without themselves being consumed or changed by the reactions, are another component of digestive system secretions (Figure 3.4). In digestion, enzymes accelerate the breakdown of food. Different enzymes are needed for the breakdown of different food components. For example, an enzyme that digests carbohydrate would have no effect on fat, and one that digests fat would have no effect on carbohydrate.

In addition to secreting substances into the lumen of the digestive tract, the digestive system secretes hormones into the bloodstream. **Hormones** are chemical messengers that are released into the blood by one organ to regulate body functions

Digestion The process of breaking food into components small enough to be absorbed into the body.

Absorption The process of taking substances into the interior of the body.

Feces Body waste, including unabsorbed food residue, bacteria, mucus, and dead cells, which is excreted from the gastrointestinal tract by passing through the anus.

Gastrointestinal tract A hollow tube consisting of the mouth, pharynx, esophagus, stomach, small intestine, large intestine, and anus, in which digestion and absorption of nutrients occur.

Lumen The inside cavity of a tube, such as the gastrointestinal tract.

Transit time The time between the ingestion of food and the elimination of the solid waste from that food.

Mucus A viscous fluid secreted by glands in the gastrointestinal tract and other parts of the body. It acts to lubricate, moisten, and protect cells from harsh environments.

Enzymes Protein molecules that accelerate the rate of specific chemical reactions without being changed themselves.

Hormones Chemical messengers that are produced in one location, released into the blood, and elicit responses at other locations in the body.

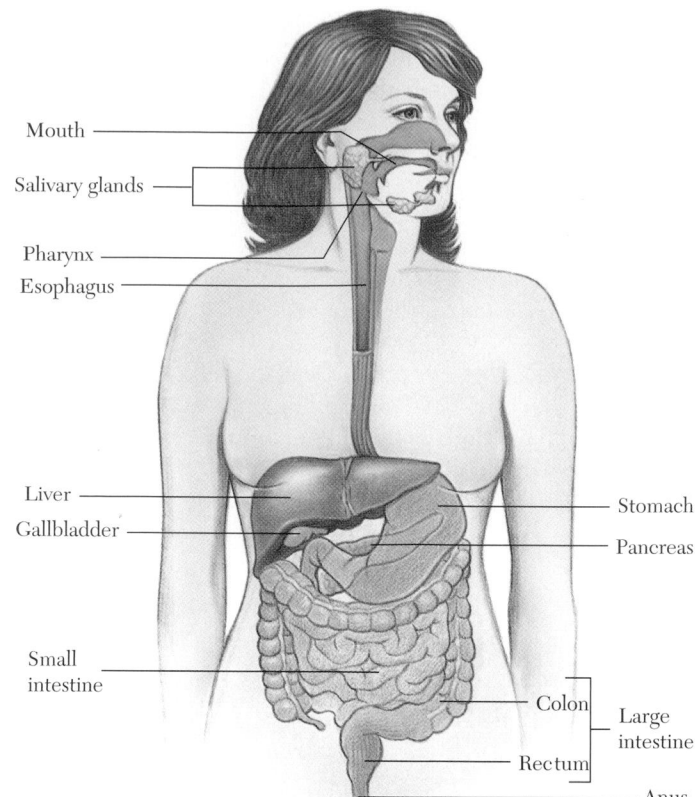

Figure 3.3

The digestive system consists of the organs of the gastrointestinal tract: the mouth, pharynx, esophagus, stomach, small intestine, large intestine, and anus, as well as a number of accessory organs: the salivary glands, liver, gallbladder, and pancreas.

Mucosa The layer of tissue lining the gastrointestinal tract and other body cavities.

elsewhere. In the gastrointestinal tract, hormones send signals that help prepare different parts of the gut for the arrival of food and thus regulate the rate that food moves through the system.

The wall of the gastrointestinal tract contains four layers of tissue (Figure 3.5). Lining the lumen is the **mucosa**, a layer of mucosal cells that secrete mucus into the lumen. The cells of the mucosa are in direct contact with churning food and harsh digestive secretions. Therefore, these cells have a short life span—only about two to five days. When these cells die, they are sloughed off into the lumen, where some components are digested and absorbed and the remainder are excreted in the

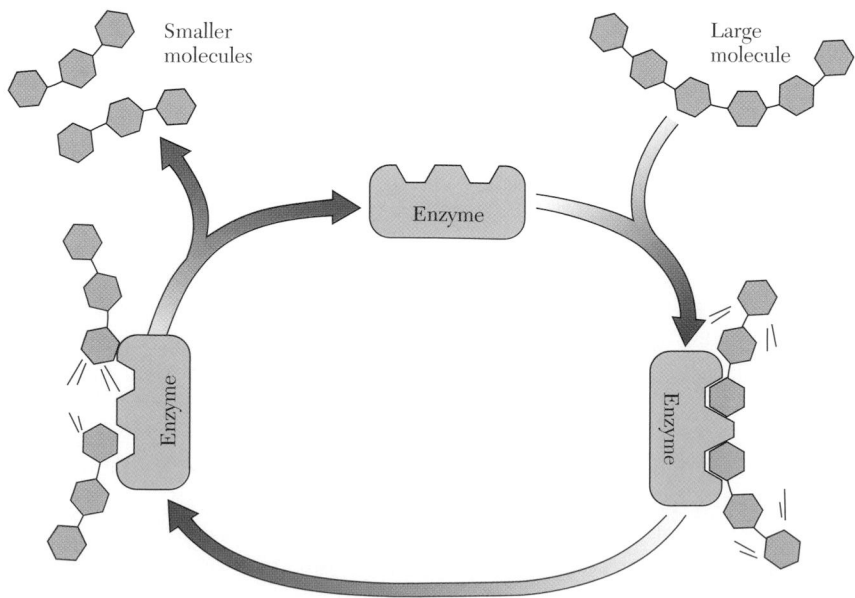

Figure 3.4

Enzymes speed up chemical reactions without themselves being altered by the reaction. In this example, an enzyme breaks a large molecule into two smaller ones.

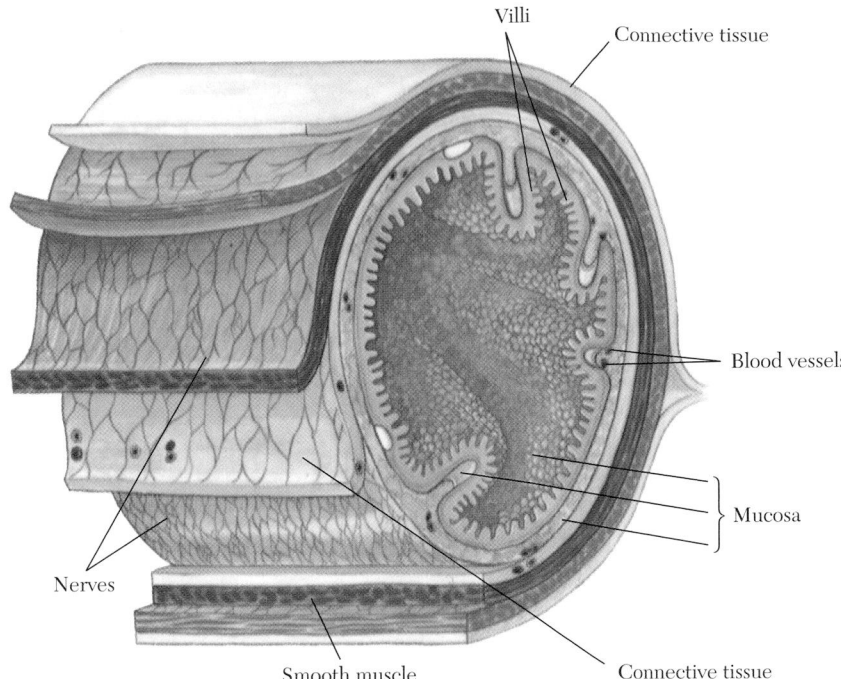

Villi
Connective tissue
Blood vessels
Mucosa
Nerves
Smooth muscle
Connective tissue

Figure 3.5

This cross section through the wall of the small intestine shows the four tissue layers: mucosa, connective tissue, smooth muscle layers, and outer connective tissue layer. (Adapted from E. P. Solomon, R. R. Schmidt, and P. J. Adragna, *Human Anatomy and Physiology*, 2nd ed. Philadelphia: Saunders College Publishing, 1990.)

feces. Because mucosal cells reproduce rapidly, the mucosa has high nutrient requirements and is therefore one of the first parts of the body to be affected by nutrient deficiencies. Surrounding the mucosa is a layer of connective tissue containing nerves and blood vessels. This layer provides support, delivers nutrients to the mucosa, and provides the nerve signals that control secretions and muscle contractions. Layers of smooth muscle—the type over which we do not have voluntary control—surround the connective tissue. The contraction of smooth muscles mixes food, breaks it into smaller particles, and propels it through the digestive tract. The final, external layer is also made up of connective tissue and provides support and protection.

• DIGESTION AND ABSORPTION

To be used by the body, food must be eaten and digested, and the nutrients must be absorbed and transported to the cells of the body. Because most foods we consume are mixtures of carbohydrate, fat, and protein, the physiology of the digestive tract is designed to allow the digestion of all of these components without competition among them. The following sections of this chapter will trace a meal through all these processes, from the body's anticipation of the meal to its elimination of the waste products.

Imagine slices of oven-roasted turkey served on fresh baked bread accompanied by an apple and a glass of lowfat milk (Figure 3.6).

Sights, Sounds, and Smells

Activity in the digestive tract begins before food even enters the mouth. As the meal is being prepared, sensory input such as the sight of a turkey being lifted out of the oven, the clatter of the table being set, and the smell of freshly baked bread may make your mouth become moist and your stomach begin to secrete digestive substances. This response occurs when the nervous system signals the digestive system to ready itself for a meal. This cephalic (pertaining to the head) response occurs as a result of external cues, such as sight and smell, even when the body is not in need of food.

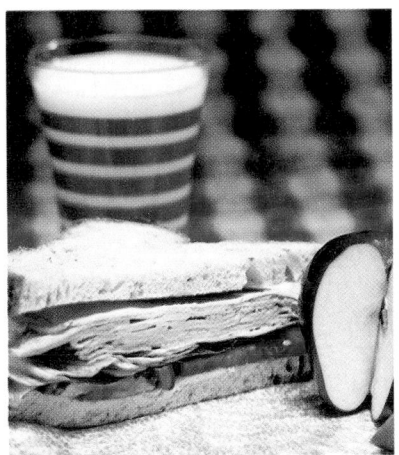

Figure 3.6

The sight, smell, and sounds of food preparation can initiate activity in the digestive tract. (Charles D. Winters)

Mouth

The mouth is the entry point for food into the digestive tract. In the mouth, the taste of food continues the processes begun by the smells, sights, and sounds of food preparation. The presence of food in the mouth stimulates the flow of **saliva** from the salivary glands located internally at the sides of the face and immediately below and in front of the ears (see Figure 3.3). Saliva contains the enzyme **salivary amylase**, which begins the digestion of carbohydrate. Salivary amylase can break the long sugar chains of starch in the bread of the turkey sandwich into shorter chains of sugars. Saliva also lubricates the upper gastrointestinal tract and moistens the food so that it can easily be tasted and swallowed.

Digestive enzymes can act only on the surface of food particles; therefore, chewing is important because it breaks food into small pieces, increasing the surface area in contact with digestive enzymes. Chewing also breaks apart fiber that traps nutrients in some foods. If the fiber is not broken, some nutrients cannot be absorbed. For example, the peel of the apple in the sample meal is a source of vitamins and minerals; however, these nutrients cannot be absorbed without first being released from the fiber in the peel. Adult humans have 32 teeth, specialized for biting, tearing, grinding, and crushing foods; thus, missing or decayed teeth can interfere with the proper digestion of food. Tooth decay, or caries, commonly called cavities, is caused by acid produced when bacteria break down carbohydrates (see Chapter 4).

Saliva A watery fluid produced and secreted into the mouth by the salivary glands. It contains lubricants, enzymes, and other substances.

Salivary amylase An enzyme secreted by the salivary glands that breaks down starch.

Pharynx

The meal that entered the mouth as a turkey sandwich, apple, and milk has now been formed into a bolus, a ball of chewed food mixed with saliva. From the mouth, the bolus moves into the **pharynx**, the part of the gastrointestinal tract responsible for swallowing. The pharynx is shared by the digestive tract and the respiratory tract: Food passes through the pharynx on its way to the stomach, and air passes here on its way to and from the lungs. During swallowing, the air passages are blocked by a valvelike flap of tissue called the epiglottis, so food passes to the stomach, not the lungs. Sometimes food can pass into an upper air passageway. It is usually dislodged with a cough, but if it becomes stuck it can block the flow of air and cause choking. A quick response is required to save the life of a person whose airway is completely blocked. The Heimlich maneuver, which forces air out of the lungs by using a sudden application of pressure to the upper abdomen, can blow an object out of the blocked air passage (Figure 3.7).

Pharynx A funnel-shaped opening that connects the nasal passages and mouth to the respiratory passages and esophagus. It is a common passageway for food and air and is responsible for swallowing.

Esophagus

The **esophagus** passes through the diaphragm, a muscular wall separating the abdomen from the cavity where the lungs are located, to connect the pharynx and stomach. The bolus of food is moved along by rhythmic contractions of the smooth muscles, a process called **peristalsis**. This contractile movement, which is controlled automatically by the nervous system, occurs throughout the gastrointestinal tract, pushing the food bolus along from the pharynx through the large intestine (Figure 3.8).

To move from the esophagus into the stomach, food must pass through a **sphincter**, a muscle that encircles the tube of the digestive tract and acts as a valve. When the muscle contracts, the valve is closed. The gastroesophageal sphincter, located between the esophagus and the stomach, normally prevents foods from moving back out of the stomach. Occasionally, materials do pass out of the stomach through this valve. Heartburn occurs when some of the acidic stomach contents leak up and out of the stomach into the esophagus, causing a burning sensation. Vomiting is the result of a reverse peristaltic wave that causes the sphincter to relax and allow the food to pass upward out of the stomach toward the mouth.

Esophagus A portion of the gastrointestinal tract that extends from the pharynx to the stomach.

Peristalsis Coordinated muscular contractions that move food through the gastrointestinal tract.

Sphincter A muscular valve that helps control the flow of materials in the gastrointestinal tract.

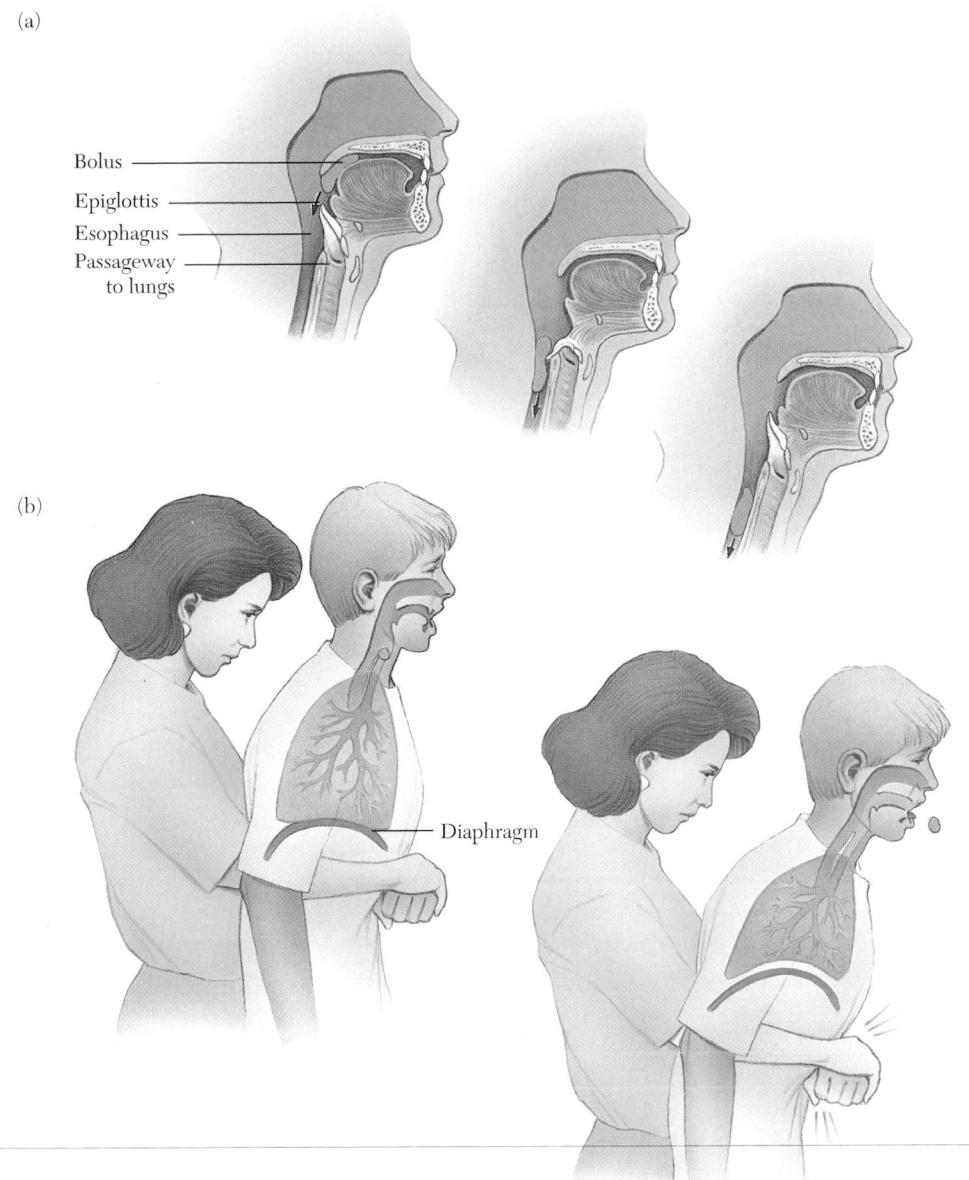

(a)

Bolus
Epiglottis
Esophagus
Passageway
  to lungs

(b)

Diaphragm

Figure 3.7
(a) When a bolus of food is swallowed, it pushes the epiglottis down over the opening to the air passageways. (b) If food does become lodged in the air passageways, it can be dislodged by the Heimlich maneuver, illustrated here.

Chyme A mixture of partially digested food and stomach secretions.

Stomach

The stomach is an expanded portion of the gastrointestinal tract that serves as a temporary storage place for food. While held in the stomach, the bolus is mixed with highly acidic stomach secretions to form a semiliquid food mass called **chyme**. The mixing of food in the stomach is aided by an extra layer of smooth muscle in the stomach wall. While most of the gastrointestinal tract is surrounded by two layers of muscle, the stomach contains a third layer, allowing for powerful contractions that thoroughly churn and mix the stomach contents. Some digestion takes place in the stomach, but, with the exception of some water, alcohol, and a few drugs such as aspirin and acetaminophen (Tylenol), very little absorption occurs here.

Regulation of Gastric Secretion Gastric or stomach secretions are regulated by both nervous and hormonal mechanisms. Signals from three different sites—the brain, stomach, and small intestine—stimulate or inhibit gastric secretion. The three phases of gastric secretion are therefore called cephalic, gastric, and

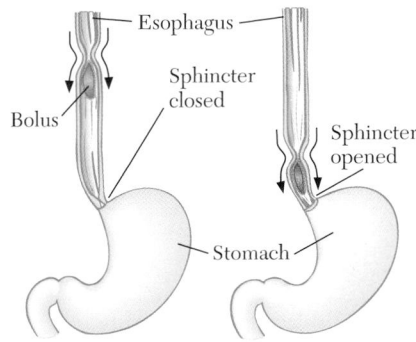

Esophagus

Sphincter
closed

Bolus

Sphincter
opened

Stomach

Figure 3.8
The rhythmic contractions of peristalsis propel food down the esophagus, through the open sphincter, and into the stomach.

Cephalic phase The phase of gastric secretion that is stimulated by the sight, smell, and taste of food.

Gastric phase The phase of gastric secretion triggered by the entry of food into the stomach.

Gastrin A hormone secreted by the stomach mucosa that stimulates the secretion of gastric juices.

Pepsin A protein-digesting enzyme produced by the stomach. It is secreted in the gastric juice in an inactive form and activated by acid in the stomach.

Peptic ulcer An open sore in the lining of the stomach, esophagus, or small intestine.

Intestinal phase The phase of gastric secretion that is begun by the entry of food into the small intestine.

intestinal. The **cephalic phase** occurs before food enters the stomach. During this phase, the thought, smell, sight, or taste of food causes the brain to send nerve signals that increase gastric secretion. This prepares the stomach to receive food (Figure 3.9).

The second phase, referred to as the **gastric phase**, begins when food enters the stomach. The presence of food in the stomach causes gastric secretion by stretching local nerves, by signaling the brain, and by stimulating the secretion of the hormone **gastrin** from the upper portion of the stomach. Gastrin triggers the release of gastric juice, which is produced by digestive glands, called gastric glands, in the lining of the stomach. One of the components of gastric juice is hydrochloric acid. Hydrochloric acid stops the carbohydrate-digesting activity of salivary amylase and helps to begin the digestion of protein. It also serves to kill most bacteria present in food. Another component of gastric juice is pepsinogen. When pepsinogen is exposed to the acidity of the stomach, it is converted into the protein-digesting enzyme **pepsin**, which breaks proteins into shorter chains of amino acids called polypeptides. Pepsin is produced in an inactive form and activated in the stomach; otherwise, its active form would digest the glands that produce it. Although salivary amylase function is stopped by the acidity of the stomach, pepsin functions best in acid. Therefore, digestion of starch from our sample meal stops in the stomach, and digestion of the protein from the turkey, milk, and bread begins. The protein of the stomach wall is protected from the acid and pepsin by a thick layer of mucus. If the mucus layer is penetrated, pepsin and acid can damage the underlying tissues and cause **peptic ulcers**, erosions of the stomach wall or some other region of the gastrointestinal tract. One of the leading causes of ulcers is acid-resistant bacteria that infect the lining of the stomach, causing damage to the gastrointestinal tract wall and destroying the protective mucosal layer.[1]

The third phase of gastric secretion, the **intestinal phase**, is begun by the passage of chyme into the small intestine. This triggers events that decrease stomach motility and secretions, and slow the release of food into the intestine. This ensures that the amount of chyme entering the small intestine does not exceed the ability of the intestine to process it.

Figure 3.9

The regulation of gastric secretion is divided into three phases. In the cephalic phase, the sight, smell, and taste of food cause the brain to signal an increase in gastric secretions. In the gastric phase, food entering the stomach stimulates gastric secretions by stretching local nerves, signaling the brain, and causing gastrin release. In the intestinal phase, food entering the small intestine inhibits gastric secretions by triggering nervous and hormonal signals. In this diagram the zigzag arrows represent nerve signals, and the dashed arrows represent hormonal signals.

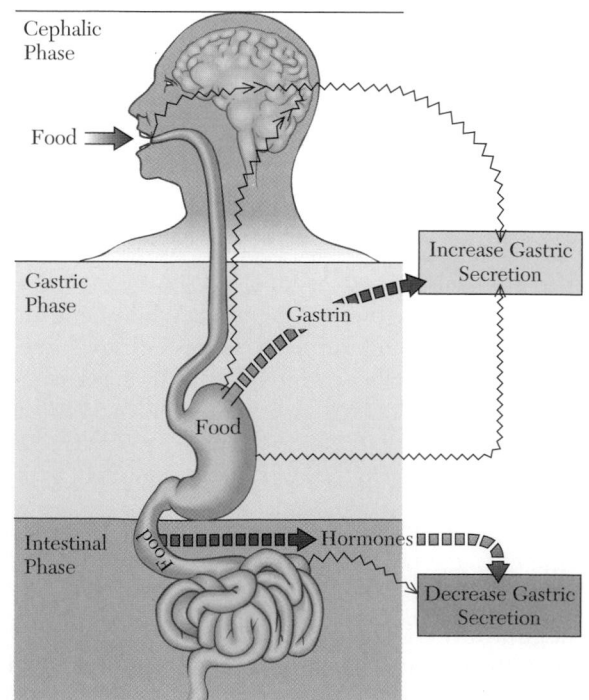

Control of Stomach Emptying Chyme normally leaves the stomach in 2 to 6 hours. The rate of stomach emptying is determined by the size and composition of the meal and controlled by signals from the small intestine. Chyme moving out of the stomach must pass through the pyloric sphincter. This sphincter helps regulate the rate at which food enters the intestine. The small intestine stretches as it fills with food. This distension inhibits stomach emptying. A large meal will take longer to leave the stomach than a small meal, and a solid meal will leave the stomach more slowly than a liquid meal. The nutritional composition of a meal also affects how long it stays in the stomach. The meal we have been following is of mixed composition. Together, the sandwich, apple, and milk contain about 25% of energy as protein, 45% as carbohydrate, and 30% as fat. The meal is partly solid and partly liquid, and so will be in the stomach for an average amount of time (about 4 hours). A high-fat meal will stay in the stomach the longest because fat entering the small intestine slows stomach emptying. A meal that is primarily protein will leave more quickly, and a meal of mostly carbohydrate will leave the fastest. The reason you are often ready to eat again soon after a meal of vegetables and rice is that this high-carbohydrate, lowfat meal leaves the stomach rapidly. Thus, what you choose for breakfast can affect when you become hungry for lunch. Toast and coffee will leave your stomach far more quickly than a larger meal with more protein and some fat, such as a bowl of cereal with lowfat milk, toast with peanut butter, and a glass of juice. Factors besides food composition also can affect gastric emptying. For example, sadness and fear tend to slow emptying, while aggression tends to increase gastric motility and speed emptying.

Small Intestine

The small intestine is a narrow tube about 20 feet in length. It is divided into three segments. The first 12 inches are the duodenum, the next 8 feet are the jejunum, and the last 11 feet are the ileum. The small intestine is the main site of digestion of food and absorption of nutrients.

Digestion in the Small Intestine In the small intestine, secretions from the **pancreas** and **gallbladder** as well as from the intestine itself aid digestion. The pancreas secretes pancreatic juice, which contains bicarbonate ions and digestive enzymes. The bicarbonate ions neutralize the acid in chyme, making the environment in the small intestine neutral rather than acidic as it is in the stomach. This neutrality allows enzymes from the pancreas and small intestine to function. Pancreatic amylase continues the job of breaking starch into sugars that was started in the mouth by salivary amylase. Pancreatic protein-digesting enzymes, including trypsin and chymotrypsin, continue to break protein into shorter and shorter chains of amino acids. Intestinal digestive enzymes, found attached to or inside the cells lining the small intestine, are involved in the digestion of sugars into single sugar units and the digestion of small polypeptides into amino acids.

The gallbladder secretes **bile**, a substance produced in the liver that is necessary for fat digestion and absorption. Bile secreted into the small intestine mixes with fat and emulsifies it, or breaks it into small droplets. These small droplets allow pancreatic enzymes, called **lipases**, to more efficiently access the fat and digest it and also facilitate fat absorption.

Hormonal Control of Secretions The release of bile and pancreatic enzymes into the small intestine is controlled by two hormones secreted by the mucosal lining of the duodenum. **Secretin** signals the pancreas to secrete bicarbonate ions and stimulates the liver to secrete bile into the gallbladder. **Cholecystokinin (CCK)** signals the pancreas to secrete digestive enzymes and causes the gallbladder to contract and release bile into the duodenum (Figure 3.10).

Pancreas An organ that secretes digestive enzymes and bicarbonate ions into the small intestine during digestion.

Gallbladder An organ of the digestive system that stores bile, which is produced by the liver.

Bile A substance made in the liver and stored in the gallbladder. It is released into the small intestine to aid in fat digestion and absorption.

Lipases Fat-digesting enzymes.

Secretin A hormone released by the duodenum that signals the pancreas to secrete bicarbonate ions and stimulates the liver to secrete bile into the gallbladder.

Cholecystokinin (CCK) A hormone released by the duodenum that signals the pancreas to secrete digestive enzymes and causes the gallbladder to contract and release bile into the duodenum.

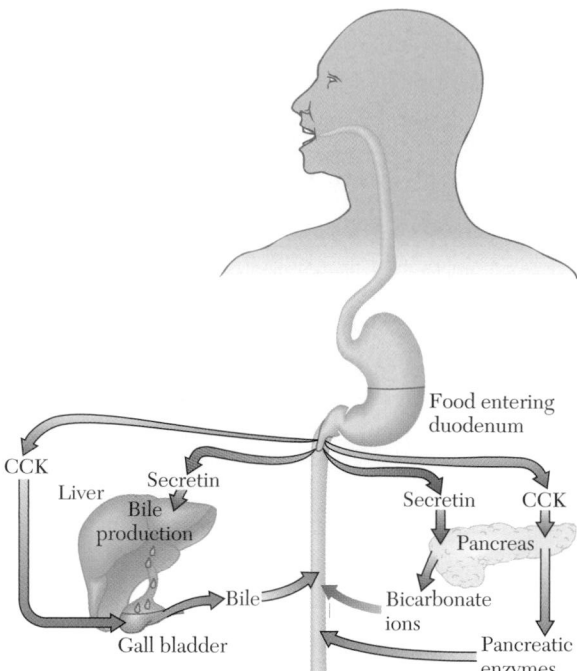

Figure 3.10

Food entering the duodenum triggers the release of the hormones secretin and cholecystokinin (CCK). Secretin increases the output of bile by the liver and the secretion of bicarbonate ions from the pancreas. CCK signals the release of bile by the gallbladder and the secretion of digestive enzymes from the pancreas.

Simple diffusion The movement of substances from an area of higher concentration to an area of lower concentration. No energy is required.

Facilitated diffusion The movement of substances across a cell membrane from an area of higher concentration to an area of lower concentration with the aid of a carrier molecule. No energy is required.

Absorption in the Small Intestine The small intestine is the primary site of absorption for water, vitamins, minerals, and the products of carbohydrate, fat, and protein digestion. Several different mechanisms are involved (Figure 3.11). Some molecules are absorbed by diffusion—the process by which a substance moves from an area of higher concentration to an area of lower concentration. Substances that move from higher to lower concentrations are said to move down their concentration gradient. When a concentration gradient exists and the nutrient can pass freely from the lumen of the GI tract across the cell membrane into the mucosal cell, the process is called **simple diffusion**. This process requires no energy. The water, small lipid molecules, and fat-soluble vitamins from the milk in our meal are absorbed by simple diffusion. Many nutrients, however, cannot pass freely across cell membranes; they must be carried by other molecules in a process called **facilitated diffusion**. Even though these nutrients are carried across the cell membrane by other molecules, they still move down a concentration gradient from an area of higher concentration to one of lower concentration without requiring energy; the sugar fructose found in the apple is absorbed by facilitated diffusion. Substances un-

Figure 3.11

Nutrients are absorbed from the lumen across the cell membrane into the cell by several mechanisms. (*a*) Simple diffusion, which requires no energy, is shown here by the purple balls that move from an area of higher concentration to an area of lower concentration. (*b*) Facilitated diffusion, which requires no energy, is shown here by the yellow cubes that move from an area of higher concentration to an area of lower concentration with the help of a carrier. (*c*) Active transport, which requires energy and a carrier, is shown here by the red pyramids that move from an area of lower concentration to an area of higher concentration.

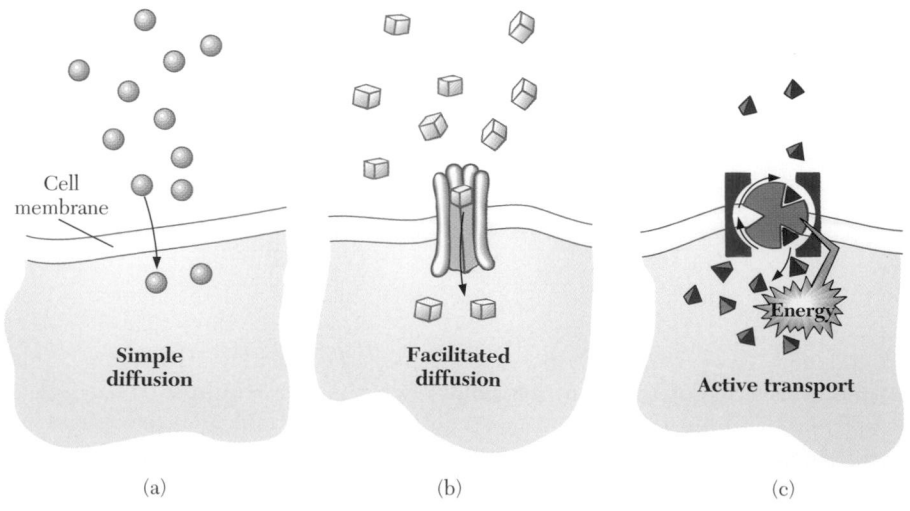

(a)   (b)   (c)

able to be absorbed by diffusion must enter the body by **active transport**, a process that requires both a carrier molecule and energy. This use of energy allows substances to be transported against their concentration gradient from an area of lower concentration to an area of higher concentration. The sugar glucose from the starch of the bread and amino acids from the protein in the milk, turkey, and bread are absorbed by active transport. This allows these nutrients to be absorbed even when they are present in higher concentrations inside the mucosal cells. More specific information about the absorption of the products of carbohydrate, fat, and protein digestion will be discussed in Chapters 4, 5, and 6, respectively.

Structure to Maximize Absorption The structure of the small intestine is specialized to allow maximal absorption of the nutrients. In addition to its length, the small intestine has three other features that increase the area of its absorptive surface (Figure 3.12). First, the intestinal walls are arranged in circular or spiral folds which increase the surface area in contact with nutrients. Second, its entire inner surface is covered with fingerlike projections called **villi** (singular, villus). And finally, each of these villi is covered with tiny **microvilli**, often referred to as the brush border. Together these features provide a surface area that is about the size of a tennis court (300 m^2 or 3229 ft^2). Each villus contains a blood vessel and a **lymph vessel** or **lacteal**, which are located only one cell layer away from the nutrients in the intestinal lumen. Nutrients must cross the mucosal cell layer to reach the bloodstream or lymphatic system for delivery to the tissues of the body.

Large Intestine

Components of chyme that are not absorbed in the small intestine pass through the ileocecal valve to the large intestine, which includes the **colon** and **rectum**. Although most absorption occurs in the small intestine, water and some vitamins

Active transport The transport of substances across a cell membrane with the aid of a carrier molecule and the expenditure of energy. This may occur against a concentration gradient.

Villi (villus) Fingerlike protrusions of the lining of the small intestine that participate in the digestion and absorption of foodstuffs.

Microvilli Minute brushlike projections on the mucosal cell membrane that increase the absorptive surface area in the small intestine.

Lymph vessel or **lacteal** A tubular component of the lymphatic system that carries fluid away from body tissues. Lymph vessels in the intestine are known as lacteals and can transport large particles such as the products of fat digestion.

Colon The largest portion of the large intestine.

Rectum The portion of the large intestine that connects the colon and anus.

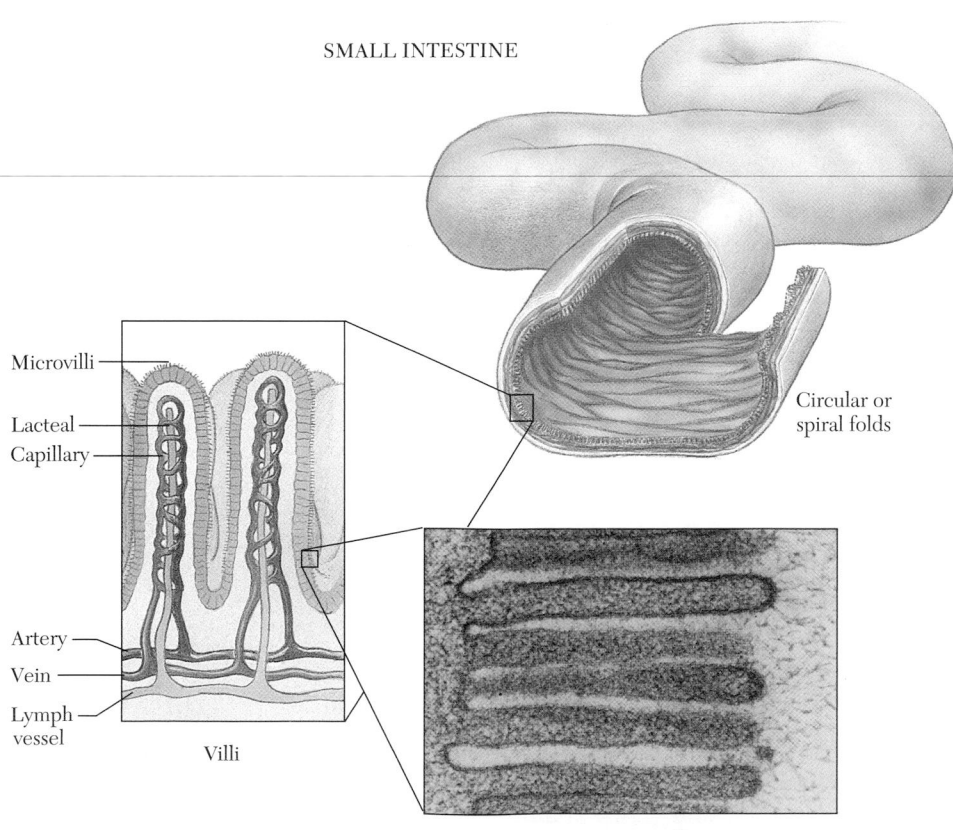

SMALL INTESTINE

Circular or spiral folds

Microvilli
Lacteal
Capillary
Artery
Vein
Lymph vessel

Villi

Microvilli

Figure 3.12
The small intestine contains folds, villi, and microvilli, which increase the absorptive surface area. (Photo, © S. Ito, D. W. Fawcett/Visuals Unlimited)

Off the Shelf

Should You Feed Your Flora?

Bacteria growing in your gut? Sounds bad, but the large intestine of a healthy adult is home to several hundred species of bacteria. The type and number of bacteria in your gastrointestinal tract are affected by both your diet and your health. In turn, the type and amount of bacteria in your GI tract can affect your health.

Most of the time the microflora in our gastrointestinal tracts have beneficial effects. They improve the digestion and absorption of essential nutrients; synthesize vitamins, some of which can be absorbed; and metabolize harmful substances, such as ammonia, thus reducing their concentration in the blood. They are important for intestinal immune function, proper growth of cells in the colon, and optimal intestinal motility and transit time.[1] A strong population of healthful bacteria can also inhibit the growth of harmful bacteria. If the wrong bacteria take over, the result could be diarrhea, infections, and perhaps an increased risk of cancer. Should we be supplementing our diet with beneficial bacteria or eating certain foods to promote their growth?

The recognition that intestinal bacteria are important to human health is not new. In the early 1900s, Nobel Prize-winning Russian scientist Eli Metchnikoff observed that Bulgarian peasants who consumed large quantities of yogurt and other fermented milk products lived long healthy lives. He proposed that the bacteria in these foods positively affected the microflora in the colon and "prevented intestinal putrification" and helped "maintain the forces of the body."[2] Modern research continues to support Metchnikoff's hypothesis

that the bacteria in fermented dairy products, which include *Bifidobacterium* and *Lactobacillus*, provide health benefits.

Today, the consumption of products, such as yogurt, that naturally contain these bacteria and supplements containing live bacteria are referred to as probiotic therapy. When eaten alive, some of these organisms survive passage through the upper GI tract and live temporarily in the colon before they are excreted in the feces. Probiotics have been hypothesized to reduce the risk of heart disease, stimulate immune function, prevent cancer, and improve the integrity of the gastrointestinal mucosa. Research has provided some support for these claims. Evidence from both human and animal studies suggests that the consumption of fermented dairy products has a moderate cholesterol-lowering effect.[3] Probiotic bacteria have also been found to have beneficial effects on immune function in the intestine,[4] and studies in animals have shown that they can prevent the formation and growth of cancerous cells in the colon.[5] Probiotics have been found to shorten the duration of diarrhea due to viral infections, and these bacteria may also be useful in treating other disorders in which the gut barrier is compromised, such as colitis.[6,7] A healthy bacterial population in the intestine may also help prevent constipation, flatulence, and excess gastric acidity.

One problem with probiotics is that when they are no longer consumed, the added bacteria are rapidly washed out of the colon. A newer approach being used to maintain a healthy microflora is to consume foods or other substances that encourage the growth of particular types of

bacteria. Substances that pass undigested into the colon and serve as food for bacteria are called prebiotics. Prebiotics can selectively stimulate the growth of certain types of bacteria. They are currently sold as dietary supplements and are added to commercially prepared tube feeding formulas to promote gastrointestinal health.

Our understanding of probiotics and prebiotics is expanding. We know that the risks of using these products are negligible, but their specific health benefits are still being investigated. Soon we may be able to take probiotics, instead of antibiotics, to eliminate hazardous bacteria in the gut. And, we may be paying attention to what we are feeding our flora—as well as ourselves.

[1]Madsen, K. L. The use of probiotics in gastrointestinal disease. *Can. J. Gastroenterol.* 15: 817–822, 2001.

[2]Metchnikoff, E. *The Prolongation of Life.* New York: G. P. Putnam's Sons, 1908.

[3]St-Onge, M-P, Farnworth, E. R., and Jones, P. J. H. Consumption of fermented and nonfermented dairy products: Effects on cholesterol concentrations and metabolism. *Am. J. Clin. Nutr.* 71: 674–681, 2000.

[4]Erickson, K. L., and Hubbard, N. E. Probiotic immunomodulation in health and disease. *J. Nutr.* 130:403S–409S, 2000.

[5]Brady, L. J., Gallaher, D. D., and Busta, F. F. The role of probiotic cultures in the prevention of colon cancer. *J. Nutr.* 130:410S–414S, 2000.

[6]De Roos, N. M., and Katan, M. B. Effects of probiotic bacteria on diarrhea, lipid metabolism, and carcinogenesis: A review of papers published between 1988 and 1998. *Am. J. Clin. Nutr.* 71:405–411, 2000.

[7]Rolfe, R. D. The role of probiotic cultures in the control of gastrointestinal health. *J. Nutr.* 130:396S–402S, 2000.

Intestinal microflora Microorganisms that inhabit the large intestine.

and minerals are also absorbed in the colon. Peristalsis here is slower than in the small intestine. Water, nutrients, and fecal matter may spend 24 hours in the large intestine, in contrast to the 3 to 5 hours it takes for chyme to move through the small intestine. This slow movement favors the growth of bacteria, referred to as **intestinal microflora**. These bacteria are permanent beneficial residents of this part of the gastrointestinal tract (see *Off the Shelf*: Should You Feed Your Flora?). The microflora act on unabsorbed portions of food, such as the fiber contained in the apple and whole grain bread, producing nutrients that they can use or, in some cases, that can be absorbed into the body. For example, the microflora synthesize small amounts of some B vitamins and vitamin K, some of which can be absorbed. One additional by-product of bacterial metabolism is gas, which causes flatulence.

Materials not absorbed are excreted as waste products in the feces. The amount of water in the feces is affected by fiber and fluid intake. Fiber retains water, so when adequate fiber and fluid are consumed, feces have a high water content and are easily passed. When inadequate fiber or fluid is consumed, feces are hard and dry, and constipation can result.

The end of the colon is connected to the rectum, where feces are stored prior to defecation. The rectum is connected to the **anus**, the external opening of the digestive tract. The rectum and anus work with the colon to prepare the feces for elimination. Defecation is regulated by a sphincter that is under voluntary control. It allows the feces to be eliminated at convenient and appropriate times. The digestion and absorption of carbohydrate, fat, and protein are summarized in Figure 3.13.

Anus The outlet of the rectum through which feces are expelled.

Digestive Problems and Solutions

Each of the organs and processes of the digestive system is necessary for the proper digestion and absorption of food. Problems at any step along the way can inhibit the ability to obtain nutrients from food and influence nutritional status. For example, dental problems can make it difficult to chew, limiting the types of food that can be consumed and reducing contact between digestive enzymes and the nutrients in

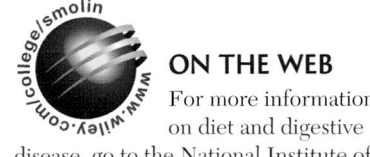

ON THE WEB
For more information on diet and digestive disease, go to the National Institute of Diabetes and Digestive and Kidney Disease at

www.niddk.nih.gov/health/digest/digest.htm/

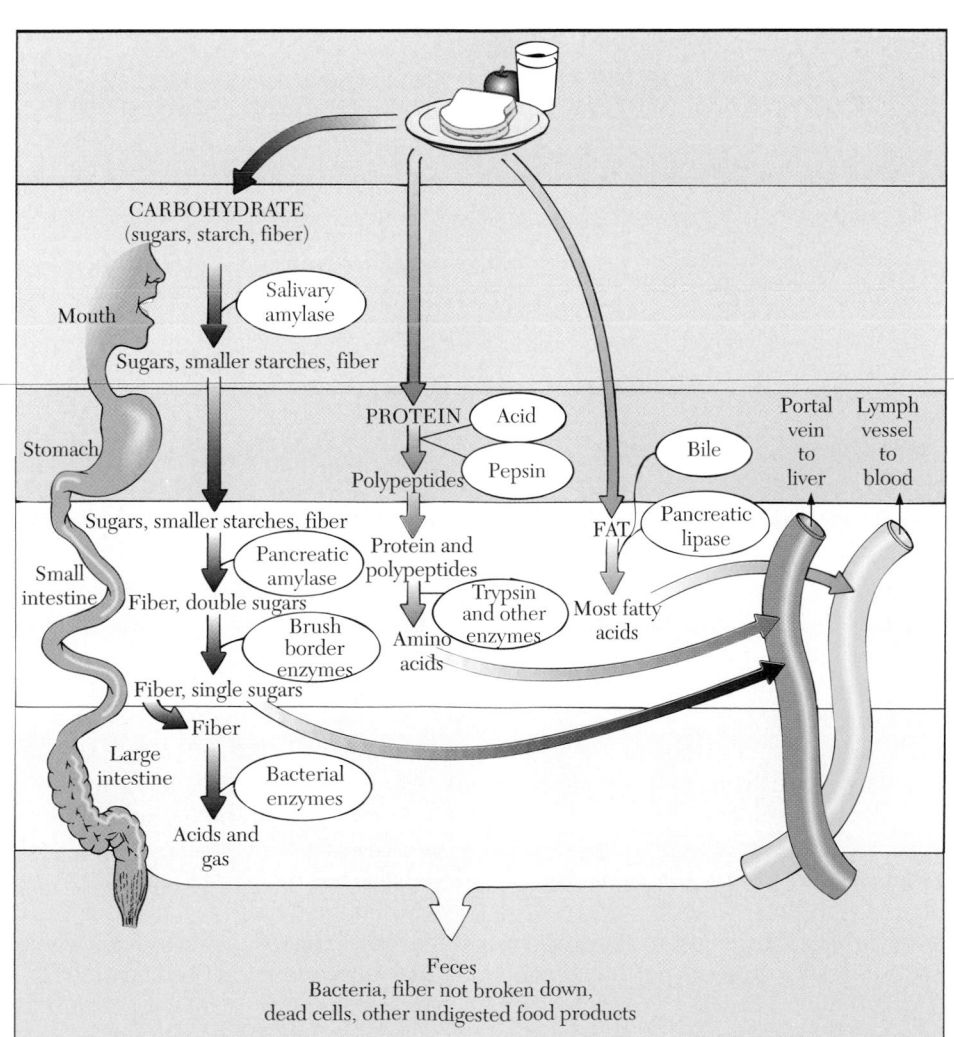

Figure 3.13

An overview of the digestion and absorption of a meal.

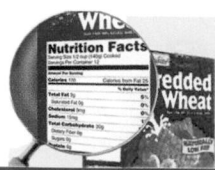

Off the Label
Antacids: Getting the Drug Facts

Medication is an often overlooked source of nutrients. In some cases, these nutrients are a welcome addition to the diet, but in others they may have a negative impact on nutritional status. Heartburn remedies, which are among the most popular over-the-counter drugs, are often a source of nutritive minerals.

Heartburn is a common minor digestive complaint that is caused by stomach acid leaking into the esophagus. The acid in stomach secretions is necessary for digestion; it enhances the absorption of certain nutrients and minimizes bacterial growth. But excess stomach acid or stomach acid that comes in contact with other parts of the gastrointestinal tract can cause pain and discomfort.

When choosing a product to help your heartburn (or any other ailment), be sure to check the label. Drug Facts labels on nonprescription drugs are designed to help consumers take medications correctly as well as understand the benefits and risks and any nutritional impact the drugs might have. The label must present information in a standardized, easy-to-follow format that is as readable and consistent as the Nutrition Facts label found on food products. Under the title "Drug Facts," the product's active ingredients must be listed first, along with the purpose for each, followed by uses, warnings, and directions, and then inactive ingredients.

The label shown here indicates that Reducid contains famotidine, a drug that works by reducing the amount of acid secreted by the stomach. It also contains calcium carbonate and magnesium hydroxide, compounds that decrease the acidity of the stomach contents as well as contribute nutrients to the diet. The label tells you that a single tablet contains 800 mg of calcium, which is 80% of the Daily Value, and 165 mg of magnesium, which is 40% of the Daily Value. Both of these nutrients are typically consumed in less than the recommended amounts in the American diet. Calcium carbonate is a good source of well-absorbed calcium. However, excess magnesium can cause diarrhea. In fact, when taken in high doses, magnesium antacids such as Milk of Magnesia can be used as laxatives.

Other antacids contain minerals that are not beneficial additions to the diet. For example, Alka-Seltzer contains sodium bicarbonate. Each tablet of Alka-Seltzer contains 567 mg of sodium, about 24% of the Daily Value. Sodium-containing antacids contribute a significant amount of sodium to any diet and would not be recommended for someone on a sodium-restricted diet. Aluminum is also found in a number of antacids. Aluminum binds to phosphate in the gut and limits phosphorus absorption. It may also cause constipation. In addition to minerals, a look at the inactive ingredients shows that many products marketed to treat heartburn contain sugar (added to make them more palatable) and starch (added as filler). The amount is small, but individuals who have diabetes or are consuming low-kcalorie diets should consider these in diet planning.

If you are looking for an over-the-counter medication to treat occasional heartburn, understanding how to read the label helps you to use it correctly and to know if the product will affect your nutritional health as well as reduce your heartburn.

[1]Nordenberg, T., New drug label spells it out simply, *FDA Consumer*, July/August 1999.

[2]Mortensen, L., and Charles, P. Bioavailability of calcium supplements and the effect of vitamin D: Comparisons between milk, calcium carbonate, and calcium carbonate plus vitamin D. *Am J. Clin. Nutr.* 63:354–357, 1996.

[3]Feldma, M. Comparison of the effects of over-the-counter famotidine and calcium carbonate antacid on postprandial gastric acid. *J.A.M.A.* 275: 1438–1441, 1996.

food. Pancreatic problems can limit the availability of enzymes needed to digest fat and protein, and gallbladder problems can interfere with fat absorption. Some digestive problems and their causes, consequences, and solutions are given in Table 3.2. Some of these problems can be treated with medications, whereas others require adaptations in the way nutrients are provided (see *Off the Label*: Antacids: Getting the Drug Facts)

For individuals who are unable to consume food or digest and absorb the nutrients needed to meet their requirements, several alternative feeding methods have been developed. People who are unable to swallow can be fed a liquid diet through a tube inserted into the stomach or intestine. Enteral or tube feeding with commercially prepared formula can provide a balanced diet containing all the essential nutrients. Tube feeding can be used in patients who are unconscious or have suffered an injury to the upper gastrointestinal tract. For individuals whose gastrointestinal tract is not functional, nutrients can be provided directly into the bloodstream. This is referred to as total parenteral nutrition (TPN). Carefully planned TPN can provide all the nutrients essential to life. When all nutrients are

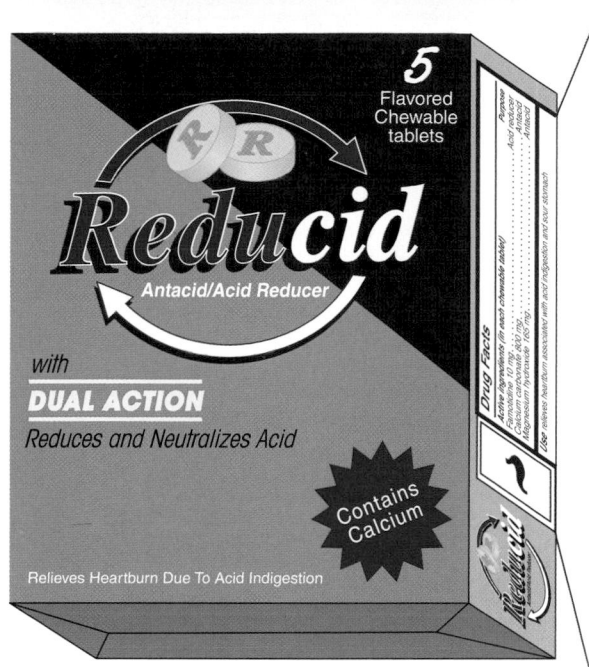

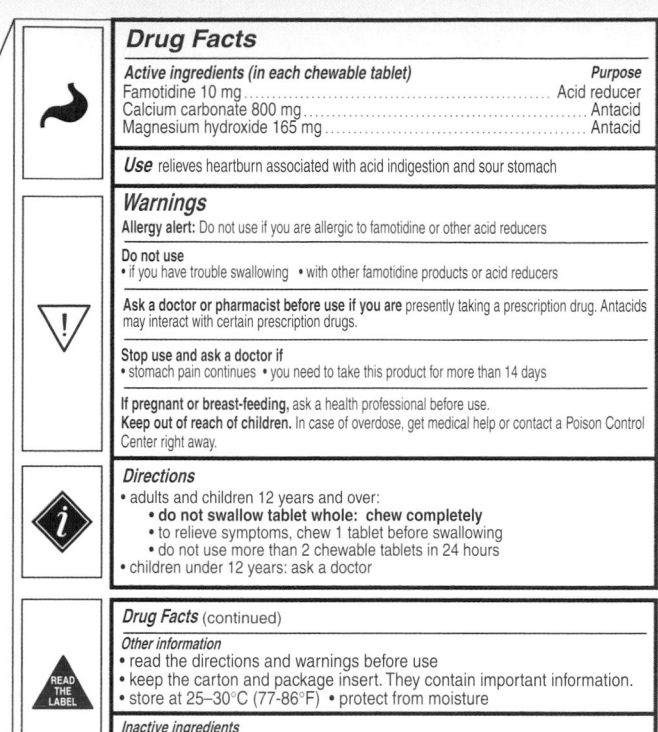

Drug Facts

Active ingredients (in each chewable tablet) — **Purpose**
Famotidine 10 mg... Acid reducer
Calcium carbonate 800 mg.................................... Antacid
Magnesium hydroxide 165 mg............................... Antacid

Use relieves heartburn associated with acid indigestion and sour stomach

Warnings

Allergy alert: Do not use if you are allergic to famotidine or other acid reducers

Do not use
• if you have trouble swallowing   • with other famotidine products or acid reducers

Ask a doctor or pharmacist before use if you are presently taking a prescription drug. Antacids may interact with certain prescription drugs.

Stop use and ask a doctor if
• stomach pain continues   • you need to take this product for more than 14 days

If pregnant or breast-feeding, ask a health professional before use.
Keep out of reach of children. In case of overdose, get medical help or contact a Poison Control Center right away.

Directions
• adults and children 12 years and over:
   • **do not swallow tablet whole: chew completely**
   • to relieve symptoms, chew 1 tablet before swallowing
   • do not use more than 2 chewable tablets in 24 hours
• children under 12 years: ask a doctor

Drug Facts (continued)

Other information
• read the directions and warnings before use
• keep the carton and package insert. They contain important information.
• store at 25–30°C (77–86°F)   • protect from moisture

Inactive ingredients
cellulose acetate, corn starch, dextrates, flavors, hydroxypropyl cellulose, hydroxypropyl methylcellulose, lactose, magnesium stearate, pregelatinized starch, red iron oxide, sodium lauryl sulfate, sugar

Questions or comments? call toll-free **1–800–555–4008**

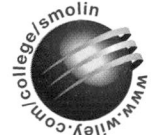

not provided in a TPN solution, nutrient deficiencies develop quickly. Inadvertently feeding patients incomplete TPN solutions has helped demonstrate the essentiality of several trace minerals.

Differences in the Digestive System Throughout Life

There are some differences in the way the digestive system functions during pregnancy and infancy and with advancing age. These changes affect the ability to ingest and digest food and absorb nutrients. However, if the diet is properly managed, nutritional status can be maintained at all stages of life.

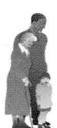

Pregnancy Physiological changes that occur during pregnancy may cause gastrointestinal problems. During the first three months, many women experience nausea, referred to as morning sickness. This term is a misnomer, because it can occur at any time of the day. Morning sickness is believed to be due to pregnancy-related hormonal changes. In most cases, it can be dealt with by eating frequent small meals

ON THE WEB
For more information on providing appropriate nutrition at all stages of life, go to the Fact sheets in the Knowledge Center of the American Dietetic Association Website at
www.eatright.org/

Table 3.2 *Digestive Problems and Nutritional Consequences*

Problem	Cause	Nutritional Consequences	Solution
Dry mouth	Disease medications	Decreased food intake due to changes in taste, difficulty chewing and swallowing, increased tooth decay, and gum disease	Change medications, use artificial saliva
Dental pain and loss of teeth	Tooth decay, gum disease	Reduced food intake due to impaired ability to chew, reduced nutrient absorption due to incomplete digestion	Change consistency of foods consumed
Heartburn	Stomach acid leaking into esophagus, caused by overeating, anxiety, stress, pregnancy, and disease processes	Pain and discomfort after eating	Reduce meal size, avoid high fat foods, consume liquids between rather than with meals, remain upright after eating
Ulcers	Infection of stomach by acid-resistant bacteria that penetrate the mucous layer and damage the epithelial lining, chronic use of drugs such as aspirin and ibuprofen that erode the mucosa	Pain, bleeding, and possible abdominal infection	Antiobiotics to treat infection, antacids, change medications
Vomiting	Bacterial and viral infections, medications, other illnesses, eating disorders	Dehydration and electrolyte imbalance; if chronic, can damage the mouth, gums esophagus, and teeth	Medications to treat infection, fluid and electrolyte replacement
Pancreatic disease	Cystic fibrosis or other chronic pancreatic diseases	Malabsorption of fat, fat soluble vitamins, and vitamin B_{12} due to reduced availability of pancreatic enzymes and bicarbonate	Oral supplements of digestive enzymes
Gallstones	Deposits of cholesterol, bile pigments, and calcium	Pain and poor fat digestion	Lowfat diet, surgery

and avoiding foods and smells that cause nausea. Eating dry crackers or cereal may also help. In severe cases where uncontrollable vomiting occurs, TPN may be needed to obtain adequate nutrition.

Later in pregnancy, the enlarged uterus puts pressure on the stomach and intestines, which can make it difficult to consume large meals. In addition, the placenta produces the hormone progesterone, which causes the smooth muscles of the digestive tract to relax. The muscle-relaxing effects of progesterone may relax the gastroesophageal sphincter enough to allow stomach contents to move back into the esophagus, causing heartburn. Symptoms of heartburn can be reduced by avoiding spicy foods; avoiding fatty foods, which slow the rate of stomach emptying; and remaining upright after eating. In the large intestine, relaxed muscles and the pressure of the uterus cause less efficient peristaltic movements and may result in constipation. Increasing water intake, eating a diet high in fiber, and exercising regularly can help relieve constipation.

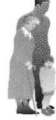 **Infancy** The digestive system is one of the last to fully mature in developing humans. At birth, the digestive tract is functional, but a newborn is not ready to consume an adult diet. The most obvious difference between the infant and adult digestive tracts is that newborns are not able to chew and swallow solid food. They are born with a suckling reflex that allows them to consume liquids from a nipple placed toward the back of the mouth. A protrusion reflex causes anything placed in the front of the mouth to be pushed out by the tongue. As head control increases, this reflex disappears, making spoon feeding possible.

Digestion and absorption also differ between infants and adults. In infants, the digestion of milk protein is aided by rennin, an enzyme produced in the infant stomach that is not found in adults.[2] The stomachs of newborns also produce the enzyme gastric lipase, which is present in adults but plays a more important role in infants where it begins the digestion of the fats in human milk. Low levels of pancreatic enzymes in infants limit starch digestion; however, enzymes at the brush border of the small intestine allow the milk sugar lactose to be digested and absorbed. The absorption of fat from the infant's small intestine is inefficient. However, the ability to absorb intact proteins is greater than that in adults. The absorption of whole proteins can cause food allergies (see Chapter 15), but it also allows infants to absorb immune factors from their mothers' milk. These proteins provide temporary immunity to certain diseases. The bacteria in the large intestine of infants are also different from those in adults because of the all-milk diet infants consume. This is the reason that the feces of breast-fed babies are almost odorless. Another feature of the infant digestive tract is the lack of voluntary control of elimination. Between the ages of two and three, this ability develops, and toilet training is possible.

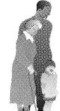 **Advanced Age** Although there are few dramatic changes in the nutrient requirements of humans as they age, changes in the digestive tract and other systems may affect the palatability of food and the ability to obtain proper nutrition. The senses of smell and taste are often diminished or even lost with age, reducing the appeal of food. A reduction in the amount of saliva may make swallowing difficult, decrease the taste of food, and also promote tooth decay. Loss of teeth and improperly fitting dentures may limit food choices to soft and liquid foods or cause solid foods to be poorly chewed. Intestinal secretions may also be reduced, but this rarely impairs absorption because the levels secreted in healthy elderly are still sufficient to break down food into forms that can be absorbed. A condition called atrophic gastritis that causes a reduction in the secretion of stomach acid is also common in the elderly. This may decrease the absorption of several vitamins and minerals and may allow bacterial growth to increase (see Chapter 16). Constipation is a common complaint among the elderly that may be caused by decreased motility and elasticity in the colon, weakened abdominal and pelvic muscles, and a decrease in sensory perception. (see *Critical Thinking*: Gastrointestinal Problems Can Affect Nutrition).

CRITICAL THINKING

Gastrointestinal Problems Can Affect Nutrition

This chapter has followed the path of a turkey sandwich, an apple, and a glass of milk through the processes of digestion and absorption. During the journey from mouth to anus, many factors affect how well these processes work. For each situation described below, think about how digestion, absorption, and the GI tract itself might be altered.

An individual is taking medication that reduces the amount of saliva produced.

What effect would this have on nutrition?
▼

When there is not enough saliva, the food is not tasted as well and it is difficult to swallow. Both of these factors are likely to decrease the appeal and therefore consumption of food. Since saliva helps protect teeth from decay, insufficient saliva also increases the likelihood of tooth decay and gum disease.

What nutrients might not be absorbed from the apple if an individual has just had some dental work done?

▼

If the food is not well chewed, digestive enzymes cannot come in contact with all components of the food. If the fiber in the apple skin is not chewed, the vitamins and minerals it contains may not be available for absorption.

After consuming the turkey sandwich, apple, and glass of milk, a large slice of high-fat cheesecake is added for dessert.

How would this affect transit time?

▼

Transit time would increase because the cheesecake is high in fat, which slows stomach emptying. The meal would take more time to pass from mouth to anus.

An individual has a disease of the pancreas that causes a deficiency of pancreatic enzymes.

What effect would this have on the digestion and absorption of the sample meal?

▼

Pancreatic enzymes are needed to digest carbohydrate, fat, and protein. If these enzymes are lacking, digestion will be incomplete, and nutrient absorption will be compromised. Carbohydrate-digesting enzymes in the mouth and intestinal brush border, as well as protein-digesting enzymes in the stomach and mucosal cells, can partially compensate for a reduction in pancreatic enzymes.

An individual has been malnourished. The malnutrition causes the intestinal villi to become flattened.

If the sample meal was consumed, how would nutrient absorption be affected?

▼

The absorption of all nutrients depends on the health of the small intestine. If the villi are flattened, the absorptive area will be decreased, so fewer nutrients will be absorbed.

An individual eats the turkey sandwich and apple but chooses not to drink the milk or consume any other fluid.

How might this affect the feces?

▼

A diet low in fluid and high in fiber could result in hard feces and constipation.

An individual has gallstones, which cause pain when the gallbladder contracts.

What type of foods should be avoided?

▼

Answer:

• PATHS OF ABSORBED NUTRIENTS

Absorbed materials are delivered to body cells by the cardiovascular system, which consists of the heart and blood vessels. The path by which nutrients enter the bloodstream varies with the nutrient. Amino acids from protein, simple sugars from carbohydrate, and the water-soluble products of fat digestion are absorbed directly into the bloodstream. The products of fat digestion that are not water soluble are taken into the lymphatic system before entering the blood.

Cardiovascular System

The cardiovascular system is a closed network of tubules through which blood is pumped. Blood carries nutrients and oxygen to the cells of all the organs and tissues of the body and removes waste products from these same cells. Blood also carries other substances, such as hormones, from one part of the body to another (Figure 3.14).

The heart is the workhorse of the cardiovascular system. It is a muscular pump with two circulatory loops—one that delivers blood to the lungs and one that delivers blood to the rest of the body. The blood vessels that transport blood and dissolved substances toward the heart are called **veins**, and those that transport blood and dissolved substances away from the heart are called **arteries**. As arteries carry blood away from the heart, they branch many times to form smaller and smaller blood vessels. The smallest arteries are called arterioles. Arterioles then branch to form **capillaries**. Capillaries are thin-walled vessels that are just large enough to allow one red blood cell to pass at a time. From the capillaries, oxygen and nutrients carried by the blood pass into the cells, and waste products pass from the cells into the capillaries. In the capillaries of the lungs, blood releases carbon dioxide to be exhaled and picks up oxygen to be delivered to the cells. In the capillaries of the GI tract, blood picks up water-soluble nutrients absorbed from the diet. Blood from capillaries then flows into the smallest veins, the venules, which converge to form larger and larger veins for return to the heart. Therefore, blood starting in the heart is pumped through the arteries to the capillaries of the lungs where it picks up oxygen. It then returns to the

Veins Vessels that carry blood toward the heart.

Arteries Vessels that carry blood away from the heart.

Capillaries Small, thin-walled blood vessels where the exchange of gases and nutrients between blood and cells occurs.

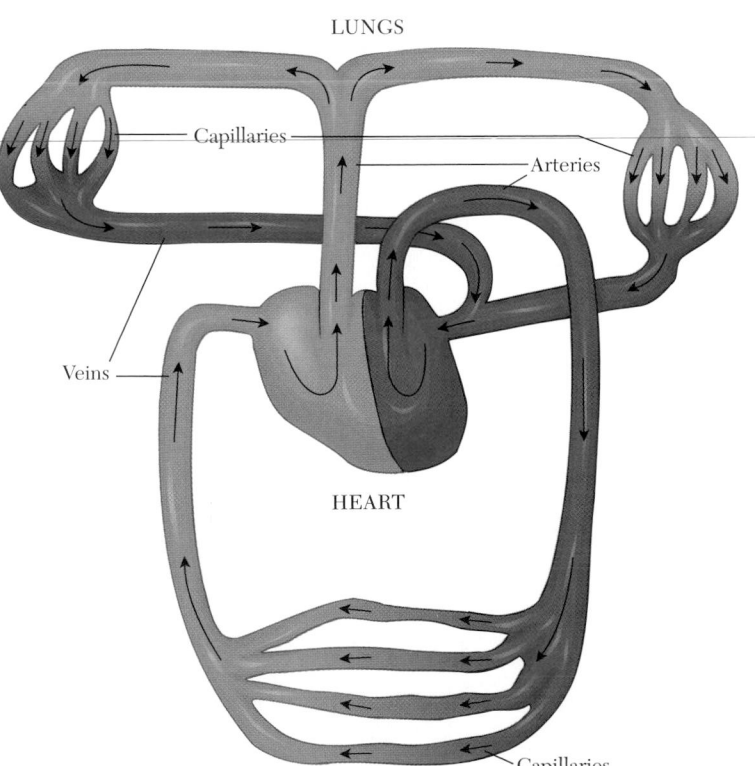

LUNGS

Capillaries

Arteries

Veins

HEART

BODY

Capillaries

Figure 3.14
Blood is pumped from the heart through the arteries to the capillaries of the lungs, where it picks up oxygen. It then returns to the heart via the veins and is pumped out again into the arteries that lead to the rest of the body. In the capillaries of the body, blood delivers oxygen and nutrients and picks up wastes before returning to the heart via the veins. In this figure, red indicates blood that is rich in oxygen, and blue represents blood that is oxygen-poor and carrying more carbon dioxide.

heart via the veins and is pumped out again into the arteries that lead to the rest of the body. In the capillaries of the body, blood delivers oxygen and nutrients and removes wastes before returning to the heart via the veins.

The volume of blood flow, and hence the amounts of nutrients and oxygen that are delivered to an organ or tissue, depends on the need. When a person is resting, about 24% of the blood goes to the digestive system, 21% to the skeletal muscles, and the rest to the heart, kidneys, brain, skin, and other organs.[3] After a large meal, a greater proportion will go to the intestines to support digestion and absorption and to transport nutrients. When a person engages in strenuous exercise, about 85% of blood flow will be directed to the skeletal muscles to deliver nutrients and oxygen and remove carbon dioxide and waste products. Attempting to exercise after a large meal creates a conflict. The body cannot direct blood to the intestines and the muscles at the same time. The muscles win, and food remains in the intestines, often resulting in cramps.

Hepatic Portal and Lymphatic Circulation

Hepatic portal circulation The system of blood vessels that collects nutrient-laden blood from the digestive organs and delivers it to the liver.

Lymphatic system The system of vessels, organs, and tissues that drains excess fluid from the spaces between cells, transports fat-soluble substances from the digestive tract, and contributes to immune function.

Hepatic portal vein The vein that transports blood from the gastrointestinal tract to the liver.

Nutrients enter the blood circulation by either the **hepatic portal circulation** or the **lymphatic system**. The villi of the intestine contain both capillaries, which are part of the portal circulation, and lacteals, which are small vessels of the lymphatic system.

The Hepatic Portal Circulation In the small intestine, water-soluble molecules, including amino acids, sugars, water-soluble vitamins, and water-soluble products of fat digestion, cross the mucosal cells of the villi and enter capillaries. These capillaries merge to form venules at the base of the villi. The venules then merge to form larger and larger veins, which eventually form the **hepatic portal vein**. The hepatic portal vein transports blood directly to the liver, where absorbed nutrients are processed before they enter the general circulation (Figure 3.15).

The liver acts as a gatekeeper between substances absorbed from the intestine and the rest of the body. Some nutrients are stored in the liver, some are changed into different forms, and others are allowed to pass through unchanged. Based on the immediate needs of the body, the liver decides whether individual nutrients will be stored or delivered directly to the cells. For example, the liver, with the help of

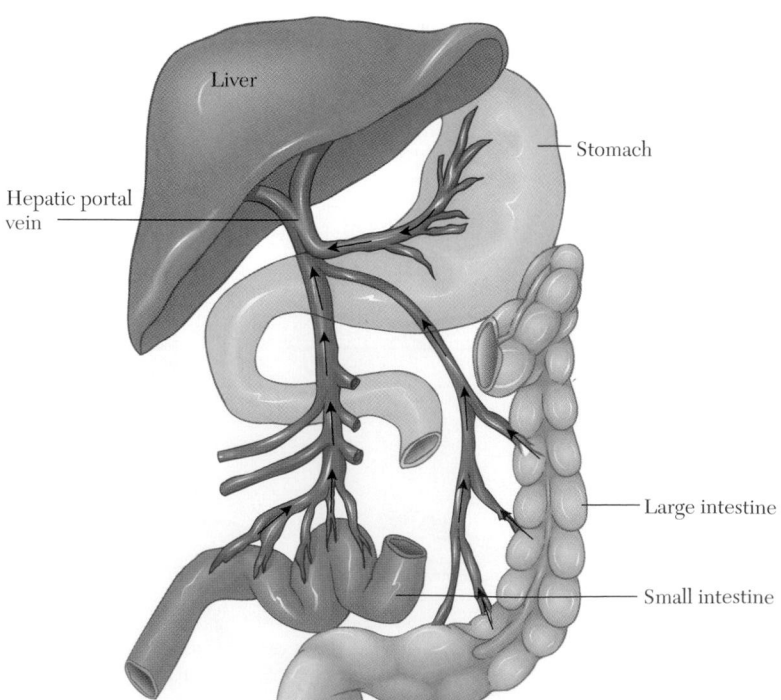

Figure 3.15

The hepatic portal circulation carries blood from the stomach and intestines to the hepatic portal vein and then to the liver.

hormones from the pancreas, keeps the concentration of sugar in the blood constant. The liver modulates blood glucose by removing absorbed glucose from the blood and storing it, by sending absorbed glucose on to the tissues of the body, or by releasing liver glucose (from stores or synthesis) into the blood. The liver is also important for the synthesis and breakdown of amino acids, proteins, and fats. It modifies the products of protein breakdown to form molecules that can be safely transported to the kidney for excretion. The liver also contains enzyme systems that protect the body from toxins that are absorbed by the gastrointestinal tract.

The Lymphatic System The lymphatic system consists of a network of tubules (lymph vessels), structures, and organs that contain infection-fighting cells. Fluid that has accumulated in tissues drains into the lymphatic system where it is filtered past a collection of infection-fighting cells. The cleansed fluid is then returned to the bloodstream. By draining the excess fluid, and any disease-causing agents it contains, away from the spaces between cells, the lymphatic system provides protection and prevents the accumulation of tissue fluid from causing swelling.

In the intestine, materials too large to enter the intestinal capillaries, such as triglycerides and fat-soluble vitamins, are transported by the lymphatic system. These pass from the intestinal mucosa into the lacteals, the smallest of the lymph vessels, which drain into larger lymph vessels. Lymph vessels from the intestine and most other organs of the body drain into the thoracic duct, which empties into the bloodstream near the neck. Therefore, substances that are absorbed via the lymphatic system do not pass through the liver before entering the blood circulation.

Destination: The Cell

For nutrients to enter a cell, they must first cross the **cell membrane**. The cell membrane maintains homeostasis in the cell by controlling what enters and what exits. It is **selectively permeable** because some substances, such as water, can pass freely back and forth, whereas the passage of others is regulated. Nutrients and other substances from the bloodstream are transported into cells by simple and facilitated diffusion and active transport. Once the nutrients have crossed the cell membrane and entered the cell, they can be broken down and used for energy, or they can be used to build the types of structural and regulatory molecules that are needed by the human body. Inside the cell membrane is the **cytoplasm**, or cell fluid that contains the cell **organelles** that perform functions necessary for cell survival. Organelles are also surrounded by membranes. The largest organelle is the nucleus, which contains the cell's genetic material (Figure 3.16).

Cell membrane The membrane that surrounds the cell contents.

Selectively permeable Describes a membrane or barrier that will allow some substances to pass freely but will restrict the passage of others.

Cytoplasm The cellular material outside the nucleus that is contained by the cell membrane.

Organelles Cellular organs that carry out specific metabolic functions.

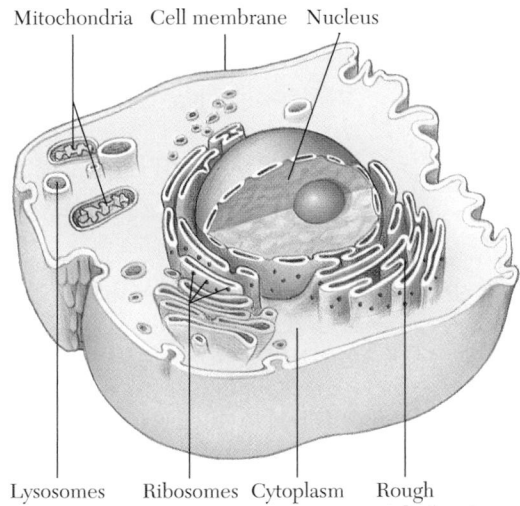

Mitochondria Cell membrane Nucleus

Lysosomes   Ribosomes Cytoplasm   Rough endoplasmic reticulum

Figure 3.16
Structure of a general animal cell. Almost all human cells contain the organelles illustrated here.

• METABOLISM: MAKING AND BREAKING MOLECULES

To stay healthy our bodies use nutrients to produce energy and to manufacture structural and regulatory molecules. The sum of the chemical reactions that occur inside body cells is collectively referred to as metabolism. If the proper amounts and types of nutrients are not delivered to cells, the reactions of metabolism cannot proceed optimally, resulting in poor health. Each nutrient plays a unique role in metabolism. The following discussion provides only a brief overview. Details about the metabolism of each nutrient will be discussed in later chapters.

Many of the reactions of metabolism occur in series known as metabolic pathways. Molecules that enter these pathways are modified at each step of the pathway with the help of enzymes. Some of the pathways are **anabolic**, using energy to build body structures, whereas others are **catabolic**, breaking large molecules into smaller ones and releasing energy. If a nutrient needed for these pathways to proceed is missing, the production of important body structures, chemical compounds, or energy may be impaired. The consequences may be as severe as a life-threatening deficiency disease or as mild as impaired athletic performance.

Anabolic and catabolic processes occur in different cellular organelles. An example of an anabolic organelle is the endoplasmic reticulum, which is a maze of internal membranes. One type of endoplasmic reticulum specializes in the synthesis of lipid-based compounds such as the sex hormones estrogen and testosterone. Another type of endoplasmic reticulum is covered with organelles called ribosomes, which are the site of protein synthesis. Proteins such as digestive enzymes are made here. Lysosomes are catabolic organelles that act as a kind of digestive system for the cell. Lysosomes contain enzymes capable of breaking down carbohydrates, fats, proteins, and other types of molecules that originate both inside and outside the cell.

The **mitochondrion** is a catabolic organelle that obtains energy from carbohydrates (Chapter 4), fats (Chapter 5), and proteins (Chapter 6) by **cellular respiration**. This process completely metabolizes these macronutrients in the presence of oxygen to produce carbon dioxide, water, and a form of energy that can be used by cells called **ATP (adenosine triphosphate)**. The chemical bonds of ATP are very high in energy, and when they break, the energy is released. The energy contained in ATP can be used to do work such as pump blood or contract muscles—or it can be used to synthesize new molecules needed to maintain and repair body tissue.

The meal consumed at the beginning of this chapter has now been delivered to the cells. The carbohydrate in the bread has been broken down into glucose. The cells can use glucose to produce ATP or to synthesize other molecules for immediate use or storage. The protein in the turkey, milk, and bread has been broken down into amino acids that can be used by cells to synthesize needed protein, make glucose if it is in short supply, or produce ATP (Figure 3.17). The fat in the milk, turkey, and mayonnaise has been broken down into fatty acids. These can be used to make ATP or to produce lipids needed for body function, or they can be stored as body fat for later use.

• ELIMINATION OF WASTES

The waste products left over from the digestion and metabolism of the meal must be removed from the body. Substances such as fiber that are not absorbed from the intestine are eliminated from the gastrointestinal tract in the feces. The waste products of cellular metabolism are eliminated by the lungs, the skin, and the kidneys. Carbon dioxide produced by cellular respiration leaves the cells and is transported to the lungs by red blood cells. At the lungs, red blood cells release their load of carbon dioxide, which is then exhaled into the environment. In addition to carbon dioxide, the lungs lose a significant amount of water by evaporation. Water, along with protein breakdown products and minerals, is also lost through the skin in perspiration or sweat.

Anabolic Energy-requiring processes in which simpler molecules are combined to form more complex substances.

Catabolic The processes by which substances are broken down into simpler molecules releasing energy.

Mitochondrion The cellular organelle responsible for generating energy in the form of ATP for cellular activities.

Cellular respiration The reactions that break down carbohydrates, fats, and proteins in the presence of oxygen to produce carbon dioxide, water, and energy in the form of ATP.

ATP (adenosine triphosphate) The high-energy molecule used by the body to perform energy-requiring activities.

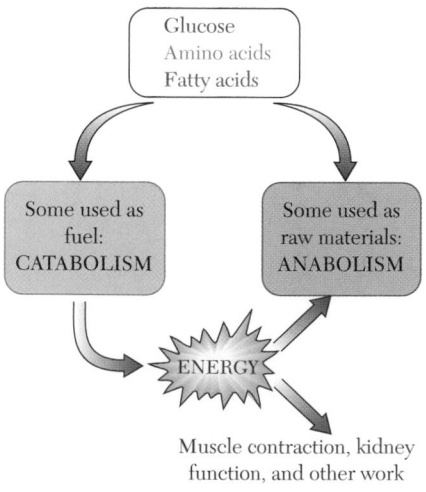

Figure 3.17
Nutrients delivered to cells can be used either to produce energy or as raw materials for the synthesis of carbohydrates, fats, and proteins in the body.

The kidney is the primary site for the excretion of water, nitrogen, and other dissolved metabolic waste products. These are excreted in the urine. The amounts of water and other substances excreted in the urine are regulated so that homeostasis is maintained (see Chapters 10 and 13).

• APPLICATIONS •

1. Imagine you wake up on a Sunday morning and join some friends for a large breakfast consisting of: a cheese omelet and sausage (foods high in fat and protein); a croissant with butter (which contains carbohydrate but is also very high in fat); and a small glass of orange juice. After the meal, you remember that you have plans to play basketball with a friend in just an hour.
   a. If you keep your plans and play basketball, what problems might you experience while exercising?
   b. Had you remembered your plans for strenuous exercise before you had breakfast, what type of meal might you have selected to ensure that your stomach would empty more quickly?

2. There are hundreds of products available to aid digestion. Go to the drug store, health food store, or search the Internet and select a product claiming to aid digestion.
   a. List the claims made for the product.
   b. Using the information in Chapter 1 on judging nutritional claims, analyze the information given.
   c. Does the product make any nutritional contributions to the diet?
   d. Does it carry any risk?
   e. Would you take it? Why or why not?

SUMMARY

1. The organization of all matter begins with the same basic structure—the atom. Atoms are linked by chemical bonds to form molecules. The cell is the smallest unit of life. Cells of similar structure and function are organized into tissues, and tissues into organs and organ systems.

2. The digestive system is the organ system primarily responsible for the movement of nutrients into the body. The digestive system provides two major functions: digestion and absorption. Digestion is the process by which food is broken down into units that are small enough to be absorbed. Absorption is the process by which nutrients are transported into the body.

3. The gastrointestinal tract consists of a hollow tube that begins at the mouth and continues through the pharynx, esophagus, stomach, small intestine, large intestine, and anus. The passage, digestion, and absorption of food in the lumen of this tube are aided by the secretion of mucus, enzymes, and hormones.

4. The processes involved in digestion begin in response to the smell or sight of food and continue as food enters the digestive tract at the mouth, where it is broken into smaller pieces by the teeth and mixed with saliva. Carbohydrate digestion is begun in the mouth by salivary amylase. From the mouth, food passes through the pharynx and into the esophagus. The rhythmic contractions of peristalsis propel it down the esophagus to the stomach.

5. The stomach acts as a temporary storage site for food. The muscles of the stomach mix the food into a semiliquid mass called chyme, and gastric juice containing hydrochloric acid and pepsin begins protein digestion. Stomach emptying is regulated by the amount and composition of food consumed and by nervous and hormonal signals from the small intestine.

6. The small intestine is the primary site of nutrient digestion and absorption. In the small intestine, bicarbonate from the pancreas neutralizes stomach acid, and pancreatic and intestinal enzymes digest carbohydrate, fat, and protein. The digestion of fat in the small intestine is aided by bile from the gallbladder. Bile helps make fat available to fat-digesting enzymes by breaking it into small droplets and also facilitates fat absorption. Secretions from the pancreas and liver are regulated by the hormones secretin and cholecystokinin, produced by the duodenum.

7. The absorption of food across the intestinal mucosa occurs by several different processes. Simple diffusion and facilitated diffusion do not require energy but depend on a concentration gradient. Active transport requires energy but can transport substances against a concentration gradient. The absorptive surface of the small intestine is increased by folds and fingerlike projections called villi, which are covered with tiny projections called microvilli.

8. Components of chyme that are not absorbed in the small intestine pass on to the large intestine, where some water and nutrients are absorbed. The large intestine is populated by bacteria that digest some of these unabsorbed materials, such as fiber, producing small amounts of nutrients and gas. The remaining unabsorbed materials are excreted in feces.

9. Absorbed nutrients are delivered to the cells of the body by the cardiovascular system. The heart pumps blood to the lungs to pick up oxygen and eliminate carbon dioxide. From the lungs, blood returns to the heart and is pumped to the rest of the body to deliver oxygen and nutrients and remove carbon dioxide and other wastes before returning to the heart. Blood is pumped away from the heart in arteries and returned to the heart in veins. Exchange of nutrients and gases occurs at the smallest blood vessels, the capillaries.

10. The products of carbohydrate and protein digestion and the water-soluble products of fat digestion enter capillaries in the intestinal villi and are transported to the liver via the hepatic portal circulation. The liver serves as a processing center, removing the absorbed substances for storage, converting them into other forms, or allowing them to pass unaltered. The liver also protects the body from toxic substances that may have been absorbed.

11. The fat-soluble products of digestion enter lacteals in the intestinal villi. The nutrients absorbed via the lymphatic system enter the blood circulation without first passing through the liver.

12. Cells are the final destination of absorbed nutrients. To enter the cells, nutrients must be transported across cell membranes. Within the cells, some organelles are catabolic, specializing in the breakdown of nutrients to produce energy. Others are anabolic, specializing in the synthesis of molecules needed by the body. The sum of all the chemical reactions of the body is called metabolism.

The reactions that completely break down macronutrients in the presence of oxygen to produce water, carbon dioxide, and energy are referred to as cellular respiration.

13. Unabsorbed materials are excreted in the feces. The waste products of metabolism are excreted by the lungs, skin, and kidneys.

REVIEW QUESTIONS

1. What is an organic molecule?

2. What is the smallest unit of plant and animal life?

3. List three organ systems involved in the digestion and absorption of food.

4. How do teeth function in digestion?

5. What is peristalsis?

6. List two functions of the stomach.

7. List three mechanisms by which nutrients are absorbed.

8. Where does most digestion and absorption occur?

9. How does the structure of the small intestine aid absorption?

10. What products of digestion are transported by the lymphatic system?

11. What path does an amino acid follow from absorption to delivery to the cell? What path does a large fatty acid follow from absorption to delivery to the cell?

12. What is the form of energy used by cells?

13. List four ways that waste products are eliminated from the body.

REFERENCES

1. McManus, T. J. Helicobacter pylori: An emerging infectious disease. *Nurse Practitioner*. 25:42–46, 2000.
2. Marieb, E. N. *Human Anatomy and Physiology*, 5th ed. Redwood City, Calif.: Benjamin/Cummings Publishing Co., 2000.
3. Rhoades, R., and Pflanzer, R. *Human Physiology*, 3rd ed. Philadelphia: Saunders College Publishing, 1996.

Carbohydrates: Sugars, Starches, and Fiber

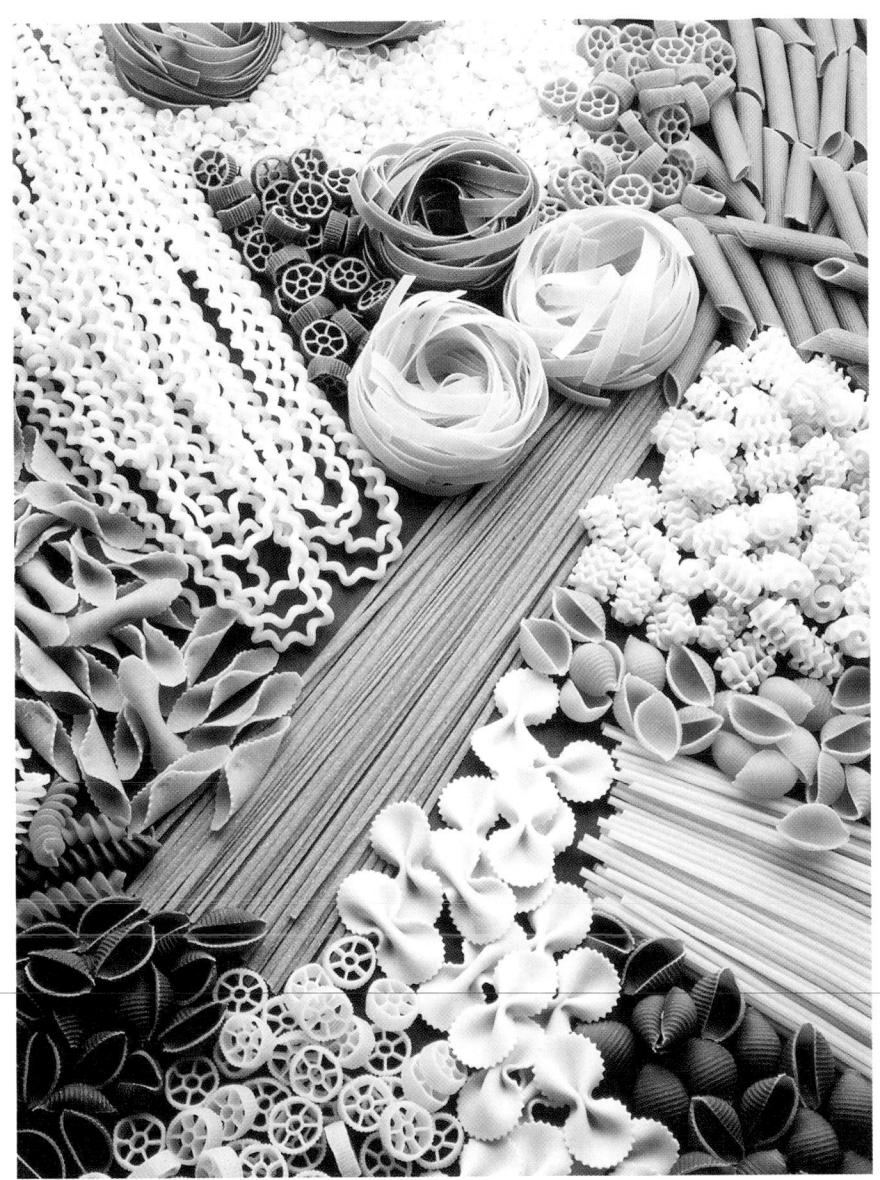

(© SUPERSTOCK)

Chapter Concepts

✔ Foods high in complex carbohydrates, such as rice, wheat, and corn, are the basis of the diet for most of the world.

✔ Carbohydrates include simple carbohydrates, such as those in table sugar and fruit, and complex carbohydrates, such as starch and fiber found in legumes and grains.

✔ Fiber is not absorbed because it cannot be broken down by human digestive enzymes.

✔ Carbohydrates provide a readily available source of energy in the body.

✔ Diabetes, which is characterized by abnormally high levels of blood glucose, is a major public health problem in the United States today.

✔ Foods high in unrefined complex carbohydrates are rich sources of other nutrients and phytochemicals.

✔ Foods high in added sugars are low in nutrient density.

✔ The typical diet in North America includes fewer whole grains and less fiber than is recommended.

✔ Carbohydrates are added in processing to sweeten, preserve, stabilize, or thicken foods.

✔ Artificial sweeteners, also called sugar substitutes, are used to reduce the sugar and energy content of foods.

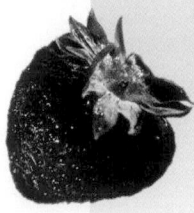

Just a Taste

Is sugar bad for you?

Are carbohydrates fattening?

Is whole wheat bread better for you than white bread?

Carbohydrate-rich foods provide the basis of the diet for most of the world. Rice is the dietary staple in much of Asia, corn in South America, and cassava, a starchy root vegetable, in parts of Africa. Although every culture eats carbohydrates, the amount and type consumed often depend on the wealth and prosperity of the society. As countries become more affluent, animal foods become more affordable, so the intake of carbohydrate from grains and vegetables typically decreases as the intake of fat and protein from animal foods increases. For example, in developing countries today, two thirds of the energy in the diet comes from carbohydrates, whereas in more economically developed countries, the typical intake of carbohydrate accounts for only about half of the energy intake.

The affluence of the society also influences the form of carbohydrate consumed. Throughout history, peasants have eaten dark breads and brown rice while the aristocracy has consumed refined white flour, white sugar, and polished rice. Is the peasant diet the one we should be following? Recommendations for a healthy diet promote diets high in whole grains, vegetables, and fruits and limited in refined carbohydrates.

• WHAT ARE CARBOHYDRATES?

Chemically, **carbohydrates** are compounds that contain carbon (carbo), as well as hydrogen and oxygen in the same proportion as in water (hydrate). They include **simple carbohydrates** also known as sugars and **complex carbohydrates**, which include starches and fibers. Carbohydrates are the primary source of energy used to fuel the body.

Carbohydrates in the Diet

Carbohydrates are found in grains, breads, legumes, fruits, vegetables, and milk, as well as in sweeteners such as honey and table sugar (Figure 4.1). Carbohydrates contribute about 50% of the energy in the American diet, with 16% coming from **added sugars**.[1] Added sugars are not nutritionally or chemically different from sugars occurring naturally in foods. The only difference is that they have been refined and thus separated from their plant sources, such as sugar cane and sugar beets. Added sugars are thought of as **empty kcalories** because they have a low nutrient density, containing energy but few other nutrients. Whole food sources of sugar, such as fruits, contain vitamins, minerals, fiber, and phytochemicals as well as energy. Therefore, they have a higher nutrient density—that is, they contain more nutrients per kcalorie than refined sugars. For example, a tablespoon of sugar contains about 50 kcalories but almost no nutrients other than sugar. A small orange also has about 50 kcalories but contributes vitamin C, folate, potassium, and some calcium as well as fiber.

Grains are the major source of complex carbohydrates in the North American diet. Grains provide a mixture of starch and fiber along with protein, lipids, vitamins, and minerals. Other plant foods such as vegetables and legumes are also sources of both fiber and starch as well as protein, vitamins, and minerals (Figure 4.2). The

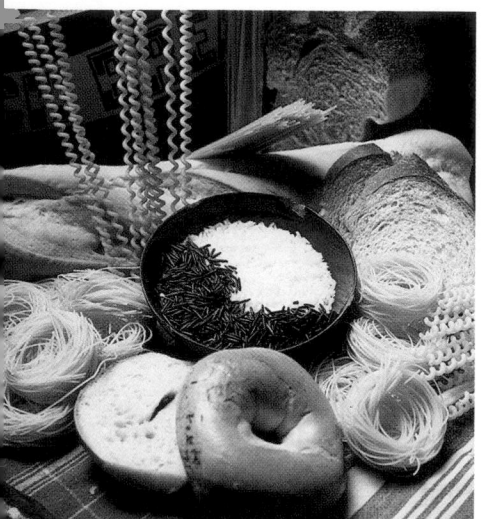

Figure 4.1
Grains, breads, and legumes are sources of dietary carbohydrate. (Charles D. Winters)

Carbohydrates Compounds containing carbon plus hydrogen and oxygen in the same proportions as in water. They include sugars, starches, and fibers.

Simple carbohydrates Carbohydrates known as sugars that include monosaccharides and disaccharides.

Complex carbohydrates Carbohydrates composed of sugar molecules linked together in straight or branching chains. They include starches and fibers.

Added sugars Sugars and syrups that have been added to foods during processing or preparation.

Empty kcalories Refers to foods that contribute energy but few other nutrients.

80

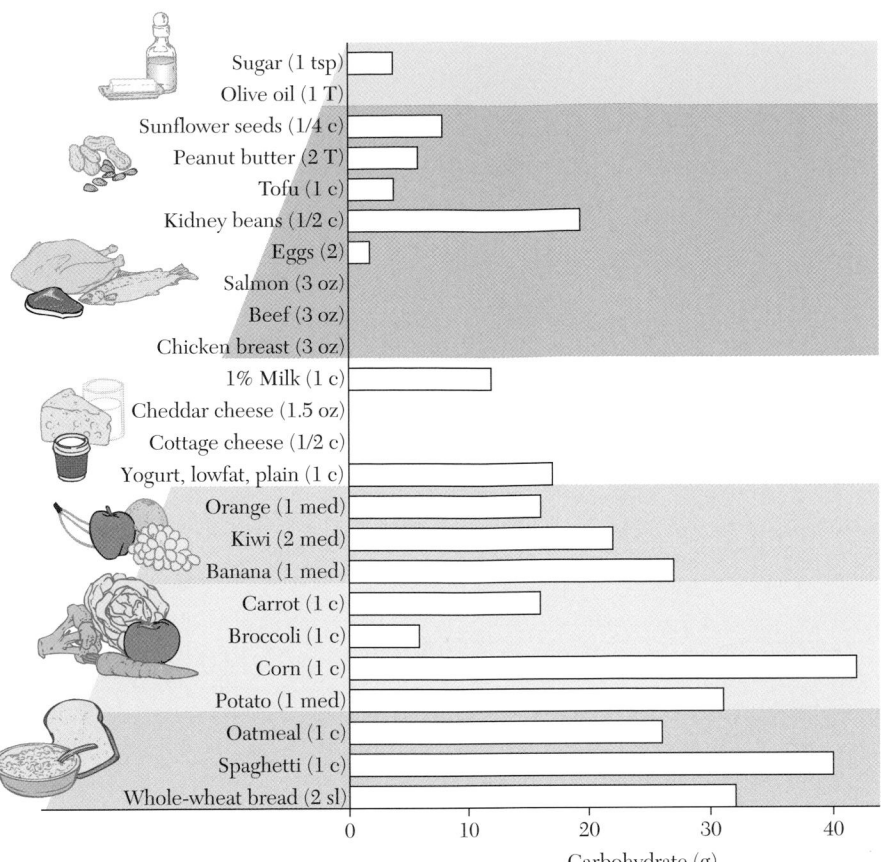

Figure 4.2

Carbohydrate content of selections from each group of the Food Guide Pyramid. The Bread, Cereal, Rice, & Pasta Group; the Vegetable Group; and legumes from the Meat, Poultry, Fish, Eggs, Dry Beans, & Nuts Group are the best sources of complex carbohydrates. The Fruit Group and the Milk, Yogurt, and Cheese Group contain good sources of naturally occurring simple carbohydrates

pulp of starchy vegetables such as potatoes provides starch, whereas the skins are a source of fiber. Dried legumes, such as pinto and kidney beans, are excellent sources of starch and fiber and are good sources of protein. Other vegetables such as green beans and broccoli are lower in starch and higher in fiber and water.

Simple Carbohydrates

The basic unit of carbohydrate is a single sugar molecule, a **monosaccharide** (*mono* means one). When two sugar molecules combine, they form a **disaccharide** (*di* means two). Monosaccharides and disaccharides are known as simple sugars, or simple carbohydrates. The three most common monosaccharides in the diet are glucose, fructose, and galactose. Each contains 6 carbon, 12 hydrogen, and 6 oxygen atoms but differs in their arrangement (Figure 4.3). **Glucose**, commonly referred to as blood sugar, is the most important carbohydrate fuel for the body. It is produced in plants by the process of **photosynthesis**, which uses energy from the sun to combine carbon dioxide and water (Figure 4.4). Glucose rarely occurs as a monosaccharide in food. It is most often found as part of a disaccharide or starch. Fructose is a monosaccharide that tastes sweeter than glucose. It is found in fruits and vegetables and makes up more than half the sugar in honey. Galactose occurs most often as a

Monosaccharide A single sugar molecule, such as glucose.

Disaccharide A sugar formed by linking two monosaccharides.

Glucose A monosaccharide that is the primary form of carbohydrate used to produce energy in the body. It is the sugar referred to as blood sugar.

Photosynthesis The metabolic process by which plants trap energy from the sun and use it to make sugars from carbon dioxide and water.

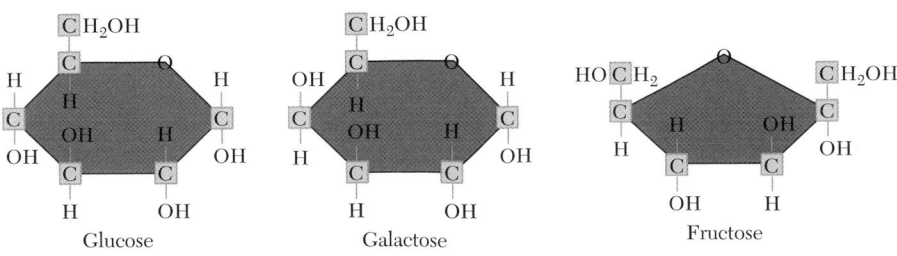

Figure 4.3

Common monosaccharides.

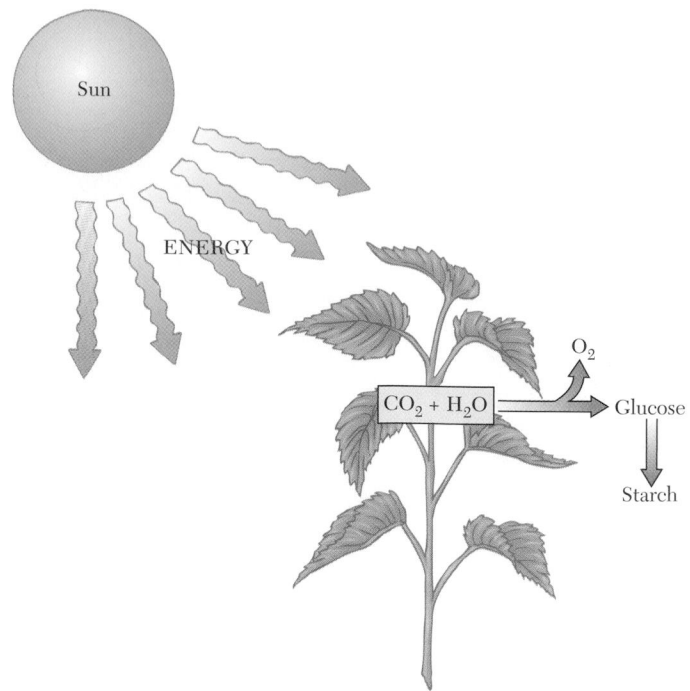

Figure 4.4

The process of photosynthesis uses energy from the sun to synthesize glucose from carbon dioxide and water. Glucose can then be stored as starch.

part of lactose, the disaccharide in milk, and is rarely present as a monosaccharide in the food supply.

Disaccharides are simple carbohydrates made up of two monosaccharides linked together (Figure 4.5). Maltose is a disaccharide consisting of two molecules of glucose. This sugar is made whenever starch is broken down. For example, it is responsible for the slightly sweet taste experienced when bread is held in the mouth for a few

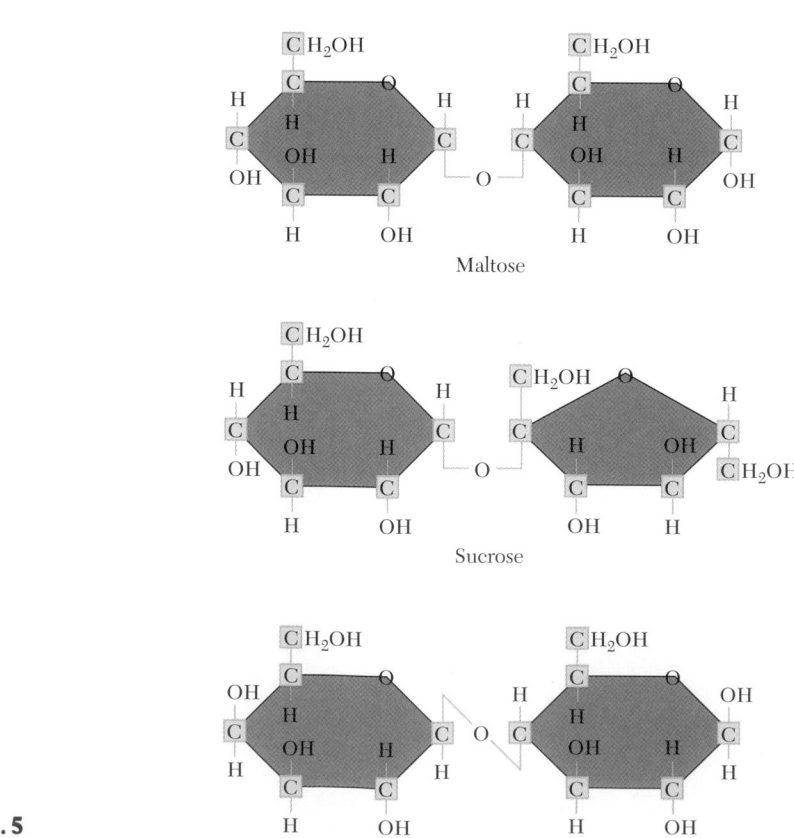

Figure 4.5

Common disaccharides.

minutes. As salivary amylase begins digesting the starch, some sweeter-tasting maltose is formed. Sucrose, or common white table sugar, is the disaccharide formed by linking glucose to fructose. It is found in sugar cane, sugar beets, honey, and maple syrup. Sucrose is the only sweetener that can be called "sugar" in the ingredient list on food labels in the United States. Lactose, or milk sugar, is glucose linked to galactose. Lactose is the only sugar found naturally in animal foods. It contributes about 30% of the energy in whole cow's milk and about 40% of the energy in human milk.

Complex Carbohydrates

Complex carbohydrates are made up of many monosaccharides linked together in chains. They are generally not sweet to the taste like simple carbohydrates. Short chains of three to ten monosaccharides are called **oligosaccharides** and longer chains are called **polysaccharides** (*poly* means many). The polysaccharides include glycogen in animals and starch and fiber in plants (Figure 4.6).

Oligosaccharides Oligosaccharides such as raffinose and stachyose are found in beans and other legumes. These cannot be digested by enzymes in the human stomach and small intestine, so they pass undigested into the large intestine. Here bacteria digest them, producing gas and other by-products. This gas produced by the intestinal microflora can cause abdominal discomfort and flatulence. Over-the-counter enzyme tablets and solutions (such as Bean-O) can be consumed to break down oligosaccharides before they reach the intestinal bacteria, thereby reducing the amount of gas produced.

Glycogen Glycogen is the storage form of carbohydrate in animals. It is made up of highly branched chains of glucose molecules. The branched structure allows it to be broken down quickly when glucose is needed. In humans, glycogen is stored in the muscles and in the liver. Muscle glycogen provides glucose to the muscle as a source of energy during activity; liver glycogen provides glucose to cells throughout the body via the bloodstream.

The amount of glycogen in the body is relatively small—about 200 to 500 grams. The amount of glycogen stored in muscle can be temporarily increased by a diet and exercise regimen called **carbohydrate loading** or **glycogen supercompensation**. This regimen is often used by endurance athletes to build up glycogen stores before an event. Extra glycogen can mean the difference between running only 20 miles or finishing a 26-mile marathon before exhaustion takes over. Glycogen supercompensation is discussed in more detail in Chapter 13.

Starches Starch is the storage form of carbohydrate in plants. It is found in two forms: amylose, which consists of long straight chains of glucose molecules, and amylopectin, which consists of branched chains of glucose molecules. Starch accumulates in roots and tubers (the underground energy storage organ of some plants)

Oligosaccharides Short chain carbohydrates containing 3 to 10 sugar units.

Polysaccharides Carbohydrates containing many sugar units linked together.

Glycogen A carbohydrate made of many glucose molecules linked together in a highly branched structure. It is the storage form of carbohydrate in animals.

Carbohydrate loading or **glycogen supercompensation** A regimen of diet and exercise that is designed to load muscle glycogen stores beyond their normal capacity.

Starch A carbohydrate made of many glucose molecules linked in straight or branching chains. The bonds that hold the glucose molecules together can be broken by the human digestive enzymes.

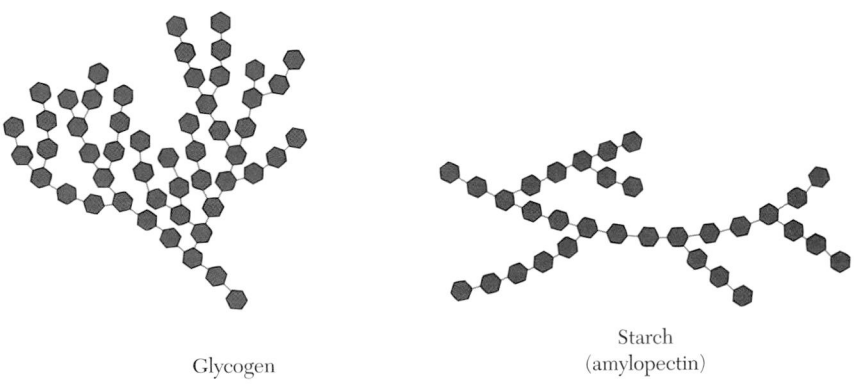
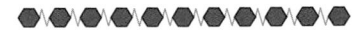

Glycogen

Starch
(amylopectin)

Cellulose

Figure 4.6
Complex carbohydrates are made up of straight or branching chains of monosaccharides.

where it provides energy for the growth and reproduction of the plant. It accumulates in seeds as an energy source for the developing plant embryo.

In our diet, we take advantage of these plant energy stores. When we eat potatoes, we are eating tubers, and when we eat sweet potatoes, yams, or cassava, a food common in West Africa, a starchy root is being used as a food source (Figure 4.7). When we eat legumes such as lentils, soybeans, and kidney beans, we are eating a starchy seed from a plant that produces seeds in a pod. When we eat products made from corn, rice, wheat, or oats, we are also eating the starch from a seed.

If we eat the entire kernel or seed from a grain we are eating a whole grain product (Figure 4.8). The outermost part of a kernel of grain, the **bran**, contains most of the fiber and is a good source of B vitamins. The **germ**, which lies at the base of the kernel, is the plant embryo where sprouting occurs. It is the source of vegetable oils such as corn or safflower oil, and is rich in vitamin E. The remainder of the kernel is the **endosperm**, which is the starchy food supply for the sprouting embryo. The endosperm is primarily starch but also contains most of the protein and some vitamins and minerals. During the milling of grain into flour, the grinding detaches the germ and bran from the endosperm. Whole grain flours such as whole wheat flour include most of the bran, germ, and endosperm. When flours are refined, these components are separated; white flour is produced from just the endosperm. Fiber and some vitamins and minerals naturally found in the whole grain are lost. In order to restore some of the lost nutrients, refined grains sold in the United States are **enriched** with some, but not all, of the nutrients lost in processing. For example, thiamin, riboflavin, niacin, and iron, which are removed by milling, are added back in the enrichment process. Vitamin E, magnesium, and vitamin B_6 are also removed by milling but are not added back (see Chapter 8).

Fiber Fibers are carbohydrates and lignins (substances in plants that are not carbohydrates but are classified as fiber) that cannot be digested by human enzymes. Since they cannot be digested, they cannot be absorbed into the body. However, fibers consumed in the diet can have beneficial health effects, from reducing constipation to lowering blood cholesterol. The term **dietary fiber** is used to refer to fibers that are found intact in plants. Fibers that have been isolated from their plant sources and have been shown to have beneficial physiological effects are called **functional fiber**. Functional fiber can be added to foods or supplements. **Total fiber** is the sum of dietary fiber and functional fiber.[1]

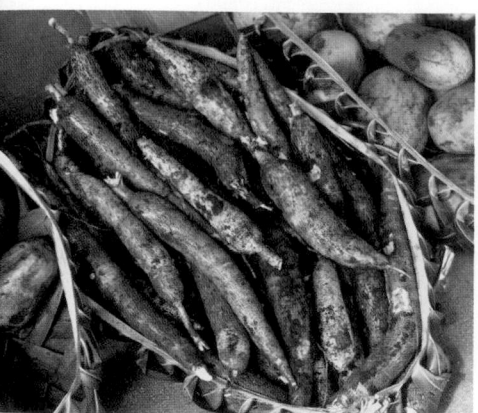

Figure 4.7
Cassava, seen in the center basket, is a starchy root vegetable that is the staple of the diet in some parts of western and central Africa. (Wolfgang Kaehler/Corbis)

Bran The protective outer layers of whole grains. It is a concentrated source of dietary fiber.

Germ The embryo or sprouting portion of a kernel of grain. It contains vegetable oil and vitamins.

Endosperm The largest portion of a kernel of grain. It is primarily starch and serves as a food supply for the sprouting seed.

Enriched The addition of nutrients lost in processing to a level equal to or higher than that originally present.

Dietary fiber Nondigestible carbohydrates and lignin that are found intact in plants.

Functional fiber Isolated nondigestible carbohydrates that have been shown to have beneficial physiological effects in humans.

Total fiber The sum of dietary fiber and functional fiber.

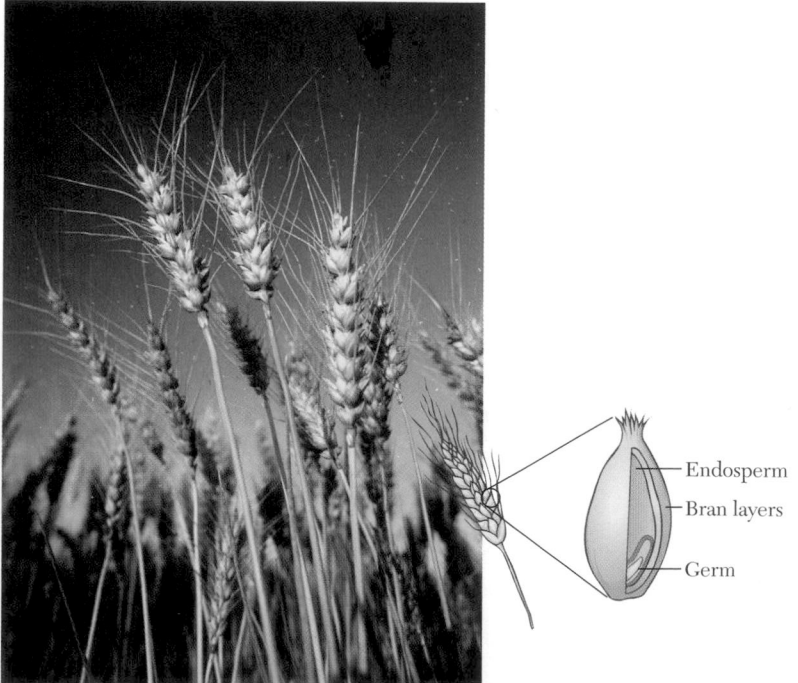

Figure 4.8
A grain of wheat contains outer layers of bran, the plant embryo or germ, and a carbohydrate-rich endosperm. (Kevin Morris/Stone)

Endosperm
Bran layers
Germ

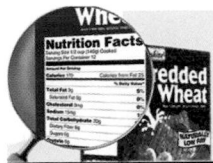

Off the Label
Fiber on Food Labels

Consumers often choose brown breads and colored pasta in an effort to increase the fiber in their diet. The color of a product, however, often reveals little about the fiber content. Better places to look are the list of ingredients and the Nutrition Facts section of the food label.

On the ingredient list of breads, cereals, pastas, crackers, and other grain products, the term "whole" before the name of the grain indicates that the bran layer is still present in the food. Wheat flour, used to describe refined white flour made from wheat, is often confused with whole wheat flour. Only when whole wheat flour is the first ingredient, as it is in the label shown here from whole wheat bread, is the product made with mostly wheat flour containing the bran layer. The first ingredient on the "wheat bread" label shown in the figure is enriched wheat flour, rather than whole wheat flour. For products containing oats, the term "rolled" indicates that the whole oat grain has been used. Fiber added to processed foods can also be identified from the list of ingredients. Insoluble fibers, such as the wheat bran added to the wheat bread shown here, are usually added to decrease the energy content of a product or to meet consumer demands for a high-fiber product. The soluble fiber oat bran is also added for these reasons, but most added soluble fibers, such as pectins and gums, are used to thicken and stabilize foods and rarely contribute a significant amount of fiber.

The Nutrition Facts section of a food label provides information about how much dietary fiber is in a product and how it fits into the recommendations for an overall diet. It lists the total amount of dietary fiber contained in a serving of the product; the amounts of soluble and insoluble fiber are not mandatory, but some manufacturers choose to include them. The percent Daily Value, based on the Daily Value for fiber of 25 grams for a 2000-kcalorie diet, is also listed. For example, the whole wheat bread shown here contains 2 grams of fiber per serving, which is 8% of the Daily Value of 25 grams. Foods that contain 20% or more of the Daily Value for fiber per serving can state on the label that they are "high in dietary fiber." Products containing 10 to 19% of the Daily Value can state that they are "a good source of dietary fiber" (see Table 4.4).

Food labels may also carry health claims related to fiber and chronic disease risk. Fiber-containing grain products, fruits, and vegetables that contain at least 2.5 grams of fiber per serving and are low in fat may claim to reduce the risk of cancer. Fruits, vegetables, and grain products that are low in total fat, saturated fat, and cholesterol and that contain at least 0.6 gram of soluble fiber per serving, and foods that contain at least 0.75 gram of soluble fiber per serving from whole oats or psyllium husks, may claim to reduce the risk of heart disease.

Although whole grain breads are usually brown in color, the dark color may also be due to ingredients such as molasses that contribute no fiber. The green, orange, and red colors of some pasta products are due to the addition of such vegetable extracts as spinach, carrot, or tomato. These vegetables may add some micronutrients but the amounts are usually too small to make a significant contribution to fiber intake. So, when looking for fiber, look beyond the color of the products you choose, and read the label.

Whole Wheat Bread

Nutrition Facts	Amount/Serving	%DV*	Amount/Serving	%DV*
Serving Size 1 Slice (27g)	**Total Fat** 1g	**2%**	**Total Carb.** 12g	**4%**
Servings Per Container 17	Sat. Fat 0g	**0%**	Dietary Fiber 2g	**8%**
Calories 70	**Cholesterol** 0mg	**0%**	Sugars 2g	
Calories from Fat 10	**Sodium** 10mg	**0%**	**Protein** 2g	

Vitamin A 0% • Vitamin C 0% • Calcium 4% • Iron 4%

Thiamin 4% • Riboflavin 2% • Niacin 4%

*Percent Daily Values (DV) are based on a 2,000 calorie diet. Your daily values may be higher or lower depending on your calorie needs:

		Calories:	2,000	2,500
Total Fat	Less than		65g	80g
Sat Fat	Less than		20g	25g
Cholesterol	Less than		300mg	300mg
Sodium	Less than		2,400mg	2,400mg
Total Carbohydrate			300g	375g
Dietary Fiber			25g	30g

NOT A SODIUM FREE FOOD

INGREDIENTS: WHOLE WHEAT FLOUR, WATER, SWEETENERS (HIGH FRUCTOSE CORN SYRUP, MOLASSES), WHEAT GLUTEN, SOYBEAN OIL, CONTAINS 2% OR LESS OF THE FOLLOWING: YEAST, DOUGH CONDITIONERS (MONO & DIGLYCERIDES, ETHOXYLATED MONO & DI-GLYCERIDES, CALCIUM STEAROYL-2-LACTYLATE), YEAST NUTRIENTS (CALCIUM SULFATE, MONO- CALCIUM PHOSPHATE), CALCIUM PROPIONATE (A PRESERVATIVE).

Wheat Bread

Nutrition Facts	Amount/Serving	%DV*	Amount/Serving	%DV*
Serving Size 1 Slice (28g)	**Total Fat** 1g	**2%**	**Total Carb.** 13g	**4%**
Servings Per Container 20	Sat. Fat 0g	**0%**	Dietary Fiber 1g	**4%**
Calories 80	**Cholesterol** 0mg	**0%**	Sugars 2g	
Calories from Fat 15	**Sodium** 190mg	**8%**	**Protein** 2g	

Vitamin A 0% • Vitamin C 0% • Calcium 4% • Iron 4%

Thiamin 4% • Riboflavin 4% • Niacin 4%

*Percent Daily Values (DV) are based on a 2,000 calorie diet. Your daily values may be higher or lower depending on your calorie needs:

		Calories:	2,000	2,500
Total Fat	Less than		65g	80g
Sat Fat	Less than		20g	25g
Cholesterol	Less than		300mg	300mg
Sodium	Less than		2,400mg	2,400mg
Total Carbohydrate			300g	375g
Dietary Fiber			25g	30g

INGREDIENTS: ENRICHED WHEAT FLOUR, (WHEAT FLOUR, BARLEY MALT, NIACIN, IRON, THIAMIN MONONITRATE, RIBOFLAVIN), WATER, WHOLE WHEAT FLOUR, SWEETENERS, (HIGH FRUCTOSE CORN SYRUP, MOLASSES, HONEY), WHEAT BRAN, YEAST, SOYBEAN OIL, CONTAINS 2% OR LESS OF THE FOLLOWING: SALT, DOUGH CONDITIONERS (MONOGLYCERIDES, SODIUM STEAROYL LACTYLATE), YEAST NUTRIENTS (AMMONIUM SULFATE, CALCIUM SULFATE), CALCIUM PROPIONATE (A PRESERVATIVE).

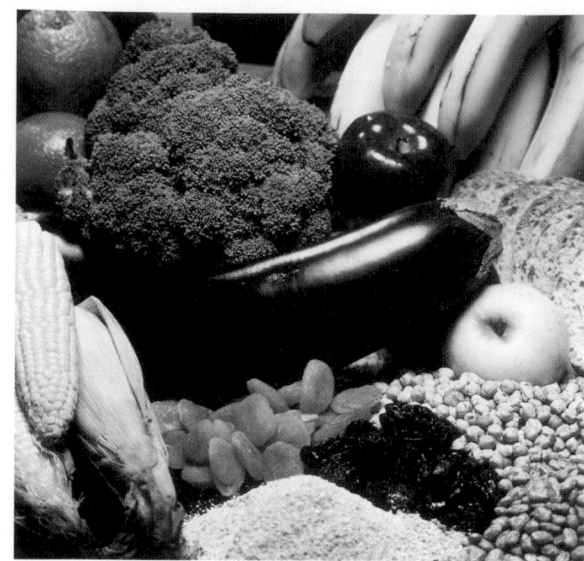

Figure 4.9
These foods are good sources of dietary fiber. (Charles D. Winters)

Soluble fiber Fiber that dissolves in water or absorbs water and can be broken down by the intestinal microflora. It includes pectins, gums, and some hemicelluloses.

Insoluble fiber Fiber that, for the most part, does not dissolve in water and cannot be broken down by bacteria in the large intestine. It includes cellulose, hemicelluloses, and lignin.

Fiber includes a number of different chemical substances that have different physical and physiological properties. Some fibers can be digested by bacteria in the large intestine, producing gas and short chain fatty acids, small quantities of which can be absorbed. These fibers also form viscous solutions when placed in water and are therefore often referred to as **soluble fibers**. Soluble fibers are found around and inside plant cells. They include pectins, gums, and some hemicelluloses. Food sources of soluble fibers include oats, apples, beans, and seaweed. Fibers that cannot be broken down by bacteria in the large intestine and do not dissolve in water are called **insoluble fibers**. They are primarily derived from the structural parts of plants, such as the cell walls, and include cellulose, some hemicelluloses, and lignins. Food sources of insoluble fiber include wheat bran, rye bran, which are mostly hemicellulose and cellulose, and vegetables such as broccoli, which contain woody fibers composed partly of lignins. Most foods of plant origin contain mixtures of soluble and insoluble fibers (Figure 4.9; *Off the Label: Fiber on Food Labels*).

• CARBOHYDRATES IN THE DIGESTIVE TRACT

The majority of disaccharide and starch digestion occurs in the small intestine. Substances that are not completely digested in the small intestine pass into the large intestine. Here the enzymes of the intestinal microflora further break down these substances. When the sugar lactose is not digested, as is the case in many people, this bacterial degradation can cause abdominal discomfort. On the other hand, when fiber passes undigested into the large intestine, as occurs in everyone, the effects are beneficial to the health of the gastrointestinal tract.

Sugars and Starches

The digestion of starch begins in the mouth, where the enzyme salivary amylase starts breaking it into shorter polysaccharides (Figure 4.10). In the small intestine, pancreatic amylases complete the job of breaking down starch. The digestion of oligosaccharides and disaccharides is completed by enzymes attached to the brush border of the villi in the small intestine. Here maltose is broken down into two glucose molecules by maltase, sucrose is broken down by the enzyme sucrase to glucose and fructose, and lactose is broken down by lactase to form glucose and galactose. The resulting monosaccharides—glucose, galactose, and fructose—are then absorbed and transported to the liver via the hepatic portal circulation.

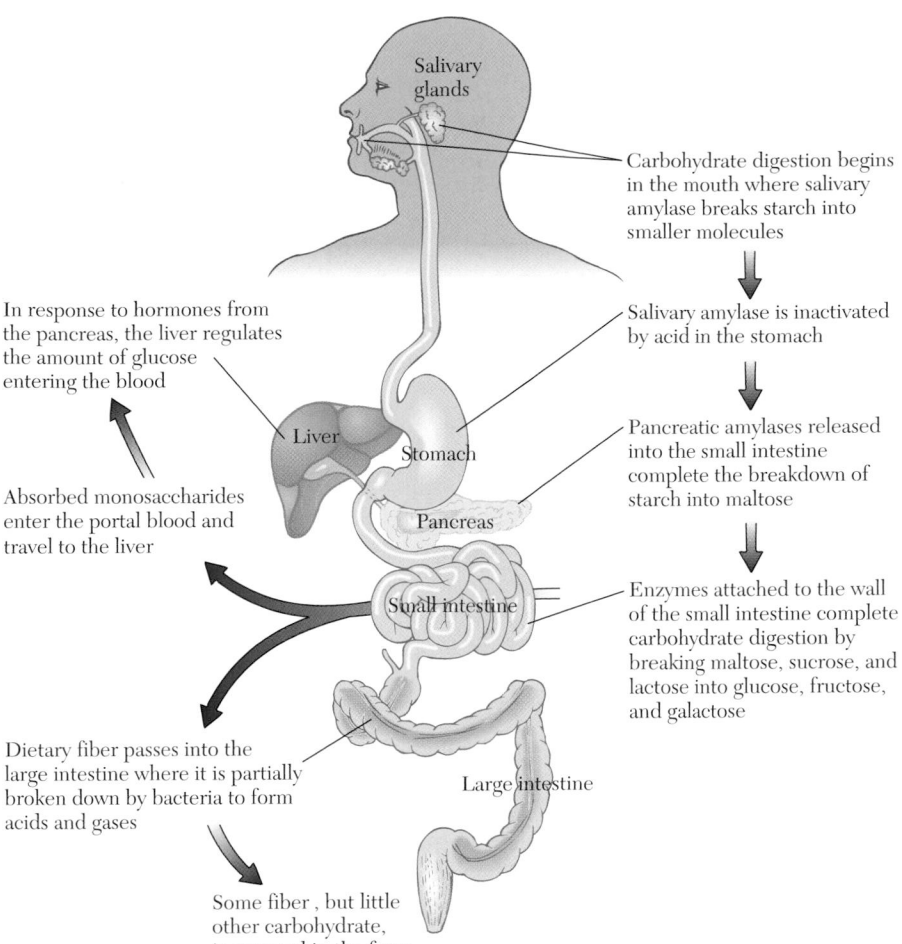

In response to hormones from the pancreas, the liver regulates the amount of glucose entering the blood

Absorbed monosaccharides enter the portal blood and travel to the liver

Dietary fiber passes into the large intestine where it is partially broken down by bacteria to form acids and gases

Some fiber , but little other carbohydrate, is excreted in the feces

Salivary glands

Liver

Stomach

Pancreas

Small intestine

Large intestine

Carbohydrate digestion begins in the mouth where salivary amylase breaks starch into smaller molecules

Salivary amylase is inactivated by acid in the stomach

Pancreatic amylases released into the small intestine complete the breakdown of starch into maltose

Enzymes attached to the wall of the small intestine complete carbohydrate digestion by breaking maltose, sucrose, and lactose into glucose, fructose, and galactose

Figure 4.10
An overview of carbohydrate digestion and absorption.

Lactose Intolerance

Lactase, needed for lactose digestion, is normally produced by all humans at birth. Lactase levels decrease with age and in many individuals decline so much that lactose cannot be completely digested. **Lactose intolerance** is a reduced ability to digest lactose. In lactose-intolerant individuals, lactose consumed in dairy products passes into the large intestine, where it is metabolized by bacteria. The undigested lactose and the acids and gas produced by the bacteria can draw water into the intestine and cause abdominal distention, flatulence, cramping, and diarrhea.

The percentage of adults with lactose intolerance ranges from a low of 5% or less in northwestern European populations to nearly 100% in Asian populations and parts of Africa.[2] In the United States, it is estimated that 30 to 50 million adults are lactose intolerant. The incidence varies enormously depending on ethnic background. For instance, 75% of African Americans and 90% of Asian Americans experience symptoms after consuming lactose.[3] Lactose intolerance may also occur as a result of an intestinal infection or other disease. It is then referred to as secondary lactose intolerance and may disappear when the other condition is resolved.

The degree of lactose intolerance varies. Some individuals cannot tolerate any lactose, whereas others can consume small amounts without symptoms. Because some of the lactose in yogurt and cheese is digested by bacteria or lost in processing, many individuals with lactose intolerance can tolerate these products. Individuals with lactose intolerance must determine their own threshold for consuming dairy products without experiencing symptoms.

Because dairy products are an important source of dietary calcium, individuals with lactose intolerance may need to consume other sources of calcium to meet their needs. In cultures where lactose intolerance is common, traditional diets provide

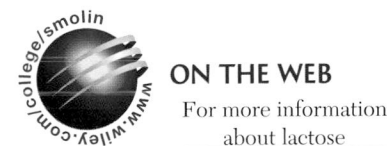

ON THE WEB

For more information about lactose intolerance, go to the National Institute of Diabetes & Digestive & Kidney Diseases at www.niddk.nih.gov/health/digest/digest.htm

Lactose intolerance The inability to digest lactose because of a reduction in the levels of the enzyme lactase. It causes symptoms including intestinal gas and bloating after dairy products are consumed.

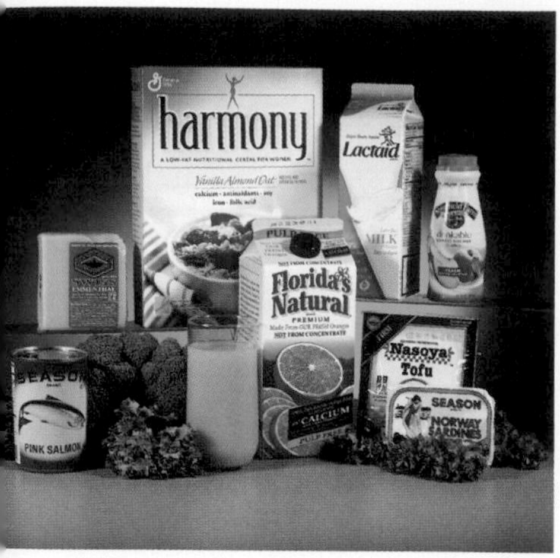

Figure 4.11

These foods are good sources of calcium and are also low in lactose. (Andy Washnik)

sources of calcium other than milk. For example, in Asia, tofu and fish consumed with bones supply calcium, and in the Near East, fermented cheese and yogurt provide much of the calcium. In the United States, milk is the most important source of calcium. The Food Guide Pyramid recommends 2 to 3 servings from the Milk, Yogurt, & Cheese Group each day. Those who can tolerate lactose in small doses can divide the 2 to 3 servings into many smaller portions. Those who cannot tolerate any lactose can meet their calcium needs with tofu, fish, calcium-rich vegetables, milk treated with the enzyme lactase, or calcium-fortified foods or supplements (Figure 4.11). Lactase tablets, which can be consumed with or before milk products, are also available. The enzyme in these tablets digests the lactose before it passes into the large intestine.

Fiber

Fiber cannot be digested by human digestive enzymes; however, fiber does have important properties that affect the digestive tract and maintain healthy bowel function. The structures of different fibers determine their physical properties and the effect they have on the digestive tract. Soluble fibers, such as pectins and gums, absorb water, forming viscous solutions in the digestive tract that slow the rate at which nutrients are absorbed. For example, in the stomach this type of fiber causes distention and slows emptying. In the small intestine, it slows the absorption of sugars and other nutrients and decreases the absorption of bile. In the colon, these fibers are fermented by the bacterial microflora producing acids and gases. Insoluble fibers, such as wheat bran, increase the amount of material in the intestine. They add bulk because they are not completely degraded by bacterial fermentation. Together, the increased bulk and the fluid drawn in by fibers result in an increased volume of material in the intestine. This allows for easier evacuation of the stool. It also promotes healthy bowel function because it stimulates peristalsis, causing the muscles of the colon to work more, become stronger, and function better. The increase in peristalsis also reduces transit time—the time it takes food and fecal matter to move through the digestive tract. In African countries, where the diet contains 40 to 150 grams of fiber per day, the transit time is 36 hours or less. In the United States, where the usual fiber intake is about 15 grams per day,[4] it is not uncommon for transit time to be as long as 96 hours.

• CARBOHYDRATES IN THE BODY

The major function of carbohydrate in the body is to provide energy. The main source of this energy is glucose. In addition, carbohydrate has several other functions. The monosaccharide galactose is an important molecule in nervous tissue. It also combines with glucose to make lactose in women who are producing breast milk. Two other monosaccharides that are of great importance to the body are deoxyribose and ribose. These sugars are components of DNA and RNA (ribonucleic acid), respectively, which contain the genetic information for the synthesis of proteins. Deoxyribose and ribose can be synthesized by the body and are not found in significant amounts in the diet. Ribose is also a component of the vitamin riboflavin. Oligosaccharides are also important in our bodies. They are found attached to proteins or lipids on the surface of cells where they help to signal information about the cells.

Carbohydrate Metabolism

Body cells receive a constant supply of glucose via the bloodstream. This supply is regulated by the liver and by hormones secreted from the pancreas. Once glucose reaches the cells, it is metabolized to produce energy.

Delivery of Glucose to Cells After a meal, monosaccharides are absorbed and travel via the hepatic portal vein to the liver where much of the fructose and galactose is metabolized for energy. The fate of the absorbed glucose depends on the energy needs of the body. If glucose is needed at the tissues, it is transported in the blood, reaching cells throughout the body. The amount of glucose in the blood is regulated at about 60 to 100 mg per 100 ml of blood (70 to 120 mg/100 ml serum). This ensures adequate glucose delivery to body cells, which is particularly important for brain and red blood cells that rely almost exclusively on glucose as an energy source. If blood glucose levels rise too high or drop too low, hormones from the pancreas act to decrease or increase levels.

Glycemic Response How quickly blood glucose levels rise after a meal, referred to as the **glycemic response**, is affected by the composition of the food or meal. Fat and protein consumed with high-carbohydrate foods cause the stomach to empty more slowly and therefore delay the rate at which glucose enters the small intestine, where it is absorbed. This causes a slower rise in blood glucose. Fiber also slows the rise in blood glucose both because foods high in fiber take longer to leave the stomach and because fiber in the small intestine slows absorption. Consuming sugar alone—for example, drinking a sugar-sweetened soft drink on an empty stomach—will cause blood glucose to increase rapidly. After a mixed meal, such as chicken, rice, and green beans, which contains starch, fat, protein, and fiber, it will take 30 to 60 minutes before blood glucose begins to rise. The **glycemic index** is a ranking of how specific foods affect blood glucose compared to the response of a reference food, such as white bread, of similar carbohydrate content.

Insulin Action A rise in blood glucose triggers the pancreas to secrete the hormone **insulin**, which allows glucose to be taken into the cells of the body (Figure 4.12). In the liver, insulin promotes the storage of glucose as glycogen and, to a lesser extent,

Glycemic response The rate, magnitude, and duration of the rise in blood glucose that occurs after a meal or food is consumed.

Glycemic index A ranking of the effect on blood glucose of a food of a certain carbohydrate content relative to an equal amount of carbohydrate from a reference food such as white bread or glucose.

Insulin A hormone made in the pancreas that allows the uptake of glucose by body cells and has other metabolic effects such as stimulating protein synthesis and the synthesis of glycogen in liver and muscle.

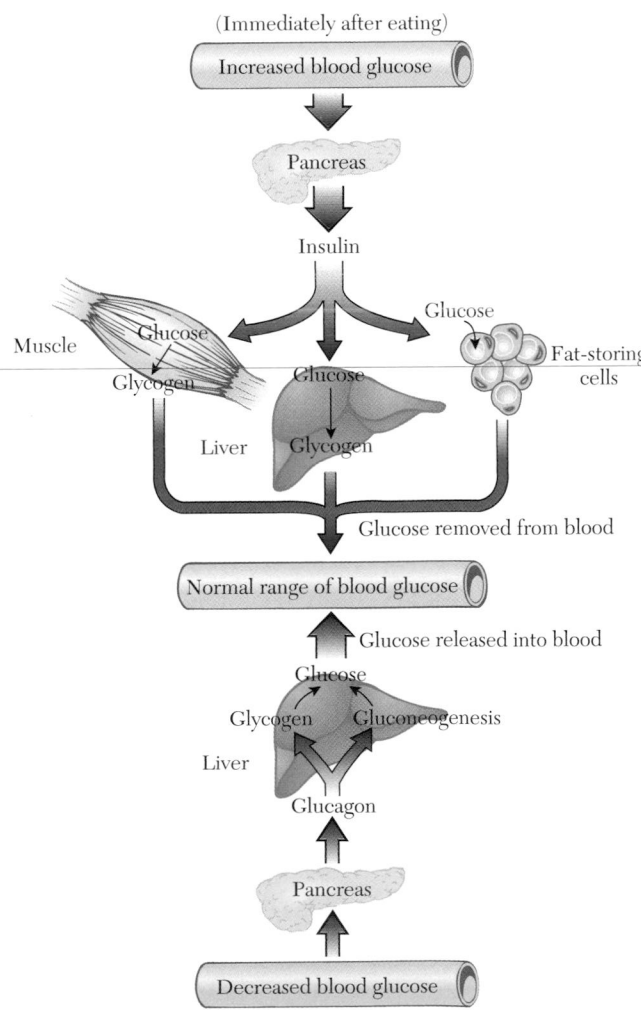

Figure 4.12

Blood glucose is regulated by hormones secreted by the pancreas. Immediately after a meal, when blood glucose increases, insulin is released and stimulates the uptake and storage of glucose. Several hours after a meal, when blood glucose levels begin to decrease, glucagon is released and stimulates the breakdown of glycogen into glucose and glucose production via gluconeogenesis.

fat. In muscle, insulin stimulates the uptake of glucose for energy production and the synthesis of muscle glycogen for energy storage. Insulin also stimulates protein synthesis and in fat-storing cells, it increases glucose uptake from the blood and stimulates lipid synthesis. These actions remove glucose from the blood, decreasing levels to the normal range.

Glucose Metabolism Once glucose has left the bloodstream and been taken up by a cell, it can be metabolized through cellular respiration to produce carbon dioxide, water, and energy in the form of ATP. Providing energy through cellular respiration involves four interconnected stages. The first takes place in the cytoplasm of the cell and is called **glycolysis** (meaning glucose breakdown). In glycolysis, the 6-carbon sugar glucose is broken into two 3-carbon pyruvate molecules. Two molecules of ATP are generated for each molecule of glucose, and high-energy **electrons** are released and passed to shuttling molecules for transport to the last stage of cellular respiration (Figure 4.13).

In the next stage, which occurs in the mitochondria, 1 carbon is removed from pyruvate, leaving 2 carbons that form acetyl-CoA. Acetyl-CoA then enters the third stage of breakdown, the **citric acid cycle**. To begin the cycle, acetyl-CoA combines with a 4-carbon molecule, oxaloacetate, derived from carbohydrate to form a 6-carbon molecule. The citric acid cycle then removes 1 carbon at a time, as carbon dioxide, from this molecule until the 4-carbon oxaloacetate is reformed. These chemical reactions produce 2 ATP molecules per glucose molecule but also remove electrons, which are passed to shuttling molecules for transport to the last stage of cellular respiration, the electron transport chain. The **electron transport chain** involves a series of molecules, most of which are proteins, associated with the inner membrane of

Glycolysis A metabolic pathway in the cytoplasm of the cell that splits glucose into two 3-carbon pyruvate molecules. The energy released from 1 molecule of glucose is used to make 2 ATP molecules.

Electrons Negatively charged high-energy particles that orbit the nucleus of an atom.

Citric acid cycle Also known as the Krebs cycle or the tricarboxylic acid cycle, this is the stage of respiration in which acetyl-CoA is broken down, releasing 2 molecules of carbon dioxide.

Electron transport chain The final stage of cellular respiration in which electrons are passed down a chain of molecules to oxygen to form water and energy is released and used to produce ATP.

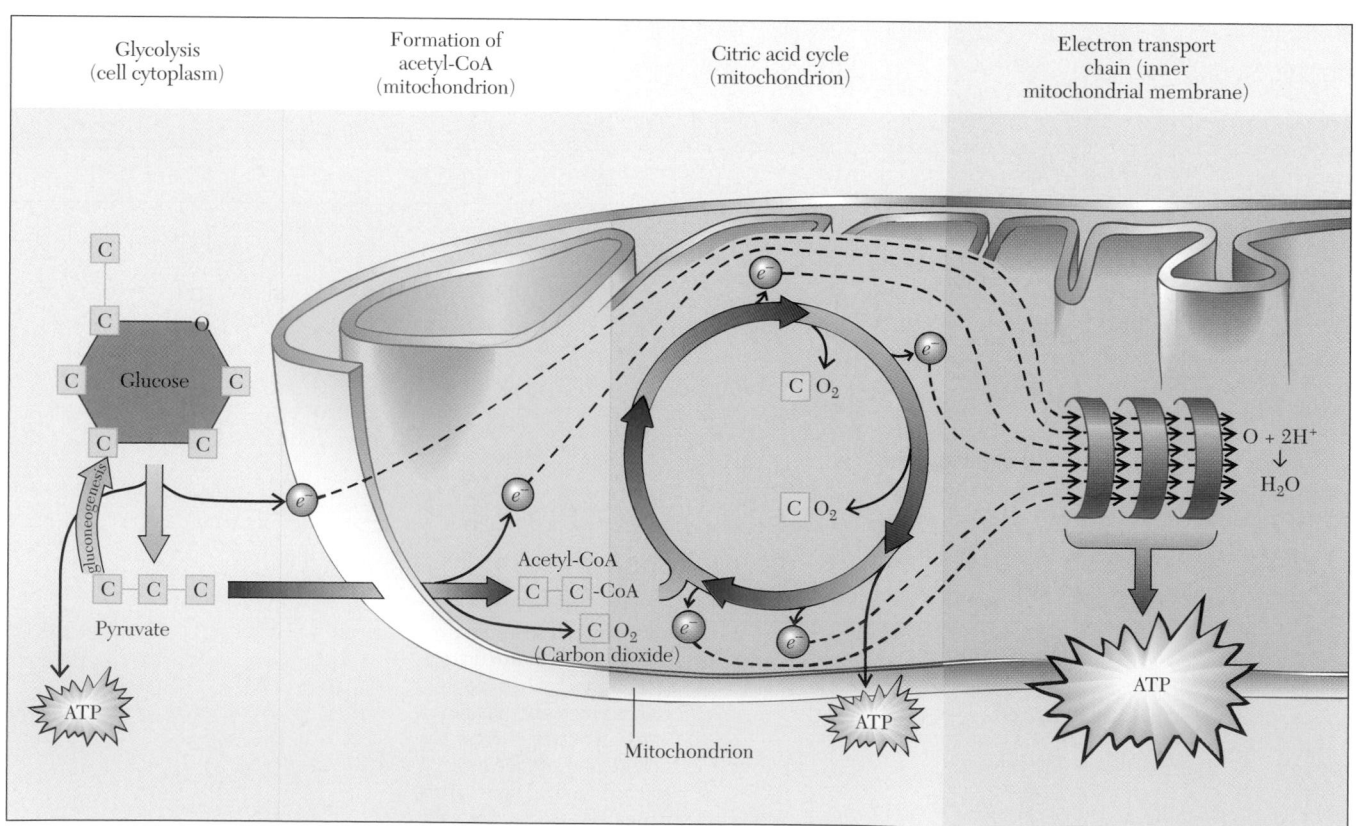

Figure 4.13

An overview of glucose metabolism. In the cytoplasm, glycolysis breaks glucose into two 3-carbon pyruvate molecules that enter the mitochondria, where they are converted into acetyl-CoA, which enters the citric acid cycle. High-energy electrons are released and transferred to the electron transport chain, where their energy is trapped to produce ATP.

the mitochondria. These molecules accept the electrons from the shuttling molecules and pass them from one to another down the chain until they are finally combined with oxygen to form water. As the electrons are passed along, their energy is trapped and used to make ATP. The reactions of cellular respiration are central to all energy-producing processes in the body.

Using Protein to Make Glucose If no carbohydrate has been eaten for a few hours, the glucose level in the blood—and consequently glucose available to the cells—begins to decrease. This triggers the pancreas to secrete the hormone **glucagon** (see Figure 4.12). Glucagon signals liver cells to break down glycogen into glucose, which is released into the bloodstream. Glucagon also stimulates the synthesis of new glucose molecules, using a pathway called **gluconeogenesis** (meaning production of new glucose). Gluconeogenesis occurs in liver and kidney cells and requires energy in the form of ATP. This pathway makes glucose from 3-carbon molecules. Three-carbon molecules come primarily from amino acids. Fatty acids cannot be used to make glucose because the reactions that break them down produce 2-carbon molecules (acetyl-CoA). Newly synthesized glucose is released into the blood to prevent blood glucose from dropping below the normal range. Gluconeogenesis can also be stimulated by the hormone epinephrine, also known as adrenaline. This hormone enables the body to respond to emergencies. For example, epinephrine is released in response to dangerous or stressful situations. It causes a rapid release of glucose into the blood to supply the energy needed for action.

Gluconeogenesis is essential for meeting the body's immediate need for glucose, particularly when carbohydrate intake is very low, but it uses protein that could be used for other essential functions such as growth and maintenance of muscle tissue. When carbohydrate is adequate in the diet, protein is not needed to synthesize glucose. Therefore, carbohydrate is said to spare protein.

Carbohydrate Is Needed to Break Down Fat To completely metabolize fat, a small amount of carbohydrate must be available. This is because fatty acids are broken into molecules of acetyl-CoA. Acetyl-CoA can be used to produce energy via the citric acid cycle only if it can combine with a 4-carbon oxaloacetate molecule derived from carbohydrate metabolism. When carbohydrate is in short supply, oxaloacetate is limited and acetyl-CoA cannot be metabolized to carbon dioxide and water. Instead, the liver converts it into compounds known as **ketones** or **ketone bodies** (Figure 4.14). The liver releases ketones into the blood. Ketones can be used for energy by tissues, such as those in the heart, muscle, and kidney. Ketone production is a normal re-

Glucagon A hormone made in the pancreas that stimulates the breakdown of liver glycogen and the synthesis of glucose to increase blood sugar.

Gluconeogenesis The synthesis of glucose from simple noncarbohydrate molecules. Amino acids from protein are the primary source of carbons for glucose synthesis.

Ketones or **ketone bodies** Molecules formed in the liver when there is not sufficient carbohydrate to completely metabolize the acetyl-CoA produced from fat breakdown.

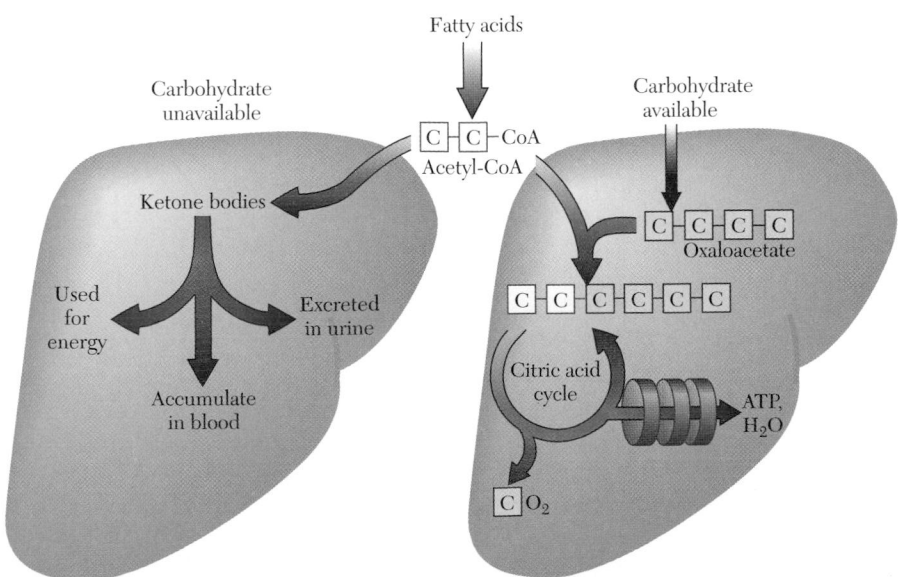

Figure 4.14
The availability of carbohydrate determines how fatty acids are metabolized. If carbohydrate is available, acetyl-CoA can combine with oxaloacetate and enter the citric acid cycle as is shown on the right side of this figure. If carbohydrate is in short supply (as shown on the left), oxaloacetate will be limited. Acetyl-CoA from fatty acid breakdown will therefore not be able to enter the citric acid cycle. Instead, the liver uses it to make ketone bodies.

sponse to starvation or a very low carbohydrate diet. Even the brain, which requires glucose, can adapt to obtain a portion of its energy from ketones. Excess ketones are excreted by the kidney in urine. However, if fluid intake is too low to produce enough urine to excrete ketones or if ketone production is high, ketones can build up in the blood, causing **ketosis**. Mild ketosis, which occurs with moderate kcalorie restriction such as that during a weight-loss diet, produces symptoms including headache, dry mouth, foul-smelling breath, and, in some cases, a reduction in appetite (see *Critical Thinking*: Losing Weight on a Low-Carbohydrate Diet). High ketone levels, such as might occur with untreated diabetes (discussion follows), increase the acidity of the blood and can result in coma and death.

Abnormal Glucose Regulation

Blood glucose levels are normally tightly controlled by insulin, glucagon, and other hormones. Abnormal blood glucose levels can result from either abnormal levels of these hormones or abnormal responses to them. When glucose homeostasis is not maintained and levels rise above the normal range, as occurs in diabetes, or drop below the normal range, as occurs in hypoglycemia, overall health can be affected.

Diabetes **Diabetes mellitus** is a major public health problem in the United States today, accounting for about $98 billion in direct medical costs and indirect costs due to disability, lost work, and premature death.[5] This disease is characterized by high blood glucose levels due to either a lack of insulin or an unresponsiveness of body cells to insulin (Figure 4.15). The elevated glucose causes damage to the large blood vessels, leading to an increased risk of heart disease and stroke. It also causes changes in small blood vessels and nerves leading to kidney failure, blindness, nerve dysfunction, and amputations. In the United States diabetes is the leading cause of

Ketosis High levels of ketones in the blood

Diabetes mellitus A disease caused by either insufficient insulin production or decreased sensitivity of cells to insulin. It results in elevated blood glucose levels.

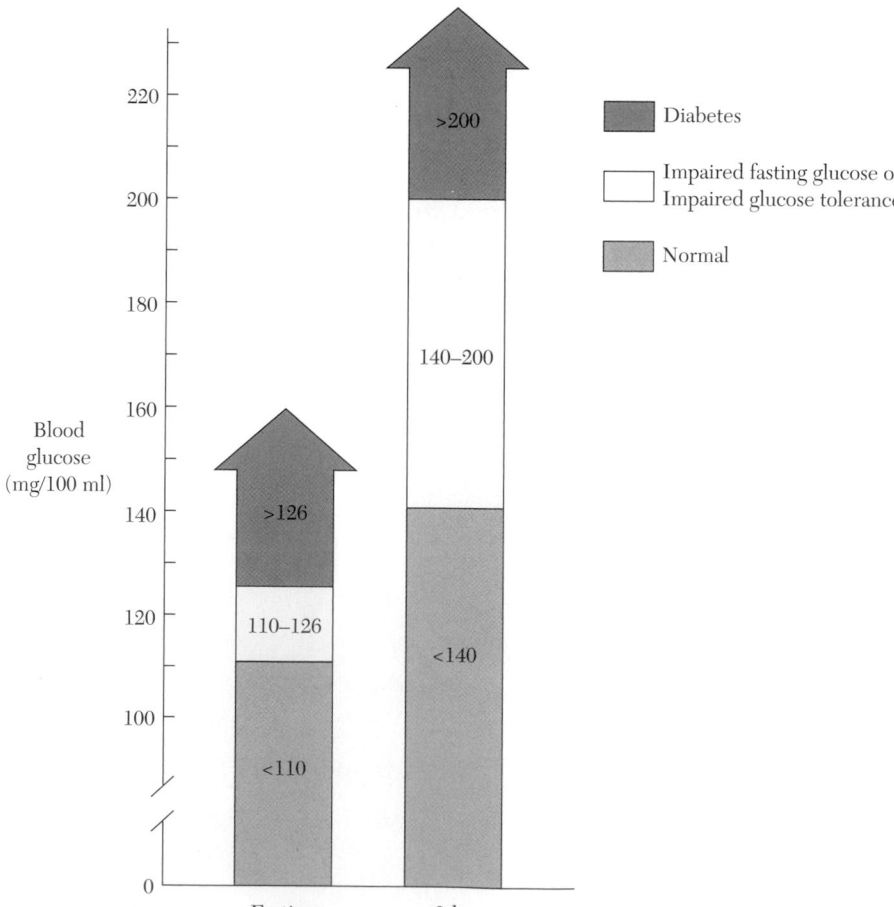

Figure 4.15

Blood glucose levels are used to diagnose diabetes. After an 8-hour fast, normal blood glucose is less than 110 mg/100 ml. Impaired fasting glucose is defined as a fasting blood glucose between 110 and 126 mg/100 ml, and diabetes is defined as a fasting blood glucose greater than 126 mg/100 ml. Blood glucose measured two hours after consuming 75 g of glucose is normally less than 140 mg/100 ml. Impaired glucose tolerance is defined as a blood glucose level between 140 and 200 mg/100 ml two hours after a glucose load and diabetes is defined as a blood glucose greater than 200 mg/100 ml two hours after a glucose load. (*American Diabetes Association at* www. diabetes.org/ diabetescare/supplement/98/s2.htm)

blindness in adults and accounts for 40% of all new cases of kidney failure and over half of all lower-limb amputations.[5]

To reduce disability and death associated with diabetes and its complications, the National Institutes of Health and the Centers for Disease Control and Prevention have established the National Diabetes Education Program. This program is designed to increase public awareness of the seriousness of diabetes, promote better management among individuals with diabetes, and improve the quality of and access to health care. There are three types of diabetes: type 1, type 2, and gestational diabetes, which occurs during pregnancy.

Type 1 Diabetes **Type 1 diabetes** is usually diagnosed before the age of 30. It accounts for only 5 to 10% of diagnosed cases.[5] What triggers the disease is unknown, but it is believed to be an **autoimmune disease** in which the immune system destroys the insulin-secreting cells of the pancreas. Because these cells have been damaged or destroyed, insulin production is reduced or absent.

Type 2 Diabetes **Type 2 diabetes** is the more common form of diabetes. It affects almost 16 million adults in the United States, and as many as two-thirds of these cases are undiagnosed.[5] The incidence is higher among minority groups, particularly African Americans, Hispanic Americans, and Native Americans.[5] Type 2 diabetes is believed to be due to a combination of genetic and lifestyle factors. Risk is increased in individuals who are overweight, in those who have a body type with more fat in the abdominal region, and in those with a family history of diabetes. This form of diabetes usually appears in persons over the age of 40, but lifestyle and dietary factors in the United States such as inactivity and excess body weight have contributed to an increasing incidence among younger individuals. In type 2 diabetes, insulin secretion may be low, normal, or even elevated, but blood glucose levels are high because body cells are insensitive to the effects of insulin. Large amounts of insulin are therefore required to allow cells to take up enough glucose to meet their energy needs.

Gestational Diabetes A third form of diabetes, called gestational diabetes, sometimes occurs in women during pregnancy. This form of diabetes may be caused by the hormonal changes that occur during pregnancy. The high levels of glucose in the mother's blood increase the risk of complications for the unborn child (see Chapter 14). Gestational diabetes usually disappears once the pregnancy is complete and hormones return to nonpregnant levels. However, individuals who have had gestational diabetes have an increased risk for developing type 2 diabetes in the future.[5]

Diabetes Symptoms The symptoms of diabetes result from the fact that without sufficient insulin, glucose cannot be used normally. Cells that require insulin to take up glucose are starved for glucose. And cells that can use glucose without insulin are exposed to damaging high levels of glucose.

The immediate symptoms of diabetes may include excessive thirst, frequent urination, blurred vision, and weight loss. Excessive thirst and frequent urination occur because blood glucose levels rise so high that the kidneys excrete glucose, drawing fluid with it and increasing the volume of urine. Blurred vision occurs when excess glucose enters the lens of the eye, causing it to swell. Weight loss and impaired growth in children occur because glucose cannot be used for energy, so the body responds as it does in starvation, breaking down fat and protein to supply fuel. With limited carbohydrate for fatty acid metabolism, ketones are formed and released into the blood. Some ketones are used as fuel by muscle and adipose tissue, but in type 1 diabetes, they are produced more rapidly than they can be used and thus accumulate in the blood. This elevation of ketones causes an increase in the acidity of the blood called **ketoacidosis**. In type 2 diabetes, ketoacidosis usually does not develop because there is enough insulin to allow some glucose to be used. Consequently, fewer ketones are produced.

Type 1 diabetes A form of diabetes that is caused by the autoimmune destruction of insulin-producing cells in the pancreas, usually leading to absolute insulin deficiency; previously known as insulin-dependent diabetes mellitus or juvenile-onset diabetes.

Autoimmune disease A disease that results from immune system reactions that destroy normal body cells.

Type 2 diabetes A form of diabetes that is characterized by insulin resistance and usually relative (rather than absolute) insulin deficiency; previously known as noninsulin-dependent diabetes mellitus or adult-onset diabetes.

Ketoacidosis Levels of ketones in the blood that are high enough to cause an increase in the acidity of the blood.

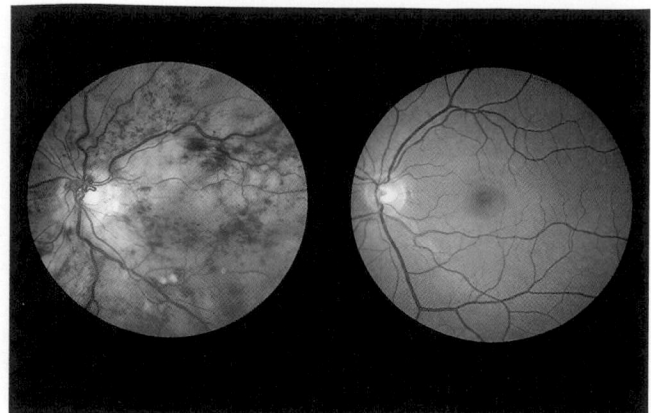

Figure 4.16
(*left*) Damaged blood vessels in the retina caused by diabetes. (*right*) Normal blood vessels in the retina of the eye. (© SBHA/Stone)

The long-term complications of diabetes include damage to the kidneys, nerves, and blood vessels and an increased risk of heart disease. The tissue damage to the kidneys, nerves, and blood vessels is thought to be a result of exposure to high levels of glucose. Cells, such as kidney and nerve cells, that do not require insulin for glucose uptake, receive too much glucose when blood levels are elevated. High levels of glucose can affect the function of peripheral nerves, and glucose can bind to proteins and alter cell function, contributing to blood vessel damage and abnormalities in blood cell function (Figure 4.16). Cardiovascular disease is a major complication and the leading cause of premature death among people with diabetes.[6]

Diabetes Treatment The goal in treating diabetes is to maintain blood glucose within the normal range to prevent tissue damage. This involves diet, exercise, and, in many cases, drug therapy. Dietary intake should be modified, based on either the Exchange Lists or a system of carbohydrate counting, to control the amount of carbohydrate consumed at any given time.[7] Recommendations consider total carbohydrate consumption—whether sucrose, fructose (which causes a smaller rise in blood glucose than sucrose), or starch. Carbohydrate consumption must be coordinated with medication and exercise schedules so that glucose and insulin are available in the proper proportions at the same time to maintain normal blood glucose levels. The diet must be adequate in energy and micronutrients, and protein should provide 10 to 20% of energy. To help delay atherosclerosis, the diet should meet the recommendations of no more than 30% of energy from fat, with 10% from saturated fat. Overweight individuals may need to restrict energy intake to promote weight loss, which can be beneficial for maintaining blood glucose levels in the normal range.[7]

Exercise is an important component of diabetes management because exercise increases the sensitivity of body cells to insulin. Because exercise can reduce blood glucose levels, individuals with diabetes are encouraged to maintain regular exercise patterns. A change in the amount of exercise an individual participates in may change the amount of insulin required.

Drug treatments include insulin injections and oral medications to lower blood glucose. In Type 1 diabetes, insulin production is low or absent, so insulin must be provided. Insulin must be injected because it is a protein that would be broken down in the gastrointestinal tract if taken orally. In type 2 diabetes, blood glucose can sometimes be normalized with diet and exercise, but when lifestyle treatments fail, medications that increase pancreatic insulin production, decrease glucose production by the liver, enhance insulin action, or slow carbohydrate digestion may be prescribed. In some cases of type 2 diabetes, injected insulin is needed to achieve normal blood glucose levels.

Blood glucose levels should be monitored frequently to assure that treatment is keeping glucose levels within the normal range. Adherence to this type of treatment regimen can reduce the incidence of elevated blood glucose levels and the complications it causes.

Hypoglycemia **Hypoglycemia** is low blood glucose that causes symptoms including irritability, nervousness, sweating, shakiness, anxiety, rapid heartbeat, headache, hunger, weakness, and sometimes seizure and coma. It can occur in diabetes as a result of over-medication. In individuals without diabetes, hypoglycemia can result from abnormalities in the production of or response to insulin or other hormones involved in blood sugar regulation.

There are two forms of hypoglycemia. Reactive hypoglycemia occurs in response to the consumption of high-carbohydrate foods. The rise in blood glucose from the carbohydrate stimulates insulin release. However, too much insulin is secreted, resulting in a rapid fall in blood glucose to an abnormally low level. The treatment for reactive hypoglycemia is a diet that prevents rapid changes in blood glucose. Small, frequent meals low in simple carbohydrates and high in protein and fiber are recommended. A second form of hypoglycemia, fasting hypoglycemia, is not related to food intake. In this disorder, abnormal insulin secretion results in episodes of low blood glucose levels. This condition is often caused by pancreatic tumors.

Hypoglycemia A low blood glucose level, usually below 40 to 50 mg of glucose per 100 ml of blood.

CRITICAL THINKING

Losing Weight on a Low-Carbohydrate Diet

John weighs about 30 pounds more than he wants to, so he decides to try a low-carbohydrate weight-loss diet. The diet allows an unlimited amount of beef, chicken, fish, and eggs as well as limited amounts of cheese and vegetables; milk, fruit, breads, grains, and cereals are not allowed. John is overjoyed with his initial rapid weight loss, but after about a week his weight loss slows and he begins to feel tired and light-headed. He is having frequent headaches and notices a funny smell on his breath.

Nutritional assessment

A nutritional assessment suggests that John needs about 2200 kcalories a day to maintain his weight. His weight-loss diet provides about 1000 kcalories from 25 grams of carbohydrate, 125 grams of protein, and 44 grams of fat per day. He consumes about 3 cups of fluid daily.

Which groups of the Food Guide Pyramid are likely to be low in John's diet?
▼

Answer:

How are John's symptoms related to his diet?
▼

John's diet is very low in energy and carbohydrate. The low-energy intake causes John to use stored fat to meet his energy needs. Because his diet does not contain enough carbohydrate to allow fat to be metabolized completely, ketones are produced and begin to accumulate in his blood. Some of the ketones are used by cells for energy; some are excreted in the urine. However, since John is not consuming much fluid, the rate of ketone production exceeds the ability of his kidneys to excrete them, and ketone levels in his blood increase. High blood ketone levels probably are causing the headaches and light-headedness he is experiencing. Some blood ketones are lost through the lungs, giving him funny-smelling breath.

Why can ketosis develop in type 1 diabetes even when plenty of carbohydrate is consumed?

▼

Answer:

• CARBOHYDRATES AND HEALTH

The consumption of carbohydrates has been blamed for a host of chronic health problems, from dental caries and hyperactivity to obesity and heart disease. Meanwhile, guidelines for a healthy diet are recommending that Americans base their diet on carbohydrate-rich foods in order to reduce their disease risk. This incongruity relates to the health effects of different forms of dietary carbohydrates: A dietary pattern that is high in unrefined carbohydrates, such as whole grains, fruits, and vegetables, has been associated with a lower incidence of a variety of chronic diseases, whereas diets high in refined carbohydrates, such as added sugars and white flour, may contribute to chronic disease risk.[8]

Dental Caries

Dental caries The decay and deterioration of teeth caused by acid produced when bacteria on the teeth metabolize carbohydrate.

The most significant health problem associated with a diet high in simple carbohydrate intake is **dental caries**, or tooth cavities. Dental caries are formed when bacteria that live in the mouth metabolize sugar from the diet and produce acid. The acid can then dissolve the enamel and underlying structure of the teeth. Simple carbohydrate, particularly sucrose, is the most rapidly utilized food source for these microbes; however, any carbohydrate-containing foods that stick to the teeth can also cause cavities. The length of time that carbohydrate is in contact with the teeth determines the likelihood that a cavity will develop. Certain foods, such as sticky candies, cereals, crackers, and cookies, tend to remain on the teeth longer, providing a continuous supply of nutrients to decay-causing bacteria. Other foods, such as chocolate, ice cream, and bananas, are rapidly washed away from the teeth. Frequent snacking also increases contact time by providing a continuous food supply for the bacteria. Limiting sugar intake can help prevent dental caries, but since starch is also eventually metabolized into acid, proper dental hygiene is important even if the diet is low in sugar.[9]

Hyperactivity

The consumption of sugary foods has also been suggested as a cause of hyperactivity in children (see Chapter 15). The increase in blood glucose after a meal high in simple carbohydrates is hypothesized to provide the energy for the excessive activity of a hyperactive child. However, research on sugar intake and behavior has failed to support the hypothesis that sugar contributes to behavioral changes.[10] Hyperactive behavior that is observed after sugar consumption is likely the result of other circumstances. For example, the excitement of a birthday party rather than the cake is more likely the cause of hyperactive behavior. Hyperactivity might also be caused by lack of sleep, overstimulation, caffeine consumption, the desire for more attention, or lack of physical activity.

Body Weight

Carbohydrates are not "fattening." They provide 4 kcalories per gram compared with 9 kcalories per gram provided by fat. This is not to say that carbohydrate consumed in excess of energy needs will not add pounds. Any energy source consumed in excess of requirements can cause weight gain. But carbohydrate is no more fattening than any other energy source. In fact, excess carbohydrate in the diet is less efficient at producing body fat than excess fat in the diet (see Chapter 7). Unrefined carbohydrates might even help reduce energy intake because the fiber in these foods adds bulk to the gastrointestinal tract and causes you to feel full after consuming less. The fats that we often add to our high-carbohydrate foods are what increases the kcalorie tally. A medium baked potato provides about 110 kcalories, but the 2 tablespoons of sour cream you add brings the total to 175 kcalories (Figure 4.17). A plate of plain pasta has about 200 kcalories, but with a high-fat sauce, the kcalories rise to 300; add sausage and the meal is now 450 kcalories.

There is some evidence that an abnormal craving for carbohydrate-rich foods is a component of a variety of disorders including obesity, premenstrual syndrome, bulimia, depression, and seasonal affective disorder.[11,12] One theory proposed to explain carbohydrate craving is that these individuals have an abnormality in the regulation of brain levels of the **neurotransmitter** serotonin. This abnormality causes them to seek carbohydrate like a drug to increase serotonin levels, which improves their mood.

Heart Disease

There is evidence that a high sugar intake can adversely affect blood lipid levels and thereby increase the risk of heart disease.[1] However, diets high in whole grains and fiber from cereals have been found to reduce the risk of heart disease.[13,14] Fiber-rich foods provide micronutrients and phytochemicals—some of which may be protective against heart disease. A diet high in fiber-rich foods may also reduce blood cholesterol levels (see Chapter 5). Studies indicate that soluble fibers from foods such as legumes, oats, guar gum, pectin, flax seed, and psyllium (a grain used in bulk-forming laxatives such as Metamucil) are more effective at lowering blood cholesterol levels than insoluble fibers such as wheat bran or cellulose.[15] This may be due to the ability of soluble fibers to bind cholesterol and **bile acids**, which are made from cholesterol, in the digestive tract. Normally, bile acids secreted into the GI tract are absorbed and reused. When bound to fiber, cholesterol and bile acids are excreted in the feces rather than being absorbed. The liver must then use cholesterol from the blood to synthesize new bile acids. This provides a mechanism for eliminating cholesterol from the body and reducing blood cholesterol levels (Figure 4.18). Soluble fiber may also reduce blood cholesterol by inhibiting cholesterol synthesis in the liver or by increasing the removal of cholesterol from the blood.[1,16] The FDA permits a health claim on food products containing either soluble fiber from psyllium seed husk or beta-glucan (found in whole oats), which states that these soluble fibers may reduce the risk of coronary heart disease.

Diabetes

A dietary pattern that is high in refined starches and added sugars causes a greater glycemic response and therefore increases the amount of insulin needed to maintain normal blood glucose levels. Evidence is emerging that long-term consumption of this dietary pattern may increase the risk of developing type 2 diabetes.[17,18] Epidemiological studies have shown that diabetes is rare in populations consuming a diet high in unrefined grains.[19] A correlation between high-fiber intake and a lower prevalence of diabetes has also been identified among individuals within a population.[18] So although a diet high in simple carbohydrates and refined starches does not cause diabetes, it does increase the demand for insulin required to maintain normal glucose levels and may increase the risk of developing diabetes.

Chronic Bowel Disorders

A diet high in fiber can relieve or prevent some chronic bowel disorders. Fiber adds bulk and absorbs water, making the feces larger and softer and reducing the amount of pressure needed for defecation. This helps to reduce the incidence of constipation and

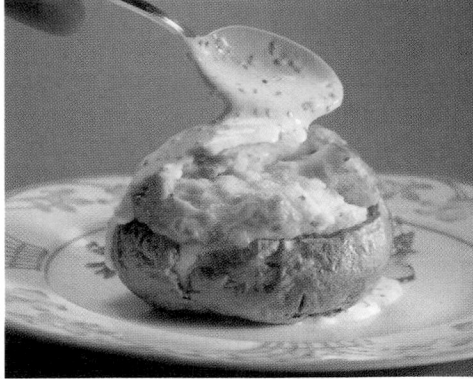

Figure 4.17
High-carbohydrate foods like baked potatoes are not high in kcalories, but the toppings used on them often are. (Michael Boys/Corbis)

Neurotransmitter A chemical substance produced by a nerve cell that can stimulate or inhibit another cell.

Bile acids Emulsifiers present in bile that are synthesized by the liver from cholesterol.

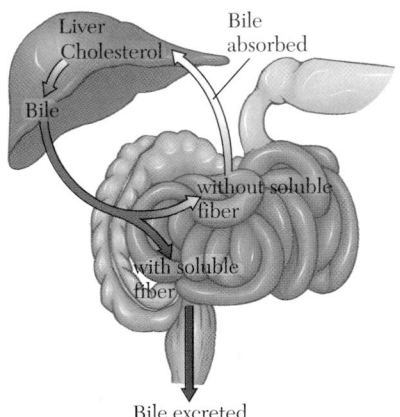

Figure 4.18
When the diet is low in soluble fiber, bile, which contains cholesterol and bile acids made from cholesterol, is absorbed and returned to the liver. When soluble fiber is present, it binds cholesterol and bile acids so they are excreted rather than absorbed.

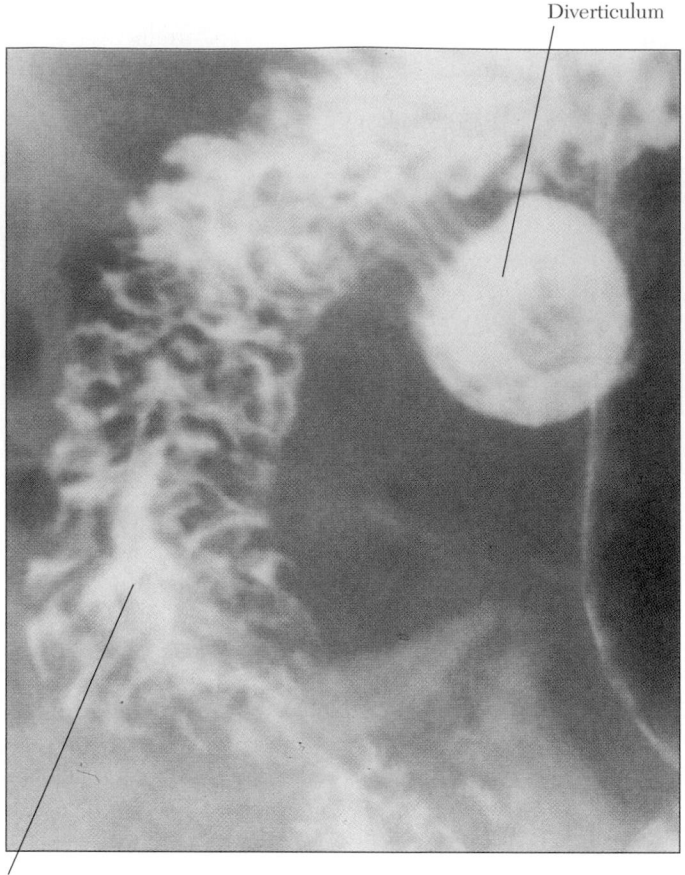

Diverticulum

Large intestine

Figure 4.19
Diverticulum in the colon. (L. V. Bergman/Project Masters)

Hemorrhoids Swollen veins in the anal or rectal area.

Diverticula Sacs or pouches that protrude from the wall of the large intestine in the disease diverticulosis. When these become inflamed, the condition is called diverticulitis.

hemorrhoids, the swelling of veins in the rectal or anal area. Reducing the pressure in the lumen of the colon can also reduce the possibility of developing diverticulosis, a condition in which the intestinal wall forms outpouches called **diverticula** (Figure 4.19). Fecal matter may occasionally accumulate in these outpouchings, causing irritation, pain, inflammation, and infection. This condition is known as diverticulitis. Treatment of diverticulitis usually includes antibiotics to reduce bacterial growth and a temporary decrease in fiber intake to prevent irritation of the inflamed tissues. Once the inflammation is resolved, however, a high-fiber intake is recommended to increase fecal bulk, decrease transit time, ease stool elimination, and reduce future attacks of diverticulitis.

Colon Cancer

In order to understand the role of fiber in cancer prevention or development, it is helpful to understand how cancer develops and spreads.

What Is Cancer? Cancer is a disease that affects the way cells behave. Different cancers originate in different parts of the body and have different causes and effects. However, all cancer cells share two traits that distinguish them from other body cells. First, they reproduce without restraint. Normal body cells reproduce only to replace lost cells or to accommodate normal growth, but cancer cells divide continuously, forming enlarged cell masses known as tumors. Second, they invade and colonize areas reserved for other cells. A normal mucosal cell in the colon will stay in the colon, but a cancerous cell could travel to the liver, bone, or other tissue and begin dividing in the new location. Therefore, cancer cells eventually crowd out the normal cells, robbing them of nourishment and preventing them from functioning properly.

Mutations Changes in DNA caused by chemical or physical agents.

Cells become cancerous as a result of **mutations** in their genetic material. The type of cancer depends on the type of cell that is originally affected—for example, lung, breast, or colon—and on how the genetic material is altered by the mutations. Most mutations are thought to be caused by environmental factors, such as diet, tobacco use, or air pollution. In the case of the colon, mutations may be caused by substances consumed in the diet or produced in the gastrointestinal tract that come in contact with mucosal cells. Any substance that causes a cell to have cancerous potential is called a **tumor initiator**. Tumor initiators sow the seeds of cancer but alone do not create cancerous cells. For the affected cell to begin growing and dividing as a cancer cell, it must be exposed to a **tumor promoter**. Although tumor promoters allow mutated cells to begin dividing, they do not cause mutations themselves.

Tumor initiator A substance that causes mutations and therefore may predispose a cell to becoming cancerous.

Tumor promoter A substance that stimulates a mutated cell to begin dividing.

The Role of Fiber Epidemiological studies have shown that the incidence of colon cancer is lower in populations consuming diets high in fiber.[4] Intervention trials have not been able to replicate these patterns by studying the effects of fiber supplements or of defined high-fiber, high-fruit and vegetable diets studied over the short term.[20,21] Nonetheless, the role of fiber in preventing the development of colon cancer may be related to its ability to decrease contact between the mucosal cells of the large intestine and the fecal contents, which may contain tumor initiators or tumor promoters. Fiber increases fecal bulk, dilutes the colon contents, and speeds transit, thereby decreasing contact time between the mucosal cells and potentially cancer-causing substances. The presence of fiber in the colon also affects the intestinal microflora and the by-products of microbial metabolism, such as fatty acids, that accumulate there. These by-products may directly affect colon cells or may cause changes in the environment of the colon that can affect the development of colon cancer. Some of the protective effect may also be due to the antioxidant vitamins and phytochemicals present in fiber-rich plant foods.

Problems with Excessive Fiber Intake

Too much fiber or a rapid increase in the fiber content of the diet can have some adverse effects. However, when consumed as part of a balanced diet, the deleterious effects are not significant in healthy individuals. Therefore, no UL has been set.[1]

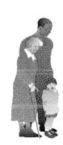

A high-fiber diet increases the volume of food needed to meet energy requirements. A person who has a small stomach capacity and consumes a diet that is very high in fiber may satisfy hunger before nutrient requirements are met. Generally, this is a problem only when the diet is low in micronutrients or when high-fiber diets are consumed by young children whose small stomachs limit the amount of food they can eat.

A high-fiber diet may decrease nutrient absorption for two reasons. First, the increased volume of intestinal contents that occurs with a high-fiber diet may prevent enzymes from coming in contact with food. If a food cannot be broken down, nutrients may not be absorbed. Second, fiber may bind some micronutrients, preventing their absorption. For instance, wheat bran fiber binds the minerals zinc, calcium, magnesium, and iron, reducing their absorption. When mineral intake meets recommendations, a reasonable intake of high-fiber foods does not compromise mineral status.

A sudden increase in the fiber content of the diet can cause abdominal discomfort, gas, and diarrhea due to the bacterial breakdown of fiber. If fluid intake is too low, fiber can also cause constipation. The more fiber there is in the diet, the more water is needed to keep the stool soft. When too little fluid is consumed, the stool becomes hard and difficult to eliminate. In severe cases when fiber intake is excessive and fluid intake is low, intestinal blockage can occur.[22] To avoid these problems, the fiber and fluid content of the diet should be increased gradually.

• CARBOHYDRATE: ONE PART OF THE TOTAL DIET

The amount and source of carbohydrate in the diet affect the healthiness of the diet as a whole. Diets that are high in complex carbohydrates from whole grains, legumes, and vegetables and in simple carbohydrates from whole foods such as fresh fruit and lowfat dairy products are high in fiber, micronutrients, and phytochemicals, and low in fat.

Recommendations for Carbohydrate Intake

The RDA for carbohydrates for adults and children has been set at 130 grams per day based on the average minimum amount of glucose used by the brain.[1] In a diet that meets energy needs, this amount will provide adequate glucose and prevent ketosis. However, carbohydrate intake is typically higher than this in order to meet energy needs and avoid excessive intakes of fat and protein. The acceptable range of carbohydrate intake for a healthy diet has been set at 45 to 65% of energy. Most of this should be from whole, unrefined sources with limited amounts of added sugar. The DRIs recommend that added sugar intake not exceed 25% of energy. During pregnancy and lactation the RDA is higher and for infants an AI has been established (see inside cover). For fiber, an AI has been set at 38 and 25 grams per day for young adult men and women, respectively, based on the amount of fiber needed to reduce heart disease risk.[1] Specific AIs for fiber have been set for different lifestage groups. No UL has been established for carbohydrate, added sugars, or fiber.

The Dietary Guidelines, Healthy People 2010, and the Food Guide Pyramid also recommend an increase in whole grains, vegetables, and fruits, and a reduction in added sugars from bakery products, candy, and soft drinks. The Food Guide Pyramid recommendations on added sugar are more restrictive, suggesting a limit of 6 to 18 teaspoons per day depending on energy intake, or about 6 to 10% of kcalories[23] (Figure 4.20; see *Critical Thinking*: Building a Healthy Base).

The typical North American diet meets some but not all of these recommendations. We consume about 50% of energy from carbohydrate but most of this comes from refined sources. Our average fiber intake is only 15 grams per day, which is well below the AI.

Determining Your Carbohydrate Intake

How does your diet compare to the recommendation of 45 to 65% carbohydrate? Table 4.1 illustrates how to calculate carbohydrate intake as a percent of energy. This same calculation can be used to determine the percent of energy as carbohydrate in individual foods. To calculate the percent of energy as carbohydrate, you need to know the amount of carbohydrate in a food or in the diet. This can be estimated from the Exchange Lists or determined using values from food labels or food composition tables (see Appendix A).

Carbohydrate Exchange Lists The Exchange Lists can be used to give a quick estimate of the total amount of carbohydrate in a food or in the diet (Table 4.2). One serving of bread or fruit provides 15 grams of carbohydrate, 1 milk serving provides 12 grams, and 1 vegetable serving provides about 5 grams. Meats and fats provide no carbohydrate. The Exchange Lists cannot be used for calculating fiber intake, but Table 4.3 offers an exchange system for estimating fiber in foods.

Carbohydrates on Food Labels Food labels list the grams of total carbohydrate, fiber, and sugars. Total carbohydrate and fiber are also listed as a percent of the Daily Value. The Daily Value for total carbohydrate is calculated as 60% of the energy. For a 2000-kcalorie diet, this represents 300 grams of carbohydrate ([2000 kcal × 0.6]/4 kcal/g of carbohydrate = 300 g). The Daily Value for fiber is 25 grams in a 2000-kcalorie diet. No Daily Value has been established for sugars, but labels can help identify products that are high in sugars. The number of grams of sugars listed in the Nutrition Facts includes all monosaccharides and disaccharides but does not distinguish between added and naturally occurring sugars. For example, the fructose found naturally in frozen strawberries, and that added as high-fructose corn syrup in soft drinks, are both listed as sugars. The list of ingredients can provide information

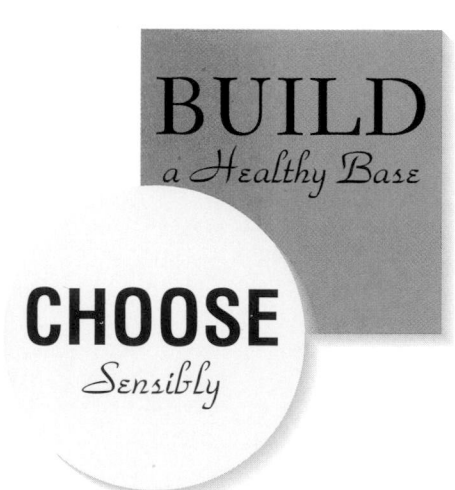

BUILD
a Healthy Base

CHOOSE
Sensibly

- Let the Pyramid guide your food choices.
- Choose a variety of grains daily, especially whole grains.
- Choose a variety of fruits and vegetables daily.
  Choose beverages and foods to moderate your intake of sugars.

Figure 4.20
The Dietary Guidelines for Americans makes recommendations about the type and amount of carbohydrate in the diet. (*USDA, DHHS, 2000*)

Table 4.1   *Calculating Percent Energy from Carbohydrate*

Determine
- The total energy (kcalorie) intake for the day
- The grams of carbohydrate in the day's diet

Calculate Energy from Carbohydrate
- Carbohydrate provides 4 kcalories per g
- Multiply grams of carbohydrate by 4 kcalories per g

$$\text{Kcalories from carbohydrate} = \text{grams carbohydrate} \times 4 \text{ kcalories/gram carbohydrate}$$

Calculate % Energy from Carbohydrate
- Divide energy from carbohydrate by total energy and multiply by 100 to express as a percent

$$\text{Percent of energy from carbohydrate} = \frac{\text{kcalories from carbohydrate}}{\text{Total kcalories}} \times 100$$

For example:

A diet contains 2500 kcalories and 350 g of carbohydrate

$$350 \text{ g of carbohydrate} \times 4 \text{ kcal/g} = 1400 \text{ kcal of carbohydrate}$$

$$\frac{1400 \text{ kcal of carbohydrate}}{2500 \text{ kcal}} \times 100 = 56\% \text{ of energy (kcal) from carbohydrate}$$

about the types of sweeteners added to foods. All added sugars are listed here and the only type of sweetener that can be called "sugar" is sucrose. Since sucrose may represent only one of many added sweeteners, consumers need to increase their carbohydrate vocabulary to recognize all the sweeteners on the label. High-fructose corn syrup, invert sugar, dextrose, lactose, honey, and mannitol are just a few (see *Off the Shelf*: Are "Natural" Sugars Better?). Nutrient claims also provide some information about whether a food contains added refined sugar. The presence of a claim such as "no added sugar" or "without added sugar" indicates that no sugars have been added in processing (Table 4.4).

Table 4.2   *Using Exchange Lists to Calculate the Carbohydrate Content of a Diet*

Exchange Groups/Lists	Serving Size	Carbohydrates (g)
Carbohydrate Group		
Starch	½ cup rice, cereal, potatoes; 1 slice bread	15
Fruit	1 small apple, peach, pear; ½ banana; ½ cup canned fruit (in juice)	15
Milk	1 cup milk or yogurt	
Nonfat		12
Lowfat		12
Reduced fat		12
Whole		12
Other carbohydrates	Serving sizes vary	15
Vegetables	½ cup cooked vegetables, 1 cup raw	5
Meat/Meat Substitute Group	1 oz meat or cheese	
Very lean		0
Lean		0
Medium-fat		0
High-fat		0
Fat Group	1 tsp butter, margarine, or oil; 1 Tbsp salad dressing	0

Table 4.3 *Fiber Content of Food Group Selections*[1]

Food Group/Serving	High Fiber	Medium Fiber	Low Fiber
Fiber per serving	4–5 g	2 g	0.5–1 g
Bread, Cereal, Rice, & Pasta Group			
Breads (1 slice)	—	Whole wheat Rye	White bread Bagel (½) Tortilla Roll (½) English muffin (½) Graham cracker
Cereals (½ cup)	All Bran Bran Buds 100% Bran Flakes	40% Bran Shredded Wheat	Cheerios Rice Krispies
Rice and pasta (½ cup)	—	Whole-wheat pasta Brown rice	Macaroni Pasta White rice
Fruit Group			
Fruits (1 medium or ½ cup)	Berries Prunes	Apple Apricot Banana Orange Raisins	Melon Canned fruit Juices
Vegetable Group			
Vegetables (½ cup)	Peas Broccoli Spinach	Green beans Carrots Eggplant Cabbage Potatoes with skin Corn	Asparagus Cauliflower Celery Lettuce Tomatoes Zucchini Peppers Potatoes without skin Onions
Dry Bean Group			
Beans (½ cup)	Pinto, red Kidney beans Blackeyed peas	—	—

[1]Adapted from Bright-See, E., Benda, C., Vartouhi, J., et al. Development and testing of a dietary fibre exchange system. *Can. Diet. Assoc. J.* 47:199–205, 1986; and Marlett, J. A. Content and composition of dietary fiber in 117 frequently consumed foods. *J. Am. Diet. Assoc.* 92:175–186, 1992.

Table 4.4 *Sugar and Fiber Content Descriptors on Food Labels*[1]

Sugar free	Product contains no amount, or a trivial amount, of sugars (less than 0.5 g per serving). Synonyms for "free" include "without," "no," and "zero."
Reduced sugar	Nutritionally altered product contains 25% less sugar than the regular or reference product.
Less sugar	Whether altered or not, a food contains 25% less sugar than the reference food. "Fewer" may be used as a synonym for "less."
No added sugars or without added sugars	No sugar or sugar-containing ingredient is added during processing.
High fiber	Food contains 20% or more of the Daily Value for fiber per serving. Synonyms for "high" include "rich in" and "excellent source of."
Good source of fiber	Food contains 10 to 19% of the Daily Value for fiber per serving. Synonyms for "good source of" include "contains" and "provides."
More fiber	Food contains 10% or more of the Daily Value for fiber per serving than an appropriate reference food. Synonyms for "more" include "added" (or "fortified" and "enriched"), "extra," or "plus."

[1]If a food is not low in total fat, the label must state total fat in conjunction with any fiber claim such as "More Fiber."

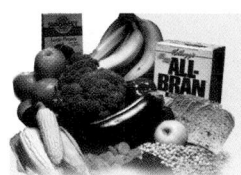

Off the Shelf

Are "Natural" Sugars Better?

Is honey healthy? Honey, blackstrap molasses, and other less-refined sugars have been promoted as healthier alternatives to table sugar since they contain some nutrients that have been processed out of pure white table sugar. Candy and baked products made with these sweeteners are marketed as more nutritious. Although these sweeteners do have more micronutrients than table sugar, the amounts are too small to add much to the diet.

Honey is derived from the nectar of flowering plants, which contains sucrose. Bees collect the nectar and convert some of the sucrose into fructose and glucose. The color, flavor, and proportions of the sugars in honey vary with the source of the nectar. Honey supplies a concentrated source of energy but only traces of vitamins and minerals, so it cannot be considered a nutrient-dense food. Since sucrose from any source is broken into glucose and fructose before it is absorbed in the small intestine, the body cannot distinguish whether the glucose and fructose it absorbs come from honey or from refined white table sugar. Honey is somewhat sweeter than sucrose, so smaller amounts

may be used for the same level of sweetness. Because honey may contain spores of the bacterium *Clostridium botulinum* (see Chapters 15 and 17), it should not be fed to infants. The benefit of honey mixed with lemon juice as a home remedy for a cough is only anecdotal.

Blackstrap molasses is a by-product of the refining of sucrose from sugar cane or sugar beets. It is a thick brown syrup that remains after the sucrose has crystallized. Refining of blackstrap molasses produces light and medium molasses. Curative properties for cancer and other disorders have been attributed to molasses, but there is no scientific support for these claims. Unlike any other concentrated nutritive sweetener, molasses does contain significant amounts of some minerals. For example, when it is made in old-fashioned iron vats with iron pipes, it is rich in iron.

Other sweeteners such as brown sugar, maple syrup, and fruit juices are also believed by some to be healthier than sucrose. In fact, most are not significantly different from sucrose. Most brown sugar is simply refined white sugar containing some molasses to color it brown. Maple syrup is formed by boiling down the sap of

maple trees. It is composed primarily of sucrose, which has been browned by the heat involved in processing. Fruit juices are also used as sweeteners. These may add small amounts of micronutrients but contribute primarily the sugar fructose to the product.

Sweeteners promoted as "natural," such as honey, molasses, brown sugar, and maple syrup, are all processed in some way, either by humans or, in the case of honey, by bees. Though these sweeteners contribute distinctive flavors to the foods to which they are added, their nutritional contribution is not significantly different from that of refined white sugar.

Foods that are high in added refined sugars provide energy but few nutrients. So, guidelines for a healthy diet recommend that refined sugars be consumed in moderation. There are some easy ways to do this—use less sugar in coffee or on cereal and reduce sweetened soft drink consumption. But finding and eliminating other sources of refined sugar in the diet isn't always easy. Consumers need to understand the information provided on food labels before they can sort out their sugar intake.

Nutritional Contributions of Various Sweeteners

	Energy (kcal)	Protein (g)	Carbohydrate (g)	Calcium (mg)	Phosphorus (mg)	Sodium (mg)	Magnesium (mg)	Potassium (mg)	Iron (mg)
Daily Value[1]	—	50	300	1000	1000	<2400	400	3500	18
Sweetener	Nutrients per Tablespoon								
Light molasses	40	0.4	10.0	25	7	2	31	138	0.6
Medium molasses	38	0.4	9.0	44	10	6	31	159	0.9
Blackstrap molasses	35	0.4	8.0	103	13	14	31	439	2.4
Honey	61	0.1	16.5	1	1	1	1	10	0.1
Brown sugar	52	0	13.4	11	5	3	9	32	0.4
White sugar	46	0	11.9	1	0	0	0	1	0

[1]Daily Value for a 2000-kcalorie diet.

Table 4.5 *Amount of Added Sugar in Common Foods*

Food	Added sugar (tsp[1])
Grains	
Bread, 1 slice	0
Doughnut, 3 inch diameter	2
Cookies, 2 medium chocolate chip	3
Frosted corn flakes, 1 oz	3
Cake, frosted, $\frac{1}{16}$ average	6
Pie, fruit, 2 crust, $\frac{1}{8}$ 8-inch pie	6
Fruit	
Fresh fruit, 1 medium	0
Fruit, canned in juice, $\frac{1}{2}$ cup	0
Fruit, canned in heavy syrup, $\frac{1}{2}$ cup	4
Milk, Yogurt. Cheese	
Milk, plain, 1 cup	0
Chocolate milk, 2%, 1 cup	3
Lowfat yogurt, plain, 1 cup	0
Lowfat yogurt, fruit, 1 cup	7
Ice cream, vanilla, $\frac{1}{2}$ cup	3
Other	
Sugar, jam, or jelly, 1 tsp	1
Syrup or honey, 1 Tbsp	3
Chocolate bar, $1\frac{1}{2}$ oz	5
Fruit sorbet, $\frac{1}{2}$ cup	3
Fruit drink, ade 12 oz	12
Cola, not diet, 12 oz can	9
Cola, not diet, 20 oz bottle	15
Cola, not diet, 32 oz fast-food portion	24

[1]1 tsp = 4 g dry weight

A Diet to Meet Recommendations: Choose More Grains, Fruits, and Vegetables

To meet the recommendations for a healthy diet, most people need to increase their fiber intake, while balancing their intake of carbohydrate, fat, and protein to stay within acceptable ranges of intake. To do this, refined carbohydrates should be replaced with complex carbohydrates from unrefined sources. For example, choosing a stir-fry meal of a few ounces of beef and plenty of vegetables on brown rice can provide the same energy but more fiber and less fat than a dinner of steak, white rice, and a small salad with dressing. To limit added sugars, foods high in added sugar should be replaced with natural sources of sugar. For example, soft drinks should be replaced with lowfat milk, and fruits should be substituted for sugary desserts (Table 4.5).

The recommendations of the Food Guide Pyramid can be used to plan a diet high in unrefined carbohydrates. A diet that follows the serving recommendations of the Pyramid will be based on plant foods with smaller proportions of animal products. Six to 11 servings should be selected from the Bread, Cereal, Rice, & Pasta Group, the base of the Pyramid. Whole grain products should be frequent choices from this group. The next level of the Pyramid contains the Vegetable Group and Fruit Group, which are also good sources of complex carbohydrates, fiber, and naturally occurring simple carbohydrates. It is recommended that 3 to 5 servings from the Vegetable Group and 2 to 4 servings from the Fruit Group be consumed each day. On the next level of the Pyramid, the Milk, Yogurt, & Cheese Group provides unrefined simple carbohydrate in the form of lactose. Many of the choices in the Meat, Poultry, Fish, Dry Beans, Eggs, & Nuts Group contain no carbohydrate. Choosing dry beans from this group will provide a protein-rich food that is also a good source of complex carbohydrates and fiber.

To emphasize moderation in the consumption of added sugar, the Food Guide Pyramid recommends that added sweeteners be used sparingly. The relative amounts of added sugar in each of the food groups are indicated by an upside-down triangle symbol (∇). The food groups that contain a higher proportion of foods with added sugar have more of these symbols. For example, the tip of the Pyramid, which includes sweets along with fats and oils, has the highest concentration of these symbols; the grain group, which includes sweetened bakery products like cakes and cookies, has a moderate concentration of symbols; and the Vegetable Group, which includes almost no foods with added sugar, has no symbols (Figure 4.21).

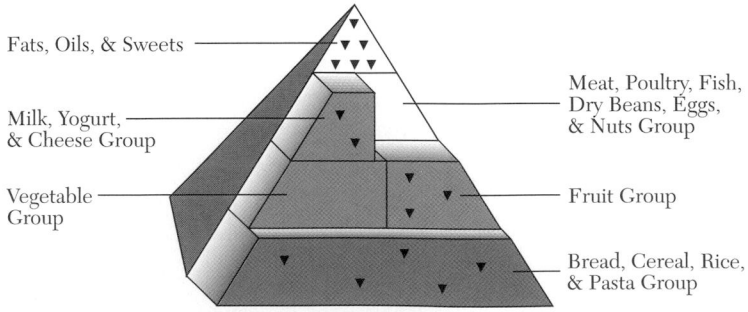

Figure 4.21

The Food Guide Pyramid groups that are sources of naturally occurring simple and complex carbohydrates are raised and colored red. The darker shades indicate groups with a greater proportion of high-carbohydrate foods. Note that the Meat, Poultry, Fish, Dry Beans, Eggs, & Nuts Group can provide complex carbohydrates if dry beans are chosen. Groups that provide good sources of fiber include the Bread, Cereal, Rice, & Pasta Group (if whole grains are chosen), the Vegetable Group, the Fruit Group, and the Meat, Poultry, Fish, Dry Beans, Eggs, & Nuts Group (if dry beans are chosen). The ∇ symbol indicates sources of added sugars.

Table 4.6 *How to Choose Carbohydrates Wisely*

1. Increase intake of whole grains, fruits, and vegetables.
2. Use whole grain products such as oatmeal, brown rice, and whole wheat bread.
3. Increase consumption of legumes such as kidney, black, and pinto beans.
4. If fresh fruits are not available, choose frozen or canned fruits without added sugar.
5. Choose packaged foods that contain 10% or more of the Daily Value for fiber.
6. When baking at home, substitute whole grain flour for one fourth to one half of the amount of flour specified in the recipe.
7. When cooking at home, use less sugar; try adding one-fourth less sugar than called for in the recipe.
8. Use less added sugar in beverages and on cereals and pancakes.
9. Eat fewer high-sugar prepared foods such as cookies and candies.
10. Read food labels to choose foods low in added sugars and high in fiber.

A diet based on the Pyramid will meet the recommendations for carbohydrate and fiber intake if care is used in choosing from the food groups. For example, switching from a breakfast of ham and eggs to one of cereal and toast will increase carbohydrate but will not add much fiber unless whole grains are chosen. Breakfast cereals all fit into the grain group, yet choosing one over another can make a big difference in sugar and fiber intake. For example, a serving of Frosted Flakes has about 120 kcalories with 1 gram of fiber and 13 grams of sugars, whereas a serving of bran flakes has about 100 kcalories but 5 grams of fiber and only 6 grams of sugars. Using fresh instead of canned fruit can also help increase fiber and decrease refined sugars. For example, half a cup of pear halves canned in heavy syrup provides 90 kcalories, 1 gram of fiber, and almost 20 grams of sugar, most of which is added in the syrup. One large fresh pear would provide 90 kcalories, 4 grams of fiber, and no refined sugar (Table 4.6). Choosing fresh fruit over juice also adds fiber. An apple provides about 80 to 90 kcalories and 2.7 grams of fiber, whereas a cup of apple juice provides the same amount of energy but almost no fiber (0.2 gram).

CRITICAL THINKING

Building a Healthy Base

Katie wants to eat a healthy diet, but she is confused about how to do this. She tries to follow the recommendations of the Food Guide Pyramid but is not sure she consumes enough high-carbohydrate foods. She records her food intake for a day and then analyzes it using a diet analysis computer program.

Diet Analysis

Katie's diet analysis indicates that she consumes about 2000 kcalories, 20% of which come from protein, 41% from fat, and 39% from carbohydrate. Her diet is higher in fat and lower in carbohydrate than recommended.

How many more grams of carbohydrate would Katie need to meet the recommendation of 45 to 65% of energy from carbohydrate?

▼

Her diet provides approximately 39% carbohydrate and 2000 kcal:

$$\frac{39 \times 2000 \text{ kcal}}{100} = 780 \text{ kcal from carbohydrate}$$

$$\frac{780 \text{ kcal from carbohydrate}}{4 \text{ kcal per gram}} = 195 \text{ grams of carbohydrate}$$

A 2000-kcalorie diet with 45% of energy from carbohydrate would provide:

$$\frac{45 \times 2000 \text{ kcal}}{100} = 900 \text{ kcal from carbohydrate}$$

$$\frac{900 \text{ kcal from carbohydrate}}{4 \text{ kcal per gram}} = 225 \text{ grams of carbohydrate}$$

Katie's diet therefore needs to provide at least 30 additional grams of carbohydrate (225 grams recommended − 195 grams consumed = 30 grams).

To increase her complex carbohydrate intake, Katie modifies her diet as shown below. She cuts down on some of her high fat choices and substitutes beans, fruits, and vegetables. The modifications decrease her fat intake and increase her carbohydrate intake to the recommended range.

Original Diet			Modified Diet	
	Carbohydrate	Fiber		Carbohydrate
Food	**(g)**	**(g)**	**Food**	**(g)**
Breakfast				
Coffee	0	0	Coffee	0
White toast (2)	30	1	White toast (2)	30
Margarine	0	0	Margarine	0
Jelly	4	0	Jelly	4
Chorizo (sausage) (2 oz)	0	0	Chorizo (sausage) (1 oz)	0
Orange juice (1 cup)	30	1	Orange juice (1 cup)	30
Lunch				
Burritos:			Burritos:	
Tortilla (2)	30	1	Tortilla (2)	30
Beef (3 oz)	0	0	Beef (3 oz)	0
Cheese (1 oz)	0	0	Beans (½ cup)	15
Milk (1 cup)	12	0	Milk (1 cup)	12
Cookies (2)	15	0.5	Cookies (2)	15
			Canned pears (1 cup)	30
Snack				
Diet soda	0	0	Diet soda	0
Pretzels (1 oz)	15	0.5	Pretzels (1 oz)	15
Dinner				
Carne asada (beef)(4 oz)	0	0	Carne asada (beef) (2 oz)	0
Potatoes (1 cup)	30	4	Potatoes (1 cup)	30
			Green beans (½ cup)	
			Salad (½ cup)	
Milk (1 cup)	12	0	Milk (1 cup)	12
Ice cream (½ cup)	15	0	Nonfat frozen yogurt (1 cup)	19
			w/ strawberries	15
Snack				
			Graham crackers (3 squares)	15
Total	193	8		282

**Are the carbohydrate-containing foods in her
modified diet from whole or refined sources?**

▼

Many of Katie's choices are refined grains. She could improve her diet by choosing whole wheat toast instead of white and a fresh pear instead of canned.

How much fiber should Katie's diet provide?

▼

The AI for fiber for a young adult woman is 25 grams per day.

**How many grams of fiber are in Katie's modified diet?
Does it meet the recommendations?**

▼

Answer:

**Does Katie's modified diet meet the recommendations
for 2–4 servings of fruits, 3–5 servings of vegetables,
and 6–11 servings of grains?**

▼

Answer:

• CARBOHYDRATES AND FOOD TECHNOLOGY

Many forms of carbohydrate are added in the manufacture of processed foods. Carbohydrates are added for sweetness, to change food texture or color, to thicken, and to preserve food. Some added carbohydrates make only a small contribution to the overall carbohydrate content of the diet, whereas others may contribute significantly.

Complex Carbohydrates as Additives

Starch is found as small granules in plants. When heated with water, these granules swell, and the solution becomes thicker. This property makes starches useful as thickeners in foods such as sauces, puddings, and gravies. As a starch-thickened mixture cools, bonds form between the molecules, creating a gel. For example, cornstarch is frequently added to thicken or gel sauces and puddings. Food manufacturers also use a product called modified starch, or modified food starch. This is starch that has been treated to cause it to form a more stable gel.

The soluble fiber pectin, common in fruits and vegetables, is also used as a thickener. Pectin forms a gel when sugar and acid are added, such as in the preparation of jams and jellies. Commercial pectin, which is sold as a thickener for home-canned fruits and jellies, is refined from citrus peels and apples. Pectin is added to thicken tomato paste and to prevent the fine particles in orange juice from settling out. Carbohydrate gums are used as thickeners and stabilizers because they combine with water to keep solutions from separating. Gravies, pie fillings, jellies, and puddings are examples of products that contain such stabilizers and thickeners. Pectins and gums are also used in reduced-fat products to mimic the texture and viscosity of fat. Gums used in food processing include gum arabic, gum karaya, guar gum, locust bean gum, xanthan gum, and gum tragacanth.

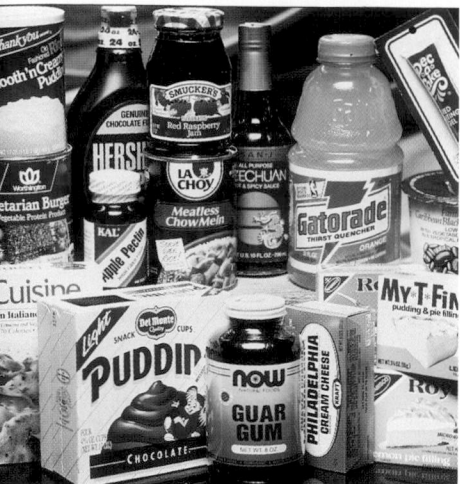

Figure 4.22
Modified food starch, pectin, and gums are used as stabilizers and thickeners in processed foods. (Charles D. Winters)

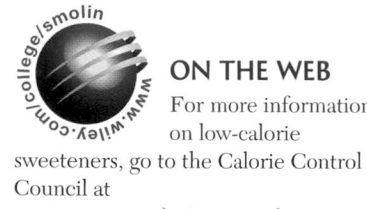

ON THE WEB
For more information on low-calorie sweeteners, go to the Calorie Control Council at
www.caloriecontrol.org/

These gums are extracted from shrubs, trees, and seed pods. Agar, carrageenan, and alginates, which come from seaweeds, are also used as thickeners and stabilizers (Figure 4.22).

Simple Carbohydrates as Additives

Americans consume about 158 pounds of sweeteners per person per year.[24] The simple carbohydrates added to foods as sweeteners include not only sucrose but also fructose, high-fructose corn syrup, corn syrup, maltose, honey, molasses, and others. They can be added in dry form or dissolved in water to form syrups. Simple carbohydrates can also be used as a preservative, as in jams and jellies, since high concentrations of sugar hold water and prevent the growth of microorganisms. They are also used to color foods, since they darken or caramelize when heated. Caramelized sugar is responsible for the brown color of caramel candy and the dark color of maple syrup.

Fructose is a component of a number of sweeteners, including sucrose, honey, and high-fructose corn syrup. High-fructose corn syrup is produced by modifying starch extracted from corn to produce a syrup that is approximately half glucose and half fructose. Fructose is sweeter and less expensive than sucrose. Therefore, it has become the most commonly used added sweetener.[7] Because fructose does not cause as great a rise in blood glucose, it is sometimes used as an alternative to sucrose in products for diabetics. However, because fructose causes an increase in blood lipids, its use should be limited.[7] Fructose consumed in fruits or juices can also cause diarrhea in children.

Artificial Sweeteners: Sugar Substitutes

America's love of sweets and the bad press surrounding sugar have driven the technological development of an increasing number of artificial and non-nutritive sweeteners. These sugar substitutes, which provide little or no energy, are added to a host of low-kcalorie and "light" foods such as yogurts, ice creams, and soft drinks. Although many sugar substitutes are technically not carbohydrates, they were developed to replace simple sugars in food products or as an alternative for table sugar at home. Artificial sweeteners are generally safe for healthy people;[25] however, to assure that they are not misused, the FDA has defined acceptable daily intakes (ADIs)—levels that should not be exceeded when using these products. The ADI is an estimate of the amount per kilogram of body weight that an individual can safely consume every day over a lifetime without risk.

The Role of Sugar Substitutes in the Diet The average American eats about 20.5 teaspoons of added sweeteners per day.[24] Replacing some of these foods with sugar-free ones will cut down on kcalories and decrease sugar intake, but it will not increase the intake of whole grains or fresh fruits and vegetables—key components of a healthy diet. Because foods that are high in added sugar tend to be nutrient-poor choices, replacing them with artificially sweetened alternatives does not increase the nutrient density of the diet. If, however, sugar substitutes and foods containing them are used in moderation as part of a diet that is based on whole grains, vegetables, and fruits, these products can be part of a healthy diet.

Artificial sweeteners have been shown to reduce the incidence of dental caries and can be helpful for managing blood sugar levels in diabetes, but their usefulness for weight loss is debatable. If individuals trying to lose weight replace sugar and high-sugar foods with artificially sweetened products, they will reduce their energy intake. When used as part of a weight control program, artificial sweeteners may facilitate weight loss and long-term weight maintenance.[26] However, despite the variety of artificial sweeteners, obesity has continued to increase in the American population. Clearly, artificial sweeteners are not the solution to the obesity epidemic.

Types of Artificial Sweeteners The main competitors in the artificial sweetener market in the United States today are saccharin, aspartame, acesulfame K (acesulfame potassium), and sucralose. These are used alone or in combination to sweeten a variety of foods (Figure 4.23). Stevia is a sugar substitute that is sold as a dietary supplement. Though it is used extensively in Japan, it cannot be sold as a sweetener in the United States because the FDA considers it an unapproved food additive. Cyclamate, an artificial sweetener that was popular in the 1960s, was banned by the FDA in 1969. It is still sold in Canada and some 50 other countries.

Saccharin Saccharin is a sweetener that is 200 to 700 times sweeter than sugar. In 1977, after large doses of saccharin were found to increase the incidence of bladder cancer in rats, the FDA proposed banning saccharin. However, the public and industry protested. In response to the outcry, a moratorium was imposed on the banning of saccharin, and all products containing saccharin were required to display a warning on the label informing the public that it may cause cancer. In May 2000, saccharin was dropped from the government's list of cancer-causing substances.

Intake of saccharin in the United States is estimated to be about 50 mg per person per day. The ADI is set at 5 mg per kg body weight per day. For a 145-pound (70-kg) individual, this would be 350 mg per day or 115 mg per day for a 50-pound (23-kg) child.[25] A 12-ounce diet beverage sweetened with saccharin alone contains about 120 mg. A packet of sweetener contains 36 mg of saccharin.

Aspartame In 1965, James Schlatter, at the pharmaceutical company G. D. Searle, was working with a chemical made up of two amino acids when he spilled some of the chemical on his fingers. Shortly afterward, he licked his finger to pick up a piece of paper and discovered an intensely sweet taste. This accidental discovery led to the development of the artificial sweetener aspartame. Since aspartame is made of two amino acids, the building blocks of protein, it is not a carbohydrate. It was approved for some uses in 1981 and for use in soft drinks in 1983. Because aspartame breaks down when heated, it works best in products that are not cooked, such as chewing gum, breakfast cereals, fruit spreads, yogurt, and beverages. Common trade names for this sweetener include NutraSweet, Equal, and NutriTaste. Each gram of aspartame contains 4 kcalories, but since it is about 200 times as sweet as sugar, only 1/200 as much of it needs to be used to achieve the same level of sweetness.

As with other artificial sweeteners, safety concerns have been raised about aspartame. It contains the amino acid phenylalanine and, therefore, can be dangerous to individuals with a genetic disorder called phenylketonuria (PKU). These individuals have an abnormality that affects the metabolism of phenylalanine. They must restrict their intake of this amino acid to prevent brain damage (see Chapter 6). There is also a concern that consuming aspartame might cause dangerously high blood phenylalanine levels in the general public. Phenylalanine occurs naturally in protein. A 4-ounce hamburger has 12 times more phenylalanine than a 12-ounce aspartame-sweetened soft drink. However, when phenylalanine is ingested without the other amino acids found in high-protein foods, blood and brain levels increase to a greater extent. There have been reports of headaches, dizziness, seizures, nausea, allergic reactions, and other side effects following ingestion of aspartame; however, double-blind placebo-controlled studies have not been able to reproduce these symptoms.[25] There has also been concern that the use of aspartame might be associated with an increased risk of brain cancer in children, but controlled studies found no evidence that aspartame is a carcinogen or that there was a correlation between aspartame use and brain cancer incidence.[27] Overall, the consensus of the scientific community is that aspartame is safe for most people.

The FDA has set an ADI of 50 mg of aspartame per kg of body weight. A packet of sweetener contains about 37 mg of aspartame. A 12-ounce soft drink sweetened with aspartame contains about 225 mg. To exceed the ADI, a 70-kg adult would have to consume almost 16 aspartame-sweetened soft drinks a day, and a 35-kg child would have to consume almost 8 soft drinks.[25]

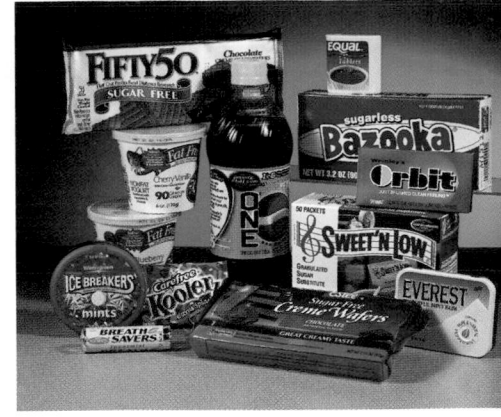

Figure 4.23
All of these products are sweetened with artificial sweeteners. (Andy Washnik)

Acesulfame K Marketed as Sunette, acesulfame potassium, or acesulfame K, is 200 times as sweet as sugar and provides no energy. It was approved for use in 1988 and is found in chewing gum, powdered drink mixes, gelatins, puddings, soft drinks, and nondairy creamers. Sold under the brand names Sunett and Sweet One, it is heat stable, so it can be used in baking. The ADI has been set at 15 mg per kg body weight. A packet of sweetener contains about 50 mg of acesulfame K.

Sucralose Sucralose (trichlorogalactosucrose) was discovered in 1976 and is the only noncaloric sweetener made from sugar. The sugar molecule is modified so it cannot be digested and passes through the digestive tract unchanged. Approved for use in the United States in 1998, it is about 600 times sweeter than sucrose. It is sold as Splenda and can be used as a tabletop sweetener that is added directly to foods. Since it is heat stable, it can be used in baked goods.[25] It is used in beverages, chewing gum, frozen desserts, puddings, jams and jellies, syrups, and many other products. It has been extensively tested for safety and found to be safe even for children and pregnant and lactating women.[28]

Sugar Alcohols Sugar alcohols such as sorbitol, mannitol, lactitol, and xylitol are chemical derivatives of sugar that are used as low-kcalorie sweeteners. Because they are not digested, absorbed, or metabolized to the same extent as monosaccharides and disaccharides, they generally provide less energy than sucrose. Maltitol provides 3 kcal per gram, lactitol 2 kcal per gram, and erythritol only 0.2 kcal per gram.

Sugar alcohols are not monosaccharides or disaccharides, so they can be used in products labeled "sugar free." Sugar-free products such as chewing gums, candies, ice creams, and baked goods sweetened with sugar alcohols may carry the health claim statement that they do not promote tooth decay. They are less likely to promote tooth decay because the bacteria in the mouth cannot metabolize sugar alcohols as rapidly as sucrose. Consumption of large amounts of sugar alcohols (more than 50 grams of sorbitol or 20 grams of mannitol per day) can cause diarrhea.

• APPLICATIONS •

1. Calculate your average carbohydrate and energy intake from the three-day diet record you kept in Chapter 2.
   a. What is the percent of energy from carbohydrate in your diet?
   b. How does this compare with the recommended 45 to 65% of energy from carbohydrate?
   c. If your diet does not meet the recommendations, suggest changes that will increase your carbohydrate intake without changing your energy intake.
   d. How does the fat content of your original diet compare with your modified diet?
   e. List some foods in your diet that are high in simple carbohydrates and some that are high in complex carbohydrates.

Classify the simple carbohydrates as either natural or added. Are the complex carbohydrates from refined or whole sources?

2. Calculate the grams of fiber in your original or modified diet from question 1 above using a computer software program or the exchanges in Table 4.3.
   a. How many grams of fiber does your diet provide?
   b. Does it meet the AI for fiber for someone of your age and gender?
   c. If your diet does not meet recommendations, modify it to meet them.

SUMMARY

1. Carbohydrates are chemical compounds that contain carbon, hydrogen, and oxygen. In food, they include sugar, starch, and fiber. Simple carbohydrates include monosaccharides and disaccharides and are found in foods such as table sugar, honey, milk, and fruit. Complex carbohydrates are oligosaccharides and polysaccharides. Polysaccharides include glycogen in animals and starch and fiber in plants. Sources of starch and fiber in the diet include whole grains, legumes, vegetables, and fruits.

2. Fiber cannot be digested by enzymes in the human stomach or small intestine and therefore is not absorbed into the body. Fiber benefits gastrointestinal function by increasing the amount of water and bulk in the intestine, which increases the ease and rate at which material moves through the gastrointestinal tract.

3. In the body, carbohydrate, primarily as glucose, provides a source of energy. Glucose is metabolized through cellular respira-

tion, involving glycolysis, which breaks glucose into pyruvate; acetyl-CoA formation; the citric acid cycle, which produces carbon dioxide and electrons; and the electron transport chain, which produces water and ATP. Several tissues, including the brain and red blood cells, require glucose as an energy source.

4. The bloodstream delivers glucose to body cells. Blood glucose levels are maintained by the hormones insulin and glucagon. When blood glucose rises, insulin is released from the pancreas to allow body cells to take up the glucose. When blood glucose falls, glucagon is released to increase blood glucose.

5. Diabetes is an abnormality in blood sugar regulation in which high blood glucose damages tissues and causes complications including heart disease, stroke, high blood pressure, kidney failure, blindness, and amputations. This occurs either because insufficient insulin is produced or because there is a decrease in the sensitivity of body cells to insulin. Treatment to maintain glucose in the normal range includes diet, exercise, and medication.

6. Hypoglycemia is a condition in which blood glucose falls to abnormally low levels, causing symptoms such as sweating, headaches, and rapid heartbeat.

7. Diets high in complex carbohydrates from whole grains, vegetables, fruits, and legumes are good sources of fiber, vitamins, minerals, and phytochemicals. Diets high in fiber may reduce the risk of chronic bowel disorders, heart disease, and colon cancer.

8. Diets high in added sugars are low in nutrient density and increase the risk of dental caries.

9. Guidelines for healthy diets recommend 45 to 65% of energy from carbohydrates with a plentiful selection of whole food sources of complex carbohydrates. Whole grains, legumes, fruits, and vegetables should be increased in the American diet, and foods high in added sugars should be consumed in moderation. Fiber intake should be increased. The AI is 38g/day for men and 25g/day for women.

10. Carbohydrates are added to foods in processing as preservatives and to provide flavor, texture, and color. Complex carbohydrates are added as thickeners and stabilizers. Simple carbohydrates are most frequently added as sweeteners.

11. Artificial sweeteners or sugar substitutes are used to replace energy-containing sweeteners. They do not contribute to tooth decay.

REVIEW QUESTIONS

1. What is the basic unit of carbohydrate?

2. List three common simple carbohydrates. In what foods are they found?

3. What is complex carbohydrate?

4. What foods are good sources of unrefined complex carbohydrates?

5. Why is added sugar considered a source of empty kcalories?

6. How much energy is provided by a gram of carbohydrate?

7. Why do we say that fiber does not provide energy?

8. Why is carbohydrate said to spare protein?

9. What is the main function of glucose in the body?

10. What is diabetes? Why is ketosis a problem only in type 1 diabetes?

11. What health benefits are associated with a diet high in unrefined carbohydrates?

12. List some functions of carbohydrates added to processed foods.

13. How can you use the information on food labels to help you identify foods that are high in added sugars? in fiber?

14. What are the risks and benefits of artificial sweeteners?

REFERENCES

1. Institute of Medicine, Food and Nutrition Board. *Dietary Reference Intakes for Energy, Carbohydrates, Fiber, Fat, Protein and Amino Acids.* Washington, D.C.: National Academy Press, 2002.

2. Lee, M. F., and Krasinski, S. D. Human adult-onset lactose decline: An update. *Nutr. Rev.* 56:1–8, 1998.

3. NIDDK Lactose Intolerance NIH Publication No. 98-2751, April 1994 e-text updated: November 1998. Available online at www.niddk.nih.gov/health/digest/pubs/lactose/lactose.htm/Accessed March 17, 2002.

4. USDA ARS Data Tables: Results from CSFII, 1996 ARS Food Surveys Research Group. Available online at www.barc.usda.bhnrc/foodsurveys/homt.htm/Accessed March 6, 2002.

5. American Diabetes Association. The Impact of Diabetes. Available online at www.diabetes.org/main/application/commerce/Accessed March 17, 2002.

6. National Diabetes Education Program. The Link between Diabetes and Cardiovascular Disease. Available online at ndep.nih.gov/control/CVD.htm/Accessed March 17, 2002.

7. American Diabetes Association. American Diabetes Association Position Statement: Evidence-based nutrition principles and recommendations for the treatment and prevention of diabetes and related complications. *J. Am. Diet. Assoc.* 102: 109–118, 2002.

8. Willett, W. C. The dietary pyramid: Does the foundation need repair? *Am. J. Clin. Nutr.* 68:218–219, 1998.

9. Konig, K. G., and Navia, J. M. Nutritional role of sugars in oral health. *Am. J. Clin. Nutr.* 62(suppl):275S–283S, 1995.

10. Wolraich, M. L., Wilson, D. B., and White, J. W. The effect of sugar on behavior or cognition in children: A meta analysis. *J.A.M.A.* 274:1617–1618, 1995.

11. Wurtman, R. J., and Wurtman, J. J. Brain serotonin, carbohydrate craving, obesity and depression. *Obes. Res.* 4:477S–480S, 1995.

12. Kurzer, M. S. Women, food, and mood. *Nutrition Reviews* 55: 268–276, 1997.

13. Jacobs, D. R., Meyer, K. A., Kushi, L. H., and Folsom, A. R. Whole-grain intake may reduce the risk of ischemic heart disease death in postmenopausal women: The Iowa Women's Health Study. *Am. J. Clin. Nutr.* 68:248–257, 1998.

14. Kushi, L. H., Meyer, K. A., and Jacobs, D. R., Jr. Cereals, legumes, and chronic disease risk reduction: Evidence from epidemiologic studies. *Am. J. Clin. Nutr.* 70(Suppl):451S–458S, 1999.

15. Food and Nutrition Board, Institute of Medicine. A Report of the Panel on the Definition of Dietary Fiber and the Standing Committee on the Scientific Evaluation of Dietary Reference Intakes Food and Nutrition Board, *Proposed Definition of Dietary Fiber.* Washington, D.C.: National Academy Press, 2002.

16. Marlett, J. A. Sites and mechanisms for the hypocholesterolemic actions of soluble dietary fiber sources. In Kritevsky, D., and Bonfield,

C., eds. *Fiber in Human Health and Disease*. New York: Plenum Press, 1997, 109–121.

17. Liu, S., Manson, J. E., Stampfer, M. J., et al. A prospective study of whole-grain intake and risk of type 2 diabetes mellitus in U.S. women. *Am. J. Public Health* 90:1409–15, 2000.

18. Meyer, K. A., Kushi, L. H., Jacobs, D. R. Jr, et al. Carbohydrates, dietary fiber, and incident type 2 diabetes in older women. *Am. J. Clin. Nutr.* 71:921–30, 2000.

19. Anderson, J. W. Nutritional management of diabetes mellitus. In *Modern Nutrition in Health and Disease*, 9th ed. Shils, M. E., Olson, J. A., Shike, M., and Ross, A. C., eds. Baltimore: Williams & Wilkins, 1999, 1365–1394.

20. Alberts, D. S., Martinez, M. E., Roe, D. J., et al. Lack of effect of a high-fiber cereal supplement on the occurrence of colorectal adenomias. *N. Engl. J. Med.* 342:1149-1155, 2000.

21. Schatzkin, A., Lanza, E., Corle, D., et al. Lack of effect of a low-fat, high-fiber diet on the recurrence of colorectal adenomias. *N. Engl. J. Med.* 342:1149–1155, 2000.

22. Miller, D. L., Miller, P. F., and Dekker, J. J. Small bowel obstruction from bran cereal. *JAMA* 263:813–815, 1990.

23. Krebs-Smith, S. M. Choose beverages and foods to moderate your intake of sugars: Measurement requires quantification. *J. Nutr.* 131: 527S–535S, 2001.

24. Coulston, A. M., and Johnson, R. K. Sugar and sugars: Myths and realities. *J. Am. Diet. Assoc.* 102:351–353, 2002.

25. American Dietetic Association. Position of the American Dietetic Association: Use of nutritive and non-nutritive sweeteners. *J. Am. Diet. Assoc.* 98:580–587, 1998.

26. Blackburn, G. L., Kanders, B. S., Lavin, P. T., et al. The effect of aspartame as part of a multidisciplinary weight-control program on short- and long-term control of body weight. *Am. J. Clin. Nutr.* 65:409–418, 1997.

27. Gurney, J. G., Pogoda, J. M., Holly, E. A., et al. Aspartame consumption in relation to childhood brain tumor risk: results from a case-control study. *J. Nat. Cancer Inst.* 89:1072–1074, 1997.

28. Calorie Control Council. Low calorie sweeteners: sucralose. Available online at www.caloriecontrol.org/sucralos.thml/Accessed March 7, 2000.

Lipids: How Much of a Good Thing? Chapter 5

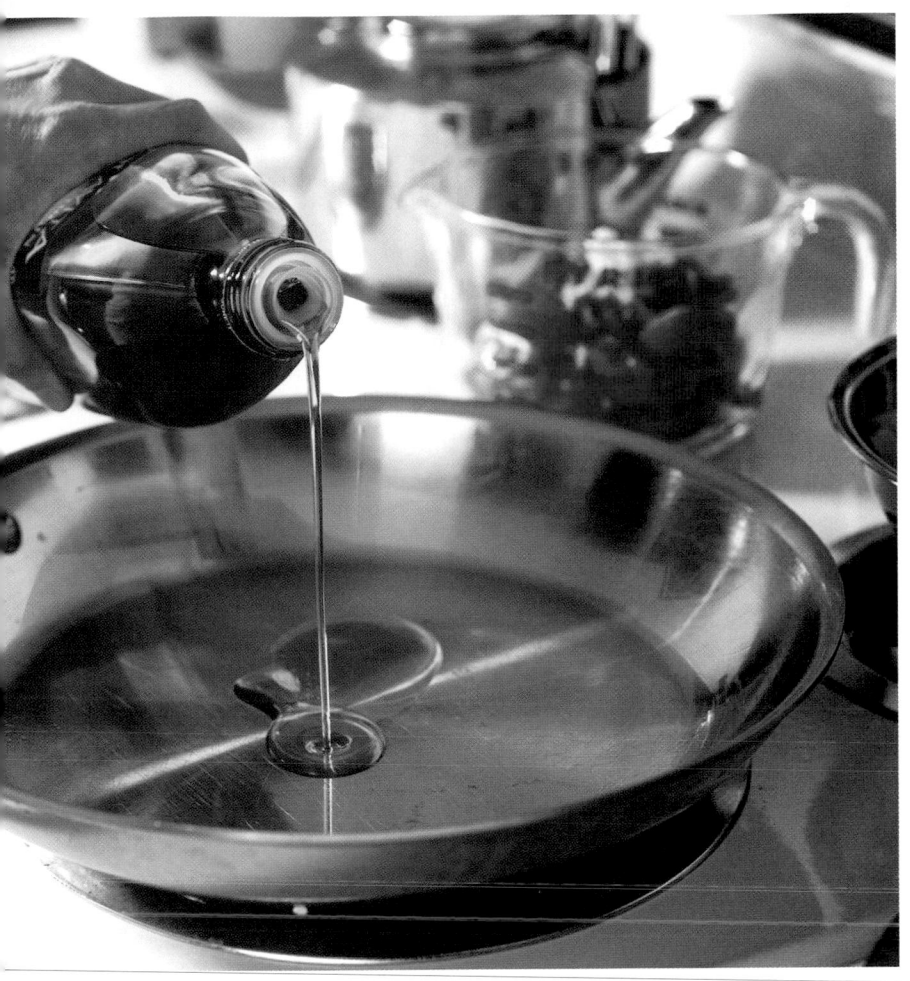

(© Benjamin F. Fink, Jr./Foodpix)

Chapter Outline

Chapter Concepts

✔ Lipids, often referred to as fats, add flavor to food and provide a concentrated source of energy.

✔ The major types of lipids in the body are fatty acids, glycerides, phospholipids, and sterols.

✔ Fatty acids are made of chains of carbons. The length of the chain and the types and locations of the carbon-carbon bonds affect their characteristics in food and functions in the body.

✔ Triglycerides (triacylglycerols) provide a concentrated source of energy in our food and in our bodies.

✔ Phosphoglycerides are important because they dissolve in both water and lipids.

✔ Cholesterol is a sterol that is both made in the body and consumed in the diet.

✔ For transport in the blood, lipids combine with protein to form lipoproteins.

✔ Diets high in some types of fat are associated with an increased risk of heart disease and cancers of the breast, colon, and prostate.

✔ To reduce the risks of developing chronic disease, public health guidelines recommend a diet moderate in fat; low in *trans* and saturated fat and cholesterol; and plentiful in grains, vegetables, and fruits.

✔ During food processing, fats may be added to foods, and the fats in food may be modified to change the stability or shelf life of the product.

✔ A number of artificial fats that provide less energy have been developed.

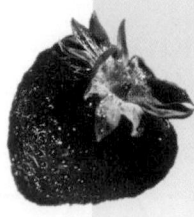

Just a Taste

Which is better for you: butter, margarine, or olive oil?

Is fat more fattening than other nutrients?

Will reducing your fat intake eliminate your risk of heart disease?

Should you put butter or margarine on your toast? Should you use canola or corn oil in cooking? There are hundreds of oils and butters and margarines from which to choose. Some are solid, some are liquid, some come from plants, some come from animals. Some are said to increase your heart disease risk while others claim to reduce risk. Which should you choose?

Epidemiological studies have shown that, in general, countries that have high intakes of fat and saturated fat tend to have higher incidences of heart disease and certain types of cancer. Yet not all countries follow this trend. Some Mediterranean countries have a high fat intake, and yet the incidence of heart disease is extremely low. How much fat and what type of fat should we be consuming?

Recommendations for a healthy diet suggest that we consume a diet moderate in fat and low in saturated fat, *trans* fat, and cholesterol. In order to follow these guidelines, consumers need to know how much and what types of fats are in the foods they choose.

• WHAT ARE LIPIDS?

Lipids A group of organic molecules, most of which do not dissolve in water. They include fatty acids, glycerides, phospholipids, and sterols.

Lipids is the chemical term for what is commonly known as fat or oil. Lipids in the diet and in our bodies provide a concentrated source of energy. Each gram of fat provides 9 kcalories, compared with only 4 kcalories per gram from carbohydrate or protein.

Lipids in the Diet

Lipids contribute to the texture, flavor, and aroma of our food. It is the high fat content of ice cream that gives it its smooth texture and rich taste. Olive oil imparts a unique taste to salads, and sesame oil gives Chinese food its distinctive aroma. The fats in foods contribute to their appeal but also increase their kcaloric content.

Some of the fat in our diets comes from obvious sources, such as the fat on the outside of a cut of meat, or a pat of butter melting on a hot baked potato (Figure 5.1). Other fats are hidden. Baked goods such as cakes and cookies are usually high in fat, as are crackers, croissants, and some muffins. Even milk and cheese can be high in fat (Figure 5.2) In all, fat contributes about 33% of the energy in the typical American diet. This is within the recommended range of 20–35% of energy as fat.[1]

Figure 5.1
Butter on a hot baked potato is a visible source of dietary fat. (© Picture Perfect)

Types of Lipids

Lipids found in the body, and in the diet include fatty acids, glycerides, phospholipids, and sterols. Each has a different structure and function in the body and their structure affects the properties they give to food.

Fatty acid An organic molecule made up of a chain of carbons linked to hydrogens with an acid group at one end.

Fatty Acids   A **fatty acid** is a chain of carbon atoms with an acid group at one end. Fatty acids are typically bound to other molecules. For example, most fatty acids in foods and in the body are bound to glycerol to form triglycerides.

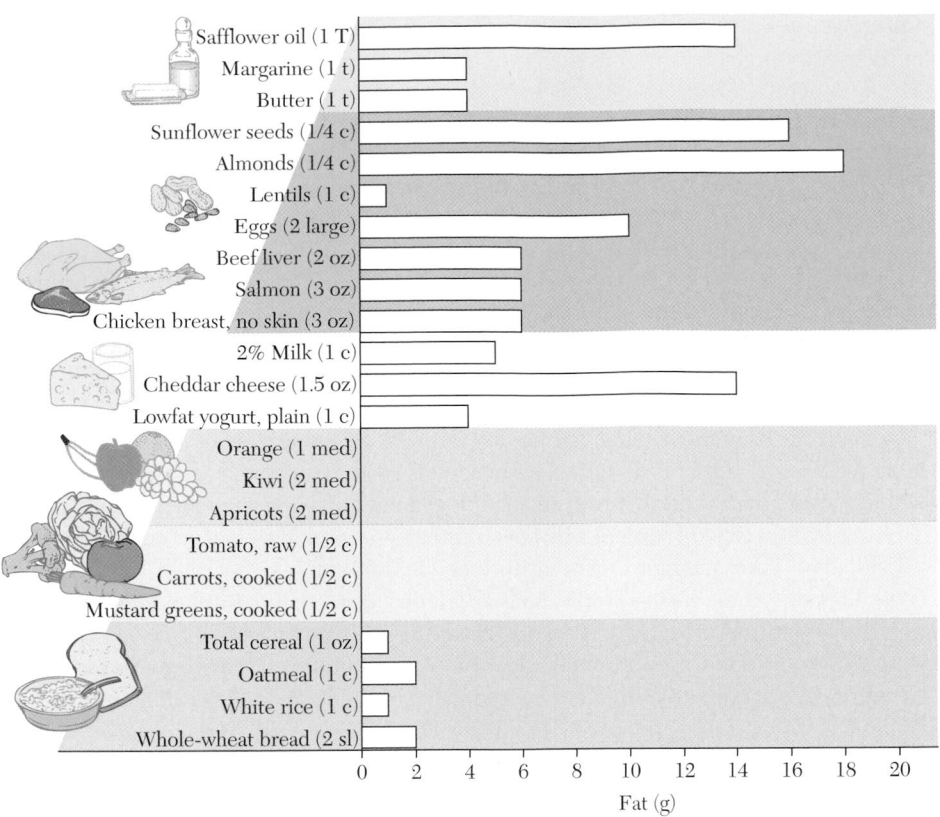

Figure 5.2

Fat content from each food group of the Food Guide Pyramid. In general, foods in the Meat, Poultry, Fish, Eggs, Dry Beans, & Nuts Group and the Milk, Yogurt, & Cheese Group are highest in fat, but fats added to vegetables and grain products also contribute a lot of fat to the diet.

The carbon chains of fatty acids vary in length from a few to 20 or more carbons. Each carbon atom forms four bonds to link it to four other atoms. If a carbon is not bound to four other atoms, double bonds are formed. At one end of the carbon chain, the omega or methyl end, the carbon atom is attached to another carbon and three hydrogens (CH_3); at the other end of the chain the acid group (COOH) is formed by joining the carbon to an oxygen by a double bond and an OH group by a single bond. Each of the carbons between is attached to two other carbons and up to two hydrogens (Figure 5.3).

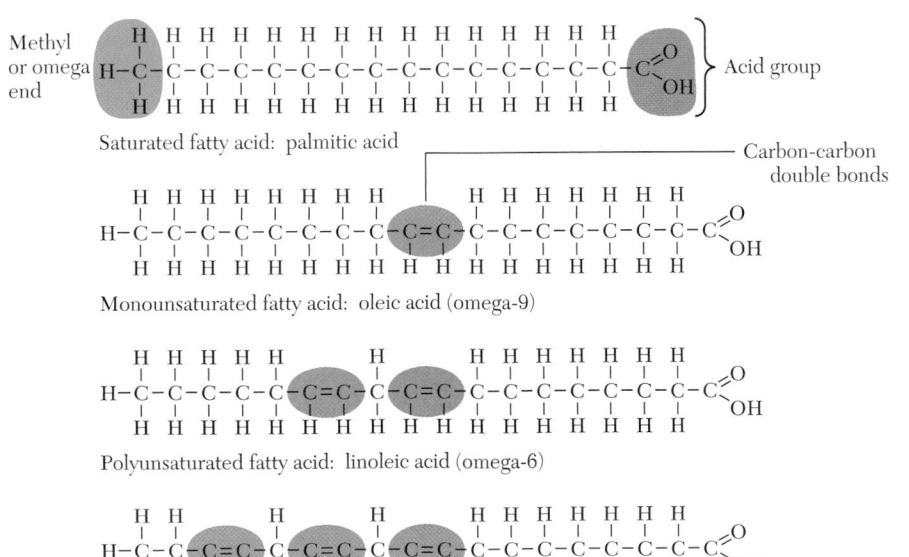

Figure 5.3

The structure of common saturated, monounsaturated, and polyunsaturated fatty acids.

Categories of Fatty Acids Fatty acids are categorized based on the number of carbons in their carbon chain as well as the types and locations of bonds between the carbons. These structural features affect their physical properties. One way to categorize fatty acids is by chain length. Short chain fatty acids range from 4 to 7 carbons in length. They remain liquid at colder temperatures. For example, the short chain fatty acids in whole milk remain liquid even in the refrigerator. Medium chain fatty acids, such as those in coconut oil, range from 8 to 12 carbons. They solidify in the refrigerator but remain liquid at room temperature. Long chain fatty acids (greater than 12 carbons), such as those in beef fat, usually remain solid at room temperature. Most fatty acids in plants and animals, including humans, contain between 14 and 22 carbons.

Fatty acids are also categorized by the types of bonds between carbons in the chain. A fatty acid in which the chain is saturated with hydrogens so that each carbon has two hydrogens bound to it is called a **saturated fatty acid**. The most common saturated fatty acids are palmitic acid, which has 16 carbons, and stearic acid, which has 18 carbons. These are found most often in animal foods such as meat and dairy products. Vegetable sources of saturated fatty acids include palm oil, palm kernel oil, and coconut oil. These are often called **tropical oils** because they are found in plants common in tropical climates. They are more resistant to rancidity and have longer shelf lives than oils containing unsaturated fats. Tropical oils are rarely added to foods at home but are used by the food industry in cereals, crackers, salad dressings, and cookies. They provide only a small proportion of the saturated fat in the American diet. However, concern about the saturated fat content of the diet has led many of the large food manufacturers to reformulate some of their products. An **unsaturated fatty acid** contains some carbons that are not saturated with hydrogens. The carbons within the chain contain double bonds formed between carbons that are bound to only one hydrogen (see Figure 5.3). A fatty acid containing one double bond in its carbon chain is called a **monounsaturated fatty acid**. In our diets, the most common monounsaturated fatty acid is oleic acid, which is prevalent in olive and canola oils. A fatty acid with more than one double bond in its carbon chain is said to be a **polyunsaturated fatty acid**. The most common polyunsaturated fatty acid is linoleic acid, found in corn, safflower, and soybean oils. Unsaturated fatty acids melt at cooler temperatures than saturated fatty acids of the same chain length. Therefore, the more unsaturated bonds a fatty acid contains, the more likely it is to be liquid at room temperature. Fats in our diets contain combinations of saturated, monounsaturated, and polyunsaturated fatty acids (Figure 5.4).

Saturated fatty acid A fatty acid in which the carbon atoms are bound to as many hydrogens as possible and which therefore contains no carbon-carbon double bonds.

Tropical oils A term used in the popular press to refer to the saturated oils—coconut, palm, and palm kernel oil—that are derived from plants grown in tropical regions.

Unsaturated fatty acid A fatty acid that contains one or more carbon-carbon double bonds.

Monounsaturated fatty acid A fatty acid that contains one carbon-carbon double bond.

Polyunsaturated fatty acid A fatty acid that contains two or more carbon-carbon double bonds.

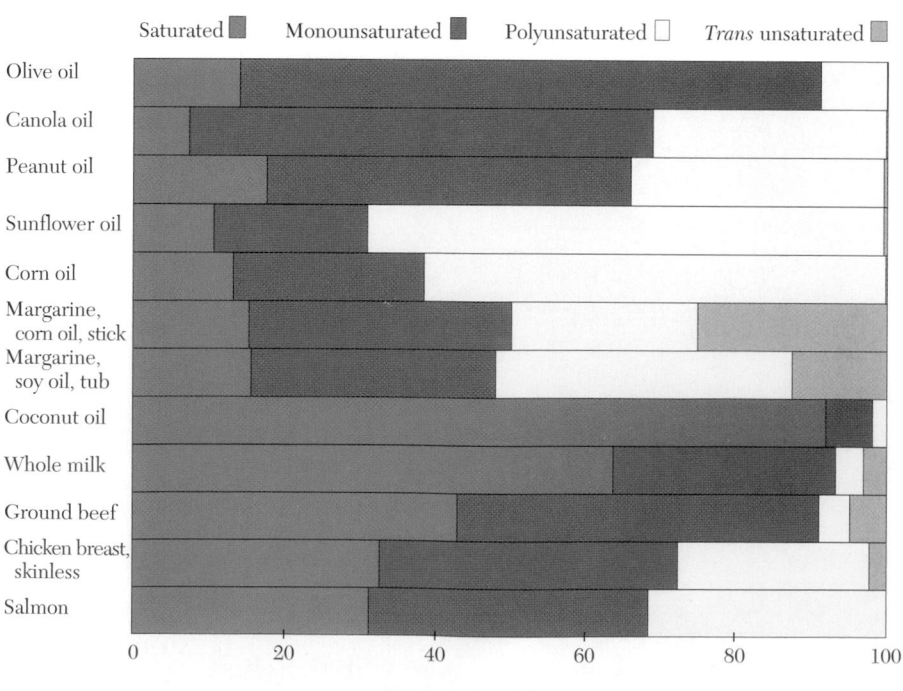

Figure 5.4
Foods contain varying amounts of saturated, monounsaturated, polyunsaturated, and *trans* unsaturated fatty acids. This graph shows the amounts of these types of fatty acids as a percentage of the total amount of fat in the product. (From USDA, ARS, Beltsville Human Nutrition Research Center, *Special Purpose Table No. 1. Fat and fatty acid content of selected foods containing* trans *fatty acids.*)

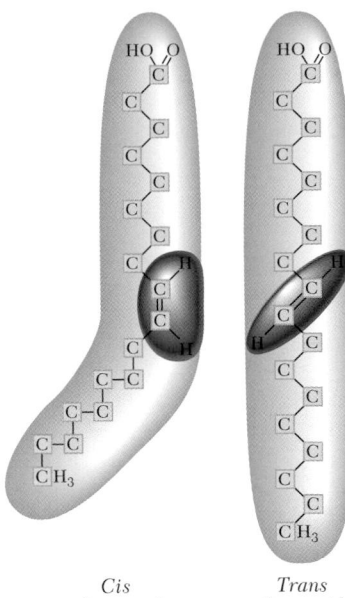

Cis
fatty acid

Trans
fatty acid

Figure 5.5

The orientation of hydrogens around the double bond distinguishes *cis* and *trans* fatty acids. In *cis* fatty acids, the hydrogens are on the same side of the double bond and cause a bend in the carbon chain. In *trans* fatty acids, the hydrogens are on opposite sides of the double bond and the carbon chain is straighter.

There are different categories of unsaturated fatty acids, depending on the location of the first double bond in the chain. If the first double bond occurs between the third and fourth carbons, counting from the omega end (CH_3) of the chain (see Figure 5.3), the fat is said to be an **omega-3 (ω-3) fatty acid**. Alpha-linolenic acid, found in vegetable oils, and eicosapentaenoic acid (EPA) and docosahexaenoic acid (DHA), found in fish oils, are omega-3 fatty acids. If the first double bond occurs between the sixth and seventh carbons (from the omega end), the fatty acid is called an **omega-6 (ω-6) fatty acid**. Linoleic acid, found in corn and safflower oils, is the major omega-6 fatty acid in the North American diet.

The position of the hydrogen atoms around a double bond is another way of classifying unsaturated fatty acids. Most unsaturated fatty acids found in nature have both hydrogen atoms on the same side of the double bond, called the *cis* configuration. When the hydrogens are on opposite sides of the double bond, called the *trans* configuration, the fatty acid is a ***trans* fatty acid** (Figure 5.5). A *trans* fatty acid has a higher melting point than the same fatty acid in the *cis* configuration. *Trans* fatty acids are found in small amounts in nature and are formed during food processing.

Essential Fatty Acids The body is capable of synthesizing most of the fatty acids it needs from glucose or other sources of carbon, hydrogen, and oxygen. Humans, however, are not able to synthesize double bonds in the omega-6 and omega-3 positions. Therefore, the fatty acids, linoleic acid (omega-6) and alpha-linolenic acid (omega-3), are **essential fatty acids**. They must be consumed in the diet to make other omega-6 and omega-3 fatty acids. Omega-6 fatty acids are important for growth, skin integrity, fertility, and maintaining red blood cell structure. Omega-3 fatty acids are important for the structure and function of cell membranes, particularly in the retina of the eye and the central nervous system. If the diet is low in linoleic acid or alpha-linolenic acid, the fatty acids synthesized from them become dietary essentials. Arachidonic acid is an omega-6 fatty acid synthesized from linoleic acid. Arachidonic acid is considered essential only when the diet is low in linoleic acid. It is found in both animal and vegetable fats. EPA and DHA are omega-3 fatty acids synthesized from alpha-linolenic acid. Arachidonic acid and DHA are necessary for normal brain development in infants and young children.

Glycerides Most fatty acids in food and in the body are found attached to a backbone of the three-carbon molecule glycerol. When three fatty acids are attached, the molecule is called a **triacylglycerol**, commonly known as a triglyceride (Figure 5.6).

Omega-3 (ω-3) fatty acid A fatty acid containing a carbon-carbon double bond between the third and fourth carbons from the omega end.

Omega-6 (ω-6) fatty acid A fatty acid containing a carbon-carbon double bond between the sixth and seventh carbons from the omega end.

***Trans* fatty acid** An unsaturated fatty acid in which the hydrogens are on opposite sides of the double bond.

Essential fatty acids Fatty acids that must be consumed in the diet because they cannot be made by the body or cannot be made in sufficient quantities to meet needs.

Triacylglycerol (triglyceride) The major form of lipid in food and in the body. It consists of three fatty acids attached to a glycerol molecule. When only one fatty acid is attached, it is a monoacylglycerol or monoglyceride, and when two are attached, it is a diacylglycerol or diglyceride.

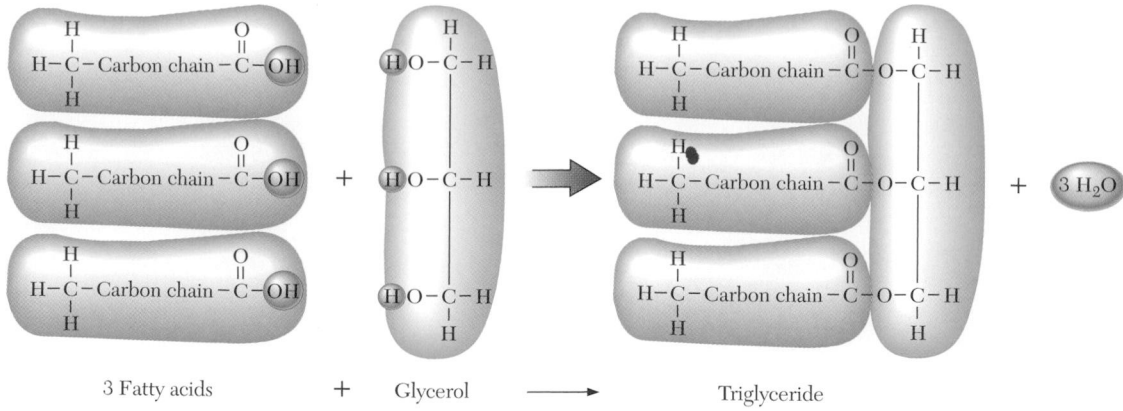

3 Fatty acids   +   Glycerol ⟶   Triglyceride

Figure 5.6
A triglyceride (triacylglycerol) is three fatty acids attached to a molecule of glycerol.

Phosphoglycerides A type of phospholipid composed of a glycerol backbone with two fatty acids and a phosphate group attached.

Emulsifiers Substances that allow water and fat to mix.

Lipid bilayer Two layers of phosphoglyceride molecules oriented so that the fat-soluble fatty acid tails are sandwiched between the water-soluble phosphate-containing heads.

Lecithin A phosphoglyceride composed of a glycerol backbone, two fatty acids, a phosphate group, and a molecule of choline.

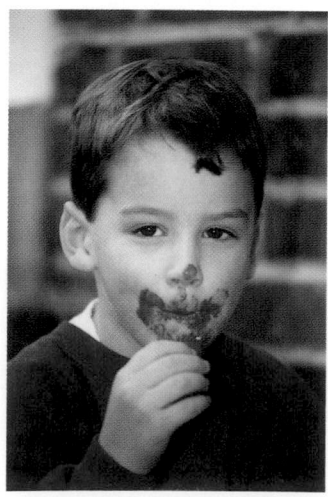

Figure 5.7
Because of its fatty acid content, chocolate is solid at cold temperatures but melts rapidly at body temperature. (George Semple)

When one fatty acid is attached, the molecule is called a monoacylglycerol, or monoglyceride, and when two fatty acids are attached, it is a diacylglycerol, or diglyceride. Triglycerides may contain any combination of fatty acids: long, medium, or short chain, saturated or unsaturated. Triglycerides make up most of the lipids in our food and in our bodies and are usually what are referred to when the term "fat" is used.

The types of fatty acids in triglycerides determine their texture, taste, and physical characteristics. For example, the triglycerides in red meat contain predominantly long chain saturated fatty acids; thus the fat on a piece of steak is solid at room temperature. The amounts and types of fatty acids in chocolate allow it to remain brittle at room temperature, snap when bitten into, and then melt quickly and smoothly in the mouth (Figure 5.7).

Phospholipids Phospholipids are lipids attached to a chemical group containing phosphorus called a phosphate group. The **phosphoglycerides** are the major class of phospholipids. Like triglycerides, they have a backbone of glycerol. However, they have only two fatty acids attached. In place of the third fatty acid is a phosphate group, which is then attached to a variety of other molecules. The fatty acid end of phosphoglycerides is soluble in fat, whereas the phosphate end is water soluble. This allows phosphoglycerides to mix in both water and fat—a property that makes them important for many functions in foods and in the body.

In foods, the ability of phospholipids to mix in water and fat allows them to act as **emulsifiers**, substances that allow water and fat to mix by breaking large fat globules into smaller ones. Egg yolk, which contains phospholipids, functions as an emulsifier in food; the egg yolk in cake batter allows the oil and water to mix. In the body, cell membranes contain phospholipids that form a **lipid bilayer**, allowing an aqueous (water) environment both inside and outside the cell with a lipid environment sandwiched between them (Figure 5.8).

The specific function of a phosphoglyceride depends on the molecule that is attached to the phosphate group. If a molecule of choline is attached, the phosphoglyceride is **lecithin**. In the body, lecithin is a major constituent of cell membranes and is required for their optimal function. It is also used to synthesize the neurotransmitter acetylcholine, which is important in the memory center of the brain. Based on these functions, lecithin is marketed to consumers as a supplement that improves memory and maintains proper cell function. However, lecithin is made in ample amounts by the body, and large doses in supplements have been shown to cause gastrointestinal upsets, sweating, and loss of appetite.[2] Eggs and soybeans are natural sources of lecithin. Lecithin is also used by the food industry as an additive in margarine, salad dressings, chocolate, frozen desserts, and baked goods to keep the oil from separating from the other ingredients.

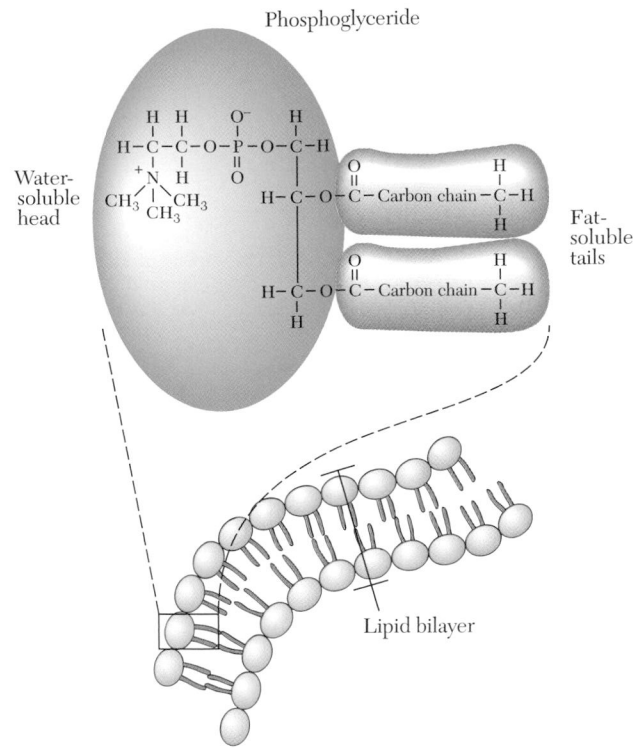

Phosphoglyceride

Water-
soluble
head

Fat-
soluble
tails

Lipid bilayer

Figure 5.8
Phosphoglycerides, such as the lecithin molecule shown here, consist of a water-soluble head containing a phosphate group and a lipid-soluble tail of fatty acids. In cell membranes, phosphoglycerides form a lipid bilayer by orienting the water-soluble portion toward the water environment.

Sterols Structurally, sterols are composed of multiple rings, which makes them very different from triglycerides and phosphoglycerides. Like other lipids, they do not dissolve well in water. **Cholesterol** is probably the best-known sterol (Figure 5.9). In the diet, cholesterol is found only in foods from animal sources. Egg yolks and organ meats such as liver and kidney are high in cholesterol. One egg yolk contains about 213 mg of cholesterol. Organ meats contain about 300 mg per 3-ounce serving. Lean red meats and skinless chicken contain about 90 mg, whereas fish contains 50 mg in 3 ounces. Plant foods do not contain cholesterol unless animal products are combined with them in cooking or processing.

Cholesterol is necessary in the body, but because it is manufactured by the liver, it is not essential in the diet. More than 90% of the cholesterol in the body is found in cell membranes. It is also part of myelin, the coating on many nerve cells. Cholesterol is needed to synthesize vitamin D in the skin; cholic acid, a component of bile; some hormones, such as testosterone and estrogen, which promote growth and the development of sex characteristics; and cortisol, which promotes glucose synthesis in the liver. The drugs known as **anabolic steroids**, which mimic the action of hormones that stimulate muscle growth, are also sterols. They have been popular among athletes trying to increase muscle strength and muscle mass; however, their use is illegal and can cause liver damage and other negative long-term health effects (see Chapter 13).

Cholesterol A lipid that consists of multiple chemical rings and is made only by animal cells.

Anabolic steroids Synthetic fat-soluble hormones used by some athletes to increase muscle mass. Their use is illegal and has dangerous side effects.

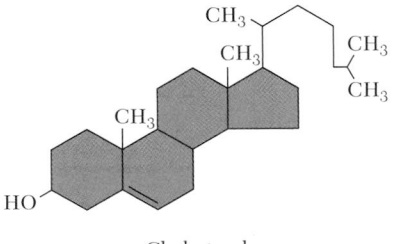

Cholesterol

Figure 5.9
Cholesterol structure. The four colored rings indicate the backbone structure common to all sterols.

• LIPIDS IN THE DIGESTIVE TRACT

Lipid digestion begins in the stomach due to the action of lipases produced in the mouth and stomach. These enzymes work best on triglycerides containing short and medium chain fatty acids such as those in milk, and so are particularly important in infants.[3] In healthy adults, most of the digestion of dietary fat takes place in the small intestine due to the action of lipases secreted by the pancreas (Figure 5.10). Here, bile from the gallbladder helps break fat into small globules, which can be accessed by enzymes that break down triglycerides into fatty acids and monoglycerides. These

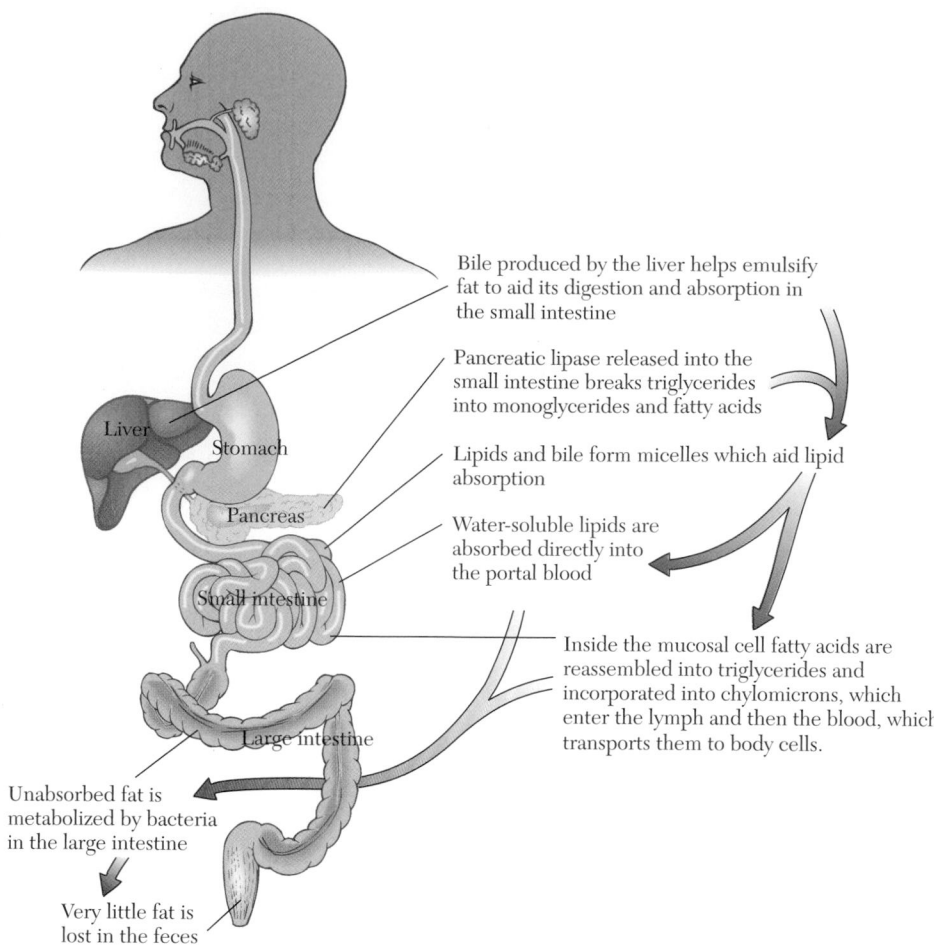

Bile produced by the liver helps emulsify fat to aid its digestion and absorption in the small intestine

Pancreatic lipase released into the small intestine breaks triglycerides into monoglycerides and fatty acids

Lipids and bile form micelles which aid lipid absorption

Water-soluble lipids are absorbed directly into the portal blood

Inside the mucosal cell fatty acids are reassembled into triglycerides and incorporated into chylomicrons, which enter the lymph and then the blood, which transports them to body cells.

Unabsorbed fat is metabolized by bacteria in the large intestine

Very little fat is lost in the feces

Liver

Stomach

Pancreas

Small intestine

Large intestine

Figure 5.10

An overview of lipid digestion and absorption.

Micelles Particles formed in the small intestine when droplets of lipid are surrounded by bile acids.

Adipose tissue Tissue found under the skin and around body organs that is composed of fat-storing cells.

Eicosanoids Regulatory molecules that can be synthesized from omega-3 and omega-6 fatty acids.

mix with bile to form smaller droplets called **micelles** (Figure 5.11). Micelles facilitate the absorption of lipids into the mucosal cells of the small intestine. When micelles come in contact with the intestinal brush border, the monoglycerides and fatty acids diffuse into the mucosal cells. Because long chain fatty acids are not soluble in water, further processing is necessary before they can be transported in the blood.

These processes, necessary for fat digestion and absorption, are also necessary for the absorption of the fat-soluble vitamins, as well as of other fat-soluble molecules present in foods, such as β-carotene. These lipid-soluble molecules must be incorporated into micelles to be absorbed, and therefore their absorption depends on the presence of dietary fat. Most of the bile acids in micelles are also absorbed and returned to the liver to be reused.

• LIPIDS IN THE BODY

In the body, lipids can be used as an immediate source of energy or stored for future use. Most lipids in the body are triglycerides stored in **adipose tissue**, which lies under the skin and around internal organs. Because triglycerides are a concentrated energy source (9 kcal/g), a large amount of energy can be stored without a great increase in body size or weight. Adipose tissue also insulates the body from changes in temperature and provides a cushion to protect against shock.

Lipids are important for lubricating body surfaces. They are also an important structural component of cells, particularly in the brain and nervous system. As components of all cell membranes, lipids protect the internal environment of cells. Lipids also have a regulatory role. Both omega-3 and omega-6 fatty acids are precursors of compounds called **eicosanoids** or prostaglandins. Eicosinoids are hormone-

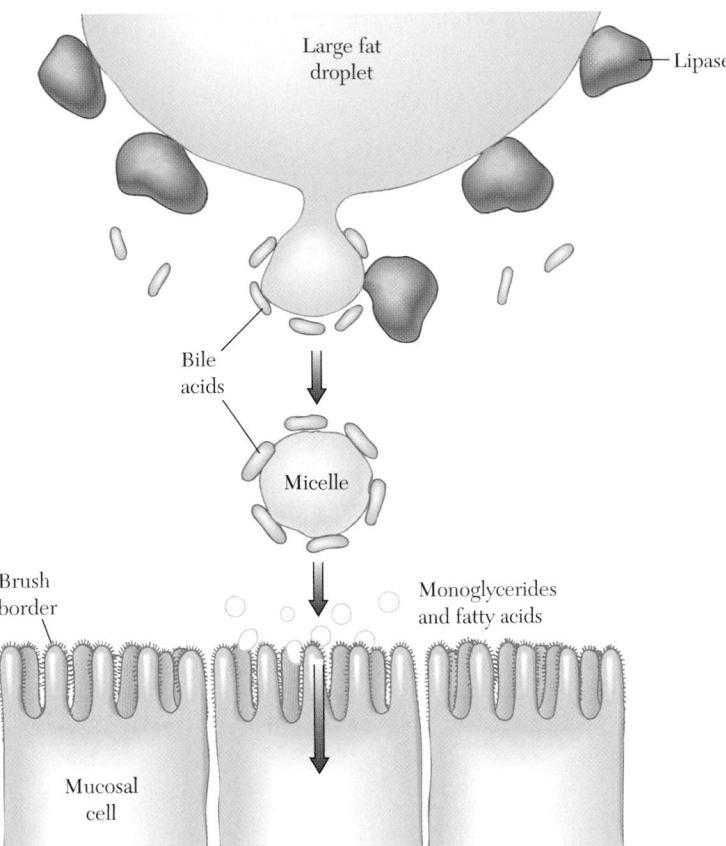

Figure 5.11
Bile acids mix with fats to form small droplets called micelles that facilitate the absorption of monoglycerides and fatty acids into the mucosal cells of the small intestine.

like compounds that help regulate blood clotting, blood pressure, immune function, and other body processes. The effect of an eicosanoid depends on the fatty acid from which it is made. For example, when the omega-6 fatty acid arachidonic acid is the starting material, the eicosanoid synthesized increases blood clotting; when the eicosanoid is made from the omega-3 fatty acid EPA, it decreases blood clotting. The correct ratio of the two is necessary to allow appropriate blood clotting and other bodily functions.

Transporting Lipids in the Body

Water-insoluble lipids are transported through the blood coated in a water-soluble envelope created when the lipids combine with phospholipids and proteins to form transport particles called **lipoproteins**. Fat-soluble vitamins are also transported in lipoproteins. Lipoproteins help transport both dietary lipids from the small intestine and stored or newly synthesized lipids from the liver.

Lipoproteins Particles containing a core of lipids surrounded by a shell of protein and phospholipid that transport lipids in blood and lymph.

Transport from the Small Intestine After absorption into the intestinal mucosal cells, lipids that are somewhat water soluble, such as short and medium chain fatty acids and phospholipids, can enter the blood. Lipids that are not soluble in water, such as long chain fatty acids and cholesterol, cannot enter the bloodstream directly. Absorbed monoglycerides and long chain fatty acids are first assembled into triglycerides by the mucosal cell. These triglycerides are then combined with cholesterol, phospholipids, and a small amount of protein to form lipoproteins called **chylomicrons**. Chylomicrons are absorbed into the lymphatic system and then enter the bloodstream without first passing through the liver.

As chylomicrons circulate in the blood, the enzyme **lipoprotein lipase**, present on the surface of the cells lining the blood vessels, breaks the triglycerides down into fatty acids and glycerol, which enter the surrounding cells. The fatty acids can be either used as fuel or resynthesized into triglycerides for storage. What remains of the

Chylomicrons Lipoproteins that transport lipids from the mucosal cells of the small intestine to other body cells.

Lipoprotein lipase An enzyme attached to cell membranes that breaks down triglycerides into fatty acids and glycerol.

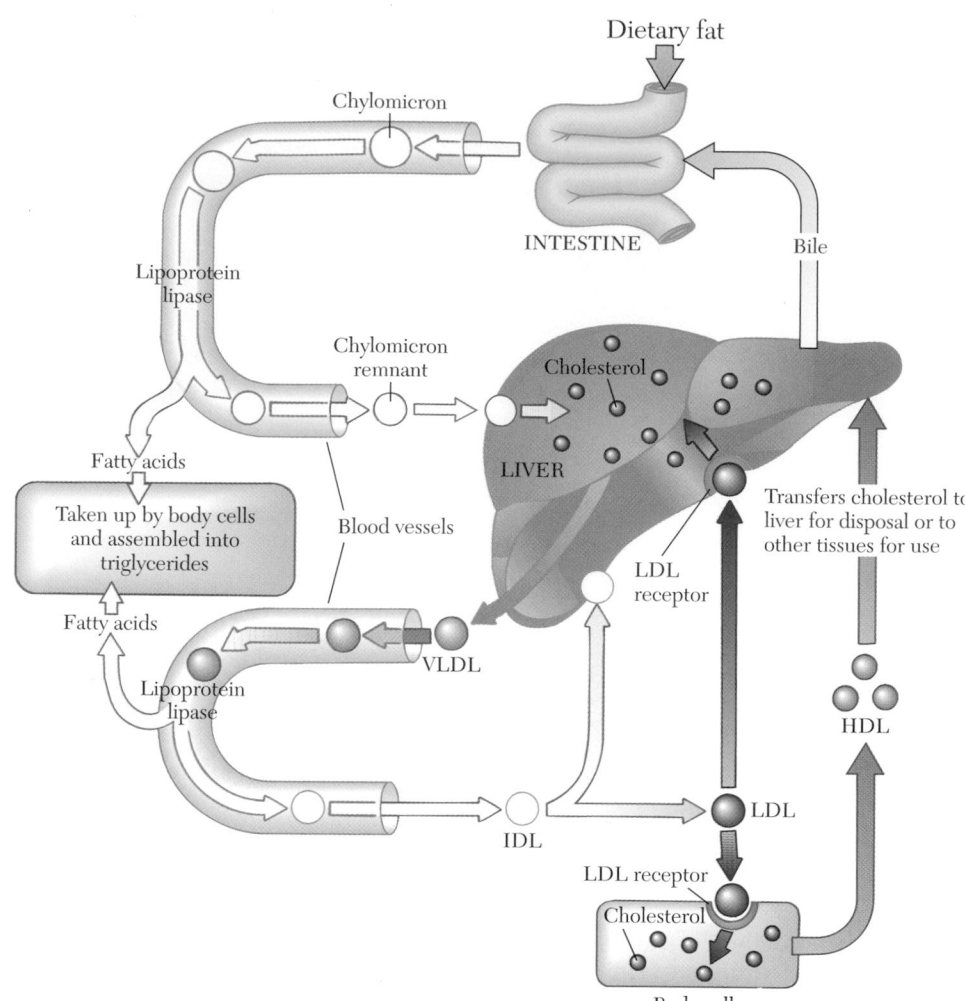

Figure 5.12
Chylomicrons carry lipids from the intestines and deliver triglycerides to body cells. VLDLs carry lipids from the liver and deliver triglycerides to body cells. LDLs are derived from IDLs and are the primary cholesterol delivery system for body cells. HDLs carry cholesterol away from cells to the liver.

Very-low-density lipoproteins (VLDLs)
Lipoproteins assembled by the liver that carry lipid from the liver and deliver triglycerides to body cells.

Low-density lipoproteins (LDLs)
Lipoproteins that transport cholesterol to cells. Elevated LDL cholesterol increases the risk of cardiovascular disease.

LDL receptor A protein on the surface of cells that binds to LDL particles and allows their contents to be taken up for use by the cell.

chylomicron is a chylomicron remnant composed mostly of cholesterol and protein. This goes to the liver and is disassembled (Figure 5.12).

Transport from the Liver The liver is the major lipid-producing organ in the body. Here excess protein, carbohydrate, or alcohol can be broken down and used to make triglycerides or cholesterol. Triglycerides made in the liver are incorporated into lipoprotein particles called **very-low-density lipoproteins (VLDLs)**. Cholesterol synthesized in the liver or returned in chylomicron remnants can also be incorporated into VLDLs or can be used to make bile. VLDLs transport lipids out of the liver and deliver triglycerides to body cells. As with chylomicrons, the enzyme lipoprotein lipase breaks down the triglycerides in VLDLs so that the fatty acids can be taken up by surrounding cells. Once the triglycerides are removed from the VLDLs, a denser, smaller, intermediate-density lipoprotein (IDL) remains. About two-thirds of the IDLs are returned to the liver, and the rest are transformed in the blood into **low-density lipoproteins (LDLs)**. LDLs contain an even higher proportion of cholesterol than VLDLs and are the primary cholesterol delivery system for cells (Figure 5.13). High levels of LDLs in the blood have been associated with an increased risk for heart disease. For LDLs to be taken up by cells, a protein on the surface of the LDL particle must bind to a receptor protein on the cell membrane, called an **LDL receptor**. This binding allows LDLs to be removed from circulation and enter cells where their cholesterol and other components can be used (see Figure 5.12).

Since most body cells have no system for breaking down cholesterol, it must be returned to the liver to be eliminated from the body. This reverse cholesterol trans-

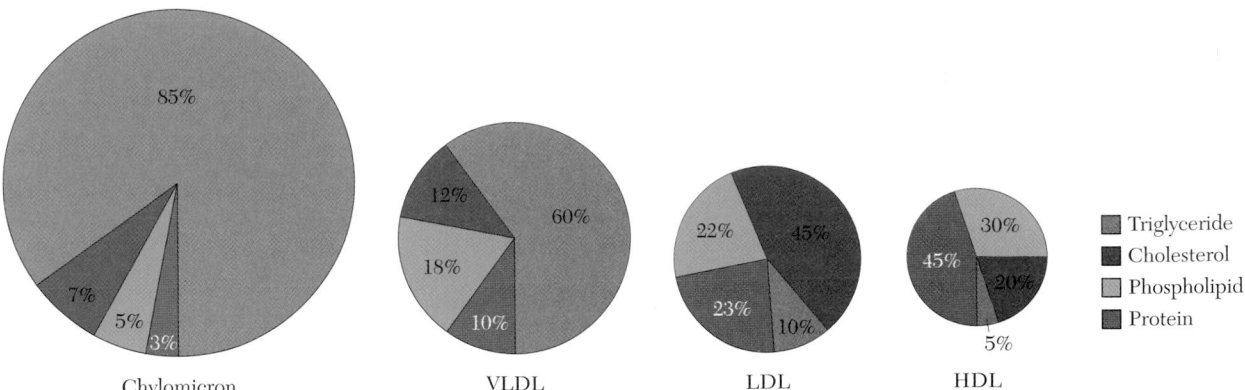

Figure 5.13

All lipoproteins consist of a shell of phospholipid, protein, and cholesterol and a center of triglycerides and cholesterol, but they vary in size and density. Particles with proportionately more triglyceride and less protein are larger and less dense. Chylomicrons are the largest, least-dense particles and contain the most triglyceride, whereas HDLs are the smallest, densest particles and have the greatest percentage of protein.

port is accomplished by the densest of the lipoprotein particles, called **high-density lipoproteins (HDLs)**. These particles originate from the intestinal tract and liver and circulate in the blood, picking up cholesterol from other lipoproteins and body cells. They function as a temporary storage site for lipid. Some of the cholesterol in HDLs is taken directly to the liver for disposal, and some is transferred to organs that have a high requirement for cholesterol, such as those involved in steroid hormone synthesis. High levels of HDL in the blood are associated with a reduction in heart disease risk.

High-density lipoproteins (HDLs) Lipoproteins that pick up cholesterol from cells and transport it to the liver so that it can be eliminated from the body. A low level of HDL increases the risk of cardiovascular disease.

Lipid Metabolism: Fat for Fuel and for Storage

Fatty acids can be used directly for energy or reassembled into triglycerides for storage. In muscle cells, fatty acids and glycerol from triglycerides are used primarily to produce ATP. The carbon chain of fatty acids is broken into two-carbon units that form acetyl-CoA and release high-energy electrons. Acetyl-CoA can then enter the citric acid cycle, which passes more high-energy electrons to the electron transport chain to generate ATP (Figure 5.14). The glycerol can also be used to produce ATP.

In adipose tissue cells, fatty acids are usually reassembled into triglycerides for storage. Throughout the day, stored triglycerides are continuously broken down and reformed depending on the immediate energy needs of the body. For example, after a meal some triglyceride will be stored; then, between meals some of the stored triglyceride will be broken down to provide energy. When the energy in the diet equals the body's energy requirements, the net amount of stored triglyceride in the body does not change.

Storing Fat for Future Use When energy is ingested in excess of needs, the excess can be converted into triglycerides and stored in adipose tissue. Excess dietary fat is transported directly to the adipose tissue in chylomicrons. Excess dietary carbohydrate and protein must first go to the liver, where they can be used, although inefficiently, to synthesize fatty acids; these fatty acids are then assembled into triglycerides, which are transported to the adipose tissue in VLDLs. Lipoprotein lipase at the membrane of cells lining the blood vessels breaks down the triglycerides from both chylomicrons and VLDLs so that the fatty acids can enter the cells, where they are reassembled into triglycerides for storage (Figure 5.15). The ability of the body to store fat is theoretically limitless. Fat cells can increase in weight by about 50 times, and new fat cells can be made when existing cells reach their maximum size (see Chapter 7).

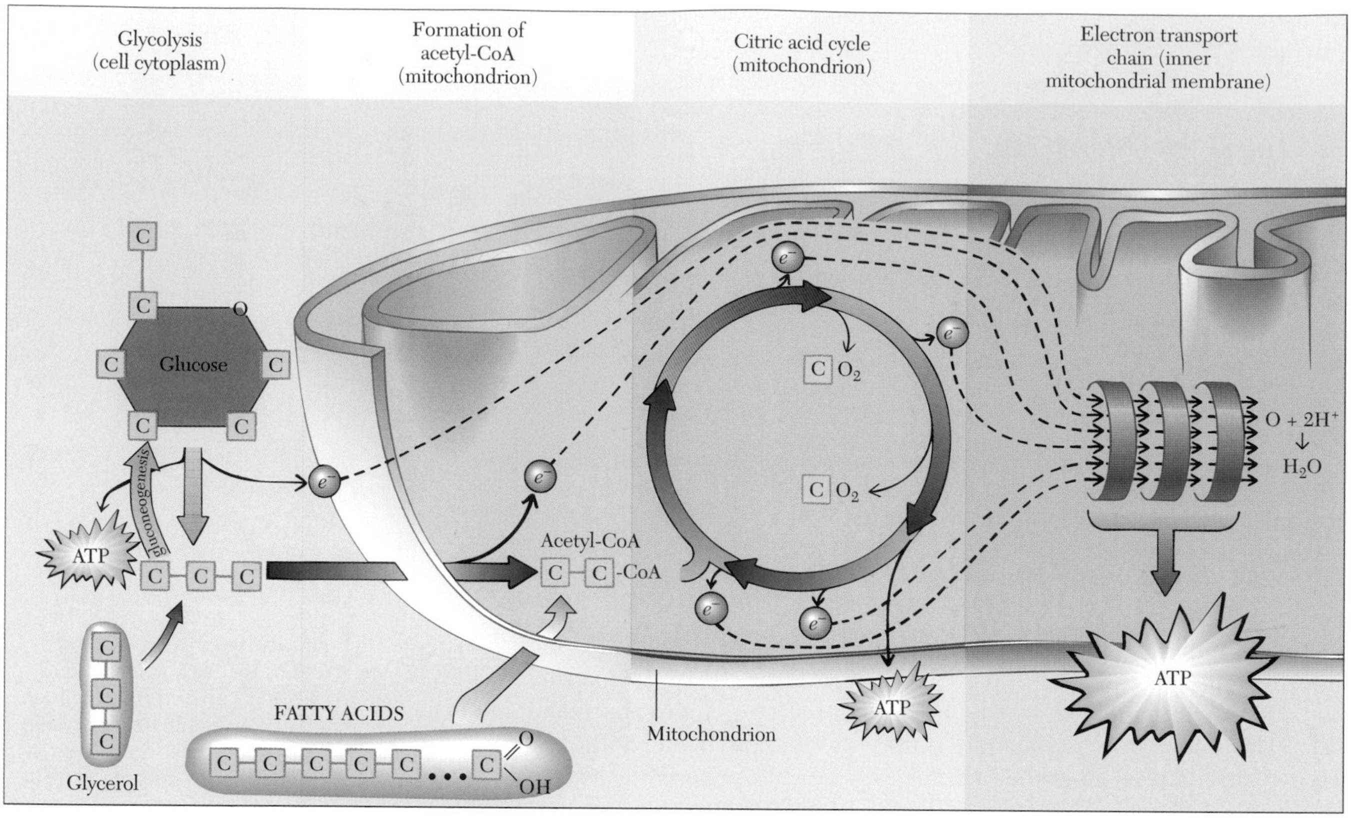

Glycolysis
(cell cytoplasm)

Formation of
acetyl-CoA
(mitochondrion)

Citric acid cycle
(mitochondrion)

Electron transport
chain (inner
mitochondrial membrane)

Glucose

ATP

Glycerol

FATTY ACIDS

Acetyl-CoA

Mitochondrion

ATP

$O + 2H^+$
$\downarrow$
H_2O

ATP

$C\ O_2$

$C\ O_2$

Figure 5.14

Triglycerides can be used to produce energy. Fatty acids break into two-carbon units and enter the citric acid cycle as acetyl-CoA. Glycerol is a three-carbon molecule that can be converted into pyruvate.

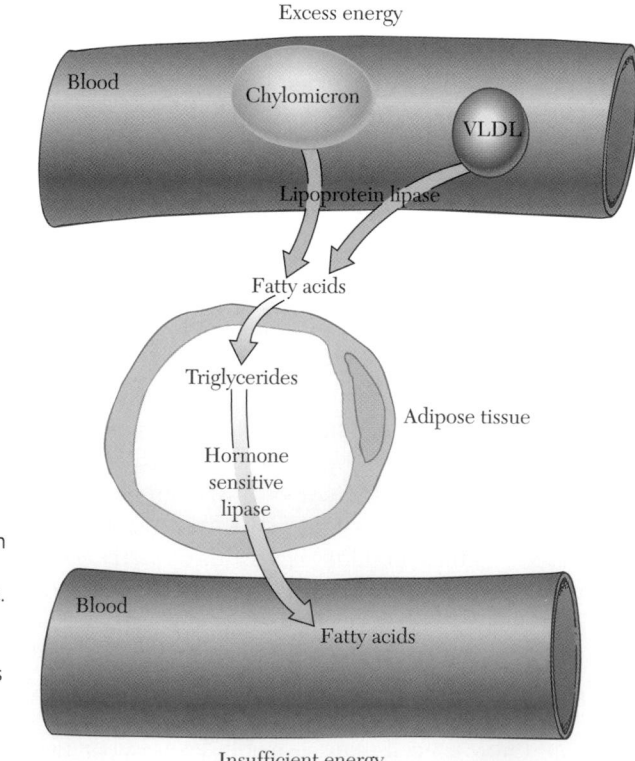

Figure 5.15

When excess dietary energy is available, lipoprotein lipase helps remove triglyceride from chylomicrons and VLDLs so it can be stored in adipose tissue. When dietary energy is insufficient, the enzyme hormone sensitive lipase helps break down stored triglycerides to make fatty acids available as an energy source.

Excess energy

Blood

Chylomicron

VLDL

Lipoprotein lipase

Fatty acids

Triglycerides

Adipose tissue

Hormone
sensitive
lipase

Blood

Fatty acids

Insufficient energy

Using Stored Fat When less energy is consumed than is needed, the body uses energy from fat stores. In this situation, the enzyme **hormone sensitive lipase** inside the fat cells receives a signal to break down stored triglycerides. The fatty acids and glycerol are released directly into the blood, where they can be taken up by cells throughout the body to produce ATP. If there is not enough carbohydrate to allow acetyl-CoA from fat breakdown to enter the citric acid cycle, it will be used to make ketones (see Chapter 4). Ketones can be used as an energy source by muscle and adipose tissue. During prolonged starvation, the brain can adapt to use ketones to meet about half of its energy needs. For the other half, it must use glucose. Fatty acids cannot be used to make glucose, and only a small amount of glucose can be made from glycerol.

Hormone sensitive lipase An enzyme present in adipose cells that responds to chemical signals by breaking down triglycerides into fatty acids and glycerol for release into the bloodstream.

• LIPIDS AND HEALTH

Adequate amounts of essential fatty acids are required in the diet to maintain normal body function. However, diets high in fat, particularly some types of fats, are associated with an increased risk for many chronic diseases. The development of **cardiovascular disease** has been linked to diets high in cholesterol, saturated fat, and *trans* fat.[4,5] And the risk of certain types of cancer, including that of the breast, colon, and prostate, has been associated with a high fat intake. Obesity is also associated with diets high in fat because these diets are usually high in energy and promote storage of body fat. Excess body fat in turn is associated with an increased risk of diabetes, cardiovascular disease, and high blood pressure.

Cardiovascular disease Any disease affecting the heart and blood vessels.

Essential Fatty Acid Deficiency

People often think of fat as unhealthy; however, if adequate amounts of linoleic and alpha-linolenic acid are not consumed, an **essential fatty acid deficiency** will result. Symptoms include scaly, dry skin, liver abnormalities, poor healing of wounds, growth failure in infants, and impaired vision and hearing. Essential fatty acid deficiency is rare because the requirement for essential fatty acids is well below the typical intake. Deficiencies have been seen in infants and young children fed lowfat diets, in individuals who are unable to absorb lipids, and in adults consuming a weight-loss diet consisting of only skim milk.

Essential fatty acid deficiency A condition characterized by dry scaly skin and poor growth that results when the diet does not supply sufficient amounts of the essential fatty acids.

Dietary Fat and Heart Disease

Over 61 million people in the United States suffer from some form of cardiovascular disease, which is any disease that affects the heart and blood vessels. It is the number one cause of death in the United States.[6] Epidemiologic studies have shown that diet and lifestyle both affect the risk of developing heart disease. The relationship between dietary fat and heart disease risk is one that has been extensively studied. In general, populations that consume high-fat diets have a higher incidence of heart disease,[5] but this does not always hold true. Populations that consume a diet high in omega-3 fatty acids, such as the Inuits in Greenland, have a low incidence of heart disease.[7] In Mediterranean countries, where the diet is high in monounsaturated fat as well as grains and vegetables, deaths from heart disease are also infrequent.[8]

ON THE WEB
The American Heart Association at www.americanheart.org/ provides information on heart disease, its risk factors, incidence, prevention, and treatment.

How Does Atherosclerosis Develop? **Atherosclerosis** is a type of cardiovascular disease in which lipids are deposited in the artery walls, reducing elasticity and eventually blocking the flow of blood. It was originally hypothesized that this was caused by dietary cholesterol transported into the bloodstream and deposited in the arteries.[9] Since this initial hypothesis, a great deal of research has been done to determine how cholesterol deposits form in arteries, how diet affects blood cholesterol levels, and whether changes in diet can decrease the risk of developing atherosclerosis.

Our current understanding of how atherosclerosis develops is based on the work of Michael Brown and Joseph Goldstein, who were awarded the Nobel Prize in 1985 for their discoveries. Their work identified LDL receptors on cells and demonstrated how they bind LDL particles in the blood, allowing them to be taken up by

Atherosclerosis A type of cardiovascular disease that involves the buildup of fatty material in the artery walls.

the cells and shutting off cholesterol synthesis in the body. When LDL particles enter body cells, the amount of LDL cholesterol in the blood is reduced. If the amount of LDL cholesterol in the blood exceeds the amount that can be taken up by cells—due to either too much LDL cholesterol or too few LDL receptors—the result is a high level of LDL cholesterol.[10] Excess LDL cholesterol in the blood can lead to the deposition of cholesterol in the artery walls, causing atherosclerosis.

The exact events that cause the buildup of cholesterol in arterial walls are still not fully understood. One theory is that an injury to the arterial wall—possibly caused by high blood pressure, high cholesterol levels, microorganisms, chemicals, or some other factor—begins the process. Once the initial injury has occurred, LDL particles, white blood cells, and blood cell fragments involved in blood clotting (called platelets) enter the artery wall. Inside the artery wall, LDL that comes in contact with highly reactive oxygen molecules is transformed into **oxidized LDL cholesterol**. Oxidized LDL cholesterol binds to scavenger receptors on the surface

Oxidized LDL cholesterol A substance formed when the cholesterol in LDL particles is oxidized by reactive oxygen molecules. It is key in the development of atherosclerosis because it is taken up by scavenger receptors on white blood cells.

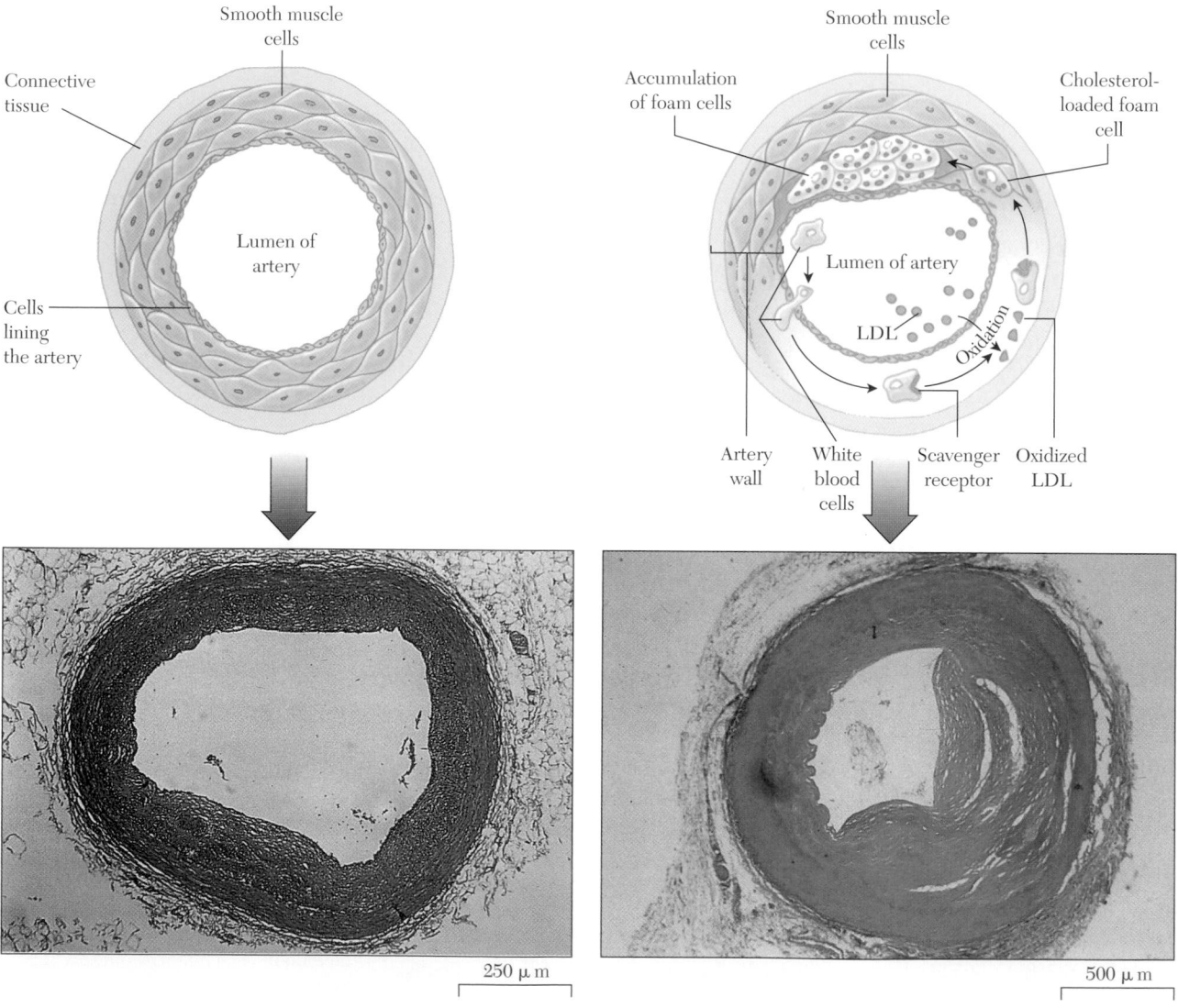

Figure 5.16

On the left are a drawing and photograph of a normal artery. On the right are a diagram showing the development of an atherosclerotic plaque and a photograph of a cross section of an artery partially blocked by atherosclerotic deposits. Plaque develops when white blood cells and LDL particles penetrate the artery wall. LDLs become oxidized and enter the white blood cells by binding to scavenger receptors. The cholesterol-filled white blood cells are transformed into foam cells that burst, depositing cholesterol in the artery wall. (*left*, © Cabisco/Visuals Unlimited; *right*, © Ober/Visuals Unlimited)

of white blood cells and is transported into these cells. As white blood cells fill with more and more oxidized LDL cholesterol, the white blood cells are transformed into cholesterol-filled foam cells. Foam cells accumulate in the artery wall and then burst, depositing cholesterol to form a fatty streak (Figure 5.16). Platelets signal muscle cells to invade the fatty streak and secrete fibrous proteins. The result is a mass of cholesterol, muscle cells, and fibrous tissue called a **plaque**. Eventually, calcium collects in the plaque and causes it to harden. Blood clots form around the plaque and it continues to enlarge, causing the artery to narrow and lose its elasticity. The buildup of material can become so large that it completely blocks the artery, or a blood clot can break loose and block an artery elsewhere. When an artery is blocked, blood can no longer move through it to supply oxygen and nutrients to the cells, and they die quickly. If blood flow to the heart muscle is interrupted, heart cells die, resulting in a heart attack or myocardial infarction. If the blood flow to the brain is interrupted, a stroke results.

Plaque The cholesterol-rich material that is deposited in the blood vessels of individuals with atherosclerosis. It consists of cholesterol, smooth muscle cells, fibrous tissue, and calcium.

Risk Factors for Heart Disease High blood pressure, diabetes, obesity, and high blood cholesterol levels directly increase the risk of developing heart disease. Other factors that affect risk include age, gender, genetics, and lifestyle factors such as smoking, exercise, and diet. These may directly affect risk or act indirectly by altering blood cholesterol levels, blood pressure, body weight, or the risk of diabetes (Table 5.1).

Diabetes, High Blood Pressure, Obesity, and Blood Cholesterol Levels Diabetes increases the risk of heart disease. The high levels of blood glucose that can occur with this disease cause damage to blood vessels. Elevated blood pressure can also increase risk by damaging blood vessels. In addition, high blood pressure forces the heart to work harder, causing it to enlarge and weaken over time. Obesity both

Table 5.1 *Factors That Affect Heart Disease Risk*

Age: Risk increases with increasing age.

Sex: Males have a higher risk until age 65; then risks do not differ between the sexes.

Disease factors:

Diabetes: fasting blood sugar greater than 126 mg/100 ml
High blood pressure: greater than 140/90
Obesity: body mass index greater than 27°
High blood lipid levels:

	Low Risk	Moderate Risk	High Risk
Total cholesterol (mg/100 ml)	< 200	200–239	≥ 240
LDL cholesterol (mg/100 ml)	< 130	130–159	≥ 160
HDL (mg/100 ml)	≥ 60	40–59	≤ 40

Lifestyle:

Risk is increased by:
  Cigarette smoking
  Stress
  A sedentary lifestyle
Risk is decreased by: regular exercise

Diet:

Risk is increased by:
  High total fat intake
  High saturated fat intake
  High cholesterol intake
  High intake of *trans* fatty acids
Risk is decreased by:
  A high intake of omega-3 fatty acids
  A high-fiber intake
  A diet high in fruits and vegetables
  A diet high in antioxidant nutrients such as vitamin E

°See Chapter 7 for information about body mass index and how it can be calculated.

increases the amount of work required by the heart and affects blood pressure, blood cholesterol levels, and the risk of diabetes. High blood cholesterol levels, and, in particular, high levels of LDL cholesterol, may also injure artery walls as well as promote plaque formation.

The desirable level for total blood cholesterol in adults is below 200 mg per 100 ml of blood. Optimal LDL levels are below 100 mg per 100 ml and risk increases as LDL levels rise. HDL cholesterol should be greater than 40 mg per 100 ml and risk decreases as HDL levels increase (see Appendix C).[11] Currently, about 51% of American adults have blood cholesterol levels of 200 or more, and 20% have values of 240 mg per 100 ml or greater.[12]

Age, Gender, Genetics, and Lifestyle Factors The risk of heart disease increases with age; four out of five people who die of heart disease are 65 or older. Men and women are both at risk, but men are generally affected a decade earlier than women. This is due in part to the protective effect of the hormone estrogen in women. As women age, the effects of menopause—including the decline in estrogen level and gain in weight—increase heart disease risk. Although it is unclear why, the incidence of heart disease among men has been declining since the 1950s, whereas the incidence among women has increased[13] (Figure 5.17).

Genetics, including ethnic background, also affect risk. Individuals with a male family member who exhibited heart disease before the age of 55 or a female family member who exhibited heart disease before the age of 65 are considered to be at greater risk. African Americans have a higher risk of heart disease than the general population because they are more likely to have high blood pressure. Mexican Americans, Native Americans and Hawaiians and some Asian Americans have higher risk, due in part to a higher incidence of diabetes and obesity in these groups.[12]

Age, gender, and genetics are risks that cannot be changed, but diet and lifestyle factors can be modified to reduce risk. Lifestyle factors that affect risk include activity level, smoking, and stress. An inactive lifestyle increases the risk of heart disease, as do cigarette smoking and stress. On the other hand, regular exercise decreases risk by promoting the maintenance of a healthy body weight, reducing the risk of diabetes, increasing HDL cholesterol, and reducing blood pressure. A number of dietary components, including the amount and type of fat, affect heart disease risk. Some dietary factors increase risk, while others offer a protective effect (see *Critical Thinking*: Dietary Fat and Heart Disease Risk).

Dietary Factors That Promote Heart Disease Excessive intake of cholesterol, saturated fat, *trans* fatty acids, and energy can increase the risk of cardiovascular disease. Some or all of their effect is due to their influence on blood cholesterol levels.

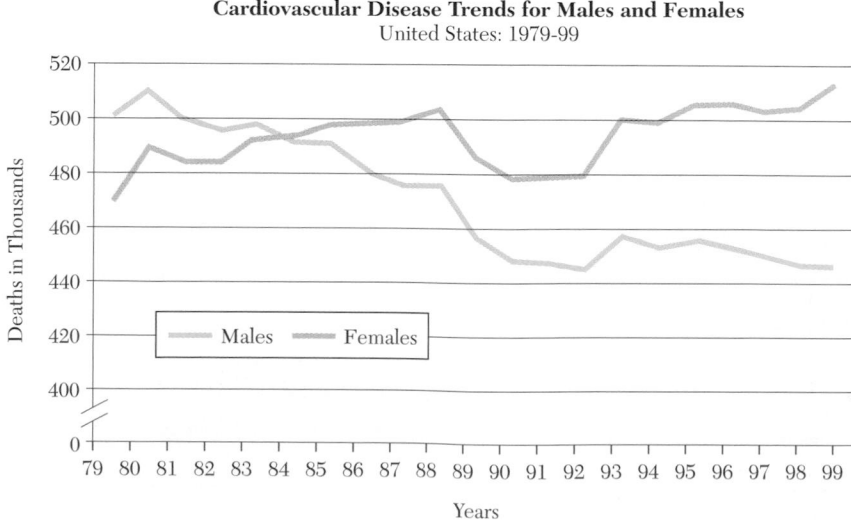

Figure 5.17

Deaths from cardiovascular disease have been decreasing for men but increasing for women. (*Source:* American Heart Association, *2002 Heart and Stroke Statistical Update.* Dallas, Tex.: American Heart Association, 2001.)

Dietary Cholesterol The extent to which cholesterol intake affects blood levels depends on an individual's genes. Cholesterol in the blood comes from cholesterol both consumed in the diet and made by the liver. Generally, about three to four times more cholesterol is made by the body than is consumed in the diet. In some individuals, as dietary cholesterol increases, liver cholesterol synthesis decreases so that blood levels do not change.[14] In others, however, liver synthesis does not decrease in response to an increase in dietary cholesterol, so blood cholesterol levels rise.

Saturated Fat Diets high in saturated fat increase LDL cholesterol in the blood. Increased LDL then increases the risk of atherosclerosis. When the diet is high in saturated fatty acids, liver production of cholesterol-carrying lipoproteins increases and the activity of LDL receptors in the liver is reduced, so that LDL cholesterol cannot be removed from the blood.[15] When the diet is low in saturated fats, lipoprotein production decreases and the number of LDL receptors increases, allowing more cholesterol to be removed from the bloodstream. There are some saturated fats, such as stearic acid found in chocolate and beef, that do not increase blood cholesterol levels. However, these may contribute to heart disease by affecting blood platelets and blood clotting, both of which are involved in plaque formation.[16]

Trans Fatty Acids Both clinical and epidemiological studies provide evidence that *trans* fatty acid intake increases the risk of heart disease. Some of the increase in risk is due to the effect of *trans* fatty acids on blood cholesterol levels. *Trans* fatty acid intake increases blood cholesterol levels less than an equivalent amount of saturated fatty acids but more than the same amount of polyunsaturated fatty acids.[17,18]

Excess Energy Excess energy intake increases the risk of heart disease because it increases body fat, which is a separate risk factor for elevated blood cholesterol levels, high blood pressure, diabetes, and heart disease in general. A reduction in body weight has been shown to reduce blood cholesterol levels, blood pressure, and heart disease risk, and to help control diabetes.

Dietary Factors That Protect Against Heart Disease Both omega-6 and omega-3 polyunsaturated fats as well as monounsaturated fat, plant foods, certain B vitamins, and moderate alcohol consumption tend to decrease the risk of heart disease. Some reduce risk by reducing LDL cholesterol and increasing HDL cholesterol. Some protect against heart disease in other ways.

Polyunsaturated Fat: Omega-6 and Omega-3 When saturated fat in the diet is replaced by any type of polyunsaturated fat, there is a beneficial decrease in LDL cholesterol.[19] However, a high intake of omega-6 polyunsaturated fatty acids may also decrease HDL cholesterol, which is undesirable in terms of heart disease risk. Omega-3 fatty acids have a similar effect on LDL levels but do not lower HDL cholesterol.[20] Studies show that replacing some of the fat in the diet with omega-3 polyunsaturated fatty acids reduces the incidence of heart disease. In addition to these effects on blood lipids, omega-3 fatty acids may reduce heart disease risk by preventing the growth of atherosclerotic plaque and by affecting blood clotting, blood pressure, and immune function.[21,22] The beneficial effects are greater when the omega-3 fatty acids are consumed in fish, such as salmon and tuna, rather than in supplements (Table 5.2).[23]

Monounsaturated Fat Populations with diets high in monounsaturated fats, such as those in Mediterranean countries where olive oil is commonly used, have a mortality rate from heart disease that is half of that in the United States. This is true even when total fat intake provides 40% or more of energy intake.[24] Substituting monounsaturated fat for saturated fat reduces LDL cholesterol without decreasing HDL cholesterol and makes LDL cholesterol less susceptible to oxidation.[20] However, the type of fat in the diet is unlikely to be the only factor responsible for the difference in the in-

Table 5.2 Omega-3 Fatty Acid Content of Fish and Seafood

Food*	Omega-3 Fatty Acids (g)
Swordfish	1.16
Salmon	1.16
Trout	1.16
Sole	0.44
Cod	0.44
Shrimp	0.27
Mussels	0.26
Clams	0.26
Tuna, canned	0.23
Lobster	0.07

*All values represent amounts in a 3-oz cooked portion.

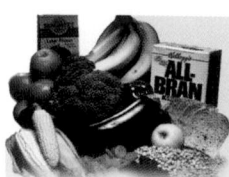

Off the Shelf
Are Supplements a Safe Way to Reduce Blood Cholesterol?

Is your blood cholesterol a little high, or are you trying to keep it from getting there? A trip to the drugstore will reveal a whole host of over-the-counter cholesterol-lowering remedies ranging from fibers and vitamins to garlic and phytochemicals. Could you benefit from one of these? Do they work? What are the risks?

Fiber Supplements The safest supplements for lowering cholesterol are probably soluble fibers such as psyllium, pectin, guar gum, or locust bean gum. Many studies have shown that fiber supplements lower total and LDL cholesterol in those with elevated levels. One study found that consumption of about 10 g of psyllium per day lowered total cholesterol by 4% and LDL cholesterol by 7% without affecting HDL cholesterol.[1] The effectiveness of a fiber supplement depends on how the fiber is processed and thus varies with the brand. An alternative to fiber supplements is to increase intake of high-fiber foods such as beans, whole oats, and fruit. These add not only soluble fiber to the diet but also the nutrients and phytochemicals present in these foods.

Niacin Niacin is a vitamin that can lower blood cholesterol. Doses of 2 to 3 g per day of a form of the vitamin called nicotinic acid have been shown to lower LDL cholesterol and raise HDL cholesterol.[2,3] But at doses this high, niacin is not really a vitamin—it is a drug. The amount used to treat high blood cholesterol is more than 50 times higher than the Tolerable Upper Intake Level (UL) of 35 mg per day that has been set for adults.[4] High doses can cause liver damage, ulcers, impaired glucose tolerance, headaches, flushing, nausea, heartburn, and diarrhea. Although readily available over the counter, niacin should not be taken at these high doses without a doctor's supervision.

Garlic Garlic has been used medicinally for centuries. Many health-promoting phytochemicals have now been identified in garlic, and today one of the promises used to market garlic supplements is that they will lower blood cholesterol. The results of studies on the effectiveness of garlic have not been consistent—some reports have found that garlic supplements are effective at reducing blood cholesterol,[5,6] whereas others have found no effect.[7,8] The doses used in these studies are equivalent to consuming one or more cloves of raw garlic daily. The primary side effect of this is a strong garlic body odor. Garlic supplements are available as capsules containing garlic extract or garlic oil and as garlic powder or garlic powder tablets. Some of these preparations are odorless.

Phytochemicals Phytosterols are phytochemicals that are marketed for their cholesterol-lowering effects. Phytosterols are plant sterols that resemble cholesterol chemically, making it difficult for the digestive tract to distinguish them from cholesterol. They are believed to lower blood cholesterol by inhibiting cholesterol absorption.[9] A Western diet provides about 200 to 400 mg of phytosterols a day from foods such as soybeans, wheat, and rice.[10] Intakes of 1500 to 3000 mg a day have been shown to reduce total cholesterol and LDL cholesterol levels in the blood and to have no effect on HDL cholesterol. A tablet of the phytosterol supplement Cholestatin contains 380 mg, so it would take four to eight tablets a day to supply the amounts that have been shown to reduce cholesterol in these studies. Phytosterols have been incorporated into several brands of margarine, including Take Control and Benecol. When sufficient quantities are consumed, these spreads lower blood cholesterol.[11] No side effects have been reported with phytosterol consumption.[9]

Phytochemicals called tocotrienols, which are related to vitamin E, have also been sold to lower cholesterol. They are found in rice, oat bran, and barley. They

cidence of heart disease between the Mediterranean countries and the United States. As already mentioned, the Mediterranean diet is higher in fruits and vegetables, lower in animal products, includes more wine, and is consumed in countries where the lifestyle includes more day-to-day activity and has fewer of the stresses of modern life. (See Appendix H for the Mediterranean Food Guide Pyramid.)

Plant Foods: Fiber and Antioxidants Epidemiology has shown that a diet high in plant foods is associated with a lower risk of heart disease. Plant foods such as fruits, vegetables, grains, and legumes are a good source of fiber, vitamins, minerals, and phytochemicals. Different types and amounts of dietary fiber can affect blood cholesterol levels. As discussed in Chapter 4, some fibers, such as those in oat bran, legumes, psyllium, pectin, and gums, have been shown to reduce blood cholesterol levels. In addition, many of the vitamins, minerals, and phytochemicals in plant foods have antioxidant functions. Antioxidants are postulated to protect against plaque formation by decreasing the formation of oxidized LDL cholesterol[25] (see *Off the Shelf*: Are Supplements a Safe Way to Reduce Blood Cholesterol?).

are believed to lower cholesterol by interfering with the liver's ability to make it. One study found that a dose of 200 mg a day for a month lowered LDL cholesterol by 13% in subjects with high cholesterol.[12] Tocotrienols have the potential to lower blood cholesterol, but obtaining these effects would require taking four to eight times the dosage recommended on supplement packages.

If You Choose to Use Supplements The use of any type of dietary supplement should be discussed with your doctor. These products are not tested as extensively as drugs, so less is known about their safety and effectiveness. In addition, they may affect other treatments. For example, Cholestin, a supplement made from Chinese red yeast rice, contains the chemical lovastatin. Lovastatin is the active ingredient in some prescription cholesterol-lowering medications. Unlike prescription lovastatin, the amount of this drug in each dose of Cholestin is not regulated and may vary. Lovastatin can cause serious side effects and should not be used by people with infections or organ transplants and by those who consume more than two alcoholic beverages a day.

Cholesterol-lowering supplements should not take the place of adequate ex-ercise and a diet low in saturated fat and cholesterol and high in fiber, fruits, vegetables, and whole grains. Most of the active ingredients contained in these supplements can be obtained from a healthy diet. This type of diet benefits not only blood cholesterol levels but blood pressure, body weight, and cancer risk as well.

[1]Anderson, J. W., Allgood, L. D., Lawrence, A., et al. Cholesterol-lowering effects of psyllium intake adjunctive to diet therapy in men and women with hypercholesterolemia: Meta-analysis of 8 controlled trials. *Am. J. Clin. Nutr.* 71:472–479, 2000.

[2]O'Connor, P. J., Rush, W. A., and Trence, D. L. Relative effectiveness of niacin and lovastatin for treatment of dyslipidemias in a health maintenance organization. *J. Fam. Pract.* 44:462–467, 1997.

[3]McKenney, J. M., McCormick, L. S., Weiss, S., et al. A randomized trial of the effects of atorvastatin and niacin in patients with combined hyperlipidemia or isolated hypertriglyceridemia. Collaborative Atorvastin Study Group. *Am. J. Med.* 104:137–143, 1998.

[4]Institute of Medicine, Food and Nutrition Board. *Dietary Reference Intakes for Thiamin, Riboflavin, Niacin, Vitamin B_6, Folate, Vitamin B_{12}, Pantothenic Acid, Biotin, and Choline.* Washington, D.C.: National Academy Press. 1998.

[5]Adler, A. J., and Holub, B. J. Effect of garlic and fish oil supplementation on serum lipid and lipoprotein concentrations in hypercholes-terolemic men. *Am. J. Clin. Nutr.* 65:445–450, 1997.

[6]Bordia, A., Verma, S. K., and Srivastava, K. C. Effect of garlic (*Allium sativum*) on blood lipids, blood sugar, fibrinogen and fibrinolytic activity in patients with coronary artery disease. *Prostaglandins Leukot. Essent. Fatty Acids* 58:257–263, 1998.

[7]Berthold, H. K., Sudhop, T., and von Bergmann, K. Effect of garlic oil preparation on serum lipoproteins and cholesterol metabolism: A randomized controlled trial. *JAMA* 279: 1900–1902, 1998.

[8]Isaacsohn, J. L., Moser, M., Stein, E. A., et al. Garlic powder and plasma lipids and lipoproteins: A multicenter, randomized, placebo-controlled trial. *Arch. Intern. Med.* 158:1189–1194, 1998.

[9]Ling, W. W., and Jones, P. J. Dietary phytosterols: A review of metabolism, benefits and side effects. *Life Sci.* 57:195–206, 1995.

[10]Jones, P. J., MacDougall, D. E., Ntanios, F., and Vanstone, C. A. Dietary phytosterols as cholesterol-lowering agents in humans. *Can J. Physiol. Pharmacol.* 75:217–227, 1997.

[11]Weststrate, J. A., and Meijer, G. W. Plant sterol–enriched margarines and reduction of plasma total- and LDL-cholesterol concentrations in normocholesterolemic and mildly hypercholesterolemic subjects. *Eur. J. Clin. Nutr.* 52:334–343, 1998.

[12]Qureshi, A. A., Bradlow, B. A., Brace, L., et al. Response of hypercholesterolemic subjects to administration of tocotrienols. *Lipids* 30:1171–1177, 1995.

B Vitamins The effect of certain B vitamins on heart disease risk is related to their effect on blood levels of the amino acid homocysteine. High homocysteine levels are associated with a higher incidence of heart disease.[26] Vitamin B_6, B_{12}, and folic acid are needed to break down homocysteine. Studies have shown that higher levels of B vitamins in the blood are related to lower levels of homocysteine. The recent fortification of the American grain supply with folic acid has shown a reduction in blood homocysteine levels in the population.[27] There is not sufficient evidence on the relationship between intake of these vitamins and homocysteine to recommend supplements, but a diet high in grains, fruits, and vegetables is recommended to assure adequate intake.

Moderate Alcohol Consumption Moderate alcohol consumption has been shown to reduce stress, to raise levels of HDL cholesterol, and to reduce blood clotting. This has a protective effect against heart disease. Some of the protection may also be due to compounds in red wine known as phenols, which are antioxidants that protect against lipoprotein oxidation, thereby preventing the development of atherosclerotic plaques.[28] The Dietary Guidelines recognize that in men over age 45 and women over age 55, moderate drinking can lower the risk of heart disease. Moderate drinking is defined as no more than one drink per day for women and two drinks per day for men. One drink is defined as 12 ounces of beer, 5 ounces of wine, or 1.5 ounces of 80-proof distilled spirits. Greater intake of alcohol increases the risk of accidental deaths, heart disease, cancer, birth defects, and drug interactions and should be avoided. Alcohol consumption is not recommended for children or adolescents, pregnant women, individuals who cannot restrict their drinking to a moderate amount, or individuals who plan to drive or perform other activities that require concentration.

Dietary Fat and Cancer

Cancer is the second leading cause of death in the United States, and it is estimated that 30 to 40% of cancers are directly linked to dietary choices.[29] As with cardiovascular disease, there is a body of epidemiological evidence correlating diet and lifestyle with the incidence of cancer. Diets high in fat and low in fiber and plant foods are correlated with an increased risk of cancer.[17] The mechanism whereby a high intake of dietary fat increases the incidence of various cancers is less well understood than the relationship between dietary fat and cardiovascular disease; however, dietary fat has been suggested to be both a tumor promoter and tumor initiator.

Dietary Fat and Breast Cancer Breast cancer is the leading form of cancer in women worldwide. In the United States, it affects 182,000 women annually. The incidence is similar among all ethnic groups, but the mortality is higher among minority women. Breast cancer is more common in postmenopausal women, in women who have had no children or who had children late in life, and in women with a family history of the disease. In populations where the diet is high in fat and low in fiber, the incidence of breast cancer is high. In populations where the typical fat intake is low, the incidence is lower and the survival rate is better in people with the disease. Currently, several major studies are under way to determine if reducing fat intake to less than 15% of energy will reduce breast cancer risk or mortality.

As is the case with heart disease, the type of fat is as important as the total amount of fat in determining risk. The incidence of breast cancer in Mediterranean women who rely on olive oil, which is high in monounsaturated fat, as a source of dietary fat is low despite a total fat intake similar to that in the United States.[30] Epidemiology also supports a protective effect from an increased intake of omega-3 fatty acids from fish, such as in the native Eskimos of Alaska and Greenland.[31] A higher intake of *trans* fatty acids found in foods such as stick margarines, however, may increase the risk of breast cancer.[32]

The mechanism by which diet affects breast cancer has been studied in laboratory animals. Since most laboratory animals do not get breast cancer tumors, studies are conducted by implanting breast tumors and examining how diet affects their growth. The tumors are more likely to grow in mice fed a high-fat diet than in those fed a lowfat diet. The type of fat also affects tumor growth; diets high in linoleic acid, which is found in polyunsaturated vegetable oils, are stronger tumor promoters than diets high in saturated fatty acids or omega-3 fatty acids.[33] However, to date, these animal studies have not been supported by human trials.[1]

Diet and Colon Cancer Epidemiology has correlated the incidence of colon cancer with high-fat, low-fiber diets. The correlation is stronger for diets high in animal fats, in particular those from red meats.[32] The connection between dietary fat and colon cancer may be related to the breakdown products of fat in the large intestine. Here, bacteria metabolize dietary fat and bile, producing substances that may cause mutations. These mutation-producing substances, or mutagens, may act as tumor initia-

ON THE WEB

For information on nutrition and cancer prevention, go to the American Cancer Society at

www2.cancer.org/

or the American Institute for Cancer Research at

www.aicr.org/

tors. A high intake of fiber tends to dilute these mutagens by increasing the volume of feces. High-fiber diets also decrease transit time. Both of these effects reduce the exposure of the intestinal mucosa to the hazardous substances (see Chapter 4).

CRITICAL THINKING

Dietary Fat and Heart Disease Risk

Rafael's mother died of a heart attack at age 60. Rafael is worried about his own heart disease risk, so he makes an appointment with his physician. He fills out a questionnaire about his medical history and lifestyle, meets with a dietitian to evaluate his diet, and has blood drawn for cholesterol analysis. The table below summarizes factors that may affect Rafael's risk of developing heart disease:

▼

Sex	Male
Age	35
Family history	Mother had heart attack at age 60.
Height/weight	68 inches/160 lb
Blood pressure	120/70
Stress level	Moderate
Smoker	Yes
Activity level	Sedentary
Blood values	
Total cholesterol	210 mg/100 ml
LDL cholesterol	160 mg/100 ml
HDL cholesterol	34 mg/100 ml
Typical daily intake from three-day food record:	
Percent energy from fat	39
Percent energy from saturated fat	17
Percent energy from polyunsaturated fat	7
Cholesterol	350 mg/day
Servings from groups of the Food Guide Pyramid:	
Bread, Cereals, Rice, & Pasta	11
Vegetable	2
Fruit	1
Milk, Yogurt, & Cheese	2
Meat, Poultry, Fish, Dry Beans, Eggs, & Nuts	4

What risk factors does Rafael have for developing cardiovascular disease?

▼

He smokes cigarettes. He is inactive.
Other answers:

What dietary and lifestyle changes would you recommend to reduce his risks?

▼

He could quit smoking.
Other answers:

If Rafael were to replace all of the added fat in his diet with olive oil, would he reduce his risk of cardiovascular disease to the level found in Mediterranean countries?

▼

Answer:

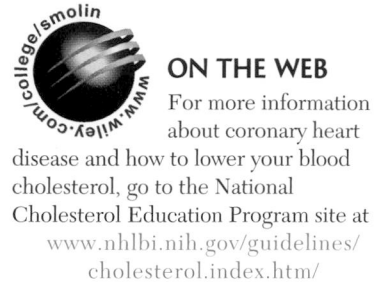

ON THE WEB

For more information about coronary heart disease and how to lower your blood cholesterol, go to the National Cholesterol Education Program site at www.nhlbi.nih.gov/guidelines/cholesterol.index.htm/

• LIPIDS: ONE PART OF THE TOTAL DIET

About 33% of the energy in the typical North American diet comes from lipids.[34] This is within the range of acceptable fat intakes for healthy adults. However, a healthy diet must also limit certain types of fats, provide adequate intakes of others, and include plenty of whole grains, vegetables, and fruits, which are high in fiber, micronutrients, and phytochemicals.

Recommendations for Fat Intake

The DRIs concluded that there is not sufficient evidence to set EAR, AI, or RDA values for total fat for adults or to establish a UL. However, an acceptable range of fat intake of 20 to 35% of energy has been recommended for adults. Specific guidelines have not been set for cholesterol, saturated fat, or *trans* fat, but it is recommended that intake of these be kept to a minimum because the risk of heart disease increases with higher intake. AI values have been established for the essential fatty acids based on the amounts consumed by the healthy U.S. population. The AI for linoleic acid is 12 grams per day for women and 17 grams per day for men. For α-linolenic acid, the AI is 1.1 grams per day for women and 1.6 grams per day for men. Rather than a UL, acceptable ranges of intake of 5 to 10% of energy for linoleic acid and 0.6 to 1.2% of energy for α-linolenic acid (with 10% or less of this as EPA and DHA) have been set.[1] These levels are consistent with the World Health Organization recommendation of a ratio of linoleic to α-linolenic acid in the diet between 5:1 and 10:1.[35]

The Dietary Guidelines also recommend a diet low in saturated fat and cholesterol and moderate in total fat (Figure 5.18). The Daily Values on food labels give more specific recommendations: less than 30% of energy as fat, no more than 300 mg of cholesterol per day, and no more than 10% of energy as saturated fat. Labels are not yet required to list *trans* fat but labeling regulations are being modified to include these.[36]

Recommendations for Special Groups In addition to these general recommendations for fat intake, some dietary recommendations are made to target specific diseases such as heart disease and cancer (see Appendix G). The National Cholesterol Education Program (NCEP) is a federally sponsored program that has developed recommendations for monitoring and controlling blood cholesterol levels. The NCEP recommends that individuals with blood cholesterol levels in the moderate risk category (see Table 5.1) and who have heart disease or two other risk factors for heart disease, begin the Step I dietary program (shown in Table 5.3).[37] If, after 6 months of consuming this diet, blood cholesterol levels have not decreased, the Step II diet is recommended. The NCEP also recommends drug therapy for individuals with extremely high cholesterol levels or for those for whom diet therapy fails. The most prominent drugs used to treat elevated cholesterol are those in the statin family, such as lovastatin (Mevacor), atorvastatin (Lipitor), and pravastatin (Pravachol). These work by blocking cholesterol synthesis in the liver and by increasing the capacity of the liver to remove cholesterol from the blood. Drugs such as cholestyramine (Questran) and colestipol (Colestid) act in the gastrointestinal tract by preventing cholesterol and bile absorption. Nictotinic acid, a form of the B vitamin niacin, can also be used to lower blood cholesterol.

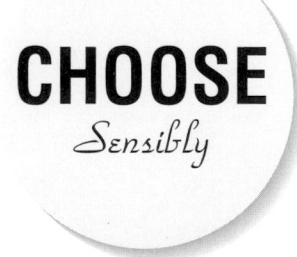

CHOOSE
Sensibly

Choose a diet that is low in saturated fat and cholesterol and moderate in total fat.

Figure 5.18

The Dietary Guidelines for Americans recommend a diet low in saturated fat and cholesterol and moderate in total fat. (USDA, DHHS, 2000)

Table 5.3 *National Cholesterol Education Program Step I and Step II Diets**

	Recommended Intake	
Nutrient	Step I	Step II
Total fat†	30% or less	30% or less
Saturated fatty acids†	8–10%	Less than 7%
Cholesterol	Less than 300 mg/day	Less than 200 mg/day
Sodium	Up to 2400 mg	Up to 2400 mg
Total energy	To achieve and maintain desired weight	To achieve and maintain desired weight

*Adapted from National Cholesterol Education Program. Available online at www.nhlbisupport.com/cgi-bin/chd1/step1intro.cgi.

†Values are % of total energy intake.

The American Heart Association has also developed a set of dietary guidelines to reduce the risk of heart disease. Many are similar to the recommendations of the NCEP, but they try to focus on foods rather than on the percentage of energy from fat or the milligrams of cholesterol. These recommend a diet rich in fruits, vegetables, legumes (beans), whole grains, lowfat dairy products, fish, lean meats, and poultry. In addition, they recommend 2 weekly servings of fatty fish, such as tuna or salmon, which are good sources of omega-3 fatty acids.[38]

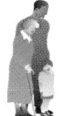 **Guidelines for Life Stages** The acceptable ranges of fat intake are higher for children than for adults: 30 to 40% of energy for ages 1 to 3 years, and 25 to 35% of energy for ages 3 to 18 years. These levels are higher than for adults because fat provides a concentrated energy source and a higher fat diet can more easily meet energy needs, especially in young children who can consume only small amounts of food. These recommendations meet the needs for growth and are unlikely to increase the risk of chronic disease. There is an AI for total fat for infants; 31 grams per day for those ages 0 to 6 months and 30 grams per day for ages 7 to 12 months, based on the amount of fat typically consumed in breast milk. AIs have been set for the essential fatty acids for each of the life stage groups in children (see inside cover). As with adults, a healthy diet that meets these needs should be based on whole grain products, fruits, vegetables, lowfat dairy products, legumes, and lean meats. The American Academy of Pediatrics specifies a lower limit of 20% of energy from total fat for children and adolescents.[39]

The acceptable ranges of fat intake are not increased during pregnancy or lactation, but the AIs for essential fatty acids are slightly higher than those for nonpregnant women. Recommendations are not different for older adults. In this population, fat intake must be carefully balanced with other nutrients to reduce the risk of malnutrition (see Chapter 16).

Determining Your Fat Intake

How does your diet compare with the recommendation of 20 to 35% of energy from fat? To calculate fat intake as a percent of energy, you need to know the number of grams of fat in the diet and how much energy is consumed (Table 5.4). The same equation can be used to calculate the percent of energy from fat in individual foods.

Databases and food composition tables provide information on the number of grams of fat contained in a wide variety of foods. Food labels provide a more accessible source of information on packaged foods (see *Off the Label*: Using Food Labels to Choose Your Fats). Unfortunately, food labels are not always available on fresh meats, which are one of the main contributors of fat in our diets.

Table 5.4 *Calculating Percent of Energy from Fat*

Determine
- The total energy (kcalorie) intake for the day
- The grams of fat in the day's diet

Calculate Energy from Fat
- Fat provides 9 kcalories per g
- Multiply grams of fat by 9 kcalories per g

$$\text{Kcalories from fat} = \text{grams fat} \times 9 \text{ kcalories/gram fat}$$

Calculate % Energy from Fat
- Divide energy from fat by total energy and multiply by 100 to express as a percent

$$\text{Percent of energy from fat} = \frac{\text{kcalories from fat}}{\text{total kcalories}} \times 100$$

For example:

A diet contains 2000 kcalories and 75 g of fat

$$75 \text{ g of fat} \times 9 \text{ kcal/g} = 675 \text{ kcalories from fat}$$

$$\frac{675 \text{ kcal from fat}}{2000 \text{ kcal}} \times 100 = 34\% \text{ of energy (kcal) from fat}$$

The Exchange Lists can be used to give a quick estimate of the total amount of fat in a food or in the diet (Table 5.5; Appendix I). An exchange of fruits, vegetables, or breads contains 1 gram or less. The amount of fat in an exchange of dairy products depends on what items you choose to consume. A serving of nonfat milk provides less than a gram of fat, but a serving of whole milk contains 8 grams. Likewise, the amount of fat in a meat exchange depends on your choice; a very lean meat such as turkey breast contains 1 gram of fat or less, whereas a serving of bologna contains 8 grams. An exchange from the fat list contains 5 grams of fat (see *Critical Thinking*: Fitting Fat into Your Diet).

Table 5.5 *Fat Content of the Exchange Lists*

Exchange Groups/Lists	Serving Size	Fat (g)
Carbohydrate Group		
Starch	½ cup pasta, rice, cereal, potatoes; 1 slice bread	0–1
Fruit	1 small apple, peach, pear; ½ banana; ½ cup canned fruit (in juice)	0
Milk	1 cup milk or yogurt	
Nonfat		0
Lowfat		2–3
Reduced-fat		5
Whole		8
Other carbohydrates	Serving sizes vary	Varies
Vegetables	½ cup cooked vegetables, 1 cup raw	0
Meat/Meat Substitute Group	1 oz meat or cheese, ½ cup legumes	
Very lean		0–1
Lean		3
Medium fat		5
High fat		8
Fat Group	1 tsp butter, margarine, or oil; 1 Tbsp salad dressing	5

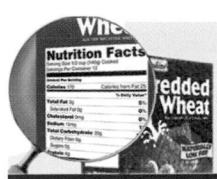

Off the Label
Using Food Labels to Choose Your Fats

The information about fat on food labels is designed to make it easier to identify the amounts and types of fat in foods. Understanding how to use this information can help consumers make more informed choices about the fats they include in their diet.

Food labels provide a number of different types of information concerning the fat in a food. The ingredient list includes the source of fat, such as corn oil, soybean oil, coconut oil, or partially hydrogenated vegetable oil, and the Nutrition Facts section provides the number of kcalories from fat, the number of grams of fat and saturated fat, and the number of milligrams of cholesterol in a serving. These are also presented as a percent of the Daily Value. Daily Values are calculated for a diet containing 2000 kcalories and are based on the recommendation that the diet should contain no more than 30% of energy from fat (about 65 grams), no more than 10% from saturated fat (20 g), and no more than 300 mg of cholesterol per day. The percent Daily Value allows consumers to tell at a glance how one food will fit into the recommendations for fat intake for the day. For example, if a serving provides 50% of the Daily Value for fat—that is, half the recommended maximum daily intake for a 2000-kcalorie diet—the rest of the day's intake will have to be carefully selected to not exceed the recommended maximum.

The amount of monounsaturated and polyunsaturated fat is voluntarily included on the labels of some products. For example, in addition to listing the 2 grams of saturated fat, the label on a bottle of olive oil may indicate that it contains 2 grams of polyunsaturated fat and 10 grams of monounsaturated fat per tablespoon. (There are no Daily Values for polyunsaturated and monounsaturated fat.) The amount of *trans* fat in a product is included in the total fat value but currently is not listed separately. Identifying foods low in *trans* fat is not easy. Some foods are labeled "*trans* free," and products likely to contain *trans* fats can be identified by looking at the ingredient list for partially hydrogenated vegetable oil. Many, but not all, partially hydrogenated oils are high in *trans* fat. At present, there is no way to determine exactly how much *trans* fat a product contains, but the FDA is in the process of revising labeling standards.

Food labels may also include terms such as "fat free," "low cholesterol," or "lean." These descriptors are added by manufacturers trying to capitalize on the public's interest in decreasing fat intake. To make these descriptors helpful to consumers as well as to manufacturers, food labeling regulations have developed standard definitions for these terms. For instance, a product labeled "lowfat" cannot contain more than 3 grams of fat in a serving (see table). So reduced-fat (2%) milk, which contains 5 grams of fat per cup, cannot be labeled as lowfat, whereas 1% milk, with only 2.5 grams per cup, does fit the definition. These terms can be used only in ways that do not confuse consumers. For instance, since saturated fat in the diet raises blood cholesterol, a food that is low in cholesterol but high in saturated fat, such as crackers containing coconut oil, cannot be labeled "low cholesterol" because it may actually raise blood cholesterol. Currently, the level of *trans* fat, a fat that increases the risk of heart disease, is considered when a food claims to be "saturated-fat free," but a product that is high in *trans* fat can claim to be "low cholesterol."

A component of food labels that may be confusing to consumers is the claim that a product is a certain percent fat free. This refers to percent by weight, not of energy. To avoid deception, labeling laws require that a product can claim to be a certain percent fat free only if it is also a fat-free or lowfat food. For example, lowfat hot dogs that are labeled 97% fat free contain 1.5 grams of fat per serving and therefore meet the definition of a lowfat food. Although packaged meats must be labeled, fresh raw meats such as steaks, which are one of the greatest contributors of fat, are not required to carry standard labels. Labels on ground beef can be particularly misleading because they may mention a certain "% lean." In this case "% lean" refers to the weight of the meat that is lean. So when the label says it is 78% lean, it means that 22% of the weight of the meat is fat, or that there are 22 grams of fat in 3.5 ounces (100 g) of raw hamburger. This works out to about 55% of energy as fat. Only ground beef that is 90% lean or greater meets the government's definition of lean—less than 10 grams of fat per serving.

Descriptors Related to Fat and Cholesterol

Descriptor	Definition
Fat free	Contains less than 0.5 gram of fat per serving.
Lowfat	Contains 3 grams or less of fat per serving.
Percent fat free	May be used only to describe foods that meet the definition of fat free or lowfat.
Reduced or less fat	Contains at least 25% less fat per serving than the regular or reference product.
Saturated fat free	Contains less than 0.5 gram of saturated fat per serving and less than 0.5 gram *trans* fatty acids per serving.
Low saturated fat	Contains 1 gram or less of saturated fat and not more than 15% of kcalories from saturated fat per serving.
Reduced or less saturated fat	Contains at least 25% less saturated fat than the regular or reference product.
Cholesterol free	Contains less than 2 mg of cholesterol and 2 grams or less of saturated fat per serving.
Low cholesterol	Contains 20 mg or less of cholesterol and 2 grams or less of saturated fat per serving.
Reduced or less cholesterol	Contains at least 25% less cholesterol than the regular or reference product and 2 grams or less of saturated fat per serving.
Lean	Contains less than 10 grams of fat, 4.5 grams or less of saturated fat, and less than 95 mg of cholesterol per serving and per 100 grams.
Extra lean	Contains less than 5 grams of fat, less than 2 grams of saturated fat, and less than 95 mg of cholesterol per serving and per 100 grams.

A Diet to Meet Recommendations: Choose Fats Wisely

Choosing a diet that limits *trans* fat, saturated fat, and cholesterol provides the AIs for essential fatty acids, and meets the recommendations for other nutrients sounds like an overwhelming task. In reality, meal planning does not need to be that difficult. Following the guidelines of the Food Guide Pyramid and checking food labels can help provide a diet that meets all of these specifications. There are also many fat-modified products on the market that may be helpful in meeting recommendations for fat intake.

Fat in the Food Guide Pyramid The concentration of high-fat choices in each of the Food Guide Pyramid groups is indicated by a circle (●) symbol (Figure 5.19). There are few of these at the base of the Pyramid. Grain products, vegetables, and fruits are naturally low in fat as long as fat is not added in preparation. The choices you make within these groups can significantly affect the fat content and nutrient density of your diet. For example, within the grain group, choosing high-fat baked goods such as doughnuts, cookies, and muffins adds more fat and energy and fewer nutrients than whole grain breads, rice, and pasta. Within the Fruit Group, fresh fruits are a lowfat choice while fruits that are baked into pies and tarts add fat and refined sugar. Most fresh vegetables have little or no fat, but fried vegetables such as french fries and fried onion rings are high in fat and energy (Table 5.6).

The food groups closer to the top of the Food Guide Pyramid—the Milk, Yogurt, & Cheese Group and the Meat, Poultry, Fish, Dried Beans, Eggs, & Nuts Group—contain more high-fat choices. The animal foods in these groups contain saturated fat and are the only source of cholesterol in the diet. To reduce your saturated fat and cholesterol intake, choose lowfat or nonfat dairy products; choose lean meats, such as chicken, turkey, flank and round steak; and use vegetable sources of protein such as legumes.

The most concentrated sources of fat—oils, butter, margarine, and salad dressings—are separated into the narrow tip of the Pyramid. These should be added sparingly to the diet. To reduce your total fat consumption, limit the amount of fat added to food at the table and in cooking. Many lowfat and nonfat salad dressings and spreads are available that offer the taste and texture of the original products with much less fat. To reduce saturated fat intake, use vegetable oils such as canola and olive oil that are high in monounsaturated fat, and corn and soybean oils that are high in polyunsaturated fat. To reduce your intake of *trans* fatty acids, consume soft margarine or liquid margarines and those that do not list partially hydrogenated fat as the first ingredient (Table 5.7).

The Role of Reduced Fat Foods There are currently a wide variety of reduced-fat and fat-free foods on the market. These products can help reduce fat intake when used in place of high-fat choices. For example, if a snack of salsa and regular tortilla

Figure 5.19

The groups that are sources of naturally occurring and added fat contain circles and are raised and colored orange. The darker the shade and the more circles, the more high-fat foods the group contains.

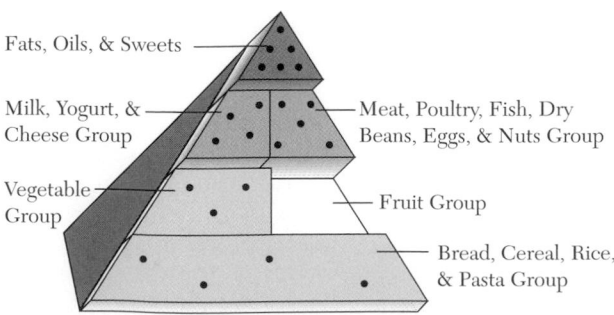

Fats, Oils, & Sweets

Milk, Yogurt, & Cheese Group

Vegetable Group

Meat, Poultry, Fish, Dry Beans, Eggs, & Nuts Group

Fruit Group

Bread, Cereal, Rice, & Pasta Group

Table 5.6   *Comparison of Lowfat and High-Fat Choices*

Food	Serving	Fat (g)	Energy (kcal)
Steak, fat trimmed	3 oz	4.2	150
Steak, not trimmed	3 oz	8.0	186
Broiled chicken breast (no skin)	3 oz	3.0	140
Fried chicken breast (with skin)	3 oz	23.0	423
Salad without dressing	1 cup	0.2	14
Salad with dressing	1 cup	3.0	45
Potato, baked	1 medium	0.1	118
Potato, baked with sour cream	1 medium	5.6	174
French fries	1 small order	10.0	202
Bagel	1 large	1.0	236
Doughnut, glazed	1 large	22.0	436
Fresh broccoli	1 cup	0.2	24
Frozen broccoli with cheese sauce	1 cup	15.0	220
Egg noodles	1 cup	2.0	213
Ramen noodles	1 cup	12.0	275
Spaghetti with tomato sauce	1 cup	1.5	216
Spaghetti with cream sauce	1 cup	19.0	385

chips is replaced with one of salsa and lowfat chips, fat and energy intake will be reduced. Used in moderation, these products can be part of a weight reduction or maintenance program. But reduced fat foods are not always low in kcalories. For instance, a brownie provides about 6.5 grams of fat and 112 kcalories. A reduced-fat brownie provides 2 grams of fat and 89 kcalories, whereas a fat-free brownie provides no fat and 76 kcalories.

A healthy diet does not need to include fat-modified foods. Likewise, using fat-modified products does not transform a poor diet into a healthy one or improve overall diet quality. If reduced-fat desserts and snack foods replace whole grains, fruits, and vegetables, the resulting diet could be low in fat but also low in fiber, vitamins, minerals, and phytochemicals—a dietary pattern that could increase the risk of chronic disease. However, if used appropriately, fat-modified foods can be part of a healthy diet.

Table 5.7   *Suggestions for Reducing Fat Intake*

1. Instead of frying, bake, broil, barbecue, roast, steam, or microwave.
2. Skip added fats like butter, margarine, mayonnaise, and salad dressing—or use lowfat or fat-free spreads and dressings.
3. Use egg whites or egg substitutes in baking.
4. Use cocoa instead of chocolate in baking.
5. Use reduced-fat milk instead of coffee creamer.
6. Use reduced-fat cheeses or limit the amounts consumed.
7. Reduce the emphasis on meat as the centerpiece of meals:
   - Base meals on whole grain products.
   - Reduce the portion size of meats served.
8. Trim visible fat from meats before cooking, and skin poultry before eating, if not before cooking.
9. Choose meats with little marbling:
   - "Prime grade" contains an abundant amount of marbled fat.
   - "Choice grade" contains a modest amount of marbling.
   - "Select grade" contains a comparatively slight amount of marbling.

CRITICAL THINKING

Fitting Fat into Your Diet

After reading about the relationship between dietary fat and chronic disease, Stella became concerned about her fat intake. She is confused by all the recommendations for different types of fat and is not sure how to change her diet. She has a busy schedule—working full-time and going to school—and has little time to cook meals at home. Currently, she relies on fast foods for breakfast and lunch and usually cooks a quick dinner when she gets home in the evening. To evaluate her new diet, she records everything that she eats for one day.

▼

Original Diet			Modified Diet		
Food	Serving	Fat (g)	Food	Serving	Fat (g)
Breakfast					
Bran muffin	1	6	Bran muffin	1	6
Margarine	1 tsp	5	Coffee	1 cup	0
Coffee	1 cup	0	Lowfat milk	1 cup	2
Whole milk	1 cup	8	Orange	1	0.2
Lunch					
Big Mac	1	25	Rice noodles	1 cup	0
French fries	20	16.6	Stir-fry vegetables	1 cup	2
			Chicken	2 oz	2.6
			in peanut oil	1 tsp	4.5
Water	1 bottle	0	Water	1 bottle	0
Snack					
Apple	1	0	Apple	1	0
			Pretzels	5	2.1
Dinner					
Fish sticks	5	17	Broiled fish	3 oz	7
Tater Tots	10	8	Rice	1 cup	0.5
			Long beans in	1 cup	1.0
			peanut oil	2 tsp	9
Cookies	2	4	Cookies	2	8
			Melon	1 cup	0.2
Tea	1 cup	0	Tea	1 cup	0
			Frozen yogurt	1 cup	6
Total		93.6			51.1

**Does Stella's original diet meet the serving recommendations
of the Food Guide Pyramid for grains, vegetables, and fruit?
Do her choices from these groups follow the selection
tips of the Food Guide Pyramid?**

▼

Answer:

A computer analysis shows that her total energy intake is 2100 kcalories. What is the percent of kcalories from fat in her original diet?

▼

Answer:

What modifications could Stella make to decrease her fat intake?

▼

A visit to her grandmother's house for dinner reminds her how much she enjoys traditional Filipino food, so she decides to incorporate these foods into her diet. For the Western foods she does not want to give up, she finds some lower-fat alternatives. She can cut her total and saturated fat intake by switching to lowfat milk. She can cut her total and *trans* fat by skipping the margarine on her bran muffin and trading her fast food lunch for leftovers. For dinner, she uses her grandmother's traditional recipes, which are low in fat and increase her servings of vegetables. Adding frozen yogurt increases her servings from the milk group. Her modified diet (shown on the right side of the table) provides comparable kcalories with less fat, *trans* fat, saturated fat, and cholesterol.

What is the percent of energy from fat in her modified diet, assuming it also contains 2100 kcalories? Does this diet meet the serving and selection recommendations of the Food Guide Pyramid for grains, vegetables, and fruit?

▼

Answer:

Hydrogenation The process whereby hydrogens are added to the carbon-carbon double bonds of unsaturated fatty acids, making them more saturated.

Partially hydrogenated vegetable oil Vegetable oil that has been modified by hydrogenation to decrease the number of unsaturated bonds, therefore raising the melting point and improving the storage characteristics.

• LIPIDS AND FOOD TECHNOLOGY

Fats may be added to foods during food processing, and the fats in food may be modified to change the stability or shelf life of the product. Which fats a product contains and how they are modified depends on the product and consumer demand.

Hydrogenated Vegetable Oils

The process of **hydrogenation** bubbles hydrogen gas into a liquid oil. This causes some of the double bonds in the oil to accept hydrogen atoms and become saturated. The resulting fat has more of the properties of a saturated fat, such as increased stability against rancidity and a higher melting point. Hydrogenated or **partially hydrogenated vegetable oils** are a primary ingredient in margarine and vegetable shortening because they raise the melting point of the products, making them more solid at room temperature. In breakfast cereals and other processed foods such as cookies, crackers, and potato chips, they are used to lengthen shelf life (Figure 5.20).

Although good for food manufacturing, the use of hydrogenated vegetable oils has created some health concerns. During hydrogenation, some of the unsaturated bonds are converted from the *cis* to the *trans* configuration. The resulting product contains more *trans* fatty acids than the original oil. Consuming a diet high in *trans* fatty acids may increase the risk of both heart disease and cancer. *Trans* fatty acids are present naturally in small amounts in animal fats, but can account for as much as

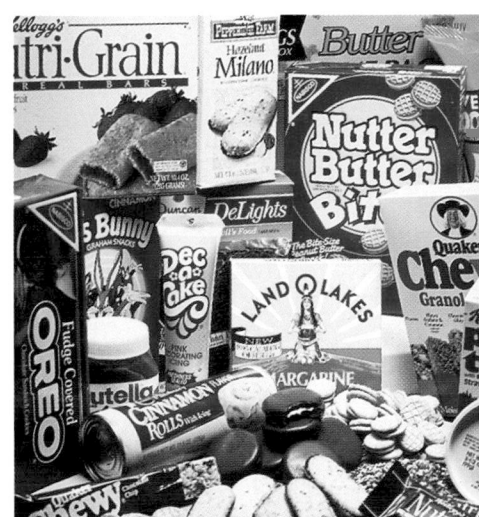

Figure 5.20

These products contain partially hydrogenated vegetable oil. (Charles D. Winters)

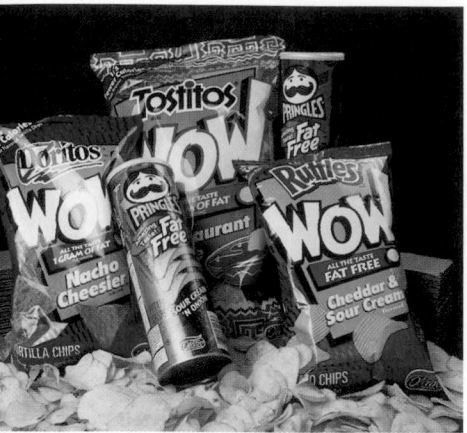

Figure 5.21
Products that contain Olestra (Olean), such as these snack chips, must carry the following health warning: "This Product Contains Olestra. Olestra may cause abdominal cramping and loose stools. Olestra inhibits the absorption of some vitamins and other nutrients. Vitamins A, D, E, and K have been added." (George Semple)

20% of the total fat in hydrogenated products such as margarine and shortening. Foods that contain *trans* fats can be identified by the presence of hydrogenated or partially hydrogenated oils in the ingredient list.

Artificial Fats

In response to consumer demand for lowfat, low-kcalorie foods, manufacturers have developed techniques for reducing the amount of fat contained in or absorbed from food. Some artificial fats replicate the taste, texture, and cooking properties of fat but are not lipids, and thus contribute less energy. Others contribute less fat and energy because they are not well absorbed from the gastrointestinal tract.[40]

Carbohydrate-based fat replacers such as various pectins and gums are often added to foods to mimic the texture that fat provides. These reduce the amount of fat in a product while adding soluble fiber. Oatrim, made from oats, and Nutrim, made from oats and barley, are carbohydrate-based fat substitutes developed by the USDA. They can provide the texture of fat in baked goods, salad dressings, sauces, and ice cream. The protein-based fat replacer Simplesse is made from egg white and milk proteins, which are modified by heating, filtering, and high-speed mixing. The resulting protein consists of millions of microscopic balls that slip and slide over each other to give it the creamy texture of fat. Because it is made from protein, it contains energy; but because the protein is mixed with water, Simplesse contains only 1.3 kcalories per gram, which is much lower than the 9 kcalories per gram in fat. It is used in frozen desserts, cheese foods, and other products, but it cannot be used for cooking because heat causes it to break down.[41]

Some fat substitutes are made from fats that have been modified to reduce how well they can be digested or absorbed. Caprenin, for example, consists of a glycerol backbone with three poorly absorbed fatty acids attached. It is digested like fat, but the fatty acids are only partially absorbed, so it provides only 5 kcalories per gram.[41] The artificial fat Olestra (sucrose polyester) is made from sucrose with fatty acids attached. Olestra cannot be digested by either the human enzymes or the bacterial enzymes in the gastrointestinal tract. It is, therefore, excreted in the feces without being absorbed. One of the problems with Olestra is that it reduces the absorption of other fat-soluble substances, including the fat-soluble vitamins A, D, E, and K. To avoid depleting these vitamins, Olestra has been fortified with them. However, it is not fortified with β-carotene and other fat-soluble substances that may be important for health. Another potential problem with Olestra is that it can cause gastrointestinal irritation, bloating, and diarrhea in some individuals because it passes into the colon without being digested. Olestra has been approved by the FDA for use in snack foods such as chips and crackers. Olestra-containing products must carry a warning label about these potential problems (Figure 5.21).

• APPLICATIONS •

1. Calculate your average fat, saturated fat, and cholesterol intake using the three-day food record you kept in Chapter 2.
   a. What is your fat intake in grams of fat, % kcalories from fat, and grams of saturated fat?
   b. How does your fat intake compare with the recommendation of 20–35% of energy from total fat?
   c. If your diet contains more than 35% of energy from fat, suggest changes that will decrease your fat intake without changing your energy intake. If your diet already contains less than 35% of energy from fat, list foods you typically consume that are high in fat and some lower-fat substitutes that you could try.
   d. Suggest food substitutions that will decrease the amount of saturated fat in your diet.
   e. How much cholesterol does your diet contain?
   f. Does your diet meet the recommendations of the Food Guide Pyramid?

2. Review all 3 days of the food record you kept in Chapter 2. Identify two foods from your diet that are sources of each of the following lipids. If your diet does not contain any foods that are sources of these, name foods that do contain them.
   a. Cholesterol
   b. Saturated fat
   c. Polyunsaturated fat
   d. Monounsaturated fat
   e. Omega-3 fatty acids
   f. *Trans* fatty acids

SUMMARY

1. Lipids are a diverse group of organic compounds, most of which do not dissolve in water. In the body, they provide a concentrated source of energy, insulate against shock and temperature changes, are a structural component of cell membranes, and are used to synthesize hormones and other molecules. In the diet, they contribute energy, texture, and flavor.

2. Fatty acids consist of a carbon chain with an acid group at one end. The length of the carbon chain and the number and position of the carbon-carbon double bonds determine the characteristics of the fat. Linoleic acid (omega-6) and alpha-linolenic acid (omega-3) are considered essential fatty acids because they cannot be synthesized by the body. In the body and in the diet, most fatty acids are found as part of triglycerides.

3. Triglycerides, commonly referred to as fat, are the storage form of fat. They consist of a backbone of glycerol with three fatty acids attached.

4. Phosphoglycerides consist of a backbone of glycerol, two fatty acids, and a phosphate group. Phosphoglycerides are an important component of cell membranes and lipoproteins because one end is water-soluble and one end is lipid-soluble.

5. Sterols, of which cholesterol is the best known, are made up of multiple chemical rings. Cholesterol is made by the body and consumed in animal foods in the diet. In the body, it is a component of cell membranes and is used to synthesize vitamin D, bile acids, and a number of hormones.

6. In the small intestine, churning and bile from the gallbladder help break large fat globules into small droplets. This allows pancreatic lipase to access these fats for digestion. The products of fat digestion, primarily fatty acids and monoglycerides, combine with bile to form micelles, which facilitate the absorption of these materials into the cells of the small intestine.

7. In body fluids, water-insoluble lipids are transported as lipoproteins. Lipids absorbed from the intestine are packaged with protein to form chylomicrons, which enter the lymphatic system before entering the blood. The triglycerides in chylomicrons are broken down by lipoprotein lipase on the surface of cells lining the blood vessels. Fatty acids are released and are taken up by surrounding cells. The chylomicron remnants that remain are returned to the liver.

8. Very-low-density lipoproteins (VLDLs) are synthesized by the liver. With the help of lipoprotein lipase, they deliver triglycerides to body cells. Once the triglycerides have been removed, intermediate-density lipoproteins (IDLs) are transformed into low-density lipoproteins (LDLs). LDLs deliver cholesterol to tissues by binding to LDL receptors on the cell surface. High levels of LDL are associated with an increased risk of cardiovascular disease. High-density lipoproteins (HDLs) are made by the liver and small intestine. They help remove cholesterol from cells for disposal and protect against cardiovascular disease.

9. After eating, chylomicrons and VLDLs deliver triglycerides to cells for energy or storage. During fasting, triglycerides stored in adipose cells are broken down by hormone sensitive lipase, and the fatty acids and glycerol are released into the blood.

10. The risk of heart disease is increased by diabetes, high blood pressure, obesity, and high blood cholesterol levels. High blood levels of total and LDL cholesterol are a risk factor for heart disease. High blood HDL cholesterol protects against heart disease.

11. Diets high in total fat, saturated fat, *trans* fatty acids, and cholesterol increase the risk of heart disease. Diets high in omega-6 or omega-3 polyunsaturated fatty acids, monounsaturated fatty acids, certain B vitamins, and plant foods containing fiber, antioxidants, and phytochemicals reduce the risk of heart disease. Diets high in fat also correlate with an increased incidence of certain types of cancer. Total dietary and lifestyle pattern is more important than any individual dietary factor in reducing heart disease risk.

12. DRI recommendations for total fat intake are given as acceptable ranges of intake (for adults 20 to 35% of energy) rather than EAR, RDA, AI, or UL values. There are no DRIs for *trans* or saturated fats or cholesterol, but the DRIs recommend reducing intakes of these. The Daily Values recommend that total fat account for no more than 30% of energy, that saturated fat account for no more than 10% of energy, that dietary cholesterol be no more than 300 mg per day.

13. AIs have been established for the essential fatty acids. For adults, the AI for linoleic acid is 12 grams per day for women and 17 grams per day for men. The acceptable range of intake is 5 to 10% of energy intake. The AI for α-linolenic acid is 1.1 and 1.6 grams per day respectively for women and men. The acceptable range is 0.6 to 1.2% of energy. Recommended values are higher for children and pregnant and lactating women.

14. Reducing fat intake requires decreasing intake of obvious sources of fat such as butter and oils, as well as baked goods, fast foods, and processed convenience foods that contain hidden fats. Saturated and *trans* fat intake can be reduced by limiting animal fats, margarine, and partially hydrogenated shortenings. To reduce health risks, the total diet, including consumption of grains, fruits, and vegetables, is as important as a moderate fat intake.

15. The types of fats used in processing depend on the desired characteristic. Partially hydrogenated vegetable oils and tropical oils are used to improve shelf life and increase the melting point.

16. Artificial fats are used to create reduced-fat products with taste and texture similar to the original. Some lowfat products are made by using mixtures of carbohydrates or proteins to simulate the properties of fat, and some use modified lipids that are not well absorbed.

REVIEW QUESTIONS

1. What is a lipid?

2. Name four types of lipids found in the body.

3. What distinguishes a saturated fat from a monounsaturated fat? From a polyunsaturated fat?

4. Name two functions of fat in foods.

5. List three functions of fat in the body.

6. In the body, what is the advantage of storing energy as fat rather than as carbohydrate?

7. What is the function of bile in fat digestion?

8. How do chylomicrons and VLDLs differ?

9. How do HDLs differ from LDLs?

10. How are blood levels of LDLs and HDLs related to the risk of cardiovascular disease?

11. What types of foods contain cholesterol?

12. What are the recommendations for dietary fat intake?

13. What is hydrogenation and how is it related to *trans* fatty acids?

14. Is essential fatty acid deficiency common in developed countries? Why or why not?

REFERENCES

1. Institute of Medicine, Food and Nutrition Board. *Dietary Reference Intakes for Energy, Carbohydrates, Fiber, Fat, Protein and Amino Acids.* Washington, D.C.: National Academy Press, 2002.

2. Wood, J. L., and Allison, R. G. Effects of consumption of choline and lecithin on neurological and cardiovascular systems. *Fed. Proc.* 41:3015, 1982.

3. Hamosh, M., Iverson, S. J., Kirk, C. L., and Hamosh, P. Milk lipids and neonatal fat digestion: Relationship between fatty acid composition, endogenous and exogenous digestive enzymes and digestion of milk fat. *World Rev. Nutr. Diet.* 75:86–91, 1994.

4. Krauss, R. M., Deckelbaum, R. J., Ernst, N., et al. Dietary guidelines for healthy American adults: A statement for health professionals from the Nutrition Committee, American Heart Association. *Circulation* 94:1795–1800, 1996.

5. Shikany, J. M., and White, G. L. Jr. Dietary guidelines for chronic disease prevention. *South Med. J.* 93(12):1138–1151, 2000.

6. American Heart Association. Heart Facts, 2002. Available online at www.americanheart.org/Accessed March 31, 2002.

7. Ascherio, A., Rimm, E. B., Stampfer, M. J., et al. Marine n-3 fatty acids, fish intake, and the risk of coronary disease among men. *N. Engl. J. Med.* 332:977–982, 1995.

8. American Heart Association. Mediterranean Diet. Available online at http://216.185.112.5/presenter.jhtml?identifier=4644/Accessed April 3, 2002

9. Gordon, T. The diet-heart idea. *Am. J. Epidemiol.* 127:220–223, 1988.

10. Brown, M. S., and Goldstein, J. L. How LDL receptors influence cholesterol and atherosclerosis. *Sci. Am.* 251:58–66, 1984.

11. National Cholesterol Education Program Adult Treatment Panel III Report, 2001. Available online at www.nhlbi.nih.gov/guidelines/cholesterol/index.htm/ Accessed Sept. 5, 2002.

12. American Heart Association, Cardiovascular Disease Statistics. Available online at www.amhrt.org/Heart_and_Stroke_A_Z_Guide/cvds.htm/ Accessed December 2, 2000.

13. Geil, P. B., Anderson, J. W., and Gustafson, N. J. Women and men with hypercholesterolemia respond similarly to an American Heart Association Step 1 Diet. *J. Am. Diet. Assoc.* 95:436–441, 1995.

14. Denke, M. A. Review of human studies evaluating individual dietary responsiveness in patients with hypercholesterolemia. *Am. J. Clin. Nutr.* 62(suppl):471S-477S, 1995.

15. Ginsberg, H. N., and Karmally, W. Nutrition, lipids, and cardiovascular disease. In *Biochemical and Physiological Aspects of Human Nutrition.* M. H. Stipanuk, ed. Philadelphia: W. B. Saunders Company, 2000, 917–944.

16. Watts, G. F., Jackson, P., Burke, V., and Lewis, B. Dietary fatty acids and progression of coronary artery disease in men. *Am. J. Clin. Nutr.* 64:202–209, 1996.

17. Lichtenstein, A. H., Ausman, L. M., Jalbert, S. M., et al. Effects of different forms of dietary hydrogenated fats on serum lipoprotein cholesterol levels. *N. Engl. J. Med.* 340:1933–1940, 1999.

18. American Heart Association. *Trans* Fatty Acids. Available online at http://216.185.112.5/presenter.jhtml?identifier=4776/ Accessed April 4, 2002.

19. Dietschy, J. M. Dietary fatty acids and the regulation of plasma low density lipoprotein cholesterol concentrations. *J. Nutr.* 128:444S–448S, 1998.

20. Katan, M. B., Zock, P. L., and Mensink, R. P. Dietary oils, serum lipoproteins, and coronary heart disease. *Am. J. Clin. Nutr.* 61(suppl):1368S–1373S, 1995.

21. Stone, N. J. Fish consumption, fish oil, lipids, and coronary heart disease. *Am. J. Clin. Nutr.* 65:1083–1086, 1997.

22. Connor, S. L., and Connor, W. E. Are fish oils beneficial in the prevention and treatment of coronary artery disease? *Am. J. Clin. Nutr.* 66(suppl):1020S–1031S, 1997.

23. Schoene, N. W., and Fitzgerald, G. A. Thrombogenic potential of dietary long-chain polyunsaturated fatty acids: session summary. *Am. J. Clin. Nutr.* 56(suppl):825S–826S, 1992.

24. Willett, W. C., Sacks, F., Trichopouluo, A., et al. Mediterranean diet pyramid: A cultural model for healthy eating. *Am. J. Clin. Nutr.* 61(suppl):1402S–1406S, 1995.

25. Kwiterovich, P. O. The effect of dietary fat, antioxidants and prooxidants on blood lipids, lipoproteins and atherosclerosis. *J. Am. Diet. Assoc.* 97(suppl): S231–S241, 1997.

26. American Heart Association. Homocysteine, Folic Acid and Cardiovascular Disease. Available online at http://216.185.112.5/presenter.jhtml?identifier=4677/Accessed April 4, 2002.

27. Selhub, J., Jacques P. F., Bostom A. G., et al. Relationship between plasma homocysteine and vitamin status in the Framingham study population. Impact of folic acid fortification. *Public Health Rev* 28:117–1145, 2000.

28. Waterhouse, A. L., German, B. L., Walzem, R. L., et al. Is it time for a wine trial? *Am. J. Clin. Nutr.* 68:220–221, 1998.

29. American Institute for Cancer Research, World Cancer Research Fund. Food, Nutrition and the Prevention of Cancer: A Global Perspective. Presented at the American Institute of Cancer Research Research Conference, October 8–10, 1997.

30. Trichopoulou, A., Katsouyanni, K., Stuver, S., et al. Consumption of olive oil and specific food groups in relation to breast cancer risk in Greece. *J. Natl. Cancer Inst.* 87:110–116, 1995.

31. Rose, D. P. Dietary fatty acids and cancer. *Am. J. Clin. Nutr.* 66(suppl):99S–1003S, 1997.

32. AHA Conference Proceedings. Summary of the Scientific Conference on Dietary Fatty Acids and Cardiovascular Health. *Circ.* 103:1034–1037, 2001.

33. Noguchi, M., Rose, D. P., Earashi, M., and Miyazaki, I. The role of fatty acids and eicosanoid synthesis inhibitors in breast carcinoma. *Oncology* 52:265–271, 1995.

34. USDA, Agricultural Service. Results from USDA's 1994–1996 Continuing Survey of Food Intakes by Individuals and 1994–1996 Health Knowledge Survey. ARS Food Surveys Research Group, 1997. Available online at www.barc.usda.gov/bhnrc/foodsurvey/home/htm/ Accessed March 6, 2002.

35. WHO and FAO Joint Consultation. Fats and oils in human nutrition. *Nutr. Rev.* 53:202–205, 1995.

36. Food and Drug Administration, Center for Food Safety and Applied Nutrition. A Food Labelling Guide. Available online at www.cfsan.fda.gov/~dms/labind.html/ Accessed February 28, 2002.

37. National Heart, Lung, and Blood Institute, National Institutes of Health, National Cholesterol Education Program. Live Healthier, Live Longer. Available online at http://rover.nhlbi.nih.gov/chd/Accessed Dec. 4, 2000.

38. Krauss R. M., Eckel R. H., Howard B., Appel L. J., et al. AHA Dietary Guidelines: Revision 2000: A statement for healthcare professionals from the Nutrition Committee of the American Heart Association. *Circulation* 102:2284–2299, 2000.

39. American Academy of Pediatrics Committee on Nutrition. Statement on cholesterol. *Pediatrics* 101:141–147, 1998

40. Sigmna-Grant, M. Can you have your low-fat cake and eat it too? The role of fat-modified products. *J. Am. Diet. Assoc.* 97(suppl):S76–S81, 1997.

41. American Dietetic Association. Position of the American Dietetic Association: Fat replacers. *J. Am. Diet. Assoc.* 98:463–468, 1998.

Protein: The Privileged Nutrient Chapter 6

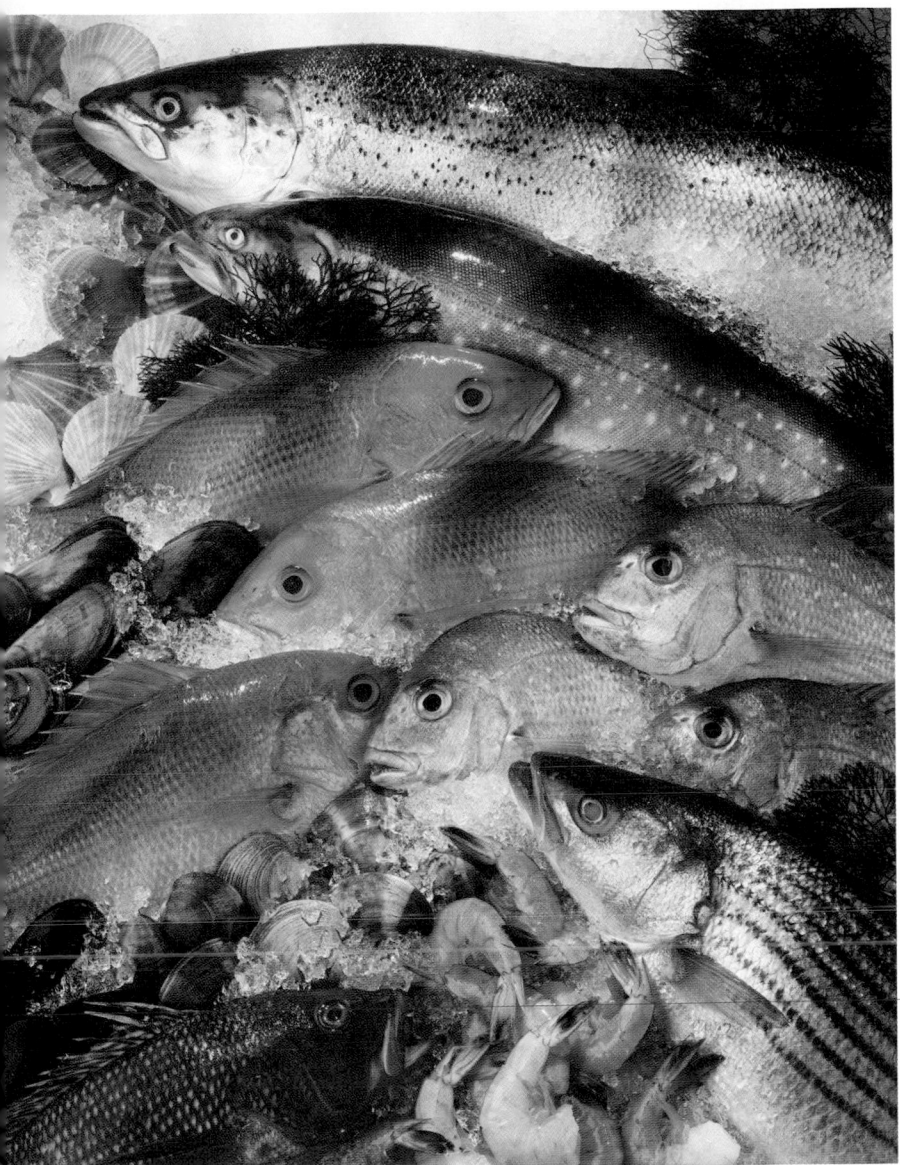

(© Lois Ellen Frank/Corbis)

Chapter Concepts

✔ Most people in economically developed countries eat more than enough protein.

✔ Protein is found in both animal and plant foods.

✔ Proteins are made up of chains of amino acids folded into three-dimensional shapes.

✔ Amino acids that cannot be made by the body in amounts sufficient to meet needs are essential in the diet.

✔ Amino acids can be used to synthesize body proteins, to synthesize nonprotein molecules, and to provide energy.

✔ Protein is necessary to allow for growth as well as to maintain structure and regulate functions in the body.

✔ The amino acid composition of a protein affects how efficiently it can be used to make body proteins. This is referred to as protein quality.

✔ Animal sources of protein are generally of higher quality than plant sources.

✔ Vegetarian diets rely on plant protein from varied sources to meet body needs.

✔ Proteins and amino acids are added to alter the texture, flavor, and nutritional characteristics of food products.

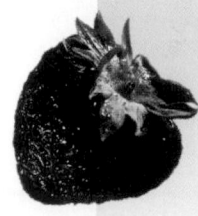

Just a Taste

Do you eat enough protein?

Does eating a high-protein diet make your muscles bigger?

Can you stay healthy eating a vegetarian diet?

Protein is a nutrient that conjures up images of vitality and strength. Unlike carbohydrate and fat, protein has had the privilege of being associated with positive effects. It has not been accused of being fattening, causing tooth decay, or increasing the risk of heart disease. It is associated with strong muscles and good health. As a result, protein is a "big seller." Protein drinks, pills, and powders fill the shelves of health food stores. Consumers often choose high-protein foods and supplements because of protein's association with good health. Is protein worthy of its lofty reputation? Do we need to worry about eating too much protein or which protein sources we choose?

Most of the world relies on plant foods such as grains and vegetables to meet their protein needs. There is growing evidence that this may be a healthier dietary pattern than one that relies heavily on animal foods. Therefore, nutritional recommendations such as the Dietary Guidelines and the Food Guide Pyramid suggest that our diets be based on whole grain products, vegetables, and fruits. Following these guidelines will decrease the amount of animal protein, and most likely total protein, in the diet. Is this a healthy dietary pattern? Does it reduce the risk of chronic disease? Or does it increase the possibility of protein and other nutrient deficiencies?

• WHAT IS PROTEIN?

Protein is a macronutrient that is distinguished from carbohydrate and lipid by the fact that it contains the element nitrogen. Protein in the diet provides the raw material to make all the various types of proteins that the body needs. These body proteins provide important structural and regulatory functions. In some circumstances protein can be used for energy, providing 4 kcalories per gram.

Protein in the Diet

In a typical day, most Americans consume about 100 grams of protein—about twice their requirement. Most of this comes from animal sources such as meat, milk, and eggs—the most concentrated sources of protein. One egg or an ounce of meat contains about 7 grams of protein, and a cup of milk contains 8 grams. But plants also provide good sources of protein (Figure 6.1). Legumes, such as lentils, soybeans, peanuts, black-eyed peas, chickpeas, red beans, pinto beans, kidney beans, and black beans, provide 6 to 10 grams of protein per half-cup serving. Nuts and seeds are also good sources of protein, providing about 5 to 10 grams per quarter cup. A half-cup serving of vegetables or grains, such as rice or pasta, provides 2 to 3 grams. Although plant proteins are not used as efficiently as animal sources to make body proteins, a diet including plant proteins from a variety of sources can easily meet most people's needs.

Proteins Are Made of Amino Acids

A protein molecule, whether found in a steak, a kidney bean, or a part of the human body, is constructed of one or more folded, chainlike strands of **amino acids**. Each different protein contains a specific number of amino acids in specific proportions

Amino acids The building blocks of proteins. Each contains a carbon atom bound to a hydrogen atom, an amino group, an acid group, and a side chain.

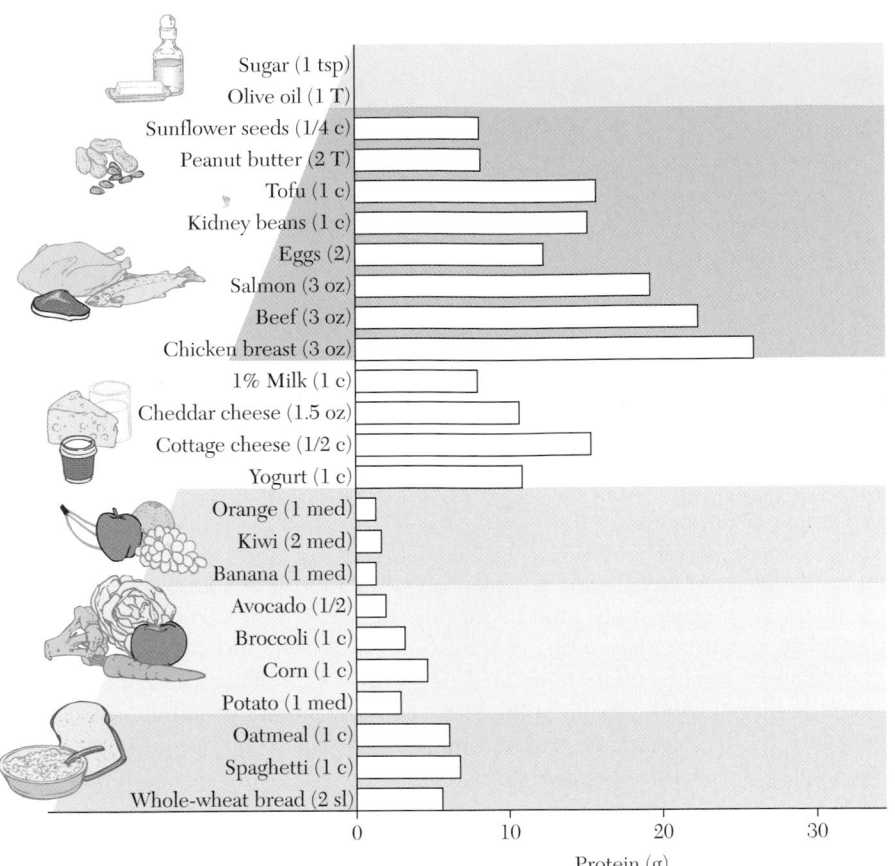

Figure 6.1

Protein content of selections from each of the Food Guide Pyramid groups. Foods in the Meat, Poultry, Fish, Dry Beans, & Nuts Group and the Milk, Yogurt, & Cheese Group contain the most protein per serving.

that are bound together in a specific order. Variations in the number, proportion, and order of amino acids allow for an infinite number of different protein structures.

There are approximately 20 amino acids commonly found in proteins. Each amino acid consists of a carbon atom bound to four chemical groups: a hydrogen atom; an amino group, which contains nitrogen; an acid group; and a fourth group called a side chain that varies in length and structure (Figure 6.2). Different side chains give specific properties to individual amino acids.

Of the 20 amino acids commonly found in protein, 9 cannot be made by the adult human body. These amino acids, called **essential** or **indispensable amino acids**, must be consumed in the diet (Table 6.1). If the diet is deficient in one or

Essential or **indispensable amino acids** Amino acids that cannot be synthesized by the human body in sufficient amounts to meet needs and therefore must be included in the diet.

Table 6.1 *Classification of Amino Acids for Adult Humans*

Essential Amino Acids	Nonessential Amino Acids
Histidine	Alanine
Isoleucine	Arginine°
Leucine	Asparagine
Lysine	Aspartic acid (aspartate)
Methionine	Cysteine (cystine)°
Phenylalanine	Tyrosine°
Threonine	Glutamic acid (glutamate)
Tryptophan	Glutamine°
Valine	Glycine°
	Proline°
	Serine

°These amino acids are also classified as conditionally essential.

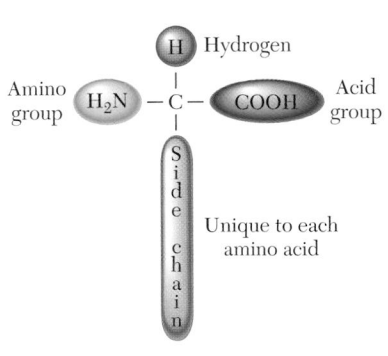

Figure 6.2

All amino acids have a similar structure, but each has a different side chain.

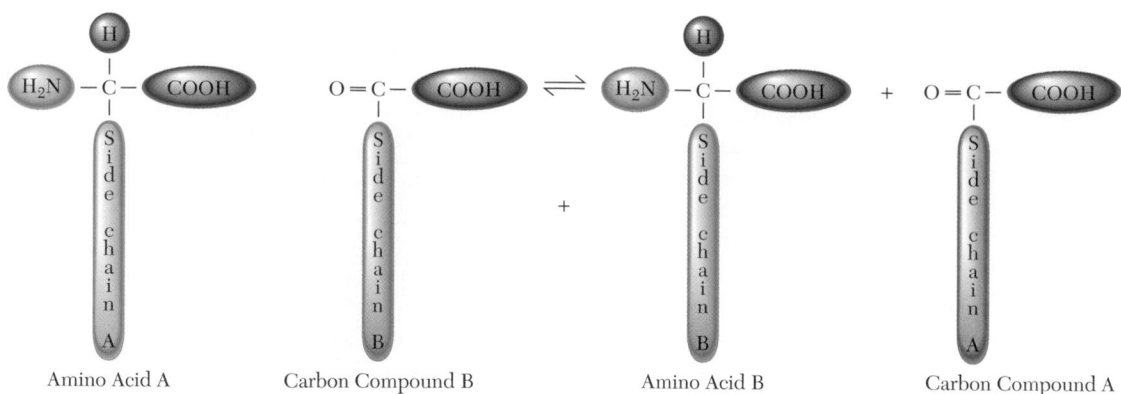

Figure 6.3

By the process of transamination, the amino group from a nonessential amino acid (Amino Acid A) is combined with a carbon compound (Carbon Compound B) to form amino acid B and carbon compound A.

Nonessential or **dispensable amino acids** Amino acids that can be synthesized by the human body in sufficient amounts to meet needs.

Transamination The process by which an amino group from one amino acid is transferred to a carbon compound to form a new amino acid.

Conditionally essential amino acids Amino acids that are essential in the diet only under certain conditions or at certain times of life.

Dipeptide Two amino acids linked by a peptide bond. A **tripeptide** is three amino acids linked by peptide bonds, and a **polypeptide** is a chain of three or more amino acids linked by peptide bonds.

more of these amino acids, new proteins containing them cannot be made without breaking down other body proteins to provide them. The 11 **nonessential** or **dispensable amino acids** can be made by the human body and are not required in the diet. When a nonessential amino acid needed for protein synthesis is not available from the diet, it can be made in the body. Most of the nonessential amino acids can be made by the process of **transamination**, in which an amino group from one amino acid is transferred to a carbon-containing molecule to form a different amino acid (Figure 6.3).

Some amino acids are **conditionally essential**. These are essential only under certain conditions. For example, the conditionally essential amino acid tyrosine can be made in the body from the essential amino acid phenylalanine. If phenylalanine is in short supply, tyrosine cannot be made and becomes essential in the diet. Likewise, the amino acid cysteine is only essential when the essential amino acid methionine is in short supply. Other amino acids may be essential under certain conditions, such as premature infancy.

Protein Structure

Amino acids are linked together to form proteins by a unique type of chemical bond called a peptide bond. This bond is formed between the acid group of one amino acid and the nitrogen atom of the next amino acid (Figure 6.4). When two amino acids are linked with a peptide bond, they are called a **dipeptide**; when three amino acids are linked, they form a **tripeptide**. Many amino acids bonded together constitute a **polypeptide**. A protein is made of one or more polypeptide chains folded into a complex three-dimensional shape. The three-dimensional shape of the protein is deter-

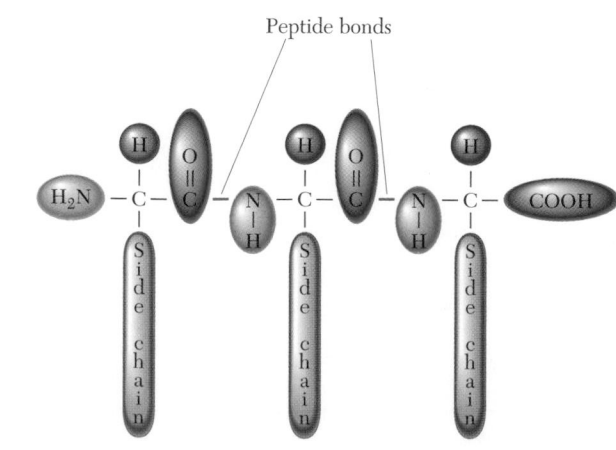

Figure 6.4

Amino acids in proteins are linked by peptide bonds.

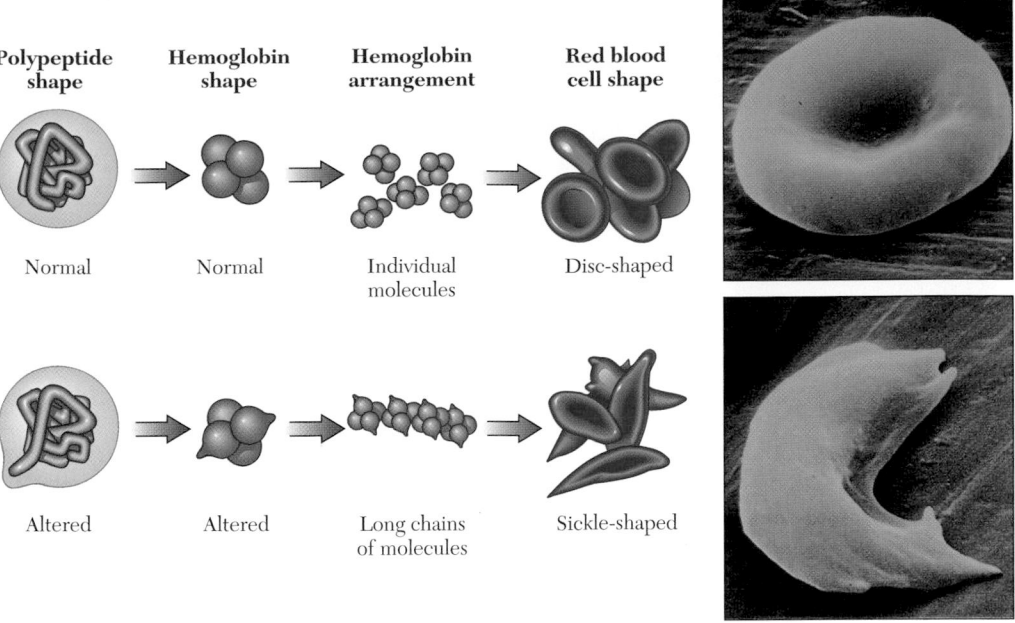

Polypeptide shape	Hemoglobin shape	Hemoglobin arrangement	Red blood cell shape
Normal	Normal	Individual molecules	Disc-shaped
Altered	Altered	Long chains of molecules	Sickle-shaped

Figure 6.5

In sickle-cell anemia, a change in the sequence of amino acids in hemoglobin causes a change in the shape and function of the protein molecule. Sickle-cell hemoglobin forms long chains that distort the shape of red blood cells. (© Stan Flegler/Visual Unlimited)

mined by the order of the amino acids, and it is the shape of a protein that determines its function.

If the shape of the protein changes, its function is altered. For example, the genetic disease sickle-cell anemia results from a change in only one of the amino acids in hemoglobin, the protein that carries oxygen in the blood. The altered amino acid chain causes the protein to change shape, which causes the characteristics of the hemoglobin molecule to change. Sickle-cell hemoglobin molecules bind together, forming long chains, whereas normal hemoglobin molecules do not bind together. A red blood cell containing normal hemoglobin is disc shaped, whereas a cell containing chains of sickle-cell hemoglobin is crescent or sickle shaped (Figure 6.5). These distorted red blood cells can block capillaries, causing inflammation and pain, and they rupture easily, leading to anemia from a shortage of red blood cells.

Changes in protein structure can also be caused by heat or acid. This change in structure is called **denaturation**, a change from the natural. In food, cooking denatures protein, thereby changing its shape and physical properties. For example, a raw egg white is clear and liquid, but once it has been denatured by cooking, it becomes white and firm (Figure 6.6).

Denaturation The alteration of a protein's three-dimensional structure.

• PROTEIN IN THE DIGESTIVE TRACT

The digestion of protein begins in the stomach, where hydrochloric acid denatures proteins, opening up their folded structure to make them more accessible to enzyme attack. The acid also activates the protein-digesting enzyme pepsin, which breaks proteins into polypeptides and amino acids. When the polypeptides enter the small intestine, they are broken into smaller peptides, tripeptides, dipeptides, and amino acids by pancreatic protein-digesting enzymes such as trypsin and chymotrypsin. The small peptides are further broken down by protein-digesting enzymes in the brush border of the small intestine. Single amino acids, dipeptides, and tripeptides can be absorbed by the mucosal cells of the small intestine. Once inside the mucosal cells, dipeptides and tripeptides are broken into single amino acids (Figure 6.7).

Amino acids cross the mucosa of the small intestine using one of several active transport systems. Amino acids with similar structures share the same transport system and therefore compete for absorption. If there is an excess of any one of the amino acids sharing a transport system, more of it will be absorbed, slowing the ab-

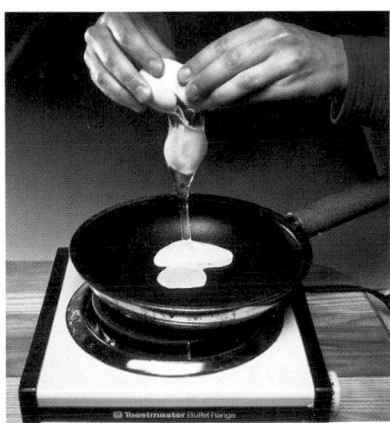

Figure 6.6

The protein in egg white is denatured by heat when the egg is cooked. (Charles D. Winters)

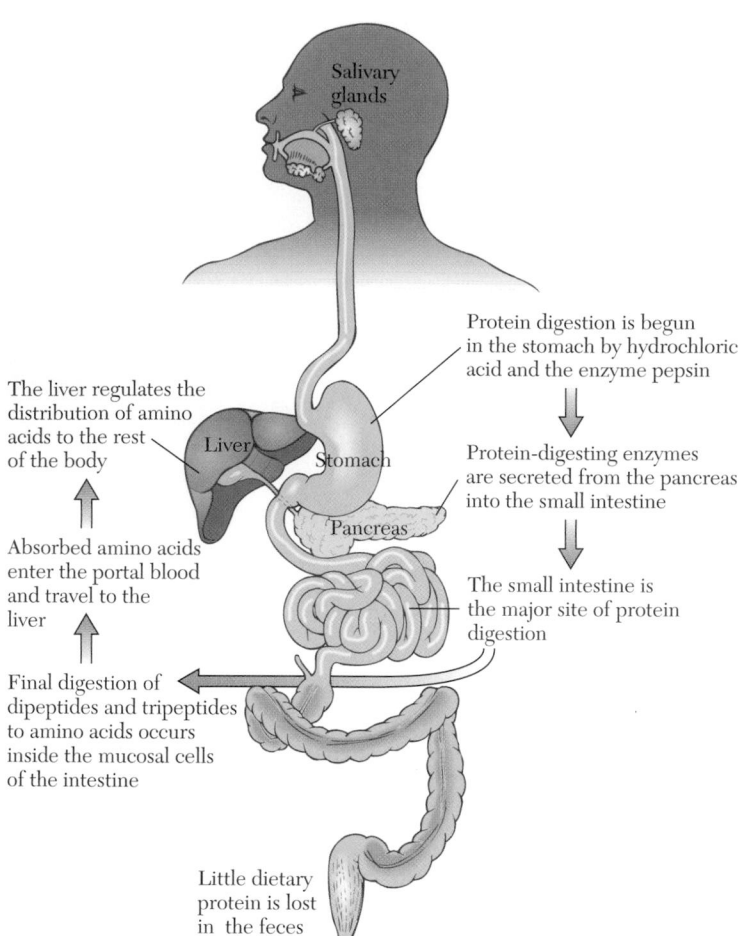

Protein digestion is begun in the stomach by hydrochloric acid and the enzyme pepsin

Protein-digesting enzymes are secreted from the pancreas into the small intestine

The small intestine is the major site of protein digestion

The liver regulates the distribution of amino acids to the rest of the body

Absorbed amino acids enter the portal blood and travel to the liver

Final digestion of dipeptides and tripeptides to amino acids occurs inside the mucosal cells of the intestine

Little dietary protein is lost in the feces

Liver

Stomach

Pancreas

Salivary glands

Figure 6.7
An overview of protein digestion and absorption.

sorption of the other competing amino acids. This is generally not a problem with foods because they contain a variety of amino acids. However, if one takes an amino acid supplement, the absorption of other amino acids that share the same transport system may be impaired (Figure 6.8). For example, weight lifters often supplement the amino acid arginine. Arginine shares the same transport system as lysine. If large doses of arginine are ingested, the absorption of lysine will be reduced.

If a protein from the diet is absorbed without being completely digested, an allergic reaction can occur (see Chapter 15). The absorbed protein is recognized as a foreign substance by the immune system, which mounts an attack. Symptoms of food allergies can include reactions of the respiratory tract (sneezing and asthma), skin (rashes or hives), nervous system (headache and dizziness), cardiovascular system (rapid heart rate), urinary tract (blood in the urine), or digestive system (vomiting and diarrhea). Allergies are most common both in people with gastrointestinal disease, because their damaged intestine allows the absorption of whole proteins, and in infants, because their immature gastrointestinal tracts are more likely to allow larger polypeptides to be absorbed. Once an infant's intestinal mucosa matures, absorption of whole proteins is less likely and food allergies usually disappear. The absorption of whole proteins by very young infants, however, can also be of benefit since antibody proteins absorbed from breast milk can provide temporary protection against certain diseases (see Chapter 14).

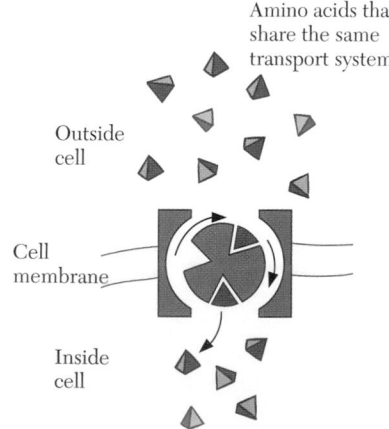

Amino acids that share the same transport system

Outside cell

Cell membrane

Inside cell

Figure 6.8
The amino acids in this figure share the same transport system, and since there are more of the purple ones than the green ones, more of the purple amino acids are able to cross the membrane into the cell.

• PROTEIN IN THE BODY

Once dietary proteins have been digested and absorbed, their amino acids become available to synthesize proteins or nonprotein molecules needed by the body or to provide energy.

Protein Metabolism: Amino Acids for Synthesis and Energy

Once amino acids are absorbed, they enter the hepatic portal vein and travel to the liver. The liver plays an important role in determining how amino acids will be used by the rest of the body. The liver can use the amino acids to synthesize blood or liver proteins, release them into the general circulation for use by other tissues, or degrade them for energy. Some amino acids are also used by the liver and other tissues to form nonprotein molecules of biological importance such as neurotransmitters, which are chemical messengers that transmit nerve signals.

Recycling Amino Acids The amino acids present in body tissues and fluids are available for use and are referred to collectively as the body **amino acid pool**. Amino acids enter this so-called pool from protein in the diet as well as from the breakdown of body proteins. Of the approximately 300 grams of protein synthesized by the body each day, only about 100 grams are made of amino acids from the diet. The other 200 grams are made from amino acids recycled from protein broken down in the body. When dietary intake of protein and energy are adequate but not excessive, most amino acids in the amino acid pool are used to synthesize body proteins and other nitrogen-containing compounds (Figure 6.9). When the diet does not provide enough total energy and when protein is consumed in excess of need, amino acids are used for energy.

Amino acid pool All of the amino acids in body tissues and fluids that are available for protein synthesis.

Protein Synthesis The amino acids used to synthesize body proteins come from the amino acid pool. The instructions that dictate which amino acids are needed, and in what order they should be combined, are contained in the stretches of DNA called **genes**. When a protein is needed, the process of protein synthesis is turned on.

The first step in protein synthesis involves transferring, or transcribing, the DNA code for the protein from the gene into a molecule of messenger RNA (mRNA). This process is called **transcription**. The mRNA then takes this information from the nucleus of the cell to ribosomes in the cytoplasm where proteins are made. Here the information in mRNA is translated via another type of RNA, called transfer RNA (tRNA). Transfer RNA reads the code and delivers the needed amino acids (Figure 6.10). This process is called **translation**. If all the necessary amino acids aren't available from the amino acid pool, the protein cannot be made.

Gene A section of DNA that codes for a protein.

Transcription The process of copying the information in DNA to a molecule of mRNA.

Translation The process of translating the RNA code into the amino acid sequence of a protein.

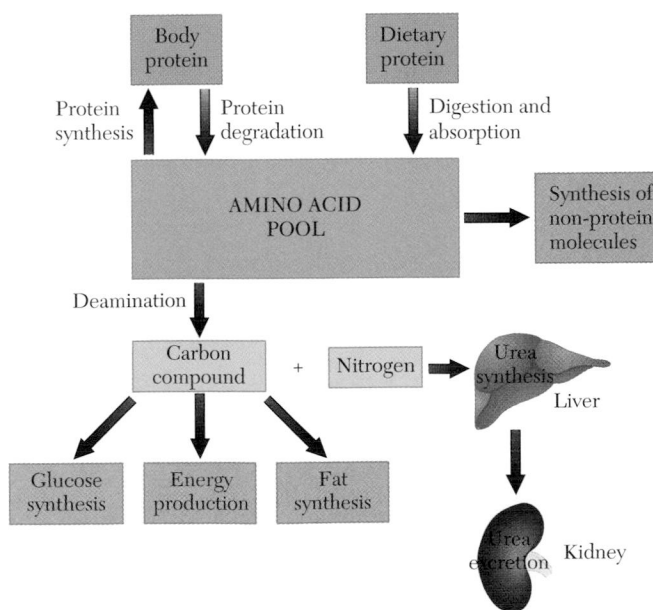

Figure 6.9
Amino acids enter the available pool from the diet and from the breakdown of body proteins. They are used to synthesize body proteins and nonprotein molecules and to provide energy.

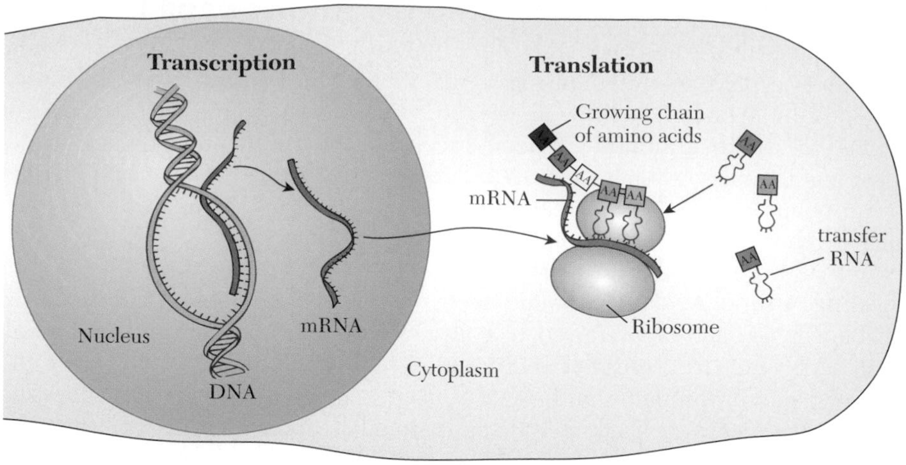

Figure 6.10

DNA in the nucleus of cells provides a blueprint for the sequence of amino acids in proteins. In the process of transcription, the information in DNA is copied into a strand of mRNA. The mRNA leaves the nucleus and travels to the cytoplasm where it binds to a ribosome. Transfer RNA molecules in the cytoplasm collect amino acids and deliver them to the mRNA strand. The sequence in the mRNA dictates which transfer RNA, and its corresponding amino acid, will be added to the growing amino acid strand. As each amino acid is added, its transfer RNA is released to collect another amino acid. As the strand grows, the ribosome moves along the mRNA to read the next part of the code.

Gene expression Refers to the events of protein synthesis in which the information coded in a gene is used to synthesize a protein.

Gene Expression When the information in a gene is used to make a protein, **gene expression** is occurring. Which proteins are made and when they are made are carefully regulated. Not all genes are expressed in all cells or at all times. For example, the hormone insulin is a protein that is made in pancreatic cells. Insulin is not made by other body cells because the gene is not expressed in cells other than those in the pancreas. The expression of some genes changes depending on the need for the protein for which they code. For example, when iron intake is high, the expression of a gene that codes for ferritin, an iron-storage protein, is turned on. This allows more of this protein to be synthesized, and the capacity to store iron is increased.[1]

Nutrients can affect how and when genes are expressed. As seen above, the amount of iron in the diet determines the amount of ferritin made. Vitamin A affects the expression of many genes involved in the maturation of cells, and vitamin D affects genes that code for calcium transport proteins (see Chapter 9). In this way, levels of nutrients can determine which proteins are made and can therefore regulate body functions. Who we are and how healthy we are depend not only on which genes we have but which genes are expressed.

Limiting Amino Acids During the construction of a protein, a shortage of one needed amino acid can stop protein synthesis. Just as on an assembly line, if one part is missing, the line stops—a different part cannot be substituted. If the missing amino acid is a nonessential amino acid, it can be synthesized in the body and protein synthesis can continue. If the missing amino acid is an essential amino acid, the body can break down its own proteins to obtain this amino acid. If an amino acid cannot be supplied, protein synthesis will stop. The essential amino acid present in shortest supply relative to need is called the **limiting amino acid**, because lack of this amino acid limits the ability to make protein. If all amino acids are present in adequate amounts at the time of synthesis, proteins will be completed and released for further processing by the cell.

Limiting amino acid The essential amino acid that is available in the lowest concentration in relation to the body's needs

Synthesis of Nonprotein Molecules Some amino acids are also used to synthesize nonprotein molecules that contain nitrogen. These include a number of neurotransmitters. For example, the amino acid tryptophan is used to synthesize the neurotransmitter serotonin, which acts in the relaxation center of the brain. The units that make up DNA and RNA are another group of nitrogen-containing compounds that are derived in part from amino acids. Other molecules synthesized from amino acids include the skin pigment melanin, the vitamin niacin, creatine needed for muscle contraction, and histamine, which causes blood vessels to dilate.

Energy Production Although carbohydrate and fat are more efficient energy sources, amino acids from dietary and body proteins are also used for energy. This use increases both when the diet does not provide enough total energy to meet needs, as in starvation, and when protein is consumed in excess of needs.

When energy is deficient, body proteins, such as enzymes and muscle proteins, are broken down into amino acids that can then be used as fuel. Before amino acids can be used for energy, the nitrogen-containing amino group must be removed in a process called **deamination**. The nitrogen is then converted by the liver into the waste product **urea**, which can be excreted by the kidneys. The carbon compounds remaining after nitrogen is removed from the amino acids can enter the citric acid cycle to produce ATP or be used to make glucose via gluconeogenesis (Figure 6.11). This provides energy in times of need, but it also robs the body of functional proteins.

Amino acids are also used for energy when protein intake exceeds protein needs. If the diet is adequate in energy and high in protein, the extra amino acids are used to produce ATP. If both energy and protein exceed needs, the extra amino acids are deaminated and converted into either glucose or fatty acids, depending on their structure, and can contribute to weight gain.

Deamination The removal of the amino group from an amino acid.

Urea A nitrogen-containing waste product that is excreted in the urine.

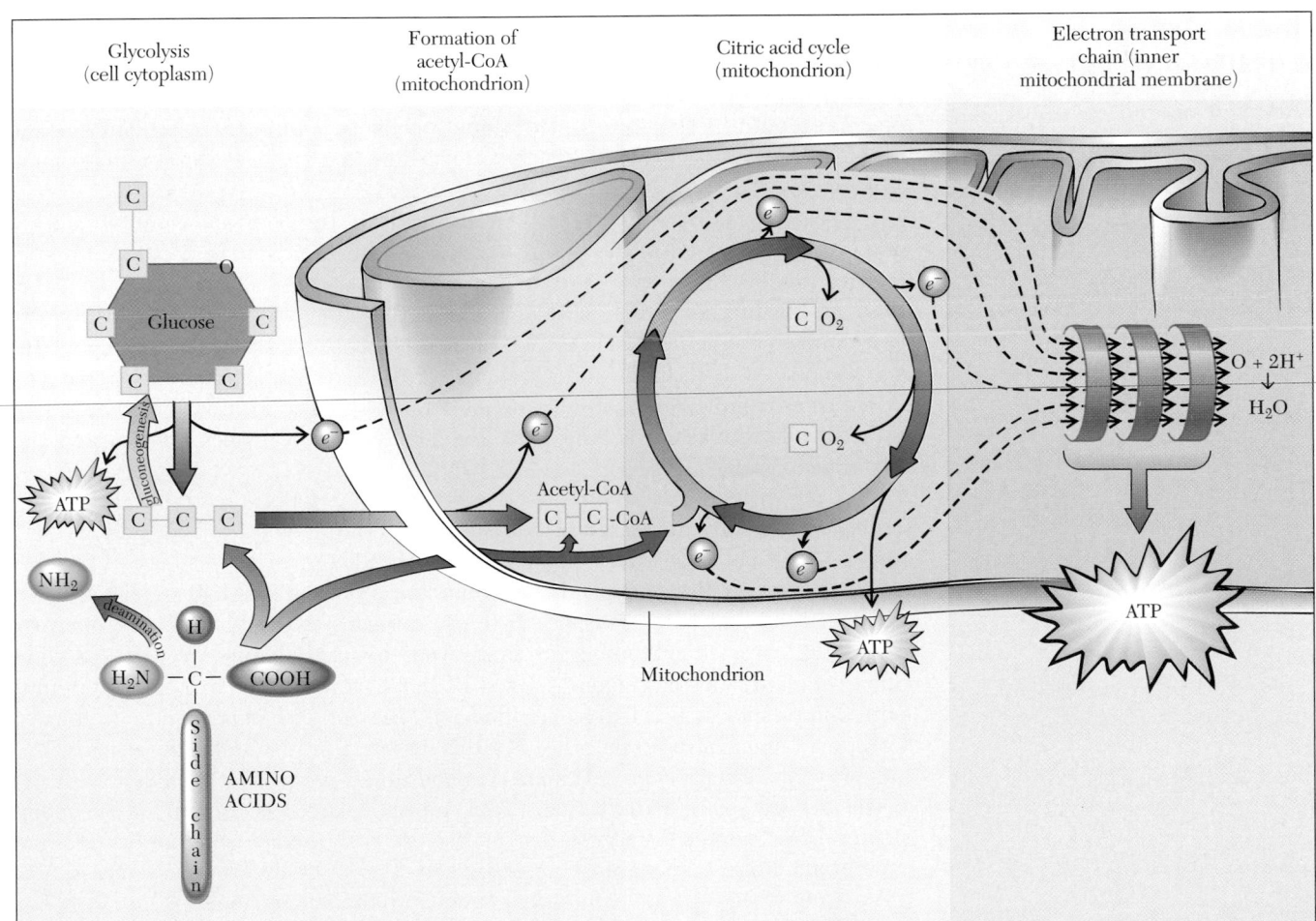

Figure 6.11
Amino acids must be deaminated to remove the nitrogen before they can be metabolized to produce energy or used to synthesize glucose.

Functions of Proteins in the Body

The number of different proteins made by the human body is vast. Each protein molecule has a specific function. Some provide structure and others help regulate body processes.

Structural Proteins Proteins provide structure to individual cells and to the body as a whole. In cells, proteins are an integral part of the cell membrane, the cytoplasm, and the organelles. Skin, hair, and muscle are composed largely of protein. Bones and teeth are made up of minerals embedded in a protein framework. When the diet is deficient in protein, these structures break down. The muscles become smaller, the skin loses its elasticity, and the hair becomes thin and can easily be pulled out by the roots. These outward signs of dietary protein deficiency have become marketing strategies for cosmetic companies. Shampoo and hand lotion manufacturers add protein to their products, suggesting that protein applied to the hair or skin will improve its structure. However, the proteins that make up hair and skin can only be made inside the body, so a healthy diet will do more for hair and skin quality than expensive protein shampoos or lotions.

Regulatory Proteins Proteins help regulate the body's many different processes to maintain homeostasis. Regulatory proteins include enzymes, transport proteins in the blood and in cells, immune system proteins, protein hormones, and proteins that aid in muscle contraction, fluid balance, and acid balance.

Enzymes Enzymes are protein molecules that speed up the metabolic reactions of the body but are not used up or destroyed in these reactions. All the reactions involved in the production of energy and the synthesis and breakdown of carbohydrates, lipids, proteins, and other molecules are expedited by enzymes. Each reaction requires a specific enzyme with a specific structure. If the structure of the enzyme molecule is changed, it can no longer function in the reaction it is designed to accelerate.

Enzymes that function in the body are made by the body and therefore do not need to be consumed in the diet. Enzymes present in foods are denatured by the cooking process and are no longer functional when eaten. When raw foods are eaten, the enzymes present are broken down during digestion and are absorbed from the gastrointestinal tract as amino acids. Purified enzymes sold as dietary supplements are also broken down in the gut. These may provide some function; for example, lactase, taken by individuals with lactose intolerance, breaks down lactose that is consumed while the lactase is in the gut. Eventually, these enzymes are digested and absorbed as amino acids.

Transport Proteins Proteins transport substances throughout the body and into and out of individual cells. Transport proteins in the blood carry substances from one organ to another. For example, hemoglobin, the protein in red blood cells, picks up oxygen in the lungs and transports it to other organs of the body. The proteins in lipoproteins are needed to transport lipids from the intestines and liver to body cells. Some vitamins, such as vitamin A, must be bound to a specific protein to be transported in the blood. When protein is deficient, the nutrients that require protein for transport cannot travel to the cells. For this reason, a protein deficiency can cause a vitamin A deficiency; even if vitamin A is consumed in the diet, it cannot be transported to the cells. At the cellular level, transport proteins present in cell membranes help move substances such as glucose and amino acids across the cell membrane. For example, transport proteins in the intestinal mucosa are necessary to absorb amino acids from the intestinal lumen into the mucosal cells.

Defense Proteins Proteins play an important role in protecting the body from injury and invasion by foreign substances. Skin, which is made up primarily of protein, is the first barrier against infection and injury. Foreign particles such as dirt or bacteria that are on the skin cannot enter the body and can be washed away. If the skin is broken and blood vessels are injured, fibrinogen and thrombin, blood-clotting proteins, help prevent too much blood from being lost. If a foreign particle such as a virus or bacterium enters the body, the immune system fights it off by synthesizing proteins called **antibodies**. Each antibody has a unique structure that allows it to attach to a specific invader. When an antibody binds to an invading substance, the production of more antibodies is stimulated, and other parts of the immune system are signaled to help destroy the invader. The next time the same type of invading bacterium or virus enters the body, the immune system is already primed to produce specific antibodies to fight off the invader. This is also how immunizations against diseases, such as measles, work. A small amount of dead or inactivated virus is injected into the body; the injected material does not cause disease, but it does stimulate the immune system to produce antibodies to the virus. The next time the body comes in contact with the virus, a large-scale immune attack is mounted and the infection is prevented. When the immune system malfunctions as a result of protein deficiency or other causes, such as HIV infection, the ability to protect the body from infection is compromised.

Antibodies Proteins produced by cells of the immune system that destroy or inactivate foreign substances in the body.

Contractile or Motile Proteins Some proteins give cells and organisms the ability to move, contract, and change shape. Actin and myosin function in the contraction of muscles. These two proteins slide past each other to shorten the muscle and cause contraction. For example, when you do a biceps curl, the muscles in your arms shorten as the alternating actin and myosin proteins slide past one another (Figure 6.12). A similar process causes contraction in the heart muscle and in the muscles that cause constriction in the digestive tract, blood vessels, and body glands. Actin and myosin can also cause contraction in nonmuscle cells. This contraction may help individual cells, such as white blood cells, change shape and move. The energy for contraction comes from ATP, which is derived primarily from the metabolism of carbohydrate and fat.

Protein Hormones Hormones are chemical messengers that are secreted into the blood by one tissue or organ and act on target cells in other parts of the body. Some hormones are made of lipid; others are made of amino acids and so are classified as peptide or protein hormones. For instance, insulin and glucagon are protein hormones.

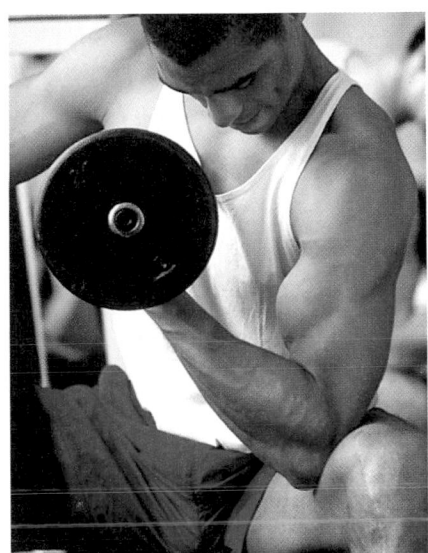

Figure 6.12
The proteins actin and myosin slide past each other to contract muscles. (© T. & D. McCarthy/Corbis Stock Market)

Proteins in Fluid Balance The distribution of fluid in body cells, in the bloodstream, and in the space between cells is important for homeostasis. Fluid moves back and forth across membranes to maintain appropriate concentrations of particles and fluids inside and outside cells and tissues (see Chapter 10). Proteins help regulate this fluid balance in two ways. First, protein pumps located in cell membranes transport particles from one side of a membrane to another. Second, large protein molecules present in the blood keep fluid in the blood both by preventing it from being forced into tissues and by attracting fluid in tissues back into blood vessels. In cases of protein malnutrition, the concentration of these large proteins in the blood decreases, so fluid is no longer held in the blood, and it accumulates in the tissues.

Proteins in Acid Balance The chemical reactions of metabolism require a specific level of acidity, or **pH**, to function properly. In the gastrointestinal tract, acidity levels vary widely. The digestive enzyme pepsin works best in the acid environment of the stomach, whereas the pancreatic enzymes operate best in the more neutral environment of the small intestine. Inside the body, large fluctuations in pH can prevent metabolic reactions from proceeding. Proteins both within cells and in the blood help prevent large changes in acidity. For instance, the protein hemoglobin in red blood cells helps neutralize acid produced when carbon dioxide, a waste product of cellular respiration, reacts with water.

pH A measure of acidity.

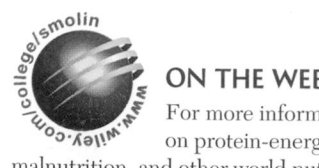

ON THE WEB

For more information on protein-energy malnutrition, and other world nutrition health issues, go to the World Health Organization at

www.who.int

Protein-energy malnutrition (PEM) A condition characterized by wasting and an increased susceptibility to infection that results from the long-term consumption of insufficient energy and protein to meet needs.

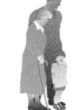

Kwashiorkor A form of protein-energy malnutrition in which only protein is deficient.

Marasmus A form of protein-energy malnutrition in which a deficiency of energy in the diet causes severe body wasting.

• PROTEIN AND HEALTH

A diet adequate in protein is essential to health. Dietary protein is needed for growth and to replace protein that is broken down and lost each day. If too little protein is consumed, the consequences can be dramatic and devastating. Too much protein, particularly if it is derived primarily from animal sources, may also have negative health implications.

Protein Deficiency

Because of the availability and variety of foods in developed countries, protein deficiency is uncommon. However, in developing nations, concerns about inadequate protein are very real. Diets deficient in protein are most often deficient in energy as well, but a pure protein deficiency can occur when food choices are extremely limited and the staple food of a population is very low in protein. The term **protein-energy malnutrition (PEM)** is used to refer to the continuum of conditions ranging from pure protein deficiency, called **kwashiorkor**, to energy deficiency, called **marasmus**.

Kwashiorkor Kwashiorkor is typically a disease of children. The word "kwashiorkor" comes from the Ga tribe of the African Gold Coast. It means the disease that the first child gets when a second child is born.[2] When the new baby is born, the older child is no longer breast-fed. Rather than receiving protein-rich breast milk, the young child is fed a watered-down version of the diet eaten by the rest of the family. This diet is low in protein and is often high in fiber and difficult to digest. The child, even if able to get adequate energy, is not able to eat a large enough quantity to get adequate protein. Because children are growing, their protein needs per unit of body weight are higher than those of adults, and the effects of a deficiency become evident much more quickly.

The symptoms of kwashiorkor can be explained by examining the roles that proteins play in the body. Because protein is needed for the synthesis of new tissue, growth in height and weight is hampered. Because proteins are important in immune function, there is an increased susceptibility to infection. There are changes in hair color because the skin pigment melanin is not made; the skin flakes because structural proteins are not available to provide elasticity and support. Cells lining the digestive tract die and cannot be replaced, so nutrient absorption is impaired. The bloated belly typical of this condition is a result of both fat accumulating in the liver because there is not enough protein to transport it and fluid accumulating in the abdomen because there is not enough protein to keep fluid in the blood (Figure 6.13*a*).

Figure 6.13
Kwashiorkor (*a*) is characterized by a bloated belly, whereas marasmus (*b*) presents as severe wasting. Most protein-energy malnutrition is a combination of the two. (*a*, Food and Agriculture Organization of the United Nations; *b*, Scott Dani Peterson/Liaison)

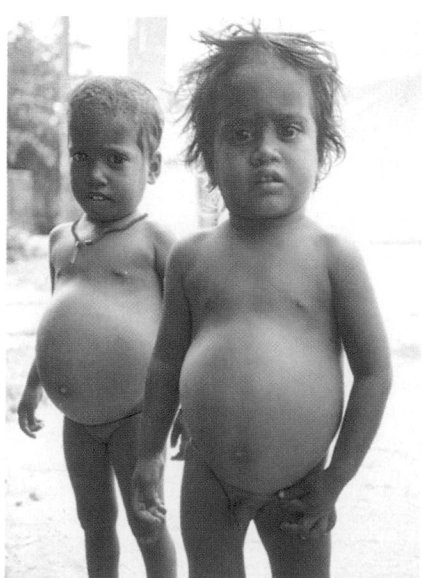

(a)

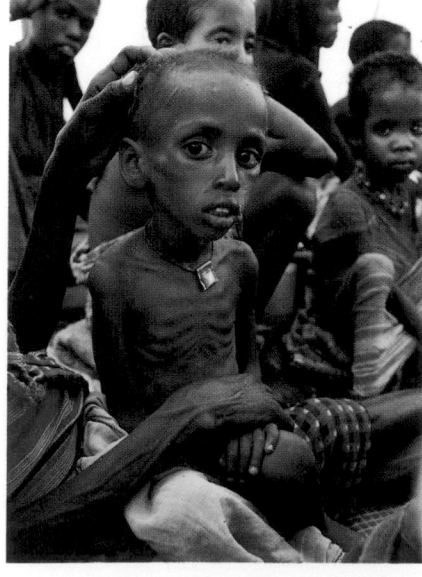

(b)

Kwashiorkor occurs most commonly in Africa, South and Central America, the Near East, and the Far East. It has also been reported in poverty-stricken areas in the United States. Although kwashiorkor is often thought of as a disease of children, it is seen in hospitalized adults who have high-protein needs due to infection or trauma and a low-protein intake because they are unable to eat.

Marasmus At the other end of the continuum of protein-energy malnutrition is marasmus, meaning to waste away. Marasmus is due to a deficiency of energy, but protein and other nutrients are usually also insufficient to meet needs. Marasmus may have some of the same symptoms as kwashiorkor, but there are also differences. In kwashiorkor, some fat stores are retained, since energy intake is adequate. Marasmic individuals appear emaciated because their body fat stores have been used to provide energy (Figure 6.13b). Since fat is a major energy source and carbohydrate is limited, ketosis may occur in marasmus. This is not so in kwashiorkor because carbohydrate intake is adequate—only protein is deficient.

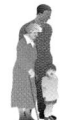

Marasmus occurs in individuals of all ages and is the form of malnutrition that occurs with eating disorders (see Chapter 7). It has devastating effects in infants and children because adequate energy is essential for growth. Because most brain growth takes place in the first year of life, malnutrition early in life causes a decrease in intelligence and learning ability that persists throughout life. Marasmus often occurs in children who are fed diluted infant formula prepared by caregivers trying to stretch limited supplies. Marasmus occurs less often in breast-fed infants.

Protein Excess

Adequate protein intake is absolutely essential to life. But is there such a thing as too much protein? Some research suggests that a high-protein diet has negative effects, while other studies find no ill effects. The only concern about high-protein diets that is not disputed is that they are usually high in foods of animal origin. Diets high in animal products are generally low in grains, vegetables, and fruits, a dietary pattern associated with a greater risk of cancer.[3] Diets high in animal protein are also typically high in saturated fat and cholesterol and, therefore, increase the risk of heart disease (see Chapter 5). Such diets are also usually high in energy and total fat, which may promote obesity (see Chapter 7).

Metabolic Effects The consumption of too much protein increases both the production of protein breakdown products and the need to eliminate them from the body. When protein is degraded, the amino groups from its amino acids are converted into urea. The kidneys must then excrete the urea. This requires more water. Although not a problem for most people, this can be a problem if the kidneys are not able to concentrate urine, as is the case with the immature kidneys of newborns. Feeding a newborn infant formula that is mixed improperly can provide excess protein, which can increase fluid losses and lead to dehydration.

Another concern with high-protein diets is that they may affect kidney and bone health. The long-term consumption of a high-protein diet may speed the progression of renal failure in individuals with kidney disease.[4] However, there is little evidence that a high-protein diet is associated with kidney disease in the healthy population.[5] Protein intake may also affect calcium balance. Protein is an important structural component of bone, but increasing protein intake increases calcium losses in the urine. High levels of protein are believed to negatively affect bone mass only if calcium intake is inadequate.[6]

Protein and Amino Acid Supplements Despite these concerns about protein excess, protein and amino acid supplements remain popular among some segments of the population. Protein is needed for proper immune function, healthy hair, and muscle growth, but supplements will affect these only if the diet is deficient in protein in the first place. Increasing protein intake above the requirement does not protect you from disease, make your hair shine, or stimulate muscle growth. Muscle

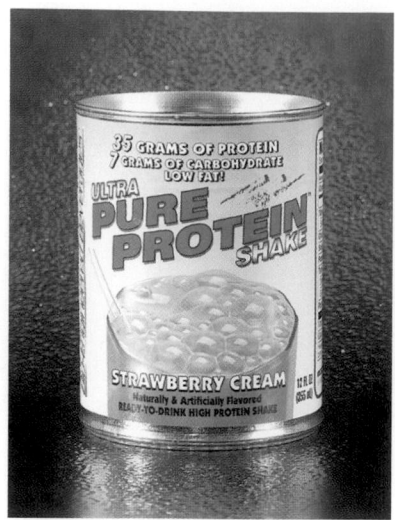

Figure 6.14
Products marketed to increase protein intake are not necessary to meet needs. (Andy Washnik)

growth occurs in response to exercise in the presence of adequate protein. Although protein supplements are not harmful for most people, they are an expensive and unnecessary way to increase protein intake. A typical protein drink provides 10 to 35 g of protein per serving, or 20 to 70% of the Daily Value (Figure 6.14). It can add about 100 to 250 kcalories to the diet and thus can contribute to weight gain. If consumed consistently, a high intake of protein from supplements or from foods may also contribute to dehydration.

Amino acid supplements are also an unnecessary and expensive addition to a healthy diet. Many of these are marketed for specific reasons; for example, ornithine, arginine, and lysine are offered to increase lean body mass. Because amino acids share transport systems, a supplement of one may impair the absorption of others that share the same transport system (see Figure 6.8).

• PROTEIN: ONE PART OF THE TOTAL DIET

In a typical North American diet, protein provides about 15% of the energy. While the recommendations do not suggest that we reduce our protein intake, there is a new emphasis on the source of protein—plant versus animal. The amount and source of dietary protein have an impact on the healthiness of the overall diet.

Recommendations for Protein Intake

Historically, recommendations for protein intake were estimated from the amount of protein consumed by healthy working men in the general population. These protein levels were often as high as 150 grams per day. Current recommendations are generally lower than this and are based on balance studies used to measure the protein needs of the body (see the following discussion). Most people in developed countries such as the United States and Canada consume more than enough protein in their diets.

The DRIs have established an RDA for protein of 0.8 gram of protein per kilogram of body weight for adults.[6] This value is calculated assuming that the diet contains high-quality plant and animal sources of protein and is set to meet the needs of the majority of the population. For a person weighing 70 kg (154 lb), the recommended intake would be 56 grams of protein per day (see Table 6.2). RDAs have also been established for each of the essential amino acids.

How Protein Requirements Are Determined Protein requirements are estimated using balance studies. Since protein is the only nutrient that contains nitrogen, the amount of protein used by the body can be calculated by comparing nitrogen intake with nitrogen loss. Nitrogen intake is calculated from dietary protein intake. Nitrogen loss or output is measured by totaling the amounts of nitrogen excreted in urine and feces and that lost from skin, sweat, hair, and nails. The majority of the nitrogen lost is excreted in the urine as urea. Comparing the amount of nitrogen consumed with the amount lost provides information about the amount of protein being synthesized and broken down within the body. An individual who is consuming enough protein to meet body needs is in protein or nitrogen balance. This means the amount of nitrogen or protein the individual consumes in the diet is enough to replace the amount that is lost from the body. If more nitrogen is lost than ingested, a negative nitrogen balance is said to exist. This indicates that more body protein is being broken down than is being consumed. This can occur when intake is too low or when the amount of protein breakdown has been increased by a stress such as injury, illness, or surgery. Positive nitrogen balance occurs when less nitrogen is lost than is ingested; this indicates that the body is using dietary protein for synthesis of new body proteins. This occurs when new tissue is synthesized, such as during growth, pregnancy, wound healing, or muscle building (Figure 6.15; see *Critical Thinking*: What Does Nitrogen Balance Tell Us?).

Table 6.2 *Calculating Protein Needs*

To determine protein requirement:

- Determine body weight. If weight is measured in pounds, convert it to kilograms by dividing by 2.2;

$$\frac{\text{weight in pounds}}{2.2 \text{ pounds/kg}} = \text{weight in kg}$$

For example:

$$\frac{150 \text{ pounds}}{2.2 \text{ pounds/kg}} = 68 \text{ kg}$$

- Determine the grams of protein required per day. Multiply weight in kg by the grams of protein per kilogram recommended for the specific gender and life-stage group.
- For example, a 23-year-old female weighing 68 kg would require 0.8 g/kg × 68 kg = 54.4 grams of protein.

Gender or Condition	Age (yrs)	RDA (g/kg)
Both sexes	0–0.5	1.52°
	0.5–1	1.5
	1–3	1.1
	4–8	0.95
	9–13	0.95
	14–18	0.85
	19 and older	0.8
Pregnancy		Nonpregnant RDA + 25 g/day
Lactation	First 6 months	Nonlactation RDA + 25 g/day

°This value is an AI.

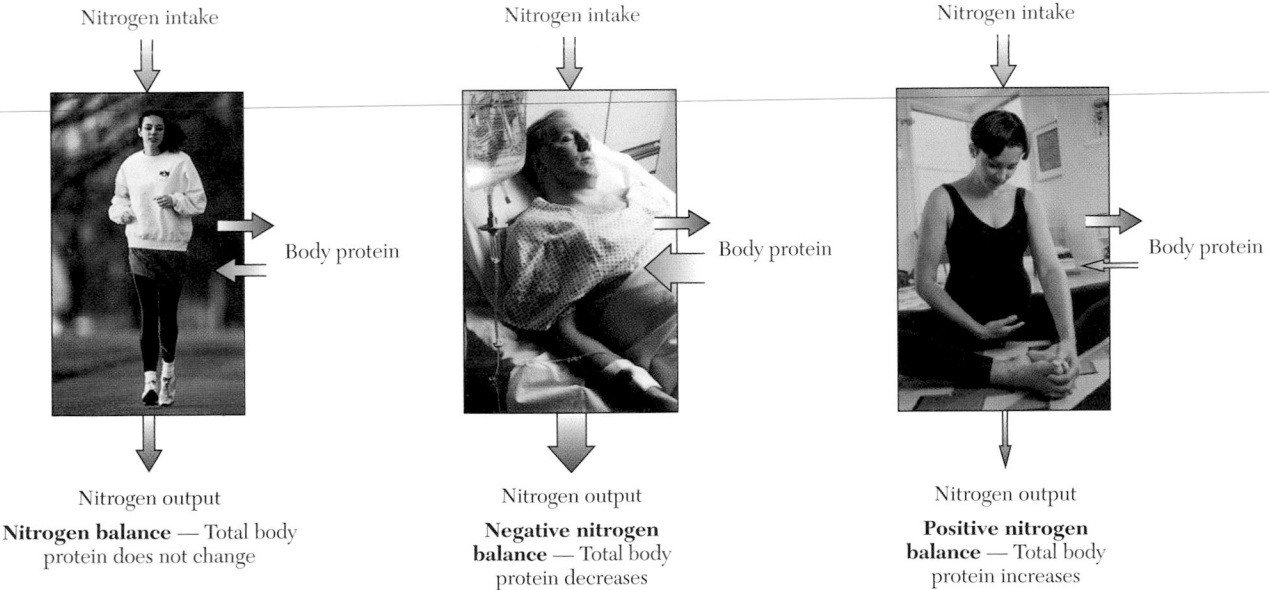

Nitrogen intake → Body protein → Nitrogen output
Nitrogen balance — Total body protein does not change

Nitrogen intake → Body protein → Nitrogen output
Negative nitrogen balance — Total body protein decreases

Nitrogen intake → Body protein → Nitrogen output
Positive nitrogen balance — Total body protein increases

Figure 6.15

In nitrogen balance, nitrogen intake is equal to the nitrogen output; in negative balance, output exceeds intake because more body proteins are broken down than synthesized and the nitrogen is excreted; in positive nitrogen balance, intake exceeds output because more protein is used to synthesize body proteins than is lost from protein breakdown. (Photos: *left*, Dennis Drenner; *center*, © Brian Yarvin/Photo Researchers, Inc.; *right*, © Donna Day/Stone)

The protein requirement of a specific individual can be determined by doing a balance study for that individual. Because this procedure cannot be done for everyone, the protein needs of populations must be estimated from balance study data. Recommendations for protein intake for the general public are actually higher than the requirements determined by balance studies for individuals. This is to allow a margin of safety that will ensure the needs of the majority of the population are met.

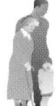 **Recommendations Throughout Life** Protein needs vary with life stage. Growth during childhood and pregnancy increases protein requirements. Lactation increases the body's protein demand, since milk is high in protein. Physical stress and exercise can also affect protein needs.

Growth During the first year of life, a large amount of protein is required to support the rapid growth rate. Thus, an AI for the first six months of life has been set at 1.52 grams per kilogram of body weight per day; for the second six months, the RDA is 1.5 grams per kilogram. As the growth rate slows, requirements per unit of body weight decrease but continue to be greater than adult requirements until 19 years of age (Figure 6.16).

Pregnancy Protein is needed in the pregnant woman's diet for the expansion of her blood volume, enlargement of her uterus and breasts, development of the placenta, and growth and development of the fetus. The RDA for pregnant women suggests an additional 25 grams per day above the nonpregnant recommendation. Most women in North America already consume this much protein in their typical diets.

Lactation The quantity of milk produced and the protein content of the milk determine the additional protein needs of lactation. The RDA recommends an additional 25 grams per day of dietary protein during lactation.

Illness and Injury Extreme stresses on the body such as infections, fevers, burns, or surgery increase protein breakdown. These losses must be replaced by dietary protein. Requirements for these types of stresses must be assessed on an individual basis, depending on the extent of the losses. For example, a severe infection increases requirements by about one-third. Burns can increase requirements to two to four times the normal level.

Exercise The marketing of protein powders and amino acid supplements to athletes might lead people to believe that protein is in short supply in the athlete's diet. In fact, athletes can obtain plenty of protein in their diets without supplements. Most athletes can meet their protein needs by consuming the RDA of 0.8 gram per kg of body weight. Those participating in endurance sports, in which protein is used for energy and to maintain blood glucose, may benefit from more protein—a total of 1.2 to 1.4 grams per kilogram per day. Strength athletes, such as weight lifters and body builders, may benefit from a total of 1.4 to 1.8 grams per kilogram per day.[7] Strength athletes require this extra protein to supply amino acids to build muscle protein; dietary protein in excess of this does not increase muscle growth. Muscle growth occurs in response to exercise, which is fueled primarily by glycogen stored in the muscles. Even endurance and strength athletes can meet their protein needs without supplements. For example, if a 200-pound (91-kg) man consumes 3600 kcal per day, 15% of which is from protein (approximately the amount contained in a typical North American diet), he will consume 135 grams of protein. This equals about 1.5 grams of protein per kilogram of body weight. The protein needs of athletes are also discussed in Chapter 13.

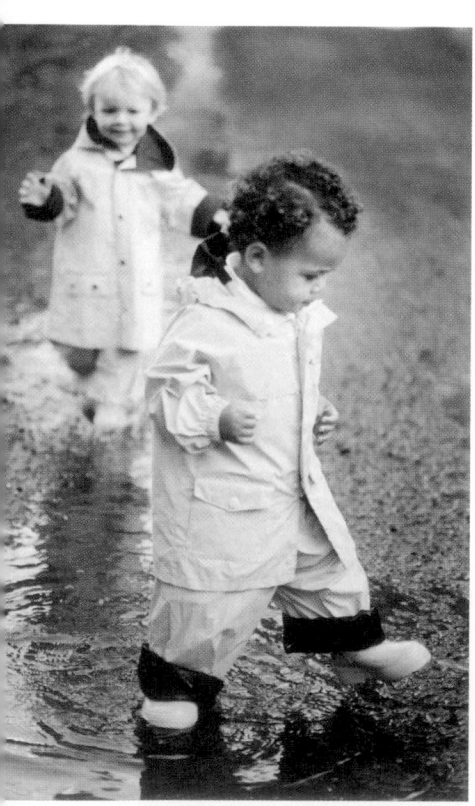

Figure 6.16
Protein needs are high in young children because of their rapid rate of growth. (Cheryl Maeder/Taxi)

CRITICAL THINKING

What Does Nitrogen Balance Tell Us?

The Amecht Company wants to include nitrogen balance studies in the assays it performs in its clinical laboratory. To test their methodology, they analyze nitrogen balance in three individuals. The technicians are given information about the daily nitrogen intake of these subjects and analyze samples of urine and feces to determine daily nitrogen losses.

$$\text{Nitrogen balance} = \text{Nitrogen In} - \text{Nitrogen Out}$$

Subject A consumed 6.4 grams of nitrogen. The laboratory determines that she lost 8.0 grams of nitrogen in her urine and feces. The nitrogen balance equation for subject A is

$$6.4\,\text{g} - 8.0\,\text{g} = -1.6\,\text{g}$$

This result of a balance of -1.6 grams per day suggests that the individual is breaking down body protein to meet her needs.

Does this make sense metabolically?
▼

Subject A is a 35-year-old woman who weighs 120 kg but is on a weight-loss diet. She is consuming only 500 kcalories and 30 grams of protein per day. To meet energy needs, her body is breaking down body protein, resulting in an increased excretion of nitrogen in the urine. A negative nitrogen balance would be expected for someone consuming such a low-energy, low-protein diet.

Subject B is a healthy 29-year-old male who weighs 82 kg and consumes an adequate diet of 2700 kcalories and 70 grams of protein a day. His nitrogen values are:

	Nitrogen In	Nitrogen Out
Subject B	11.2 g	11.2 g

What is his nitrogen balance?
▼

Answer:

Does his nitrogen balance make sense metabolically?
▼

Yes. He is in nitrogen balance. This means his protein intake meets his needs, and he is neither retaining protein for growth or repair of tissues nor breaking down body protein for energy.

Subject C is a 31-year-old pregnant woman of average prepregnancy weight who is consuming 2500 kcalories and 80 grams of protein a day. Her nitrogen values are:

	Nitrogen In	Nitrogen Out
Subject C	12.8 g	10.4 g

What is her nitrogen balance?
▼

Answer:

Does her nitrogen balance make sense metabolically?
▼

Answer:

Determining Your Protein Intake

To determine if your protein intake meets recommendations, the protein content of your diet can be calculated using food composition tables or databases, the information on food labels, or Exchange Lists. Food composition tables and databases contain information on all types of foods and supplements. Food labels provide a more readily available source of information; however, since the labeling of raw meats and fish is voluntary, many of the greatest sources of protein in the diet do not carry food labels. Another way to estimate protein in the diet is to use the exchanges shown in Table 6.3. According to the Exchange Lists, a 1-ounce serving of meat (28 g) provides 7 grams of protein. One cup of milk provides 8 grams, and grains and vegetables provide 2 to 3 grams per serving. For diets based primarily on plant proteins, **protein quality** must also be considered.

Protein quality A measure of how efficiently a protein in the diet can be used to make body proteins.

Protein Quality The recommendations for protein intake assume that the diet contains proteins of various quality. Protein quality is a measure of how useful a protein in the diet is for building body protein. Animal proteins usually contain a pattern of

Table 6.3 *Using Exchange Lists to Calculate the Protein Content of a Diet*

Exchange Groups/Lists	Serving Size	Protein (g)
Carbohydrate Group		
Starch	½ cup rice, cereal, potatoes; 1 slice bread	3
Fruit	1 small apple, peach, pear; ½ banana; ½ cup canned fruit (in juice)	0
Milk	1 cup milk or yogurt	
Nonfat		8
Lowfat		8
Reduced fat		8
Whole		8
Other carbohydrates	Serving sizes vary	Varies
Vegetables	½ cup cooked vegetables, 1 cup raw	2
Meat/Meat Substitute Group	1 oz meat or cheese, ½ cup legumes	
Very lean		7
Lean		7
Medium fat		7
High fat		7
Fat Group	1 tsp butter, margarine, or oil; 1 Tbsp salad dressing	0

amino acids closer to that needed by the body than do plant proteins. Therefore, they are said to be of higher quality. Plant proteins are limited in one or more amino acids and are therefore said to be of lower quality. Since foods with high-quality protein provide more of the essential amino acids in the proportions needed by the body than do foods with low-quality protein, less total protein is needed when the diet contains high-quality protein.

Measuring Protein Quality Protein quality is evaluated experimentally in a number of ways (see Table 6.4). One way is to compare the amino acid pattern of the food being evaluated with that found in a reference protein known to be of high quality, such as egg protein. A **chemical** or **amino acid score** is calculated by comparing the amount of the limiting amino acid in the test protein with the amount of that amino acid in egg protein. In this analysis, proteins with the most desirable proportions of amino acids will have the highest scores. Another factor that must be considered when assessing how well protein is used by the body is digestibility. A measure that considers both amino acid composition and digestibility is the **protein digestibility-corrected amino acid score**. This method is currently used to assess the protein quality of foods for humans and is required by the FDA to assess the protein quality for food labels on products intended for people over one year of age. Other methods of evaluating protein quality include the **protein efficiency ratio**, which measures how well a protein promotes growth in animals, and **net protein utilization** and **biological value**, which measure how well a protein is used by the body for growth and maintenance.

Each of these measures has scientific advantages and drawbacks. They are useful for determining the dietary protein quality available to populations. For example, the quality of protein in a dietary staple such as corn or cassava is extremely important in a country where both food and protein are scarce. In industrialized countries, where protein is usually not scarce, measuring protein quality is less crucial and is generally too cumbersome to be used for diet planning.

A more appropriate way of evaluating protein quality in an individual diet is to look at the sources of the protein. Foods of animal origin, because they supply essential amino acids in the proper proportions for human use, are sources of **complete dietary protein**. Plant foods, on the other hand, contain proteins that do not provide all the amino acids in the proper proportions required for protein synthesis in humans and are therefore said to be incomplete. If the protein in a diet comes from both complete and incomplete sources, it most likely contains adequate amounts of all the essential amino acids needed for protein synthesis. If the protein in a diet comes only from incomplete sources, different types of incomplete protein must be combined so the amino acids provided complement each other to supply all the essential amino acids.

Chemical or **amino acid score** A measure of protein quality determined by comparing the amount of the limiting amino acid in a food with that in a reference protein.

Protein digestibility-corrected amino acid score A measure of protein quality that is calculated by adjusting the amino acid score for digestibility.

Protein efficiency ratio A measure of protein quality determined by comparing the weight gain of a laboratory animal fed a test protein with the weight gain of an animal fed a reference protein.

Net protein utilization A measure of protein quality determined by comparing the amount of nitrogen retained in the body with the amount eaten in the diet.

Biological value A measure of protein quality determined by comparing the amount of nitrogen retained in the body with the amount absorbed from the diet.

Complete dietary protein Protein that provides essential amino acids in the proportions needed to support protein synthesis.

Table 6.4   *Measures of Protein Quality*

Chemical or Amino Acid Score =
$$\frac{\text{mg of limiting amino acid per g of test protein}}{\text{mg of limiting amino acid per g of reference protein}} \times 100$$

Protein Digestibility-Corrected Amino
Acid Score (PDCAAS) = amino acid score $\times$ digestibility factor

Protein Efficiency Ratio (PER) =
$$\frac{\text{wt gain when fed test protein}}{\text{wt gain when fed reference protein}}$$

Net Protein Utilization (NPU) =
$$\frac{\text{nitrogen retained}}{\text{nitrogen intake}} \times 100$$

Biological Value (BV) =
$$\frac{\text{nitrogen retained}}{\text{nitrogen absorbed}} \times 100$$

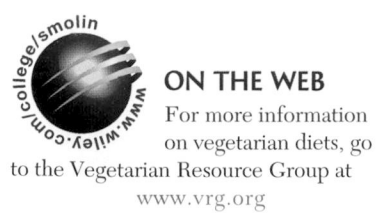

ON THE WEB
For more information
on vegetarian diets, go
to the Vegetarian Resource Group at
www.vrg.org

Vegetarianism A pattern of food intake that eliminates some or all animal products.

Vegan A pattern of food intake that eliminates all animal products.

Protein complementation Combining proteins from different sources so that they collectively provide the proportions of amino acids required to meet needs.

A Diet to Meet Recommendations: Vegetarian or Not?

Populations around the world meet their protein requirements with different types and amounts of protein. In the United States, two-thirds of the dietary protein comes from animal sources—meat, poultry, fish, eggs, and dairy products—but in many cultures smaller amounts of animal proteins are used.[8] To meet requirements, plant proteins must be combined with small amounts of animal proteins or with other plant proteins containing different limiting amino acids. Plant protein-based or vegetarian diets have evolved mostly out of necessity because animal sources are unavailable physically or economically. In affluent societies, vegetarian diets are followed for a variety of reasons other than economics, such as health, religion, personal ethics, or environmental awareness.

Traditionally, **vegetarianism** is defined as abstinence from meat, fish, and fowl. The current interpretation of vegetarianism includes a wide variety of eating patterns depending on the degree of abstinence from animal products. Semivegetarians are those who avoid only certain types of red meat, fish, or poultry—for example, individuals who avoid all red meat but continue to consume poultry and fish. Lacto-ovo vegetarians are those who eat no animal flesh but do eat eggs and dairy products such as milk and cheese; lacto vegetarians are those who avoid animal flesh and eggs but do consume dairy products; and **vegans** are those who avoid all food of animal origin.

Protein Complementation Vegetarian diets meet protein needs by using **protein complementation**, a technique for combining foods containing different limiting amino acids in order to improve the protein quality of the diet as a whole. By eating plant proteins with complementary amino acid patterns, essential amino acid requirements can be met without consuming any animal proteins. The amino acids that are most often limited in plant proteins are lysine, methionine, cysteine, and tryptophan. As a general rule, legumes are deficient in methionine and cysteine but high in lysine. Grains and nuts and seeds are deficient in lysine but high in methionine and cysteine. Corn is deficient in lysine and tryptophan but is a good source of methionine. Consuming a diet containing foods from various categories improves the amino acid composition of the diet as a whole. For example, when rice, which is limited in the amino acid lysine but high in methionine, is eaten with beans, which are high in lysine but limited in methionine, the combination will provide a much higher quality protein than if either is eaten alone.

Common combinations of grains and legumes that have become cultural staples include beans and rice or beans and wheat or corn tortillas in Central and South America; rice and tofu in China and Japan; rice and lentils in India; rice and black-eyed peas in the southern United States; and peanut butter (peanuts are legumes) and bread throughout the United States (Figure 6.17). Plant proteins can also be complemented with animal protein in order to meet the need for essential amino acids. For example, in Asia rice is often flavored with a small amount of spiced beef, chicken, or fish. Although it is not necessary to consume complementary proteins at each meal, the entire day's diet should include proteins from complementary sources in order to satisfy the daily need for amino acids.[9]

Benefits and Pitfalls of Vegetarian Diets The health benefits of vegetarian diets have made them increasingly popular in affluent societies as people strive to adopt health-promoting lifestyles. Vegetarians have been shown to have lower risks for obesity, diabetes, cardiovascular disease, high blood pressure, and some types of cancer.[9,10] Studies of Seventh-Day Adventists, a religious group that espouses a diet containing no animal products as well as abstinence from alcohol consumption and cigarette smoking, found that the incidence of heart disease is about half that of non–Seventh-Day Adventists living in the same area.[11] Even when lifestyle factors other than diet, such as abstinence from alcohol use and cigarette smoking, were

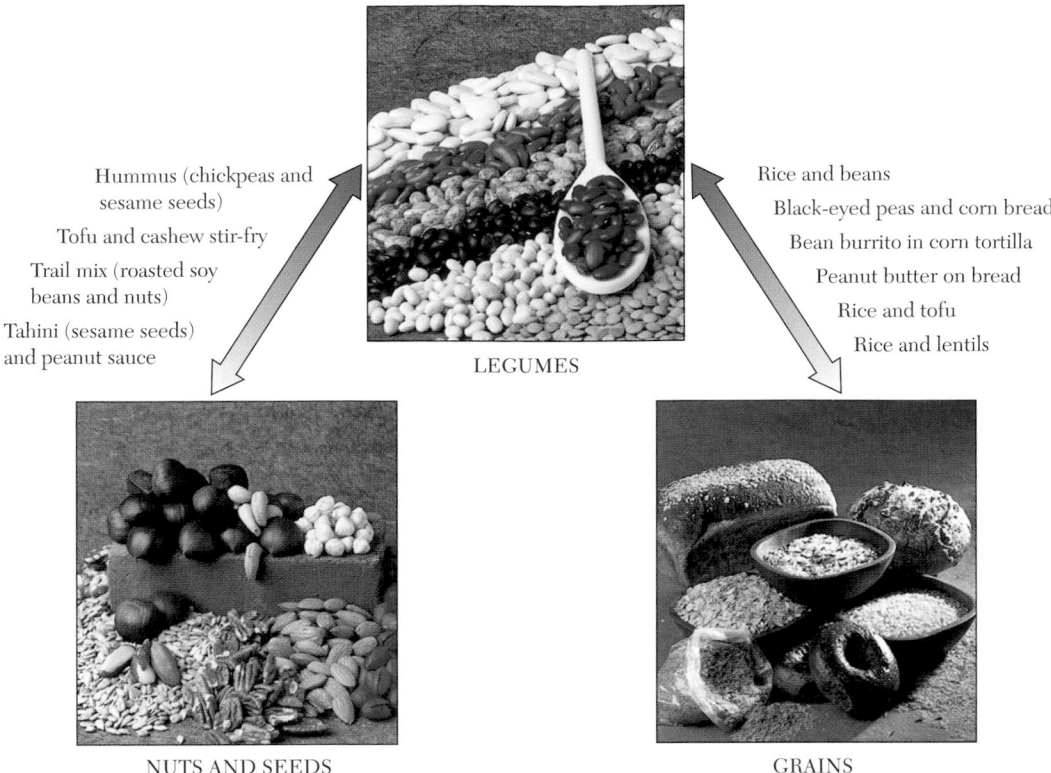

Hummus (chickpeas and
sesame seeds)

Tofu and cashew stir-fry

Trail mix (roasted soy
beans and nuts)

Tahini (sesame seeds)
and peanut sauce

Rice and beans

Black-eyed peas and corn bread

Bean burrito in corn tortilla

Peanut butter on bread

Rice and tofu

Rice and lentils

LEGUMES

NUTS AND SEEDS

GRAINS

Figure 6.17

Combining complementary sources of incomplete plant proteins can provide a diet containing
enough of all the essential amino acids. (George Semple)

kept constant by comparing Seventh-Day Adventists who do not consume vegetarian
diets with their vegetarian counterparts, eating meat was associated with a higher incidence of heart disease and certain types of cancer.[12] Because vegetarian diets eliminate or limit the intake of animal foods, they are lower in saturated fat, cholesterol,
and animal protein. The increased intakes of grains, legumes, vegetables, and fruits
add fiber, vitamins (including antioxidant vitamins), minerals, and phytochemicals to
the diet. It is not known whether the reduction in chronic disease is due to the
amount and type of fat in the diet, the source of the protein, or the increase in fiber,
micronutrients, and phytochemicals. It is likely that the total dietary pattern rather
than a single factor alone is responsible (see *Off the Shelf*: Soy Protein for Your
Health?).

In addition to reducing disease risks, diets that rely more heavily on plant
proteins are more economical. A meal based on rice, pasta, or beans with a small
serving of meat costs less and can provide plenty of protein with less fat than a
meal based on a large serving of meat. For example, a dinner of stir-fried vegetables and rice with a small amount of meat costs about half as much as a meal of
steak and potatoes. Yet both meals provide a significant portion of the day's protein requirement.

Despite the health and economic benefits, nutrient deficiencies can be a problem for people consuming unsupplemented vegetarian diets, particularly vegan
diets. Most people can easily meet their protein needs with lacto and lacto-ovo vegetarian diets. These diets contain high-quality animal proteins from eggs or milk,
which complement the limiting amino acids in the plant proteins. Protein deficiency
is a potential risk when vegan diets, which contain little high-quality protein, are
consumed by small children and adults with increased protein needs, such as pregnant women and those recovering from illness or injury. These individuals must consume carefully planned diets to meet their protein needs.

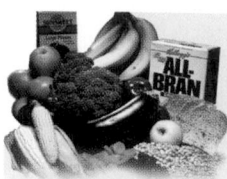

Off the Shelf

Soy Protein for Your Health?

Soy products have long been a major protein source in Asian diets, and their popularity is soaring in the United States. Sales of soy products were almost a billion dollars in 1992 and are projected to exceed $3 billion in 2002.[1] Why has soy increased in popularity? Soy is a high-quality plant protein that is low in fat and high in phytochemicals. Its popularity, however, is more likely to be due to claims that it can reduce the risk of heart disease and cancer, and lessen the symptoms of menopause. Does soy live up to its healthy reputation? Should we be eating more?

The evidence that the consumption of soybeans and products made from soybeans may reduce the risk of heart disease is convincing. Compared to animal protein, soy is low in fat and saturated fat and contains no cholesterol. When soy protein is substituted for animal protein in the diet, it lowers blood levels of LDL (bad) cholesterol and either increases or causes no change in HDL (good) cholesterol levels.[2] Support for soy's beneficial effects on heart disease risk is strong enough for the FDA to allow the use of a health claim on the labels of foods that are low in saturated fat and cholesterol and provide at least 6.25 g of soy protein per serving. In addition, the American Heart Association has recommended that patients with elevated cholesterol include soy foods in their diets.[3]

Investigators are still not sure what component of the soybean is responsible for heart-protective effects. Most research has concerned phytochemicals in soybeans called isoflavones, which are also known as plant estrogens or phytoestrogens. When soy isoflavones are consumed in food, they reduce cholesterol levels, but when they are consumed as supplements, they do not affect cholesterol levels.[4] Because data on the benefits of soy for heart health are

Products Made from Soybeans

Food	Amount	Energy (kcal)	Protein (g)	Fat (g)
Soy milk, regular	1 cup	150	4	8
Soy milk, fat free	1 cup	89	4	0
Tofu, regular	1 oz	22	2.3	1.4
Tofu, lowfat	1 oz	10	1.7	0.3
Miso	1 Tbsp	35	2	1
Tempeh	1 Tbsp	21	2	1
Roasted soybeans	1/4 cup	203	15	11
Soybean sprouts	1 cup	85	9	4
Texturized soy protein (TSP)	1 oz	42	9	0.4
Veggie dogs	1 serving	112	10	6
Soy veggie burger	3 oz	120	15	5
Tofutti frozen dessert, regular	1/2 cup	120	2	2
Tofutti frozen dessert, lowfat	1/2 cup	87	2	0.2
Soy flour, regular	1 Tbsp	23	2	1
Soy flour, fat free	1 Tbsp	21	3	0

strongest when the complete protein is consumed, the FDA health claim is only for whole foods such as tofu and soy milk that contain soy protein—it does not apply to supplements of isoflavones.

There is also evidence that soy may protect against cancer. Isoflavones are chemically similar to the hormone estrogen and may protect against hormone-related cancers, such as cancers of the breast and prostate.[5,6,7] The high intake of soy in traditional Asian diets has been hypothesized to be one reason that Asian women have a relatively low breast cancer incidence.[8] However, there is some evidence that isoflavones may stimulate cancer growth in women who already have breast cancer.[7]

In addition to reducing the risks of heart disease and cancer, soy may reduce some of the symptoms of menopause. Soy isoflavones have been shown to have a small effect on short-term menopausal symptoms such as hot flashes.[9] They may also have long-term benefits on the risk of osteoporosis, which increases after menopause. Epidemiologic evidence suggests that populations who consume a large amount of soy have a lower incidence of osteoporosis.[10] When compared to a soy-free diet, women consuming a soy-containing diet show an increase in bone mineral density, supporting the suggestion that soy may help prevent osteoporosis. A synthetic isoflavone, called ipriflavone, is even used to treat women with osteoporosis.[11] All other factors being equal, these data suggest, but by no means prove, that replacing some animal protein with soy protein would have a desirable effect on bone health.

Deficiencies of some vitamins and minerals are a greater risk for vegetarians than protein deficiency. Vitamin B_{12} is found almost exclusively in animal products; therefore, supplements or fortified foods must be used in vegan diets to meet needs. The major source of calcium in the North American diet is dairy products, so again, vegan diets must be carefully planned to meet calcium needs. Likewise, most dietary vitamin D comes from fortified dairy products, so vegans must get their vitamin D from sunshine (see Chapter 9) or consume other sources of this vitamin such as for-

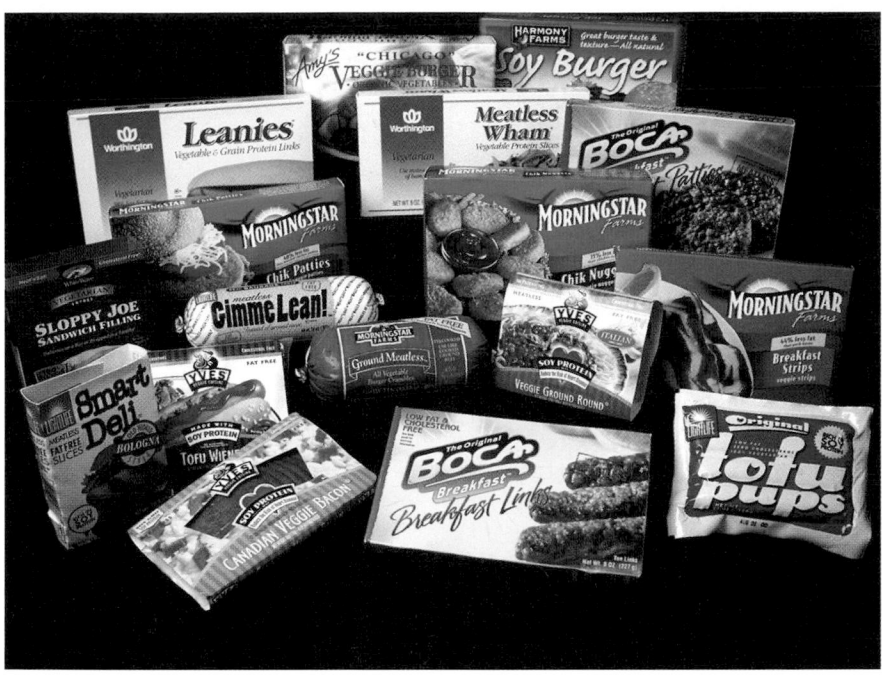

Courtesy www.soyfoods.com

Based on all of these findings, the American public may benefit from an increase in soy protein consumption. How much do you need to eat to achieve these benefits? The health claim allowed on food labels states that "25 g of soy protein a day, as part of a diet low in saturated fat and cholesterol, may reduce the risk of heart disease." But there is evidence that consuming only 10 grams of soy protein per day (the amount provided by Asian diets) may decrease the risks of coronary heart disease and certain cancers, and improve bone health.

How can you increase your intake of soy protein? Soy-based foods are available in many forms. Soybeans can be eaten boiled or roasted. Soybean sprouts can be added to salads. Tofu, also known as bean curd, is a soft cheeselike product made by curdling fresh hot soy milk. It can be consumed cooked or raw. Miso and tempeh are fermented soybean products that are used in soups and mixed dishes. Soy flour can be incorporated into baked goods. It is also used to make texturized soy protein (TSP). TSP is used to make vegetarian burgers and hot dogs. Although the evidence supporting the health-promoting effects of soy is strong, simply including soy-based foods, or any single food, in the diet is not the answer to good health. Replacing some of the animal sources of protein with soy protein may help protect your health, but other dietary and lifestyle factors also influence your overall risk. "Soy by itself is not a magic food," says Christine Lewis of the Center for Food Safety and Applied Nutrition. "But rather it is an example of the different kinds of foods that together in a complete diet can have a positive effect on health."[11]

[1]Henkel, J. Soy: Health claims for soy protein, questions about other components. *FDA Consumer*, May–June 2000.

[2]Anthony, M. S. Soy and cardiovascular disease: Cholesterol lowering and beyond. *J. Nutr.* 130:662S–663S, 2000.

[3]Krauss, R. M., Eckel, R. H., Howard, B., et al. AHA dietary guidelines: Revision 2000: A statement for healthcare professionals from the Nutrition Committee of the American Heart Association. *Circulation* 102:2284–2299, 2000.

[4]Sirtori, C. R., and Lovati, M. R. Soy proteins and cardiovascular disease. *Curr. Atheroscler. Rep.* 3:47–53, 2001.

[5]Adlercreutz, H., Mazur, W., Bartels, P., et al. Phytoestrogens and prostate disease. *J. Nutr.* 130:658S–659S, 2000.

[6]Goodman, M. T., Wilkens, L. R., Hankin, J. H., et al. Association of soy and fiber consumption with the risk of endometrial cancer. *Am. J. Epidemiol.* 146:294–306, 1997.

[7]Kurzer, M. S. Supplement: Fourth Int'l Symposium on the Role of Soy in Preventing and Treating Chronic Disease. Hormonal Effects of Soy in Premenopausal Women and Men. *J. Nutr.* 132:570S–573S, 2002.

[8]Stoll, B. A. Eating to beat breast cancer: potential role for soy supplements. *Ann. Oncol.* 8:223–225, 1997.

[9]Vincent, A. and Fitzpatrick, L. A. Soy isoflavones: Are they useful in menopause? *Mayo Clin. Proc.* 75:1174–1184, 2000.

[10]Adlercreutz, H., and Mazur, W. Phytoestrogens and Western disease. *Ann. Med* 29:95–120, 1997.

[11]Potter, S. M., Baum, J. M., Teng, H., et al. Soy protein and isoflavones: Their effects on blood lipids and bone density in postmenopausal women. *Am. J. Clin. Nutr.* 68(suppl):1375S–1379S, 1999.

tified soy milk. Iron and zinc may be deficient in vegetarian diets because the best sources of these minerals are red meats and these minerals are poorly absorbed from plant sources. Since iron and zinc are low in dairy products, lacto-ovo and lacto vegetarians as well as vegans are at risk for deficiencies. A separate RDA for iron has been established for vegetarians. Vegetarian sources of these nutrients are listed in Table 6.5 and discussed in Chapters 8 to 11 (see *Critical Thinking*: Choosing a Vegetarian Diet).

Table 6.5 *Sources of Essential Nutrients Potentially Lacking in Vegan Diets*

Nutrient	Sources in Vegan Diets
Protein	Soy-based products, legumes, seeds, nuts, grains, and vegetables
Vitamin B_{12}	Products fortified with B_{12} such as soy beverages and cereals, vitamin supplements
Calcium	Tofu processed with calcium, broccoli, kale, bok choy, legumes, and products fortified with calcium such as soy beverages, grain products, and orange juice
Vitamin D	Sunshine, products fortified with vitamin D such as soy beverages and margarine
Iron	Legumes, tofu, green leafy vegetables, dried fruit, whole grains, iron-fortified cereals and breads (absorption is improved by vitamin C found in citrus fruit, tomatoes, strawberries, and dark green vegetables)
Zinc	Whole grains, legumes, nuts, tofu, and fortified cereals

Choosing a Diet to Meet Needs A simple way to ensure an adequate protein intake from a combination of plant and animal proteins is to follow the recommendations of the Food Guide Pyramid. The groups in the Food Guide Pyramid that are highest in protein are the Milk, Yogurt, & Cheese Group and the Meat, Poultry, Fish, Dry Beans, Eggs, & Nuts Group. These two food groups are in the upper sections of the Pyramid, indicating that these foods should make up a relatively small proportion of

Table 6.6 *Selecting a Vegetarian Diet Using the Food Guide Pyramid[a]*

Food Group	Suggested Number of Servings	Serving Sizes
Bread, Cereal, Rice, & Pasta Group	6–11	1 slice bread 1 oz cold cereal ½ cup rice, pasta, or cooked cereal
Vegetable Group[b]	3–5	½ cup cooked 1 cup raw leafy
Fruit Group	2–4	1 medium apple, orange, or banana ½ cup chopped or canned ¾ cup juice ¼ cup dried
Dry Beans, Nuts, Seeds, Eggs, & Meat Substitutes Group	2–3	1½ cups cooked dry beans 4–6 Tbsp nuts, seeds, or peanut butter 1 cup soy milk ½ cup tofu 2–3 eggs[c]
Milk, Yogurt, & Cheese Group[d]	0–3	1 cup milk 1.5 oz cheese 1 cup yogurt
Fats, Oils, and Sweets	Use sparingly	Candy Butter Oil Salad dressing

[a]For vegan diets vitamin B_{12} supplements or vitamin B_{12}-fortified foods are necessary to meet needs.

[b]Include 1 cup of dark green leafy vegetables daily to help meet iron and calcium needs.

[c]Lacto vegetarians and vegans may eliminate this choice.

[d]Vegetarians who choose not to use milk need to select milk substitutes fortified with calcium and vitamin D, such as fortified soy milk, and other foods rich in calcium such as dark green leafy vegetables. At least two servings of calcium-rich foods should be consumed daily.

Modified from the National Center for Nutrition and Dietetics, the American Dietetic Association; based on the USDA Food Guide Pyramid, © ADAF, 1997.

the day's intake. Two to three servings per day are recommended from each. Two 8-ounce glasses of milk and two 2-ounce servings of meat provide about 44 grams of protein. Consuming the minimum recommended servings from the Bread, Cereal, Rice, & Pasta Group and the Vegetable Group, 6 and 3 servings respectively, would bring the total to 71 grams of protein—more than enough to meet most people's needs.

Vegetarians can meet their needs by modifying their selections from the traditional Food Guide Pyramid (see Table 6.6). The food choices and recommended number of servings from the grains, vegetables, and fruit are the same. The groups in the next level of the traditional Pyramid (meat and milk) include foods of animal origin. Vegetarians can choose 2 to 3 servings of dry beans, nuts, seeds, eggs, and meat substitutes. Lacto vegetarians (those who consume dairy products) should also consume 2 to 3 servings from the milk group. Vegans (those who do not consume any animal foods) should consume milk substitutes fortified with calcium and vitamin D, or other foods high in these nutrients. To obtain adequate vitamin B_{12}, vegans must take B_{12} supplements or use products fortified with vitamin B_{12}.

A Food Guide Pyramid designed specifically for vegetarian diets is shown in Figure 6.18.[13] It includes five major plant-based food groups in the bottom portion of the pyramid. All vegetarians should consume selections from these groups, which include whole grains, legumes, fruits, vegetables, and nuts and seeds. The four food groups in the smaller upper portion of the pyramid are optional. These include dairy, eggs, vegetable oils, and sweets. One or more of these optional food groups can be included in the diet depending on the philosophical values and health beliefs of the individual. Although the dairy group is optional, the nutrients provided by this group are not, and adequate calcium and vitamin D must be obtained from other sources if no selections are made from this group. If no animal products are consumed, a reliable source of vitamin B_{12} must be included. In addition to providing for the dietary needs of vegetarians with diverse eating patterns, this Vegetarian Food Guide Pyramid also considers lifestyle factors. Moderate exposure to sunlight is important to ensure adequate vitamin D. Adequate physical activity and water intake are also important for health.

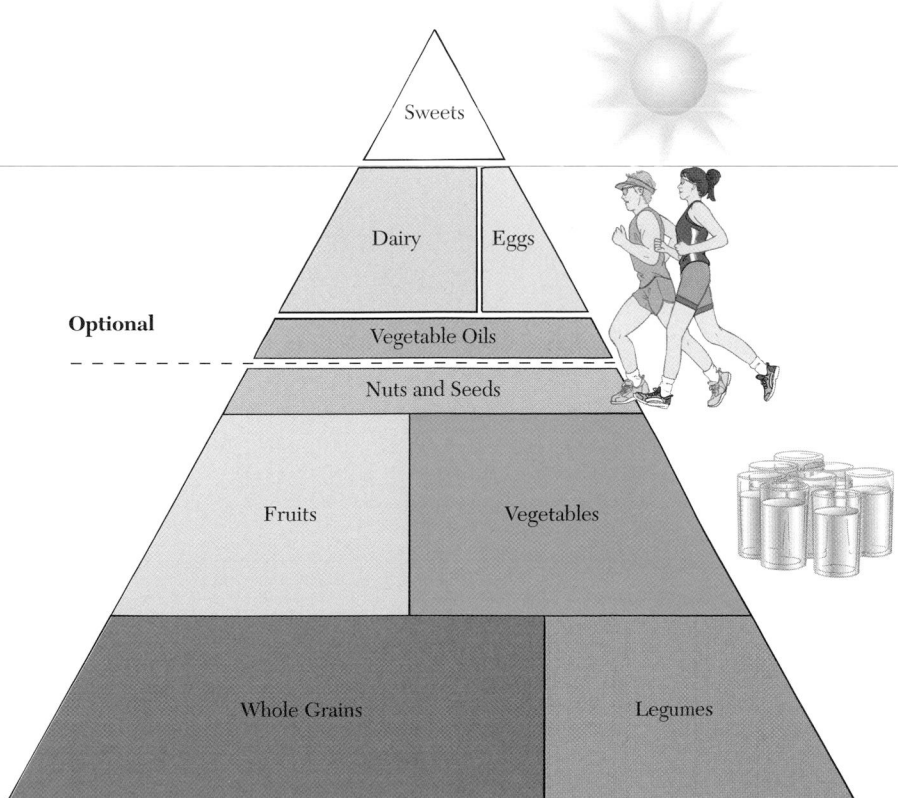

Note: A reliable source of vitamin B_{12} should be included if no dairy or eggs are consumed.

Figure 6.18
This Vegetarian Food Guide Pyramid can be used to select a diet that meets nutrient needs without including animal foods. All vegetarians should make selections from the five plant-based groups in the lower trapezoid-shaped portion of the pyramid. Depending on the type of vegetarian diet, additional selections can be made from one or more of the four groups in the upper portion of the pyramid. For example, a lacto-vegetarian would include selections from the dairy group. This pyramid also emphasizes the importance of moderate exposure to sunlight to ensure adequate vitamin D, physical activity, and adequate water consumption for health. (Source: Haddad, E.H., Sabate, J., and Whitten, C.G. Vegetarian food guide pyramid: A conceptual framework. *Am. J. Clin. Nutr.* 70 (suppl): 615S–619S, 1999. Available online at www.llu.edu/llu/nutrition/vegguide.html.)

CRITICAL THINKING

Choosing a Vegetarian Diet

A year ago Ajay decided to stop eating meat. While studying protein in his nutrition class, he became concerned that his diet did not correctly complement protein sources. Ajay is 26 years old and weighs 154 pounds. Does his diet meet his protein needs?

What is the RDA for protein for someone of his age and weight?

▼

$$\frac{154 \text{ lb}}{2.2 \text{ lb/kg}} = 70 \text{ kg}$$

RDA for adults = 0.8 g protein per kg body weight

$$70 \text{ kg} \times \frac{0.8 \text{g}}{\text{kg}} = 56 \text{ g of protein}$$

He records his food intake for one day and then uses diet analysis software to calculate his protein intake.

▼

Food	Amount	Protein (g)
Breakfast		
Grape Nuts	3 Tbsp	2.4
Milk, lowfat	½ cup	4
Orange juice	½ cup	0.8
Toast, wheat	2 slices	5
Peanut butter	1 Tbsp	4
Coffee	1 cup	0
Lunch		
Dahl (lentil soup)	1 cup	9
Rice	1 cup	6
Banana	1	1
Apple juice	1 cup	0
Dinner		
Green salad	1 cup	1
with dressing	1 Tbsp	0
Rice	1 cup	6
Curried potatoes	½ cup	1.5
and chickpeas	⅓ cup	5
Yogurt	1 cup	13
Poori (fried bread)	2 pieces	5
Ice cream	½ cup	2
Total		**65.7**

His diet provides 65.7 grams of protein, which exceeds his calculated RDA of 56 grams.

Do Ajay's food choices include complementary proteins?

▼

At breakfast, Ajay has milk, which is a high-quality protein, and bread and peanut butter, which contain proteins that complement each other (see Figure

6.17). At lunch, the protein in the dahl complements the protein in the rice. At dinner, he has chickpeas, which complement both the rice and the wheat protein in the poori. He also has yogurt and ice cream, which provide high-quality proteins.

How much protein would this diet provide if he decided to eliminate dairy products?
▼

Answer:

How would eliminating dairy products affect his calcium and vitamin D intake?
▼

The major source of calcium in his diet is dairy products, so he would have to carefully plan his diet to include other calcium sources. Likewise, most of his dietary vitamin D comes from fortified dairy products, so he would need to be sure to get his vitamin D from sunshine or other fortified foods. Vegetarian sources of these nutrients are listed in Table 6.5 and discussed in Chapters 8 to 11.

Does his diet meet the Food Guide Pyramid recommendations for vegetarians?
▼

Answer:

• PROTEINS, AMINO ACIDS, AND FOOD TECHNOLOGY

Protein in foods provides more than nutrients; it contributes to the taste, texture, shape, and color of food. It is the protein in grains that provides the structure of breads and baked goods. Egg protein gives custard stability. The protein in cream allows it to be whipped into whipped cream; and myoglobin, the iron-carrying protein in muscle, gives meat its red color. These chemical and physical properties of proteins have made them important additives in processed foods.

Proteins in Processed Foods

Many proteins are added to foods in purified forms in order to contribute taste and texture. The milk protein casein (sodium caseinate) is used in coffee whiteners and frozen dessert toppings. The casein in these products helps simulate the taste and texture of cream. Gelatin, a protein derived from animal connective tissue, is used to gel yogurt; to whip foams such as cupcake fillings; to clear fruit juices, wines, and beer; to increase viscosity; and to prevent the growth of ice crystals in frozen desserts. Gelatin, although it is derived from an animal protein, is completely deficient in the essential amino acid tryptophan and low in other essential amino acids, so though a useful additive for the food industry, it is not a good source of high-quality dietary protein. **Protein hydrolysates** or **hydrolyzed proteins** are also frequently added to foods. They are proteins that have been treated with acid or enzymes to break them down into amino acids and small peptides. They are used as flavorings, flavor enhancers, stabilizers, or thickening agents in foods such as packaged rice and potato products.

Protein hydrolysates or hydrolyzed proteins Mixtures of amino acids or amino acids and polypeptides produced when a protein is completely or partially broken down by treatment with acid or enzymes.

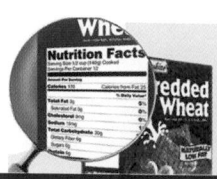

Off the Label
Identifying Protein Sources

Food labels provide information about the composition of foods and the contribution they make toward meeting daily nutrient intake recommendations. Since protein is a nutrient that is adequate in the diet of most Americans, the protein content of foods is listed but not emphasized on most food labels. For some individuals, however, such as those with allergies to certain proteins and those who wish to avoid specific foods for religious, ethical, or other reasons, food labels are an important source of information that can help identify foods appropriate for their diets.

Like other nutrients, information on protein is listed in the Nutrition Facts section of the food label as well as in the ingredient list. The Nutrition Facts section lists the number of grams of protein per serving. However, the percent Daily Value is required only on foods that contain protein of very low quality. When listed, the percent Daily Value is adjusted for protein quality. For example, a food that contains 10 grams of high-quality protein supplies 20% of the Daily Value for protein, whereas a food that contains 10 grams of a low-quality protein may indicate that it provides only 5% of the Daily Value for protein. Only the latter must list the percent Daily Value on the label.

The ingredient list indicates the source of protein in foods. For individuals who restrict their intake of certain proteins, this information can be invaluable. If an individual's religion prohibits the consumption of pork, the ingredient list is needed to determine if a packaged food, such as frozen egg rolls, contains pork. For a child who is allergic to peanut protein, the ingredient list can be lifesaving. Because peanut allergy can be so severe, even products that do not intentionally contain peanuts may include them at the end of the ingredient list or provide a special warning if there is a potential for cross-contamination from equipment or foods made in the same facility. When foods contain isolated proteins such as the milk protein casein, determining the source of the protein is more challenging. For example, if someone who is allergic to casein wanted to use powdered creamer in his coffee, he might select a brand labeled nondairy creamer. Reading the ingredient list would show that the product does contain casein, along with the statement that casein is a milk derivative. If he selected a brand that does not claim to be nondairy, casein would be listed without the statement that it is a milk derivative.

Even products that typically contain little or no protein may have small amounts of protein hydrolysates added to them. To help individuals avoid specific proteins, foods containing protein hydrolysates are required to list the source of the hydrolysate. For example, the spaghetti sauce mix whose label is shown here contains so little protein that the Nutrition Facts section lists the grams of protein as zero. The ingredient list, however, shows that the product contains hydrolyzed corn gluten, soy protein, and wheat gluten protein. An individual with an allergy to soy should avoid this product and all products listing soy or hydrolyzed soy protein as an ingredient. This information is also helpful to vegetarians who restrict animal proteins.

Individual amino acids added to foods are also included in the ingredient list. For instance, some people try to avoid consuming the amino acid glutamate (glutamic acid) because they experience MSG symptom complex. Glutamate in the form of MSG is used as a flavor enhancer in foods such as potato chips and other snack foods; canned soups, meats, and fish; packaged meals such as frozen seafood, chicken, and other entrees;

Soy proteins are used in processed foods for many reasons. Soy protein concentrate is a derivative of soybeans that is used to aid in emulsification and provide texture in products such as canned gravies and candy bars. Soy protein isolates and texturized vegetable protein are types of soy protein that can be formed into chunks, woven or spun into fibers, or otherwise shaped and flavored to form meat substitutes. They are used to make imitation hot dogs, meatballs, chicken, and veal, or they can be added to animal protein as an extender or filler. Soy is a legume so it is low in the sulfur amino acids, methionine and cystine, but it is so high in easily digestible protein that it is nearly equivalent to animal protein in quality.

An addition to the array of proteins used in processed foods is the fat substitute Simplesse. Simplesse is made from egg white and milk proteins that are modified by heating, filtering, and high-speed mixing. The resulting protein consists of millions of microscopic balls that slip and slide over one another, providing the slippery texture of fat. Despite its "fatty" texture, Simplesse is made from protein and water and so contains a little more than 1 kcalorie per gram, compared with 9 kcalories per gram for fat.

Amino Acids Added to Foods

The amino acid composition of foods is also sometimes changed by genetic engineering and food processing. For example, the amino acid composition of plant procured meats and lunch meats; and foods of many international cuisines. When added, it must appear on the label in the ingredient list as monosodium glutamate or potassium glutamate, as shown in the figure. Seasonings that contain MSG include Accent, Ajinomoto, Zest, Vestin, Gourmet Powder, Subu, Chinese seasoning, Glutavene, Glutacyl, RL-50 Kombu extract, and Meijing or Wei-jing. Glutamate may also be added to food as a component of a protein hydrolysate. Foods containing ingredients that are sources of glutamate, such as hydrolyzed protein, may not state "no MSG" or "no added MSG" on the label.[1]

Food labels generally focus on providing information to help the population meet the current recommendations for maintaining health and preventing disease. In the case of protein, which is not a focus of public health guidelines in the United States, the information is helpful to individuals who have special needs.

[1]U.S. Food and Drug Administration. FDA and monosodium glutamate (MSG). *FDA Backgrounder,* August 31, 1995. Available online at www.fda.gov/opacom/backgrounders/msg.htm/ Accessed April 3, 2002.

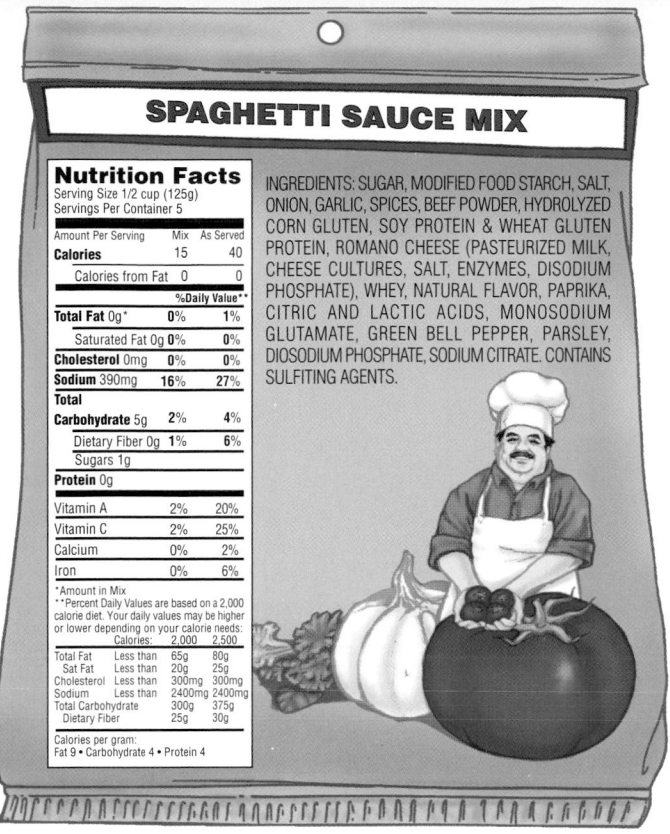

teins can be modified by genetic engineering to produce a higher quality protein, such as a variety of corn that is higher in lysine. In processed foods, limiting amino acids can be supplemented to enhance the quality of vegetable protein. Amino acids are also added to provide flavor. Two examples are the low-kcalorie sweetener aspartame and the flavor enhancer monosodium glutamate (MSG).

Aspartame Aspartame is a dipeptide composed of the amino acids aspartic acid and phenylalanine. Aspartame is used in a wide variety of foods, including carbonated beverages, gelatin desserts, and chewing gum (Figure 6.19). It cannot be used in cooked products because it breaks down when heated, losing its sweet taste.

Aspartame contains the amino acid phenylalanine and therefore can be dangerous to individuals with a genetic disorder called **phenylketonuria (PKU)**. In individuals with PKU, an enzyme needed to metabolize the amino acid phenylalanine does not function properly, leaving them unable to convert the essential amino acid phenylalanine to the semiessential amino acid tyrosine. Instead, phenylalanine is converted to compounds called phenylketones, which build up in the blood. High phenylketone levels can interfere with brain development, causing mental retardation. To prevent mental retardation, infants and children with PKU must consume a diet with just enough phenylalanine to meet the body's need for protein synthesis

Phenylketonuria (PKU) An inherited disease in which the body cannot metabolize the amino acid phenylalanine. If the disease is untreated, toxic by-products accumulate in the blood.

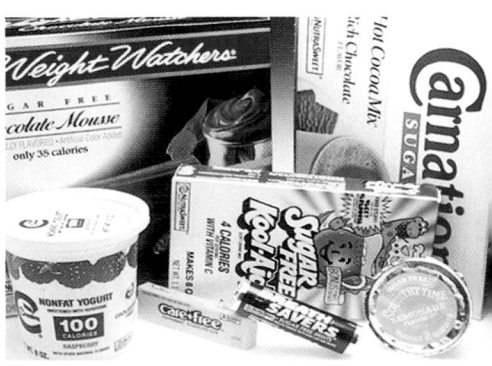

Figure 6.19
Aspartame is used to sweeten a variety of products. (Charles D. Winters)

but not so much that the buildup of phenylketones occurs. The diet must also provide sufficient tyrosine, because the disease prevents conversion of phenylalanine to tyrosine. PKU afflicts about 1 in 12,000 newborn infants.[14] Infants are tested for this disorder at birth. Special low-phenylalanine or phenylalanine-free formulas are manufactured for infants with this disease. Pregnant women with PKU must be especially careful to consume a low-phenylalanine diet in order to protect their unborn children from high phenylketone levels and the mental retardation and other birth defects they cause.[15] Because these individuals must restrict their phenylalanine intake, warnings for individuals with PKU are included on the labels of all products containing aspartame, though few of them specify the actual amount of the sweetener contained in the product.

Monosodium Glutamate Monosodium glutamate (MSG) is a flavor enhancer best known for its use in Chinese cooking. It is added to a variety of packaged foods and sold as a powder for use in home cooking. It consists of the amino acid glutamic acid (or glutamate) bound to sodium. Some people report adverse reactions including a flushed face, tingling or burning sensations, headache, rapid heartbeat, chest pain, and general weakness after consuming MSG.[16] These symptoms are referred to as MSG symptom complex, commonly termed Chinese restaurant syndrome, and are most likely to occur within an hour after eating about 3 grams or more of MSG on an empty stomach (see *Off the Label:* Identifying Protein Sources). However, a typical serving of foods containing MSG includes only about 0.5 mg of MSG. Controlled studies have not been able to consistently document reactions to MSG.[17] Because glutamate is a neurotransmitter, some brain researchers are concerned that very high dietary intakes of glutamate could be toxic to nerves in humans. However, a review of scientific data has found no evidence that dietary MSG causes brain lesions or damages nerve cells in humans. The FDA has therefore maintained glutamate on the list of substances generally recognized as safe (see Chapter 17).[18]

• APPLICATIONS •

1. Calculate your average protein intake using the three-day food record you kept in Chapter 2.
   a. What is your average daily protein intake in grams?
   b. Is your intake higher or lower than the RDA for protein for someone of your weight, age, and life stage?
   c. If you consumed more than the RDA for protein, do you think you should decrease your protein intake? Why or why not?
   d. If you consumed less than the RDA for protein, suggest changes that will increase your protein intake to meet needs. How did these changes affect the amount of fat in your diet?

2. Using the three-day record you kept in Chapter 2, compare your protein and fat intake for each day.

	Protein (g)	Fat (g)
Day 1		
Day 2		
Day 3		

   a. What is the relationship between the fat and protein in your diet?

   b. Look at the three foods that contribute the most protein to your diet each day. Are they animal or plant foods?
   c. What percentage of your total fat for that day do these provide?

3. Imagine that you have decided to become a lacto vegetarian. Make a list of the nondairy animal foods in your diet and then list plant foods you could substitute. Use protein complementation (see Figure 6.17) to be sure that you meet your need for essential amino acids.
   a. Does your modified diet meet the serving recommendations in Table 6.6? If not, what changes would you suggest?
   b. How much protein is in your lacto vegetarian diet? Does it meet the RDA for protein for someone in your age and gender group?
   c. If you already consume a lacto vegetarian diet, design a vegan diet by substituting plant sources of protein for dairy products. Make sure the diet includes at least 2 servings of calcium-rich foods.

4. Assume you are a vegetarian and you will be hosting Thanksgiving dinner for your family. Use a vegetarian cookbook or information on the Internet to design a vegetarian menu that will provide complementary proteins as well as provide a festive holiday meal.

SUMMARY

1. Dietary protein comes from both animal and plant sources. In developed countries, protein intakes are usually well above needs.

2. Proteins are made of amino acid chains that fold over on themselves to create unique three-dimensional structures. The shape of a protein determines its function. Amino acids consist of a carbon atom with a hydrogen atom, a nitrogen-containing group, an acid group, and a unique side chain attached. The amino acids that the body is unable to make in sufficient amounts are essential amino acids and must be consumed in the diet.

3. Digestion breaks dietary protein into small peptides and amino acids, which are absorbed. Amino acids can be used for the synthesis of protein and other nitrogen-containing molecules and can be deaminated and used for energy or to synthesize glucose or fatty acids.

4. The amino acids used by cells to synthesize proteins come from both dietary protein and the degradation of body proteins.

5. DNA in the nucleus of cells contains the information needed to make body proteins. These proteins then provide structure, regulate body functions as enzymes and hormones, transport molecules in the blood and in cells, function in the immune system, and aid in muscle contraction, fluid balance, and acid balance.

6. Protein-energy malnutrition is a public health concern, primarily in developing countries. Kwashiorkor occurs when the protein content of the diet is deficient. It is most common in children. Marasmus occurs when total energy intake is deficient.

7. For healthy adults, the RDA for protein is 0.8 gram per kilogram of body weight. Growth, pregnancy, lactation, illness, and injury can increase requirements. Certain types of physical activity may also increase protein needs.

8. Animal proteins contain a pattern of amino acids that matches the needs of the human body more closely than the pattern of amino acids in plant proteins. Animal proteins are therefore said to be of higher quality than plant proteins.

9. Diets that include little or no animal protein can provide adequate protein if the sources of protein are complemented to supply enough of all the essential amino acids.

10. Proteins and amino acids can be used in the preparation of processed foods to enhance nutritional value and to change texture and flavor.

REVIEW QUESTIONS

1. List some good sources of plant protein.

2. What are amino acids?

3. What is an essential amino acid?

4. What is the "amino acid pool"?

5. List six functions of proteins in the body.

6. Why is protein deficiency most common in infants and children?

7. How does the typical protein intake in North America compare to recommendations?

8. What effect does moderate exercise have on protein needs?

9. What does nitrogen balance suggest about the balance between protein synthesis and protein breakdown in the body?

10. What is protein quality?

11. What is protein complementation?

12. List some uses of proteins and amino acids in processed foods.

REFERENCES

1. Kuhn, L. C. Iron and gene expression: Molecular mechanisms regulating cellular iron homeostasis. *Nutr. Rev.* 56(II):S11–S19, 1998.

2. Williams, C. D. Kwashiorkor: Nutritional disease of children associated with maize diet. *Lancet* 2:1151–1154, 1935.

3. van't Veer, P., Jansen, M. C., Klerk, M., and Kok, F. J. Fruits and vegetables in the prevention of cancer and cardiovascular disease. *Public Health Nutr.* 3:103–107, 2000.

4. Maroni, B. J., and Mitch, W. E. Role of nutrition in prevention of the progression of renal disease. *Annu. Rev. Nutr.* 17:435–455, 1997.

5. Millward, D. J. Optimal intakes of protein in the human diet. *Proc. Nutr. Soc.* 58:403–413, 1999.

6. Institute of Medicine, Food and Nutrition Board. *Dietary Reference Intakes for Energy, Carbohydrates, Fiber, Fat, Protein and Amino Acids.* Washington, D.C.: National Academy Press, 2002.

7. American Dietetic Association. Nutrition and athletic performance. Position of the American Dietetic Association, the Canadian Dietetic Association and the American College of Sports Medicine. *J. Am. Diet. Assoc.* 100:1543–1556, 2000.

8. Smit, E., Nieto, F. J., Crespo, C. J., and Mitchell, P. Estimates of animal and plant protein intake in U.S. adults: Results from the Third National Health and Nutrition Examination Survey, 1988–1991. *J. Am. Diet. Assoc.* 99:813–820, 1999.

9. Messina, V. K., and Burke, K. I. Position of the American Dietetic Association: Vegetarian diets. *J. Am. Diet. Assoc.* 97:1317–1321, 1997.

10. Walter, P. Effects of vegetarian diets on aging and longevity. *Nutr. Rev.* 55(II):S61–S68, 1997.

11. Fonnebo, V. The healthy Seventh-Day Adventist. *Am. J. Clin. Nutr.* 59(suppl):1124S–1129S, 1994.

12. Fraser, G. Associations between diet and cancer, ischemic heart disease, and all-cause mortality in non-Hispanic white California Seventh-Day Adventists. *Am. J. Clin. Nutr.* 70(suppl):532S–538S, 1999.

13. Haddad, E. H., Sabaté, J., and Whitten, C. G. Vegetarian food guide pyramid: A conceptual framework. *Am. J. Clin. Nutr.* 70(suppl):615S–619S, 1999.

14. Seymour, C. A., Cockburn, F., Thomason, M. J., et al. Newborn screening for inborn errors of metabolism: A systematic review. *Health Technol. Assess.* I:1–95, 1997.

15. Brown, A. Barriers to control among pregnant women with phenylketonuria—United States 1998–2000. *MMWR* February 15, 2002.

16. Walker, R., and Lupien, J. R. The safety evaluation of monosodium glutamate. *J. Nutr.* 130:1049S–1052S, 2000.

17. Geha, R. S., Beiser, A., Ren, C., et al. Review of alleged reaction to monosodium glutamate and outcome of a multicenter double-blind placebo-controlled study. *J. Nutr.* 130:1058S–1062S, 2000.

18. U.S. Food and Drug Administration. FDA and monosodium glutamate (MSG). *FDA Backgrounder,* August 31, 1995. Avalable online at www.fda.gov/opacom/backgrounders/msg.html/ Accessed April 3, 2002.

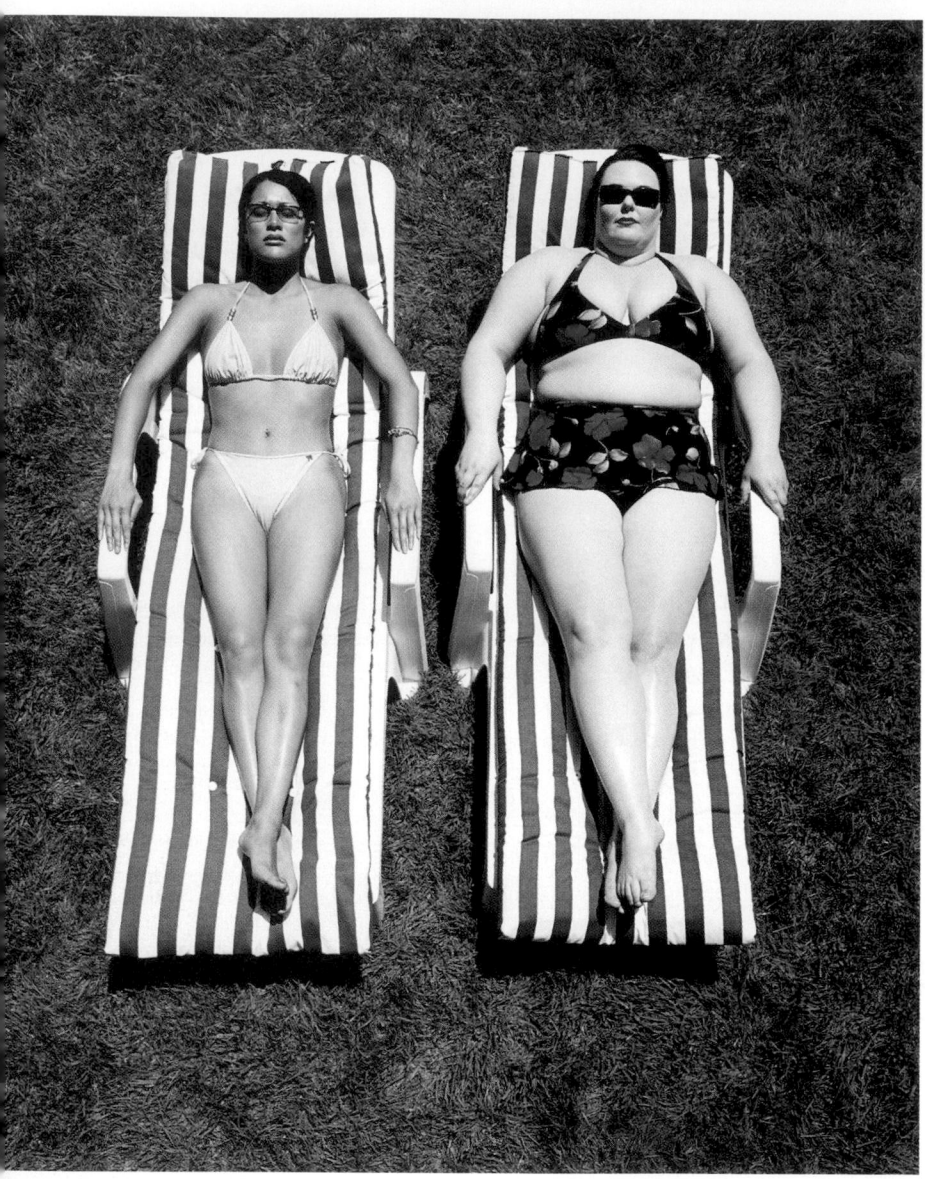

(© Robert Daily/Stone.)

Chapter Concepts

✔ Energy in food and the body is measured in kcalories or kjoules.

✔ Body weight is maintained by balancing energy intake with output—the principle of energy balance.

✔ Energy is needed for basal functions, fueling activity, and processing the nutrients from food.

✔ Energy consumed in excess of needs is stored primarily as fat.

✔ Excess body fat, or obesity, is a disease that increases the risk of other chronic diseases and early death.

✔ Body Mass Index (BMI) is currently the accepted standard for assessing body fatness.

✔ The propensity for storing excess body fat is genetic, but our food intake and activity level affect what we actually weigh.

✔ The goal of weight management is to reduce body fat to a healthy level and maintain that level throughout life.

✔ Weight loss requires reducing food intake, increasing activity, and/or changing eating habits.

✔ Eating disorders are psychological disorders that involve abnormal eating behaviors due to a pathological concern with body size and weight.

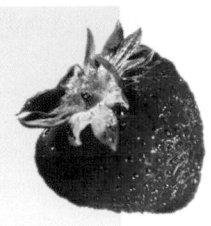

Just a Taste

Do overweight people consume more kcalories than thin people?

Is obesity inherited?

Are weight-loss drugs a safe approach to weight loss?

Our society puts a high value on physical appearance. Being thin is considered attractive and being fat is not. Overweight individuals face discrimination just about everywhere—in school, in the workplace, even on public transportation. Excess body fat also increases the risk of developing chronic diseases such as diabetes, heart disease, and cancer. Nevertheless, about 61% of adults in the United States are either overweight or obese.[1] This percentage has risen dramatically over the last 20 years. Between 1980 and 1999 the incidence of obesity increased from about 15% to an estimated 27%.[1] Why are we getting fatter when society and health promotion messages tell us to be thin?

It is not easy to lose weight. Although thousands of Americans diet every year, many never lose any weight at all, and most people who lose weight eventually regain it. This creates a ready supply of customers for the thousands of weight-loss plans offered by commercial ventures, physicians, and support groups. A tour of any bookstore will reveal a mind-boggling assortment of diet books. Weight-loss choices range from liquid diets and unusual food combinations to drug therapy and stomach bypass surgery.

The increasing prevalence of obesity and the failure of most attempts at weight loss have created a major public health problem. Estimates suggest that the annual health-care costs of obesity are about $99.2 billion,[2] more than the health-care costs of daily smokers and heavy drinkers.[3] Why are we overweight, and how can we reduce this growing trend?

Energy The capacity to do work.

Kilojoule (kjoule) The amount of work required to move an object weighing 1 kilogram a distance of 1 meter under the force of gravity.

Kilocalorie (kcalorie) The amount of heat required to raise the temperature of 1 kilogram of water 1° Celsius.

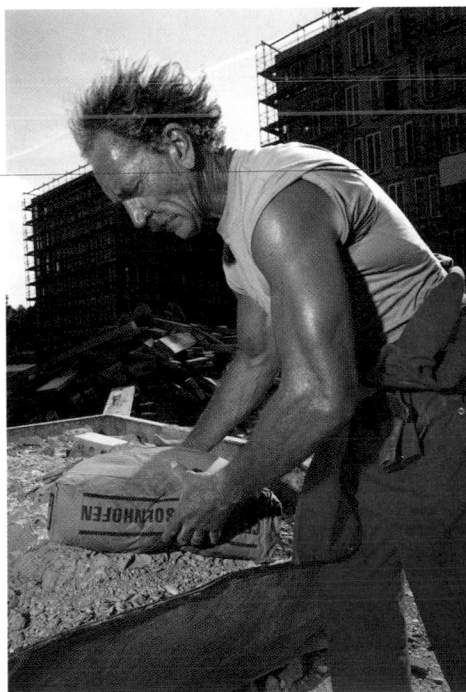

Figure 7.1
The energy in the food we eat can be used by the body to produce ATP, which can then be used for muscle contraction. (Thomas Hoeffgen/Stone)

• WHAT IS ENERGY?

Energy is the ability to do work. It exists in many forms that can be converted from one to another. For example, the energy in flowing water can be converted into electrical energy, which can then be converted into the light energy emitted by a light bulb. In the human body, energy is obtained from the energy-yielding nutrients in food and from energy stored in body tissues. Cellular respiration converts the energy stored in carbohydrate, fat, protein, and alcohol into the high-energy compound ATP. The energy in ATP can be used to maintain the internal environment of the body, synthesize new molecules, and power activity (Figure 7.1).

In the context of human activity, energy is measured in **kilojoules (kjoules)**, which are units of work, and in **kilocalories (kcalories)**, which are units of heat. A kjoule is the amount of work required to move an object weighing 1 kilogram a distance of 1 meter under the force of gravity. In Europe, the kjoule is the standard measure of energy in food and the body. Kcalories are the measure most commonly used in the United States and Canada. Technically, a kcalorie is the amount of heat required to raise the temperature of 1 kilogram of water 1° Celsius. In practical terms, a kcalorie is a measure of the amount of energy in food that can be supplied to the body. We don't eat kcalories; we eat food, which provides energy measured in kcalories. Individuals who struggle with weight loss often think of kcalories as an enemy—something to be avoided. However, food and the energy it provides are

177

essential to maintain life. Just as gasoline is necessary to run an engine, kcalories are necessary to run the body.

The amount of energy consumed and the amount used are the critical components of **energy balance**. When the amount of energy—or number of kcalories—consumed is equal to the amount of energy that is used, body weight is maintained. If excess energy is consumed, the excess will be stored for later use, mostly as fat, and weight will increase. If too little energy is consumed, stored energy will be used to fuel the body and weight will be lost. Energy balance can be achieved at any weight—fat, thin, or in between. Being in a state of energy balance simply means that the energy consumed is equal to the energy expended.

Energy balance A state in which body weight remains stable because the amount of energy consumed in the diet equals the amount expended.

• ENERGY INTAKE

The energy needed to fuel the body comes from the food we eat and the energy stored in our bodies. Carbohydrate, fat, protein, and alcohol in food provide energy (Figure 7.2). The amount of energy taken in depends on the total amount of food consumed and the nutrient composition of the food.

The Energy in Food

Bomb calorimeter An instrument used to determine the energy content of food. It measures the heat energy released when a food is combusted.

The energy content of food can be measured by using a **bomb calorimeter**, which consists of a chamber surrounded by a jacket of water (Figure 7.3). Food is dried, placed in the chamber, and burned. As the food combusts, heat is released, raising the temperature of the water. The increase in water temperature can be used to calculate the amount of energy in the food based on the fact that 1 kcalorie is the amount of heat needed to increase the temperature of 1 kilogram of water by 1° Celsius. This method determines the total amount of energy contained in foods. However, because the body cannot completely digest, absorb, and utilize all of the substances in a food, bomb calorimeter values are slightly higher than the amount of energy the body can obtain from that food.

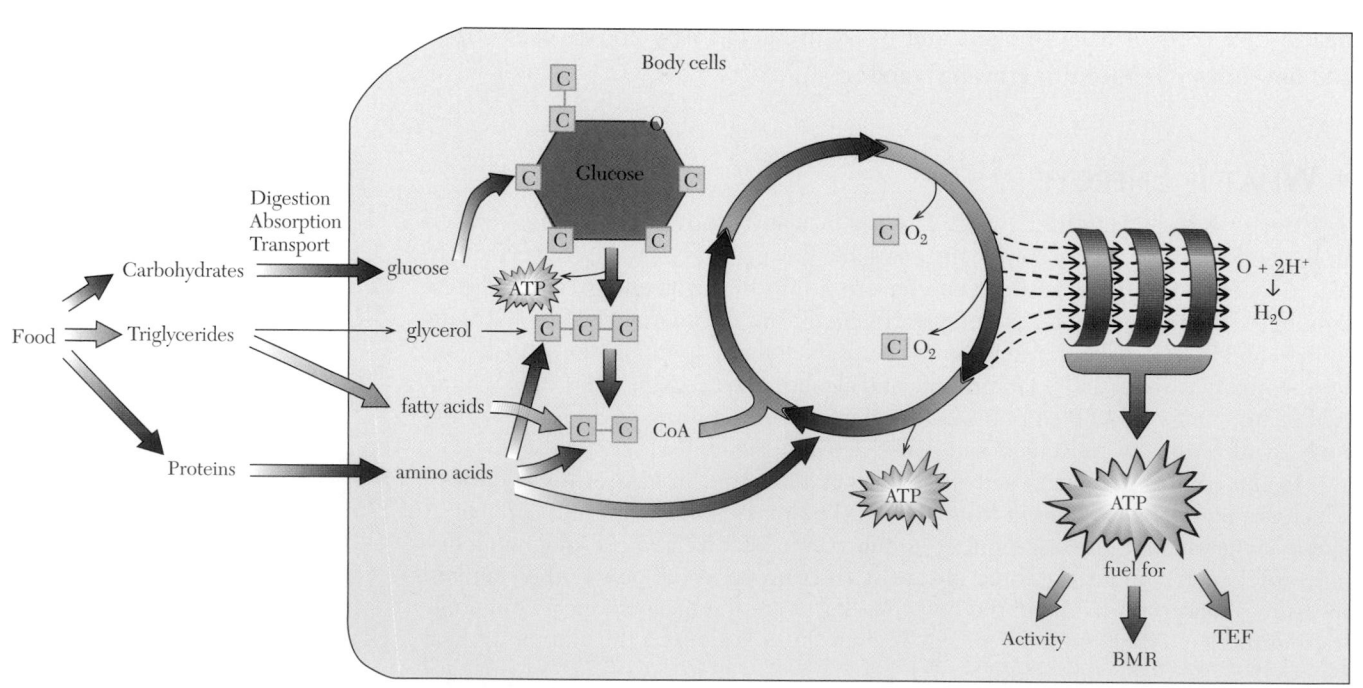

Figure 7.2

Energy is consumed in carbohydrates, triglycerides, and proteins, which can be metabolized to produce ATP. The energy in ATP can be used for activity, basal metabolic rate (BMR), and the thermic effect of food (TEF).

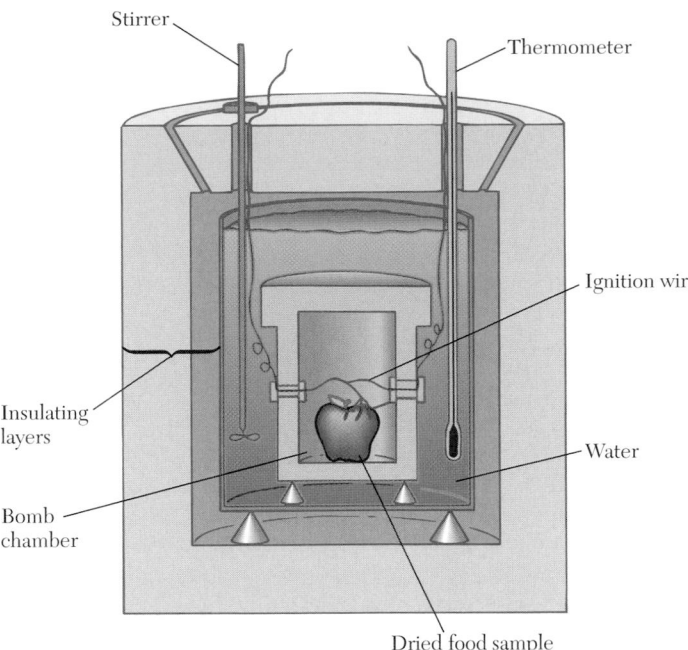

Stirrer

Thermometer

Ignition wire

Insulating layers

Water

Bomb chamber

Dried food sample

Figure 7.3
When dried food is combusted inside the chamber of a bomb calorimeter, the rise in temperature of the surrounding water can be used to determine the energy content of the food.

Information on the energy content of foods can be found in food composition tables and databases and on food labels. The Nutrition Facts portion of food labels lists the total kcalories in a serving of food (see *Off the Label*: Knowing Your Kcalories). The energy content of foods in a diet can also be estimated from the Exchange Lists shown in Table 7.1. For example, one starch exchange, whether a slice of bread, one-half cup (100 g) of cereal, or six saltines, provides about 80 kcalories.

Table 7.1 *Using Exchange Lists to Calculate the Energy Content of a Diet*

Exchange Groups/Lists	Serving Size	Energy (kcal)
Carbohydrate Group		
Starch	1/2 cup rice, cereal, potatoes; 1 slice bread	80
Fruit	1 small apple, peach, pear; 1/2 banana; 1/2 cup canned fruit (in juice)	60
Milk	1 cup milk or yogurt	
Nonfat		90
Lowfat		110
Reduced fat		120
Whole		150
Other carbohydrates	Serving sizes vary	Varies
Vegetables	1/2 cup cooked vegetables, 1 cup raw	25
Meat/Meat Substitute Group	1 oz meat or cheese; 1/2 cup legumes	
Very lean		35
Lean		55
Medium fat		75
High fat		100
Fat Group	1 tsp butter, margarine, or oil; 1 Tbsp salad dressing	45

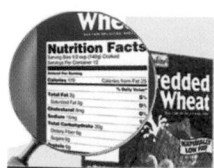

Off the Label
Knowing Your Kcalories

If you are trying to maintain a healthy weight by choosing foods that are low in kcalories, where should you start? When selecting packaged foods, start with the label. But be sure you know what the terms mean.

The Nutrition Facts portion of a food label lists the kcalories per serving, but it is important to check the serving size. Food labels are required to use standard serving sizes, but their "standard" may be different from the consumer's. For instance, the standard serving of cookies is usually one ounce, or about three cookies. If you consume 12 cookies, you are consuming four times more energy than is listed on the label.

Nutrient content descriptors such as "low calorie," "calorie free," "reduced calorie," and "light" may also be helpful in selecting foods that are low in energy. These terms all have standard definitions. A food labeled "low calorie" must have no more than 40 kcalories per serving. A product labeled "calorie free," must contain fewer than 5 kcalories in a serving. "Reduced calorie" or "fewer calories" on the label means the product contains at least 25% fewer calories per serving than a reference food. "Light" or "lite" may be used to describe foods that contain one-third fewer kcalories or half the fat of a comparable product. For example, the label on "lite" microwave popcorn or "light" corn chips must state both the number of kcalories per serving and the fact that this is 30% fewer than the regular product. The terms "light" and "lite" are also used to describe food properties such as texture and color. For example, a label that says "light in texture" means just that; it does not mean that the kcalories are reduced. The term "light"

may also appear without explanation on foods like brown sugar, cream, or molasses, which have traditionally included the term as part of their name.

Lowfat and reduced fat products are a popular choice among dieters. People associate lowfat with low calorie. When fat is removed from baked goods, it is often replaced with carbohydrate. Although carbohydrate contains less energy per gram than fat, it still contributes kcalories to the food. Use the labels shown here to compare the kcalories in a serving of reduced fat cookies to the kcalories in regular cookies. By how many kcalories will your intake be reduced if you replace a serving of regular cookies with the reduced fat variety?

The bottom line on using food labels is to read and understand the entire label before assuming that you are making the best choice.

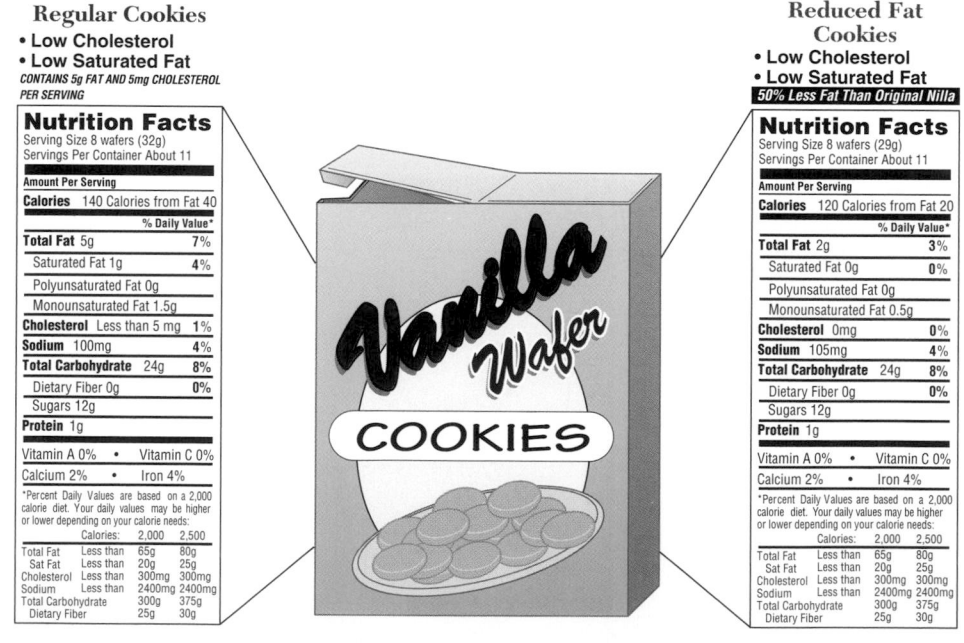

Regular Cookies
- Low Cholesterol
- Low Saturated Fat

CONTAINS 5g FAT AND 5mg CHOLESTEROL PER SERVING

Nutrition Facts
Serving Size 8 wafers (32g)
Servings Per Container About 11

Amount Per Serving	
Calories 140	Calories from Fat 40

	% Daily Value*
Total Fat 5g	7%
Saturated Fat 1g	4%
Polyunsaturated Fat 0g	
Monounsaturated Fat 1.5g	
Cholesterol Less than 5 mg	1%
Sodium 100mg	4%
Total Carbohydrate 24g	8%
Dietary Fiber 0g	0%
Sugars 12g	
Protein 1g	

Vitamin A 0%	•	Vitamin C 0%
Calcium 2%	•	Iron 4%

*Percent Daily Values are based on a 2,000 calorie diet. Your daily values may be higher or lower depending on your calorie needs:

	Calories:	2,000	2,500
Total Fat	Less than	65g	80g
Sat Fat	Less than	20g	25g
Cholesterol	Less than	300mg	300mg
Sodium	Less than	2400mg	2400mg
Total Carbohydrate		300g	375g
Dietary Fiber		25g	30g

Reduced Fat Cookies
- Low Cholesterol
- Low Saturated Fat

50% Less Fat Than Original Nilla

Nutrition Facts
Serving Size 8 wafers (29g)
Servings Per Container About 11

Amount Per Serving	
Calories 120	Calories from Fat 20

	% Daily Value*
Total Fat 2g	3%
Saturated Fat 0g	0%
Polyunsaturated Fat 0g	
Monounsaturated Fat 0.5g	
Cholesterol 0mg	0%
Sodium 105mg	4%
Total Carbohydrate 24g	8%
Dietary Fiber 0g	0%
Sugars 12g	
Protein 1g	

Vitamin A 0%	•	Vitamin C 0%
Calcium 2%	•	Iron 4%

*Percent Daily Values are based on a 2,000 calorie diet. Your daily values may be higher or lower depending on your calorie needs:

	Calories:	2,000	2,500
Total Fat	Less than	65g	80g
Sat Fat	Less than	20g	25g
Cholesterol	Less than	300mg	300mg
Sodium	Less than	2400mg	2400mg
Total Carbohydrate		300g	375g
Dietary Fiber		25g	30g

When the nutrient composition of a food is known, totaling the energy from the carbohydrate, fat, and protein in the food can approximate the energy content. Carbohydrate and protein provide about 4 kcalories per gram. So, 5 grams of sugar, which is almost pure carbohydrate, contains about 20 kcalories (5 g × 4 kcal/g). Fat, the most concentrated source of energy, provides 9 kcalories per gram, and alcohol provides 7 kcalories per gram. Five grams of corn oil, which is almost pure fat, contains about 45 kcalories (5 g × 9 kcal/g). Vitamins, minerals, and water, though essential nutrients, do not provide energy to the body. Most foods are of mixed composition; for instance, a half-cup (100 g) serving of macaroni and cheese contains 8 grams of protein, 20 grams of carbohydrate, and 11 grams of fat (Figure 7.4). Its energy content is therefore:

$$(4 \text{ kcal/g} \times 8 \text{ g protein}) + (4 \text{ kcal/g} \times 20 \text{ g carbohydrate})$$
$$+ (9 \text{ kcal/g} \times 11 \text{ g fat}) = 211 \text{ kcal}$$

Energy Stores in the Body

Energy is stored in the body primarily as fat in the form of triglyceride; some is also stored as glycogen. These stores accumulate when energy consumed in the diet is not used to meet immediate energy needs. This stored energy can be used when intake is less than needs, whether this occurs between meals or over the long term.

Using Body Stores The body must have a steady supply of energy, and some of it must come from glucose. As we eat, energy is supplied by the diet. Between meals the breakdown of stored glycogen provides glucose, and the breakdown of stored fat meets other energy needs. Typically, these stores are then replaced by energy consumed in the next meal so that there is no net change in the amount of stored energy. However, if energy stores are not replenished, the amount of stored energy—and hence, body weight—will decrease.

If no food is eaten for more than several hours, the body must shift the way it uses energy to ensure that glucose continues to be available. Glycogen stores are limited so glucose is also supplied by the breakdown of small amounts of body protein, primarily muscle protein, to yield amino acids. Amino acids can then be used to make glucose via gluconeogenesis (see Chapters 4 and 6). Once glycogen stores are depleted all of the glucose must come from gluconeogenesis. Because protein is not stored in the body, the breakdown of protein to provide energy and glucose results in the loss of functional body proteins.

Energy for tissues that don't require glucose is provided by the breakdown of stored fat. If the supply of glucose is limited, such as during starvation, fatty acids delivered to the liver cannot be completely broken down, so ketones are produced (see Chapter 4). Ketones can be used as an energy source by many tissues. After about 3 days of starvation, even the brain adapts to meet some of its energy needs from ketones (see Chapter 5). This reduces the amount of glucose needed and, therefore, slows the rate of protein breakdown.

During prolonged energy restriction, substantial amounts of fat are used to provide energy and protein is degraded to provide glucose. This results in weight loss. The amount of weight lost depends on the degree of energy deficit and the length of time over which it occurs.

Building Body Stores People typically eat three to six times during the day. The sum of the intake for all of these meals and snacks must meet energy needs for weight to remain stable, but at each occasion more energy is likely to be consumed than is needed at that moment in time. When excess energy is consumed, we generally say this excess is stored as fat. This is an oversimplification of a complex situation. After eating, the body prioritizes how nutrients are used based on its needs, which nutrients can be stored, and how efficiently they can be stored. Amino acids from dietary protein are used to meet needs for the synthesis of body proteins and nonprotein molecules; any excess is then broken down because there is no mechanism for storing them as amino acids or proteins. Carbohydrate is used to maintain blood glucose and to build glycogen stores. Once glycogen stores are full, the remaining carbohydrate is used for energy. The body is capable of converting carbohydrate and amino acids into fat for storage. However, this rarely occurs because it is energetically costly, requiring numerous metabolic reactions.[4] Most of the fat that is stored in the body comes from dietary fat. Fat, unlike carbohydrate and protein, is not a unique fuel source or needed to build tissues and can be stored in the body in virtually unlimited amounts.

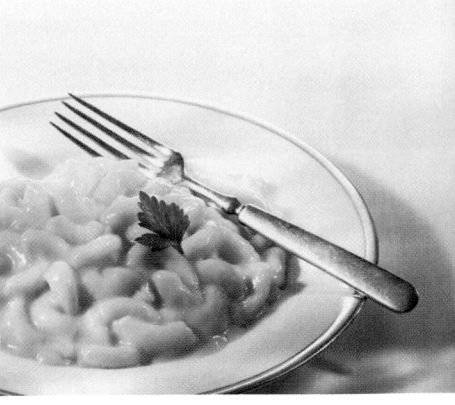

Figure 7.4
The carbohydrate, protein, and fat in macaroni and cheese contribute to its energy content. (Judd Pilosoff/Foodpix)

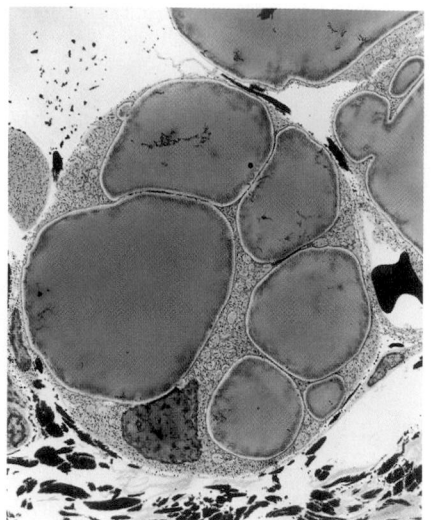

Figure 7.5
Adipocytes contain droplets of fat surrounded by other cell components. As body fat is gained, the size of the fat droplets increases. (© Ed Reschke/Peter Arnold, Inc.)

Adipocytes Fat-storing cells.

Basal energy expenditure (BEE) The energy expended per day needed to maintain awake resting body.

Basal metabolic rate (BMR) The rate of energy expenditure under resting conditions. It is measured after 12 hours without food or exercise.

Resting metabolic rate (RMR) The rate of energy expenditure at rest. It is measured after 5 to 6 hours without food or exercise.

Lean body mass Body mass attributed to nonfat body components such as bone, muscle, and internal organs. It is also called fat-free mass.

In addition, the metabolic cost of converting dietary fat to stored body fat is very small. Therefore, dietary fat is preferentially stored unless carbohydrate and protein do not meet immediate energy needs. In this situation, enough fat is metabolized to meet immediate energy needs, and any remaining dietary fat is stored as triglycerides, primarily in adipose tissue.

Adipose tissue is made up of fat cells, or **adipocytes**. Adipocytes store triglycerides that they pick up from the blood with the help of the enzyme lipoprotein lipase (LPL). These cells grow in size as they accumulate more fat (Figure 7.5). The greater the number of adipocytes an individual has, the greater the ability to store fat. Most adipocytes are formed between infancy and adolescence. In adulthood, only excessive weight gain can cause the production of new fat cells.

• ENERGY OUTPUT

The energy used by the body, or energy output, is determined primarily by the amount of energy needed to maintain basic body functions to fuel physical activity, and to process the nutrients consumed in food.

Basal Needs

About 60 to 75% of the body's total energy requirement is for the maintenance of basic body functions such as breathing and circulating blood. This **basal energy expenditure (BEE)** is defined as the amount of energy needed to keep an awake, resting body alive. The rate at which energy is used for these basic functions is called the **basal metabolic rate (BMR)** and is often expressed in kcalories per hour. Basal needs include the energy necessary for essential metabolic reactions and life-sustaining functions but do not include the energy needed for physical activity or for the digestion and absorption of food. Therefore, to minimize residual energy being used for activity or processing food, BMR is measured in the morning in a warm room before the subject rises and at least 12 hours after food intake or activity. Because of the difficulty of achieving these conditions, measures are often made after about 5 to 6 hours without food or exercise. When done under these conditions the rate of energy expenditure determined is referred to as **resting metabolic rate (RMR)** or resting energy expenditure (REE). RMR values are about 10% or 20% higher than BMR.[5]

BMR is affected by body weight, **lean body mass**, gender, and age. BMR increases with increasing body weight, and so is higher in heavier individuals. It also rises with increasing lean body mass; BMR is generally higher in men than in women because men have greater lean body mass. BMR decreases with age, partly due to a decrease in lean body mass that usually occurs in older adults.

Basal needs can be altered by certain abnormal conditions. An elevation in body temperature, such as that which occurs with a fever, increases energy needs. It is estimated that for every 1° Fahrenheit above normal body temperature, there is a 7% increase in BMR. This extra energy use explains why weight loss can occur with fever. Abnormal levels of thyroid hormones can also affect basal needs. Individuals with an overproduction of these hormones require more energy, and those with underproduction require less energy. The fact that thyroid hormones, produced by the thyroid gland, affect energy expenditure is the reason obesity was once explained as a glandular problem. It is now known that obesity due to a lack of thyroid hormone is rare. Energy needs may also be affected by low-energy diets; BMR decreases when energy intake remains below needs.[6] This drop in BMR decreases the amount of energy needed to maintain weight. It is a beneficial adaptation in starvation, but it makes intentional weight loss more difficult.

Physical Activity

Physical activity is the second major component of energy expenditure. It includes the energy needed for exercise as well as for performing the activities of daily life, such as cooking, gardening, and walking the dog. In most cases, activity accounts for 15 to 30%

of energy requirements, but this varies greatly among individuals. Because it takes more energy to move a heavier object, the amount of energy expended for many activities increases as body weight increases. The energy required for an activity depends on how strenuous the activity is and the length of time it is performed. For example, walking at a speed of 3 to 4 mph requires a moderate degree of exertion and uses about 60 kcal/mile for a 70 kg individual. The energy required increases progressively as the walking speed and the body weight of the exerciser increase. In addition to the energy expended during exercise, there is a small increase in energy expenditure for a period of time after exercise has been completed. To maintain health, people today need to consciously increase their physical activity. This does not mean you have to run marathons. Choosing to take the stairs rather than the elevator, walking rather than taking the bus, and riding a bike rather than driving to the store all increase activity (Figure 7.6). The energy costs of specific activities are listed in Appendix K.

The Thermic Effect of Food

The **thermic effect of food (TEF)** is the energy expended above BMR for the digestion of food and the absorption, metabolism, and storage of nutrients. This causes body temperature to rise slightly for several hours after eating. The energy required for TEF is estimated to be about 10% of energy intake but can vary depending on the amounts and types of nutrients consumed. Because it takes energy to store nutrients, TEF increases with the size of the meal. The composition of meals also affects TEF. A meal that is high in fat has a lower TEF than a meal high in carbohydrate or protein because dietary fat can be efficiently stored as body fat. This difference in the energy cost of storing energy means a diet high in fat may produce more body fat than a diet high in carbohydrate.[7]

• ENERGY REQUIREMENTS

The energy requirements of the body include those for basal functions, activity, and processing food. During growth and pregnancy, they also include the energy cost of depositing new tissues; during lactation, they include the energy needed to produce milk. There is also a small amount of energy needed to maintain body temperature in a cold environment. The total amount of energy required by the body, or **total energy expenditure (TEE)**, can be assessed in a number of ways. These measures are then used to develop recommendations for energy intakes that will meet the needs of the general population for maintenance and growth.

Measuring Energy Expenditure

Historically, the amount of energy used by the body was measured in a process called calorimetry. **Direct calorimetry** measures heat production. Combusting food in a bomb calorimeter is a type of direct calorimetry. In humans, direct calorimetry measures the amount of heat given off by the body; the heat produced is proportional to the amount of energy used. This heat is generated by metabolic reactions that both convert food energy into ATP and use ATP for body processes. Direct calorimetry is an accurate method for measuring energy expenditure, but it is expensive and impractical because it requires that the individual being assessed remain in an insulated chamber throughout the evaluation.

Indirect calorimetry, which estimates energy use by assessing nutrient utilization, is somewhat less cumbersome than direct calorimetry. It measures the amounts of oxygen consumed and carbon dioxide expired by the body. The body's energy use can be calculated from these values because the burning of fuels by the body in cellular respiration uses oxygen and produces carbon dioxide. Oxygen use and carbon dioxide production can be measured by analyzing the difference between inhaled and exhaled air.

Measuring respired gases requires that one breathe into a mask or ventilated hood so that the expired air be measured (Figure 7.7). This method can be used to measure the energy used for individual components of expenditure, such as physical activ-

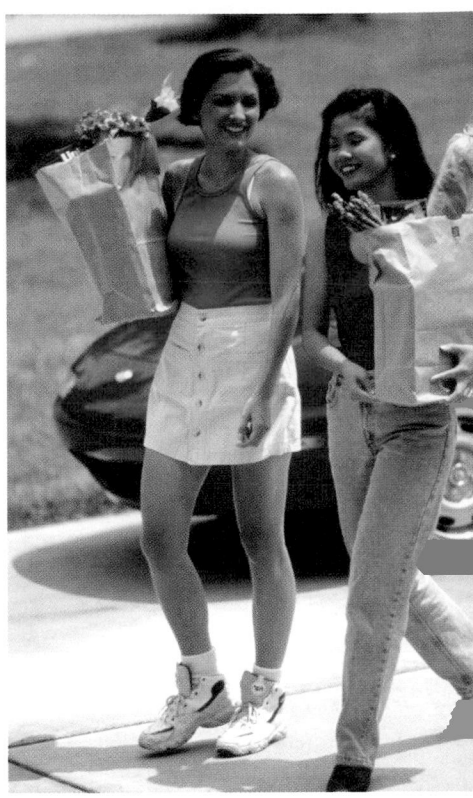

Figure 7.6
Even small changes in daily activity, such as walking or riding your bike to the grocery store instead of driving can affect energy balance. (Novastock/PhotoEdit)

Thermic effect of food (TEF) The energy required for the digestion, absorption, metabolism, and storage of food. It is equal to approximately 10% of daily energy intake.

Total energy expenditure (TEE) The sum of basal energy expenditure, TEF, and the energy used in physical activity, regulation of body temperature, deposition of new tissue, and production of milk.

Direct calorimetry A method of determining energy use that measures the amount of heat produced by the body.

Indirect calorimetry A method of estimating energy use that compares the amount of oxygen consumed with the carbon dioxide expired.

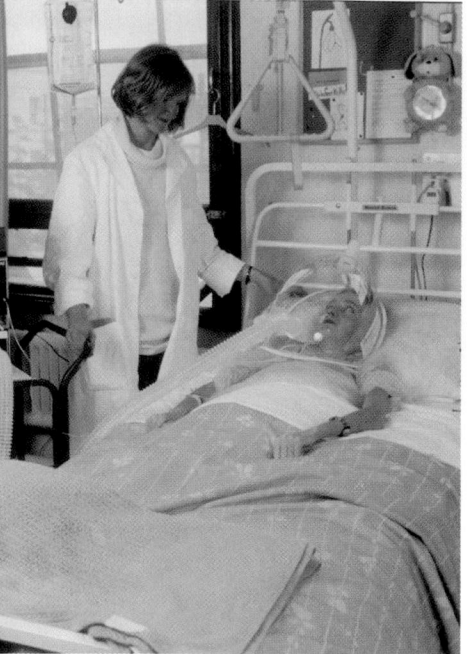

Figure 7.7
Measuring expired gases by having the subject breathe into a hood is an easy way to assess BMR, but it cannot easily be used to measure the energy costs of daily living. (St. Bartholomew's Photo Library/Custom Medical Stock Photo)

Doubly labeled water technique A technique for determining energy expenditure based on measuring the distribution of isotopes of hydrogen and oxygen in body fluids after administration of a defined amount of water labeled with both isotopes.

Isotope An alternative form of an element that has a different atomic mass, which may or may not be radioactive.

ity or BMR. It can also be used to estimate total energy needs, but it is not practical in free-living individuals because the equipment is inappropriate for long-term use.

Current energy intake recommendations are based on measurements made using the **doubly labeled water technique**. This involves having the individual ingest or be injected with water labeled with **isotopes** of oxygen and hydrogen. The labeled oxygen and hydrogen are used by the body in metabolism. By measuring the rate at which labeled oxygen and labeled hydrogen disappear from body water, the amount of carbon dioxide produced by the energy-requiring reactions in the body can be estimated. The doubly labeled water technique does not require the individual to carry any equipment and can be used to measure expenditure in free-living subjects for periods up to 2 weeks. Doubly labeled water is now the preferred method for determining the total daily energy expenditures in both healthy and clinical populations.[8] However, it is not helpful in determining the proportion of energy used for BMR, physical activity, or TEF.

Estimated Energy Requirements (EER)

The current recommendations for energy intake in the United States are the **estimated energy requirements (EER)** established by the DRIs.[5] An EER is the amount of energy predicted to maintain energy balance in a healthy person of a defined age, gender, weight, height, and level of physical activity.* These values were determined from studies that used doubly labeled water to measure energy expenditure. Equations developed from this data can be used to calculate an individual's EER. No specific RDAs or ULs have been established.

Calculating EERs EER calculations take into account age, gender, height, weight, life stage, and level of physical activity (Table 7.2 or inside cover). Four physical ac-

Table 7.2 *Calculating Estimated Energy Requirements*

To determine EER:

- Determine weight in kilograms (kg) and height in meters (m)

$$\text{Weight in kg} = \text{weight in pounds}/2.2 \text{ pounds per kg}$$

$$\text{Height in meters} = \text{height in inches} \times 0.0254 \text{ inches per m}$$

For example: 160 pounds = 160 lbs/2.2 lbs/kg = 72.7 kg

5 feet 9 inches = 69 inches × 0.0254 in/m = 1.75 m

- Determine PA (physical activity) by estimating the amount of physical activity per day and using Table 7.4 to find the PA value. For example, a 19-year-old male who performs 40 minutes of vigorous activity a day is in the active category and has a PA of 1.25.
- Use the appropriate EER prediction equation to find the EER (see below or inside cover):
  For example: for an active 19-year-old male,

$$\text{EER} = 662 - (9.53 \times \text{age in yrs}) + \text{PA}\,[(15.91 \times \text{weight in kg}) + (539.6 \times \text{height in m})]$$

Where age = 19 yr, weight = 72.7 kg, height = 1.75 m, active PA = 1.25

$$\text{EER} = 662 - (9.53 \times 19) + 1.25([15.91 \times 72.7] + [539.6 \times 1.75]) = 3107 \text{ kcal/day}$$

Life Stage	EER Prediction Equation
Boys 9–18 yr	EER = 88.5 − (61.9 × age in yrs) + PA [(26.7 × weight in kg) + (903 × height in m)] + 25
Girls 9–18 yr	EER = 135.3 − (30.8 × age in yrs) + PA [(10.0 × weight in kg) + (934 × height in m)] + 25
Men ≥ 19 yr	EER = 662 − (9.53 × age in yrs) + PA [(15.91 × weight in kg) + (539.6 × height in m)]
Women ≥ 19 yr	EER = 354 − (6.91 × age in yrs) + PA [(9.36 × weight in kg) + (726 × height in m)]

*EERs are defined as values for normal weight individuals. Equations that predict the amount of energy needed for weight maintenance are available for overweight and obese individuals.

Table 7.3 *How Activities Contribute to Physical Activity Level*

Category	Examples
Activities of Daily Living	Gardening (no lifting), watering plants, raking leaves, mowing the lawn, household tasks, mopping, vacuuming, walking from the house to car or bus, loading/unloading the car, walking the dog. It is assumed that we spend about 2.5 hours per day in these types of activities.
Moderate	Calisthenics (light, no weights), cycling (leisurely, 6–7 mph), golf (without cart), swimming (slow), walking (3 mph, 20 min/mile), walking (4 mph, 15 min/mile), or other activities that expend about 250 to 350 kcal/hr for a 70 kg individual.
Vigorous	Aerobics (moderate to heavy), ballet, climbing (hills or mountains), cycling (moderate or higher, greater than 10 mph), dancing (square dancing or fast ballroom), ice skating, jogging (12 min/mile or faster), roller skating, rope jumping, skiing (water, downhill, or cross country), squash, swimming (moderate to fast), tennis, walking (5 mph, 12 min/mile), or other activities that expend more than 350 kcal/hr for a 70 kg individual.

tivity levels have been defined: sedentary, low active, active, and very active.[5] A "sedentary" individual is one who does not participate in any activity beyond that required for daily independent living, such as housework, homework, yard work, gardening, and walking the dog (Table 7.3). To move into the "low active" category, an adult weighing 70 kg would need to expend an amount of energy equivalent to walking 2.2 miles at a rate of 3 to 4 miles per hour in addition to the activities of daily living. To be "active," an individual would need to perform daily exercise equivalent to walking 7 miles at a rate of 3 to 4 miles per hour, and to be "very active," an individual would need to perform the equivalent of walking 17 miles at this rate in addition to the activities of daily living. In order to maintain a healthy weight and reduce the risk of chronic disease, physical activity at the "active" level is recommended.

Estimating Physical Activity Level An individual can estimate their activity level by keeping a daily log of their activities and recording the amount of time spent in each. Activities can then be categorized as activities of daily living, moderate, or vigorous (Table 7.3). Activity level can be estimated based on the time spent in each category of activity (Table 7.4). Each physical activity level is assigned a numerical PA value that can then be used in the EER calculation. Activity level has a significant effect on EER. For example, a 30-year-old woman who is 5 feet 5 inches tall and weighs 130 pounds has an EER of 1898 kcal/day if she is sedentary. If she increases her activity to "active," the level recommended by the DRIs, her EER increases to 2370 kcal/day.

Table 7.4 *Levels of Physical Activity with PA Values*

	PA Values			
	3–18 years		**≥ 19 years**	
Physical Activity Level	**Boys**	**Girls**	**Men**	**Women**
Sedentary: Engages only in the activities of daily living and no moderate or vigorous activities	1.00	1.00	1.00	1.00
Low active: Daily activity equivalent of at least 30 minutes of moderate activity and a minimum of 15 to 30 minutes of vigorous activity depending on the intensity of the activity.	1.13	1.16	1.11	1.12
Active: Engages in at least 60 minutes of moderate activities or a minimum of 30 to 60 minutes of vigorous activity depending on the intensity of the activity.	1.26	1.31	1.25	1.27
Very Active: Engages in at least 2.5 hours of moderate activity or a minimum of 1 to 1.75 hours of vigorous activity depending on the intensity of the activity.	1.42	1.56	1.48	1.45

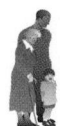

EERs for Different Lifestages The EER values for infants, children, and adolescents include the energy used to deposit tissues associated with growth. Beginning at age 3, there are separate EER equations for boys and girls because of differences in growth and physical activity. The EER for pregnancy is determined as the sum of the total energy expenditure of a nonpregnant woman plus the energy needed to maintain pregnancy and deposit maternal and fetal tissue. During lactation, EER is the sum of the total energy expenditure of nonlactating women and the energy in the milk produced, minus the energy mobilized from maternal tissue stores.

• BODY WEIGHT AND HEALTH

To maintain energy balance, energy intake must equal energy output. If excess energy is consumed, it will be stored, mostly as body fat. Some fat storage is essential. Individuals who have little stored fat have a greater risk for illness than individuals whose body fat is within the normal range. However, excess stored body fat can increase the risk of illness and can create psychological and social problems.

Overweight and **obesity** are a major public health problem in the United States, affecting over 60% of all adult Americans.[1] Weight problems are also increasing among children and adolescents.

Overweight A BMI of 25 to 29.9 kg/m² or a body weight 10 to 19% above the healthy body weight standard.

Obesity A condition characterized by excess body fat. It is defined as a body mass index of 30 kg/m² or greater or a body weight that is 20% or more above the healthy body weight standard.

What's Wrong with a Few Extra Pounds?

High blood pressure, heart disease, high blood cholesterol, diabetes, stroke, gallbladder disease, arthritis, sleep disorders, respiratory problems, and cancers of the breast, uterus, prostate, and colon all occur more frequently in overweight individuals.[1] And, the presence of these diseases increases the risk of illness and premature death that is associated with being overweight. Obesity can also affect other aspects of health. It increases the incidence and severity of infectious disease and has been linked to poor wound healing and surgical complications. It increases pregnancy risks both for the mother and child. People who gain excess weight at a young age and remain overweight throughout life have greater health risks. In addition to the amount of excess fat, the distribution of the fat affects the risk of developing many of these diseases.

Psychological and social problems are also associated with being overweight. Overweight children are often teased and ostracized. They frequently find themselves isolated socially from their peers. If obese children grow into obese adolescents and adults, and most of them do, they may experience discrimination in college admissions and in the job market. Obese individuals of every age are more likely to experience depression, a negative self-image, and feelings of inadequacy. The physical health risks of obesity may not manifest themselves as disease for years, but the psychological and social problems experienced by the obese are felt every day.

A Few Pounds Too Few?

If excess body fat is bad for you, what's wrong with being lean? Research has suggested that being on the low side of the body weight standard may reduce the risk of diabetes and may even increase longevity.[9,10] However, some body fat is essential as an insulator and as a reserve for periods of illness. Substantial reductions in body weight have been shown to decrease the ability of the immune system to fight disease, and very low body weight is associated with an increased risk of early death.[11] In developed countries, socioeconomic conditions may create isolated pockets of undernutrition, but severe cases of wasting are usually a result either of self-starvation due to eating disorders, such as anorexia nervosa, or of a disease process, such as AIDS or cancer.

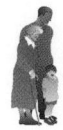

Too little body fat causes problems at all stages of life. Low weight gains during pregnancy are correlated with an increase in low-birth-weight infants, who are at a higher risk of health complications and death (see Chapter 14). For teenage girls, too little body fat can delay sexual development. In healthy but very lean female athletes, menstrual irregularities are common, increasing the risk of developing osteoporosis (see Chapters 10 and 13).[12] Too little body fat in the elderly increases the risk of malnutrition.

Guidelines for Healthy Body Weight

Body weight includes the weight of body fat as well as lean tissue. There are many ways to evaluate desirable levels of body weight and fat. Some rely on measures of weight in relation to height, and others use methods that approximate the proportion of body weight that is fat.

Body Mass Index Body mass index (BMI) is an index of body weight in relation to height. Although BMI is not actually a measure of body fat, it correlates well with body fat and has become the medical standard for assessing whether an individual is

Body mass index (BMI) An index of weight in relation to height that is used to compare body size with a standard.

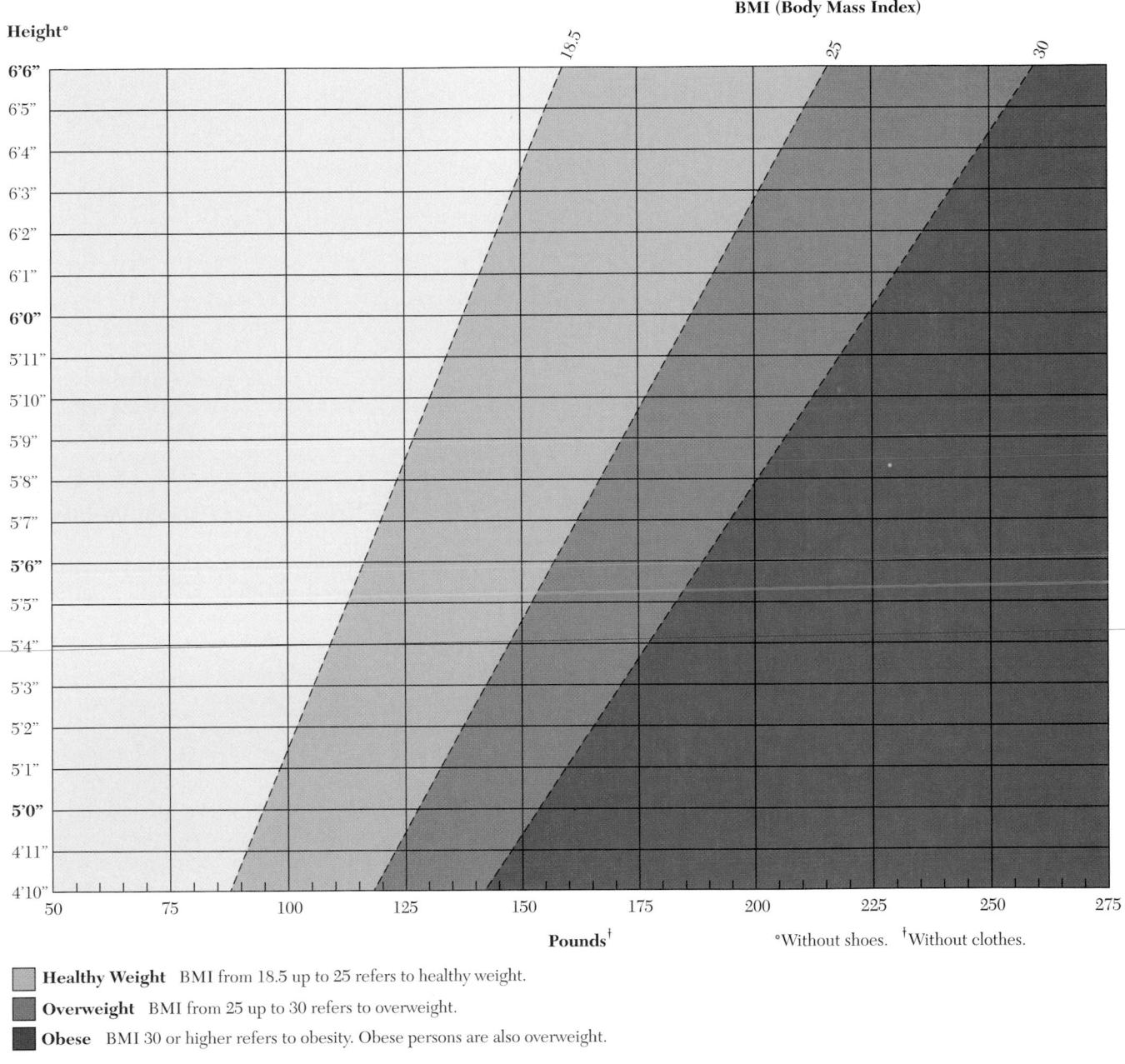

Healthy Weight BMI from 18.5 up to 25 refers to healthy weight.

Overweight BMI from 25 up to 30 refers to overweight.

Obese BMI 30 or higher refers to obesity. Obese persons are also overweight.

Figure 7.8

To determine your BMI range, locate the point that lines up with your weight (in pounds) on the bottom scale and draw a vertical line up from this point. Locate your height (in feet and inches) on the left-hand scale and draw a horizontal line that extends into the graph. The point where these two lines meet indicates your BMI status. (*Report of the Dietary Advisory Committee on the Dietary Guidelines for Americans, 2000.*)

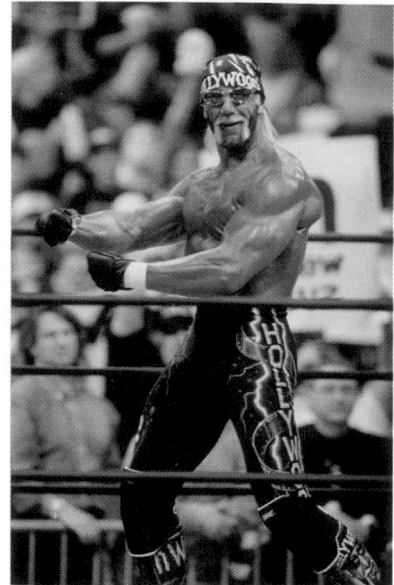

Figure 7.9
Wrestler/actor Hulk Hogan, at 6 feet 8 inches tall and 275 pounds, has a BMI of 30.3, which falls into the category of obese. However, it is unlikely that his high BMI is due to excess body fat or that it indicates an increased risk of disease. (Duomo/Corbis Images)

Underweight A BMI of less than 18.5 kg/m² or a body weight 10% or more below the healthy body weight standard.

Extreme or **morbid obesity** A condition in which body weight is 100 pounds (45.5 kg) above healthy body weight or BMI is greater than 40 kg/m².

Frame size An estimate of the proportion of body weight that is due to bone.

at a healthy body weight. BMI is calculated from the ratio of weight to height according to the following equation:

$$BMI = \text{weight in kg}/(\text{height in m})^2$$

$$\text{or, } BMI = \text{weight in pounds}/(\text{height in inches})^2 \times 704.5°$$

For example, someone who is 6 feet (72 inches) tall and weighs 180 pounds has a body mass index of 24.5 kg/m² (180/72² × 704.5).

A healthy body weight is defined as a BMI between 18.5 and 24.9 kg/m². In general, people with a BMI within this range have the lowest health risks.[13] **Underweight** is defined as a body mass index of less than 18.5 kg/m², overweight is defined as 25 to 29.9 kg/m², and obese as 30 kg/m² or greater.[14] A BMI of 40 or over is classified as **extreme** or **morbid obesity**. Figure 7.8 can be used to determine if one's BMI falls in the healthy weight category.

Even though BMI correlates well with body fat, it is not a perfect tool for evaluating the health risk associated with obesity. An individual with a BMI in the overweight range who consumes a healthy diet and exercises regularly may be more fit than an individual with a BMI in the healthy range who is sedentary and eats a poor diet. Or an individual may have a high BMI but not have excess body fat. For example, body builders may have a high body weight and BMI because they have a large amount of lean body mass. Although BMI is high, body fat and hence disease risk is low (Figure 7.9).

Weight-for-Height Tables Weight-for-height tables that list ranges of healthy weight for height are still used in some settings to evaluate body weight. The most commonly used weight tables are the Metropolitan Life Insurance Company tables. These present healthy weight ranges based on height, sex, and **frame size**, which is an approximation of weight due to bone mass (see Appendix B). The Metropolitan Life Insurance tables were developed by determining the weight at which individuals of a given age, sex, and height live the longest. Unfortunately, these tables were developed using weights recorded at the time individuals purchased insurance. Because there was no follow-up to determine if the individuals' weights had changed by the time of death, the weights in the table may not represent the healthiest weights. In addition, because they are based only on people who bought insurance, the values may underrepresent lower socioeconomic and minority groups who could not afford insurance.

Body Fat Distribution The distribution of body fat affects the health risks of being overfat. Fat that is located under the skin, called subcutaneous fat, carries less risk than fat that is deposited around the organs, called visceral fat. An increase in visceral fat is associated with a higher incidence of heart disease, high blood pressure, stroke, diabetes, and breast cancer. Generally, fat in the hips and lower body is subcutaneous, whereas fat deposited around the waist in the abdominal region is primarily visceral fat. Therefore, people who carry their excess fat around and above the waist have more visceral fat. Those who carry their extra fat below the waist in the hips and thighs have more subcutaneous fat. These body types have been dubbed apples and pears, respectively, by the popular literature (Figure 7.10).

Where an individual deposits body fat is determined primarily by genetics.[15] For example, African American women, who have an incidence of obesity that is 50% higher than that of Caucasian women, store less visceral fat.[16] Gender, age, and environment also influence where fat is stored.[17] Visceral fat storage is more common in men than women. But after menopause, visceral fat increases in women. Stress, tobacco, and alcohol consumption predispose people to visceral fat deposition, whereas activity reduces it.[18]

°The multiplier 704.5 is used by the National Institutes of Health. Other organizations may use a slightly different multiplier; for example, the American Dietetic Association suggests multiplying by 700. The variation in outcome is insignificant.

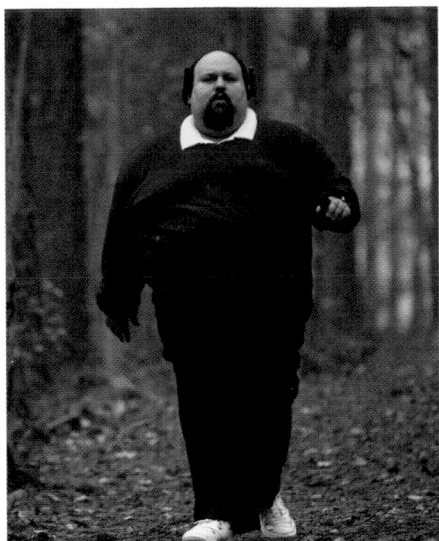 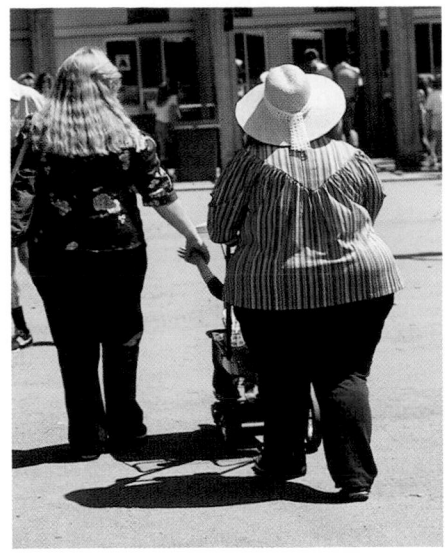

Figure 7.10

(*a*) Overweight individuals with apple-shaped body types deposit fat in the abdominal region and are at greater risk of developing heart disease and diabetes. (*b*) Overweight individuals with pear-shaped body types deposit fat in the hips and thighs where it is primarily subcutaneous. (*a*, Corbis; *b*, © Tom McHugh/Photo Researchers, Inc.)

Distinguishing the relative amounts of visceral and subcutaneous fat requires sophisticated imaging techniques. However, the risk associated with visceral fat deposition can be estimated by measuring waist circumference. For males, a BMI of 25 to 34.9 kg/m² and a waist circumference greater than 40 inches is associated with increased risk. For females in this BMI range, waist circumference of greater than 35 inches increases risks (Table 7.5). In individuals under 5 feet in height or with a BMI greater than or equal to 35 these cut-off points do not predict risk. In order to monitor body weight and risk, the Dietary Guidelines for Americans, 2000, recommend that all Americans keep track of their weight and their waists and avoid increases in both.

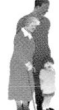

Body Composition Body composition—that is, the proportion of weight that is lean tissue versus fat—is affected by gender and life stage. At birth the percentage of body fat is about 12% and increases in the first year of life. During childhood, muscle mass increases and body fat decreases. During adolescence, females gain proportionately more fat and males gain more muscle mass. As adults, women continue to have more stored body fat than men. A healthy level of body fat for a young adult fe-

Table 7.5 *BMI, Waist Circumference, and Disease Risk*

| | BMI (kg/m²)* | Disease Risk† | |
		Men, waist ≤ 40 inches, and women, waist ≤ 35 inches	Men, waist > 40 inches, and women, waist > 35 inches
Underweight	< 18.5		
Normal weight	18.5–24.9		
Overweight	25.0–29.9	Increased	High
Obesity (class I)	30.0–34.9	High	Very high
Obesity (class II)	35.0–39.9	Very high	Very high
Extreme or morbid obesity (class III)	≥ 40	Extremely high	Extremely high

*BMI = body weight (kg)/ height squared (m²)

†Disease risk for type 2 diabetes, hypertension, and cardiovascular disease relative to individuals with a normal weight and normal waist circumference. National Institutes of Health, National Heart, Lung, and Blood Institute. Clinical Guidelines on the Identification, Evaluation, and Treatment of Overweight and Obesity in Adults. Executive summary, June 1998. Available online at: www.nhlbi.nih.gov/guidelines/obesity/ob_home.htm/.

male is between 20 and 30% of total weight; for young adult males, it is between 12 and 20%.[13] There is an increase in body fat during pregnancy to provide energy stores for the mother and fetus. With aging, lean body mass decreases and body fat increases even if body weight remains the same. Some of this change may be prevented by physical activity.

Measures of body composition are more cumbersome than simply measuring height and weight, but these measures are important because it is the amount of fat, not weight, that correlates with the risk of chronic disease.

Underwater Weighing An accurate noninvasive technique for assessing body composition is **underwater weighing**, which involves weighing an individual both on land and in the water (Figure 7.11). The difference between these two weights can be used to determine body volume. The percentage of body fat can then be determined using standardized equations. Although this method is accurate, it requires special equipment and cannot be used for some groups such as small children or frail adults. A newer method for estimating body composition measures air displacement rather than water displacement to calculate body fat. The individual is placed in an air-filled chamber (known as the BOD POD) rather than in water. It is accurate and more convenient than underwater weighing.[19]

Circumference and Skinfold Thickness Measurements of circumference and **skinfold thickness** at various locations on the body can be used to assess body composition. Skinfold thickness measures the fat under the skin, or subcutaneous fat, and assumes that it is representative of the total body fat. It is measured at one or more locations using a caliper. The most common sites for skinfold measurements are triceps (the area over muscles on the back of the upper arm) and subscapular (just below the shoulder blade) (Figure 7.12). Either a nomogram or mathematical equations are then used to estimate percent body fat from these measurements. These measurements provide accurate estimates of body fat in normal-weight individuals but are difficult to perform and less accurate in obese and elderly subjects.

Bioelectric Impedance Analysis **Bioelectric impedance analysis** estimates body fat by measuring current flow through the body. A painless, low-energy electrical current is directed through the body by electrodes placed on the hands and feet. Because fat is a poor conductor of electricity, it offers resistance to the current. The percentage of the body that is fluid and allows current flow is estimated, and the remainder is assumed to be body fat. Bioelectric impedance techniques assume a standard amount of body water. Therefore, measurements should be done when the gastrointestinal (GI) tract and bladder are empty and hydration is normal. For example, measurements are not accurate if done within 24 hours of a strenuous bout of exercise because body water has been lost in sweat.

Isotopic Methods Because water is present primarily in lean tissue and not in fat, a water-soluble isotope can be ingested or injected into the bloodstream and allowed to mix with the water throughout the body. The concentration of the isotope in a sample of body fluid, such as blood, can then be measured. The extent to which the isotope has been diluted can be used to calculate the amount of lean tissue in the body, and body fat can then be calculated by subtracting lean weight from total body weight. Another technique measures a naturally occurring isotope of potassium. Because potassium is found primarily in lean tissue, a measure of the amount of this isotope in the body can be used to determine the total amount of body potassium, which can then be used to estimate the amount of lean tissue. Isotopic techniques are expensive and usually require injections. They are used primarily for research purposes.

Radiologic Methods Radiologic methods for assessing body composition are less invasive than isotopic methods. Computerized tomography (CT), generally used as a diagnostic technique, can be used to visualize fat and lean tissue. CT is particularly

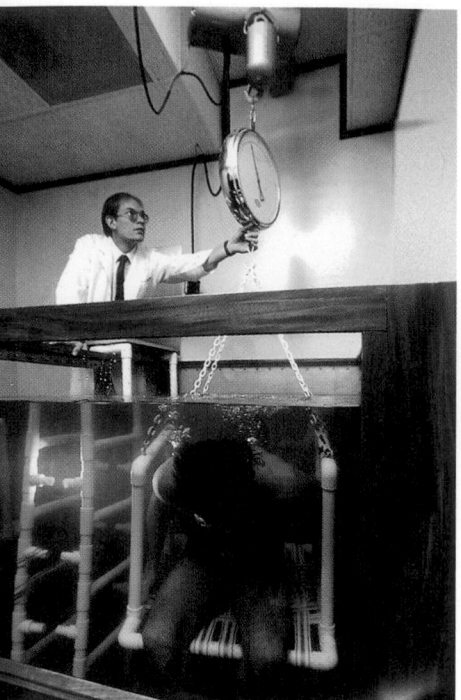

Figure 7.11
To determine the percent of body weight that is due to fat, body weight on land and weight in water (with all air expelled from the lungs) can be used. (© Jim Olive/Peter Arnold, Inc.)

Underwater weighing A technique that uses the difference between body weight under water and body weight on land to estimate body composition.

Skinfold thickness A measurement of subcutaneous fat used to estimate total body fat.

Bioelectric impedance analysis A technique for estimating body composition that measures body water by directing electric current through the body and calculating resistance to flow.

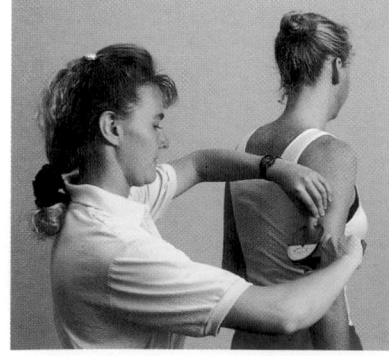

Figure 7.12
The triceps skinfold is measured at the midpoint of the back of the arm. This measure of the thickness of the fat layer under the skin can be used to estimate body fat. (David Young-Wolff/PhotoEdit)

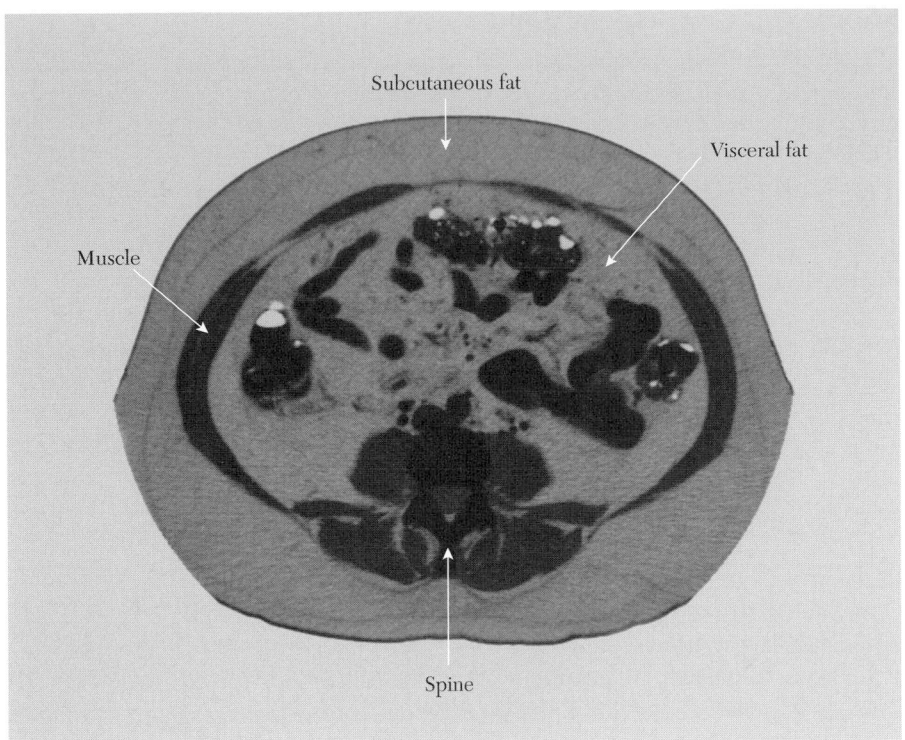

Subcutaneous fat

Visceral fat

Muscle

Spine

Figure 7.13

As shown in this CT scan taken at waist level in an overweight female, fat in the abdominal region is located both under the skin (subcutaneous) and around the internal organs (visceral). (Courtesy of Michael F. Smolin, M.D.)

useful for measuring the amount of visceral adipose tissue (Figure 7.13).[20] Dual-energy X-ray absorptiometry (DEXA) is another method that uses low-energy X-rays for assessing body composition. A single investigation can accurately determine total body mass, bone mineral mass, and percent body fat, but it does not distinguish between visceral and subcutaneous fat. Another method, magnetic resonance imaging (MRI), uses magnetic fields to create an internal body image. MRI can be used to accurately estimate the amount of abdominal fat, which is associated with the risk of heart disease and other chronic diseases.

• HOW IS BODY FATNESS REGULATED?

In most people, body fat and weight remain remarkably constant over long periods despite fluctuations in food intake and activity level. The reason is that body weight, like body temperature, is believed to be regulated to remain at a particular level or set point. When energy intake or activity level changes, the body compensates to prevent a significant change in weight or fat.[21]

The set point for body fatness is determined by genetics. In an obese individual, body fat is set to remain at a higher level or set point than it is in a lean individual. When people lose weight, regardless of whether they are lean or obese at the outset, metabolic signals are generated to decrease energy output and increase energy intake in order to return their weight to its set point.[21] As anyone who had tried to lose weight can attest, it is difficult to decrease body weight, and most people who lose weight eventually regain all they have lost.

However, the mechanisms that defend body weight are not absolute. Changes in physiological, psychological, and environmental circumstances do cause the level at which body weight is regulated to change, usually increasing it over time. For example, body weight increases in most adults between the ages of 30 and 60 years, and after having a baby, most women return to a weight that is 1 to 2 pounds higher than their prepregnancy weight. This suggests that the mechanisms that defend against weight loss are stronger than those that prevent weight gain.[22]

Short- and Long-Term Regulation

The mechanisms that regulate the set point for body weight and fatness must respond both to changes in the intake of nutrients that occur over a short time frame as well as to more long-term changes in the amount of body fat. Signals related to food intake affect hunger or satiety over a short period of time—from meal to meal—whereas signals from the adipose tissue trigger the brain to adjust both food intake and energy expenditure for long-term regulation.

Meal-to-Meal Food Intake   The short-term regulation of energy balance involves the control of food intake from meal to meal. We eat in response to **hunger**, which is the physiological drive to consume food. We stop eating when we experience **satiety**, the feeling of fullness and satisfaction that follows food intake. But what, when, and how much we eat are also affected by **appetite**, the drive to eat specific foods that is not necessarily related to hunger. Signals to eat or stop eating can be external, originating from the environment, or they can be internal, originating from the GI tract, circulating nutrients, or higher centers in the brain.[23]

External factors that motivate eating include the sight, taste, and smell of food, the time of day, cultural and social conventions, the appeal of the foods available, and ethnic and religious rituals.[24,25] Some people eat lunch at noon out of social convention, not because they are hungry. We eat turkey on Thanksgiving because it is a tradition. We eat cookies or cinnamon rolls while walking through the mall because the smell entices us to buy them. Likewise, external factors such as religious dietary laws or negative experiences associated with certain foods can signal us to stop eating.

Internal signals that promote hunger and satiety originate both before and after food is absorbed. The simplest type of signal about food intake comes from local nerves in the walls of the stomach and small intestine that sense the volume or pressure of food and send a message to the brain to either start or stop food intake. The presence of glucose, fat, and amino acids in the GI tract also sends information directly to the brain and triggers the release of GI hormones such as cholecystokinin, which causes satiety.[26] Absorbed nutrients may also send information to the brain to modulate food intake. Circulating levels of nutrients, including glucose, amino acids, ketones, and fatty acids, are monitored by the brain and may trigger signals to eat or not to eat.[27] Nutrients that are taken up by the brain may affect neurotransmitter concentrations, which then affect the amount and type of nutrients consumed. For example, some studies suggest that when brain serotonin is low, carbohydrate is craved, but when it is high, protein is preferred.[27] The liver may also be involved in signaling hunger and satiety by monitoring changes in fuel metabolism. Changes in liver metabolism, in particular the amount of ATP, are believed to modulate food intake.[24] The pancreas is also involved in food intake regulation because it releases insulin, which may affect hunger and satiety by lowering the levels of circulating nutrients. Insulin may also be involved in long-term regulation of body fat.

Psychological factors can also affect eating behavior. Psychological distress may come from events in the external environment, but the processing of these events occurs in the higher centers of the brain. The effect that emotions have on appetite depends on the individual. Some people eat for comfort and to relieve stress. Others may lose their appetite when these same emotions are felt.

Signals Related to Body Fatness   Short-term regulators of energy balance affect the size and timing of individual meals. If a change in input is sustained over a long period, however, it can affect long-term energy balance and, hence, body weight and fatness. To regulate body fatness at a set level, the body must be able to monitor how much body fat is present. Some of this information comes from hormones, such as insulin and leptin, that are secreted in proportion to the amount of body fat.[26] Insulin is secreted from the pancreas when blood glucose levels rise; its circulating concentration is proportional to the amount of body fat. Insulin can affect food intake and body weight by sending signals to the brain and by affecting the amount of

Hunger The desire to acquire and consume food that occurs in response to physiological signals.

Satiety The feeling of fullness and satisfaction, caused by food consumption, that eliminates the desire to eat.

Appetite The desire to consume specific foods that is independent of hunger.

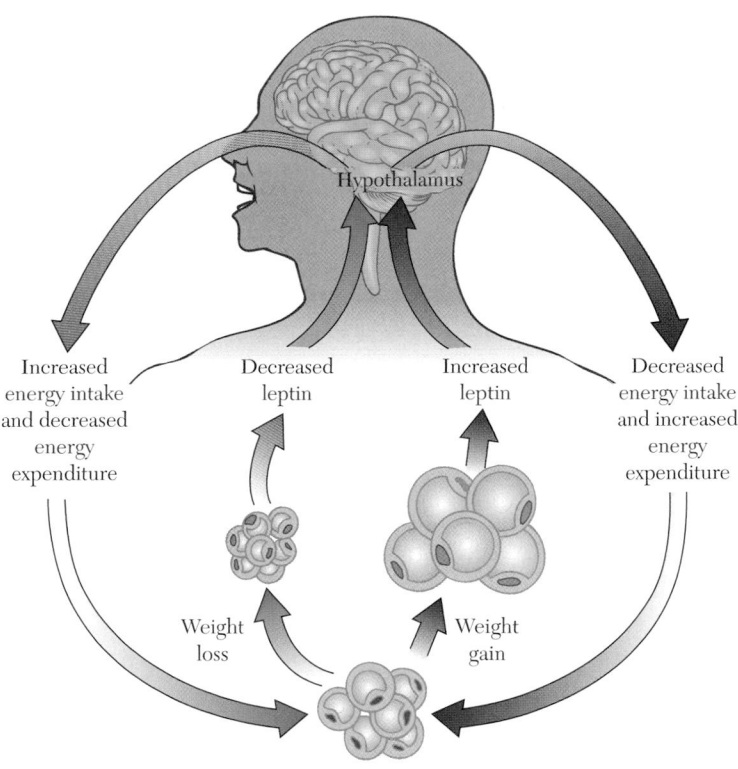

Figure 7.14
Leptin helps maintain body fat at a preset level. When adipocytes gain fat, more leptin is released, triggering events that decrease food intake and increase energy expenditure. When fat is lost, less leptin is released, causing an increase in food intake and a decrease in energy expenditure.

leptin produced and secreted.[23] **Leptin** is a hormone produced by the adipocytes, and the amount of leptin produced is proportional to the size of adipocytes, so more leptin is released as fat stores grow. Leptin travels in the blood to a part of the brain called the **hypothalamus** where it binds to proteins called leptin receptors. When leptin levels are high, mechanisms that cause an increase in energy expenditure and a decrease in food intake are stimulated, and pathways that promote food intake and, hence, weight gain are inhibited. When fat stores shrink, less leptin is released. Low leptin levels in the brain allow pathways that decrease energy expenditure and increase food intake to become active.[28] Thus, leptin acts like a thermostat or lipostat to keep body fatness from changing (Figure 7.14).

Heredity Versus Environment

Excess body fat accumulates when energy intake exceeds energy output. Traditionally, the explanation for why some people are fat and others are not has focused on external factors such as excessive food intake or lack of exercise. However, this theory did not explain why children have body shapes, sizes, and compositions similar to those of their parents. Some of us inherit tall, slender bodies with long, thin bones (Figure 7.15). Others inherit stocky bodies with short bones, wide hips, and stubby fingers. Heredity also plays a role in how much body fat we accumulate and where it is deposited. But environmental and behavioral factors, such as what we eat and how much we exercise, also affect how much body fat we carry.

Heredity and Body Weight If one or both of your parents is obese, your risk of becoming obese is increased. Individuals with a family history of obesity are two to three times more likely to be obese, and the risk increases with the magnitude of the obesity.[29]

Obesity is passed from parent to child because the information that regulates energy balance, body size, and body shape is contained in **genes**. A gene is a segment of DNA that provides the code or blueprint for the synthesis of a protein. Some proteins are involved in sending signals about food intake and energy expendi-

Leptin A protein hormone produced by adipocytes that signals information about the amount of body fat.

Hypothalamus The region of the brain that monitors and regulates conditions and activities in the body, including food intake and energy expenditure.

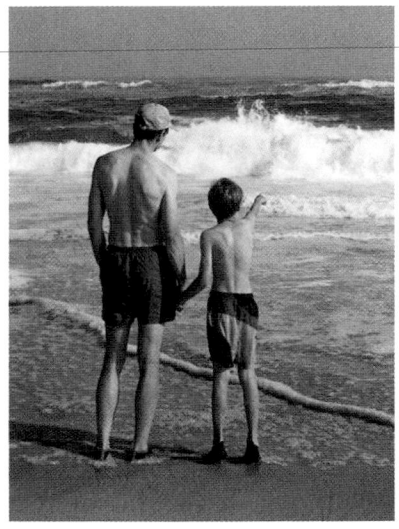

Figure 7.15
The genes we inherit from our parents are important determinants of our body size and shape. (Lori Smolin)

gene A length of DNA that contains the instructions for making a protein.

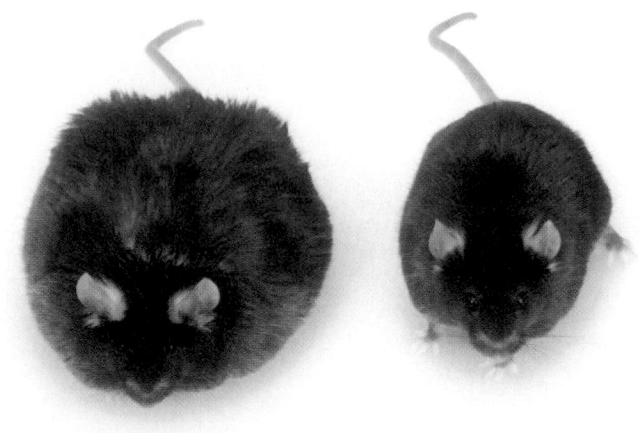

Figure 7.16

A mouse with a defect in the leptin gene (*ob*) may weigh three times as much as a normal mouse. Both of these mice have defective (*ob*) genes but the one on the right was treated with leptin injections (Courtesy John Sholtis, Rockefeller University, New York/© 1995 Amgen, Inc.)

ture to the brain, particularly to the hypothalamus. The hypothalamus monitors, integrates, and organizes these signals and then sends messages to other parts of the body to control food intake and energy expenditure. When a gene is defective, the protein it codes for is not made or is made incorrectly. When an obesity gene, such as the gene for leptin, is defective, the signals to decrease food intake and/or increase energy expenditure are not received, and weight gain results. A few cases of human obesity have been linked directly to defects in the genes for leptin and for leptin receptors.[30] But mutations in single genes such as these are not responsible for most human obesity. Rather, variations in many genes interact with one another and the environment to regulate body shape and size as well as energy intake and expenditure. A host of genes involved in the regulation of body weight have been identified in rodents, and similar genes have been found in humans, but we do not know how all the proteins made by these genes affect body weight (Figure 7.16).[31]

Environment and Body Weight Having obese parents increases one's risk of obesity not only genetically but also because obese families typically consume more energy and expend less through exercise than leaner families.[32] An individual with a genetic predisposition to obesity who has a limited supply of food or who engages in strenuous physical labor may never be obese, but someone with no genetic tendency toward obesity who consumes a high-energy diet and gets little exercise may accumulate too much body fat.

The typical lifestyle in the United States today, which fosters increased food intake and discourages physical activity, has been proposed as a major reason for the increasing numbers of obese people.[33] Supermarkets, fast-food restaurants, and all-night convenience marts provide ready access to food throughout the day and night. Bigger is marketed as better in terms of portion sizes; super-size beverages may contain over 600 kcalories (Figure 7.17). Along with the increase in energy intake, there has been a decrease in the amount of energy used in the activities of daily life. A farmer in 1900 did not have to plan an exercise program to increase his physical activity; his day-to-day life was active. Advances in technology have brought tractors, automobiles, elevators, and vacuum cleaners, which allow people to work without being as physically active; television, electronic games, and computers have given us sedentary ways to spend our leisure time. Socioeconomic status can also affect body weight. Education, income, and occupation influence behaviors that affect energy consumption and expenditure.

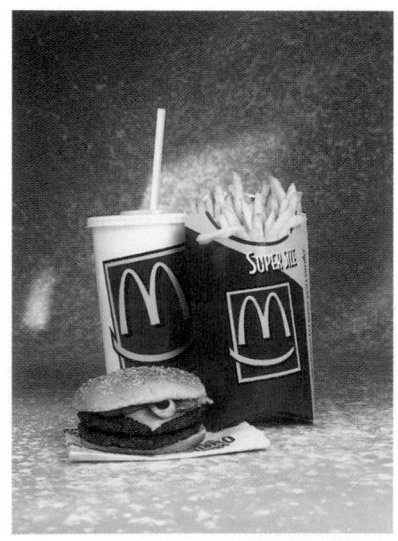

Figure 7.17

A supersized fast-food meal can contribute as much as 1500 kcalories and 55 grams of fat to daily intake. (© George Semple)

Interactions of Genes and Environment It is unlikely that the increasing incidence of obesity in the United States is due to genetics because it takes many generations to change the genes present in a population.[1] Therefore, nongenetic factors such as increased energy intake and decreased physical activity are thought to be the major contributors to our increasing in body weight. When genetically susceptible individuals find themselves in an environment where food is appealing and plentiful and physical activity is easily avoided, obesity is a likely outcome. An example of human obesity that clearly demonstrates the interaction of a genetic predisposition and an environment that is conducive to obesity is the Pima Indian tribe living in Arizona. More than 75% of this population is obese. Genetic analysis has identified a number of genes that may be responsible for this group's tendency to store more body fat.[34] Typically, Pimas have low energy requirements per unit of fat-free mass, which, coupled with a low level of physical activity and a high intake of an energy-dense diet, has caused body fat to be maintained at a high level. A group of Pima Indians living in Mexico is genetically the same as those in the United States, but they are farmers who consume the food they grow and have a high level of physical activity.[35] They still have higher rates of obesity than would be predicted from their diet and exercise patterns, suggesting genes that favor high body weight. However, they are significantly less obese than the Arizona Pima Indians.

Although genes seem to affect almost every behavior, including how much we exercise and what we eat,[17] the genes you inherit do not have the final say in whether you walk or take the bus or in how much ice cream you have for dessert. A genetic predisposition to obesity makes maintaining desirable body weight more difficult but not impossible.

Do Obese People Eat More?

Many overweight people contend that they eat very few kcalories and yet continue to gain weight. This would imply that their energy expenditure is less than in normal-weight individuals. One possible explanation for this is that overweight individuals use energy very efficiently so that more of the energy they consume is converted into ATP or deposited in energy stores than in someone with a less efficient metabolism. They would therefore need to eat less to maintain body weight. But actual studies of energy intake in overweight individuals have been inconclusive, in part because determining energy intake is difficult. Overweight individuals are more likely to underreport their energy intake than their lean counterparts.[8] Studies using doubly labeled water have shown that energy expenditure increases with increasing body weight, suggesting that obese individuals need to eat *more* than lean controls to maintain their higher body weight.[8] Although some individuals may need fewer kcalories than others, there is little evidence that an efficient metabolism is a factor in the majority of human obesity.

Do Obese Individuals Expend Less Energy? Although energy expenditure may be greater in obese individuals, they do not expend enough to keep their body fat in a healthy range. This may be due to mechanisms that regulate basal energy expenditure or to their level of physical activity.

Adaptive Thermogenesis In studies that control food intake, RMR decreases in both lean and obese subjects when food intake is restricted and increases during overconsumption.[21] Some studies found the drop in RMR seen with weight reduction was greater in obese than in lean subjects, and the increase in RMR seen with weight gain was less in obese than in lean subjects.[21] Changes in the amount of energy expended in response to changes in circumstance, such as over- or under-feeding, changes in temperature, or trauma, are referred to as **adaptive thermogenesis**. Increased energy expenditure through adaptive thermogenesis may prevent some of the weight gain that accompanies an increase in energy intake.[36,37]

Adaptive thermogenesis The change in energy expenditure induced by factors such as changes in ambient temperature and food intake.

Several biochemical mechanisms have been proposed to explain adaptive thermogenesis. The first is substrate cycling or futile cycling, which wastes energy by allowing opposing biochemical reactions to occur simultaneously. For example, a molecule is formed and then broken down. The result is that energy is consumed, but there is no net change in the number of molecules in the body and, therefore, no

Brown adipose tissue A type of fat tissue that has a greater number of mitochondria than the more common white adipose tissue. It can waste energy by producing heat and is believed to be responsible for some of the change in energy expenditure in adaptive thermogenesis in rodents.

storage of energy as fat. A second way that excess energy might be dissipated is by separating or uncoupling the electron transport chain from the production of ATP. When this occurs, energy is lost as heat. For example, the increase in energy expenditure that occurs when mice are injected with leptin is hypothesized to be due to the stimulation of receptors on a specialized type of adipose tissue called **brown adipose tissue**. Brown adipose tissue can waste energy as heat. It contains many more mitochondria than other adipose tissue, and these mitochondria can be uncoupled from the electron transport chain to release the energy in food as heat. In rats, brown adipose tissue generates heat to prevent weight gain during overfeeding and to provide warmth when the ambient temperature is low. Except for newborns, humans have only a very small amount of brown adipose tissue, but humans may be able to dissipate energy in other tissues. Several proteins that uncouple the electron transport chain from the production of ATP have been identified in human muscle, white adipose tissue, lung, spleen, white blood cells, bone marrow, and stomach.[38] It is hypothesized that these proteins may be involved in increasing energy output to regulate body weight in humans.

Physical Activity The amount of energy an individual expends depends primarily on metabolic rate and activity. Genetics determine our metabolic rate. Activity level is affected by genetics and individual choices. When the energy expended for physical activity is compared with the amount of body fat, it is found that individuals with the most body fat have the lowest levels of physical activity, supporting the hypothesis that obesity is associated with a lower level of physical activity.[39] This does not mean that reduced physical activity necessarily causes obesity. The reduction in activity may occur as a result of the obesity. Excess weight makes it more difficult to exercise or even to perform simple daily activities. A 230-pound man walking a mile is carrying the same weight as a 200-pound man walking a mile carrying a 30-pound suitcase. This extra burden reduces the inclination to increase activity. In addition to the physical stress, obese individuals often shy away from exercise because they don't want to be compared with their leaner counterparts. Obese children may avoid athletic activities to escape being teased about their weight.

We tend to think of physical activity as the amount of planned exercise we engage in, but energy is also expended in involuntary exercise, such as fidgeting, maintenance of posture, and the other small movements that occur during daily living. A study that overfed nonobese individuals found there was a 10-fold variation in the amount of fat gained. Some subjects were able to increase energy expenditure to a greater extent and so gained less fat. About two-thirds of the increase in energy expenditure that occurred with overfeeding was found to be due to an increase in involuntary exercise.[40] Individuals who gained little weight had a greater level of involuntary exercise than those who gained more weight. It is still not known what mechanisms control why some people respond to excess energy by becoming restless and fidgeting more while others remain lethargic in their daily activities (see *Critical Thinking*: Balancing Intake and Expenditure).

CRITICAL THINKING

Balancing Intake and Expenditure

April is unhappy about the 10 pounds she gained during her freshman year at college. Her parents are both obese, and she is worried that she too will become obese. She is 5 feet 4 inches tall, 23 years old, and weighs 140 pounds. She would like to weigh 130 pounds.

In analyzing why she gained weight, April realizes that, with her busy college schedule, she gets less exercise than she used to and often eats candy bars from the vending machine while studying late at night. By recording and analyzing her food intake for 3 days, she determines that she eats about 2450 kcalories per day. To see how this compares to her recommended intake, she calculates her EER. By keeping an activity log, she estimates that a typical day includes 30 minutes of moderate activity. This puts her activity level in the "low active" category.

What is her EER?
▼

April's EER =

(*Hint:* Use the EER equation in Table 7.2 and the low-active PA value in Table 7.4 for a 23-year-old woman.)

How does her EER compare to her intake?
▼

Answer:

April realizes she needs to either increase her output or decrease her intake in order to lose weight. She decides to start by increasing her activity level. She loves to play tennis and so plans to add two hours of tennis a day to her schedule. Tennis is a vigorous activity so playing 2 hours per day would move her into the "very active" category.

What would her EER be with the added 2 hours of tennis per day?
▼

Answer:

Is this a reasonable plan?
▼

Although April loves tennis and this level of activity would allow her to lose weight, she probably won't play for two hours each day. A more reasonable approach might be to plan on playing tennis three days a week while also adding some moderate activity such as riding her bike to and from class, using the stairs instead of the elevator, and going dancing some evenings with friends. She is more likely to keep up this schedule and this amount of activity will put her in the "active" category, which is the level recommended to maintain health.

To lose weight, April must also change her diet. She eats many high-kcalorie, high-fat foods such as cheese Danish, chicken nuggets, and candy bars. Replacing these with lower kcalorie options, such as bagels, broiled chicken and fruit, will reduce her energy intake.

Is she destined to become obese?
▼

Answer:

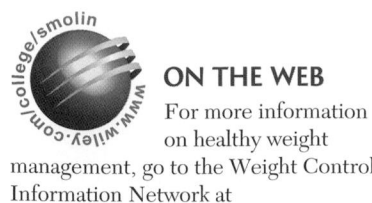

ON THE WEB

For more information on healthy weight management, go to the Weight Control Information Network at www.niddk.nih.gov/health/nutrit/htm/.

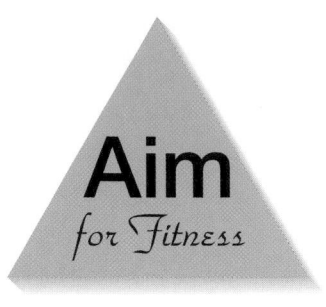

▲ Aim for a healthy weight

Figure 7.18

The Dietary Guidelines for Americans, 2000 advises us to "Aim for a healthy weight."

Weight cycling The cycle of repeatedly losing and regaining weight.

• ACHIEVING A HEALTHY WEIGHT

Rather than focusing on weight loss, which is unlikely to be successful in the long term, weight problems should be viewed in terms of weight management. One goal of weight management is to prevent excess body weight gain. Healthy eating habits and active lives that promote the maintenance of a healthy weight should be developed in childhood and maintained throughout life (Figure 7.18). Just as a family history of heart disease or an increase in blood cholesterol should set in motion dietary and lifestyle changes to maintain health, a family history of obesity or an increase in body weight should trigger dietary and lifestyle changes that maintain weight at a healthy level. For those who are already overweight, the goal of weight management is to reduce body fat to a healthy level that can be maintained over a lifetime.[41]

Weight-Loss Guidelines

For most people, a loss of 5 to 15% of body weight, most of which is fat, will significantly reduce disease risk.[42] The initial goal of weight loss should, therefore, be to reduce body weight by approximately 10% over a period of about 6 months.[14] After this initial weight loss, risks can be reassessed to determine if additional weight loss would be beneficial. A slow loss of 10% of body weight is considered achievable for most individuals and is easier to maintain than larger weight losses. Most people who lose large amounts of weight or lose weight rapidly eventually regain all that they have lost. Repeated cycles of weight loss and regain, referred to as **weight cycling**, increase the proportion of body fat with each successive weight regain and cause a decrease in BMR, making subsequent weight loss more difficult (Figure 7.19).[43] Even if an individual has lost and regained weight in the past, weight loss is recommended if they are still obese or overweight and have two or more conditions that increase the health risks associated with obesity.[42]

In order to decrease body fat, energy intake must be less than energy output. It is estimated that a pound of body fat provides 3500 kcalories. Therefore, to lose a pound of fat, one must decrease energy intake by this amount or increase energy output by this amount. To lose a pound in a week, one must shift energy balance by 500 kcalories per day (3500 kcal ÷ 7 days = 500 kcal/day). This is the predicted average weight loss at this energy deficit. However, the actual amount of weight lost per week may vary over time. To promote the loss of fat and not lean tissue, a weight-loss program should encourage the loss of only 1/2 to 2 pound per week.[42] If weight is lost more rapidly, the loss is less likely to be maintained, and the additional loss will be from fluid, muscle and liver glycogen, and muscle protein.

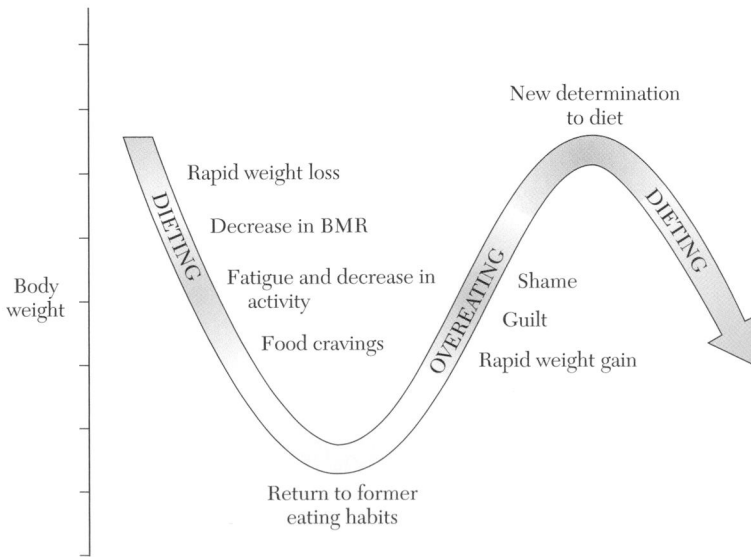

Figure 7.19

Weight cycling is the repeated loss and regain of body weight.

Approaches to Weight Management

Although the arithmetic is simple, achieving a reduction in body weight is not easy. There are regulatory mechanisms at work to keep body weight stable. There are environmental and emotional motivators to increase food intake and reduce the inclination to exercise. Nonetheless, reductions in intake, increases in activity, and changes in behavior can promote weight loss and long-term weight management.

Decreasing Energy Intake For safe and effective weight loss, the diet must be low in energy but provide for all the body's nutrient needs. Nutrient density becomes more important as energy intake is reduced. Choosing foods that are low in fat and added sugars will increase the nutrient density of the diet. With energy intakes less than 1200 kcalories per day, it is difficult to meet the requirements for micronutrients, so a multivitamin and mineral supplement is recommended. Medical supervision is recommended if intake is 800 kcalories per day or less.

Increasing Physical Activity Physical activity is an important component of any well-designed weight-management program. Exercise promotes fat loss and weight maintenance. It increases energy expenditure, so if intake remains the same, energy stored as fat is used for fuel. An increase in activity of 200 kcalories five times a week will result in the loss of a pound in about three and a half weeks. Exercise also promotes muscle development. This is important during weight loss because muscle is metabolically active tissue. Increasing muscle mass helps to prevent the drop in BMR that occurs as body weight decreases. Weight loss is also better maintained when physical activity is included in the weight-management program.[44] In addition, physical activity improves overall fitness and relieves boredom and stress. The benefits of exercise are discussed in Chapter 13.

Modifying Behavior In order to keep weight at a new lower level, food consumption and exercise patterns must be changed for life. Changing these behaviors requires identifying the old patterns that led to weight gain and replacing them with new ones to maintain weight loss. This can be accomplished through a process called **behavior modification**, which is based on the theory that behaviors involve (1) antecedents or cues that lead to the behavior, (2) the behavior itself, and (3) consequences of the behavior. These are referred to as the ABCs of behavior modification.

The first step in a behavior modification program is to identify cues that lead to eating. This is usually done by keeping a log of all food consumed, where it was consumed, what other activities were involved, and what motivated the eating. The log can then be analyzed to determine what led to the behavior (in this case, eating), and what the consequences of the behavior were. The key to modifying the behavior is to recognize the antecedent so that the behavior and consequences can be changed. For instance, sitting in front of the television and mindlessly demolishing a bag of potato chips may leave you feeling bad because you consumed the extra kcalories. In this case, the antecedent is watching TV, the behavior is mindlessly eating the chips, and the consequence is feeling remorse and gaining weight. The key to modifying this behavior is to recognize the antecedent, change the behavior, and replace the negative consequence with a positive one. For example, never taking food with you to the television, or taking only the portion of food you want to consume, eliminates the antecedent and the behavior. The consequence is that you have consumed only the food you planned, you do not gain weight, and you feel a sense of accomplishment. Applying behavior modification techniques to change eating behaviors has been shown to improve long-term weight maintenance.

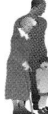

Weight Loss at Life Stages Obesity and overweight is a growing problem among children (Figure 7.20). It is estimated that 13 percent of children ages 6 to 11 years old and 14% of adolescents ages 12 to 19 years old are overweight.[45] This is the result of both excessive intake of foods high in fat and energy and inadequate physical

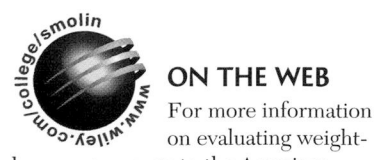

ON THE WEB
For more information on evaluating weight-loss programs, go to the American Dietetic Association at
www.eatright.org/
and search for weight loss.

Behavior modification A process used to gradually and permanently change habitual behaviors.

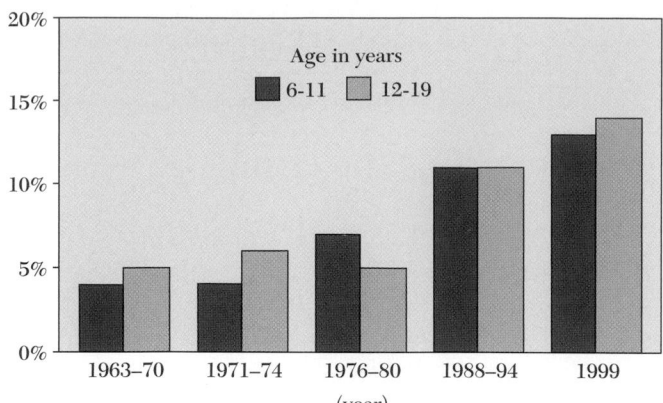

Figure 7.20
The prevalence of obesity among children and adolescents in the United States has increased over the last 30 years. (Source: National Center for Health Statistics. Prevalence of Overweight Among Children and Adolescents: United States, 1999, www.cdc.gov/nchs/products/pubs/pubd/hestats/overwght99.htm)

activity. However, strict weight-loss diets are generally not recommended for children or adolescents because a reduction in intake can interfere with growth. A better approach is to encourage physical activity, along with a moderate energy-intake restriction, allowing the child to grow in height with little additional weight gain (see Chapter 15).

Weight-loss diets are also not recommended during pregnancy. Even women who are overweight at the start of pregnancy should gain at a slow, steady rate to accumulate about 15 to 25 pounds over the course of pregnancy. A weight-loss program can be initiated after the baby is born and the mother has recovered (see Chapter 14). Slow weight loss is appropriate during lactation, but rapid weight loss can decrease milk production.

For older adults, the risks associated with excess body fat are lower than they are for younger adults.[46] However, the decision to treat obesity should not be based on age alone. Weight loss can enhance day-to-day functioning and improve cardiovascular disease risk factors at all ages.[14] Older people tend to lose muscle and replace it with fat; therefore, weight-training activities are an important part of a weight loss program in the elderly (see Chapter 16).

Suggestions for Weight Gain As difficult as weight loss is for some people, weight gain can be equally elusive for underweight individuals (see Table 7.6). The first step toward weight gain is a medical evaluation to rule out medical reasons for low body weight. This particularly important when weight loss occurs unexpectedly. If the low body weight is due to low intake or high expenditure, gradually increasing consumption of energy-dense foods is suggested. More frequent meals and high-kcalorie snacks such as peanut butter or milkshakes between meals can help increase

Table 7.6 *Principles of Food Selection for Weight Loss, Weight Gain, or Weight Maintenance*

Starches are not high in energy. Remember, carbohydrate has only 4 kcalories per gram. It is usually the fats added to starches that add the energy.

Foods high in fat are high in energy. These include obvious fats, like butter and margarine, and hidden fats in fried foods and baked goods.

Foods high in fiber are relatively low in energy. Fiber cannot be absorbed, and fiber is filling, so high-fiber foods make us feel full longer.

Foods high in simple sugars, like soda, provide energy without many other nutrients.

All essential nutrients must be considered when designing a weight-loss diet.

When planning a diet, start by recording your typical food intake.

Start by making small, reasonable changes in your current diet.

Make changes that are likely to last a lifetime.

energy intake. Replacing low-kcalorie fluids like water and diet beverages with fruit juices and milk may also help. To encourage a gain in muscle rather than fat, strength-training exercise should be a component of any weight gain program. This approach requires extra kcalories to fuel the activity needed to build muscles. These recommendations apply to individuals who are naturally thin and have trouble gaining weight on the recommended energy intake. This dietary approach may not promote weight gain for those who limit intake because of an eating disorder.

• OPTIONS FOR REDUCING ENERGY INTAKE

Overweight people, desperate to lose weight, are prey to all sorts of products and procedures that promise quick fixes. They have their jaws wired shut, eat a single-food for days at a time, select foods based on special fat-burning qualities, and consume odd combinations of foods at specific times of the day. Jaw-wiring is a temporary procedure that restricts intake to liquids that can be taken through a straw. Fad diets, such as those that emphasize eating primarily a single food, special foods, or specific combinations of foods, may promote weight loss over the short term, but since they are not nutritionally sound, they cannot be consumed safely for long periods. These fads do not encourage exercise or promote the changes in eating behavior that affect body weight over the long term.

An ideal weight-management program should provide for a reduction in energy intake along with education about meeting nutrient needs, an increase in energy expenditure, and lifestyle modifications to change the patterns that led to weight gain. Prescription medications and surgery may also be acceptable weight-management tools for obese individuals when conventional methods fail. When selecting an approach to weight management, an individual should find a plan that is based on sound nutrition and exercise principles, suits their individual food preferences, promotes long-term lifestyle changes, and meets their needs for structure and social support (Table 7.7). If the program's approach is not one that can be followed for a lifetime, it is unlikely to promote successful weight management. Cost, convenience, and the time commitment required by the program are also important considerations.

Table 7.7   What to Look for in a Weight-Management Program

A healthy dietary pattern that can be followed for life

Does the diet plan meet all nutrient needs?

Can the diet plan meet individual health needs? (For example, can it be used by someone who has diabetes or high blood cholesterol?)

Does the program include an education component to teach participants how to make healthy food choices?

Does the program take into consideration a participant's eating habits and preferences?

Is the diet plan flexible enough to be followed in different settings and on different occasions?

Does the diet require the purchase of special foods or supplements?

Reasonable weight loss

Does the program set realistic weight-loss goals in the range of 1/2 to 2 pounds per week?

Physical activity

Does the program stress the need to increase physical activity?

Behavior change

Does the program include some type of social support?

Does the program promote changes in behavior that can be maintained over the long term?

Scientifically sound

Is the program based on sound scientific principles?

Are the personnel monitoring the weight management program health professionals?

Adapted from the American Heart Association's Web site at www.amhrt.org/Health/Risk_Factors/Overweight/Fad_Diets/fadguide.html.

The following sections discuss some of the more common methods for reducing energy intake. The advantages and disadvantages of a number of commercial weight-management programs are given in Table 7.8. Pharmaceutical and surgical approaches to reducing intake are also discussed.

Low-Kcalorie Diets

Weight-loss plans based simply on reducing energy intake are the most common. Some recommend energy reduction without restricting the types of foods selected, some use exchange systems to plan energy and nutrient intake, and others provide low-kcalorie packaged meals and formulas.

Free-Choice Diets Free choice diets allow dieters to choose the foods they eat as long as energy intake is reduced. They offer flexibility and variety, and can suit different food preferences. The disadvantage is that these diets may not meet nutrient needs unless they are based on some type of food selection guidelines. The Food Guide Pyramid can provide the structure necessary to plan a balanced low-kcalorie diet. A diet with as few as 1200 kcalories can be planned by using the low end of the range of suggested servings and making low-kcalorie choices. Food labels can be

Table 7.8 *Advantages and Disadvantages of Some Commercial Weight-Management Programs*

Program	Approach	Advantages	Disadvantages
Weight Watchers	Low energy, social support	Safe, inexpensive, flexible	Requires group participation
Jenny Craig	Low energy	Safe, convenient	Expensive; relies on purchase of special foods
SlimFast	Low energy	Safe	Does not promote long-term behavior change
The New Beverly Hills Diet	Specific timing and combinations of foods	Inexpensive	Based on unsound principles; does not promote long-term behavior change; nutritionally unsound
Optifast	Very low-kcalorie formula	Rapid weight loss	Expensive; dangerous if does not include medical supervision
Fit or Fat	Increased exercise	Safe, inexpensive	No social support
The Zone (and Mastering the Zone) Diet	Low carbohydrate (40% of energy)	Inexpensive, flexible	Based on questionable principles; no social support
Eating Thin for Life	Moderation—written as weight-loss success stories, recipes, and menu ideas	Inexpensive	No social support
Dieting with the Duchess	Simple nutrition and exercise tips	Inexpensive, flexible	No social support
Cabbage Soup Diet	Unlimited amounts of cabbage soup, fruit, coffee, and tea	Rapid weight loss	No social support; does not promote long-term behavior change; lack of variety
Grapefruit diet	Some foods have special qualities that burn fat	Inexpensive	Based on unsound principles
Sugar Busters	Eliminates sugar; low kcalorie—1200 kcal a day	Inexpensive	No social support; based on unsound principles; insufficient carbohydrate
Volumetrics Weight Control Plan	Emphasizes foods high in water, fiber, and air to promote fullness with few kcalories	Safe, inexpensive	No social support or exercise component
Atkins' Diet	Very low carbohydrate	Inexpensive; rapid initial weight loss	Based on unsound principles; no social support; insufficient carbohydrate

used to help select packaged foods that are appropriate for a low-kcalorie diet (see *Off the Label*: Knowing Your Kcalories).

Exchange Plans Some diet plans use exchanges to assure nutritional adequacy along with reduced energy. They may use either the Exchange Lists (see Table 7.1 and Appendix I) or similar plans that recommend a set number of servings from each of several food lists. These diets are more likely to meet nutrient needs than free-choice plans and still offer variety from meal to meal and from day to day. In addition, they teach meal-planning skills that are easy to apply away from home and can be used over the long term.

Fixed Meal Plans Fixed meal plans allow only a defined set of foods. Some plans sell prepackaged meals, and others provide defined lists of foods allowed at each meal. For instance, a fixed meal plan might specify a cup of corn flakes with a banana for breakfast, ham salad and an apple for lunch, and broiled chicken with broccoli for dinner. These diets are easy to follow but can be boring and are not practical in the long term; they don't teach food selection skills because the meals are standardized. Plans that sell prepackaged meals can be expensive, and they are difficult to follow when traveling or eating out.

Liquid Formula Diets Liquid diets can make dieting easier for some people because the problem of choosing a low-energy diet is eliminated. Liquid weight-loss diets that are available over-the-counter recommend a combination of food and formula to provide a daily energy intake of about 800 to 1200 kcalories. These formulas can be effective as long as the foods eaten with them are low in kcalories. Although over-the-counter formulas are easy to use and relatively inexpensive, they do little to change eating habits for life (Figure 7.21). Most diet programs that rely exclusively on liquid formulas have high dropout rates and poor long-term weight-maintenance results. Weight-loss regimens that rely exclusively on liquid formulas are not recommended without medical supervision.

Very-Low-Kcalorie Diets **Very-low-kcalorie diets** are defined as those containing fewer than 800 kcalories per day. They became popular in response to a desire for rapid weight loss. These diets are generally a variation of the **protein-sparing modified fast**, a diet providing little energy and a high proportion of protein. The concept behind this is that the protein in the diet will be used to meet the body's protein needs and will, therefore, prevent excessive loss of body protein. Frequently, very-low-kcalorie diets are offered as a liquid formula. These formulas provide from 300 to 800 kcalories and 50 to 100 g of protein per day and meet all other nutrient needs.

Initial weight loss is rapid with very-low-kcalorie diets—3 to 5 pounds per week. This can provide a psychological boost and motivate the dieter to continue losing weight; however, in most cases, almost 75% of this initial weight loss is from water loss. Once the initial water loss ends, weight loss slows. The dieter's BMR decreases to conserve energy, and physical activity decreases because the dieter often does not have the energy to continue their typical level of physical activity.

Very-low-kcalorie diets are no more effective than other methods in the long term and carry more risks. At these low-energy intakes, body protein is broken down and potassium is excreted. Depletion of potassium can result in an irregular heartbeat and is potentially deadly. Other side effects include gallstones, fatigue, nausea, cold-intolerance, light-headedness, nervousness, constipation or diarrhea, anemia, hair loss, dry skin, and menstrual irregularities. These diets are not recommended for people who are less than 30 to 40% above their healthy body weight, for pregnant or breast-feeding women, or for children, adolescents, or those with severe medical problems.[47] Since 1984, the FDA has required that all very-low-kcalorie diet formulas carry a warning that they can cause serious illness and should be used only under medical supervision.

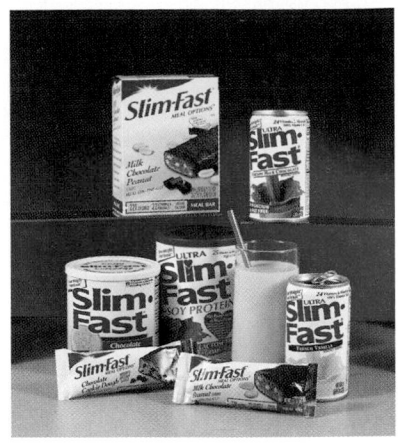

Figure 7.21
Liquid diet products such as these eliminate food choices and may result in weight loss but do nothing to change eating habits. (© Andy Washnik)

Very-low-kcalorie diet A weight-loss diet that provides fewer than 800 kcalories per day.

Protein-sparing modified fast A very-low-kcalorie diet of high protein content designed to maximize the loss of fat and minimize the loss of protein from the body.

Diets That Modify Macronutrient Intake

Rather than focusing on counting kcalories as a way of reducing body weight, some diets concentrate on modifying the proportions of energy-containing nutrients.

Lowfat Diets Because fat is high in kcalories, consuming a lowfat diet typically reduces energy intake. Lowfat diets provide more food for the same amount of energy than high-fat diets and may satisfy hunger after less energy is consumed. Differences in the way dietary fat and dietary carbohydrate are used by the body also explain why lowfat diets are more effective for weight loss. Excess dietary fat kcalories are stored more efficiently than excess carbohydrate kcalories, so consuming excess energy from fat leads to a greater accumulation of body fat than consuming excess energy as carbohydrate.[48]

Despite the advantages, lowfat diets are not always low in energy; even a diet low in fat will result in weight gain if energy intake exceeds energy output. This is illustrated by the fact that the percent of kcalories as fat in the typical American diet has decreased while the number of people who are overweight continues to increase.

Low-Carbohydrate Diets A number of different low-carbohydrate weight-loss diets have been promoted over the last 30 years. Some of these diets severely restrict carbohydrate intake by prohibiting foods such as breads, grains, and fruits, and limiting vegetable intake while allowing unlimited quantities of meat and high-fat foods that are low in carbohydrate. Others are less restrictive and suggest a moderate reduction in carbohydrate intake to about 40% of energy. These diets are all based on the premise that a high carbohydrate intake causes an increase in insulin levels, which promotes the storage of body fat. Restricting carbohydrate intake is hypothesized to reduce insulin, thereby reducing fat storage and promoting fat loss. Unfortunately, the relationship between carbohydrate intake, insulin levels, and body fat is not that simple.

Blood insulin levels rise when carbohydrate is consumed, but not all high-carbohydrate foods cause a sharp rise in insulin. Whole grains and vegetables that are high in fiber do not increase insulin nearly as much as refined carbohydrates such as white flour and sugar. So, the type of carbohydrate consumed may be as important as the amount. Restricting the consumption of whole grains and vegetables reduces the intake of fiber and micronutrients and has only a modest effect on insulin levels.

When carbohydrate is severely restricted, there is an initial rapid weight loss, most of which is water. This occurs because when carbohydrate intake is low, glycogen stores, along with the water they hold, are lost quickly. Ketones are produced because fat is not completely broken down in the absence of carbohydrate. Excretion of these ketones causes additional water loss. In addition, there is evidence that ketones in the blood suppress appetite, making it easier to reduce food intake.

The bottom line is that weight loss occurs on low-carbohydrate diets because total energy intake is reduced. This may be due in part to a decrease in hunger associated with a reduction in insulin levels, but it is also because the total amount of food allowed by many of these diet plans is limited or because dieters reduce their food intake out of boredom with the limited food choices. Although weight loss will occur with low carbohydrate diets, restricting a single nutrient is unlikely to solve the obesity epidemic. In addition, a diet that severely restricts carbohydrate will be higher in fat and protein than is recommended. More research is needed to determine the health consequences of long-term consumption of very low-carbohydrate diets (see *Critical Thinking:* Do You Think This Diet Will Work?).

Weight-Loss Drugs

There are a variety of drug therapies available to promote weight loss. Some are well studied and offer legitimate aids to weight loss; others offer little more than water loss. An ideal drug treatment for obesity would permit an individual to lose weight and maintain the loss, be safe when used for long periods of time, have no side effects, and not be addictive. Many attempts have been made to develop such a drug, but weight loss drugs still carry risks. In 1997, a drug combination called fen-phen (fenfluramine and phentermine) that was being used to reduce food intake was linked to serious heart valve damage. As a result, fenfluramine and the related drug dexfenfluramine were withdrawn from the market.[49]

Currently, drug treatment is only recommended for those whose health is seriously compromised by their body weight. It should be considered in individuals with a BMI greater than 30 with no obesity related risk factors or diseases and in those with a BMI greater than or equal to 27 who have risk factors or diseases.[14]

Prescription Medications There are a number of prescription drugs on the market that promote weight loss by reducing energy intake. Sibutramine (Meridia) decreases food intake by affecting the activity of brain neurotransmitters that regulate food intake. Orlistat (Xenical) reduces fat absorption and, therefore, energy intake by blocking fat-digesting enzymes in the intestine. Although many drugs have shown promise at promoting weight loss in the short term, weight is regained when the drugs are discontinued. There are also a number of drugs in various stages of development that may someday help reduce body weight by increasing energy expenditure, by increasing the release of fat from adipose tissue, or by decreasing fat synthesis.[50]

Products Available without a Prescription Products sold over-the-counter to promote weight loss include nonprescription medications and dietary supplements. Some may be moderately effective, but, as with prescription medications, the weight is usually regained when the product is no longer taken.

Nonprescription medications are regulated by the U.S. Food and Drug Administration (FDA) and must adhere to strict guidelines regarding the dose per pill and the effectiveness of the ingredients. The FDA does not regulate dietary supplements for weight loss unless they claim to be a substitute for a drug or claim to perform a drug action or therapy (see Chapter 12). Weight-loss supplements often include herbal sources of compounds contained in prescription medications. Some of these are powerful drugs with dangerous side effects. Because they are not strictly regulated, their safety and effectiveness may not have been carefully tested, and doses may vary from tablet to tablet and brand to brand. It cannot be assumed that a product is safe simply because it is labeled "herbal" or "all natural."

Over-the-Counter Medications Only a limited number of substances have been approved by the FDA for sale as nonprescription weight-loss medications. Fibers such as methylcellulose and glucomannan are used in weight-loss products because they absorb water to create a feeling of fullness; pills containing them claim to fill the stomach with indigestible bulk so that one feels sated and eats less. The anesthetic benzocaine is included in weight-loss products because it numbs the tongue, making eating a less pleasurable experience. Caffeine, which is a stimulant and a diuretic, is used in many weight-loss products. Stimulants tend to blunt the appetite, and diuretics cause the kidneys to increase fluid excretion, resulting in weight loss from water loss. These same effects can be derived from caffeine-containing beverages like coffee, tea, and some soft drinks.

Dietary Supplements Common ingredients in weight-loss dietary supplements include the amino acids arginine and ornithine, chromium, and a variety of herbs. Arginine and ornithine are hypothesized to burn fat during sleep because they stimulate the release of growth hormone. Although growth hormone promotes fat loss and muscle growth, research has not found any relationship between body weight and the levels of growth hormone. The mineral chromium is usually included as chromium picolinate. It is claimed to decrease body fat and increase the proportion of lean tissue, but human trials have not consistently demonstrated an effect of supplemental chromium picolinate on body composition or body weight.[51]

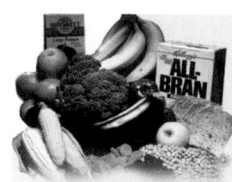

Off the Shelf

Fat Burners: The Hot and the Cold

Do you have an extra ten pounds that you'd rather not carry around with you? You start an exercise program and lose a few pounds, but as weight loss slows, so does your motivation and soon the weight is back? Wouldn't it be nice if there were a pill that you could take to increase your metabolism without breaking a sweat? There are many dietary supplements that claim to do just this—but do they work and are they safe?

Weight-loss supplements that claim to increase metabolism are called fat burners or thermogenic stimulators. They promise to boost metabolism, prevent loss of lean muscle tissue, suppress appetite, and increase the burning of stored fat. Most of these products contain some vitamins, minerals, and amino acids along with central nervous system stimulants such as ephedrine (ephedra) and methylxanthines (compounds such as caffeine found in coffee and theophylline found in tea). Many also contain aspirin.

Do they really boost metabolism? Ephedrine is a decongestant and a central nervous system stimulant that increases heart rate and blood pressure. It stimulates nerves called adrenergic neurons that (among other effects) inhibit hunger and stimulate energy expenditure, fat breakdown, and fat oxidation. There are different types of adrenergic neurons with different effects. Stimulation of a combination of adrenergic neurons can increase energy expenditure by 5 to 10% and increase the relative proportion of fat that is burned. This may be the mechanism responsible for the weight loss caused by agents such as ephedrine plus caffeine.[1] Research supports the claim that the combination of ephedrine and caffeine increases thermogenesis, depresses appetite, and enhances fat loss when compared to a placebo.[2] The

addition of aspirin to this combination does not appear to further increase the thermic effect.[3] A mixture of ephedrine, caffeine, and theophylline was also shown to increase energy expenditure, particularly in individuals predisposed to obesity.[4] The results of this study suggested that dietary methylxanthines may work mainly by increasing the thermogenic response to food in individuals predisposed to obesity.[4]

Are fat burners the magic bullet that will help keep Americans slim? Despite evidence that they do increase energy expenditure, the cost to overall health may be higher than that of the extra pounds. Ephedrine is a powerful drug with dangerous side effects. Between 1993 and 1995, the Texas Department of Health received 500 reports of adverse effects, including eight deaths, in people who consumed dietary supplements containing ephedrine and substances related to ephedrine.[5] Side effects range from nervousness, dizziness, headache, gastrointestinal distress, and changes in blood pressure and heart rate to chest pain, heart attack, hepatitis, stroke, seizures, psychosis, and death. Combinations of caffeine and ephedrine cause side effects that are more severe than those caused by either compound alone. These symptoms have occurred in young, otherwise healthy individuals as well as those with other confounding conditions such as hypertension.

What if the supplement is "all natural"? Aspirin, ephedrine, and caffeine sound more like drugs than natural ingredients, and they are. But supplements can contain these compounds and still claim to be "all natural" by using herbal sources. For example, *Citrus aurantium* is an herb that contains a chemical derivative of ephedrine called synephrine; ma huang is a Chinese herb that contains ephedrine;

gaurana extract is an herbal source of caffeine; and white willow bark extract contains salicin, a compound similar to aspirin. Just because these compounds are added as components of herbs does not mean they are any less biologically active or cause fewer side effects than when they are present in over-the-counter or prescription medications.

So, should you take a fat burner or keep up your routine at the gym? The risks of ephedrine-containing supplements are very real, and there is no evidence of long-term benefits. Boosting metabolism may cause short-term weight loss, but eventually intake is likely to catch up with expenditure, causing weight loss to slow or stop. The weight may be regained even with the supplement. Losing weight and keeping it off requires changes in lifestyle and the behaviors that led to the accumulation of extra pounds in the first place.

[1]Astrup, A., and Lundsgaard, C. What do pharmacological approaches to obesity management offer? Linking pharmacological mechanisms of obesity management agents to clinical practice. *Exp. Clin. Endocrinol. Diabetes* 106 (Suppl. 2):29–34, 1998.

[2]Astrup, A., Toubro, S., Christensen, N. J., and Quaade, F. Pharmacology of thermogenic drugs. *Am. J. Clin. Nutr.* 55 (1 Suppl.):246–248S, 1992.

[3]Horton, T. J., and Geissler, C. A. Postprandial thermogenesis with ephedrine, caffeine and aspirin in lean, an predisposed obese and obese women. *Int. J. Obes. Relat. Metab. Disord.* 20:91–97, 1996.

[4]Dulloo, A. G., and Miller, D. S. The thermogenic properties of ephedrine/methylxanthine mixtures: human studies. *Int. J. Obes.* 10:467–481, 1986.

[5]MMWR August 16, 1996: Adverse events associated with ephedrine-containing products—Texas, December 1993–September 1995. Available online at vm.cfsan.fda.gov/~dms/ephedrin.html/ Accessed April 25, 2000.

Ma huang is an herb that is used in supplements known as herbal fat burners. Ma huang is an herbal source of Ephedra (also called ephedrine, or synphedrine), a central nervous system stimulant that reduces appetite. Ephedra is approved by the FDA for use as a decongestant but not for use in over-the-counter weight-loss medications. Ephedra can be effective at increasing metabolic rate and suppressing appetite, but serious side effects have been reported with its use, particularly in individuals with high blood pressure, diabetes, or thyroid conditions (see *Off the Shelf*: Fat Burners: The Hot and the Cold).

Other types of herbal products marketed for weight loss are teas and supplements that contain plant-derived laxatives such as senna, aloe, buckthorn, rhubarb root, cascara, and castor oil. Cascara, senna, and castor oil are approved by the FDA and regulated as drugs for use in nonprescription laxatives. These cause weight loss by inducing diarrhea, which causes water loss. They don't lead to fat loss, however, because they do not significantly reduce nutrient absorption. This is because they act in the colon, not in the small intestine, where most absorption occurs. Overuse of herbal laxatives can cause serious side effects, including nausea, diarrhea, vomiting, stomach cramps, chronic constipation, fainting, and severe electrolyte imbalances leading to cardiac arrhythmia and death.[52]

Weight-Loss Surgery

A more drastic method of weight management is surgery. Obesity surgery is recommended in cases where the risk of dying from obesity and its complications is great. It is appropriate only for individuals with a BMI greater than or equal to 40 kg/m^2 (extreme obesity) and in those with a BMI between 35 and 40 kg/m^2 who have other life-threatening conditions that could be remedied by weight loss.[14] The success of weight-loss surgery, as with other treatment, depends on the motivation and behavior of the patient. The appropriateness of surgery has to be evaluated on a case-by-case basis by considering the individual's potential risks and benefits.

Currently, the most popular surgical approaches to treat obesity are gastroplasty and gastric bypass. Gastroplasty involves stapling off the top part of the stomach to make it smaller. Gastric bypass involves bypassing part of the stomach by connecting the intestine to the upper portion of the stomach. In both cases, food intake is reduced because the now smaller stomach becomes full with less food. Significant weight loss is usually achieved 18 to 24 months after surgery. Some weight regain is common after two to five years. The success rate is lower with gastroplasty because the staples can be broken by consumption of large meals. Both of these procedures have short-term surgical risks and a long-term risk of nutrient deficiencies, particularly of vitamin B$_{12}$, folate, and iron.[53] To be successful, even such surgical procedures must be accompanied by behavior modification, diet programs, and exercise.

Another surgical approach, liposuction, is primarily a cosmetic procedure that will not significantly reduce overall body weight but may alter fat distribution. This procedure involves inserting a large hollow needle under the skin into a localized fat deposit and literally vacuuming out the fat. It is often advertised as a way to remove cellulite, which is just fat that has a lumpy appearance because of the presence of connections to the tissue layers below.

CRITICAL THINKING

Do You Think This Diet Will Work?

FAT-AWAY DIET MEAL PROGRAM:

A Fast, Sensible, Three-Step Approach to Weight Loss

Step 1: Replace breakfast and lunch with a scrumptious, nutrient-dense chocolate, vanilla, peach, or strawberry shake. Each shake provides 200 kcalories, 15 grams of protein, and 50% of the Daily Value for vitamins and minerals.

Step 2: For dinner, eat a well-balanced meal, limiting kcalories to 500, including 3 ounces of lean meat, 1 cup of nonfat milk, and 1/2 cup each of starchy foods, fruits, and vegetables.

Step 3: Before going to bed, take Fat-Away's unique nighttime complex of amino acids. They help convert fat into energy, curb cravings for carbohydrate, and control appetite and satisfy hunger during the day.

Following these easy steps should result in a weight loss of 3 to 5 pounds per week and costs only $39.95 for one week's supply. You should consult your physician before trying this or any other diet.

Does this diet meet all nutritional needs except energy?
▼

Probably. The combination of the nutritionally fortified shake and a variety of solid foods for one meal a day can provide a diet adequate in protein, vitamins, and minerals, although it is probably low in fiber and phytochemicals. Most diets providing fewer than 1200 kcalories do not meet micronutrient needs. This diet can because it includes the nutrient-fortified liquid meal.

Does the program provide a wide variety of obtainable foods with no special products to buy?
▼

No. Although variety is encouraged in the one 500-kcalorie meal, the dieter is required to purchase the powdered meal formula as well as an amino acid supplement at a cost of about $5.70 per day.

Does the plan offer a reasonable rate of weight loss?
▼

No. It promises a weight loss of 3 to 5 pounds per week. At this rate, muscle as well as fat will probably be lost.

Is the diet flexible enough to account for individual tastes, and is it adaptable to social settings?
▼

Possibly. This plan allows some flexibility because individuals are free to choose what they will eat for one meal a day. However, it is not flexible enough for occasions such as holidays when traditional foods are served at more than one meal.

Is the diet based on scientifically sound principles?
▼

Not entirely. Reducing energy intake below needs will result in weight loss, but there is little evidence that an amino acid supplement will help to curb appetite or convert fat into energy as you sleep.

Does this program include an exercise component?
▼

Answer:

Does the program promote changes in eating habits and lifestyle that will encourage achieving and maintaining a healthy weight?
▼

Answer:

• EATING DISORDERS

Eating disorders are a group of conditions that share a pathological concern with body weight and shape. According to mental health guidelines, there are three categories of eating disorders: **anorexia nervosa**, **bulimia nervosa**, and eating disorders not otherwise specified, which includes **binge-eating disorder** (Table 7.9).[54] At the mild end of this spectrum is the individual with binge-eating disorder who buys a box of donuts and cannot stop eating until they are gone. That person's weight may range from normal to obese. Individuals suffering from bulimia nervosa are more frequent binge eaters who are driven by compulsive behavior to consume extremely large amounts of high-kcalorie foods. They then experience depression and guilt and use behaviors such as self-induced vomiting to rid the body of the extra energy. At the far end of the spectrum are individuals with anorexia nervosa who use self-starvation and excessive exercise to reduce weight or prevent weight gain. If untreated, eating disorders can seriously affect health and even be fatal. In the United States, anorexia, bulimia, and binge-eating disorder affect about 5% of girls and women and 1% of boys and men.[55,56]

What Causes Eating Disorders?

In the search for the cause of eating disorders, sociocultural, psychological, and biological factors have been examined. Certain personality characteristics and psychological problems are common among individuals with eating disorders; the typical picture is an intelligent, adolescent female overachiever who feels ineffective and has low self-esteem.[57]

There is some evidence that biology may play a role. Much of the risk of developing anorexia and bulimia, as well as personality traits that predispose one to these

ON THE WEB

For more information on eating disorders, go to the National Eating Disorders Association at www.nationaleatingdisorders.org/, or to the National Institutes of Mental Health Web site at www.nimh.nih.gov/

Anorexia nervosa An eating disorder characterized by self-starvation, a distorted body image, and low body weight.

Bulimia nervosa An eating disorder characterized by the consumption of large amounts of food at one time (binge eating), followed by purging behavior such as vomiting and the use of laxatives to eliminate food from the body.

Binge-eating disorder An eating disorder characterized by recurrent episodes of binge eating in the absence of purging behavior.

Table 7.9 *Diagnostic Criteria for Eating Disorders*

Anorexia Nervosa

Refusal to maintain body weight at or above 85% of normal weight for age and height.

Intense fear of gaining weight or becoming fat, even though underweight.

Disturbance in the way body weight or shape is experienced or denial of the seriousness of the current low body weight.

Absence of at least three consecutive menstrual cycles without other known cause.

Bulimia Nervosa

Recurrent episodes of binge eating.

Recurrent inappropriate compensatory behavior to prevent weight gain, such as self-induced vomiting; misuse of laxatives, diuretics, enemas, or other medications; fasting; or excessive exercise.

Occurrence, on average, of binge eating and inappropriate compensatory behaviors at least twice a week for three months.

Undue influence by body shape and weight on self-evaluation.

Disturbance does not occur exclusively during episodes of anorexia nervosa.

Eating Disorders Not Otherwise Specified

Criteria for anorexia nervosa are met except the individual menstruates regularly.

Criteria for anorexia nervosa are met except that, despite substantial weight loss, the individual's current weight is in the normal range.

Criteria for bulimia nervosa are met except binges occur at a frequency of less than twice a week and for a duration of less than three months.

Inappropriate compensatory behavior after eating small amounts of food in individuals of normal body weight.

Regularly chewing and spitting out, without swallowing, large amounts of food.

Binge-Eating Disorder

Recurrent episodes of binge eating in the absence of the regular use of inappropriate compensatory behaviors characteristic of bulimia.

From American Psychiatric Association. *Diagnostic and Statistical Manual*, 4th ed. Washington, D.C.: American Psychiatric Association, 1994.

disorders, appears to be inherited.[58] Abnormalities in the levels of neurotransmitters such as serotonin and their metabolites and in levels of the hormone leptin have been hypothesized to contribute to the behaviors typical of anorexia and bulimia.[58]

Eating disorders most commonly begin in adolescence when physical, psychological, and social development is occurring rapidly. While they are more common in young women, males make up 5 to 10% of individuals with eating disorders; male athletes in weight-regulated activities like wrestling are at particular risk. Eating disorders are typically associated with Caucasians of higher socioeconomic class, but in reality they occur in all ethnic and socioeconomic groups.[56] They are as common among Hispanic as Caucasian females and are more frequent among Native Americans and less frequent among African and Asian American females.[59]

Eating disorders are more prevalent in groups concerned with weight and body image.[60] The incidence is very low in underdeveloped countries and increases in certain subcultures in developed countries, such as professional dancers and models. In North America, young women in particular are concerned with body image. Being thin is associated with beauty, success, intelligence, and vitality. Being plump, on the other hand, is associated with failure, stupidity, and clumsiness. What young woman would want to be plump? A young woman facing a future where she must be independent, have a prestigious job, maintain a successful love relationship, bear and nurture children, manage a household, and stay in fashion can become overwhelmed. Unable to master all these roles, she may look for some aspect of her life that she can control. Food intake and body weight are natural choices, since being thin brings the societal associations of success. Young women today often aspire to the adage that you can never be too rich or too thin.

Anorexia Nervosa

Anorexia nervosa is a life-threatening disorder. It is characterized by extreme weight loss due to behaviors such as self-starvation and excessive exercise, an overwhelming fear of gaining weight, and use of body weight and shape as a means of self-evaluation (see Table 7.9). Anorexia nervosa was originally described over a century ago. The name anorexia, which means lack of appetite, is a misnomer because it is a desire to be thin rather than a lack of appetite that causes individuals with this disorder to decrease their food intake (Figure 7.22). Anorexia nervosa affects 1% of female adolescents in the United States.[61] The average age of onset is 17. There is a 5% death rate in the first two years, and this can reach 20% in untreated individuals.[62]

Although anorexia is a psychological disorder, many of the problems associated with it are nutrition related. Individuals with anorexia may be unable to maintain a minimally healthy body weight; thus show dramatic weight loss, have a fear of gaining weight even when underweight, and display abnormal food consumption patterns. Disturbances in their perception of body size prevent anorexics from seeing themselves as underweight, so they continue to use diets, exercise, or **purging** to remain thin or lose more weight. They often develop a personal diet ritual, limiting certain foods and eating them in specific ways. Anorexics spend an enormous amount of time thinking about food, talking about food, and preparing food for others. Instead of eating, they move the food around the plate and cut it into tiny pieces. Those who use exercise to increase energy expenditure do not stop when they are tired; instead, they train compulsively beyond reasonable endurance. It is estimated that 50% of people with anorexia use purging as a means of weight control.[63]

Physiological State The first obvious physical symptom of anorexia is weight loss. As weight loss becomes severe, symptoms of starvation begin to appear. Starvation affects mental function, causing anorexics to become apathetic, dull, exhausted, and depressed. Physical symptoms include fat-store depletion; muscle wasting; inflammation and swelling of the lips; dry, peeling, flaking skin; abnormal hair growth on the body; and dry, thin, brittle hair on the head that may fall out. In females, estro-

Purging Behaviors such as self-induced vomiting and misuse of laxatives and diuretics to rid the body of energy.

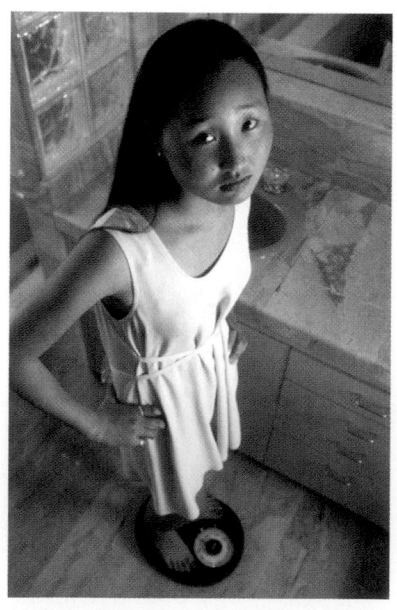

Figure 7.22
A person with anorexia nervosa carefully regulates what they eat to maintain a very low body weight. (David Young Wolff/PhotoEdit)

gen levels drop, and menstruation becomes irregular or stops. This affects sexual maturation and can have long-term effects on bone density. In males, testosterone levels decrease. In the final stages of starvation, there are abnormal electrolyte balance, dehydration, edema, cardiac abnormalities, absence of ketones due to fat-store depletion, and infection, which further increases nutritional needs.

Treatment of Anorexia Nervosa Early treatment of anorexia is important because starvation may cause irreversible damage. The goal of treatment is to help resolve psychological and behavioral problems while providing for nutritional rehabilitation. The goal of nutrition intervention is to promote weight gain by increasing energy intake and expanding dietary choices.[64] Nutritional rehabilitation in mild cases involves learning about nutrition and meal planning in order to develop healthy eating patterns. In more severe cases, anorexics are hospitalized, and their food intake and exercise behaviors are carefully controlled. Total parenteral nutrition (TPN) may be necessary to keep the individual alive. Some anorexics make full recoveries but about half have poor long-term outcomes—remaining irrationally concerned about weight gain and never achieving normal body weight.

Bulimia Nervosa

Bulimia nervosa is a disorder that involves frequent episodes of **binge eating** or **binging** that are almost always followed by purging and other inappropriate compensatory behaviors. A diagnosis of bulimia is based on the frequency with which episodes of binge eating and inappropriate compensatory behaviors occur (see Table 7.9). Bulimia is subdivided into nonpurging and purging types. Nonpurging bulimics use behaviors such as fasting or excessive exercise to prevent weight gain. Purging bulimics regularly engage in behaviors that may include self-induced vomiting and misuse of enemas, laxatives and diuretics, or other medications.

During a food binge, a bulimic experiences a sense of lack of control. While a normal teenager may consume 2000 to 3000 kcalories per day, a bulimic may consume over 3400 kcalories in under 2 hours, and some consume up to 20,000 kcalories in binges lasting as long as 8 hours.[65] A binge usually occurs in secrecy and stops only when pain, fatigue, or an interruption intervenes. Binging and purging are then followed by intense feelings of guilt and shame.

Bulimia was recognized as a separate eating disorder in the late 1970s. It currently occurs in 2 to 5% of the population.[56] Individuals suffering from bulimia are not necessarily underweight and may even be slightly overweight. Bulimia shares with anorexia a preoccupation with body weight and shape. As with anorexics, bulimics have a negative body image accompanied by a distorted perception of their body size. They are preoccupied with the fear that once they start eating they will not be able to stop (Figure 7.23).

Physiological State It is the purging of the binge-purge cycle that is most hazardous to health in bulimia nervosa. Purging by vomiting brings stomach acid into the mouth. Frequent vomiting affects the gastrointestinal tract by causing tooth decay, sores in the mouth and on the lips, swollen jaws and salivary glands, irritation of the throat, esophageal inflammation, and changes in stomach capacity and stomach emptying.[66] It also causes broken blood vessels in the face from the force of vomiting, electrolyte imbalance, dehydration, muscle weakness, and menstrual irregularities. Laxative and diuretic abuse can also cause dehydration and electrolyte imbalance. Rectal bleeding may occur from laxative overuse.

Treatment of Bulimia Nervosa The overall goal of therapy for people with bulimia nervosa is to separate eating from their emotions and from their perceptions of success and to promote eating in response to hunger and satiety. Psychological issues

Binge eating or bingeing The rapid consumption of a large amount of food in a discrete period of time associated with a feeling that eating is out of control.

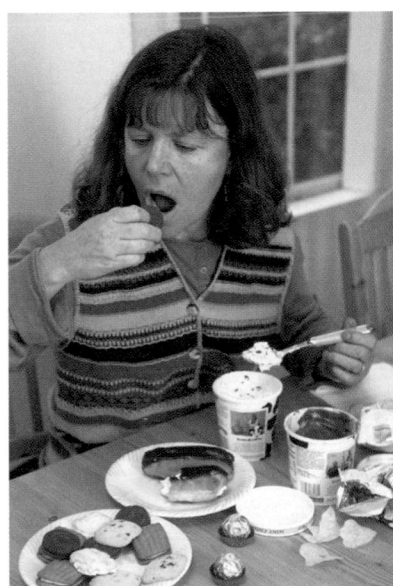

Figure 7.23
Bulimia is characterized by binge eating followed by purging. (David Young Wolff/ PhotoEdit)

related to body image and a sense of lack of control over eating must be resolved. Nutritional therapy must address physiological imbalances caused by purging episodes as well as provide education on nutrient needs and how to meet them. Antidepressant medications have also been shown to reduce the frequency of binge episodes. Treatment has been found to speed recovery, but for some women this disorder may remain a chronic problem throughout life.[67]

Other Eating Disorders

A third class of eating disorders, termed "eating disorders not otherwise specified or EDNOS," includes conditions such as weight loss that is less severe than the diagnostic criteria for anorexia (that is, 15% below desirable body weight) or binging and purging that is less frequent than the diagnostic criteria for bulimia.

Binge-Eating Disorder Individuals who suffer from binge-eating disorder engage in recurrent episodes of binge eating but do not regularly engage in purging behaviors such as vomiting, fasting, or excessive exercise. These individuals are likely to have above-normal body weights and may seek help for treatment of obesity rather than for their binge-eating behavior.[56] About one-quarter to one-third of individuals who attend weight-loss clinics meet the criteria for binge-eating disorder.[58]

Fad Bulimia Because of the desire of some to have their cake and eat it too, bulimia is "catching on." To those who are concerned about being 10 pounds heavier than they were when they started college, but who don't want to miss out on the food at social gatherings, bulimia may seem like the perfect solution. This type of bulimia, often termed *fad bulimia*, takes place among friends and is common among female college students, particularly sorority members.[68] It is also common among male athletes who participate in sports with competitive weight categories, such as body building and wrestling.

Despite the attractiveness of being able to eat all you want without gaining weight, purging rituals do not eliminate all the kcalories. Vomiting eliminates 70 to 80% of the ingested energy. The use of laxatives affects the colon, not the small intestine where food is absorbed, so water is lost but most of the energy is not. Diuretics also result in the loss of water, not energy.

The quantities of food consumed by fad bulimics are usually smaller than those in severe forms of bulimia, and the individuals engaged in these activities do not exhibit the serious emotional disturbances and shame about the bulimic practices that true bulimics do. Still, fad bulimia is dangerous. If an individual is predisposed to developing an eating disorder, this type of behavior may evolve into a more severe eating disorder. Even individuals not predisposed to an eating disorder may learn to use this behavior as a way of dealing with anxiety. The physical damage caused is the same in both fad bulimia and bulimia nervosa. (See Table 7.10 for information on how to help someone suspected of having an eating disorder.)

Table 7.10 *Eating Disorders: How to Help*

- Get the person to a doctor; the sooner the illness is treated, the more likely there will be a successful outcome.
- Talk to the family (parents, spouse).
- Explain your concerns and the potential hazards of the disease.
- Do not expect the person to cooperate; denial is common.
- If you work with the person, contact your employee assistance program.

Adapted from Lifescape.com, Toby Goldsmith, M.D. Department of Psychiatry, University of Florida Brain Institute. Available online at www.lifescape.com/.

• APPLICATIONS •

1. Use Figure 7.8 to determine if you are in the healthy weight range?
   a. Measure your waist circumference. Does it indicate a risk due to visceral fat storage?
   b. Even if you are not overweight, answer the following questions to see how many factors you have that may increase your risk of obesity-related complications if you become overweight.

   Do you have a personal family history of heart disease? _____

   Are you a male older than age 45? _____

   Are you a postmenopausal female? _____

   Do you smoke cigarettes? _____

   Do you have a sedentary lifestyle? _____

   Do you have high blood pressure? _____

   Do you have high LDL cholesterol, low HDL cholesterol, or high triglycerides? _____

   Do you have diabetes? _____

2. Using the three-day food record you kept in Chapter 2, calculate your average energy intake.

   a. Keep an activity log for several days. Use Tables 7.3 and 7.4 to determine your physical activity level and PA value. Calculate your EER. (See Table 7.2.)
   b. How does your EER compare with your energy intake?
   c. If you consumed and expended this amount of energy every day, would your weight increase, decrease, or stay the same?
   c. If intake does not equal EER, how much would you gain or lose in a month? (Assume that a pound of fat is equal to 3500 kcal.)
   e. If your energy intake does not equal your EER, list some specific changes you could make in your diet or the amount of activity you get to make the two balance.

3. Go to the grocery store and select five to ten products labeled "light," "reduced-calorie," "low-calorie," or "calorie-free." Record the number of kcalories and the amount of fat per serving.
   a. Would any of these products be useful for someone on a weight-loss diet?
   b. Can they be consumed in unlimited amounts without significantly increasing energy intake?
   c. Rate these foods in terms of their nutrient density.

SUMMARY

1. Energy is the ability to do work. It is measured in kcalories or kjoules. A kcalorie is the amount of heat needed to raise the temperature of 1 kilogram of water 1° Celsius.

2. The principle of energy balance states that if energy intake equals energy needs, body weight will remain constant.

3. Energy is provided to the body by protein and carbohydrate, which each provide 4 kcalories per gram, fat, which provides 9 kcalories per gram, and alcohol, which provides 7 kcalories per gram.

4. When energy in the diet does not meet needs, body energy stores are used. When excess energy is consumed, it is stored for later use. Fat is preferentially stored, while carbohydrate is used for energy and amino acids are used to meet protein needs.

5. In the adult body, energy is required for basal metabolism, activity, and the thermic effect of food. Basal energy expenditure is the largest component of energy output. It differs with body size, body composition, age, and gender. The energy needed for activity accounts for 15 to 30% of energy needs. The thermic effect of food (TEF) is equal to about 10% of energy consumed. The energy needs of healthy people can be predicted by calculating estimated energy requirements (EER).

6. Excess body fat increases the risk of chronic diseases such as diabetes, heart disease, high blood pressure, and certain types of cancer. Too little body fat is also unhealthy.

7. Body weight and fat can be measured in many ways. BMI is the currently accepted standard for assessing body fatness. It correlates better with body fat than does comparing weight for height. Techniques that measure body composition, including skinfold thickness, underwater weighing, isotope dilution techniques, and imaging, can be used to assess the amount and distribution of body fat.

8. Body fatness is regulated by internal mechanisms. Signals from the gastrointestinal (GI) tract, hormones, and circulating nutrients regulate short-term hunger and satiety. Signals such as the release of leptin from fat cells regulate long-term energy intake and expenditure.

9. Although what we weigh is greatly affected by genetics, environmental factors such as the availability of high kcalorie foods and labor saving devices, as well as personal choices concerning the amount and type of food consumed and activity level also affect energy balance.

10. More than half of adult Americans are overweight. Most people succeed in short-term weight loss but, in the long term, regain all the weight they have lost.

11. Weight management involves adjusting energy intake and expenditure and modifying long-term behaviors. To lose a pound of fat, expenditure must be increased or intake decreased by approximately 3500 kcalories. Slow, steady weight loss of 1/2 to 2 pound per week is more likely to be maintained than rapid weight loss.

12. There are thousands of programs and techniques for weight management. All involve a decrease in energy intake and/or an increase in energy expenditure. An ideal program involves a decrease in intake, an increase in expenditure, and behavior modification to reduce body weight and maintain the loss.

13. Drug therapy and surgery may be effective approaches to weight management in certain obese individuals. However, these methods do not foster development of long-term maintenance behaviors.

14. Eating disorders are psychological disorders in which the perception of body size is altered. Anorexia nervosa is characterized by self starvation and an abnormally low body weight. Bulimia nervosa is characterized by repeated cycles of binge eating followed by purging and other behaviors to prevent weight gain. Treatment involves supplying an adequate diet and psychological counseling to change body image and improve eating habits.

REVIEW QUESTIONS

1. What is energy balance?

2. What is a kcalorie?

3. Which nutrients provide energy?

4. List three components of energy expenditure.

5. What is basal metabolic rate?

6. What is EER and what factors are used in its calculation?

7. What health problems are associated with excess body fat?

8. What is the accepted standard for assessing body weight?

9. How does the distribution of body fat affect the risks of excess weight?

10. List some environmental factors that affect energy balance and discuss how these might interact with an individual's genetic predisposition to a particular weight.

11. Define what is meant by a healthy weight.

12. Describe three approaches to reducing energy intake.

13. What is the best approach to weight management? Why?

14. What are the characteristics of anorexia nervosa and bulimia nervosa?

15. How is nutrition involved in the treatment of eating disorders?

REFERENCES

1. Obesity and Overweight: A Public Health Epidemic, Centers for Disease Control and Prevention, Available Online at www.cdc.gov/nccdphp/dnpa/obesity/epidemic.htm/ Accessed March 20, 2002.

2. Statistics Related to Overweight and Obesity, National Institutes of Diabetes and Digestive and Kidney Diseases, Weight Control Information Network. Available online at www.niddk.nih.gov/health/nutrit/pubs/statobes.htm#cost/ Accessed April 1, 2002.

3. Sturm, R. The effects of obesity, smoking, and problem drinking on chronic medical problems and health care costs. *Health Affairs.* 21:245–253, 2002.

4. Hellerstein, M. K. De novo lipogenesis in humans: metabolic and regulatory aspects. *Eur. J. Clin. Nutr.* 53 (Suppl. 1):S53–S65, 2000.

5. Institute of Medicine, Food and Nutrition Board, *Dietary Reference Intakes for Energy, Carbohydrate, Fiber, Fat, Protein and Amino Acids.* Washington, D.C.: National Academy Press, 2002.

6. Wadden, T. A., Foster, G. D., Letizia, K. A., and Muller, J. L. Long-term effects of dieting on resting metabolic rate in obese patients. *JAMA* 264:707–711, 1990.

7. Horten, T. S., Drougas, H., Brachey, A., et al. Fat and carbohydrate overfeeding in humans: Different effects on energy storage. *Am. J. Clin. Nutr.* 62:19–29, 1995.

8. Schoeller, D. A. Recent advances from application of doubly-labeled water to measurement of human energy expenditure. *J. Nutr.* 129:1765–1768, 1999.

9. Williamson, D. F. Intentional weight loss: Patterns in the general population and its association with morbidity and mortality. *Int. J. Obes. Relat. Metab. Disord.* 21(Suppl.): S14–S19, 1997.

10. Bosello, O., Armellini, S., Zamboni, M., and Fitchet, M. The benefits of modest weight loss in type II diabetes. *Int. J. Obes. Relat. Metab. Disord.* 21(Suppl):S10–S13, 1997

11. Katzmarzyk, P. T., Craig, C. L., and Bouchard, C. Underweight, overweight and obesity: Relationships with mortality in the 13-year follow-up of the Canada Fitness Survey, *J. Clin. Epidemiol.* 54:916–920, 2001.

12. Arena, B., Maffulli, N., Maffulli, F., and Morleo, M. A. Reproductive hormones and menstrual changes with exercise in female athletes. *Sports Med.* 19:278–287, 1995.

13. Abernathy, R. P., and Black, D. R. Healthy body weights: an alternative perspective. *Am. J. Clin. Nutr.* 63(Suppl):448S–451S, 1996.

14. National Institutes of Health; National Heart, Lung, and Blood Institute. Clinical guidelines on the identification, evaluation, and treatment of overweight and obesity in adults. Executive summary, June 1998. Available online at www.nhlbi.nih.gov/guidelines/obesity/ob_home.htm/ Accessed Jan 5, 2001.

15. Bouchard, C., Tremblay, A., Després, J.-P., et al. The response to long term feeding in identical twins. *N. Engl. J. Med.* 322:1477–1482, 1990.

16. Conway, J. M. Ethnicity and energy stores. *Am. J. Clin. Nutr.* 62(Suppl): 1067S–1071S, 1995.

17. Albu, J., Allison, D., Boozer, C. N., et al. Obesity solutions: Report of a meeting. *Nutr. Rev.* 55:150–156, 1997.

18. Dietz, W. H. Periods of risk in childhood for the development of adult obesity—what do we need to learn? *J. Nutr.* 127:1884S–1886S, 1997.

19. Fields, D. A., Hunter, G. R., and Goran, M. I. Validation of the BOD POD with hydrostatic weighing: Influence of body clothing. *Int. J. Obes. Relat. Metab. Disord.* 24:200–205, 2000.

20. Plourde, G. The role of radiologic methods in assessing body composition and related metabolic parameters. *Nutr. Rev.* 55:289–296, 1997.

21. Leibel, R. L., Rosenbaum, M., and Hirsch, J. Changes in energy expenditure resulting from altered body weight. *N. Engl. J. Med.* 332: 622–628, 1995.

22. Peters, J. C., Kriketos, A. D., and Hill, J. O. Control of energy balance. In *Biochemical and Physiological Aspects of Human Nutrition.* Stipanuk, M. H., ed. Philadelphia: W. B. Saunders Company, 2000, 425–438.

23. Schwartz, M. W., Baskin, D. G., Kaiyala, K. J., and Woods, S. C. Model for the regulation of energy balance and adiposity by the central nervous system. *Am. J. Clin. Nutr.* 69:584–596, 1999.

24. Friedman, M. I. Control of energy intake by energy metabolism. *Am. J. Clin. Nutr.* 62(suppl):1096S–1100S, 1995.

25. Smith, G. P. Control of food intake. In *Modern Nutrition in Health and Disease*, 9th ed. Shils, M. E., Olson, J. A., Shike, M., and Ross, A. C., eds. Baltimore: Williams & Wilkins, 1999. 631–644.

26. Woods, S. C., Seeley, R. J., Porte, D., and Schwartz, M. W. Signals that regulate food intake and energy homeostasis. *Science* 280: 1378–1383, 1998.

27. Anderson, G. H. Regulation of food intake. In *Modern Nutrition in Health and Disease*, 8th ed. Shils, M. E., Olson, J. A., and Shike, M., eds. Philadelphia: Lea & Febiger, 1994. 524–536.

28. Friedman, J. M. The alphabet of weight control. *Nature* 385:119–120, 1997.

29. Bouchard, C. Genetics of human obesity: Recent results from linkage studies. *J. Nutr.* 127:1887S–1890S, 1997.

30. Tsigos, C., Kyrou, I., and Raptis, S. A. Monogenic forms of obesity and diabetes mellitus. *J. Pediatr. Endocrinol. Metab.* 15:241–253, 2002.

31. Friedman, J. M. Obesity in the new millennium. *Nature* 404:632–634, 2000.

32. Moore, L. L., Lombardi, D. A., White, M. J., et al. Influence of parents' physical activity levels on activity levels of young children. *J. Pediatr.* 118:215–219, 1991.

33. Hill, J. O., and Peters, J. C. Environmental contributions to the obesity epidemic. *Science* 280:1371–1374, 1998.

34. Norman, R. A., Thompson, D. B., Foroud, T., et al. Genomewide search for genes influencing percent body fat in Pima Indians: Suggestive linkage at chromosome 11q21-q22. *Am. J. Human Genet.* 60:166–173, 1997.

35. Esparza, J., Fox, C., Harper, I. T., et al. Daily energy expenditure in Mexican and USA Pima Indians: Low physical activity as a possible cause of obesity. *Int. J. Obes. Relat. Metab. Discord.* 24:55–59, 2000.

36. Tremblay, A., Després, J-P., Thriault, G., et al. Overfeeding and energy expenditure in humans. *Am. J. Clin. Nutr.* 56:857–862, 1992.

37. Diaz, E. O., Prentice, A. M., Goldberg, G. R., et al. Metabolic response to experimental overfeeding in lean and overweight healthy volunteers. *Am. J. Clin. Nutr.* 56:641–655, 1992.

38. Gura, T. Uncoupling proteins provide new clues to obesity's causes. *Science* 280:1369–1370, 1998.

39. Lisette, C. P., de Groot, G. M., and van Staveren, W. A. Reduced physical activity and its association with obesity. *Nutr. Rev.* 53:11–18, 1995.

40. Levine, J. A. , Eberhardt, N. L., and Jensen, M. D. Role of nonexercise activity thermogenesis in resistance to fat gain in humans. *Science* 283:212–214, 1999.

41. Robison, J. I., Hoeer, S. L., Petersmarck, K. A., and Anderson, J. V. Redefining success in obesity intervention: The new paradigm. *J. Am. Diet. Assoc.* 4:422–423, 1995.

42. U.S. Department of Agriculture, U.S. Department of Health and Human Services. *Nutrition and Your Health: Dietary Guidelines for Americans*, 5th ed. Home and Garden Bulletin No. 232. Hyattsville, Md.: U.S. Government Printing Office, 2000.

43. American Dietetic Association. Position of the American Dietetic Association: Weight management. *J. Am. Diet. Assoc.* 97:71–74, 1997.

44. Wilmore, J. H. Increasing physical activity: alterations in body mass and composition. *Am. J. Clin. Nutr.* 63(suppl):456S–460S, 1996.

45. National Center for Health Statistics. Prevalence of Overweight Among Children and Adolescents: United States, 1999. Available online at www.cdc.gov/nchs/products/pubd/hestats/overwght99.htm/ Accessed April 4, 2002.

46. Stevens, J., Cai, J., Pamuk, E. R., et al. The effect of age on the association between body mass index and mortality. *N. Engl. J. Med.* 338:1–7, 1998.

47. American Dietetic Association. Position of the American Dietetic Association: Very-low-calorie weight-loss diets. *J. Am. Diet. Assoc.* 94:722–726, 1990.

48. Horten, T. S., Drougas, H., Brachey, A., et al. Fat and carbohydrate overfeeding in humans: Different effects on energy storage. *Am. J. Clin. Nutr.* 62:19–29, 1995.

49. Frackelmann, K. Diet drug debacle: How two federally approved weight-loss drugs crashed. *Science News* 152:252–253, 1997.

50. Campfield, L. A., Smith, F. J., and Burn, P. Strategies and potential molecular targets for obesity treatment. *Science* 280:1383–1387, 1998.

51. Anderson, R. A. Effects of chromium on body composition and weight. *Nutr. Rev.* 56:266–270, 1998.

52. Kurtzweil, P. Dieter's brews make tea time a dangerous affair. *FDA Consumer* 31: July–August, 1997. Available online at www.fda.gov/fdac/features/1997/597_tea.html/ Accessed February 18, 2001.

53. Flancbaum, L., and Choban, P. S. Surgical implications of obesity. *Ann. Rev. Med.* 49:214–234, 1998.

54. American Psychiatric Association. *Diagnostic and Statistical Manual*, 4th ed. Washington, D.C.: American Psychiatric Association, 1994.

55. National Eating Disorders Association. Statistics: Eating disorders and their precursors. Available online at www.edap.org/edinfo/stats2.html/ Accessed April 2, 2002.

56. American Dietetic Association. Position of the American Dietetic Association. Nutrition intervention in the treatment of anorexia nervosa, bulimia nervosa, and eating disorder not otherwise specified (EDNOS). *J. Am. Diet. Assoc.* 101:810–819, 2001.

57. Leon, G. R., Keel, P. K., Klump, K. L., and Fulkerson, J. A. The future of risk factor research in understanding the etiology of eating disorders. *Psychopharmacol. Bull.* 33:405–411, 1997.

58. Walsh, B. T., and Devlin, M. J. Eating disorders: Progress and problems. *Science* 280:1387–1390, 1998.

59. Crago M., Shisslak, C. M., and Estes, L. S. Eating disturbances among American minority groups: A review. *Int. J. Eat. Disord.* 19:239–248, 1996.

60. Hsu, L. K. Epidemiology of the eating disorders. *Psychiatr. Clin. North Am.* 19:681–700, 1996.

61. ANRED. Anorexia Nervosa and Related Eating Disorders, Inc. Statistics: How Many People Have Eating Disorders? Available online at www.anred.com/stats.html/ Accessed April 2, 2002.

62. Foreyt, J. P., Poston, W. S. C., II, and Goodrick, G. K. Future directions in obesity and eating disorders. *Addict. Behav.* 21:767–778, 1996.

63. Medical Sciences Bulletin. Seratonin and eating disorders. Available online at www.pharminfo.com/pubs/msb/serotonin.html/ Accessed April 18, 2000.

64. Rock, C. L., and Curran-Celentano, J. Nutritional management of eating disorders. *Psychiatr. Clin. North Am.* 19:701–713, 1996.

65. Farley, D. Eating disorders require medical attention. *FDA Consumer* 26:27–29, March 1992.

66. Anderson, L., Shaw, J. M., and McCargar, L. Physiological effects of bulimia nervosa on the gastrointestinal tract. *Can. J. Gastroenterol.* 11:451–459, 1997.

67. Keel, P. K., and Mitchell, J. E. Outcome in bulimia nervosa. *Am. J. Psychiatry* 154:313–321, 1997.

68. Crandall, C. S. Societal contagion of binge eating. *J. Pers. Soc. Psychol.* 55:589–599, 1988.

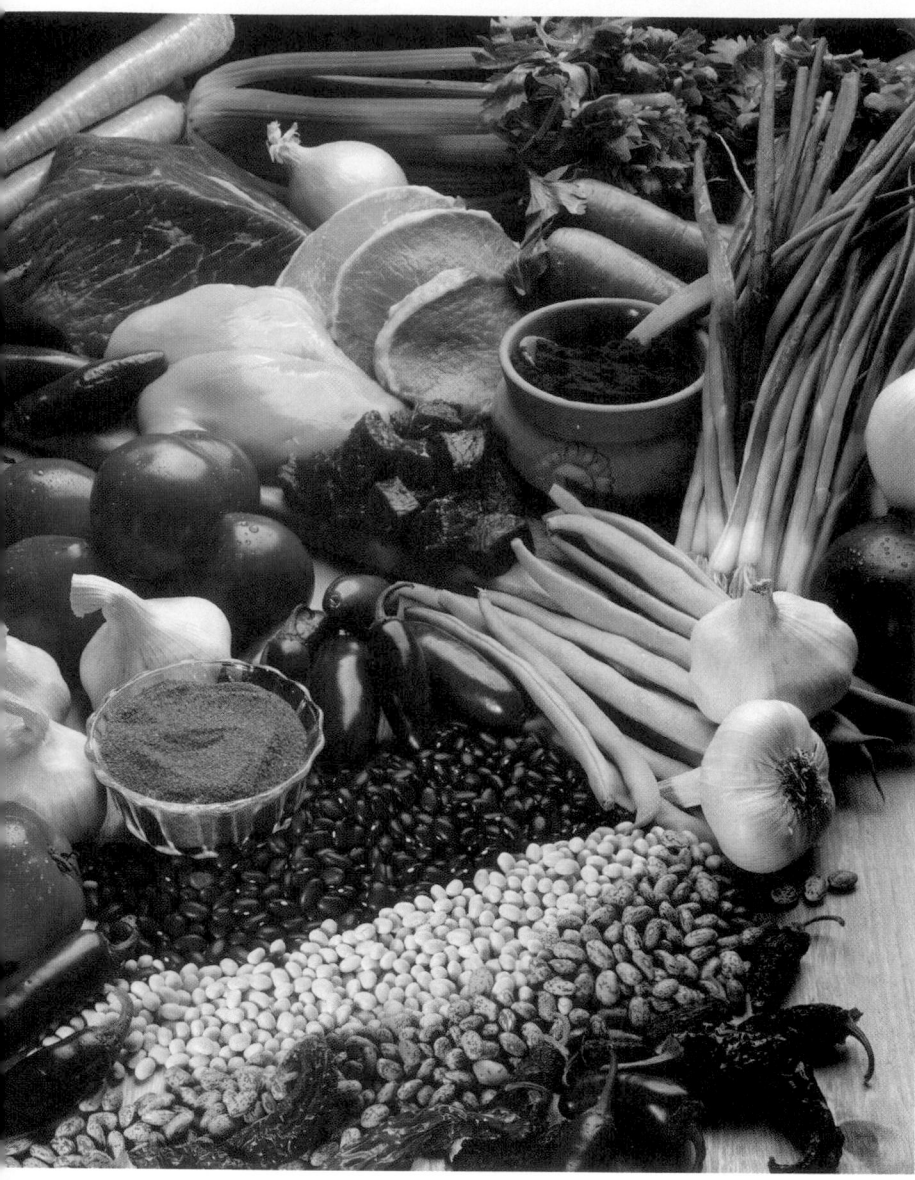

(© Gale Beery/Index Stock)

Chapter Concepts

✔ Vitamins are essential organic nutrients that provide no energy but that are needed in small amounts in the diet to allow for growth, reproduction, and the maintenance of health.

✔ Vitamins are found in almost all foods. The amount of a vitamin that is available to the body depends on how much of it is consumed, absorbed, transported, activated, stored, and excreted.

✔ For most individuals, a carefully planned diet can provide an adequate intake of vitamins.

✔ A lack of a vitamin results in deficiency symptoms, whereas excesses of some can be toxic.

✔ Thiamin, riboflavin, niacin, biotin, and pantothenic acid function as coenzymes in reactions that produce energy from carbohydrate, fat, and protein, as well as alcohol.

✔ Vitamin B₆ is a coenzyme essential for amino acid metabolism.

✔ Folate is a coenzyme that is needed for cell division.

✔ Vitamin B₁₂ is needed to maintain nerve cells and for the metabolism of folate and methionine.

✔ Vitamin C is an antioxidant and is needed for the synthesis of collagen, neurotransmitters, and hormones.

✔ Choline has not been defined as a vitamin but may be essential at some stages of life.

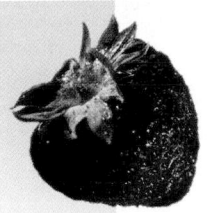

Just a Taste

Can vitamins give you extra energy?

Should everyone take folic acid supplements?

Does vitamin C cure the common cold?

Folic acid prevents birth defects! Vitamin E protects your heart! Vitamin A prevents cancer! The significance of vitamins in health promotion and disease prevention stimulates intrigue and excitement. A century ago, discoveries related to food, vitamins, and health were just as tantalizing. At that time, a number of diseases that seemed incurable, and that were often fatal, were cured by changes in diet. In 1885 it was discovered that beriberi, a disease that killed thousands of sailors in the Orient, could be prevented by adding meat and whole grains to the usual shipboard diet. In 1913, a fat-soluble factor that allowed animals to grow better was identified in butter, and in 1915, pellagra, a disease that filled psychiatric hospitals in the southern United States, was cured by adding meat to the diet. Discoveries such as these helped scientists connect specific diseases with dietary deficiencies. The existence of and need for vitamins were recognized because of the symptoms that occurred when they were absent. Even before the chemistry of these substances was determined, the civilized world was enchanted with the magic of vitamins. There was hope that incurable diseases could be remedied by simple dietary additions.

Today, the vitamin deficiency diseases of the early 20th century are rare in the United States, but interest in vitamins as factors that protect against chronic disease, slow aging, and enhance performance is thriving. A knowledge of what vitamins do and how much of each we need is necessary to evaluate the information that promotes vitamins as magic bullets.

• WHAT ARE VITAMINS?

Vitamins are organic compounds that are essential in the diet in small amounts to promote and regulate body functions necessary for growth, reproduction, and the maintenance of health. An organic compound is classified as a vitamin if a lack of the compound in the diet results in deficiency symptoms that are relieved by its addition to the diet. Although vitamins do not provide energy, many aid in the chemical reactions that produce energy from carbohydrate, fat, protein, and alcohol.

The term "vitamin" was coined in 1912 by Polish biochemist Casimir Funk, who originally used the word "vitamine" to refer to substances that are *amines* (compounds containing an amino group NH_2) and are vital to life (vital + amine). Today we know vitamins are vital to life, but they are not all amines, so the "e" has been dropped, and the term "vitamin" refers to all these substances. Initially, the vitamins were named alphabetically in approximately the order in which they were identified: A, B, C, D, and E. The B vitamins were first thought to be one chemical substance but were later found to be many different substances, so the alphabetical name was broken down by numbers. Vitamins B_6 and B_{12} are the only ones that are still commonly referred to by their numbers. Thiamin, riboflavin, and niacin were originally referred to as vitamin B_1, B_2, and B_3, respectively.

Vitamins have traditionally been grouped based on their solubility in water or fat. This chemical characteristic allows generalizations to be made about how they

Vitamins Organic compounds needed in the diet in small amounts to promote and regulate the chemical reactions and processes needed for growth, reproduction, and maintenance of health.

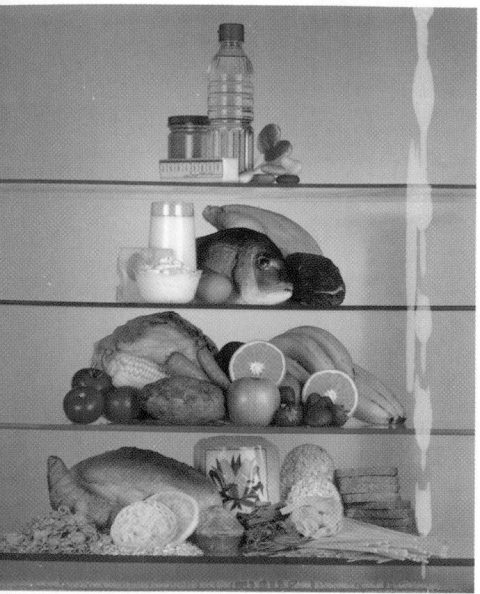

Figure 8.1
All the food groups contain choices that are good sources of vitamins. (© Topic Photo Agency)

Water-soluble vitamins Vitamins that dissolve in water.

Fat-soluble vitamins Vitamins that dissolve in fat.

Fortification A term used generally to describe the addition of nutrients to foods, such as the addition of vitamin D to milk.

Enrichment A term used to describe the addition of nutrients to a food in order to restore those lost in processing to a level equal to or higher than that originally present.

Bioavailability A general term that refers to how well a nutrient can be absorbed and used by the body.

are absorbed, transported, excreted, and stored in the body. The **water-soluble vit-amins** include the B vitamins and vitamin C. The **fat-soluble vitamins** include vita-mins A, D, E, and K (see Chapter 9.)

Vitamins in the Diet

Almost all foods contain some vitamins (Figure 8.1). Grains are good sources of thi-amin, niacin, riboflavin, pantothenic acid, and biotin. Meat and fish are good sources of all of the B vitamins. Milk provides riboflavin and vitamins A and D; leafy greens provide folate, vitamin A, vitamin E, and vitamin K; citrus fruit provides vitamin C; and vegetable oils are high in vitamin E.

The vitamin content of foods can be affected by cooking, storage, and process-ing. The vitamins naturally found in foods can be washed away during preparation or destroyed by cooking. Exposure to light and oxygen can also cause vitamin losses. Processing can both cause nutrient losses and add nutrients to food. The addition of nutrients to foods is called **fortification**. The added nutrients may or may not have been present in the original food. **Enrichment** is a type of fortification in which nu-trients are added for the purpose of restoring those lost in processing to the same or a higher level than originally present. The milling of whole grain wheat to make white flour results in the loss of the nutrients contained in the bran and germ. En-richment adds back the vitamins thiamin, niacin, and riboflavin and the mineral iron. Not all the nutrients lost in processing are restored by enrichment (Figure 8.2). Foods that are staples of the diet are often fortified to prevent vitamin or mineral de-ficiencies and promote health in the population (see Chapter 12). For example, milk is fortified with vitamin D to promote bone health, and grains are fortified with folic acid to reduce the incidence of birth defects. Some foods are fortified because they are used in place of other foods that are good sources of an essential nutrient. For example, margarine is fortified with vitamin A because it is often used instead of but-ter, which naturally contains vitamin A.

Supplements are another source of vitamins. While supplements provide spe-cific nutrients, they do not provide all the benefits of foods. A pill that meets vita-min needs does not provide the energy, protein, minerals, fiber, or phytochemicals that would have been supplied by food sources of these vitamins (Figure 8.3). Supplements are discussed with each nutrient and in greater depth in Chapter 12.

Vitamins in the Digestive Tract

About 40 to 90% of the vitamins in food are absorbed, primarily in the small intes-tine (Figure 8.4). The composition of the diet and conditions in the body, however, may influence **bioavailability**—the amount of a nutrient that can be absorbed and utilized by the body. The bioavailability of a specific nutrient may also be affected by other foods and nutrients in the diet. For example, the amount of fat in the diet af-

Figure 8.2
Many of the nutrients in whole grains are lost in refining, but only a few are added back in enrichment. This figure compares the amounts of some nutrients found in enriched and unenriched white flour with the amount in the whole wheat grain. The nutrients present in whole durum wheat are represented as 100%. Values for folate are included because enriched grains are also fortified with folic acid.

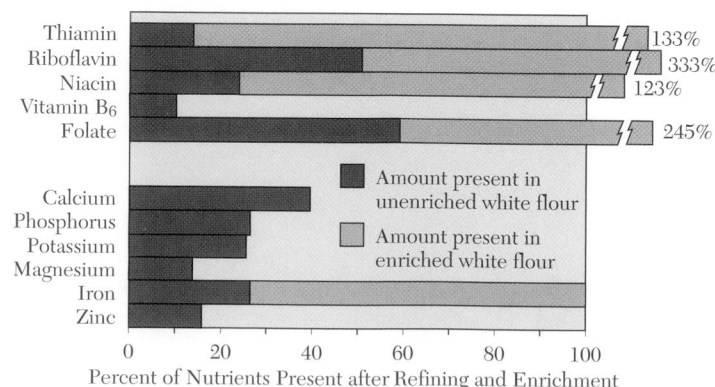

fects the bioavailability of fat-soluble vitamins because they are absorbed along with dietary fat. Fat-soluble vitamins are poorly absorbed when the diet is very low in fat. The mechanism by which vitamins are absorbed also determines the amount that enters the body. Fat-soluble vitamins are easily absorbed by simple diffusion. Many of the water-soluble vitamins depend on energy-requiring transport systems or binding molecules in the gastrointestinal tract in order to be absorbed. For example, thiamin and vitamin C are absorbed by energy-requiring transport systems, riboflavin and niacin require carrier proteins for absorption, and vitamin B_{12} must be bound to a protein produced in the stomach before it can be absorbed in the intestine.

Some vitamins are absorbed in inactive **provitamin** or **vitamin precursor** forms that must be converted into active vitamin forms once inside the body. How much of each provitamin can be converted into the active vitamin and the rate at which this occurs affect the amount of a vitamin available to function in the body.

Vitamins in the Body

Vitamins promote and regulate body functions. For instance, vitamin C is essential for the synthesis of neurotransmitters, hormones, and a protein vital to the structure of connective tissue. Vitamin E functions as an antioxidant, vitamin A is needed for vision and affects cell maturation by altering how genes are expressed, vitamin D affects bone health, and vitamin K is needed for blood clotting. The B vitamins act as **coenzymes**, which are organic nonprotein substances that bind to enzymes to promote their activity (Figure 8.5). As coenzymes, B vitamins are essential to the proper functioning of numerous enzymes involved in the metabolism of the energy-yielding nutrients.

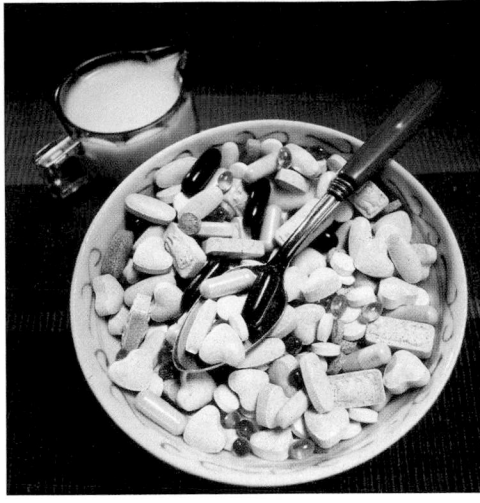

Figure 8.3
Vitamin supplements cannot take the place of a balanced diet. (Charles D. Winters)

Provitamin or **vitamin precursor** A compound that can be converted into the active form of a vitamin in the body.

Coenzymes Small nonprotein organic molecules that act as carriers of electrons or atoms in metabolic reactions and are necessary for the proper functioning of many enzymes.

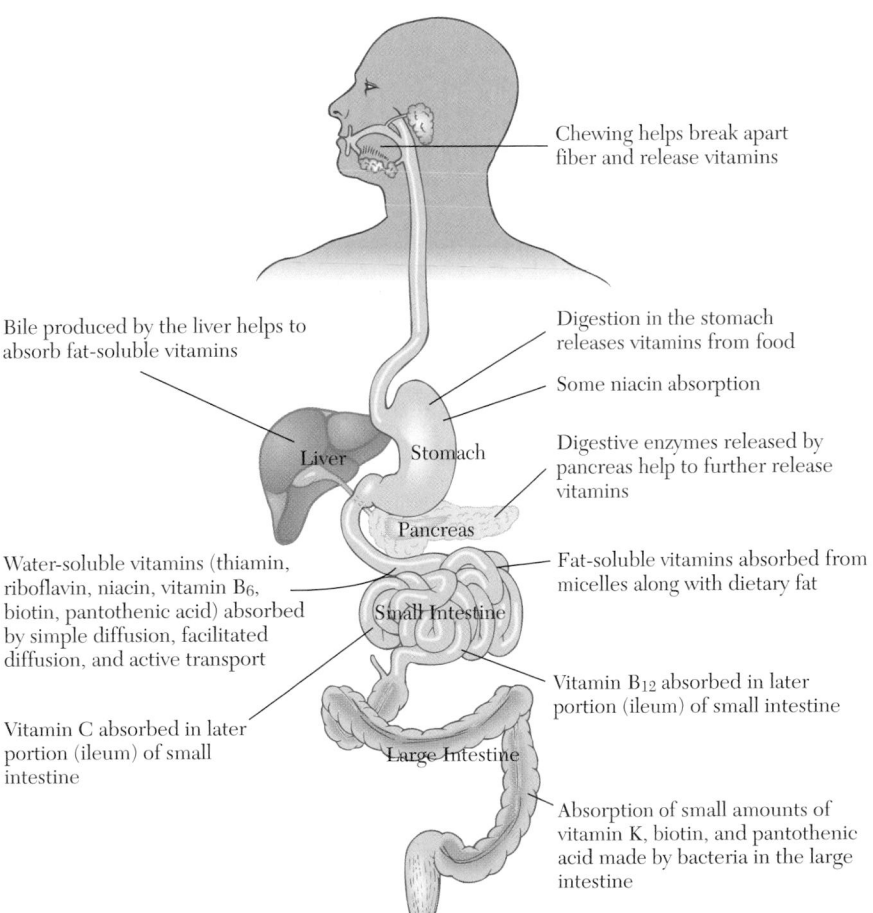

Chewing helps break apart fiber and release vitamins

Digestion in the stomach releases vitamins from food

Some niacin absorption

Digestive enzymes released by pancreas help to further release vitamins

Bile produced by the liver helps to absorb fat-soluble vitamins

Liver

Stomach

Pancreas

Fat-soluble vitamins absorbed from micelles along with dietary fat

Water-soluble vitamins (thiamin, riboflavin, niacin, vitamin B_6, biotin, pantothenic acid) absorbed by simple diffusion, facilitated diffusion, and active transport

Small Intestine

Vitamin B_{12} absorbed in later portion (ileum) of small intestine

Vitamin C absorbed in later portion (ileum) of small intestine

Large Intestine

Absorption of small amounts of vitamin K, biotin, and pantothenic acid made by bacteria in the large intestine

Figure 8.4
An overview of vitamins in the digestive tract.

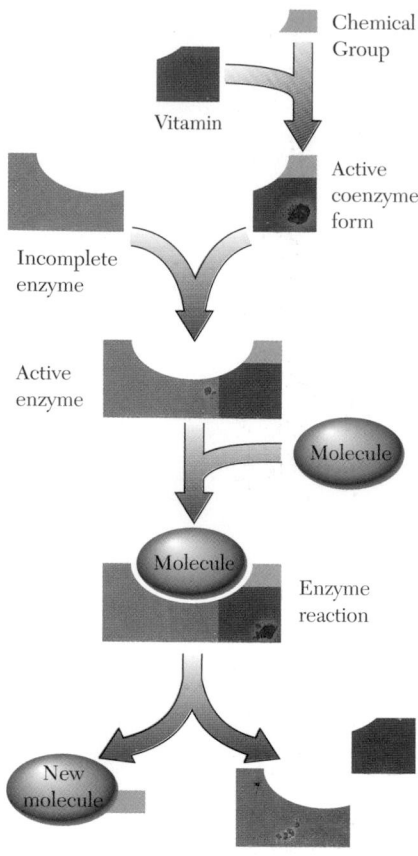

Figure 8.5

The B vitamins serve as coenzymes. The active coenzyme form of the vitamin is necessary for enzyme activity and acts as a carrier of chemical groups or electrons in the reaction.

Delivering Vitamins to Cells Once absorbed into the blood, vitamins must be transported to the cells. Despite their solubility in water, most of the water-soluble vitamins are bound to blood proteins for transport. Fat-soluble vitamins must be incorporated into lipoproteins or bound to transport proteins in order to be transported in the aqueous environment of the blood. For example, vitamins A, D, E, and K are all incorporated into chylomicrons for transport from the intestine. Vitamin A is stored in the liver, but it must be bound to a specific transport protein to be transported in the blood to other tissues; therefore, the amount delivered to the tissues depends on the availability of the transport protein.

Excretion of the Vitamins The ability to store and excrete vitamins helps to regulate the amount present in the body. With the exception of vitamin B_{12}, the water-soluble vitamins are easily excreted from the body in the urine. Because they are not stored to any great extent, supplies of water-soluble vitamins are rapidly depleted and they must be consumed regularly in the diet. Nevertheless, it takes more than a few days to develop deficiency symptoms, even when these vitamins are completely eliminated from the diet. Fat-soluble vitamins, on the other hand, are stored in the liver and fatty tissues and cannot be excreted in the urine. In general, because they are stored to a larger extent, it takes longer to develop a deficiency of fat-soluble vitamins when they are no longer provided by the diet.

How Much of Each Vitamin Do We Need?

Recommendations for vitamin intake for healthy populations in the United States and Canada are made by the Dietary Reference Intakes (DRI) (see Chapter 2). Before a recommendation (Estimated Average Requirement (EAR) and Recommended Dietary Allowance (RDA) or an Adequate Intake (AI)) can be established, specific criteria upon which to base the adequacy of the nutrient are selected. These may include any parameter related to health and nutrient function, such as the amount of a nutrient or metabolite excreted in the urine, the level of a nutrient in the blood, or the activity of an enzyme dependent on that nutrient. The role of the nutrient in reducing disease risk is also taken into account. For example, the amount of a vitamin considered adequate may be defined as the amount that maintains normal blood levels and provides protection from a chronic condition such as cardiovascular disease. The requirements of each life stage and gender are considered separately.

EARs are developed using the criteria of adequacy and information about the vitamins' bioavailability. The EAR value is an estimate of the average requirement for the population. The RDA is a goal for intake of individuals set to meet the needs of 97 to 98% of the healthy population. If sufficient information is not available to determine an EAR, an AI is set based on observed or experimentally determined estimates of the average intake in the healthy population. Therefore, for each vitamin and life stage, the DRIs include either an RDA value, when sufficient information is available, or an AI, when a recommendation is estimated from population data. Either of these values can be used as a goal for dietary intake by individuals. The DRIs also establish Tolerable Upper Intake Levels (ULs) as a guide to the maximum amount of a vitamin that is unlikely to cause adverse health effects (see Appendix G).

Vitamins and Health

Even though the last of the 13 compounds recognized as vitamins today was characterized in 1948, vitamin deficiencies remain a major public health problem in many parts of the world. Thousands of children in developing nations go blind due to vitamin A deficiency and have malformed bones from vitamin D deficiency. In industrialized countries, a more varied food supply, along with the fortification and enrichment of foods, has almost eliminated vitamin deficiency diseases in the majority of the population. Concern in these countries now focuses on meeting the needs of high-risk groups such as children and pregnant women, evaluating the effects of marginal deficiencies such as the effect of low B vitamin intake on heart disease risk, and assessing the risk of consuming toxic amounts from fortified foods and supplements.

• THE B VITAMINS AND ENERGY METABOLISM

Thiamin, riboflavin, niacin, pantothenic acid, and biotin all serve as coenzymes for reactions that release energy from carbohydrate, fat, and protein as well as alcohol (Figure 8.6). They are grouped together in this section because of this common role.

Thiamin

More than 4000 years ago, affluent members of Far Eastern societies began the practice of removing the outer hulls of rice to produce white or "polished" rice. As polished rice became the staple of the diet, the prevalence of the disease **beriberi** increased. A connection between diet and beriberi was not made until the late 19th century, when a surgeon in the Japanese navy demonstrated that shipboard beriberi could be prevented by the addition of sources of thiamin such as meat and whole grains to the diet.

Beriberi The disease resulting from a deficiency of thiamin.

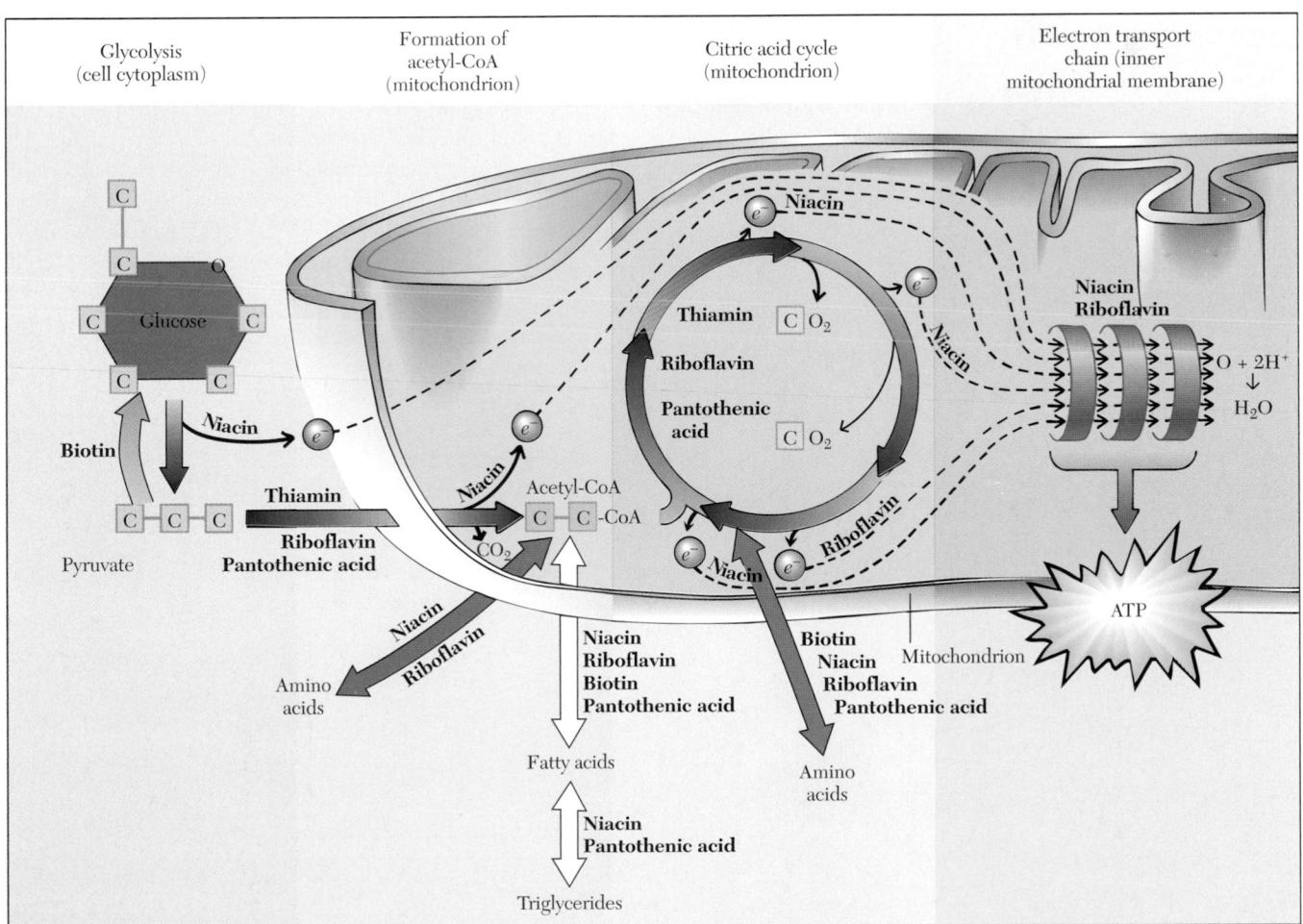

Figure 8.6

These are examples of metabolic reactions that require the vitamins thiamin, riboflavin, niacin, biotin, or pantothenic acid as coenzymes. These reactions are particularly important for the production of energy from carbohydrate, fat, and protein.

Thiamin in the Diet Thiamin is widely distributed in foods (Figure 8.7). A large proportion of the thiamin consumed in the United States comes from enriched grains used in foods such as breakfast cereals and baked goods. Pork, whole grains, legumes, nuts, seeds, and organ meats (liver, kidney, heart) are also good sources.

Thiamin in foods may be destroyed during cooking or storage because it is sensitive to heat, oxygen, and low-acid conditions. Thiamin availability is also affected by the presence of antithiamin factors that destroy the vitamin. For instance, there are enzymes in raw shellfish and freshwater fish that degrade thiamin during food storage and preparation and during passage through the gastrointestinal tract. These enzymes are destroyed by cooking so they are only a concern in foods consumed raw. Other antithiamin factors that are not inactivated by cooking are found in tea, coffee, betel nuts, blueberries, and red cabbage. Because these make thiamin unavailable to the body, habitual consumption of foods containing antithiamin factors increases the risk of thiamin deficiency.[1]

Thiamin in the Body Thiamin does not provide energy, but it is important in the energy-producing reactions in the body. The active form, thiamin pyrophosphate, is a coenzyme in reactions in which carbon dioxide is lost from larger molecules. For instance, the reaction that forms acetyl-CoA from pyruvate and one of the reactions of the citric acid cycle require thiamin pyrophosphate (see Figure 8.6). Thiamin is therefore essential to the production of energy from glucose.

Thiamin is also needed for the metabolism of other sugars and certain amino acids; the synthesis of the neurotransmitter acetylcholine; and the production of the sugar ribose, which is needed to synthesize RNA (ribonucleic acid).

How Much Thiamin Do We Need? The RDA for thiamin for adult men age 19 and older is set at 1.2 mg per day and for adult women 19 and older, at 1.1 mg per day. The RDA is based on the amount of thiamin needed to achieve and maintain normal activity of a thiamin-dependent enzyme found in red blood cells and normal urinary thiamin excretion.[2] For an average adult, half of the RDA can be obtained from 4 ounces of pork or one-quarter cup of shelled sunflower seeds.

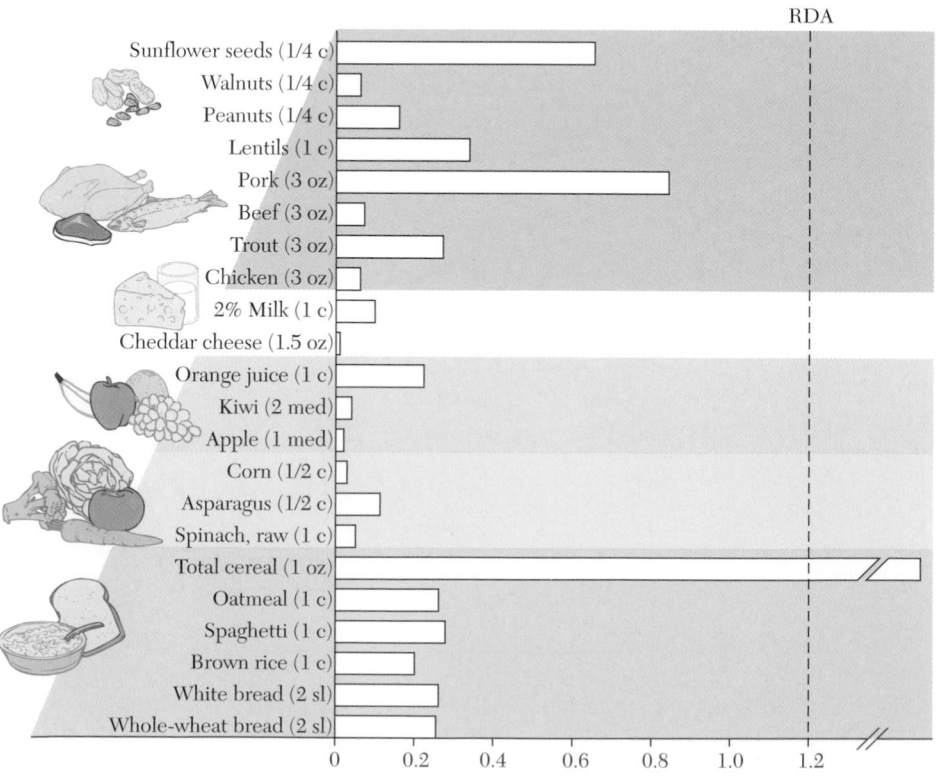

Figure 8.7

Thiamin content of selections from each group of the Food Guide Pyramid. The dashed line represents the RDA for adult men. Pork is a better source of thiamin than other meats. Whole and fortified grains are also good sources.

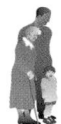

The requirement for thiamin is increased during pregnancy to accommodate the needs of growth and energy utilization, and during lactation to meet the need for both increased energy for milk production and to replace the thiamin secreted in milk. There is not enough information to establish an RDA for infants, so an AI has been set based on the thiamin intake of infants fed human milk.

Thiamin Deficiency Thiamin deficiency results in the disease beriberi. In Sri Lanka, the word "beriberi" literally means "I cannot," describing the extreme weakness and lassitude that occurs with this disease and reflecting the importance of this vitamin in energy metabolism.

Beriberi affects the nervous and cardiovascular systems. Some, but not all, of these symptoms can be explained by the roles of thiamin in glucose metabolism and in the synthesis of the neurotransmitter acetylcholine. The earliest symptoms, depression and weakness, which occur after only about ten days on a thiamin-free diet, are probably related to the inability to completely use glucose. Since brain and nerve tissue rely on glucose for energy, the inability to form acetyl-CoA rapidly affects nervous system activity. Poor coordination, tingling in the arms and legs, and paralysis may also be caused by the lack of acetylcholine. It is not clear why thiamin deficiency causes cardiovascular symptoms such as heart failure.

Overt beriberi is rare in North America today, but thiamin deficiency does occur in alcoholics. They are particularly vulnerable because thiamin absorption is decreased due to the effect of alcohol on the gastrointestinal tract. In addition, the liver damage that occurs with chronic alcohol consumption reduces conversion of thiamin to active coenzyme forms; thiamin intake also may be low due to a diet high in alcohol and low in nutrient-dense foods.[1] Thiamin-deficient alcoholics may develop a neurological condition known as the Wernicke-Korsakoff syndrome. It is characterized by mental confusion, psychosis, memory disturbances, and coma.

Thiamin Toxicity Since no toxicity has been reported when excess thiamin is consumed from either food or supplements, not enough information is available to establish a UL for thiamin intake.[2] This does not mean that high intakes are necessarily safe. Intakes of thiamin above the RDA have not been shown to provide health benefits.

Thiamin Supplements Thiamin supplements containing up to 50 mg per day are widely available and are marketed with the promise that they will provide "more energy." Although thiamin is needed to produce energy, it does not stimulate energy production. Unless thiamin is deficient, increasing thiamin intake does not increase the ability to produce energy. Because thiamin deficiency causes mental confusion and damages the heart, supplements often promise to improve mental function and prevent heart disease. However, in the absence of a deficiency, supplements do not have these effects.

A summary of the sources, recommended intakes, functions, deficiencies, and toxicities of thiamin and other water-soluble vitamins is provided in Table 8.1.

Riboflavin

While searching for a cure for beriberi, scientists also isolated riboflavin and several other B vitamins as well as thiamin. This occurred because the extracts they made from vegetables and grains could be separated into two components: One contained thiamin, the antiberiberi factor they sought, and cured beriberi; the other was a mix of B vitamins that was later determined to contain riboflavin along with vitamin B_6, niacin, and pantothenic acid.

Riboflavin in the Diet Milk is the best source of riboflavin in the North American diet. Other major sources include liver, red meat, poultry, fish, and whole grains and enriched breads and cereals. Vegetable sources include asparagus, broccoli, mushrooms, and leafy green vegetables such as spinach (Figure 8.8). Because riboflavin is

Table 8.1 *A Summary of the Water-Soluble Vitamins and Choline*

Vitamin	Sources	Recommended Intake for Adults	Major Functions	Deficiency Diseases and Symptoms	Groups at Risk	Toxicity	Tolerable Upper Intake Levels (UL)
Thiamin (vitamin B$_1$, thiamin mononitrate)	Pork, sunflower seeds, whole and enriched grains, legumes	1.1–1.2 mg	Coenzyme in acetyl-CoA formation, citric acid cycle; nerve function	Beriberi: nerve tingling, poor coordination, weakness, heart changes	Alcoholics, those in poverty	None reported	ND
Riboflavin (vitamin B$_2$)	Milk, leafy greens, enriched grains	1.1–1.3 mg	Coenzyme in citric acid cycle, fat metabolism, electron transport chain	Inflammation of mouth and tongue	None	None reported	ND
Niacin (nicotinamide, nicotinic acid)	Enriched grains, peanuts, tuna, chicken, beef	14–16 mg NE	Coenzyme in glycolysis, electron transport chain, fat metabolism	Pellagra: dermatitis, diarrhea, dementia	Those consuming a limited diet high in corn products, alcoholics	Flushing, nausea, rash, tingling extremities	35 mg/d†
Biotin	Liver, egg yolks, synthesized in the gut	30 µg°	Coenzyme in glucose production and fat synthesis	Dermatitis, nausea, depression, hallucinations	Those consuming large amounts of raw egg whites	Unknown	ND
Pantothenic acid (calcium pantothenate)	Meat, whole grains, legumes	5 mg°	Coenzyme in citric acid cycle, fat metabolism	Fatigue, rash	Alcoholics	Diarrhea, water retention	ND
Vitamin B$_6$ (pyridoxine, pyridoxine HCl, pyridoxal phosphate, pyridoxamine)	Meat, legumes, seeds, leafy greens, whole grains	1.3–1.7 mg	Coenzyme in protein metabolism, neurotransmitter and hemoglobin synthesis	Headache, neurologic symptoms, nausea, poor growth, anemia	Women, alcoholics	Nerve destruction	100 mg/d
Folate (folic acid, folacin)	Leafy greens, organ meats, legumes, orange juice	400 µg DFE	Coenzyme in DNA synthesis and amino acid metabolism	Macrocytic anemia, inflammation of tongue, diarrhea, poor growth, neural tube defects	Pregnant women, alcoholics	Masks B$_{12}$ deficiency	1000 µg/d†
Vitamin B$_{12}$ (cobalamin, cyanocobalamin)	Animal products	2.4 µg	Coenzyme in folate metabolism; nerve function	Pernicious anemia, macrocytic anemia, poor nerve function	Vegans, elderly, those with stomach or intestinal disease	None reported	ND
Vitamin C (ascorbic acid, ascorbate)	Citrus fruit, broccoli, strawberries, greens	75–90 mg	Collagen synthesis, hormone and neurotransmitter synthesis, antioxidant	Scurvy: poor wound healing, bleeding gums	Alcoholics, elderly men	GI distress, diarrhea	2000 mg
Choline	Egg yolks, organ meats, leafy greens, nuts	425–550 mg°	Synthesis of cell membranes and the neurotransmitter acetylcholine	Liver dysfunction	None	Sweating, reduced growth, low blood pressure, liver damage	3500 mg/d

°Adequate Intake (AI).

†UL considers amounts from fortified foods and supplements.

ND—insufficient data to determine a UL.

destroyed by exposure to light, poor handling decreases a food's riboflavin content. This is a problem when milk is stored in clear containers and exposed to light. Cloudy plastic milk bottles block some light, partially protecting the riboflavin, but cardboard milk containers are better at preventing losses.[3]

Riboflavin in the Body Riboflavin forms the active coenzymes flavin mononucleotide (FMN) and flavin adenine dinucleotide (FAD). FAD functions in the citric acid cycle and is important for the breakdown of fatty acids. Both FMN and FAD function as electron carriers in the electron transport chain (see Figure 8.6). Therefore, adequate riboflavin is crucial in producing energy from carbohydrate, fat, and protein. Riboflavin

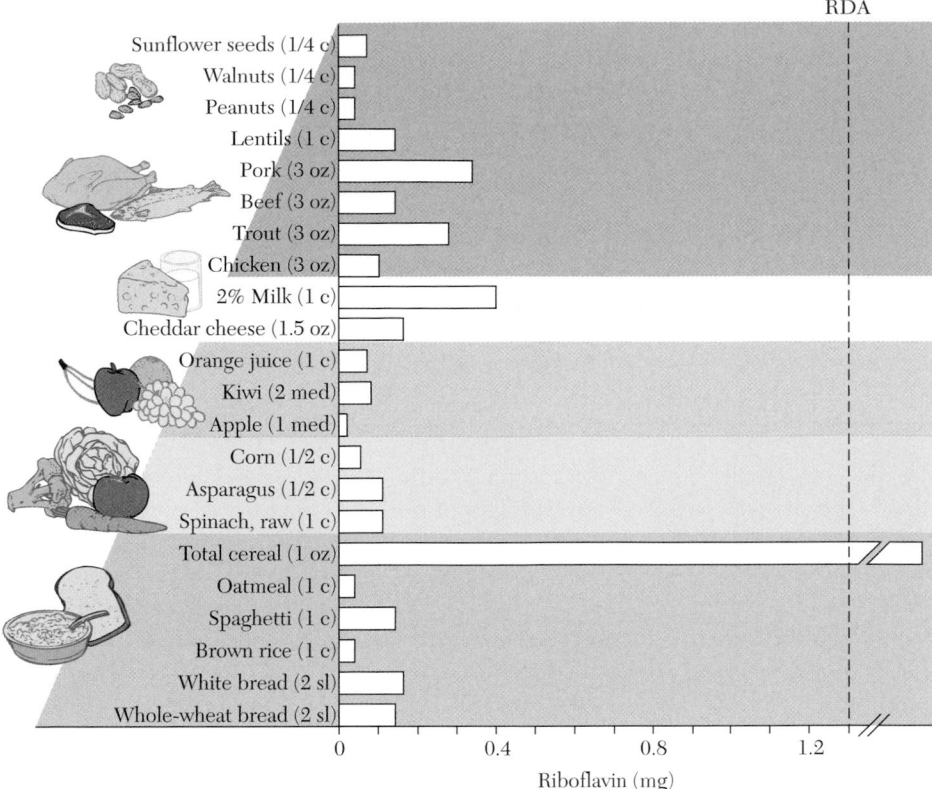

RDA

Figure 8.8
Riboflavin content of selections from each group of the Food Guide Pyramid. The dashed line represents the RDA for adult men. Milk and fortified cereals are exceptionally good sources of riboflavin.

is also involved directly or indirectly in converting a number of other vitamins, including folate, niacin, vitamin B_6, and vitamin K, into their active forms.

How Much Riboflavin Do We Need? The RDA for riboflavin for adult men age 19 and older is 1.3 mg per day and for adult women 19 and older, 1.1 mg per day. This recommendation is based on the amount of riboflavin needed to maintain normal activity of a riboflavin-dependent enzyme in red blood cells and normal riboflavin excretion in the urine.[2] Two cups of milk provide about half the amount of riboflavin recommended for a typical adult. The recommended intake can be met without milk if the daily diet includes two to three servings of meat and four to five servings of enriched grain products and high-riboflavin vegetables, such as spinach.

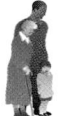

Additional riboflavin is recommended during pregnancy to support growth and increased energy utilization, and during lactation to allow for the riboflavin secreted in milk. There is not enough information to establish an RDA for infants, so an AI has been set based on the amount of riboflavin consumed by infants fed human milk.

Riboflavin Deficiency When riboflavin is deficient, injuries heal poorly because new cells cannot grow to replace the damaged ones. Tissues that grow most rapidly, such as the skin and the linings of the eyes, mouth, and tongue, are the first to be affected by a deficiency. Symptoms of riboflavin deficiency, called **ariboflavinosis**, include inflammation of the eyes, lips, mouth, and tongue; scaly, greasy skin eruptions; cracking of the tissue at the corners of the mouth; and confusion. Deficiency symptoms may develop after approximately two months on a riboflavin-poor diet.

A deficiency of riboflavin is rarely seen alone. It usually occurs in conjunction with deficiencies of other B vitamins. One reason is that the food sources of B vitamins are similar (see Table 8.1). Therefore, a deficiency due to poor diet will likely lead to multiple vitamin deficiencies. Because riboflavin is needed to convert other vitamins into their active forms, some of the symptoms seen with riboflavin deficiency are actually due to deficiencies of these other nutrients.

Ariboflavinosis The condition resulting from a deficiency of riboflavin.

Riboflavin Toxicity No adverse effects have been reported from overconsumption of riboflavin from foods or supplements, and there are not sufficient data to establish a UL for this vitamin. Large doses of riboflavin are not well absorbed, and it is readily excreted in the urine. A harmless side effect of high riboflavin intakes, such as may be obtained from over-the-counter supplements, is bright yellow urine.

Riboflavin Supplements As with thiamin, the role of riboflavin in energy production has led to claims that supplements containing riboflavin will provide an energy boost. Although riboflavin is needed for energy production, it does not provide energy. Since a deficiency causes skin and eye symptoms, riboflavin has also been suggested as a cure for eye diseases and skin disorders. However, in the absence of a deficiency, supplementation does not affect the eyes or skin.

Niacin

Pellagra The disease resulting from a deficiency of niacin.

In the early 1900s, psychiatric hospitals in the southeastern United States were filled with patients in the advanced stages of **pellagra**, the disease resulting from a deficiency of niacin. These individuals were institutionalized with dementia, a late symptom of pellagra, which led to a diagnosis of mental illness. In response to the pellagra epidemic, in 1909 the U.S. Public Health Service sent Dr. Joseph Goldberger to investigate. Goldberger believed that pellagra was due to a nutritional deficiency. To prove this, he conducted a study in which 12 convicts, promised pardons for their cooperation, were fed diets suspected of causing pellagra; 6 developed the disease. Proof that pellagra was not an infectious disease was provided by Goldberger and his coworkers, who tried to infect themselves with pellagra by ingesting blood, nasal secretions, feces, and urine from patients with the disease. None of them contracted pellagra. Goldberger was able to prevent and cure pellagra by improving the diets of patients in mental institutions. Nevertheless, pellagra remained a common problem among the southern poor who consumed a diet of primarily corn meal, molasses, and fatback or salt pork—all poor sources of niacin. A federally sponsored program was begun in 1941 to enrich grains, including corn meal, with niacin, thiamin, and riboflavin. This helped eliminate the pellagra epidemic in the United States.[4]

Niacin in the Diet Meat and fish are good sources of niacin (Figure 8.9). Other sources include legumes, mushrooms, wheat bran, asparagus, and peanuts. Niacin added to enriched flours and baked goods provides much of the usable niacin in the North American diet. Niacin can also be synthesized in the body from the essential amino acid tryptophan. In a diet that contains high-protein foods such as milk and eggs, which are poor sources of niacin but good sources of tryptophan, much of the need for niacin can be met by tryptophan. Tryptophan, however, is only used to make niacin if enough is available to first meet the needs of protein synthesis. When the diet is low in tryptophan, it is not used to synthesize niacin. Food composition tables and databases list only preformed niacin in a food, not the amount of niacin that can be made from tryptophan contained within the food.

Historically, the appearance of niacin deficiency has been associated with a predominantly corn diet. This has been attributed to the low-tryptophan content of corn and the fact that the niacin found naturally in corn (and to a lesser extent in other cereal grains) is bound to other molecules and therefore not well absorbed. The treatment of corn with lime water (water and calcium hydroxide), as is done in Mexico and Central America during the making of tortillas, enhances the availability of niacin (Figure 8.10). As a result, populations that consume corn treated with lime water rarely suffer from pellagra. Today, pellagra remains common in India and parts of China and Africa. Efforts to eradicate this deficiency include the development of new varieties of corn that provide more available niacin and more tryptophan than traditional varieties.

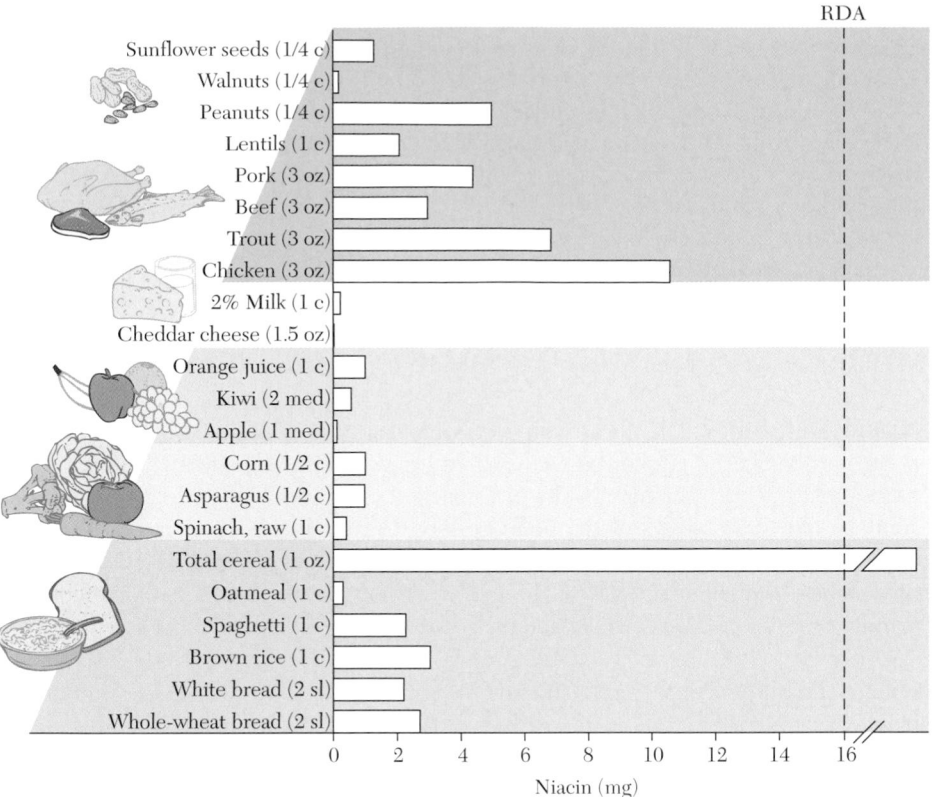

Figure 8.9
Niacin content of selections from each group of the Food Guide Pyramid. The dashed line represents the RDA for adult men. Meat, legumes, and whole and fortified grains are good sources of the vitamin.

Niacin in the Body Niacin is important in the production of energy from the energy-yielding nutrients as well as in reactions that synthesize other molecules. There are two forms of niacin: nicotinic acid and nicotinamide. Either form can be used by the body to make the two active coenzymes nicotinamide adenine dinucleotide (NAD) and nicotinamide adenine dinucleotide phosphate (NADP). NAD functions in glycolysis and the citric acid cycle, accepting released electrons and passing them on to the electron transport chain where ATP is formed (see Figure 8.6). NADP acts as an electron carrier in reactions that synthesize fatty acids and cholesterol. The need for niacin is so widespread in metabolism that a deficiency causes major changes throughout the body.

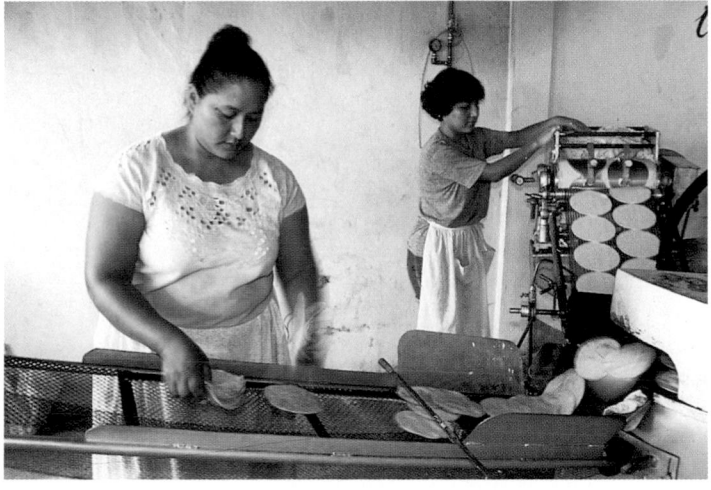

Figure 8.10
The treatment of corn with lime water during the preparation of tortillas makes niacin available and has prevented pellagra in Mexico and other Latin American countries. (© Jeff Greenberg/Photo Researchers, Inc.)

Niacin equivalents (NEs) The measure used to express the amount of niacin present in food, including that which can be made from its precursor, tryptophan. One NE is equal to 1 mg of niacin or 60 mg of tryptophan.

How Much Niacin Do We Need? The RDA for niacin is expressed as **niacin equivalents (NEs)**. One NE is equal to 1 mg of niacin or 60 mg of tryptophan. This allows for the fact that some of the requirement for niacin can be met by the synthesis of niacin from tryptophan. Approximately 60 mg of tryptophan is needed to make 1 mg of niacin. To estimate the niacin contributed by high-protein foods, protein is considered to be about 1% tryptophan. The criterion used to estimate the average niacin requirement is urinary excretion of niacin metabolites. The RDA for adult men and women of all ages is 16 and 14 mg NE per day, respectively.[2] A medium chicken breast and a cup of steamed asparagus provides this amount.

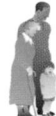

Niacin needs are increased in pregnancy to account for the increase in energy expenditure, and in lactation to account for both the increase in energy expenditure and the niacin secreted in milk. There is not enough information to establish an RDA for infants, so an AI has been set based on the amount of niacin found in human milk.

Niacin Deficiency The early symptoms of pellagra include fatigue, decreased appetite, and indigestion, followed by the three Ds: dermatitis, diarrhea, dementia. If left untreated, niacin deficiency results in a fourth D—death. The dermatitis resembles sunburn and strikes parts of the body exposed to sunlight, heat, or injury. Gastrointestinal symptoms include a bright-red tongue and may include vomiting, constipation, or diarrhea. Mental symptoms begin with irritability, headaches, loss of memory, insomnia, and emotional instability and progress to psychosis and acute delirium.

Niacin Toxicity There is no evidence of any adverse effects from consumption of niacin naturally occurring in foods, but supplements can be toxic. The adverse effects of high intakes of niacin include flushing of the skin, a tingling sensation in the hands and feet, a red skin rash, nausea, vomiting, diarrhea, high blood sugar levels, abnormalities in liver function, and blurred vision.[5] Since flushing is the first toxicity symptom to appear as the dose is increased, the UL for adults was set at 35 mg, the highest level that is unlikely to cause flushing in the majority of healthy people. This value applies to the forms of niacin contained in supplements and fortified foods, but does not include niacin naturally occurring in foods.

Niacin Supplements Niacin deficiency is no longer of public health concern in the United States, and excessive intakes of niacin can be toxic. Despite this, niacin is a commonly used vitamin supplement. High doses of niacin supplements are used to treat elevated blood cholesterol. When vitamins are taken in large doses to treat diseases that are not due to vitamin deficiencies, they are really being used as drugs rather than vitamins.

Doses of 50 mg per day or greater of the nicotinic acid form of niacin have been found to decrease blood levels of LDL cholesterol and triglycerides and increase HDL cholesterol. They are also associated with a reduction in recurrent heart attacks and deaths in individuals with cardiovascular disease[6,7] Supplements containing high doses of niacin should be used only with medical supervision.

Biotin

Biotin was discovered when rats fed protein derived from raw egg white developed a syndrome of hair loss, dermatitis, and neuromuscular dysfunction. This deficiency of biotin was caused by a protein in raw egg white, called avidin, that tightly binds biotin and prevents its absorption.

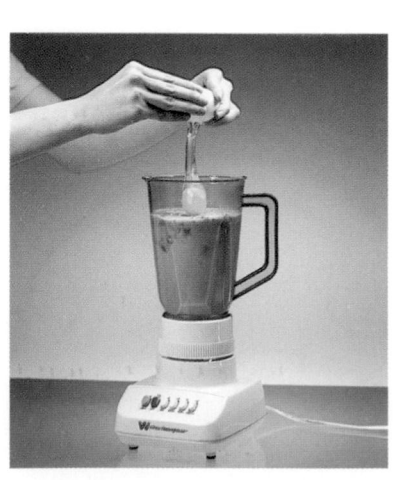

Figure 8.11
Raw eggs are often used to make high-protein shakes. This is not recommended because raw eggs may contain bacteria that cause food-borne illness, and raw egg whites contain a protein that binds biotin and makes it unavailable. (Charles D. Winters)

Biotin in the Diet Good sources of biotin include liver, egg yolks, yogurt, and nuts. Fruit and meat are poor sources. Foods containing raw egg whites should be avoided not only because avidin binds biotin and prevents its absorption, but because raw eggs also may be contaminated with bacteria that can cause food-borne illness (Figure 8.11). Thoroughly cooking eggs destroys bacteria and denatures avidin so that it cannot bind biotin.

Biotin in the Body Biotin is a coenzyme for a group of enzymes that add the acid group COOH to molecules. It functions in energy production because it is needed to make a 4-carbon molecule necessary in the citric acid cycle and in glucose synthesis. It is also important in the metabolism of fatty acids and amino acids (see Figure 8.6).

How Much Biotin Do We Need? It is difficult to estimate a biotin requirement because some biotin is produced by bacteria in the gastrointestinal tract and absorbed into the body. No RDA could be determined for biotin, but an AI of 30 μg per day has been established for adult men and women based on the amount of biotin found in a typical North American diet.

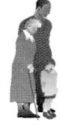

No additional biotin is recommended for pregnancy, but the AI is increased during lactation to account for the amount secreted in milk. The AI for infants is based on the amount of biotin consumed by infants fed human milk.

Biotin and Health Although biotin deficiency is uncommon, it has been observed in people with malabsorption or protein-energy malnutrition, those receiving tube feedings or total parenteral nutrition without biotin, those taking anticonvulsant drugs for long periods, and those frequently consuming raw egg whites.[2] When biotin intake is deficient, symptoms including nausea, thinning hair, loss of hair color, a red skin rash, depression, lethargy, hallucinations, and tingling of the extremities gradually appear.

No toxicity has been reported in patients given 200 mg per day of biotin to treat various disease states, and sufficient data are not available to establish a UL.

Pantothenic Acid

Pantothenic acid, which gets its name from the Greek word *pantos* (meaning "from everywhere"), is widely distributed in foods.

Pantothenic Acid in the Diet Pantothenic acid is particularly abundant in meat, eggs, whole grains, and legumes. It is found in lesser amounts in milk, vegetables, and fruits.

Pantothenic Acid in the Body Pantothenic acid is part of coenzyme A (CoA), which is part of acetyl-CoA, a molecule formed during the breakdown of carbohydrates, fatty acids, and amino acids. Pantothenic acid is also needed to produce acyl carrier protein needed for the synthesis of cholesterol and fatty acids (see Figure 8.6).

How Much Pantothenic Acid Do We Need? There is no RDA for pantothenic acid, but an AI of 5 mg per day has been recommended for adult men and women.[2] This value is based on the intake of pantothenic acid sufficient to replace urinary losses. The AI is increased to 6 and 7 mg per day to meet the needs of pregnancy and lactation, respectively.

Pantothenic Acid and Health The wide distribution of pantothenic acid in foods makes deficiency rare in humans. A deficiency of this vitamin alone has not been reported, but it may occur as part of a multiple B vitamin deficiency resulting from malnutrition or chronic alcoholism.

Pantothenic acid is relatively nontoxic. No toxic symptoms were reported in a study that fed young men 10 grams of pantothenic acid per day for 6 weeks. Another study found that doses of 10 to 20 grams per day may result in diarrhea and water retention.[2] Data are not sufficient to establish a UL for pantothenic acid.

• VITAMIN B$_6$ AND PROTEIN METABOLISM

Vitamin B$_6$ was identified only when a deficiency syndrome was discovered that did not respond to thiamin or riboflavin supplementation. The important role of vitamin B$_6$ in amino acid metabolism distinguishes it from the other B vitamins.

Vitamin B₆ in the Diet

Vitamin B₆ is found in both animal and plant foods. Animal sources include chicken, fish, pork, and organ meats. Good plant sources include whole wheat products, brown rice, soybeans, sunflower seeds, and some fruits and vegetables such as bananas, broccoli, and spinach (Figure 8.12). Vitamin B₆ is easily destroyed in processing. It is not added back in the enrichment of grain products, but fortified breakfast cereals make an important contribution to vitamin B₆ intake.[8]

Vitamin B₆ in the Body

Pyridoxine The chemical term for vitamin B₆.

Vitamin B₆, also known as **pyridoxine**, comprises a group of compounds including pyridoxal, pyridoxine, and pyridoxamine. All three forms can be converted into the active coenzyme form, pyridoxal phosphate. Pyridoxal phosphate is needed for the activity of more than 100 enzymes involved in the metabolism of carbohydrate, fat, and protein. It is particularly important for protein and amino acid metabolism (Figure 8.13). Without pyridoxal phosphate, the nonessential amino acids cannot be synthesized and the conditionally essential amino acid cysteine cannot be synthesized from methionine. Pyridoxal phosphate is needed to synthesize hemoglobin, the oxygen-carrying protein in red blood cells. Pyridoxal phosphate is important for the immune system because it is needed to form white blood cells. It is also needed for the conversion of tryptophan to niacin, the metabolism of glycogen, the synthesis of certain neurotransmitters, and the synthesis of the lipids that are part of the myelin coating on nerves.

How Much Vitamin B₆ Do We Need?

The RDA for vitamin B₆ is 1.3 mg per day for both adult men and women 19 to 50 years of age.[2] This is the amount needed to maintain adequate blood concentrations of the active coenzyme pyridoxal phosphate. In adults 51 years and older, the RDA is increased to 1.7 mg per day in men and 1.5 mg per day in women to maintain normal blood pyridoxal phosphate. A 3-ounce (85-g) serving of chicken, fish, or pork, or half

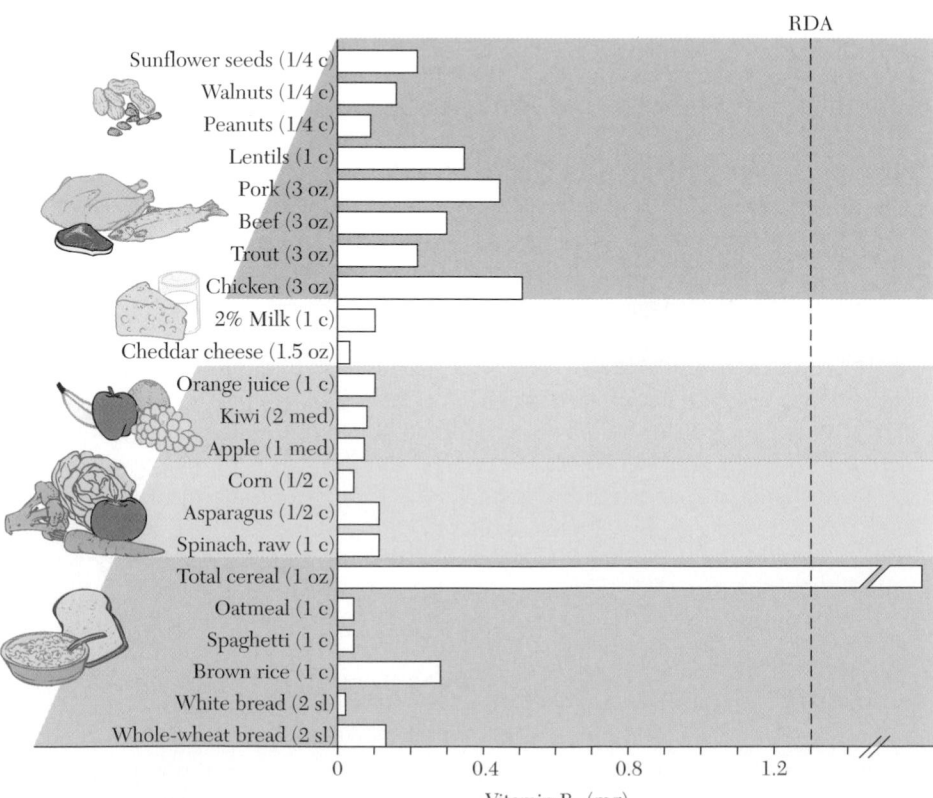

Figure 8.12
Vitamin B₆ content of selections from each group of the Food Guide Pyramid. The dashed line represents the RDA for men and women up to 50 years of age. The best sources are meats, legumes, and whole and fortified grains.

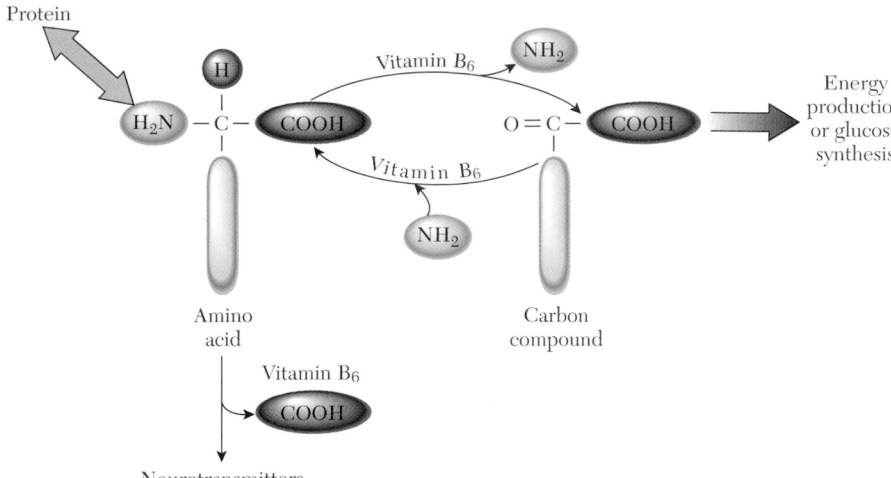

Figure 8.13
Vitamin B$_6$ is needed to synthesize nonessential amino acids by transamination, to remove the amino group so amino acids can be used to produce energy or to synthesize glucose, to remove the COOH group from amino acids for the synthesis of neurotransmitters, and for many other reactions of amino acid metabolism.

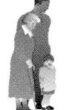

a baked potato, provides about a quarter of the RDA for an average adult; a banana provides about one-third.

The RDA for vitamin B$_6$ is increased during pregnancy to allow for metabolic needs and growth of the mother and fetus. Because the vitamin B$_6$ concentration in breast milk is dependent on the mother's intake, the RDA is increased during lactation to assure adequate levels are supplied to the infant. There is no RDA for infants, but an AI has been established based on the vitamin B$_6$ content of human milk.

Vitamin B$_6$ and Health

A vitamin B$_6$ deficiency syndrome was defined in 1954 when an infant formula was overheated in manufacture, destroying the vitamin B$_6$. The infants who consumed only this formula developed abdominal distress, convulsions, and other neurological symptoms.[9] No adverse effects have been associated with high intakes of vitamin B$_6$ from foods, but large doses found in supplements can cause serious toxicity symptoms.

Vitamin B$_6$ Deficiency Vitamin B$_6$ deficiency causes neurological symptoms including depression, headaches, confusion, numbness and tingling in the extremities, and seizures. These may be related to the the role of vitamin B$_6$ in neurotransmitter synthesis and myelin formation. Anemia also occurs in vitamin B$_6$ deficiency due to impaired hemoglobin synthesis; red blood cells are small (microcytic) and pale (hypochromic) due to the lack of hemoglobin. Other deficiency symptoms such as poor growth, skin lesions, and decreased antibody formation may occur because vitamin B$_6$ is important in protein and energy metabolism. Since vitamin B$_6$ is needed for amino acid metabolism, the onset of a deficiency can be hastened by a diet that is low in vitamin B$_6$ but high in protein.

Vitamin B$_6$ status in the body can be affected by a number of drugs, including alcohol and oral contraceptives. Alcohol decreases the formation of the active coenzyme pyridoxal phosphate and makes it more susceptible to breakdown. Oral contraceptive use has been associated with small decreases in blood levels of pyridoxal phosphate. But vitamin B$_6$ supplements are not routinely recommended for women taking oral contraceptives.[2]

Vitamin B$_6$ and Cardiovascular Disease? It has been hypothesized that vitamin B$_6$ affects the risk of heart disease through its role in the breakdown of homocysteine, an intermediate in methionine metabolism (Figure 8.14). Individuals with a rare genetic disorder that causes chronically high blood levels of homocysteine develop atherosclerosis at an early age. Large doses of vitamin B$_6$ (100–1000 mg/day) have been successfully used to reduce elevated homocysteine and the risk of atherosclerosis in these patients.[10]

Figure 8.14

B vitamins, including vitamin B_6, B_{12}, and folate, are needed to maintain normal homocysteine levels. Vitamin B_6 is needed to convert homocysteine to cysteine. Vitamin B_{12} and folate are needed to convert homocysteine to methionine. A deficiency of any of these can lead to the accumulation of homocysteine, which is associated with an increased risk of cardiovascular disease.

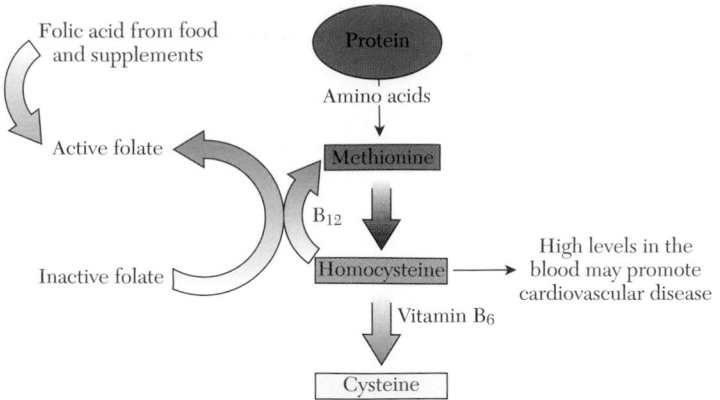

In the normal population, a mild elevation in blood homocysteine has been shown to be a risk factor for cardiovascular disease.[11] It has been proposed that a deficiency of vitamin B_6, vitamin B_{12}, or folate, the latter two of which are also involved in homocysteine metabolism, may cause homocysteine accumulation and eventually lead to atherosclerosis. A study that examined the effect of folate and vitamin B_6 intake in women found that those with the highest levels of folate and vitamin B_6 in their diets had about half the risk of coronary heart disease as women with the lowest levels.[12] Supplements of all three of these vitamins have been used to reduce homocysteine levels in individuals with mild homocysteine elevation.[13] At this time, however, the DRI panel believes that it is premature to conclude that increased intakes of vitamin B_6, vitamin B_{12}, or folate could decrease the risk of cardiovascular disease.[2]

Vitamin B_6 Toxicity In the 1980s, there were reports of severe nerve impairment in individuals taking 2 to 6 grams of pyridoxine per day.[14] Some subjects were unable to walk. These symptoms improved when the pyridoxine supplements were stopped. The UL is based on an amount that will not cause nerve damage in the majority of healthy people. For adults it is set at 100 mg per day from food and supplements.[2] Since high-dose supplements of vitamin B_6 containing 100 mg per dose (5000% of the Daily Value) are available over the counter, it is easy to obtain a dose that exceeds the UL.

Vitamin B_6 Supplements Supplements of vitamin B_6 are marketed to help a wide variety of ailments ranging from carpal tunnel syndrome to premenstrual syndrome (PMS) and poor immune function. Some of these marketing claims are founded in science, but others are exaggerated to sell products.

A Cure for Carpal Tunnel Syndrome? Vitamin B_6 has been suggested to be useful in treating a condition called carpal tunnel syndrome, in which pressure on the nerves in the hand causes pain and weakness. Studies have not found a relationship between carpal tunnel syndrome and vitamin B_6 status.[15] In some patients, supplements have been found to reduce pain, but there is little evidence to support the use of vitamin B_6 supplements as a treatment for carpal tunnel syndrome.

The PMS Promise? Premenstrual syndrome (PMS) causes mood swings, food cravings, bloating, tension, depression, headaches, acne, breast tenderness, anxiety, temper outbursts, and over 100 other symptoms. The proposed connection between these symptoms and vitamin B_6 is the fact that the vitamin is needed for the synthesis of the neurotransmitters serotonin and dopamine. Insufficient vitamin B_6 has been suggested to reduce levels of these neurotransmitters and cause the anxiety, irritability, and depression associated with PMS. A review of published studies evaluating the effect of vitamin B_6 supplements on PMS suggests that low-dose supplements may be effective in reducing symptoms.[16]

Immune System Improver? Immune function can be impaired by a deficiency of any nutrient that hinders cell growth and division. Therefore, one of the most common claims for vitamin supplements in general is that they improve immune function. Vitamin B$_6$ is no exception. Vitamin B$_6$ supplements have been found to improve immune function in older adults.[17] However, since the elderly frequently have low intakes of vitamin B$_6$, it is unclear whether the beneficial effects of supplements are due to an improvement in vitamin B$_6$ status or immune system stimulation.

• FOLATE, VITAMIN B$_{12}$, AND CELL DIVISION

The B vitamins folate and vitamin B$_{12}$ have overlapping roles in the synthesis of DNA, which is required for cells to divide. Therefore, some of the same symptoms are seen in severe deficiency of either vitamin—most notably anemia. This type of anemia occurs because developing red blood cells cannot divide. Marginal deficiencies of these nutrients are a modern concern, particularly for two life-stage groups—women of childbearing age and the elderly.

Folate or Folic Acid

It has been known for over a hundred years that anemia often occurs during pregnancy. In 1937, anemia in a pregnant woman was successfully treated with a yeast preparation named *Wills Factor*, after Dr. Lucy Wills who treated this patient. The Wills Factor was later isolated from spinach and named *folate*, after the Latin word for foliage.

Folate is a general term for the many chemical forms of this vitamin. Most folate in food is bound to a string of glutamate molecules that must be removed before the vitamin can be absorbed. Folic acid is a stable form of folate that rarely occurs naturally in food but is used in supplements and fortified foods. It is more easily absorbed because it is only bound to a single glutamate molecule.

Folate in the Diet Excellent food sources of folate include liver, yeast, asparagus, oranges, and legumes. Fair sources include vegetables such as corn, snap beans, mustard greens, and broccoli, as well as some nuts. Small amounts are found in meats, cheese, milk, fruits, and other vegetables (Figure 8.15). Since 1998, grain products, including enriched breads, flours, corn meal, pasta, grits, and rice, have been fortified with folic acid. The bioavailability of the synthetic folic acid added to grain products and used in supplements is about twice that of the folate naturally found in food.

Folate in the Body There are a number of different active coenzyme forms of folate that are involved in reactions that transfer chemical groups containing a single carbon atom. Folate coenzymes are needed for the synthesis of DNA and the metabolism of some amino acids. Before a cell divides, its DNA must replicate. Therefore, the role of folate in DNA synthesis makes it particularly important in tissues where cells are rapidly dividing, such as bone marrow, where red blood cells are made, intestines, and skin, and during periods of rapid growth, such as early in embryonic life. Insufficient folate in early pregnancy has been related to **neural tube defects**.

How Much Folate Do We Need? The adult RDA for folate is set at 400 μg **dietary folate equivalents (DFEs)** per day for adult men and women. One DFE is equal to 1 μg of food folate, 0.6 μg of synthetic folic acid from fortified food or supplements consumed with food, or 0.5 μg of synthetic folic acid consumed on an empty stomach. In order to reduce the risk of neural tube defects, a special recommendation is made for women capable of becoming pregnant. A daily intake of 400 μg of synthetic folic acid from fortified foods and/or supplements is recommended in addition to the food folate consumed in a varied diet. Therefore, the total folate intake of this group should exceed the RDA.

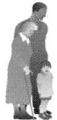

The RDA for folate during pregnancy is increased to 600 μg per day due to the increase in cell division. Although this level can be met by a carefully selected diet, folate is typically supplemented during pregnancy. The RDA is increased during lacta-

Neural tube defects Abnormalities in the brain or spinal cord that result from errors that occur during prenatal development.

Dietary folate equivalents (DFEs) The unit used to express the amount of folate present in food. One DFE is equivalent to 1 μg of folate naturally occurring in food, 0.6 μg of synthetic folic acid from fortified food or supplements consumed with food, or 0.5 μg of synthetic folic acid consumed on an empty stomach.

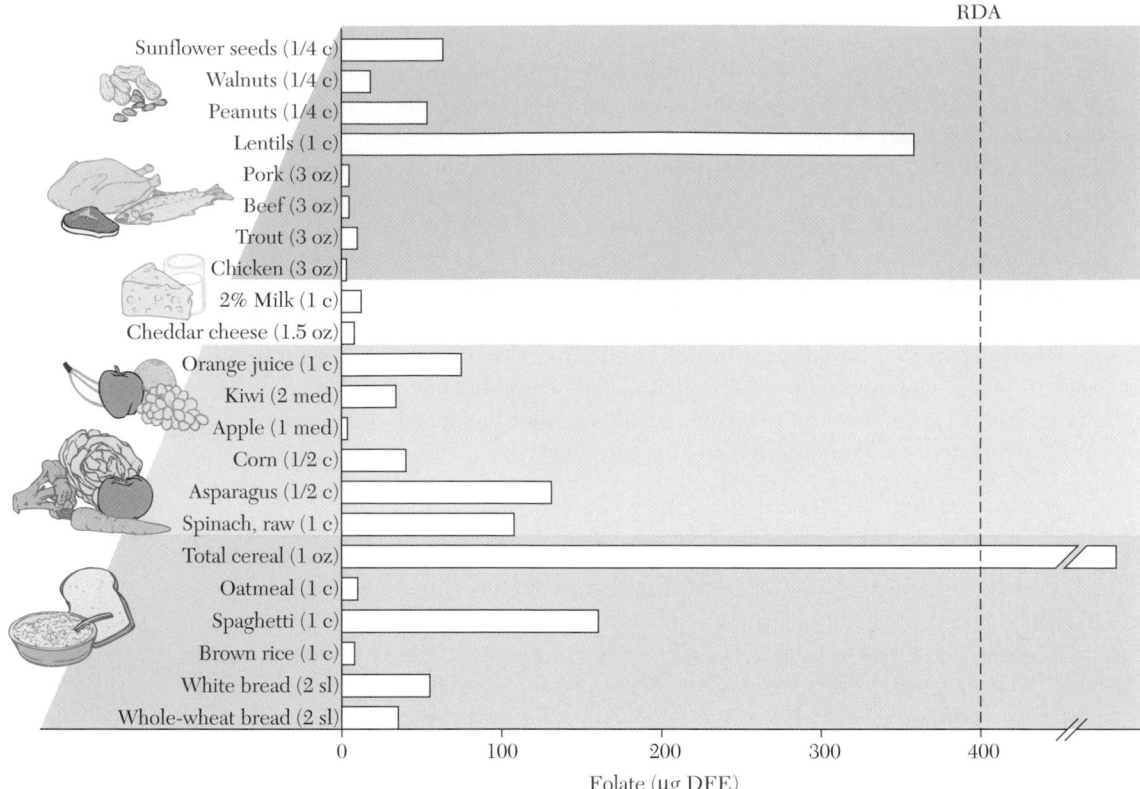

Figure 8.15
Folate content of selections from each group of the Food Guide Pyramid. The dashed line represents the RDA for adults. Legumes, fortified foods, and some fruits and vegetable are good sources.

tion to account for folate secretion in milk. Needs are higher for infants and children than for adults because of their rapid growth. Human and cow's milk provide enough folate to meet infant needs, but goat's milk does not. Infants and children given goat's milk may not receive adequate folate unless it is provided from other sources.

Folate and Health A severe deficiency of folate results in anemia, but low intakes of folate have been associated with an increased risk of neural tube defects, heart disease, and certain types of cancer. An excess of folate can mask the symptoms of vitamin B_{12} deficiency.

Folate Deficiency Folate deficiency symptoms include poor growth, problems in nerve development and function, diarrhea, inflammation of the tongue, and anemia. Anemia results when folate is deficient because the bone marrow cells that develop into blood cells cannot duplicate their DNA and so cannot divide. Instead, they just grow bigger. These large immature cells are known as **megaloblasts** and can be converted into large red blood cells called **macrocytes**. The result is that fewer mature red cells are produced, and the oxygen-carrying capacity of the blood is reduced. This condition is called **megaloblastic** or **macrocytic anemia** (Figure 8.16).

Groups at risk of folate deficiency include pregnant women and premature infants because of their rapid rate of cell division and growth; the elderly because of their limited intake of foods high in folate; alcoholics because alcohol inhibits folate absorption; and tobacco smokers because smoke inactivates folate in the cells lining the lungs.[2]

Folate and Neural Tube Defects Neural tube defects, such as spina bifida and other birth defects that affect the brain and spinal cord (Figure 8.17), are not true folate deficiency symptoms because not every pregnant woman with inadequate folate lev-

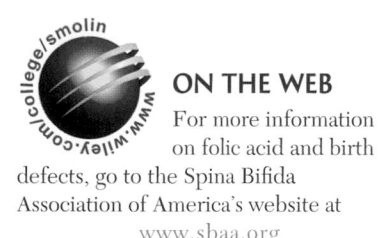

ON THE WEB
For more information on folic acid and birth defects, go to the Spina Bifida Association of America's website at
www.sbaa.org

Megaloblasts Large, immature red blood cells that are formed when developing red blood cells are unable to divide normally.

Macrocytes Larger-than-normal mature red blood cells that have a shortened life span.

Megaloblastic or **macrocytic anemia** A condition in which there are abnormally large immature and mature red blood cells and a reduction in the total number of red blood cells.

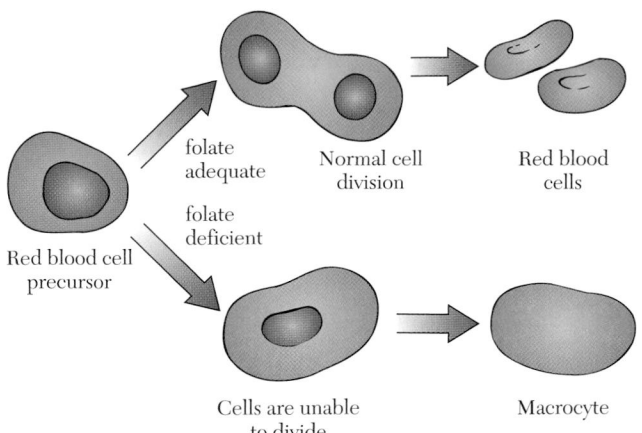

Figure 8.16
Macrocytic anemia occurs when blood cells are unable to divide, leaving large immature red blood cells (megaloblasts) and large mature red blood cells (macrocytes).

els will give birth to a child with a neural tube defect. Instead, neural tube defects are probably due to a combination of factors that include low folate levels and a genetic predisposition. The exact role of folate in neural tube development is not known, but it is necessary for a critical step called neural tube closure. Neural tube closure occurs only 28 days after conception; therefore, folate status should be adequate even before a pregnancy begins (see Chapter 14). Studies in which supplemental folic acid was given to women before and during early pregnancy showed that 360 to 800 μg per day of synthetic folic acid in addition to food folate was associated with a reduced incidence of neural tube defects.[2] Because it is not known whether a diet naturally rich in folate offers the same protection as folic acid supplements, and because folate must be adequate before most women are aware that they are pregnant, folic acid from supplements or fortified foods is recommended for all women of childbearing age. The fortification of grain products in 1998 made it easier for women to meet this recommendation. Since then, the incidence of neural tube defects has decreased by 19%.[18]

Folate and Heart Disease Folate's effect on heart disease risk is related to its role in the metabolism of the amino acid methionine. When folate is lacking, homocysteine, produced during methionine metabolism, accumulates because it cannot be converted back to methionine (see Figure 8.14). The risk of cardiovascular disease increases with elevated homocysteine levels and homocysteine level increases with folate deficiency (see preceding discussion of vitamin B$_6$ and cardiovascular disease). Homocysteine levels and the risk of cardiovascular disease are reduced by increasing intakes of folate.[12,13]

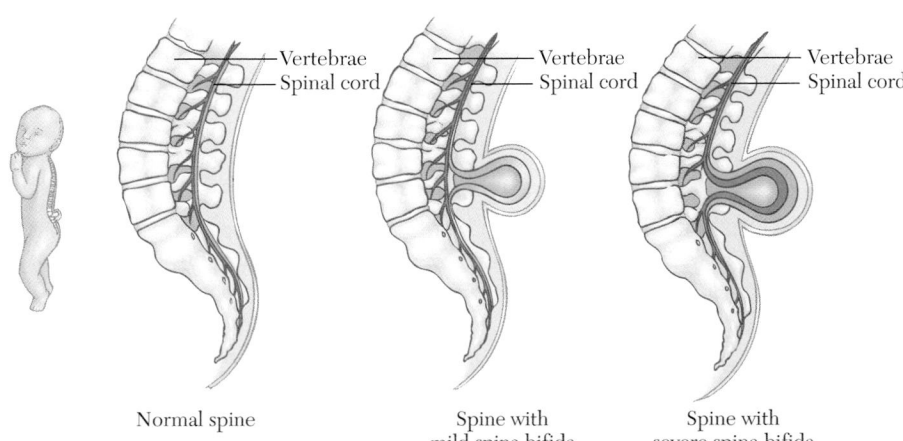

Figure 8.17
The neural tube develops into the brain and spinal cord. If folate is inadequate during neural tube closure, neural tube defects such as spina bifida, shown here, occur more frequently.

Folate and Cancer Low folate status increases the risk of developing forms of cancer that affect epithelial tissues such as the uterus, cervix, lung, stomach, esophagus, and colon. Although folate deficiency does not cause cancer, it has been hypothesized that low folate intake enhances an underlying predisposition to cancer. Data supporting the effects of folate intake on cancer risk are strongest for colon cancer.[19] Alcohol consumption greatly increases the cancer risk associated with a low folate diet.[20]

Folate Toxicity Although there is no known folate toxicity, a high intake may mask the early symptoms of vitamin B_{12} deficiency, allowing irreversible nerve damage to occur. The UL for folic acid for adults is set at 1000 μg per day from supplements and/or fortified foods. This value was determined based on the progression of neurological symptoms seen in patients who are deficient in vitamin B_{12} and taking folic acid supplements.

Meeting Folate Needs with Food and Supplements Adult women in the United States consume an average of 400 μg DFE of folate from natural and fortified foods daily. This meets the RDA but falls short of the recommendation for women of childbearing age to consume 400 μg DFE from fortified foods and supplements in addition to food folate. Depending on food choices, including 400 μg DFE of synthetic folic acid from fortified foods would mean eating about 1 to 4 servings of fortified breakfast cereal or 4 to 6 servings of other fortified grain products each day. If it is not possible to meet recommendations from fortified foods, supplements should be used (see *Critical Thinking:* Four Hundred of Fortified Folate).

Because the fortification of grain products with folic acid is relatively recent, there are some discrepancies in how folate values are expressed. Food composition databases may provide fortified values for some products but not for others. Adding to the confusion is the fact that the Daily Values on food labels and values in some food composition tables are listed as μg total folate, not as μg DFE. The term μg DFE was developed to correct for differences in the bioavailability of different forms of folate. For foods that are natural sources of folate, the folate content can be determined by multiplying the Daily Value (400 μg) by the % Daily Value listed on the label (see *Off the Label:* Figuring Micronutrients from Food Labels). So to calculate the folate in a package of frozen spinach that provides 25% of the Daily Value, multiply 400 μg folate × 25% = 100 μg DFE. In foods fortified with folic acid, the amount of folate indicated by the % Daily Value must be multiplied by 1.7 to account for the greater availability of folic acid.

Vitamin B_{12}

Pernicious anemia An anemia resulting from vitamin B_{12} deficiency that occurs when dietary vitamin B_{12} cannot be absorbed due to a lack of intrinsic factor. If not treated with vitamin B_{12} injections or large oral doses, the condition will result in nerve damage.

In 1820, **pernicious anemia**, a fatal form of anemia that did not respond to iron supplementation, was described. Pernicious anemia is caused by an inability to absorb sufficient vitamin B_{12}. In 1926, Drs. Minot and Murphy were awarded the Nobel Prize for curing the disease with a diet containing large quantities of liver, which is a good source of vitamin B_{12}. Today, concern focuses on the effects of marginal deficiencies of this vitamin and the potential masking of B_{12} deficiency by high intakes of folic acid.

Vitamin B_{12} in the Diet In our diet, vitamin B_{12} is found almost exclusively in animal products (Figure 8.18). Vitamin B_{12} can be made by bacteria, fungi, and algae but not by plants and animals. It accumulates in animal tissue from the diet or from synthesis by bacterial microflora. Microorganisms in the human colon produce B_{12}, but it cannot be absorbed. Vitamin B_{12} is not supplied by plant products unless they have been contaminated with bacteria, soil, insects, or other sources of B_{12}, or have been fortified with vitamin B_{12}. Diets that do not include animal products must include supplements or foods fortified with vitamin B_{12} in order to meet needs.[21]

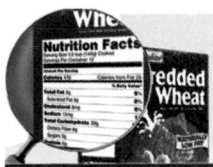

Off the Label
Figuring Micronutrients from Food Labels

How much vitamin C is in your orange juice? How much folate is in your breakfast cereal? And how much iron is in a box of raisins? Micronutrients are important in your diet, but with the exception of sodium it may be difficult to tell from the label exactly how much is in a food.

It is easy to find out how much sodium is in a bag of potato chips. The number of milligrams per serving is listed in the Nutrition Facts section of the food label. But the amounts of other micronutrients in foods are listed only as a percent of the Daily Value. Food labels are required to provide the % Daily Values for vitamin A, vitamin C, iron, and calcium. In order to determine the amount of one of these nutrients of a food, you need to know its Daily Value. The Daily Values for micronutrients are equal to the Reference Daily Intake values given in Table 2.4. Once you know the Daily Value, you can multiply it by the % Daily Value on the label to determine the amount in a serving of the food.

You can now calculate the amounts of micronutrients from food labels, but even if you don't look up the Daily Value and do the math, the % Daily Value on the food label tells you how the amount of the micronutrients listed fits into your daily diet. Foods with only a small % of the Daily Value contribute only a small amount of that nutrient to the daily diet. If the % Daily Value is 10 to 19%, the food is a good source of that nutrient. If the % Daily Value is 20% or more, the food is an excellent source of that nutrient.

Calculating Vitamin and Mineral Content from Food Labels

1. Look up the Daily Value for the nutrient of interest (see Table 2.4).
2. Find the % Daily Value for that nutrient on your food label.
3. Multiply the % Daily Value by the Daily Value to determine the amount of the nutrient in a serving.
   Example: The Daily Value for vitamin C is 60 mg
   A fruit snack has 2% of the Daily Value for vitamin C
   60 mg × 2% of Daily Value = 60 × 0.02 = 3 mg vitamin C
4. Be sure to consider how many servings you plan to eat.

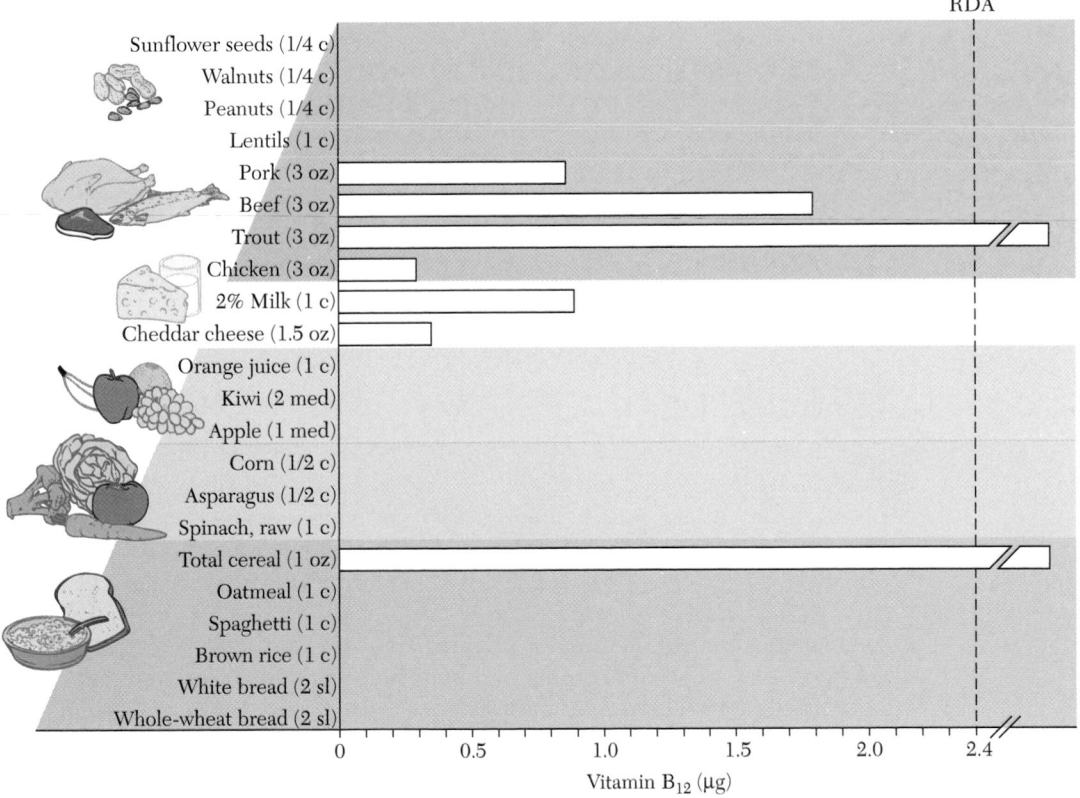

Figure 8.18

Vitamin B$_{12}$ content of selections from each food group of the Food Guide Pyramid. The dashed line represents the RDA for adult men and women. Vitamin B$_{12}$ is only found in foods of animal origin or foods that have been fortified with the vitamin.

Intrinsic factor A protein produced in the stomach that is needed for the absorption of adequate amounts of vitamin B_{12}.

Parietal cells Large cells in the stomach lining that produce and secrete intrinsic factor and hydrochloric acid..

Cobalamin The chemical term for vitamin B_{12}

Vitamin B_{12} in the Digestive Tract Naturally occurring vitamin B_{12} is bound to protein in food and must be released before it can be absorbed. It is released in the stomach by stomach acid and pepsin. The released vitamin B_{12} then binds to special proteins called R proteins, present in saliva, gastric juice, and other body fluids. The R protein-bound vitamin B_{12} travels to the small intestine where pancreatic enzymes free it from the R proteins so it can bind to **intrinsic factor**. Intrinsic factor is a protein secreted by the **parietal cells** in the lining of the stomach. It binds to vitamin B_{12} and allows the vitamin to be absorbed in the ileum of the small intestine (Figure 8.19). Only a small amount of vitamin B_{12} can be absorbed without intrinsic factor. Vitamin B_{12} absorption can be disrupted by reduced stomach acid, insufficient pancreatic secretions, and low levels of intrinsic factor. Vitamin B_{12} also enters the digestive tract in bile. Most of the B_{12} secreted in bile is reabsorbed. Because of this efficient recycling, it can take many years of a deficient diet before the symptoms of vitamin B_{12} deficiency appear.

Vitamin B_{12} in the Body The terms vitamin B_{12} and **cobalamin** refer to members of a group of cobalt-containing compounds. Vitamin B_{12} is necessary for the maintenance of myelin, which insulates nerves and is necessary for nerve transmission. Vitamin B_{12} can be converted into either of two active cobalamin coenzyme forms that function in several reactions. One B_{12}-dependent reaction rearranges carbon atoms so that the breakdown products of fatty acids can be used to generate energy via the citric acid cycle. A second reaction synthesizes the amino acid methionine from homocysteine. This reaction also regenerates the active coenzyme form of folate that functions in DNA synthesis (see Figure 8.14). Because of the need for vitamin B_{12} in folate metabolism, a deficiency of vitamin B_{12} can cause a secondary folate deficiency and, consequently, megaloblastic anemia. If individuals with vitamin B_{12} deficiency consume enough folate, they will not develop anemia, but more serious symptoms, such as nerve damage will be allowed to progress. Although the fortification of grain

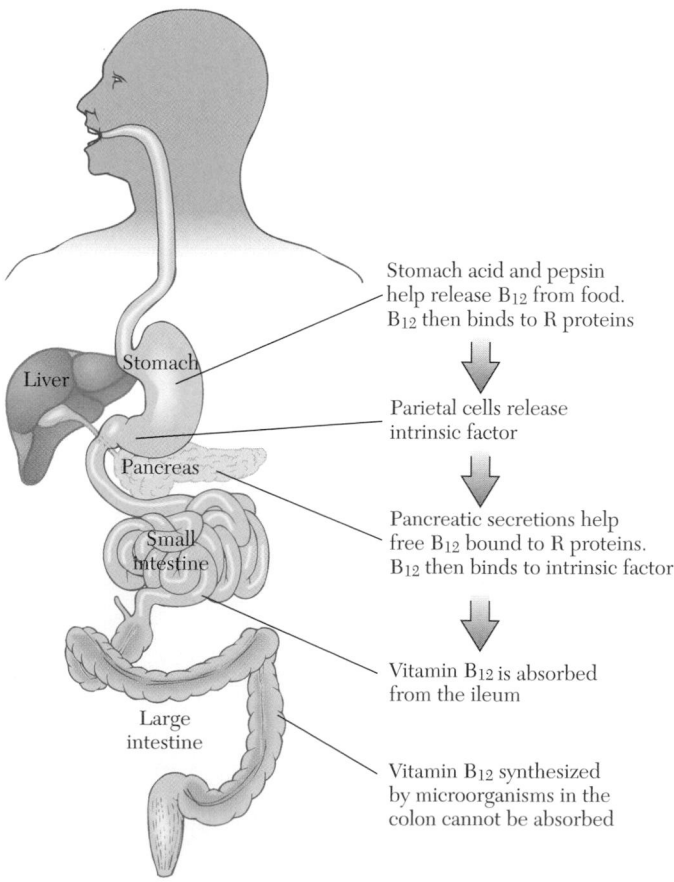

Stomach acid and pepsin help release B_{12} from food. B_{12} then binds to R proteins

Parietal cells release intrinsic factor

Pancreatic secretions help free B_{12} bound to R proteins. B_{12} then binds to intrinsic factor

Vitamin B_{12} is absorbed from the ileum

Vitamin B_{12} synthesized by microorganisms in the colon cannot be absorbed

Liver   Stomach   Pancreas   Small intestine   Large intestine

Figure 8.19
The absorption of vitamin B_{12} involves the stomach, pancreas, and small intestine.

products with folate has raised concern that additional folate in the food supply could delay diagnosis of vitamin B$_{12}$ deficiency, the amount consumed from a typical diet is unlikely to be high enough to cause problems. However, the amounts of folate in supplements may be high enough to mask a vitamin B$_{12}$ deficiency.[22]

How Much Vitamin B$_{12}$ Do We Need? The RDA for adults of all ages for vitamin B$_{12}$ is 2.4 μg per day.[2] This is the amount needed to maintain normal red blood cell parameters and blood vitamin B$_{12}$ concentrations. It is assumed that only 50% of the vitamin B$_{12}$ ingested is absorbed. Average intake in the U.S. population exceeds the RDA for both adult men and women.

The RDA for vitamin B$_{12}$ is increased during pregnancy, even though absorption is increased. The RDA during lactation is increased to account for the amount secreted in milk. Pregnant and lactating vegans, like anyone who does not eat animal products, are advised to take a supplement or consume fortified foods to obtain the recommended intake for vitamin B$_{12}$.

Vitamin B$_{12}$ and Health Blatant deficiencies of vitamin B$_{12}$ are rare because the body stores and reuses it. However, marginal vitamin B$_{12}$ status is of public health concern particularly for older adults and vegetarians who consume no animal products.

Vitamin B$_{12}$ Deficiency Symptoms of vitamin B$_{12}$ deficiency include an increase in blood homocysteine levels and a macrocytic, megaloblastic anemia that is indistinguishable from that seen in folate deficiency. Neurological symptoms include numbness and tingling, abnormalities in gait, memory loss, and disorientation due to degeneration of the myelin that coats the nerves, spinal cord, and brain. If not treated, this eventually causes paralysis and death. Pernicious anemia, a disease in which the parietal cells that produce intrinsic factor are destroyed, is the major cause of severe B$_{12}$ deficiency. Without intrinsic factor, vitamin B$_{12}$ cannot be absorbed normally. This anemia must be treated with injections of the vitamin or with oral megadoses, some of which can be absorbed by passive diffusion.

About 10 to 30% of individuals over 50 years of age are unable to absorb food-bound vitamin B$_{12}$ normally because they have a condition called **atrophic gastritis**, which reduces stomach acid secretion and allows microbial overgrowth. When stomach acid is reduced, the enzymes that release protein-bound vitamin B$_{12}$ cannot function properly and the bound vitamin B$_{12}$ cannot be released and absorbed. In addition, microbes in the gut reduce absorption by competing for available vitamin B$_{12}$. It is recommended that individuals over the age of 50 meet their RDA for vitamin B$_{12}$ by consuming fortified foods such as breakfast cereals or soy-based products or by taking a vitamin B$_{12}$-containing supplement. Because the form of the vitamin in these products is not bound to proteins, it is absorbed even when stomach acid is low.

Vitamin B$_{12}$ deficiency is also a concern among vegan vegetarians since vitamin B$_{12}$ is only found in foods of animal origin. Severe deficiency has been observed in breast-fed infants of vegan women, but marginal deficiency is a concern for all vegans if supplements or fortified foods are not included in the diet.

Vitamin B$_{12}$ Toxicity No toxic effects have been reported with excess vitamin B$_{12}$ intakes of up to 100 μg per day from food or supplements. There are not sufficient data to establish a UL for vitamin B$_{12}$.

Vitamin B$_{12}$ Supplements Supplements of vitamin B$_{12}$ are available as cyanocobalamin in both oral and injectable forms. Because vitamin B$_{12}$ deficiency causes anemia, supplements of the vitamin, particularly as injections, have been promoted as a pick-me-up for tired, run-down individuals. However, there are no proven benefits of vitamin B$_{12}$ supplementation in individuals who are not vitamin B$_{12}$ deficient. Oral supplements may be of benefit for those at risk for vitamin B$_{12}$ deficiency, such as vegans and individuals over 50 who may poorly absorb vitamin B$_{12}$ from foods.

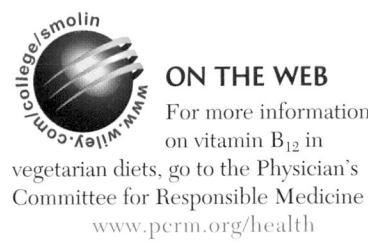

ON THE WEB
For more information on vitamin B$_{12}$ in vegetarian diets, go to the Physician's Committee for Responsible Medicine
www.pcrm.org/health

Atrophic gastritis An inflammation of the stomach lining. It causes a reduction in stomach acid and allows bacterial overgrowth.

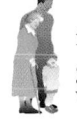

CRITICAL THINKING

Four Hundred of Fortified Folate

Marcia is considering having a child and wants to be sure she is in the best shape possible before trying to conceive. She consults her physician who gives her a clean bill of health but suggests she evaluate the amount of folate in her diet.

Why is folate a concern for women capable of becoming pregnant?

▼

Research has shown that women of childbearing age who consume extra folic acid have a reduced risk of a type of birth defect called a neural tube defect that affects the brain or spinal cord. For the extra folic acid to be beneficial, it must be consumed for at least a month before conception and continued for a month after. Since many pregnancies are not planned, it is recommended that 400 μg of folic acid from fortified foods or supplements be included routinely in the diets of women of childbearing age.

Marcia records her food intake for one day to determine her folate intake:

Food	Servings	Total Folate (μg)
Breakfast		
Corn flakes	1 cup	100
Milk, reduced fat	1 cup	12
Banana	1 medium	22
Orange juice	8 oz (240 ml)	75
Coffee	1 cup	0
Lunch		
Hamburger	1	11
Hamburger bun	1	32
French fries	20 pieces	24
Coke	12 oz	0
Apple	1 medium	4
Dinner		
Chicken	3 oz	4
Refried beans	1/2 cup	106
Rice	1 cup	80
Roll	1	60
Margarine	2 tsp	1
Salad	1 cup	64
Salad dressing	1 Tbsp	1
Milk, reduced fat	1 cup	12
Cake	1 piece	32
Total		**640**

Does her folate intake meet the RDA?

▼

Yes. She consumes 640 μg of folate, which is greater than the RDA of 400 μg DFE, but her doctor reminds her that women who are capable of becoming pregnant should consume 400 μg of folic acid from fortified foods or supplements each day in addition to the folate found in a varied diet.

Why not set the RDA at 800 μg DFE?

▼

Prevention of neural tube defects was not used as a criterion of adequacy for the RDAs for several reasons. First of all, only women who actually become pregnant would benefit from this amount. In addition, the period of time that this intake is beneficial is short (about one month before to one month after conception). Finally, the studies that showed a reduced risk of neural tube defects were done using folic acid supplements in addition to other dietary folate. It is uncertain whether folate found naturally in foods will have the same effect.

What foods in Marcia's diet are natural sources of folate? Which are fortified with folic acid?

▼

The best sources of naturally occurring folate are the orange juice and the beans. Other fruits, vegetables, and dairy products contribute smaller amounts. Meats contribute little folate. Together, these foods provide 336 μg of folate. The grain products in her diet, including the cereal, hamburger bun, roll, rice, and cake, are all fortified and together contribute about 304 μg of folate. Some of this is from the folate naturally found in these grains but most is from folic acid added in fortification. Fortified foods can be identified because folic acid is included on food labels in the ingredient list. Many products also list the amount of folate as a percent of the Daily Value, which can be used to calculate the μg of folate per serving.

List some substitutions that would increase Marcia's intake of naturally occurring folate and of folic acid from fortified foods.

▼

Answer:

Would you recommend Marcia take a folate supplement?

▼

Answer:

• VITAMIN C

Vitamin C deficiency has been the scourge of armies, navies, and explorers throughout history. This deficiency, known as **scurvy**, was described by ancient Greeks, Egyptians, and Romans. In the mid-1500s, the Indians of eastern Canada knew that an extract from white cedar needles would cure the disease. In the 17th century, Sir Richard Hawkins observed on his voyage to the South Seas that this sickness could be cured by including citrus fruit in the diet. Despite his observation, 10,000 British sailors died of scurvy that same year. Over 100 years later, James Lind, a Scottish physician serving in the British navy, tested various agents for their effectiveness at curing scurvy and reported that two patients given citrus fruits recovered within six days. However, it was another 48 years before it was required that lime or lemon juice be included in the rations of the mercantile service, earning British sailors the name *limeys.* Unfortunately, the rest of the world did not heed the lesson of the limeys. In the mid-19th century, during the American Civil War, scurvy was rampant.

Scurvy A vitamin C deficiency disease.

Vitamin C in the Diet

Citrus fruits, such as oranges, lemons, and limes, are an excellent source of vitamin C. Other fruits that are high in vitamin C include strawberries and cantaloupe. Vegetables in the cabbage family, such as broccoli, cauliflower, bok choy, and brussels sprouts, as well as green leafy vegetables, green and red peppers, okra, tomatoes, and potatoes, are good sources (Figure 8.20). Meat, fish, poultry, eggs, dairy products, and grains are poor sources. The amount of vitamin C in packaged foods must be listed on food labels as a percentage of the Daily Value. Vitamin C is unstable and is destroyed by oxygen, light, and heat, so it is readily lost in cooking. This loss is accelerated by contact with copper or iron cooking utensils and by low-acid conditions.

Vitamin C in the Body

Ascorbic acid or **ascorbate** The chemical term for vitamin C.

Vitamin C, known as **ascorbic acid** or **ascorbate**, is a water-soluble vitamin that donates electrons in biochemical reactions, including those needed for the synthesis and maintenance of connective tissue. Vitamin C also has a more general role as an antioxidant that protects the body from reactive oxygen molecules, helps maintain the immune system, and aids in the absorption of iron.

Collagen The major protein in connective tissue.

Reactions Requiring Vitamin C: Connective Tissue Many of the reactions requiring vitamin C add a hydroxyl group (OH) to other molecules. Two such reactions are essential for the formation of **collagen**, the protein that forms the base of all connective tissue in the body. The hydroxyl groups are necessary for the formation of chemical bonds that crosslink strands of collagen to give it strength (Figure 8.21). Vitamin C also serves in reactions needed for the synthesis of other cell compounds, including neurotransmitters, hormones such as the thyroid and steroid hormones, bile acids, and carnitine needed for fatty acid breakdown.

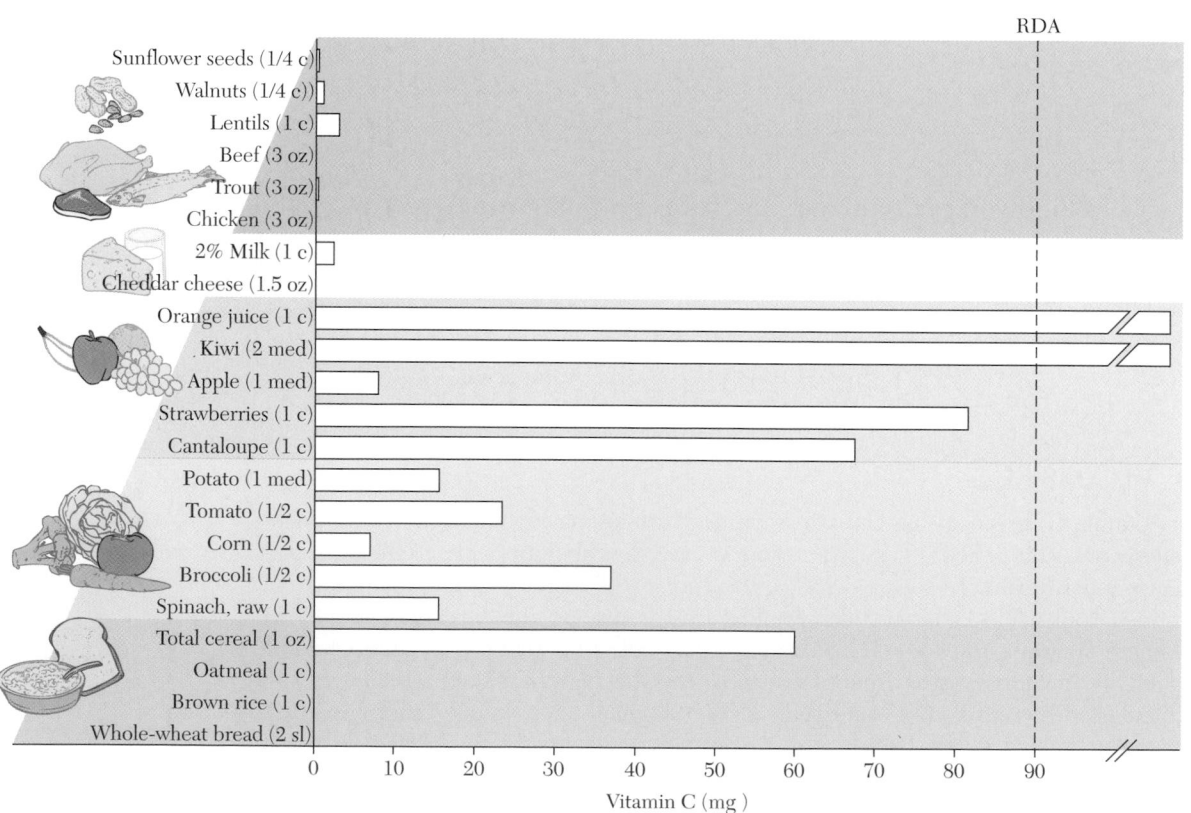

Figure 8.20

Vitamin C content of selections from each food group of the Food Guide Pyramid. The dashed line represents the RDA for adult men. Fruits and vegetables are the best sources of vitamin C.

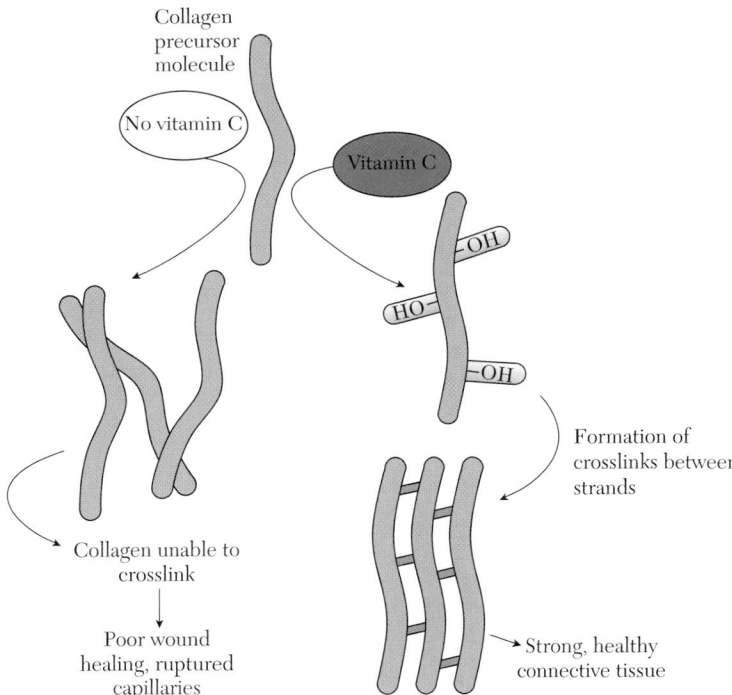

Collagen precursor molecule

No vitamin C

Vitamin C

—OH

HO—

—OH

Formation of crosslinks between strands

Collagen unable to crosslink

Poor wound healing, ruptured capillaries

Strong, healthy connective tissue

Figure 8.21
Vitamin C is needed for the formation of chemical bonds that link collagen molecules together to give connective tissue strength and stability.

Vitamin C as a General Antioxidant Vitamin C also functions as an **antioxidant**. Antioxidants are substances that protect against **oxidative damage**, which is damage caused by reactive oxygen molecules. **Oxidative stress** refers to a serious imbalance between the amounts of reactive oxygen molecules and the amounts of antioxidant defenses available. Oxidative stress has been related to the aging process as well as to the development of cancer and heart disease. Agents that can induce oxidative stress by causing an increase in reactive oxygen molecules, a decrease in antioxidant defenses, or an increase in oxidative damage are called **pro-oxidants**.

How Do Antioxidants Work? Reactive oxygen molecules such as **free radicals** can be generated by normal oxygen-requiring reactions inside the body or can come from environmental sources such as air pollution or cigarette smoke. Free radicals cause damage by snatching electrons from DNA, proteins, carbohydrates, or unsaturated fatty acids. This results in changes in the structure and function of these molecules. DNA damage is hypothesized to be a major reason for the increase in cancer incidence that occurs with age. And free radical damage to lipoproteins and lipids in membranes is implicated in the development of atherosclerosis.[23]

Antioxidants act by destroying reactive oxygen molecules before they can do damage. Some directly destroy free radicals, while others neutralize superoxide radicals or hydrogen peroxide, which are other reactive molecules, before they can form free radicals. Some antioxidants are produced in the body; others are consumed in the diet. Vitamin C, vitamin E, and the mineral selenium have been classified as **dietary antioxidants** (see Chapter 9, *Off the Shelf*: Will Antioxidant Supplements Keep Us Healthy?).[24]

The Role of Vitamin C Vitamin C acts as an antioxidant in the blood and other body fluids. It can destroy superoxide radicals and free radicals before they can damage lipids and DNA (Figure 8.22). Vitamin C has also been shown to scavenge reactive oxygen molecules in white blood cells, the lungs, and the stomach mucosa.[24] The antioxidant properties of vitamin C can affect other nutrients. It regenerates the active antioxidant form of vitamin E and enhances iron absorption by keeping iron in its

Antioxidant A substance that is able to neutralize reactive oxygen molecules and thereby reduce oxidative damage.

Oxidative damage Damage caused by highly reactive oxygen molecules that steal electrons from other compounds, causing changes in structure and function.

Oxidative stress A condition that occurs when there are more reactive oxygen molecules than can be neutralized by available antioxidant defenses. It occurs either because excessive amounts of reactive oxygen molecules are generated or because antioxidant defenses are deficient.

Pro-oxidant A substance that promotes oxidative damage.

Free radical One type of highly reactive molecule that causes oxidative damage.

Dietary antioxidant A substance in food that significantly decreases the adverse effects of reactive species on normal physiologic function in humans.

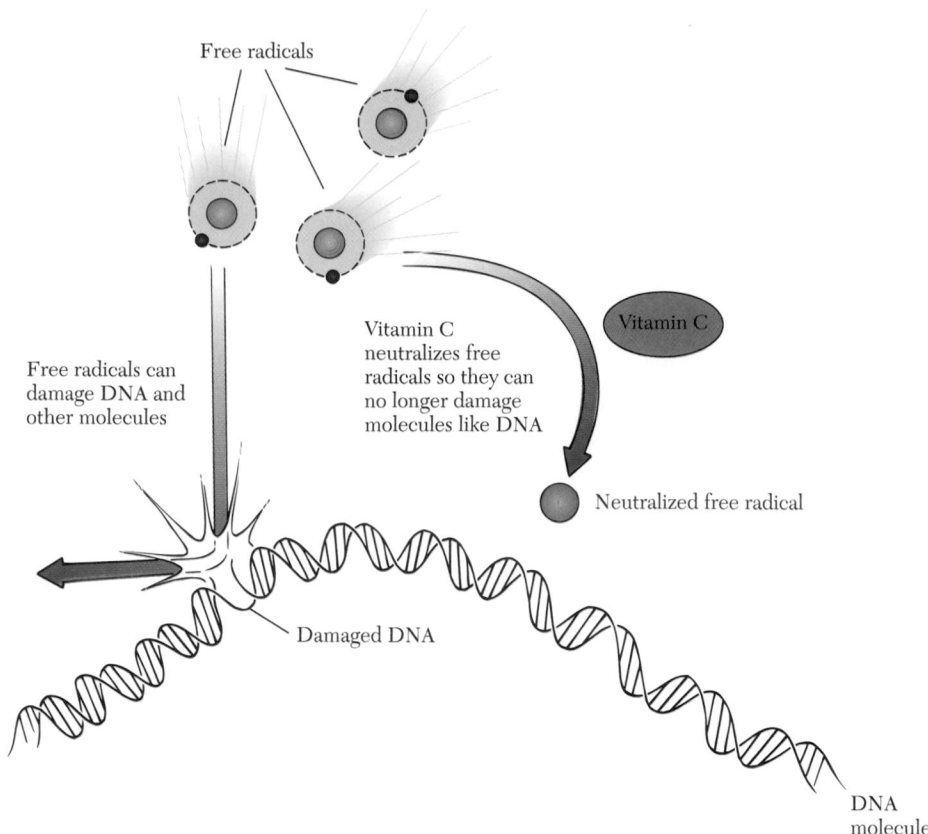

Figure 8.22
Vitamin C functions as an antioxidant, neutralizing free radicals so that they are no longer damaging.

more readily absorbed reduced form (Fe^{+2}). When about 50 mg of vitamin C—the amount contained in 3.5 ounces of orange juice—is consumed in a meal containing iron, iron absorption is enhanced (see Chapter 11).

Vitamin C may also act as a pro-oxidant by converting iron and copper to reduced forms that can then generate free radicals. There is some evidence that vitamin C supplements could lead to oxidative damage to DNA. However, studies of the pro-oxidant effects of vitamin C are inconsistent.[25] More research is needed to determine what factors influence whether the antioxidant or pro-oxidant properties of vitamin C predominate.

How Much Vitamin C Do We Need?

Humans are one of only a few animal species that require vitamin C in the diet. Most animals can synthesize vitamin C in their bodies. For example, a pig makes 8 grams a day. The recommendations for vitamin C intake are based on the amount needed to minimize excretion of the vitamin in the urine and maximize concentrations in neutrophils, a type of white blood cell. The RDA is 90 mg per day for men and 75 mg per day for women. This amount is easily obtained by drinking an 8-ounce glass of orange juice.

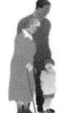

The RDA for vitamin C is increased during pregnancy and lactation. The recommendation for infants is based on the vitamin C content of human milk. The recommended intake for vitamin C is not increased in older adults. Cigarette smoking increases the requirement for vitamin C because vitamin C is used to break down compounds in cigarette smoke. It is recommended that cigarette smokers consume an extra 35 mg of vitamin C daily.

Vitamin C Deficiency

When vitamin C intake is below 10 mg per day, the symptoms of scurvy may appear. These symptoms reflect the role of vitamin C in the maintenance of collagen and blood-vessel integrity. Without vitamin C, the bonds holding adjacent collagen molecules together cannot be formed and maintained, resulting in poor wound healing, the reopening of previously healed wounds, bone and joint aches, bone fractures, and improperly formed and loose teeth. Due to weakened blood vessels and ruptured capillaries, small skin discolorations appear, the gums bleed, and bruising occurs easily. Anemia may also occur from impaired iron absorption. The psychological manifestations of scurvy include depression and hysteria.

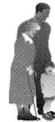

Two centuries ago, fruits containing vitamin C saved the lives of thousands of sailors. Today, marginal vitamin C deficiency is a concern for individuals who consume few fruits and vegetables, but severe vitamin C deficiency leading to scurvy is uncommon. Scurvy can occur in infants fed diets consisting exclusively of cow's milk and in alcoholics and elderly individuals consuming nutrient-poor diets.

Vitamin C Toxicity

Vitamin C is generally considered nontoxic. Large increases in intake do not cause large increases in the amount of vitamin C in body fluids. This is because the percentage of the dose absorbed decreases as the size of the dose increases and because vitamin C absorbed in excess of need is excreted by the kidney. The most common symptoms that occur with consumption of vitamin C doses of 1 gram or more are diarrhea, nausea, and abdominal cramps. These are caused when unabsorbed vitamin C draws water into the intestine. Another concern with vitamin C supplements is damage to tooth enamel. Vitamin C is an acid that is strong enough to dissolve tooth enamel when vitamin C tablets are chewed.

High intakes of vitamin C should be avoided by individuals prone to kidney stones because it can increase stone formation, by individuals who are unable to regulate iron absorption because it increases absorption, and by those with sickle-cell anemia because it can worsen symptoms. Other potential problems associated with vitamin C intakes greater than 3 grams per day include interference with drugs prescribed to slow blood clotting and, because the structure of vitamin C is similar to that of glucose, interference with urine tests used to monitor glucose levels. The UL for vitamin C has been set at 2000 mg/day from food and supplements.

Vitamin C Supplements

One-third of the population of the United States takes supplements of vitamin C in the hope that it will prevent or reduce symptoms of the common cold. More recently, however, the role of vitamin C as an antioxidant has been used to promote vitamin C supplements as protection against cardiovascular disease and cancer.

Vitamin C and the Common Cold Studies examining the relationship between vitamin C and the common cold date back to the 1930s. A review of placebo-controlled trials that supplemented diets with 1 gram (or more) per day found that vitamin C did not reduce the incidence of colds but did cause a reduction in the duration and severity of cold symptoms.[26] The effect of vitamin C on cold symptoms may be due to its direct antiviral effect, its antioxidant effect, its role in stimulating various aspects of immune function, its ability to increase the breakdown of histamine (a molecule that causes inflammation), or a combination of these.[27,28]

Vitamin C and Cardiovascular Disease Vitamin C supplements have been suggested to reduce the risk of cardiovascular disease by reducing blood pressure, blood cholesterol levels, and the formation of oxidized LDL cholesterol. Several studies have suggested that blood pressure is inversely related to vitamin C status; however, the data are not conclusive.[29] It has been hypothesized that vitamin C reduces blood cholesterol because it is involved in the synthesis of bile acids from cholesterol in the liver. Adequate vitamin C allows cholesterol to be used for bile synthesis and therefore may reduce the amount of cholesterol in the blood. In addition, vitamin C is an antioxidant that may delay atherosclerosis by preventing the oxidation of LDL cholesterol (see Chapter 5).[29] Despite these important roles of vitamin C in modulating blood cholesterol levels and protecting LDL cholesterol from oxidation, data thus far from epidemiology and human intervention trials have provided little evidence to support the use of vitamin C supplements in preventing atherosclerosis in humans.[30]

Vitamin C and Cancer It has been suggested that high doses of vitamin C both treat and prevent cancer. Although controlled trials have not found any benefits of vitamin C in the treatment of patients with advanced cancer,[31] there is evidence supporting a role for vitamin C in cancer prevention. Epidemiological studies have found inverse relationships between dietary vitamin C intake and cancers of the cervix, breast, rectum, lungs, stomach, mouth, and pancreas.[32] As an antioxidant, vitamin C may protect against cancers caused by oxidative damage. In the case of gastrointestinal cancers, vitamin C may prevent cancer by inhibiting the formation of carcinogenic nitrosamines (see Chapter 17). Despite the association between higher intakes of vitamin C and a lower incidence of various cancers, these studies cannot rule out factors other than vitamin C found in fruits and vegetables that might be responsible for the protective effect.[33]

• CHOLINE: IS IT A VITAMIN?

Choline is needed to synthesize a number of important molecules, including a phospholipid found in cell membranes, the neurotransmitter acetylcholine, and the methyl donor betaine. It is also an important source of carbon atoms in biochemical reactions. Choline can be synthesized to a limited extent by humans and is not currently classified as a vitamin. However, there is evidence that it is essential in healthy men. There is not enough information to determine if choline is also essential in the diets of women, infants, children, and older adults.[2]

Choline is widely distributed in foods. Particularly good sources include egg yolks, organ meats, spinach, nuts, and wheat germ. Average daily choline intake is estimated to be about 600 to 1000 mg per day. An AI of 550 mg per day for men and 425 mg per day for women has been established based on the amount needed to prevent liver damage. There are few data to assess whether dietary choline is needed at all stages of life. At some stages, requirements may be met by synthesis in the body. Choline deficiency causes liver abnormalities. Deficiency is unlikely in healthy humans, but it has been observed in individuals fed a choline-deficient diet and in those receiving total parenteral nutrition without choline.[2] Choline is required by human cells grown in culture, and prolonged deficiency in animals leads to fat accumulation in the liver and may contribute to liver cancer.

Intakes of choline that are much higher than can be obtained from foods can cause body odor, sweating, reduced growth rate, low blood pressure, and liver damage. A UL for adults of 3.5 g per day has been set based on the occurrence of low blood pressure.

• APPLICATIONS •

1. Use your food intake record from Chapter 2 to answer the following:
   a. How much folate does your diet contain?
   b. How does your intake compare with the RDA?
   c. If your diet doesn't meet recommendations, suggest modifications to meet the RDA for folate.
   d. List some natural sources of folate in your diet and some foods fortified with folic acid.
2. Evaluate each of the following supplements:
   Pyridoxine: 100 mg dose
   Stress tab: pyridoxine, 35 mg; thiamin, 1 mg; riboflavin, 1.1 mg; niacin, 30 mg; choline, 500 mg
   Folic acid: 800 μg dose

   a. Do any of them create a risk for toxicity? Which ones and why?
   b. Would you recommend them for everyone? For a specific group? Why or why not?
3. Using the Internet, find a website for a nutritional supplement manufacturer. What is the highest dose of pyridoxine that you see included in one of its products? Is this a safe dose? What advertising promises are included with supplements containing pyridoxine? Evaluate these claims for accuracy. What forms of niacin are in supplements marketed by this company? How much niacin is included per dose? Is this a safe level of intake?

SUMMARY

1. Vitamins are essential organic nutrients that do not provide energy and are required in small quantities in the diet to promote and regulate body activities needed for growth, reproduction, and tissue maintenance. They are classified by their solubility in either water or fat.

2. We consume vitamins that are naturally present in foods, added to foods by fortification and enrichment, and contained in supplements.

3. The amount of a vitamin that is available to the body is regulated by vitamin absorption, transport, activation, storage, and excretion.

4. Vitamin deficiencies remain a major health problem worldwide. In industrialized countries, marginal dietary deficiencies and toxicities from supplements are a growing concern.

5. Recommended intakes for vitamins are expressed as RDAs or AIs. UL values estimate the highest dose that is unlikely to cause toxicity.

6. The active forms of thiamin, riboflavin, niacin, biotin, and pantothenic acid function as coenzymes in reactions involved in the metabolism of carbohydrate, fat, and protein.

7. Thiamin is required for the generation of energy from carbohydrate, fat, and protein and for the synthesis of the neurotransmitter acetylcholine. The best food sources are lean pork, legumes, and whole or enriched grains. Thiamin deficiency, or beriberi, causes nervous system abnormalities. Deficiencies are common in alcoholics. No toxicity has been identified.

8. Riboflavin coenzymes are needed for the generation of energy. Riboflavin deficiency is rarely seen alone because food sources of riboflavin are also sources of other B vitamins and because riboflavin is needed for the utilization of several other vitamins. Milk, meat, and enriched grain products are the best food sources. No toxicity has been identified.

9. Niacin coenzymes are important in the breakdown of carbohydrate, fat, and protein and in the synthesis of fatty acids and sterols. A deficiency results in pellagra, which is characterized by dermatitis, diarrhea, dementia, and finally, if untreated, death. Beef, chicken, turkey, fish, and enriched grain products are the best food sources. The amino acid tryptophan can be converted into niacin, so dietary tryptophan can meet some of the niacin requirement. Supplements of the nicotinic acid form of niacin can lower elevated blood cholesterol but frequently cause toxicity symptoms such as flushing, tingling sensations, nausea, and a red skin rash.

10. Biotin is needed for the synthesis of glucose and fatty acids, and the metabolism of certain amino acids. An RDA has not been established because some of our biotin need is met by bacterial synthesis in the gastrointestinal tract. However, an AI has been set. Liver and egg yolks are good sources. Toxicity has not been reported.

11. Pantothenic acid is part of coenzyme A (CoA), which is required for the production of energy from carbohydrate, fat, and protein and the synthesis of cholesterol and fat. It is abundant in the food supply, and deficiency is rare. There is no RDA, but an AI has been established.

12. Pyridoxal phosphate, the coenzyme form of vitamin B_6, is needed for the activity of more than 100 enzymes involved in the metabolism of carbohydrate, fat, and protein. Vitamin B_6 is particularly important for amino acid metabolism. Food sources include chicken, fish, liver, eggs, and whole grains. Large doses of vitamin B_6 can cause nervous system abnormalities.

13. Folate is necessary for the synthesis of DNA, so it is especially important for rapidly dividing cells. Folate deficiency results in macrocytic anemia. Low levels of folate before and during early pregnancy are associated with an increased incidence of neural tube defects in the offspring. It is recommended that women of child-bearing age consume 400 μg of folic acid from fortified foods and supplements in addition to the folate found in a varied diet. Food sources include liver, legumes, oranges, leafy green vegetables, and fortified grains. A high intake of folate can mask the early symptoms of vitamin B_{12} deficiency.

14. Vitamin B_{12} is needed for the metabolism of folate and fatty acids and to maintain the insulating layer of myelin surrounding nerves. Deficiency results in anemia and permanent nerve damage. Vitamin B_{12} is found almost exclusively in animal products. The absorption of vitamin B_{12} from food requires adequate levels of stomach acid, intrinsic factor, and pancreatic secretions. Marginal deficiency is a concern in vegans, who consume no animal products, and in older individuals in whom stomach acid secretion is reduced.

15. Vitamin C is necessary for the synthesis and maintenance of connective tissue and for the synthesis of hormones and neurotransmitters. Vitamin C deficiency, called scurvy, is characterized by poor wound healing, bleeding, and other symptoms related to the improper formation and maintenance of collagen. The best food sources are citrus fruits. Vitamin C supplements are the most commonly taken vitamin supplements and are usually used to reduce the symptoms of the common cold.

16. Vitamin C is a water-soluble antioxidant. Antioxidants protect the body from reactive oxygen molecules such as free radicals. These molecules are generated from normal body reactions and come from the environment. They cause damage by stealing electrons from DNA, proteins, carbohydrates, and unsaturated fatty acids.

17. Choline is a substance necessary for metabolism and is not currently classified as a vitamin. It may be required in the diet at certain stages of life, so an AI has been established.

REVIEW QUESTIONS

1. What is a vitamin?

2. List four factors that affect how much of a vitamin is available to the body.

3. What do enrichment and fortification mean?

4. List a function common to all of the B vitamins.

5. Why is thiamin deficiency a concern in alcoholics?

6. Why should milk be packaged in opaque containers?

7. What is pellagra?

8. How is vitamin B_6 involved in protein metabolism?

9. Why is low folate intake of particular concern for women of childbearing age?

10. Why would someone who has had his stomach removed (or had gastric bypass surgery) need to receive injections of vitamin B_{12} to meet his needs?

11. Why are vegans at risk for vitamin B_{12} deficiency? the elderly?

12. Why does vitamin C deficiency cause poor wound healing?

13. What are reactive oxygen molecules, and how do they cause damage?

14. What is the role of antioxidants and pro-oxidants in oxidative stress?

15. Does choline fit the definition of a vitamin? Why or why not?

REFERENCES

1. Tanphaichitr, V. Thiamin. In *Modern Nutrition in Health and Disease*, 9th ed. Shils, M. E., Olson, J. A., Shike, M., and Ross, A. C., eds. Baltimore: Williams & Wilkins, 1999, 381–389.

2. Institute of Medicine, Food and Nutrition Board. *Dietary Reference Intakes for Thiamin, Riboflavin, Niacin, Vitamin B-6, Folate, Vitamin B-12, Pantothenic Acid, Biotin, and Choline.* Washington, D.C.: National Academy Press, 1998.

3. Potter, N. N., and Hotchkiss, J. H. *Food Science*, 5th ed. New York: Chapman & Hall, 1995.

4. Syndenstricker, V. P. The history of pellagra, its recognition as a disorder of nutrition and its conquest. *Am. J. Clin. Nutr.* 6:409–441, 1958.

5. Morgan, J. M., Capuzzi, D. M., and Guyton, J. R. A new extended-release niacin (Niaspan): Efficacy, tolerability, and safety in hypercholesterolemic patients. *Am. J. Cardiol.* 8229U–8234U, 1998.

6. Guyton, J. R., Blazing, M. A., Hagar, J., et al. Extended-release niacin vs gemfibrozil for the treatment of low levels of high-density lipoprotein cholesterol. Niaspan-Gemfibrozil Study Group. *Arch. Intern. Med.* 160:1177–1184, 2000.

7. Gibbons, K. W., Gonzales, V., Gordon, N., and Grundy, S. The prevalence of side effects with regular and sustained release nicotinic acid. *Am. J. Med.* 99:378–385, 1995.

8. USDA Agricultural Research Service. Results from USDA 1994–1996 CSFII. 1997.

9. Bessey, O. A., Adam, D. J., and Hansen, A. E. Intake of vitamin B_6 and infantile convulsions: a first approximation of requirements of pyridoxine in infants. *Pediatrics* 20:33–44, 1957.

10. Wilcken, D. E., and Wilcken, B. The natural history of vascular disease in homocystinuria and the effects of treatment. *J. Inherit. Metab. Dis.* 20:295–300, 1997.

11. Ford, E. S., Smith, S. J., Stroup, D. F., et al. Homocyst(e)ine and cardiovascular disease: a systematic review of the evidence with special emphasis on case-control studies and nested case-control studies. *Int. J. Epi.* 31:59–70, 2002.

12. Rimm, E. B., Willett, W. C., Hu, F. B., et al. Folate and vitamin B_6 from diet and supplements in relation to risk of coronary heart disease among women. *JAMA* 279:359–364, 1998.

13. Schnyder, G., Roffi, M., Pin, R., et al. Decreased rate of coronary restenosis after lowering of plasma homocysteine levels. *N. Engl. J. Med.* 345:1593–1600, 2001.

14. Schaumburg, H., Kaplan, J., Windebank, A., et al. Sensory neuropathy from pyridoxine abuse. *N. Engl. J. Med.* 309:445–448, 1983.

15. Keniston, R. C., Nathan, P. A., Leklem, J. E., and Lockwood, R. S. Vitamin B6, vitamin C, and carpal tunnel syndrome. A cross-sectional study of 441 adults. *J. Occup. Environ. Med.* 38:949–959, 1997.

16. Wyatt, K. M., Dimmock, P. W., Jones, P. W., and Shaughn O'Brien, P. M. Efficacy of vitamin B-6 in the treatment of premenstrual syndrome: Systematic review. *B.M.J.* 318:1375–1381, 1999.

17. Lesourd, B. M., Mazari, L., and Ferry, M. The role of nutrition in immunity in the aged. *Nutr. Rev.* 56(II):S113–S125, 1998.

18. Honein, M., Paulozzi, L., Mathews, T., et al. Impact of folic acid fortification in the US food supply on the occurrence of neural tube defects. *JAMA* 285:2981–2986, 2001.

19. Prinz-Langenohl, R., Fohr, I., and Pietrzik, K. Beneficial role for folate in the prevention of colorectal and breast cancer. *Eur. J. Nutr.* 40:98–105, 2001.

20. Su, L. J., and Arab, L. Nutritional status of folate and colon cancer risk: Evidence from NHANES I epidemiologic follow-up study. *Ann. Epidemiol.* 11:65–72, 2001.

21. Messina, V. K., and Burke, K. I. Position of the American Dietetic Association: Vegetarian diets. *J. Am. Diet. Assoc.* 97:1317–1321, 1997.

22. Keohler, K. M., Pareo-Tubbeh, S. L., Romero, L. J., et al. Folate nutrition and older adults: challenges and opportunities. *J. Am. Diet. Assoc.* 97:167–173, 1997.

23. Halliwell, B. Antioxidants and human disease: a general introduction. *Nutr. Rev.* 55:(II)S44–S52, 1997.

24. Food and Nutrition Board, Institute of Medicine. *Dietary Reference Intakes for Vitamin C, Vitamin E, Selenium, and Carotenoids.* Washington, D.C.: National Academy Press, 2000.

25. Carr, A., and Frei, B. Does vitamin C act as a pro-oxidant under physiological conditions? *FASEB J.* 13:1007–24, 1999.

26. Hemilä, H. Does vitamin C alleviate the symptoms of the common cold? A review of current evidence. *Scand. J. Infect. Dis.* 26:1–6, 1994.

27. Jari, R. J., and Harakeh, S. Antiviral and immunomodulatory activities of ascorbic acid. In *Subcellular Biochemistry*, vol. 25: *Ascorbic Acid: Biochemistry and Biomedical Cell Biology*. Harris, J. R., ed. New York: Plenum Press, 1996, 215–231.

28. Johnston, C. S. The antihistamine action of ascorbic acid. In *Subcellular Biochemistry*, vol. 25: *Ascorbic Acid: Biochemistry and Biomedical Cell Biology*. Harris, J. R., ed. New York: Plenum Press, 1996, 189–213.

29. Lynch, S. M., Gaziano, M., and Frei, B. Ascorbic acid and atherosclerotic cardiovascular disease. In *Subcellular Biochemistry*, vol. 25: *Ascorbic Acid: Biochemistry and Biomedical Cell Biology*. Harris, J. R., ed. New York: Plenum Press, 1996, 331–367.

30. Lonn, E. M., and Yusuf, S. Is there a role for antioxidant vitamins in the prevention of cardiovascular diseases? An update on epidemiological and clinical trials data. *Can. J. Cardiol.* 13:957–965, 1997.

31. Shklar, G., and Schwartz, J. L. Ascorbic acid and cancer. In *Subcellular Biochemistry*, vol. 25: *Ascorbic Acid: Biochemistry and Biomedical Cell Biology*. Harris, J. R., ed. New York: Plenum Press, 1996, 233–247.

32. Head, K. A. Ascorbic acid in the prevention and treatment of cancer. *Altern. Med. Rev.* 3:174–186, 1998.

33. van Poppel, G., and van den Berg, H. Vitamins and cancer. *Cancer Lett.* 19:195–202, 1997.

The Fat-Soluble Vitamins Chapter 9

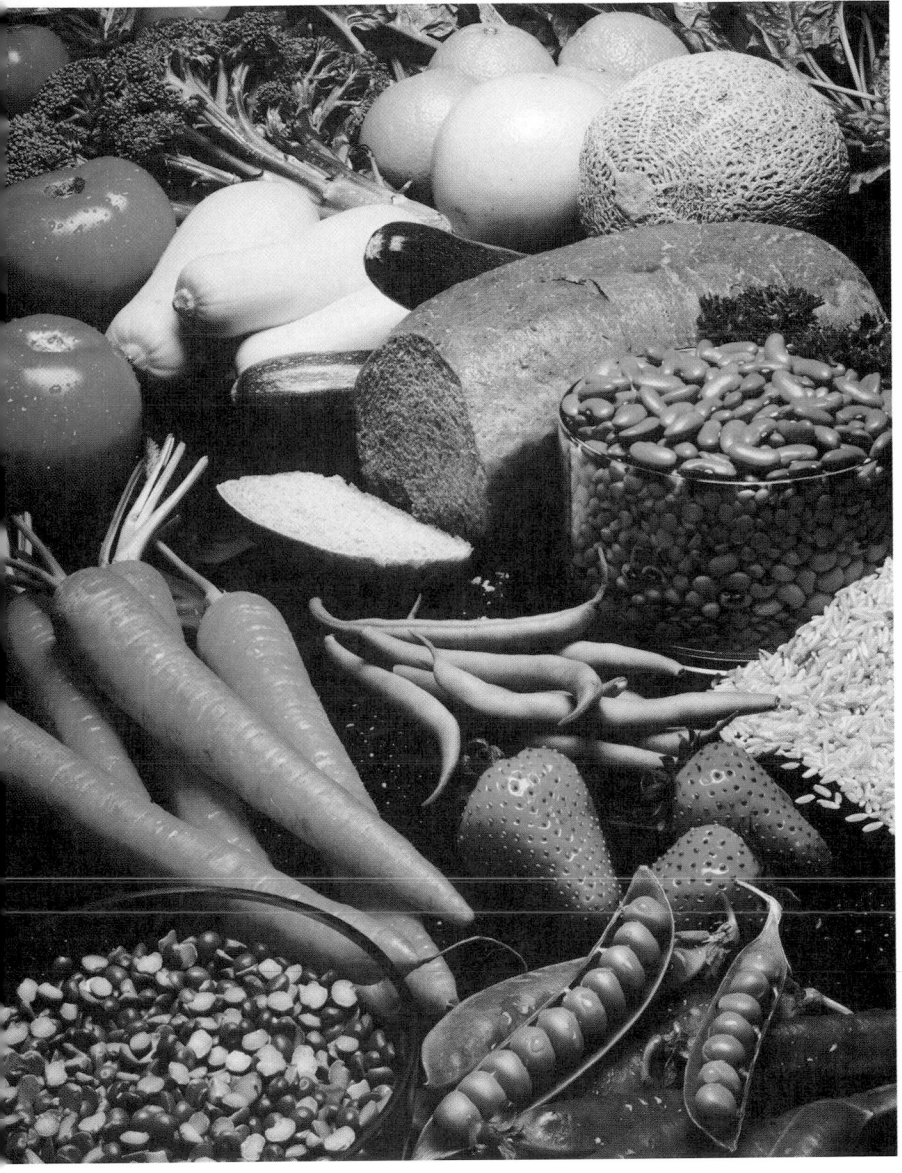

(© Nathan Benn/Corbis)

Chapter Outline

Chapter Concepts

✔ The fat-soluble vitamins are grouped together because of their solubility, but each has unique functions.

✔ Vitamin A is essential for vision, and it regulates cell differentiation and growth by affecting gene expression.

✔ β-carotene and some other carotenoids are vitamin A precursors and also act as antioxidants.

✔ When exposure to sunlight is limited, vitamin D is a dietary essential. It acts by affecting gene expression and is necessary for the formation and maintenance of bone.

✔ Vitamin E is an antioxidant that protects lipid membranes.

✔ Vitamin K is necessary for blood clotting.

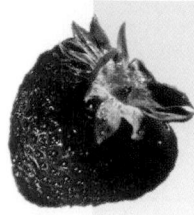

Just a Taste

Does eating carrots improve your vision?

Will vitamin E prevent heart disease?

Can you get vitamins from the sun?

Each of the fat-soluble vitamins has a unique and unrelated function. Vitamin A keeps our eyes healthy, vitamin D keeps our bones strong, vitamin K allows our blood to clot, and vitamin E protects us from oxidative damage. Unlike the water-soluble vitamins, many of which have similar sources and overlapping functions, the fat-soluble vitamins are marked by contrasts—contrasts in their functions and in how deficiencies and excesses affect health. Vitamins A and D are among the most toxic of the vitamins, yet diets deficient in these affect the health of millions, especially children. The deficiency symptoms that occur with these two vitamins are dramatic and life-threatening yet the symptoms of vitamin E deficiency are so subtle that for a time it was thought of as a vitamin in search of a disease because no specific human deficiency disease could be identified. Vitamin K deficiency causes uncontrolled bleeding, but drugs to inhibit vitamin K and prevent blood from clotting save thousands of lives every year. The four fat-soluble vitamins are so different from each other that the DRI committees have evaluated their requirements in three different nutrient groups—Vitamin D with minerals involved in bone formation, vitamin E with antioxidants, and vitamin A and K with an assortment of trace minerals.

• VITAMIN A: A VITAMIN THAT TURNS ON OUR GENES

Are carrots really good for your eyes? Carrots are high in a precursor of vitamin A, and vitamin A is important for vision. This connection between vision and foods that we now know are high in vitamin A has been known for centuries. In ancient times, the Egyptians knew that eating liver could treat night blindness, a difficulty in adjusting from bright light to dim light, such as when a bright light strikes your eyes at night. In 1968, George Wald earned the Nobel Prize in medicine for identifying the mechanism by which vitamin A is involved in vision. Although this is a key function of vitamin A, attention today is focused more on how vitamin A interacts with genes to regulate growth and **cell differentiation**. Despite our expanding understanding of the functions of vitamin A, deficiency remains a world health problem.

Vitamin A in the Diet

Vitamin A is found preformed and in precursor or provitamin forms in our diet. Preformed vitamin A compounds are known as **retinoids**. The retinoids include retinal, retinol, and retinoic acid. They are found in animal foods such as liver, fish, egg yolks, and dairy products. Margarine and nonfat and reduced-fat milk are fortified with vitamin A because they are often consumed in place of butter and whole milk, which are good sources of this vitamin.

Plant sources of vitamin A, including carrots, cantaloupe, apricots, mangoes, and sweet potatoes, contain yellow-orange pigments called **carotenoids**. About 50 of the 600 carotenoids that have been isolated provide vitamin A activity. **Beta-carotene (β-carotene)**, the most potent precursor, is plentiful in carrots, squash, and other red and yellow vegetables and fruits as well as in leafy greens where the yellow pig-

Cell differentiation Structural and functional changes that cause cells to mature into specialized cells.

Retinoids The chemical forms of preformed vitamin A: retinol, retinal, and retinoic acid.

Carotenoids Natural pigments synthesized by plants and many microorganisms. They give yellow and red-orange fruits and vegetables their color.

Beta-carotene (β-carotene) A carotenoid that has more provitamin A activity than other carotenoids. It also acts as an antioxidant.

250

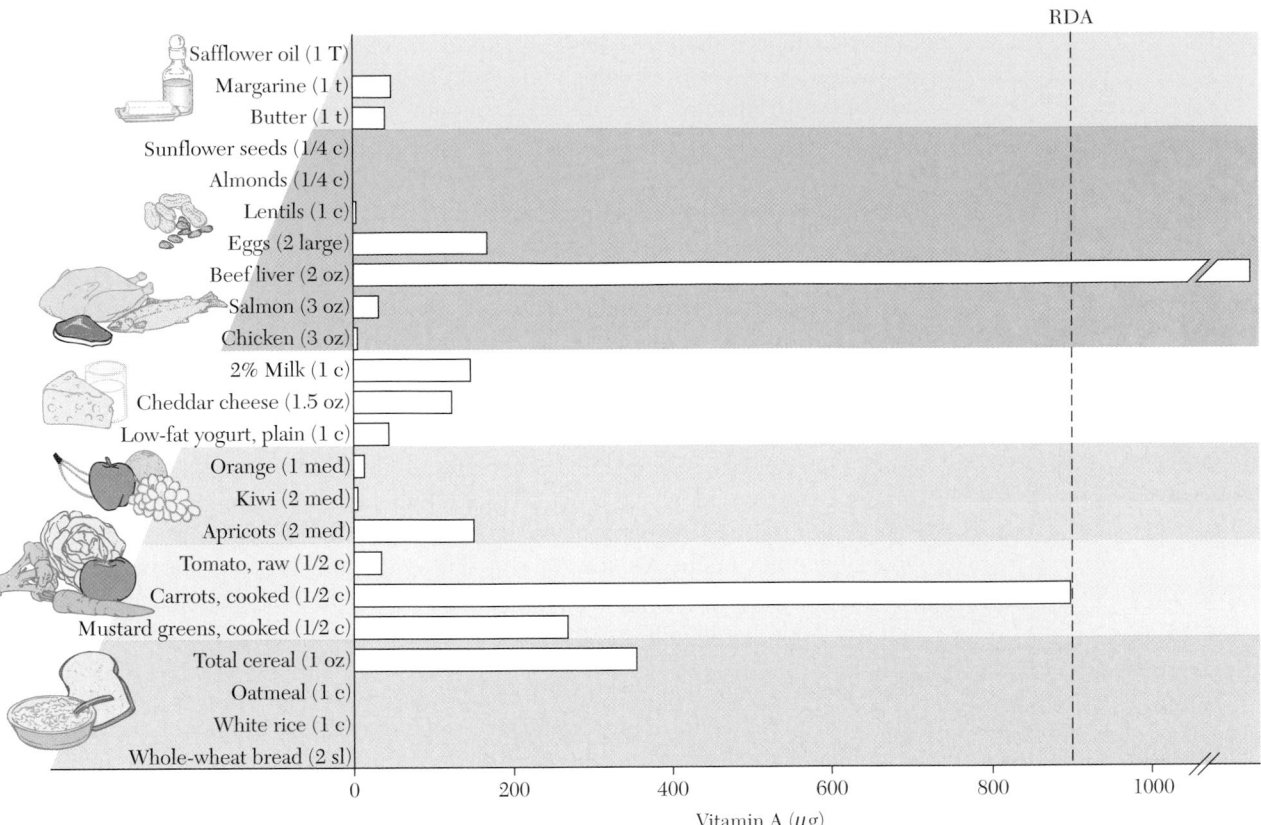

Figure 9.1
Vitamin A content of selections from each food group of the Food Guide Pyramid. The dashed line represents the RDA for adult men. Both plant and animal foods are good sources of vitamin A.

ment is masked by green chlorophyll (Figure 9.1). Other carotenoids that provide some provitamin A activity include α-carotene found in leafy green vegetables, carrots, and squash, and β-cryptoxanthin found in corn, green peppers, and lemons.[1] Lutein, lycopene, and zeaxanthin are carotenoids with no vitamin A activity.

To help consumers identify food sources of vitamin A, labels on packaged foods must list the vitamin A content as a percentage of the Daily Value. All forms of vitamin A in the diet are fairly stable when heated but may be destroyed by exposure to light and oxygen.

Vitamin A in the Digestive Tract

Both retinoids and carotenoids are bound to proteins in foods. To be absorbed, they must be released from the protein by pepsin and other protein-digesting enzymes. Then the released carotenoids and retinoids must combine with bile acids and other fat-soluble food components to form micelles, which facilitate their diffusion into mucosal cells. Absorption of preformed vitamin A is efficient—70 to 90% of what is consumed. Carotenoids are less well absorbed, and absorption decreases as intake increases.[2] Once inside the mucosal cells, much of the β-carotene is converted to retinal and then retinol.

Insufficient fat intake (less than 10 g/day) can reduce vitamin A absorption. This is rarely a problem in industrialized countries, where typical fat intake ranges from 50 to 100 grams per day. However, in populations with low dietary fat intakes, vitamin A deficiency may occur due to poor absorption. Diseases that cause fat malabsorption can also interfere with vitamin A absorption and cause a deficiency.

Consumption of large amounts of the artificial fat Olestra (sucrose polyester) interferes with vitamin A absorption. Olestra cannot be digested and absorbed in the human digestive tract. As it passes through the intestine, it takes fat-soluble substances with it. It therefore decreases the absorption of the fat-soluble vitamins A, D, E, and K, as well as β-carotene and other carotenoids. Foods containing Olestra are fortified with vitamins A, D, E, and K, but not with carotenoids.

Vitamin A in the Body

Retinol-binding protein A protein that is necessary to transport vitamin A from the liver to other tissues.

Retinoids and carotenoids are transported from the intestine in chylomicrons. These lipoproteins deliver the retinoids and carotenoids to body tissues such as bone marrow, blood cells, spleen, muscles, kidney, and liver. In the liver, some carotenoids can be converted into retinol. To move from liver stores to the tissues, preformed vitamin A must be bound to **retinol-binding protein**. There is no specific blood transport protein for carotenoids, but since they are fat soluble, they are incorporated into lipoproteins to travel in the bloodstream.

The different forms of vitamin A have different functions. Retinol and retinal can be interconverted from one to the other. Retinal is the form that is important for vision. Retinoic acid, which is made from retinol or retinal, cannot be used in the visual cycle (see next section) but is the form that affects gene expression and is responsible for vitamin A's role in cell differentiation, growth, and reproduction.[3] Carotenoids that are not converted to retinoids may act as antioxidants or provide other biological functions.

Rhodopsin A light-sensitive compound found in the retina of the eye that is composed of the protein opsin loosely bound to retinal.

The Visual Cycle Vitamin A is involved in the perception of light (Figure 9.2). In the eye, the retinal form of the vitamin combines with the protein opsin to form the visual pigment **rhodopsin**. Rhodopsin helps transform the energy from light into a nerve impulse that is sent to the brain. This nerve impulse allows us to see.

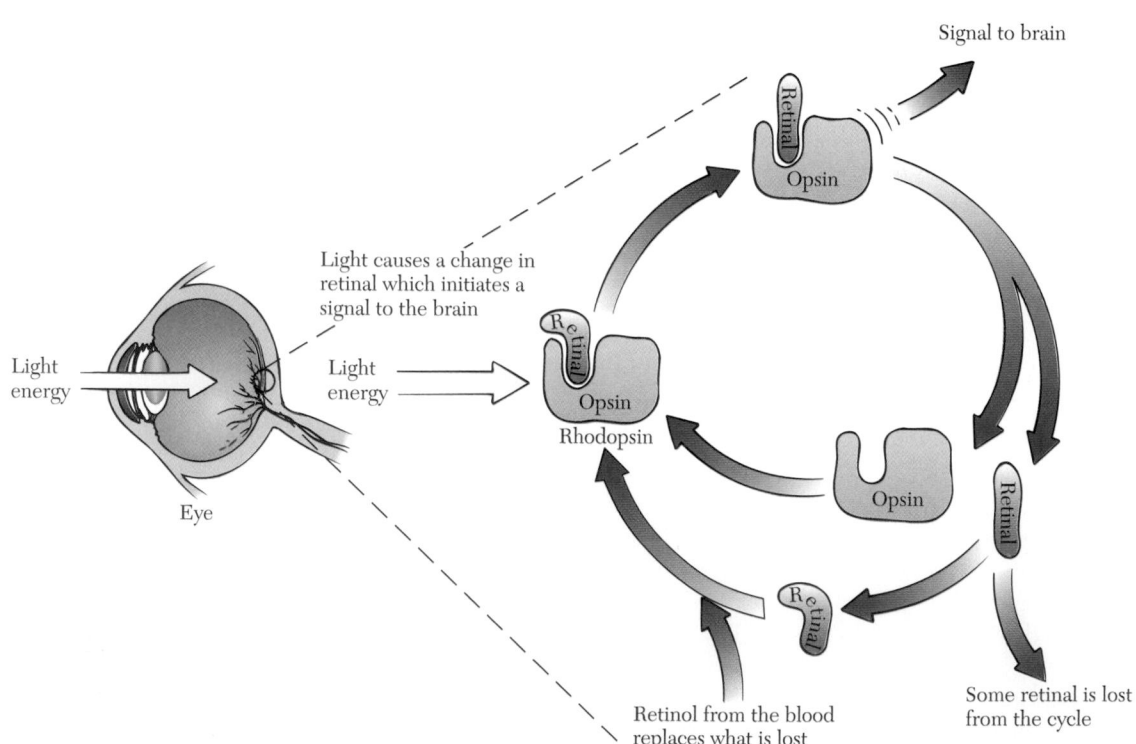

Figure 9.2

In the visual cycle in the eye, retinal binds to the protein opsin to form rhodopsin. When light strikes rhodopsin, it causes a change in retinal that sends a nerve signal to the brain and causes retinal to be released from opsin. Some retinal returns to its original form and binds opsin to begin the cycle again. Some retinal is lost, and retinol from the blood must be converted to replace it.

The visual cycle begins when light passes into the eye and strikes rhodopsin. The light changes retinal in rhodopsin from a curved molecule to a straight one by converting a *cis* double bond in retinal to a *trans* double bond. This change in shape initiates a series of events causing a nerve signal to be sent to the brain and retinal to be released from opsin. After the light stimulus has passed, the *trans* retinal is converted back to its original *cis* form and recombined with opsin to regenerate rhodopsin. Each time this cycle occurs, some retinal is lost and must be replaced by retinol from the blood. The retinol is converted into retinal in the eye. When vitamin A is deficient, there is a delay in the regeneration of rhodopsin, which causes difficulty in adapting to dim light after experiencing a bright light—a condition called night blindness. Night blindness is one of the first and more easily reversible symptoms of vitamin A deficiency.

Regulating Gene Expression: Cell Differentiation Cell differentiation is the process whereby immature cells change in structure and function to become specialized. For instance, in the bone marrow, some cells differentiate into white blood cells, whereas others differentiate to form red blood cells. Vitamin A affects cell differentiation through its effect on gene expression. This means that it can turn on or turn off the production of certain proteins that regulate functions within cells and throughout the body. By affecting gene expression, vitamin A can also determine what type of cell an immature cell will become.

In order to affect gene expression, the retinoic acid form of vitamin A enters specific target cells. Inside the nucleus of these target cells, retinoic acid binds to protein receptors; this retinoic acid-protein receptor complex then binds to regulatory regions of DNA. This binding changes the amount of messenger RNA (mRNA) that is made by the gene. The change in mRNA changes the amount of the protein that is produced (Figure 9.3). This turning on (or turning off) of the gene increases (or decreases) the production of proteins and thereby affects various cellular functions. For example, vitamin A turns on a gene that makes an enzyme in liver cells, which enables the liver to make glucose by gluconeogenesis.

Maintenance of Epithelial Tissue Vitamin A is necessary for the maintenance of epithelial tissue. This type of tissue covers external body surfaces and lines internal cavities and tubes. It includes the skin and the linings of the eyes, intestines, lungs, vagina, and bladder. When vitamin A is deficient, epithelial cells do not differentiate normally because vitamin A is not there to turn on or turn off the production of particular proteins. For example, the epithelial tissue on many body surfaces contains

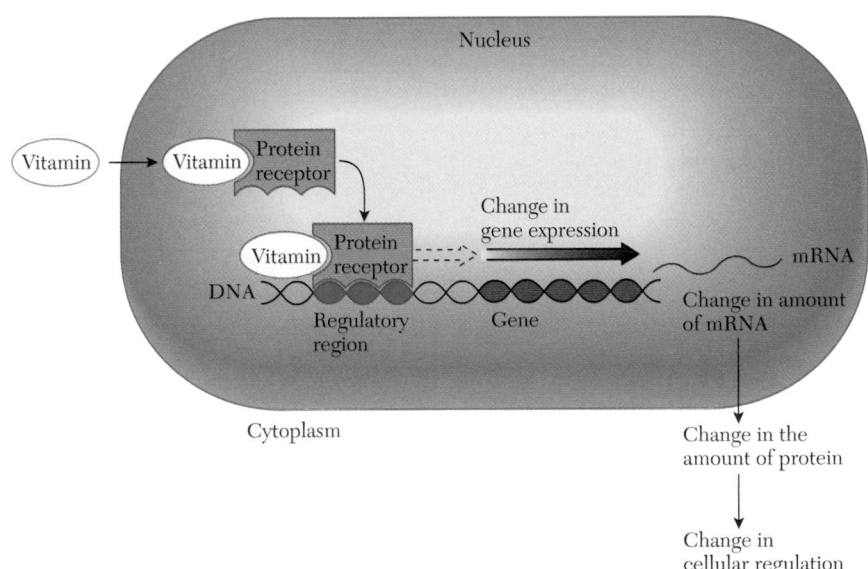

Figure 9.3

The retinoic acid form of vitamin A (shown as the yellow vitamin) functions by entering the nucleus and binding to a protein receptor. The complex then binds to a regulatory region of DNA to change the expression of a gene and hence the amount of a protein synthesized as well as the cellular functions and body processes that are affected by this protein.

Keratin A hard protein that makes up hair and nails.

cells that produce mucus for lubrication. When mucus-secreting cells die, new cells differentiate into mucus-secreting cells to replace them. When vitamin A is deficient, the new cells do not differentiate properly and instead become cells that produce a protein called **keratin**. Keratin is the hard protein that makes up hair and fingernails. As the mucus-secreting cells die and are replaced by keratin-producing cells, the epithelial surface becomes hard and dry. This process is known as keratinization. The hard, dry surface does not have the protective capabilities of normal epithelium and increases the likelihood of infection. The risk of infection is compounded by the fact that vitamin A deficiency also decreases immune function.

All epithelial tissues are affected by vitamin A deficiency, but the eye is particularly susceptible to damage. The mucus in the eye normally provides lubrication, washes away dirt and other particles, and also contains a protein that helps destroy bacteria. When vitamin A is deficient, the lack of mucus and the buildup of keratin cause the cornea to dry and leave the eye open to infection. A spectrum of eye disorders known as **xerophthalmia** is associated with vitamin A deficiency. In the early stages, xeropthalmia can be treated by increasing vitamin A intake but if left untreated, it can result in a softening of the cornea, called keratomalacia, and permanent blindness.

Xerophthalmia A spectrum of eye conditions resulting from vitamin A deficiency that may lead to blindness. An early symptom is night blindness, and as deficiency worsens, lack of mucus leaves the eye dry and vulnerable to cracking and infection.

Reproduction, Growth, and Immunity The ability of vitamin A to regulate the growth and differentiation of cells makes it essential throughout life for normal reproduction, growth, and immune function. In reproduction, vitamin A is hypothesized to play a role during early embryonic development by directing cells to form the shapes and patterns needed for a completely formed organism.[4] Poor overall growth is an early sign of vitamin A deficiency in children. Vitamin A affects the activity of cells that form and break down bone, and a deficiency early in life can cause abnormal jawbone growth, resulting in crooked teeth and poor dental health. In the immune system, vitamin A is needed for the differentiation that produces the different types of immune cells. When vitamin A is deficient, the activity of specific immune cells cannot be stimulated. This impaired immune function increases the risk of illness and infection due to defective epithelial tissue barriers.

β-carotene: A Vitamin A Precursor and an Antioxidant Some carotenoids, particularly β-carotene, can be converted to vitamin A in the intestinal mucosa. Unconverted carotenoids also reach the blood and tissues where they may function as antioxidants, a role independent of any conversion to vitamin A. β-carotene and other carotenoids are fat-soluble antioxidants that may play a role in protecting cell membranes from damage by free radicals. The antioxidant properties of carotenoids have stimulated interest in their ability to protect against diseases in which oxidative processes play a role, such as cancer, heart disease, and impaired vision due to macular degeneration and cataracts. However, currently the evidence for their roles in the living body is not strong enough for the DRIs to categorize them as dietary antioxidants.[2]

How Much Vitamin A Do We Need?

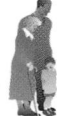

The recommended intake for vitamin A is based on the amount needed to maintain normal body stores. The RDA is set at 900 μg of vitamin A per day for men and 700 μg per day for women (Table 9.1).[2] There is no recommendation to increase intake above this level for older adults. The RDA is increased in pregnancy to account for the vitamin A that is transferred to the fetus and during lactation to account for the vitamin A lost in milk. The RDA for children is set lower than that for adults based on their smaller body size. For infants, an AI has been set based on the amount of vitamin A consumed by an average healthy breastfed infant.

Recommendations for vitamin A intake are expressed in μg of retinol. This can be supplied by both retinol and carotenoids in the diet. No quantitative recommendations have been made for intakes of β-carotene or other carotenoids alone. Their intake is considered only with regard to the amount of retinol they provide. Because

Table 9.1 *A Summary of the Fat-Soluble Vitamins*

Vitamin	Sources	Recommended Intake for Adults	Major Functions	Deficiency Diseases and Symptoms	Groups at Risk	Toxicity	Tolerable Upper Intake Level (UL)
Vitamin A (vitamin A acetate, vitamin A palmitate, retinol, retinal, retinoic acid, retinyl palmitate, provitamin A, carotene, β-carotene, carotenoids)	Liver, fish, carrots peaches, leafy greens, fortified milk, sweet potatoes, broccoli	700–900 μg	Vision, growth, cell differentiation, reproduction, immune function	Night blindness, xerophthalmia, poor growth, dry skin, impaired immunity	Those who live in poverty (particularly children and pregnant women), those consuming very lowfat or low-protein diets	Headache, vomiting, hair loss, liver damage, skin changes, birth defects, bone pain	3000 μg/day preformed vitamin A
Vitamin D (cholecalciferol, ergocalciferol)	Egg yolk, liver, fish oils, tuna, salmon, fortified margarine and milk, sunlight	5-15 μg°	Absorption of calcium and phosphorus, maintenance of bone	Rickets in children, osteomalacia in adults	Breast-fed infants, children and elderly (especially with dark skin and little sun exposure), people with kidney disease	Calcium deposits in the soft tissues, growth retardation, kidney damage	50 μg/day
Vitamin E (alpha-tocopherol acetate, alpha-tocopherol	Vegetable oils, leafy greens, nuts, peanuts	15 mg	Antioxidant, protects cell membranes	Hemolyzed red blood cells, nerve damage	Those with poor fat absorption, premature infants	Inhibition of vitamin K activity	1000 mg/day from supplemental sources
Vitamin K (phylloquinone, menaquinone)	Vegetable oils, leafy greens, intestinal bacteria	90–120 μg°	Blood clotting	Hemorrhage	People on long-term antibiotics, newborns (especially premature)	Anemia, brain damage	ND

°Adequate Intake (AI).

ND = Insufficient evidence to set a UL

carotenoids are less well absorbed and not completely converted to vitamin A, a correction factor, referred to as **retinol activity equivalents (RAE)**, must be applied to carotenoids to determine the amount of usable vitamin A they provide. Twelve μg of β-carotene provide 1 RAE of vitamin A, and 24 μg α-carotene or β-cryptoxanthin provide 1 RAE.[2]

As our understanding of vitamin A has increased, the units in which recommended intakes have been expressed have changed. These older values are still found in food composition databases and tables. The 1989 RDAs used values called retinol equivalents (RE) to account for differences in absorption between retinoids and carotenoids. Prior to 1980, vitamin A was also expressed in international units (IUs). Values for converting REs and IUs to usable vitamin A are given in Table 9.2.

Retinol activity equivalent (RAE) The amount of retinol, β-carotene, α-carotene, or β-cryptoxanthin that provides vitamin A activity equal to 1μg of retinol.

Vitamin A and Health

Vitamin A deficiency is a world health problem responsible for growth failure, increased susceptibility to infection, blindness, and death. Consumption of too much preformed vitamin A, however, can also be deadly. A low intake of carotenoids is not associated with any specific deficiency disease as long as sufficient preformed vitamin A is supplied in the diet.

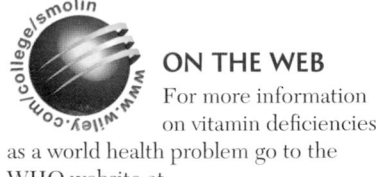

ON THE WEB
For more information on vitamin deficiencies as a world health problem go to the WHO website at
www.who.int

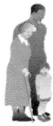

Vitamin A Deficiency: A World Health Problem Vitamin A deficiency is a threat to the health, sight, and lives of millions of children in the developing world.[5] Children deficient in vitamin A have poor appetites, are anemic, and have an increased

Table 9.2 *Converting Vitamin A Units into μg Vitamin A*

Form and source	Amount equal to 1 μg retinol
Preformed vitamin A in food or (supplements)	1 μg
	1 RAE
	1 μg RE
	3.3 IU
β-carotene in food°	12 μg
	1 RAE
	2 μg RE
	20 IU
α-carotene or β-cryptoxanthin in food	24 μg
	1 RAE
	2 μg RE
	40 IU

°Beta-carotene in supplements may be better absorbed than β-carotene in food and so provides more vitamin A activity. It is estimated that 2 μg of β-carotene dissolved in oil provides 1 μg of vitamin A activity.

susceptibility to infections, including measles, and are more likely to die in childhood.[6] It is estimated that over 3 million children worldwide have xerophthalmia and that 250 to 500 million children go blind annually due to vitamin A deficiency.[2] It is most common in India, Africa, Latin America, and the Caribbean (Figure 9.4).

Vitamin A deficiency can be caused by insufficient intakes of vitamin A, fat, protein, or the mineral zinc. Without fat, vitamin A cannot be absorbed, so a diet very low in fat can cause a deficiency by reducing vitamin A absorption. Protein deficiency can cause vitamin A deficiency because the retinol-binding protein needed to transport vitamin A cannot be made in sufficient quantities. The importance of zinc for vitamin A utilization is believed to be due to its role in protein synthesis. When zinc is deficient, proteins needed for vitamin A transport and metabolism are lacking.

Vitamin A deficiency is not common in developed countries, but intakes below the RDA may be caused by poor food choices. In the United States the intake of fresh fruits and vegetables, many of which are excellent sources of provitamin A, does not meet recommendations. A typical fast-food meal of a hamburger and french fries provides almost no vitamin A (see *Critical Thinking*: How Much Vitamin A Is in Your Fast-Food Meal?).

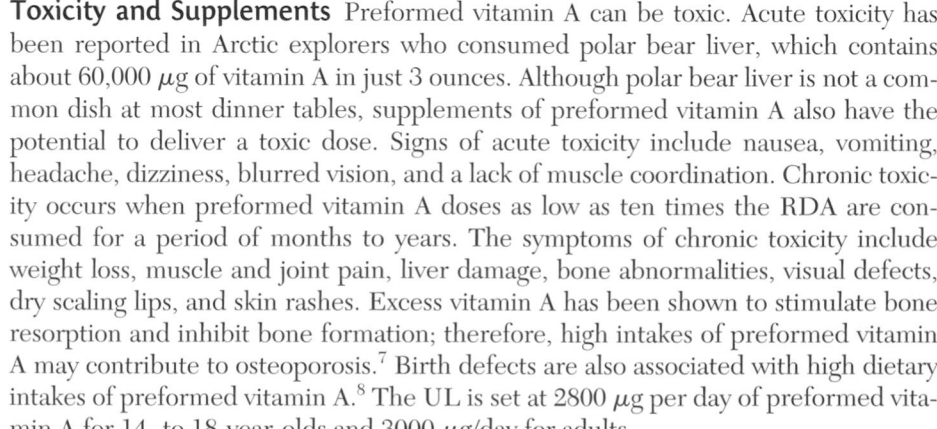

Toxicity and Supplements Preformed vitamin A can be toxic. Acute toxicity has been reported in Arctic explorers who consumed polar bear liver, which contains about 60,000 μg of vitamin A in just 3 ounces. Although polar bear liver is not a common dish at most dinner tables, supplements of preformed vitamin A also have the potential to deliver a toxic dose. Signs of acute toxicity include nausea, vomiting, headache, dizziness, blurred vision, and a lack of muscle coordination. Chronic toxicity occurs when preformed vitamin A doses as low as ten times the RDA are consumed for a period of months to years. The symptoms of chronic toxicity include weight loss, muscle and joint pain, liver damage, bone abnormalities, visual defects, dry scaling lips, and skin rashes. Excess vitamin A has been shown to stimulate bone resorption and inhibit bone formation; therefore, high intakes of preformed vitamin A may contribute to osteoporosis.[7] Birth defects are also associated with high dietary intakes of preformed vitamin A.[8] The UL is set at 2800 μg per day of preformed vitamin A for 14- to 18-year-olds and 3000 μg/day for adults.

Because of the toxicity of preformed vitamin A, most supplements contain carotenoids as a source of vitamin A. Carotenoids are not toxic because their absorption from the diet decreases at high doses, and once in the body, their conversion to active vitamin A is limited. Large daily intakes of carotenoids—usually in the form of

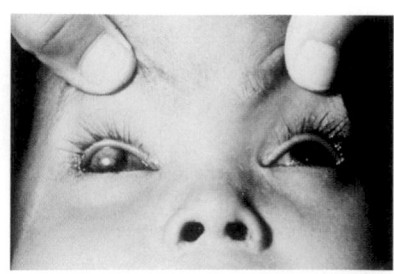

Figure 9.4
Vitamin A deficiency is a major cause of blindness worldwide. (L.V. Bergman/The Bergman Collection)

carrot juice or β-carotene supplements—do, however, lead to a condition known as **hypercarotenemia**. In this condition, the carotenoids stored in the adipose tissue make the skin look yellow-orange. This is particularly apparent on the palms of the hands and the soles of the feet. It is not known to be dangerous, and when intake decreases, the skin returns to its normal color.

Carotenoid supplements may be harmful to cigarette smokers. Two clinical research trials found an increased incidence of lung cancer in cigarette smokers who took β-carotene supplements.[9,10] Even though other trials have not shown this effect, until more information is available, smokers are advised to avoid β-carotene supplements and to rely on food sources to obtain carotenoids in their diet. The small amounts found in standard strength multivitamin supplements are not likely to be harmful for any group. The DRIs evaluated the risks associated with consumption of high doses of carotenoids, but did not set a UL.

Hypercarotenemia A condition caused by an accumulation of carotenoids in the adipose tissue, causing the skin to appear yellow-orange.

CRITICAL THINKING

How Much Vitamin A Is in Your Fast-Food Meal?

John lives on his own, goes to school, and works part time. He eats breakfast at home and usually brings a sandwich for lunch, but dinner is always a fast-food meal. He recently heard a report indicating that fast-food was low in some vitamins, particularly vitamin A. To explore this issue, John uses the Internet to look up the nutrient composition of his favorite fast-food meals.

Food		Vitamin A (μg)	% Daily Value
McDonalds	Big Mac	89	8.9
	Fries	2	0.2
Pizza Hut	Pepperoni Pizza	358	35.8
KFC	Chicken leg and breast	24	2.4
	Mashed potatoes and gravy	14	1.4

What is the best choice if he wants to increase the amount of vitamin A he gets in his fast-food meals?
▼

The pizza is the best choice. It is a good source of vitamin A because the tomato sauce is high in provitamin A carotenoids and the cheese is a source of preformed vitamin A. The hamburger and chicken meals provide little vitamin A.

In researching vitamin A, John discovers that much of the vitamin A we get in our diet comes from vitamin A precursors found in fruits and vegetables. Fast food is generally low in fruits and vegetables, so he looks at his other meals for sources of vitamin A. For breakfast he has cereal, toast, and coffee, and for lunch he packs a ham and cheese sandwich, potato chips, an apple, and a soda.

Use the Food Guide Pyramid to suggest foods that John could add to improve his diet. Be sure to select foods high in vitamin A or vitamin A precursors.
▼

Answer:

John's meals are also low in vitamin C. What foods could he add to his diet to increase his intake of vitamin C?

▼

Answer:

• VITAMIN D: THE SUNSHINE VITAMIN

Vitamin D is known as the sunshine vitamin because it can be produced in the skin by exposure to ultraviolet light. Because vitamin D can be made in the body, there is a long-standing debate as to whether vitamin D is a vitamin or a hormone. By definition, vitamins are dietary essentials. However, vitamin D can be formed in the skin, so it is only essential in the diet when exposure to sunlight is limited or the body's ability to synthesize the vitamin is reduced. Vitamin D acts like a hormone because it is produced in one organ, the skin, and affects other organs, primarily the intestine and bone.

Vitamin D in the Diet

Cholecalciferol The chemical name for vitamin D_3. It can be formed in the skin of animals by the action of sunlight on a form of cholesterol called 7-dehydrocholesterol.

Only a few foods are natural sources of vitamin D. These include liver, fatty fish such as salmon, and egg yolks (Figure 9.5). These foods contain **cholecalciferol**, or vitamin D_3. Cholecalciferol is the form of vitamin D that is made in the skin of animals by the action of sunlight on a compound made from cholesterol, called 7-dehydrocholesterol. Foods fortified with vitamin D include milk and margarine. These may contain vitamin D_3 or vitamin D_2, another active form of the vitamin.

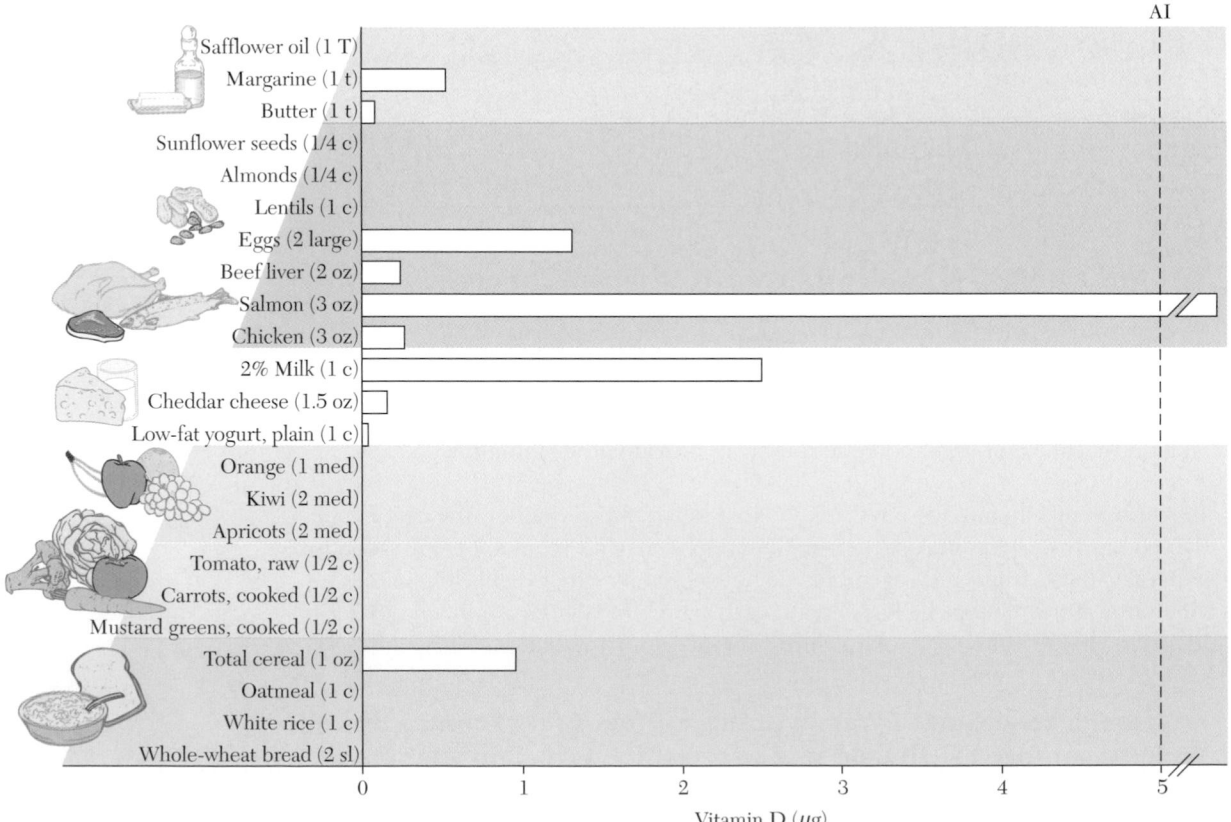

Figure 9.5

Vitamin D content of selections from each food group of the Food Guide Pyramid. The dashed line represents the AI for adults 19 through 50 years of age. Only a few foods, such as salmon and eggs, are natural sources of vitamin D; others are fortified with the vitamin.

Vitamin D in the Body

Vitamin D from the diet and from synthesis in the skin is inactive until it is chemically altered in the liver and then the kidney. In the liver, a hydroxyl group (OH) is added to vitamin D to form 25-hydroxy vitamin D_3, which then travels to the kidney where another hydroxyl group is added to make the active form of vitamin D: 1,25-dihydroxy vitamin D_3 (Figure 9.6).

The principal function of vitamin D is to maintain normal blood levels of calcium and phosphorus. When blood calcium levels drop too low, the parathyroid gland releases **parathyroid hormone (PTH)**. PTH release stimulates enzymes in the kidney to convert 25-hydroxy vitamin D_3 to the active form of the vitamin.

Active vitamin D regulates calcium and phosphorus balance by altering gene expression in cells at the intestine and bone. At the intestine, vitamin D increases the absorption of calcium and phosphorus. This occurs because vitamin D increases the

Parathyroid hormone (PTH) A hormone released by the parathyroid gland that acts to increase blood calcium levels.

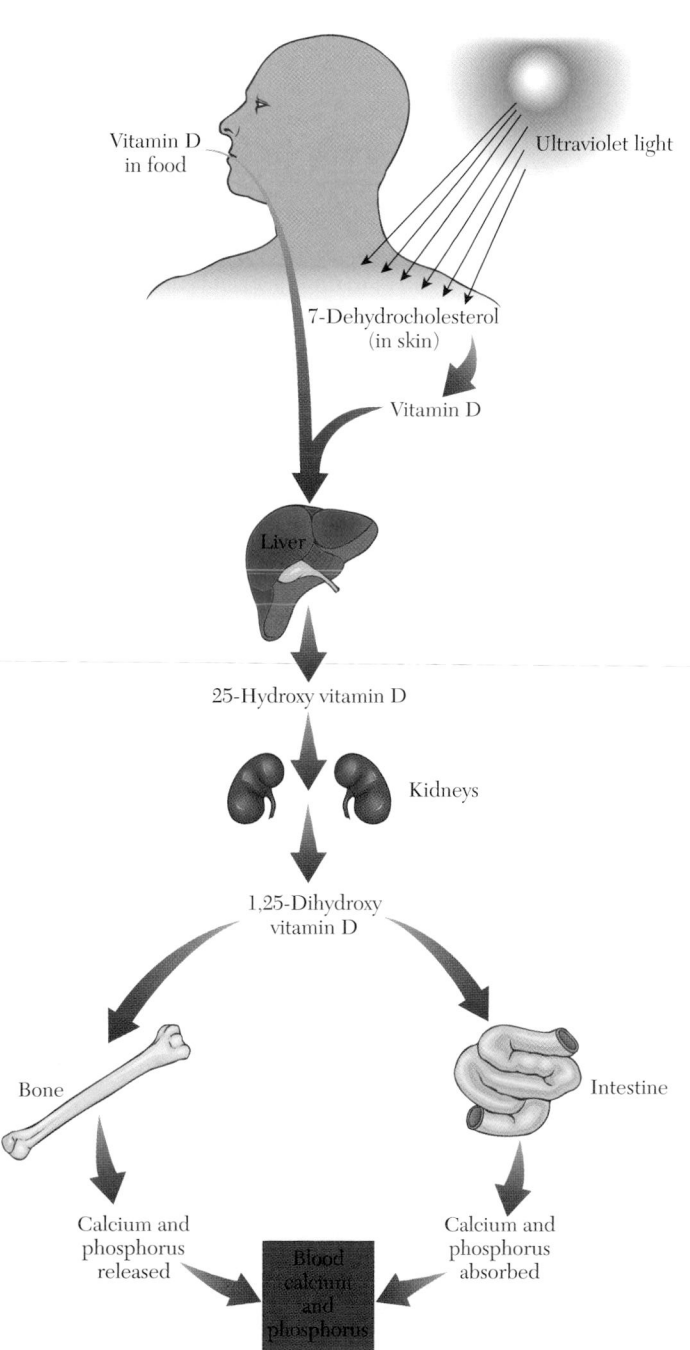

Figure 9.6

Vitamin D comes from food and from synthesis in the skin. In order to function, it must have hydroxyl groups (OH) added at the liver and kidney. Active vitamin D then functions in maintaining calcium and phosphorus balance by stimulating the release of these minerals from bone and their absorption from the intestine.

expression of genes that code for intestinal calcium transport proteins (see Figure 9.3). At the bone, vitamin D works in conjunction with PTH to increase bone break-down, releasing calcium and phosphorus into the blood. This occurs because vitamin D causes precursor cells in the bone to differentiate into cells that break down bone.[11] Vitamin D also acts with PTH to increase the amount of calcium retained by the kidneys. In addition to bone, intestine, and kidney, receptors for active vitamin D have been found in the pancreas, parathyroid gland, cells of the immune system, reproductive organs, and skin.[12] The effect of vitamin D in these tissues is under investigation.

How Much Vitamin D Do We Need?

The recommended intake of vitamin D is based on the amount needed in the diet to maintain normal blood levels of 25-hydroxy vitamin D_3. The AI for adult men and women is set at 5 μg per day.[13] The AI is expressed in μg, but the vitamin D content of foods and supplements may also be given as International Units (IUs); one IU is equal to 0.025 μg of vitamin D_3 (40 IU = 1 μg of vitamin D). The AI for vitamin D for adults is contained in about 2 cups of vitamin D-fortified milk (see Table 9.1).

The AI is based on the assumption that no vitamin D is synthesized in the skin. This assumption is made because of the variation in the extent to which synthesis from sunlight meets the requirement. If there is sufficient sun exposure, dietary vitamin D is not needed. The amount synthesized in the skin is affected by skin pigmentation, climate, season, clothing, the presence of pollution and tall buildings that block sunlight, and the use of sunscreens. Although sunscreens prevent the formation of vitamin D in the skin, children and active adults usually spend enough time outdoors without sunscreens to provide for their vitamin D requirement.

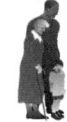

Despite the smaller body size of infants and children, the AI for vitamin D for this age is the same as that for adults. This is to allow sufficient vitamin D for bone development during periods of rapid growth. Although breast milk is low in vitamin D, infants who are exposed to sunlight for about half an hour per day do not require supplemental vitamin D. The AI for adults 50 to 70 years of age is 10 μg per day to prevent bone loss during periods of low sun exposure. In adults 70 and older the AI is 15 μg per day to maintain blood levels of vitamin D and prevent skeletal fractures. The AI for pregnancy and lactation is not increased above young adult levels.

Vitamin D and Health

Vitamin D is essential for bone health. A deficiency causes improper bone development in children and weakened bones in adults. However, too much vitamin D can be toxic.

Vitamin D Deficiency When vitamin D is deficient, dietary calcium cannot be absorbed efficiently. As a result, calcium is not available for proper bone mineralization and abnormalities in bone structure occur.

In children who are deficient in vitamin D, bones are weak because they do not contain enough calcium and phosphorus. This syndrome, called **rickets**, is characterized by bone deformities such as narrow rib cages known as pigeon breasts and bowed legs (Figure 9.7). The legs bow because the bones are too weak to support the weight of the body. Rickets was common in 17th- to 19th-century Europe. The incidence increased during the Industrial Revolution when large numbers of poorly nourished children lived under a layer of smog in the newly industrialized cities. Even though the fortification of milk with vitamin D has helped to greatly reduce rickets in most developed countries, it is still a problem in inner-city children who have a poor diet and whose exposure to sunlight is limited.[14] Dark-skinned children are more likely to be vitamin D deficient than those with lighter skin because dark skin pigment prevents the UV light rays from penetrating into the dermis of the skin, thereby reducing the formation of vitamin D. Rickets is also seen in children with disorders that affect fat absorption and in vegetarian children who do not drink milk.

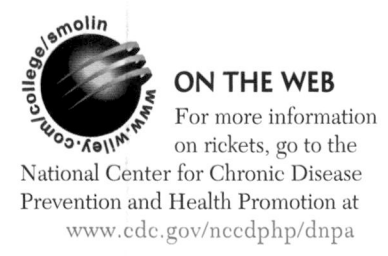

ON THE WEB
For more information on rickets, go to the National Center for Chronic Disease Prevention and Health Promotion at
www.cdc.gov/nccdphp/dnpa

Rickets A vitamin D deficiency disease in children that is characterized by poor bone development because of inadequate calcium deposition.

In adults, the vitamin D deficiency disease comparable to rickets is called **osteomalacia**. Because bone growth is complete in adults, osteomalacia does not cause deformities, but bones are weakened because not enough calcium is available to form the mineral deposits needed to maintain healthy bone. Insufficient bone mineralization leads to fractures of the weight-bearing bones such as those in the hips and spine. A more common cause of fractures is a condition called osteoporosis, which is a loss of total bone mass, not just minerals (see Chapter 10). Osteomalacia is common in adults with kidney failure because the conversion of vitamin D from inactive to active forms is reduced. The elderly are at risk for vitamin D deficiency because the ability to produce vitamin D in the skin decreases with age and older adults typically cover more of their skin with clothing and spend less time in the sun than their younger counterparts.[15] In addition, the elderly tend to have a lower intake of dairy products.

Vitamin D Toxicity and Supplements Consumption of unfortified foods does not cause vitamin D toxicity. And synthesis of vitamin D from exposure to sunlight does not produce toxic amounts because vitamin D formation is carefully regulated. However, oversupplementation and overfortification do pose a risk. One case of accidental overfortification of milk resulted in the hospitalization of 56 individuals and the death of 2.[16] Symptoms of vitamin D toxicity include high blood and urine calcium concentrations, deposition of calcium in soft tissues such as the blood vessels and kidney, and cardiovascular damage. A UL of 50 μg has been established for adults.

• VITAMIN E: A FAT-SOLUBLE ANTIOXIDANT

Vitamin E is a fat-soluble vitamin with an antioxidant function. It was first identified as a fat-soluble component of grains that was necessary for fertility in laboratory rats. It took almost 30 years to isolate this vitamin and to determine that it is also necessary for reproduction in humans. The chemical name for vitamin E, **tocopherol**, is from the Greek *tos*, meaning childbirth, and *phero*, meaning to bring forth. Vitamin E has been promoted as a cure for infertility, an antiscar medication, a defense against air pollution, and a fountain of youth. Today we continue to explore the role of this antioxidant in protecting us from chronic disease (see *Off the Shelf*: Will Antioxidant Supplements Keep Us Healthy?).

Vitamin E in the Diet

There are several naturally occurring forms of vitamin E in food, but only the **alpha-tocopherol (α-tocopherol)** form can meet vitamin E requirements in humans. The other forms do not meet vitamin E needs because they are not converted to α-tocopherol in humans and cannot be transported by the α-tocopherol transfer protein.

There are also differences between natural α-tocopherol and the synthetic form found in dietary supplements and fortified foods. Synthetic α-tocopherol is composed of eight different **isomers**. Only half of these are active in the body. Therefore, synthetic α-tocopherol provides half of the biological activity of natural α-tocopherol; 10 mg of synthetic α-tocopherol provides the function of 5 mg of natural α-tocopherol.

The discovery that only the alpha form of tocopherol provides vitamin E activity is relatively recent. Prior to this finding, all forms of tocopherol were included when calculating vitamin E content. Vitamin E content was expressed as either International Units (IUs) or α-tocopherol equivalents (α-TEs). An IU is defined as 1 mg of synthetic α-tocopherol. Alpha-TEs expressed the amounts of other tocopherols as fractions of α-tocopherol. Most nutrient databases and nutrition labels still use these older units and may therefore overrepresent the amount of functional vitamin E in foods. To correct for this, formulae have been developed to convert IUs and α-TEs into mg of α-tocopherol (Table 9.3). Dietary sources of vitamin E include nuts and peanuts; plant oils, such as soybean, corn, and sunflower oils; leafy green vegetables; wheat germ; and fortified breakfast cereals (Figure 9.8).

Osteomalacia A vitamin D deficiency disease in adults characterized by a loss of minerals from bones. It causes weak bones and an increase in bone fractures.

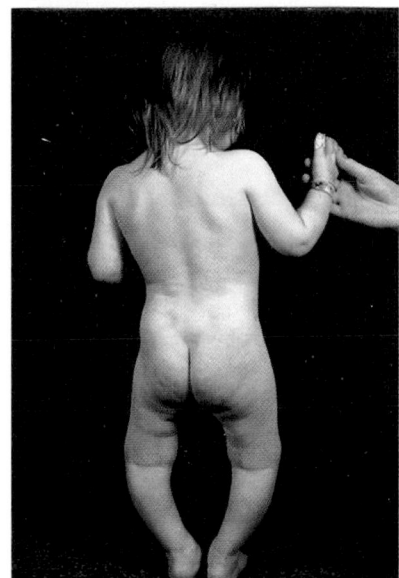

Figure 9.7
Bowed legs are characteristic of rickets. (© Biophoto Associates/Photo Researchers, Inc.)

Tocopherol The chemical name for vitamin E.

Alpha-tocopherol (α-tocopherol) The only form of tocopherol that provides vitamin E activity in humans.

Isomers Molecules with the same molecular formula but a different arrangement.

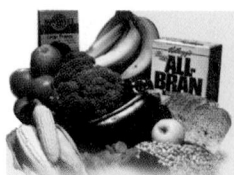

Off the Shelf
Will Antioxidant Supplements Keep Us Healthy?

Many vitamins, minerals, and enzymes are marketed as antioxidant supplements. These are suggested to boost our antioxidant defenses and keep us healthy by protecting us from heart disease, cancer, and even aging. Although antioxidant nutrients are an important part of our defense system, they are not the only source of antioxidant protection, and more is not always better.

The rationale for needing extra antioxidants is based on the fact that we are constantly bombarded with damaging reactive molecules called free radicals. Free radicals contain unpaired electrons and include peroxide, superoxide, and hydroxyl radicals. Free radicals and other reactive molecules are generated from reactions inside our body and come from environmental sources such as air pollution and cigarette smoke. If the body's antioxidant defense mechanisms become overwhelmed, oxidative stress occurs. Sometimes a cell in oxidative stress adapts and increases the production of antioxidant defenses, making it more resistant. However, if the stress is too great or lasts too long, oxidative damage to DNA, proteins, carbohydrates, and lipids occurs and cell death can result. The cumulative effect of oxidative stress is believed to play a role in the aging process and in the development of chronic diseases.

To protect us from oxidative damage, the body is equipped with many types of antioxidant defenses. Some of these are vitamins or vitamin precursors—vitamin C, vitamin E, and β-carotene. Others are enzymes—catalase, glutathione peroxidase, and superoxide dismutase. These enzyme systems rely on minerals, including zinc, copper, manganese, iron, and selenium, for activity.

Can supplements of nutrients or enzymes boost our antioxidant defenses? Each antioxidant in the body acts in different locations under specific conditions to destroy particular types of reactive oxygen compounds (see figure). Vitamin C can inactivate free radicals, singlet oxygen, and hydrogen peroxide in blood and other body fluids. Vitamin E and β-carotene can inactivate free radicals to protect lipids in cell membranes. Selenium is a part of the antioxidant enzyme glutathione peroxidase, which neutralizes peroxides in the cytoplasm and mitochondria before they can form dangerous free radicals. Catalase is an iron-containing enzyme that can also destroy peroxides. Zinc, copper, and manganese are necessary for forms of the enzyme superoxide dismutase, which destroys superoxide radicals.

Although scientific evidence confirms the role of certain nutrients as antioxidants, we do not know the optimum dose of each for maximum antioxidant protection. The amounts needed will vary depending on environmental conditions and the health and genetic makeup of the individual. In addition, many of the antioxidant nutrients interact. Therefore, a deficiency of one of these nutrients could increase the need for another, and an excess of one may create a deficiency of another. For instance, vitamin C is necessary to regenerate the active form of vitamin E, selenium helps prevent vitamin E deficiency, and excesses of zinc can cause copper deficiency. Some antioxidants such as vitamin C can also act as pro-oxidants under certain conditions. Therefore it is possible for the wrong amounts to promote rather than prevent oxidative damage.

If antioxidant vitamins and minerals are deficient in the diet, increasing their intake will enhance antioxidant defenses. But whether consumption of these nutrients above the recommended intake will further improve the body's antioxidant defenses is still under investigation. Taking a supplement that contains an antioxidant enzyme like catalase, superoxide dismutase, or glutathione peroxidase will not boost antioxidant defenses because it will not increase the amount of enzyme in the body. Enzymes supplied in the diet, whether in food or in supplements, are broken down to amino acids and peptides in the gastrointestinal tract before they can be absorbed.

Your overall diet is probably more important in protecting you from oxidative damage than any of these nutrients alone. Some of the antioxidants present in foods are phytochemicals with no vitamin activity. Other components of the diet, such as fat and fiber intake, may be just as important as vitamins and minerals at protecting us from chronic disease. Based on our current understanding, it is best to boost antioxidant nutrients by eating more fruits and vegetables that are high in vitamin C, vitamin E, and phytochemicals, and by including foods containing iron, copper, selenium, manganese, and zinc in your diet.

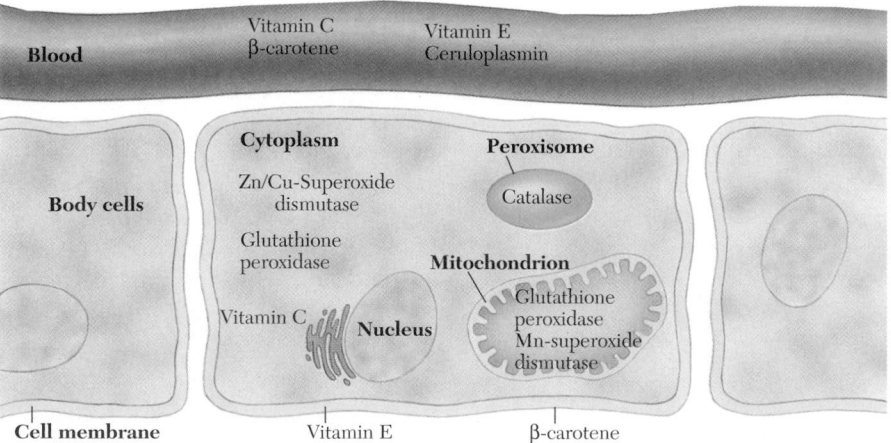

Each of the antioxidant defenses functions in specific locations in the body and protects against specific types of damaging reactions.

Table 9.3 Converting Vitamin E Values into mg α-Tocopherol

To estimate the α-tocopherol intake from foods:

- If values are given as mg α-TEs:

$$\text{mg } \alpha\text{-TE} \times 0.8^\circ = \text{mg } \alpha\text{-tocopherol}$$

- If values are given as IUs:

  First, determine if the source of the α-tocopherol is natural or synthetic.

  - For natural α-tocopherol:

  $$\text{IU of natural } \alpha\text{-tocopherol} \times 0.67 = \text{mg } \alpha\text{-tocopherol}$$

  - For synthetic α-tocopherol (dl-α-tocopherol):

  $$\text{IU of synthetic } \alpha\text{-tocopherol} \times 0.45 = \text{mg } \alpha\text{-tocopherol}$$

°Based on dietary data from the NHANES III study, approximately 80% of the α-tocopherol equivalents from food are from α-tocopherol and can thus contribute to the body's requirement for vitamin E.

Because vitamin E is sensitive to destruction by oxygen, metals, light, and heat, some is lost during food processing, cooking, and storage. Although it is relatively stable at normal cooking temperatures, the high temperatures used in deep-fat frying and the repeated use of the same oil tend to destroy most of the vitamin E.

Vitamin E in the Body

Vitamin E functions primarily as an antioxidant. It neutralizes reactive oxygen compounds before they damage unsaturated fatty acids in cell membranes (Figure 9.9). By protecting cell membranes, vitamin E is important in maintaining the integrity of red blood cells, cells in nervous tissue, and cells of the immune system. A number of vitamin E's roles are hypothesized to reduce the risk of heart disease. As an antioxidant, it helps protect LDL cholesterol from oxidation.[17] It may also inhibit an enzyme

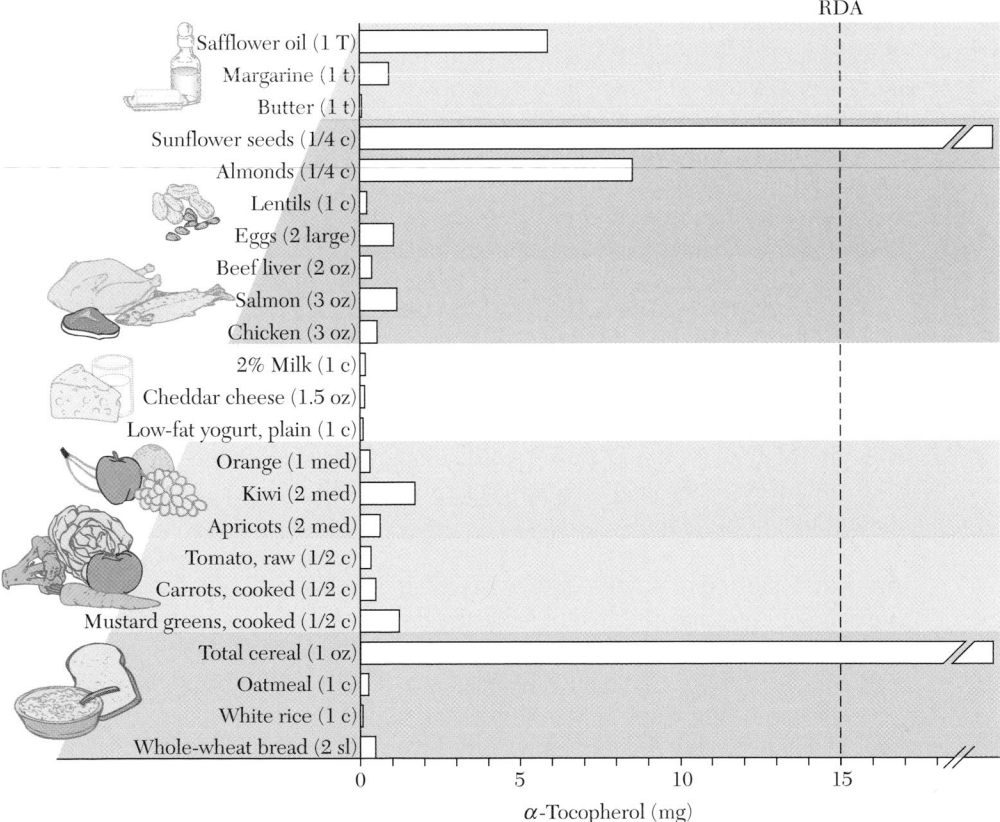

Figure 9.8
Vitamin E content of selections from each food group of the Food Guide Pyramid. The dashed line represents the RDA for adults. Vitamin E is found in plant oils, nuts and seeds, leafy green vegetables, and fortified cereals.

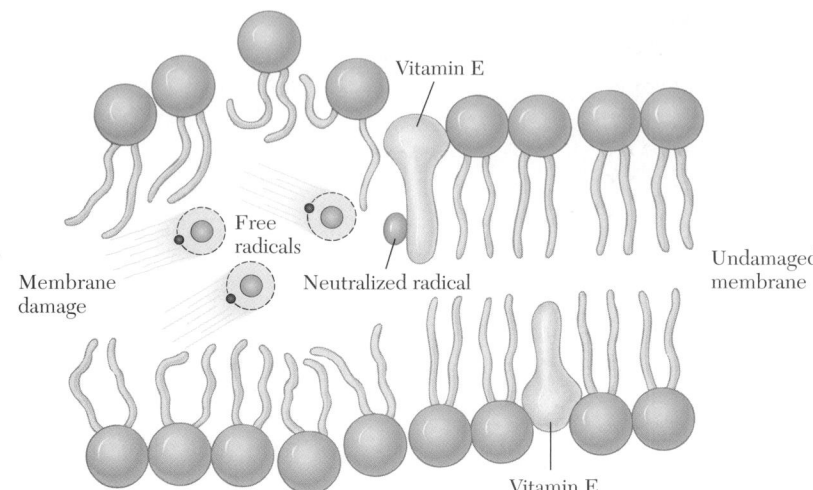

Figure 9.9
Vitamin E functions as an antioxidant that protects the unsaturated fatty acids in cell membranes by neutralizing free radicals.

that allows the buildup of atherosclerotic plaque and increase the synthesis of an enzyme needed to produce eicosinoids that help lower blood pressure and reduce blood clot formation.[18,19] Vitamin E can also defend cells from damage by heavy metals, such as lead and mercury, and toxins, such as carbon tetrachloride, benzene, and a variety of drugs. It also protects against some environmental pollutants such as ozone. After vitamin E is used to eliminate free radicals, its antioxidant function can be restored by vitamin C. Because polyunsaturated fats are particularly susceptible to oxidative damage, the vitamin E requirement increases as polyunsaturated fat intake increases.

How Much Vitamin E Do We Need?

The recommendation for vitamin E intake is based on the amount needed to maintain plasma concentrations of α-tocopherol that protect red blood cells from breaking. The RDA for adult men and women is set at 15 mg/day of α-tocopherol. The RDA does not change with advancing age.

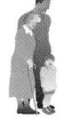

For infants, an AI for vitamin E has been set based on the amount consumed by infants fed principally with human milk. EARs and RDAs for children and adolescents have been estimated from adult values. The RDA for pregnancy is not increased above nonpregnant levels. To estimate the requirement for lactation, the amount secreted in human milk is added to the requirement for nonlactating women.

Vitamin E and Health

Although vitamin E deficiency is uncommon, supplements are promoted to grow hair; restore, maintain, or increase sexual potency and fertility; alleviate fatigue; maintain immune function; enhance athletic performance; reduce the symptoms of PMS and menopause; slow aging; prevent heart disease and cancer; and treat a host of other medical problems.

Vitamin E Deficiency Vitamin E protects membranes; therefore a deficiency can cause membrane changes. Red blood cells and nerve tissue are particularly susceptible. For example, when vitamin E is deficient, red blood cell membranes are damaged and may rupture. Vitamin E deficiency is rare because vitamin E is plentiful in the food supply and is stored in many of the body's tissues. Deficiencies have been identified in premature infants, and in individuals with genetic abnormalities, protein-energy malnutrition, and fat malabsorption. In individuals with cystic fibrosis, a condition that reduces fat absorption, deficiency can develop rapidly, causing serious neurological problems, which, if untreated, can become permanent.

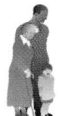

All newborn infants have low blood tocopherol levels because there is little transfer of vitamin E from mother to fetus until the last weeks of pregnancy. The levels are lower in premature infants, who are born before much vitamin E is transferred from the mother. In these infants, ruptured red blood cells may cause a type of anemia called hemolytic anemia. Infant formula for premature newborns is supplemented with higher amounts of vitamin E than formula for full-term infants.

Vitamin E Toxicity Vitamin E is relatively nontoxic. The UL is 1000 mg/day from supplemental sources. Vitamin E supplements should not be taken by individuals taking blood-thinning medications because it reduces blood clotting and interferes with the action of vitamin K. There is no evidence of adverse effects from consuming large amounts from food.

Vitamin E Supplements: Do They Protect Your Heart? In epidemiological studies, intakes of vitamin E greater than 100 IU per day have been associated with a reduced risk of heart disease in both men and women.[20,21] However, the results of human intervention trials that supplemented vitamin E are mixed. One study, which was done in patients with proven coronary artery disease, demonstrated a significant reduction in heart attacks.[22] In contrast, The Heart Outcomes Prevention Evaluation Study, which examined nearly 10,000 adults 55 years or older who were at high risk for heart attack or stroke, found that after $4\frac{1}{2}$ years there was no difference in the rate of stroke or heart attack between controls and subjects given vitamin E supplements.[23] The results of intervention trials are inconsistent, and the association between vitamin E intake and heart disease observed in epidemiological studies may be due to substances in the diet other than vitamin E. Therefore, additional studies are needed before vitamin E supplements can be recommended to the general public to decrease the risk of heart disease.

• VITAMIN K: COAGULATION

Vitamin K is one of the few vitamins about which extravagant claims are not made. Like the other fat-soluble vitamins, it was discovered inadvertently by feeding animals a fat-free diet. In this case, researchers in Denmark noted that chicks fed this diet developed a type of bleeding disorder that was cured by feeding them a fat-soluble extract from green plants. Vitamin K was named for *koagulation*, the Danish word for **coagulation**, or blood clotting.

Coagulation The process of blood clotting.

Vitamin K in the Diet

As with all the fat-soluble vitamins, vitamin K is found in several forms. **Phylloquinone** is the form found in plants and the primary form in the diet. A group of vitamin K compounds, called **menaquinones**, are found in fish oils and meats and are synthesized by bacteria, including those in the human intestine. Menaquinones are the form found in supplements. Only a small number of foods provide significant amounts of vitamin K. Liver and leafy green vegetables such as spinach, broccoli, brussels sprouts, kale, and turnip greens provide about half of the vitamin K in a typical North American diet.[24] Some vegetable oils are also good sources (Figure 9.10). Some of the vitamin K produced by bacteria in the human gastrointestinal tract is also absorbed.

Phylloquinone The form of vitamin K found in plants.

Menaquinones The forms of vitamin K synthesized by bacteria and found in animals.

Vitamin K in the Body

Vitamin K is needed for the production of the blood-clotting protein **prothrombin** and other specific blood-clotting factors. These proteins are needed to produce fibrin, the protein that forms the structure of a blood clot (Figure 9.11). Injuries as well as the normal wear and tear of daily living produce micro tears in blood vessels. To prevent blood loss, these tears must be repaired with blood clots. Other roles for vitamin K are less well understood. For example, there are several vitamin K-dependent proteins in bone that may be involved in bone mineralization and demineralization.[25]

Prothrombin A blood protein required for blood clotting.

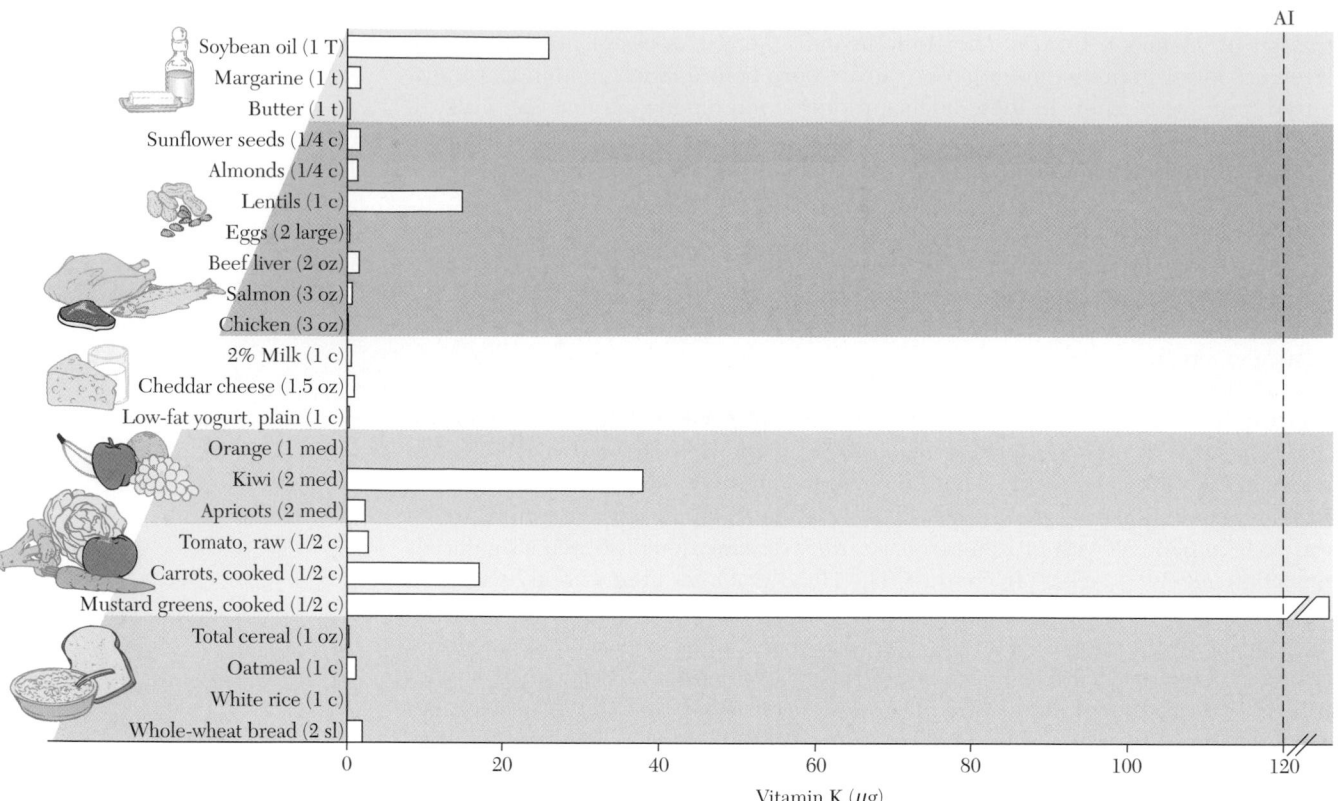

Figure 9.10

Vitamin K content of selections from each food group of the Food Guide Pyramid. The dashed line represents the AI for adult men. The best sources of vitamin K are leafy green vegetables and some plant oils.

How Much Vitamin K Do We Need?

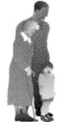

Unlike other fat-soluble vitamins, vitamin K is used rapidly by the body, so a constant supply is necessary. An AI for vitamin K has been set at about 120 μg day for men and 90 μg/day for women (see Table 9.1). Typical intakes in North America are close to this amount.[26] Additional vitamin K is provided by bacteria in the gastrointestinal tract. Although the form produced by intestinal bacteria is less well absorbed than that from plant sources and alone is not enough to meet needs, it is an important source of this vitamin. The AI is not increased for pregnancy or lactation. An AI for infants was set based on the amount typically consumed in breast milk.

Vitamin K and Health

The inability to form blood clots due to vitamin K deficiency or drugs that interfere with vitamin K activity can cause death from excess blood loss. Conversely, blood clots causing heart attacks and strokes are responsible for killing about a half-million Americans annually.

Vitamin K Deficiency Abnormal blood coagulation is the major symptom of vitamin K deficiency. A deficiency is very rare in the healthy adult population, but it may result from fat malabsorption syndromes or the long-term use of antibiotics. The antibiotics kill the bacteria in the gastrointestinal tract that are a source of the vitamin. In combination with an illness that reduces the dietary intake of vitamin K, this may precipitate a deficiency. Injections of vitamin K are typically administered before surgery to aid in blood clotting.

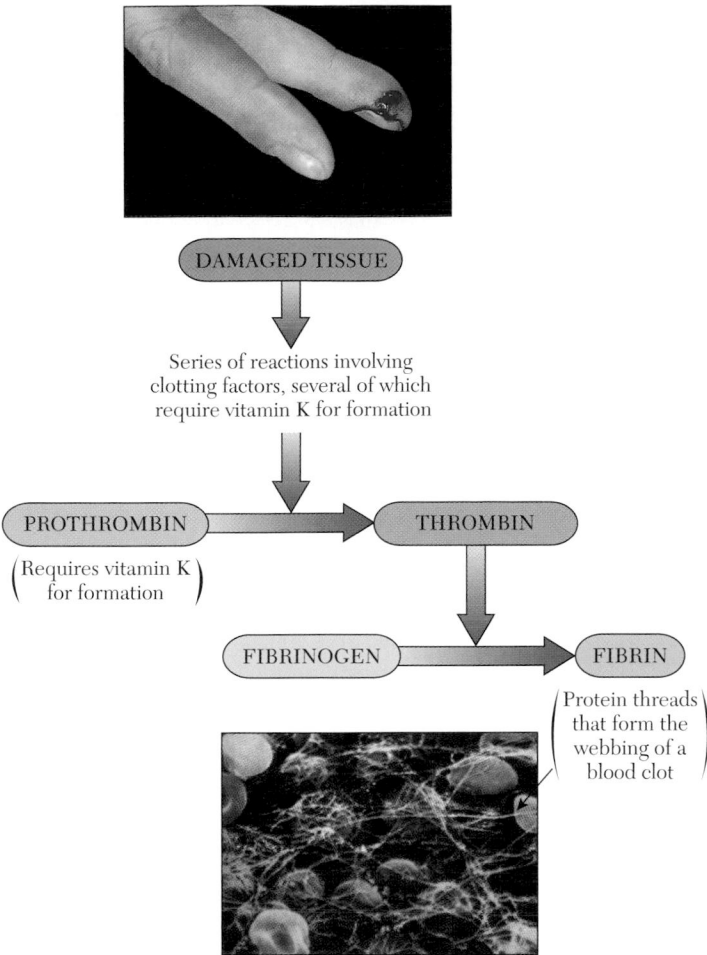

Figure 9.11
Blood clotting involves a number of substances called clotting factors. Several of these, including prothrombin, require vitamin K for synthesis. Without them, fibrinogen cannot be converted into its active form, fibrin, which is a structural component of blood clots. (*top*, © Amethyst/Custom Medical Stock Photo; *bottom*, CNRI/Science Photo Library/Custom Medical Stock Photo)

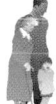 Vitamin K deficiency is most common in newborns. There is little transfer of this vitamin from mother to fetus, and because the infant gut is free of bacteria, none is made there. Further, breast milk is low in vitamin K. Therefore, to prevent uncontrolled bleeding, infants are typically given a vitamin K injection within 6 hours of birth.

Of Cows and Clover: The Value of Medically Induced Vitamin K Deficiency

In 1933, a disgruntled farmer delivered a bale of moldy clover hay, a pail of unclotted blood, and a dead cow to the laboratory of Dr. Carl Link at the University of Wisconsin. Six years and many bales of moldy clover later, Link and colleagues had isolated the **anticoagulant** dicumarol from moldy clover. Dicumarol is a derivative of coumarin, which gives clover its sweet scent; mold converts coumarin to dicumarol. Cows fed moldy clover consume dicumarol, which interferes with vitamin K activity. It inhibits their blood from clotting, and they bleed to death from minor cuts and scratches. Within a few years of its discovery, dicumarol was widely used to treat heart attack victims and others at risk for blood clots. Further work with this anticoagulant led Link to propose the use of a more potent derivative, called warfarin, as rat poison. When rats consume the odorless, colorless warfarin, their blood fails to clot, and they bleed to death. Warfarin is now also used as a blood thinner to save the lives of heart attack victims.

Anticoagulant A substance that delays or prevents blood coagulation.

Vitamin K Toxicity and Supplements

A UL has not been established for vitamin K because there are no well-documented side effects, even with intakes up to 370 μg/day from food and supplements. Because vitamin K functions in blood clotting, high doses can interfere with anticoagulant drugs. Therefore, individuals prescribed these medications should consult with their physicians before taking supplements containing vitamin K.

• APPLICATIONS •

1. Using the three-day food intake record you kept in Chapter 2:
   a. Calculate your average daily intake of vitamin A.
   b. How does your vitamin A intake compare to the RDA for someone of your age and sex?
   c. What are three major food sources of vitamin A in your diet?
   d. Do the major food sources of vitamin A in your diet contain preformed vitamin A or provitamin A carotenoids?

2. Using the food intake record you kept in Chapter 2:
   a. Calculate your average intake of vitamin E.
   b. How does your intake of vitamin E compare with the RDA?
   c. If your diet does not meet the RDA, make modifications that will add enough vitamin E to your diet to meet the RDA without increasing your energy intake.

SUMMARY

1. The fat-soluble vitamins A, D, E, and K each have unique functions in the body.

2. Vitamin A is needed for vision and for the growth and differentiation of cells. It affects epithelial tissue, reproduction, and immune function by altering gene expression. It is found in the diet both preformed as retinoids and in precursor forms called carotenoids. Vitamin A deficiency is a world health problem that causes blindness and death. Preformed vitamin A can be toxic at doses as low as ten times the RDA and can increase the risk of birth defects. The major food sources of preformed vitamin A include liver, eggs, fish, and fortified dairy products.

3. Some carotenoids are precursors of vitamin A. The most potent is β-carotene. Carotenoids are found in yellow-orange fruits and vegetables such as mangoes and carrots and in leafy greens. β-carotene functions as an antioxidant, a role that is independent of its conversion to vitamin A. Carotenoids are not toxic, but a high intake can give the skin a yellow appearance.

4. Vitamin D can be made in the skin by exposure to sunlight, so dietary needs vary depending on the amount synthesized. Vitamin D is found in fish oils and fortified milk. It is essential for maintaining proper levels of calcium and phosphorus in the body. It promotes calcium and phosphorus absorption from the intestines and release from bone. A deficiency in children results in a condition called rickets; in adults, vitamin D deficiency causes osteomalacia.

5. Vitamin E functions primarily as a fat-soluble antioxidant. It is necessary for reproduction and protects cell membranes from oxidative damage. Since polyunsaturated fats are particularly susceptible to oxidative damage, the requirement for vitamin E increases as the polyunsaturated fat content of the diet increases. It is found in nuts, plant oils, green vegetables, and fortified cereals.

6. Vitamin K is essential for blood clotting. Since vitamin K deficiency is a problem in newborns, they are routinely given vitamin K injections at birth. Dicumarol, a substance that inhibits vitamin K activity, is used medically as an anticoagulant. Vitamin K is found in plants and is synthesized by bacteria in the gastrointestinal tract.

REVIEW QUESTIONS

1. List two food sources of preformed vitamin A and two of provitamin A.
2. List three functions of preformed vitamin A.
3. What is β-carotene?
4. What are the symptoms of vitamin A deficiency?
5. Is vitamin A toxic? Is β-carotene toxic?
6. Why is vitamin D called the sunshine vitamin?
7. Name two sources of vitamin D in the diet.
8. What is the function of vitamin D?
9. Explain how vitamin A and vitamin D can affect the amount of a protein that is produced.
10. What is the function of vitamin E?
11. Name two sources of vitamin E in the diet.
12. What is the main function of vitamin K?

REFERENCES

1. Clinton, S. K. Lycopene: Chemistry, biology, and implications for human health and disease. *Nutr. Rev.* 56(I):35–51, 1998.
2. Food and Nutrition Board, Institute of Medicine. *Dietary Reference Intakes: Vitamin A, Vitamin K, Arsenic, Boron, Chromium, Copper, Iodine, Iron, Manganese, Molybdenum, Nickel, Silicon, Vanadium, and Zinc.* Washington, D.C.: National Academy Press, 2001.
3. Ross, A.C. Vitamin A and retinoids. In *Modern Nutrition in Health and Disease*, 9th ed. Shils, M. E., Olson, J. A., Shike, M., and Ross, A. C., eds. Baltimore: Williams & Wilkins, 1999. 305–327.
4. Maden, M. Vitamin A in embryonic development. *Nutr. Rev.* 52:S3–S12, 1994.
5. Ross, D. A. Vitamin A and public health. Proc. *Nutr. Soc.* 57:159–165, 1998.
6. Underwood, B. A. Micronutrient malnutrition: Is it being eliminated? *Nutr. Today* 33:121–129, 1998.
7. Binkley, N., and Krueger, D. Hypervitaminosis A and Bone. *Nutr. Rev.* 58:138–144, 2000.
8. Collins, M. D., and Mao, G. E. Teratology of retinoids. *Annu. Rev. Pharmacol. Toxicol.* 39:399–430, 1999.
9. Cooper, D. A., Eldridge, A. L., and Peters, J. C. Dietary carotenoids and lung cancer: a review of recent research. *Nutr. Rev.* 57:133–145, 1999.
10. Pryor, W. A., Stahl, W., and Rock, C. L. Beta-carotene: From biochemistry to clinical trials. *Nutr. Rev.* 58(I):39–53, 2000.
11. Holick, M. F. Vitamin D. In *Modern Nutrition in Health and Disease*, 9th ed. Shils, M. E., Olson, J. A., Shike, M., and Ross, A. C., eds. Baltimore: Williams & Wilkins, 1999. 329–345.
12. DeLuca, H. F., and Zierold, C. Mechanisms and functions of vitamin D. *Nutr. Rev.* 56(II):S4–S10, 1998.

13. Food and Nutrition Board, Institute of Medicine. *Dietary Reference Intakes: Calcium, Phosphorus, Magnesium, Vitamin D, and Fluoride.* Washington, D.C.: National Academy Press, 1997.

14. Pugliese, M. T., Blumberg, D. L., Hludzinski, J., and Kay, S. Nutritional rickets in suburbia. *J. Am. Coll. Nutr.* 17:637–641, 1998.

15. Jacques P. F., Felson, D. T., Tucker K. L., et al. Plasma 25-hydroxyvitamin D and its determinants in an elderly population sample. *Am. J. Clin. Nutr.* 66:929–936, 1997.

16. Blank, S., Scanlon, K. S., Sinks, T. H., and Falk, H. An outbreak of hypervitaminosis D associated with the overfortification of milk from a home-delivery dairy. *Am. J. Public Health* 85:656–659, 1995.

17. Abbey, M. The importance of vitamin E in reducing cardiovascular risk. *Nutr. Rev.* 53:S28–S32, 1995.

18. Steiner, M. Vitamin E, a modifier of platelet function: Rationale and use in cardiovascular and cerebrovascular disease. *Nutr. Rev.* 57:306–309, 1999.

19. Emmert, D. H., and Kirchner, J. T. The role of vitamin E in the prevention of heart disease. *Arch. Family Med.* 8:537–542, 1999.

20. Rimm, E. B., Stampfer, M. J., Ascherio, A., et al. Vitamin E consumption and the risk of heart disease in men. *N. Engl. J. Med.* 328:1450–1456, 1993.

21. Stampfer, M. J., Hennekens, C. H., Manson, J. E., et al. Vitamin E consumption and the risk of heart disease in women. *N. Engl. J. Med.* 328:1487–1489, 1993.

22. Stephens, N. G., Parsons, A., Schofield, P. M., et al. Randomized controlled trial of vitamin E in patients with coronary disease: Cambridge Heart Antioxidant Study (CHAOS). *Lancet* 347:781–786, 1996.

23. Yusuf, S. Vitamin E supplementation and cardiovascular events in high-risk patients. The Heart Outcomes Prevention Evaluation Study Investigators. *N. Engl. J. Med.* 342:154–160, 2000.

24. Booth, S. L., Pennington, J. A. T., and Sadowski, J. A. Food sources and dietary intakes of vitamin K_1 (phylloquinone) in the American diet: Data from the FDA Total Diet Study. *J. Am. Diet. Assoc.* 96:149–154, 1996.

25. Olson, R. E. Vitamin K. In *Modern Nutrition in Health and Disease*, 9th ed. Shils, M. E., Olson, J. A., Shike, M., and Ross, A. C., eds. Baltimore: Williams & Wilkins, 1999. 363–380.

26. Booth, S. L., and Suttie, J. W. Dietary intake and adequacy of vitamin K. *J. Nutr.* 128:785–788, 1998.

The Internal Sea: Water and the Major Minerals

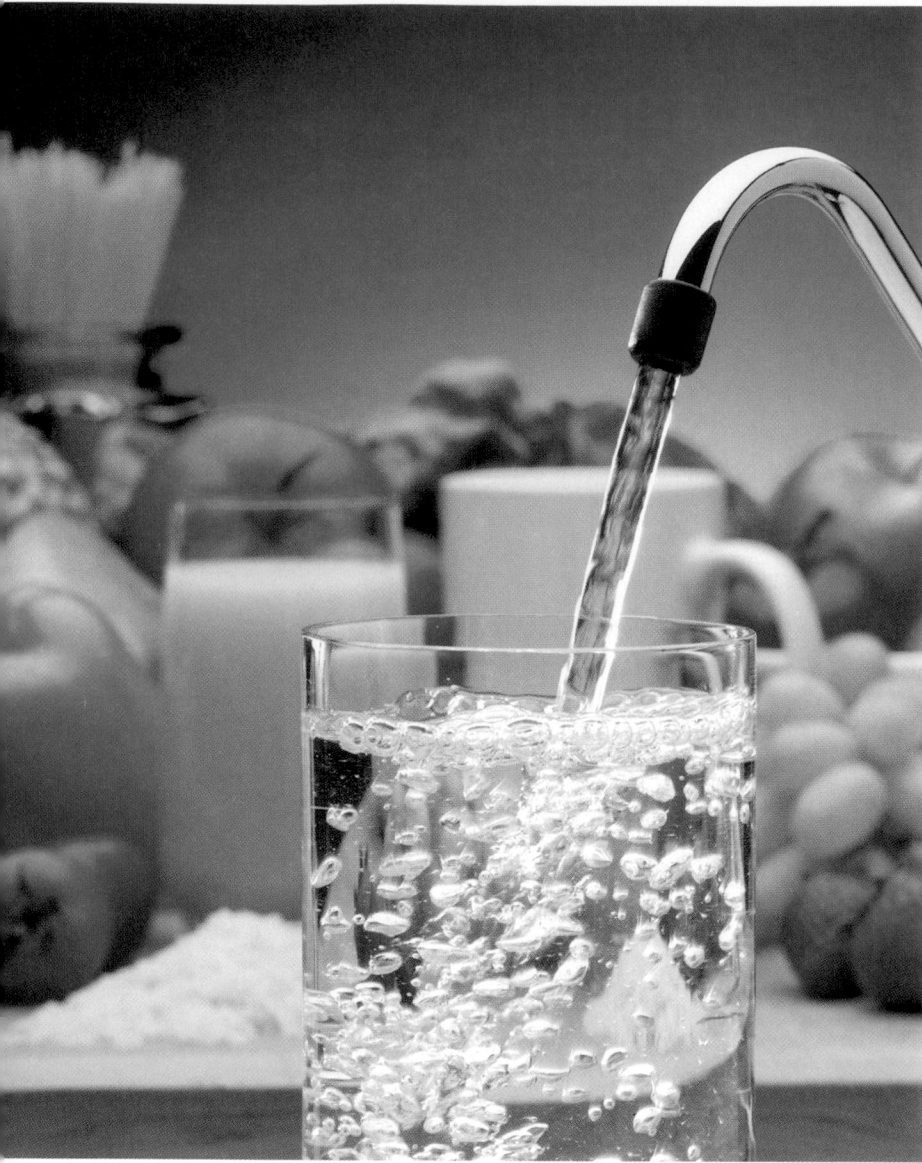

(© Jackson Vereen/Foodpix)

Chapter Concepts

✔ Water is an essential macronutrient that cannot be stored; to maintain fluid balance, intake must equal losses.

✔ Nutritionally, minerals are inorganic molecules needed in the diet that function as structural components and regulators of the chemical reactions and body processes needed to maintain health.

✔ Sodium, chloride, and potassium, referred to as the electrolytes, regulate fluid balance and function in nerve conduction and muscle contraction.

✔ Hypertension, or high blood pressure, a major public health problem in the United States, can be affected by

the intake of specific nutrients as well as the dietary pattern as a whole.

✔ Bone is a metabolically active tissue that is constantly being broken down and reformed.

✔ Calcium provides structure to bones and teeth and is essential for nerve conduction, muscle contraction, blood clotting, and blood pressure regulation.

✔ Phosphorus provides structure to bones and teeth and is important in acid-base balance.

✔ Magnesium is important to bone structure and functions as a cofactor in many enzymatic reactions.

✔ Sulfur is important in the structure of some proteins and vitamins and in the regulation of acid-base balance.

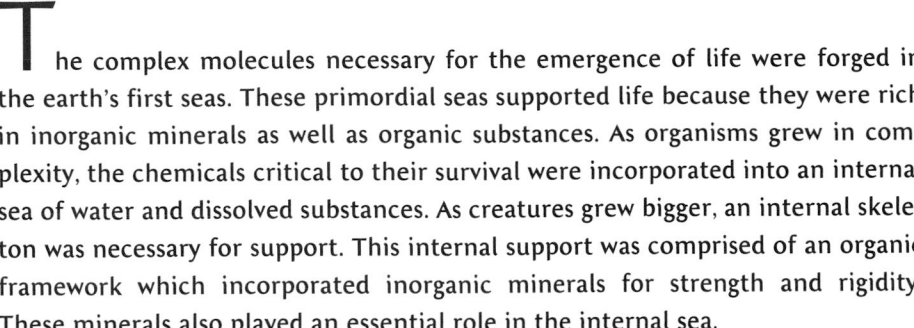

Just a Taste

How long can a person survive without water?

Does reducing salt intake reduce blood pressure?

Does drinking milk build strong bones?

The complex molecules necessary for the emergence of life were forged in the earth's first seas. These primordial seas supported life because they were rich in inorganic minerals as well as organic substances. As organisms grew in complexity, the chemicals critical to their survival were incorporated into an internal sea of water and dissolved substances. As creatures grew bigger, an internal skeleton was necessary for support. This internal support was comprised of an organic framework which incorporated inorganic minerals for strength and rigidity. These minerals also played an essential role in the internal sea.

Just as the right combination of water, organic molecules, and minerals was necessary for the beginning of life, the right combination is necessary in the body for the maintenance of life. Scientists are still researching the exact mixture of minerals and other substances necessary for this internal sea to sustain life. We understand the function of some minerals, such as the importance of calcium in bone, but our understanding of the amounts needed for optimal health is still evolving. For other minerals, such as nickel and arsenic, essentiality is just now being established and there is not enough information to determine recommended intakes.

• WATER: THE INTERNAL SEA

Water is essential to survival. Without food, an average individual can live for about eight weeks, but a lack of water reduces survival to only a few days. Although the amount and distribution of body water are regulated, water cannot be stored. Even minor changes in the amount and distribution of body water can be life threatening. When water losses are increased, as they are in hot weather and with exercise, intake must increase to maintain homeostasis.

Water in the Diet

Most of the water in the body comes from the diet—not only as water we drink but from other liquids and solid food (Figure 10.1). Milk is 90% water, apples are about 85% water, and roast beef is about 50% water. A small amount of water is generated inside the body by metabolism, but this is not significant in meeting body water needs (see *Off the Shelf*: Is Bottled Water Better?).

Water in the Body

In adults, about 60% of body weight is water. The percentage is higher in infants and then decreases with age in adulthood primarily due to a decline in muscle mass. Water is found in varying proportions in all the tissues of the body; blood is about 90% water, muscle about 75%, and bone about 25%. About two-thirds of body water is found inside cells; this is known as **intracellular fluid**. The remaining one-third is outside cells, as **extracellular fluid**. Extracellular fluid includes primarily blood plasma, lymph, and the fluid between cells, called **interstitial fluid**. The concentration of substances dissolved in body water, or **solutes**, varies

Intracellular fluid The fluid located inside cells.

Extracellular fluid The fluid located outside cells. It includes fluid found in the blood, lymph, gastrointestinal tract, spinal column, eyes, joints, and that found between cells and tissues.

Interstitial fluid The portion of the extracellular fluid located in the spaces between cells and tissues.

Solutes Dissolved substances.

271

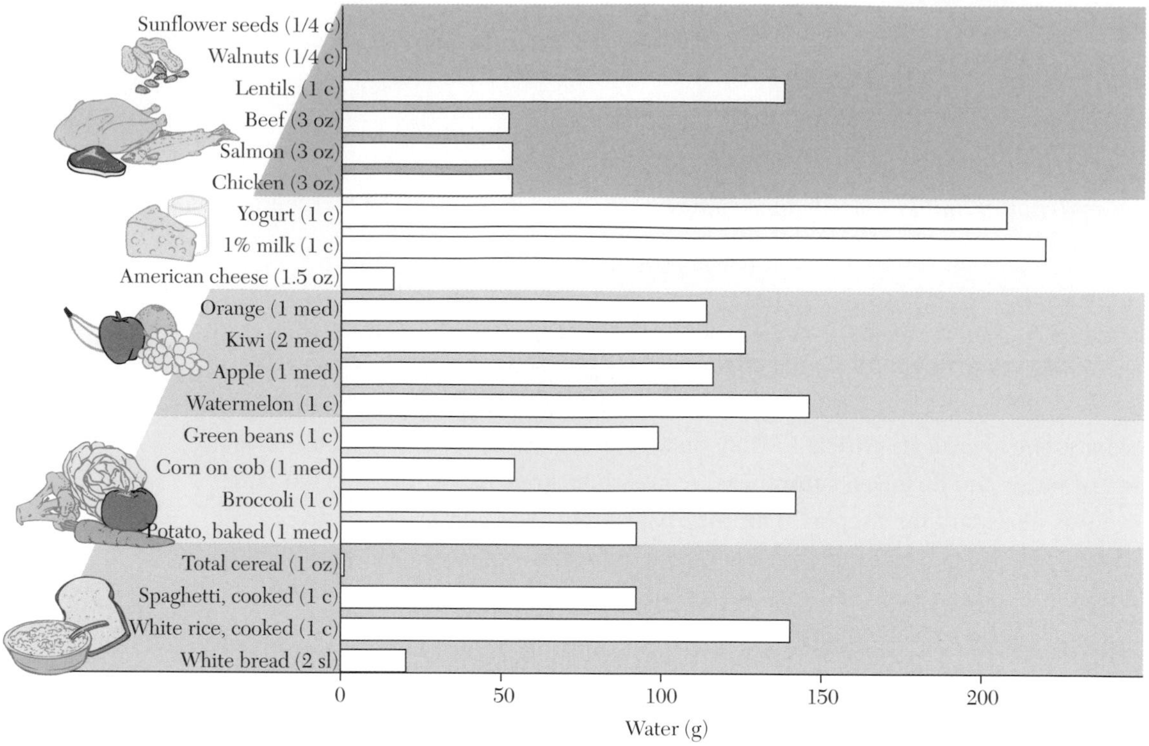

Figure 10.1

The body's need for water is met by the water consumed in fluids and food. Fruits and vegetables as well as many choices from other food groups have a high water content.

among these body compartments. The concentration of protein is highest in intracellular fluid, lower in extracellular fluid, and even lower in interstitial fluid. Extracellular fluid has a higher concentration of sodium and chloride and a lower concentration of potassium, and intracellular fluid is higher in potassium and lower in sodium and chloride.

The movement of water from one compartment to another depends on fluid pressure and on the concentration of solutes in each compartment. The fluid pressure of blood against the blood vessel walls, or **blood pressure**, causes water to move from the blood into the interstitial space. The difference in the concentration of solutes between the capillaries and the interstitial space causes much of this water to re-enter the capillaries. When the concentration of solutes in one compartment is higher than in another, water will move to equalize the solute concentration. This diffusion of water across a membrane from an area with a lower solute concentration to an area with a higher solute concentration is called **osmosis**. Osmosis occurs when there is a selectively permeable membrane, such as a cell membrane, which allows water to pass freely but regulates the passage of other substances. Water moves across this membrane in a direction that will equalize the concentration of solutes on both sides. For example, when sugar is sprinkled on fresh strawberries, the water inside the strawberries moves across the skin of the fruit to try to equalize the sugar concentration on each side, causing the fruit to shrink (Figure 10.2). The body can regulate the amount of water in each compartment by adjusting the concentration of solutes and relying on osmosis to move water.

Regulating Water Intake A constant supply of water without excess or deficiency is needed in the body. Water intake must equal water loss in order to maintain water balance. The desire to drink, or thirst, is triggered by the thirst center in the brain when it senses a decrease in blood volume and an increase in the concentration of

Blood pressure The amount of force exerted by the blood against the artery walls.

Osmosis The passive movement of water across a membrane to equalize the concentration of solutes on both sides.

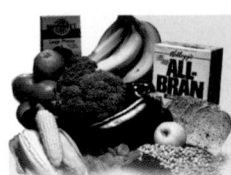

Off the Shelf

Is Bottled Water Better?

We need to consume water to survive. We want it to be safe and taste good. In general the water supply in the United States is safe; but water is not risk free. Our drinking water is potentially exposed to hundreds of different contaminants including pesticides, nitrates from fertilizers, microorganisms, metals such as lead and iron, and radioactive compounds. Sometimes a problem arises because contamination has entered a municipal water supply, and sometimes the source of contamination is an individual well or household. For example, in one community, *Cryptosporidium*, a parasite that is commonly found in rivers and lakes, found its way into a municipal water supply and caused an outbreak of gastrointestinal illness.[1] Well water can be contaminated with pesticides and fertilizers from agricultural runoff, and lead, leaching from old household plumbing, can contaminate water after it enters the home. Although water contamination is rare, stories such as these have created concern about the safety of the water supply and prompted many consumers to purchase bottled water. But is bottled better?

By definition, bottled water is water that is intended for human consumption sealed in bottles or other containers with no added ingredients except safe and suitable antimicrobial agents.[2] It comes in many forms—spring water, drinking water, purified water, well water. There are over 700 different brands of bottled water available in the United States. Consumers who assume that buying water in a bottle is a guarantee of purity may be wasting their money. In reality, the jug at the water cooler and the Evian that you guzzle at the gym may not be any safer than tap water. Standards for the purity of municipal water systems are set by the Environmental Protection Agency (EPA). These standards are used by the FDA to ensure that the minimum quality of bottled water is comparable with that of tap water.[3] Because the standards that regulate bottled water are no more rigid than those regulating tap water, it is not surprising that some bottled water actually is tap water.

About 75% of bottled water comes from protected wells and springs, but the other 25% is from municipal water supplies. To help consumers identify the source of their bottled water and make labeling consistent from state to state, the FDA established standard definitions for all bottled water products.[4] Under these regulations, bottled water that comes from tap water must be clearly labeled as such. However, water that has been taken from a municipal water supply and then treated— for example, filtered or disinfected—need not indicate that it is tap water. "Distilled water" and "purified water," are examples of water taken from municipal water supplies and then treated. If you want water that did not come from the tap, select artesian water, spring water, well water, or mineral water. These come from underground water sources.

Water from all of these sources, as well as the water used in certain types of flavored bottled waters, must comply with the bottled water standards set by the FDA. Products labeled as carbonated water, seltzer water, soda water, and tonic water are considered soft drinks and so are regulated as food, not as water.

Individuals who are concerned about their tap water, but who do not want to carry water home from the grocery store, may choose a home water-treatment system. There are many different kinds. Faucet filters remove chlorine and other substances that make the water taste bad. More elaborate filter units, distillation units, and water softeners remove contaminants but may also change the mineral content of the water. For example, an ion exchange unit, or water softener, removes some minerals, mainly calcium and magnesium, from water and replaces them with sodium. Since minerals in hard water stain tubs, clog water heaters, and cause soap to form a film that is difficult to remove from laundry, softened water makes life easier at home. But, there may be health benefits to hard water. The incidence of heart attacks is lower in areas of the country that have hard water.[5] In addition, softened water has about twice the amount of sodium— about 94 mg per liter. If you are following a sodium-restricted diet, you may need to bypass the water softener when it comes to drinking water.

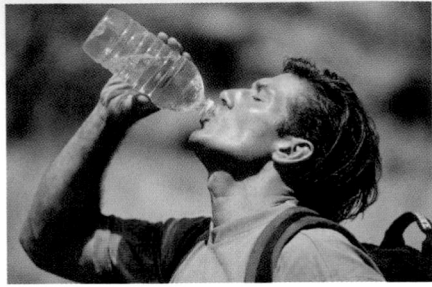

(© Ron Chappel/Getty Images)

When choosing your water, you must weigh the benefits against the risks. Bottled water and water-treatment systems cost money and whether you are drinking your tap water straight, filtering it with a home water-treatment system, or buying bottled water off the shelf, contamination is possible. The safest alternative is to buy distilled water. In the distillation process, nonvolatile chemicals are removed, and the heat destroys bacteria and other biological contaminants. The resulting water is probably free of contaminants, but it is tasteless and lacking in essential dietary minerals that water usually supplies. Before making a choice, take a look at the results of water-monitoring tests your water company is required to perform and compare them with the legal limits of contaminants set by the EPA. This should help you decide. For information, call the FDA, the International Bottled Water Association, or the EPA Hotline or look for their sites on the World Wide Web.

[1] EPA and CDC Office of Ground Water and Drinking Water. Guidance for people with severely weakened immune systems. June 17, 1998. Available online at www.epa.gov/safewater/crypto.html/ Accessed January 14, 2001.

[2] Requirements of laws and regulations enforced by the U.S. Food and Drug Administration. Available online at www.fda.gov/opacom/morechoices/smallbusiness/blubook.htm#btlwater.html/ Accessed January 14, 2001.

[3] Notebook. *FDA Consumer* 29:27, March 1995.

[4] FDA Talk Paper No. 2 (T95–59), November 7, 1995.

[5] Rubenowitz, E., Axelsson, G., and Rylander, R. Magnesium in drinking water and death from acute myocardial infarction. *Am. J. Epidemiol.* 143:456–462, 1996.

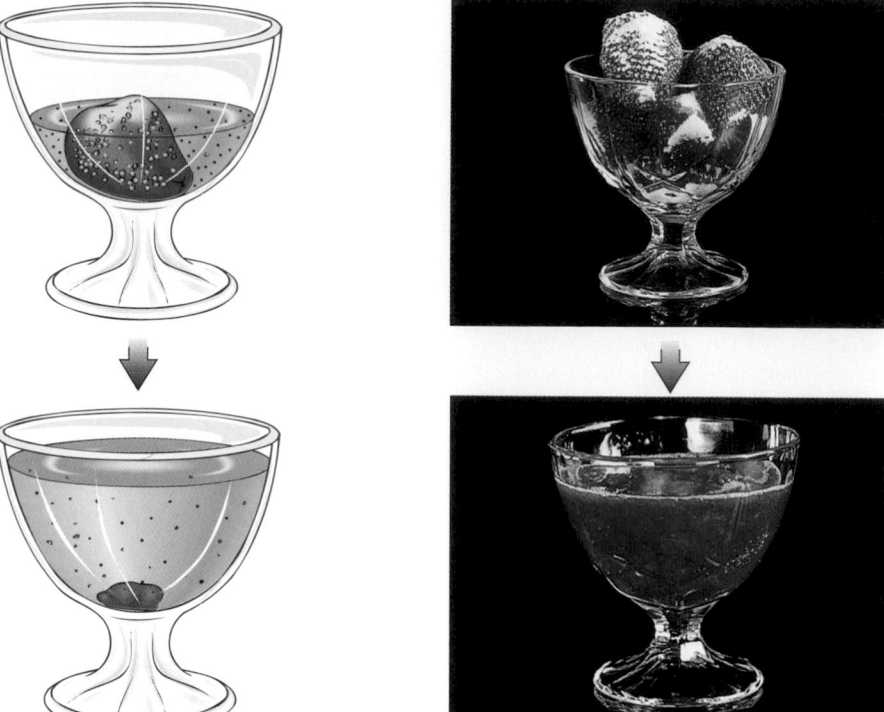

Figure 10.2
Osmosis is the process by which water moves across a membrane from an area of lower solute concentration to an area of higher solute concentration. When sugar is sprinkled on strawberries, osmosis draws water out of the strawberries to dilute the concentrated sugar solution on the surface. (Photos, Dennis Drenner)

dissolved substances in the blood. A decrease in the amount of water in the blood also decreases saliva secretion. Together, signals from the brain and a dry mouth motivate the consumption of fluid. However, these signals to consume water are not perfect regulators of water intake. Thirst is quenched almost as soon as fluid is consumed and long before water balance is restored. Also, the sensation of thirst often lags behind the need for water. For example, athletes exercising in hot weather lose water rapidly but do not experience intense thirst until they have lost so much body water that their physical performance is compromised.[1] A person with fever, vomiting, or diarrhea may also be losing water rapidly and thirst mechanisms may not be 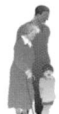 adequate to replace the fluid. In the elderly, the thirst mechanism often becomes unreliable, so an individual may not be thirsty even though body water is depleted. Also, being thirsty does not mean that the individual will take a drink. Since people cannot and do not always respond to thirst, water loss from the body is regulated to prevent dehydration.

Water Loss from the Body Water is lost from the body in urine, in feces, and through evaporation from the lungs and skin. As shown in Figure 10.3, a typical young man loses 2.75 liters of water daily through urine, feces, and evaporation. This amount must be replaced through consumption of food and fluids in order to maintain water balance.

Typical urine output is 1 to 2 liters per day, but this varies depending on the amount of fluid consumed and the amount of waste to be excreted. The waste products that must be excreted in urine include urea and other nitrogen-containing products from protein breakdown, ketones from fat breakdown, phosphates, sulfates, and other minerals. The amount of urea that must be excreted is increased when dietary or body protein breakdown is increased. Ketone excretion is increased when body fat is broken down. In both cases, the need for water increases in order to produce more urine to excrete the extra wastes.

The amount of water lost in the feces is usually small, only about 200 ml per day (less than a cup). This is remarkable because every day about 9 liters of fluid

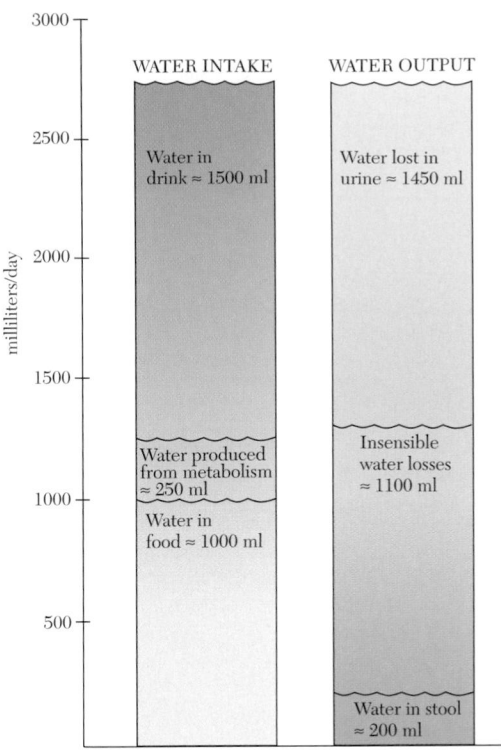

Figure 10.3

To maintain water balance, intake must equal output. This figure approximates the sources of water intake and output in a 70-kg adult who is not losing water in sweat.

enter the gastrointestinal tract via food, water, and secretions. Under normal conditions, more than 95% is reabsorbed before the feces are eliminated. However, in cases of severe diarrhea, large amounts of water can be lost through the gastrointestinal tract.

Water loss due to evaporation from the skin and lungs occurs without the individual being aware that it is occurring; such losses are therefore referred to as **insensible losses**. An inactive person at room temperature loses about 1 liter per day through insensible losses but the amount varies depending on body size, environmental temperature and humidity, and physical activity. For example, a very dry environment, such as in an airplane or in the desert, increases evaporative losses.

Water lost in sweat is distinct from insensible losses because it is a detectable loss. The amount of water lost through sweat is extremely variable depending on the individual as well as their activity level and environment. An individual doing light work at a temperature of about 84°F will lose about 2 to 3 liters of sweat per day. Strenuous exercise in a hot environment can cause water losses in sweat to be as high as 2 to 4 liters in an hour.[2] Adequate water intake is essential to compensate for these losses. Endurance athletes can estimate water loss by weighing themselves before and after exercise. Lost weight should then be replaced by consuming at least the equivalent weight in fluids. For instance, an athlete who loses 2 pounds during a workout should consume at least an extra 2 pints or a liter of fluid (1 lb = 1 pint = $\frac{1}{2}$ liter (see Chapter 13).

Kidneys Regulate Water Excretion The kidneys serve as a filtering system that regulates the amount of water and dissolved substances retained in the blood and excreted in urine. As blood flows through the kidneys, water and small molecules are filtered out of the blood vessels. Some of the water and molecules are reabsorbed and the rest are excreted in the urine. The amount of water that is reabsorbed depends on conditions in the body. When the concentration of solutes in the blood is high, **antidiuretic hormone (ADH)**, which is secreted from the pituitary gland, signals the kidneys to reabsorb water to reduce the amount lost in the urine. This

Insensible losses Fluid losses that are not perceived by the senses, such as evaporation of water through the skin and lungs.

Antidiuretic hormone (ADH) A hormone secreted by the pituitary gland that increases the amount of water reabsorbed by the kidney and therefore retained in the body.

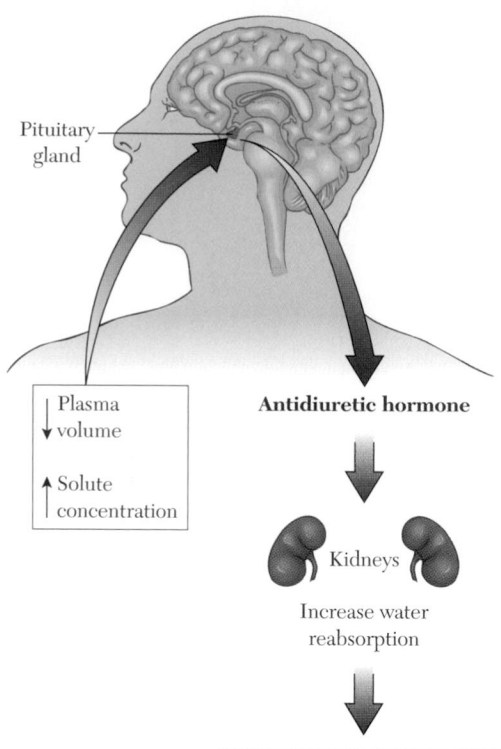

Figure 10.4
When an individual hasn't consumed enough fluid, the volume of plasma (the liquid portion of the blood that remains when the blood cells are removed) decreases and solute concentration increases, signaling the pituitary gland to secrete antidiuretic hormone, which acts on the kidneys to increase water reabsorption, thereby decreasing water losses.

reabsorbed water is returned to the blood, decreasing the solute concentration in the blood to normal (Figure 10.4). When the solute concentration in the blood is low, ADH levels decrease so less water is reabsorbed and more is excreted in the urine, allowing blood solute concentration to increase to normal. The amount of sodium in the blood, blood volume, and blood pressure also play a role in regulating body water.

Functions of Water in the Body In the body, water serves as a medium in which chemical reactions take place; it also transports nutrients, provides protection, helps regulate temperature, and participates in chemical reactions and acid base balance (Table 10.1).

Solvent A fluid in which one or more substances dissolve.

Polar Used to describe a molecule that has a positive charge at one end and a negative charge at the other.

Electrons Negatively charged particles.

Ion An atom or group of atoms that carries an electrical charge.

Dissociate To separate two charged ions.

Water as a Solvent One of the key functions of water in the body is as a **solvent**, which is a fluid in which solutes can dissolve to form a solution. Water is an ideal solvent for some substances because it is **polar**; that is, the two sides or poles of the water molecule have different electrical charges. The polar nature of water comes from its structure, which consists of two hydrogen atoms and one oxygen atom. These atoms, like all atoms, are made up of a positively charged central core, or nucleus, with negatively charged **electrons** orbiting around it. To form a water molecule, the two hydrogen atoms move close enough to share their electrons with an atom of oxygen. But the sharing is not equal. The shared electrons spend more time around the oxygen atom than around the hydrogen atoms, giving the oxygen side of the molecule a slightly negative charge and the hydrogen side a slightly positive charge. This polar nature of water allows it to surround other charged molecules and disperse them. Table salt, which dissolves in water, consists of a positively charged sodium **ion** bound to a negatively charged chloride ion. When placed in water, the sodium and chloride ions move apart, or **dissociate**, because the positively charged sodium ion is attracted to the negative pole of the water

Table 10.1 A Summary of Water and the Major Minerals

Nutrient	Sources	Recommended Intake for Adults	Major Functions	Deficiency Diseases and Symptoms	Groups at Risk	Toxicity	Tolerable Upper Intake Levels (UL)
Water	Food and beverages	1 ml/kcal	Solvent, reactant, protector, transporter, temperature regulator	Thirst, weakness, poor endurance, confusion, disorientation	Infants, those with fever and diarrhea, elderly, athletes	Unlikely, confusion, coma, convulsions	NA
Sodium	Table salt, processed foods	500–2400 mg	Major extracellular ion, nerve transmission, muscle extraction, fluid balance	Muscle cramps	Those consuming a severely sodium-restricted diet	High blood pressure in sensitive individuals	NA
Potassium	Fruits, vegetables, grains	At least 1600–3500 mg	Major intracellular ion, nerve transmission, muscle contraction	Irregular heartbeat, fatigue, muscle cramps	Those consuming diets high in processed foods, those taking thiazide diuretics	Abnormal heartbeat	NA
Chloride	Table salt	750–3400 mg	Major extracellular ion	Unlikely	None	None likely	NA
Calcium	Dairy products, bony fish, leafy green vegetables	1000–1200 mg°	Bone and tooth structure, nerve transmission, muscle contraction, blood clotting, blood pressure regulation, hormone secretion	Increased risk of osteoporosis	Postmenopausal women, children, adolescents, elderly, those with kidney disease	Kidney stones in susceptible individuals	2500 mg
Phosphorus	Meat, dairy, cereals, and baked goods	700 mg	Structure of bones, teeth, membranes, ATP and DNA, buffer	Bone loss, weakness, lack of appetite	Premature infants, alcoholics, elderly	Calcium resorption from bone	4000 mg
Magnesium	Nuts, greens, whole grains, seeds	310–420 mg	Bone structure, ATP reactions, nerve and muscle function	Nausea, vomiting, weakness, heart changes	Alcoholics, those with kidney and gastrointestinal disease	Nausea, vomiting, low blood pressure	350 mg (nonfood)
Sulfur	Protein foods, preservatives	None specified	Part of amino acids and vitamins, buffer	None when protein needs are met	None	None likely	NA

°Adequate intake (AI).

NA—No UL established at time of publication.

molecule and the negatively charged chloride ion is attracted to the positive pole (Figure 10.5). Substances like sodium chloride that dissociate in water to form positively and negatively charged ions are known as **electrolytes**. Electrolytes got their name because they are capable of conducting an electrical current when dissolved in water.

Water as Transport Blood, which is 90% water, transports oxygen and nutrients to cells. It then carries carbon dioxide and waste products away from the cells. Water in urine transports waste products, such as urea and ketones, out of the body.

Water as Protection Water functions as a lubricant and cleanser. Watery tears lubricate the eyes and wash away dirt, synovial fluid lubricates the joints, and saliva lubricates the mouth, making it easier to chew and swallow food. Water inside the eyeballs and spinal cord acts as a cushion against shock. Similarly, during pregnancy, water in the amniotic fluid provides a protective cushion for the fetus.

Water as a Regulator of Temperature Body temperature is closely regulated to maintain a normal level of around 98.6°F (37°C). If the body temperature rises

Electrolytes Substances that separate in water to form positively and negatively charged ions. In nutrition this term refers to sodium, potassium, and chloride.

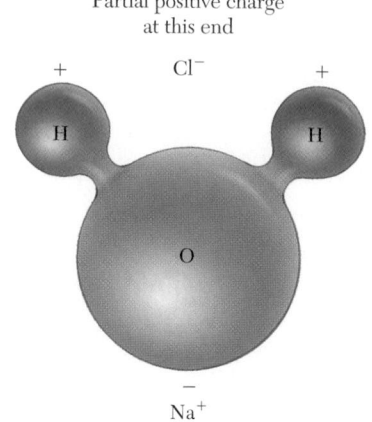

Partial positive charge
at this end

Partial negative charge
at this end

Figure 10.5

Two hydrogen atoms share electrons with one oxygen atom to form a molecule of water. The electrons spend more time around the oxygen atom, giving it a slightly negative charge, while the side of the molecule with the two hydrogens has a slightly positive charge. When salt (sodium chloride) is added to water, the positive sodium ion is attracted to the negative pole of the water molecule and the negative chloride ion is attracted to the positive pole.

pH A measure of the level of acidity or alkalinity of a solution.

above 108°F or falls below 80°F, death is likely. The fact that water changes temperature slowly in response to changes in the external environment helps the human body resist temperature change when the outside temperature fluctuates. The water in blood actively regulates body temperature. When body temperature starts to rise, the blood vessels in the skin dilate, causing blood to flow close to the surface of the body and release some of the heat to the environment. This occurs with fevers as well as when environmental temperature rises. In a cold environment, blood vessels in the skin constrict, restricting the flow of blood near the surface and conserving body heat. The most obvious way that water helps regulate body temperature is through the evaporation of sweat. When body temperature increases, the sweat glands in the skin secrete this watery substance. As the sweat evaporates from the skin, heat is lost.

Water in Chemical Reactions Water is involved in chemical reactions in the body. Hydrolysis reactions break large molecules into smaller ones by the addition of water. For example, water is added in the reaction that breaks a molecule of maltose into two glucose molecules. Water is also involved in reactions that join two molecules. These reactions are referred to as condensation reactions. The formation of a dipeptide from two amino acids requires the removal of a water molecule.

Regulation of Acid-Base Balance The chemical reactions that occur in the body are very sensitive to acidity. Acidity is expressed in units of **pH**. The range of pH units is from 1 to 14, with 1 being very acidic, 14 being very basic, and 7 being neutral. Most reactions in the body occur in slightly basic solutions, around pH 7.4. If body solutions become too acidic or too basic, chemical reactions cannot proceed efficiently (Figure 10.6). Water and the dissolved substances it contains are important for main-

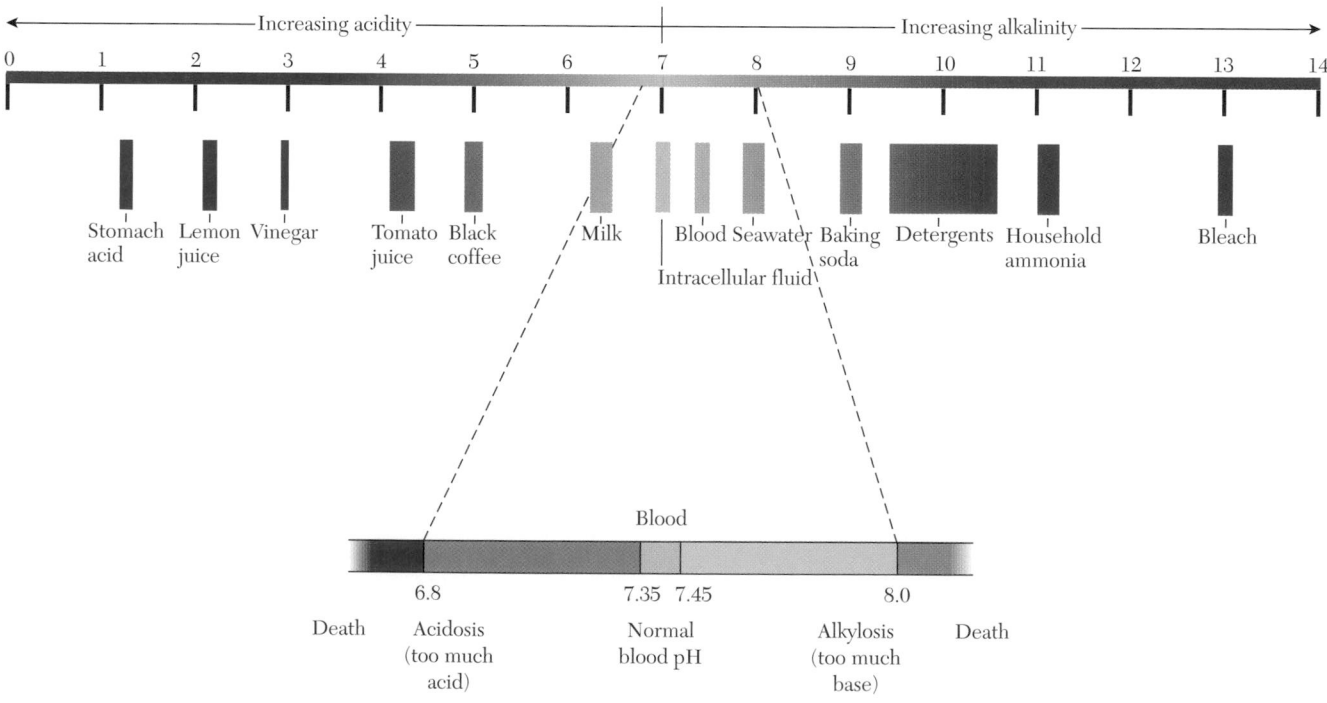

Figure 10.6

The pH values for some common fluids. Fluctuations from the normal blood pH range of between 7.35 and 7.45 lead to acidosis (too much acid) or alkylosis (too much base) and, if severe, can be fatal.

taining the proper level of acidity. Water serves as a medium for the chemical reactions that prevent changes in pH and it participates in some of these reactions. Water is also needed as a transport medium to allow the respiratory tract and kidneys to regulate acid-base balance.

How Much Water Do We Need?

Adults need about 1 ml of water per kcalorie of energy requirement, or about 2 to 3 liters per day. This amount is sufficient under average conditions, but needs can be increased by variations in activity, environment, and diet. For instance, a person exercising in a hot climate can require an additional 4 liters or more per day to replace water lost through sweating (Figure 10.7). Water needs are also affected by the composition and adequacy of the diet. A low-energy diet increases water needs because water losses increase to excrete the ketones produced by fat breakdown. A high-protein diet increases the amount of nitrogenous waste that must be excreted. A high-sodium diet increases water needs because the excess salt must be excreted in the urine. Caffeine is a diuretic, so a diet that is high in caffeine increases water loss from the kidneys and therefore increases water needs. A high-fiber diet also increases water needs because more fluid is retained in the gastrointestinal tract.

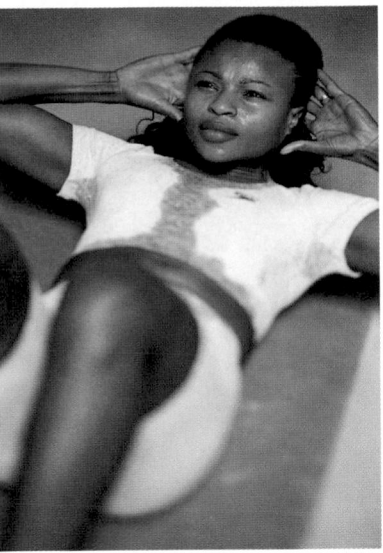

Figure 10.7

Exercise in a hot environment can dramatically increase water losses from sweat. (© Lori Adamski Peek/Getty Images)

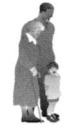

Water needs also increase during pregnancy and lactation. In pregnancy, water is needed to increase blood volume, produce amniotic fluid, and nourish the fetus. During lactation, the fluid secreted in milk, about 750 ml or 3 cups per day, must be replaced by the mother's fluid intake.

The fluid requirements for infants are proportionately higher than those for adults. One reason is that the infant's kidneys cannot concentrate urine as efficiently as adult kidneys, so water loss is greater. Moreover, insensible losses are proportionally greater in infants and children because body surface area relative to body weight is much greater than in adults. In addition to having greater water needs, infants are susceptible to dehydration because they cannot ask for a drink when they are thirsty. The recommended intake is 1.5 ml per kcalorie of energy expenditure, or about 3 cups (750 ml) per day for a six-month-old infant. This is the water-to-energy ratio in human milk.

Water and Health

When water loss exceeds water intake, dehydration results. Dehydration occurs when the drop in body water is great enough for blood volume to decrease, thereby reducing the ability to deliver oxygen and nutrients to cells and remove waste products. Even mild dehydration—a body water loss of 1 to 2% of body weight—can impair physical and cognitive performance.[3] Early symptoms of dehydration include headache, fatigue, loss of appetite, dry eyes and mouth, and dark-colored urine. A loss of 5% body water can cause nausea and difficulty concentrating. Confusion and disorientation can occur when water loss approaches 7%. A loss of about 10 to 20% can result in death (Figure 10.8).

Young athletes involved in sports with weight classes, such as wrestling and boxing, sometimes use dehydration to reduce their body weight so they can compete in a lower weight class. Being at the high end of the lower weight class is thought to provide an advantage over smaller opponents in that class.[4] However, when this is accomplished through even mild dehydration, exercise performance can be impaired (see Chapter 13).

An excess of water, or water toxicity, is rare because of the kidneys' ability to regulate how much water is excreted. However, it can occur due to illness or improper administration of intravenous fluids. Symptoms of water toxicity include mental dulling, confusion, coma, convulsions, and even death.

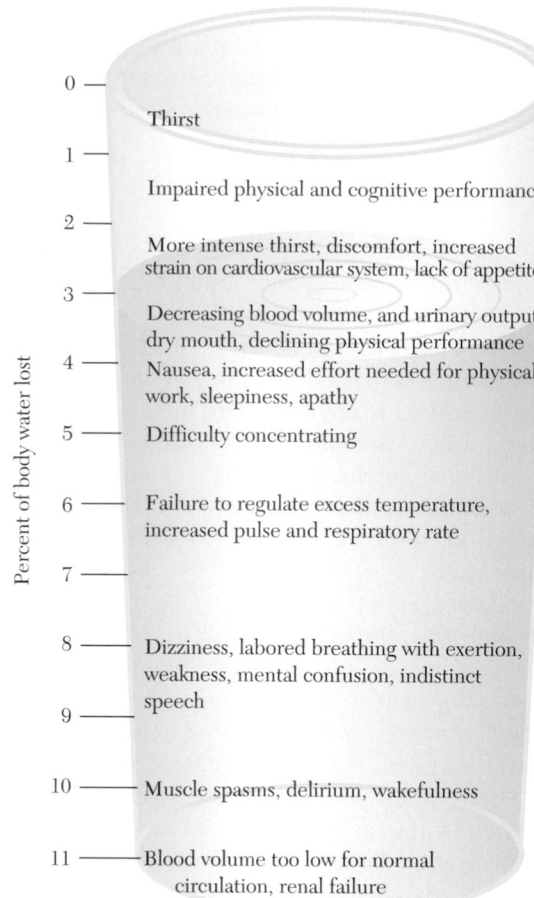

Figure 10.8
As the degree of dehydration increases, the adverse effects of dehydration increase in severity. This can occur rapidly if water losses are excessive, as may occur with profuse sweating, vomiting, or diarrhea.

Percent of body water lost

- 0 — Thirst
- 1
- — Impaired physical and cognitive performance
- 2 — More intense thirst, discomfort, increased strain on cardiovascular system, lack of appetite
- 3 — Decreasing blood volume, and urinary output, dry mouth, declining physical performance
- 4 — Nausea, increased effort needed for physical work, sleepiness, apathy
- 5 — Difficulty concentrating
- 6 — Failure to regulate excess temperature, increased pulse and respiratory rate
- 7
- 8 — Dizziness, labored breathing with exertion, weakness, mental confusion, indistinct speech
- 9
- 10 — Muscle spasms, delirium, wakefulness
- 11 — Blood volume too low for normal circulation, renal failure

• WHAT ARE MINERALS?

Minerals are inorganic elements needed by the body as structural components and regulators of body processes. Minerals may combine with other elements in the body, but they retain their chemical identity. Unlike vitamins, they are not destroyed by heat, oxygen, or acid. The ash that remains after a food is combusted in a bomb calorimeter contains the minerals that were present in that food. Minerals have tra-

Figure 10.9
Minerals are chemical elements found in the periodic table. The major minerals are shown in purple, and the trace elements are shown in blue.

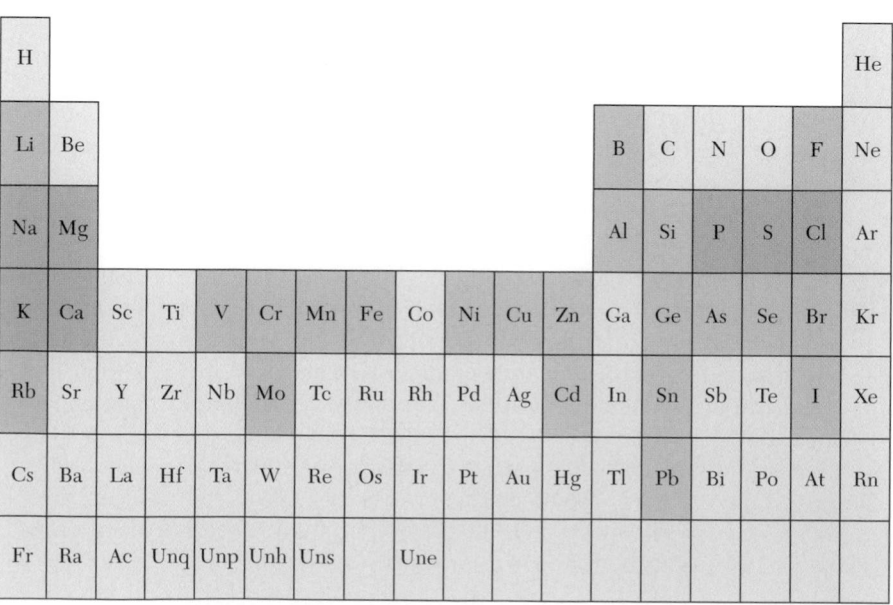

ditionally been divided into **major minerals**, or those needed in the diet in amounts greater than 100 mg per day or present in the body in amounts greater than 0.01% of body weight, and **trace elements**, which are minerals required by the body in an amount of 100 mg or less per day or present in the body in an amount of 0.01% or less of body weight (Figure 10.9).

Minerals in the Diet

Minerals in the diet come from both plant and animal sources. In some foods, the amounts of minerals are predictable because the minerals are regulated components of the plant or animal. For instance, iron is a component of muscle tissue; therefore, it is found in consistent amounts in meat. Magnesium is a component of chlorophyll, so it is found in consistent amounts in leafy greens. The amounts of some trace minerals in food vary depending on the mineral concentration in the soil and water at the food's source (Figure 10.10). For example, the soil content of iodine is high near the ocean but usually quite low in inland areas. Therefore, foods grown near the ocean are better sources of iodine than those grown inland. In developed countries, modern transportation systems make foods produced in many locations available, so the diet is unlikely to be deficient in trace elements. In countries where the diet consists predominantly of locally grown foods, individual trace element deficiencies and excesses are more likely to occur.

Food processing and refining also affect the mineral content of foods. When the skins of produce and the bran and germ of grains are removed, trace elements are lost. For example, iron, selenium, zinc, and copper are lost when flour is refined. But only iron is replaced by enrichment. Processing tends to decrease the potassium content of foods and increase the sodium content. Some minerals are added inadvertently through contamination. For example, the iodine content of dairy products is increased by contamination from the cleaning solutions used in milking machines. Other minerals are added intentionally. For example, the fortification of breakfast cereals can add calcium and other minerals. The mineral content of the diet can be maximized by eating a variety of foods, including many unprocessed or less processed foods such as fresh fruits, vegetables, and whole grains and cereals (Figure 10.11).

Minerals in the Digestive Tract

The degree to which minerals are absorbed from the digestive tract varies dramatically. Almost 100% of the sodium consumed in the diet is absorbed, whereas calcium absorption is typically about 25% and iron absorption may be as low as 5%. For some minerals the amount absorbed depends primarily on the amount that is consumed. For others, the composition of the diet as well as the nutritional status and life stage of the consumer affect absorption and bioavailability.

Some dietary components decrease mineral bioavailability. Mineral ions that carry the same charge compete for absorption in the gastrointestinal tract. Calcium, magnesium, zinc, copper, and iron all carry a 2^+ charge, and a high intake of one may reduce the absorption of others. For example, a high intake of calcium in a meal containing iron may reduce the absorption of iron. Mineral bioavailability is also affected by the binding of minerals to other substances in the gastrointestinal tract. **Phytic acid**, or **phytate**—an organic compound containing phosphorus that is found in whole grains, bran, and soy products—binds calcium, zinc, iron, and magnesium, limiting their absorption. Phytic acid can be broken down by yeast, so the bioavailability of minerals is increased in yeast-leavened foods such as breads. **Tannins**, found in tea and some grains, can interfere with iron absorption, and **oxalates**, which are organic acids found in spinach, rhubarb, beet greens, and chocolate, have been found to interfere with calcium and iron absorption (Figure 10.12). Dietary fiber also interferes with mineral absorption. Although North Americans generally do not consume enough of any of these components to cause trace element deficiencies, problems may occur in developing countries. For example, in some populations

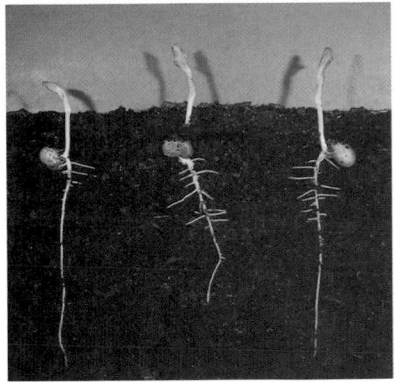

Figure 10.10
The mineral content of some plants varies with the mineral content of the soil in which they are grown. (Stephen J. Krasemann/Peter Arnold, Inc.)

Major minerals Minerals needed in the diet in amounts greater than 100 mg per day or present in the body in amounts greater than 0.01% of body weight.

Trace elements Minerals required in the diet in amounts of 100 mg or less per day or present in the body in amounts of 0.01% of body weight or less.

Phytic acid, or phytate An inorganic phosphorus storage compound found in seeds and grains that can bind minerals and decrease their absorption.

Tannins Substances found in tea and some grains that can bind certain minerals and decrease their absorption.

Oxalates Organic acids found in spinach, rhubarb, and other leafy green vegetables that can bind certain minerals and decrease their absorption.

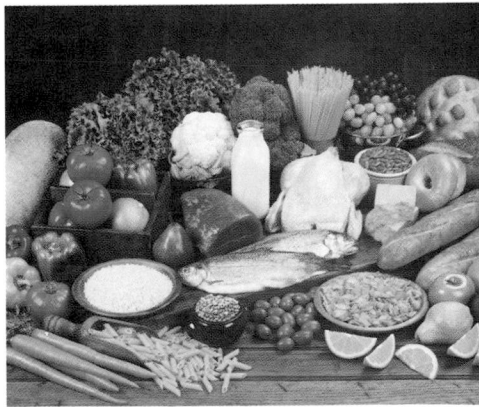

Figure 10.11
The trace element content of the diet can be maximized by eating a variety of nutrient-dense foods. (© PhotoDisc, Inc.)

the intake of phytate (which decreases zinc absorption) is high enough to increase the requirement for zinc.

There are also substances in the diet that promote mineral absorption. For example, when iron is consumed with acidic foods, the low pH helps to keep it in its more absorbable chemical form. Vitamin C in the diet enhances the absorption of iron both because it is an acid and because it forms a complex with iron that makes the iron more easily absorbed.

Nutritional status and life stage can also affect mineral bioavailability. For example, when iron stores are low, the ability of the body to transport iron from mucosal cells to body tissues increases, but when iron stores are high, iron stays in the mucosal cells and is lost when they die. During pregnancy, increased calcium needs are met by an increase in absorption.

Minerals in the Body

Minerals are transported in the blood bound to plasma proteins or specific transport proteins. The binding of minerals to transport proteins helps regulate their absorption and prevents reactive minerals from forming free radicals that could cause oxidative damage.

Minerals perform a wide range of vital structural and regulatory roles in the body. For example, calcium, phosphorus, magnesium, and fluoride affect the structure and strength of bones. Iodine is a component of the thyroid hormones, which regulate metabolic rate; chromium plays a role in regulating blood glucose levels; and zinc plays an important role in gene expression. Many of the minerals serve as **cofactors** necessary for enzyme activity. Selenium, copper, zinc, iron, and manganese each function as a cofactor for antioxidant enzyme systems.

Some minerals interact in their structural and regulatory functions. For example, calcium and phosphorus are both needed to mineralize bone, and blood levels of one can influence how the other is used. Sodium and potassium ions, which both carry a 1^+ charge, are exchanged across cell membranes to regulate fluid balance and the electrical charge of the membrane.

How Much of Each Mineral Do We Need?

The DRI recommendations for mineral intakes are based on evidence from many types of research studies, ranging from laboratory studies done with animals and clinical trials with humans to epidemiological observations—and in some cases the study of rare diseases and inadvertent outcomes of medical interventions.

Depletion-repletion studies are often used to assess mineral essentiality and determine mineral requirements. Minerals, like other nutrients, are considered essential if a deficiency consistently results in less than optimal biological function and is preventable or reversible by supplementation of that nutrient at levels similar to those found normally in the diet. In a depletion-repletion study, the subject is depleted of a nutrient until symptoms of a deficiency appear; then the nutrient is repleted to a level at which symptoms resolve. However, because of the many potential interactions among minerals and other dietary components, the need for any one mineral must be examined within the context of the total diet, and thus studied along with known amounts of other dietary components that interact with it. Depletion-repletion studies are particularly difficult with trace elements because requirements are so small that trace elements present in the environment and those already in the body can meet needs and obscure experimental results.

In addition to planned experiments, information about trace element needs has come from the study of diseases affecting trace element utilization and from the study of deficiency symptoms in individuals fed solely by **total parenteral nutrition (TPN)** solutions for long periods of time (Figure 10.13). For example, much of our knowledge about copper comes from studying Menkes kinky hair syndrome, an inherited condition in which copper absorption and metabolism are abnormal. The symptoms of this syndrome are manifestations of a copper deficiency. Observations of

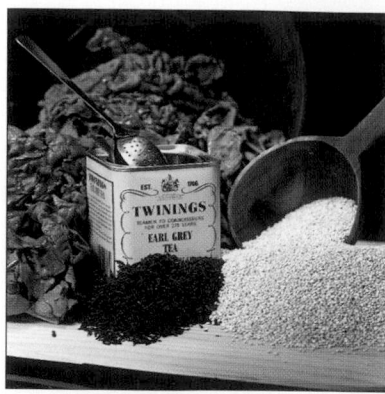

Figure 10.12
Compounds such as phytic acid, oxalates, and tannins found in these foods decrease mineral absorption. (Charles D. Winters)

Cofactor An inorganic ion or coenzyme required for enzyme activity.

Total parenteral nutrition A method of providing complete nutrition by infusing nutrients into a large central vein.

a patient receiving a TPN solution deficient in selenium helped establish the essentiality of this mineral. The patient developed symptoms that resolved when selenium was added to the solution.

As with other nutrients, when no other data are available, mineral needs can be estimated by evaluating the intake in a healthy population. It is assumed that if there are no deficiency symptoms, the diet must meet the requirement for that nutrient. One problem with this approach, however, is that deficiency symptoms may become apparent only when the deficiency is severe. Subtle signs of a mineral deficiency in a population may be difficult to detect.

Minerals and Health

The right amount of each mineral is needed in the correct proportion in order to maintain health. Both deficiencies and excesses cause changes in body function. For some minerals, too much or too little causes obvious symptoms that impact short-term health. For others, underconsumption or overconsumption has few immediate symptoms but may affect the risk of chronic disease later in life. Due to the many interactions among minerals, an excess or deficiency of one can affect the status of another.

Deficiency Deficiencies of the minerals iron, iodine, and calcium are world health problems. Iron deficiency affects people in both developed and the developing world. Only a few months of inadequate iron intake can cause a decrease in the number and size of red blood cells, reducing the blood's capacity to deliver oxygen. Iodine deficiency disorders are a problem primarily in developing countries, where they impact individuals at every stage of life. Like iron deficiency, iodine deficiency causes problems over a relatively short period of time. Low calcium intake poses a problem in both developed and developing countries. There are no short-term consequences, but a diet deficient in calcium can reduce bone density and impact bone health later in life.

Deficiencies of other minerals are rare, occurring only when the food supply is particularly limited. For example, in certain rural areas of China, selenium deficiency may occur because the selenium content of the soil is extremely low and the diet is based on locally grown food.

Toxicity Mineral toxicity occurs most often as a result of environmental pollution or excessive use of supplements. For example, environmental lead from old chipped lead paint, lead pipes, and soil and air contamination is a risk to small children. Chronic exposure can cause growth retardation and learning disabilities (see Chapter 15). Trace element supplements may pose a risk of toxicity because elements that are essential in small doses may be toxic when consumed in larger amounts. For instance, iron is essential, yet can be deadly at high doses.

Mineral supplements may also cause problems because of the complex interactions among minerals. Taking high doses of one can compromise the bioavailability of others, creating a mineral imbalance that can interfere with functions essential to human health. The body's regulatory mechanisms control the absorption and excretion of minerals but have evolved to deal with the amounts of these elements that occur naturally in the diet. Large doses of mineral supplements may override this regulation, causing toxicity.

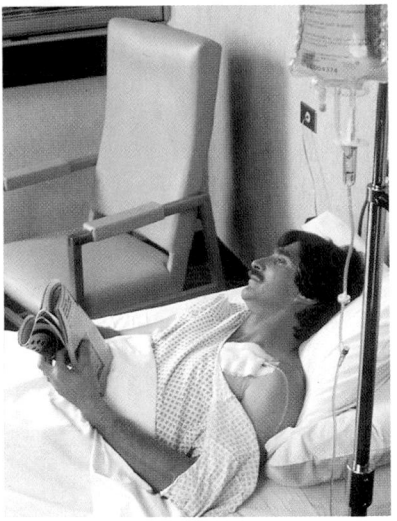

Figure 10.13
Trace element deficiencies can occur if incomplete TPN solutions are administered long-term.
(© W. L. Steinmark/Custom Medical Stock Photo)

• ELECTROLYTES: SALTS OF THE INTERNAL SEA

Electrolytes are elements that conduct electricity when dissolved in water. In nutrition, the term is used to refer to the minerals sodium, potassium, and chloride—the principal electrolytes in body fluids. The modern diet is typically low in potassium and high in sodium and chloride, which are generally consumed together as sodium chloride, or table salt. This is a change from the diets of prehistoric hunter-gatherers, which consisted of plant foods such as nuts, berries, roots, and greens that are high in potassium and low in salt. Most of this change is due to the use of salt as a food additive. Salt is used as a preservative in food because it inhibits bacterial growth; it is also used to add flavor and to heighten existing flavors. It was highly prized by ancient cultures in Asia, Africa, and Europe, where it was used in rituals as well as in the preservation of food. Roman soldiers were paid in *sal*, the Latin word for salt from which we get our word *salary*.

Today, rather than a prized commodity, salt is a substance we attempt to limit in the diet. The reason for restricting salt is that diets high in salt have been implicated as a risk factor for **hypertension**.

Hypertension Blood pressure that is consistently elevated to 140/90 mm of mercury or greater.

Electrolytes in the Diet

The typical American diet contains about 9 grams of salt. Salt is 40% sodium and 60% chloride by weight, so 9 grams contains 3.6 grams of sodium ($9 \times 40\% = 3.6$ g) and 5.4 grams of chloride. Most of the salt in the Western diet comes from processed foods. Only 10% comes from salt found naturally in food; 15% is from that added in cooking and at the table, and 75% is from that added during processing and manufacturing. Most of the sodium in processed foods is from sodium chloride, but other sodium salts, such as sodium bicarbonate, sodium citrate, and sodium glutamate, are used as food additives and contribute to the sodium content of the diet. These sodium-containing additives are used as preservatives and leavening agents. Drinking water from community water supplies contributes less than 10% of our sodium intake.[5] Softened water or mineral water is often higher in sodium than tap water and, if consumed in large quantities, can contribute significantly to daily sodium intake.

In contrast to sodium and chloride, the richest sources of potassium are unprocessed foods such as fruits, vegetables, whole grains, and fresh meats. Bananas, oranges, potatoes, and tomatoes are some of the best sources. Processed foods are generally lower in potassium (Figure 10.14).

Electrolytes in the Body

Almost all of the sodium, chloride, and potassium consumed in the diet is absorbed. Despite large variations in dietary intake, homeostatic mechanisms act to regulate the concentrations of these electrolytes in the body where they help regulate fluid balance and are important for nerve conduction and muscle contraction.

Electrolytes and Fluid Balance Electrolytes and other solutes cannot move freely back and forth across cell membranes, but water can. The movement of water between intracellular and extracellular compartments, therefore, depends on the concentrations of sodium and potassium and other solutes in these compartments. For example, if the concentration of electrolytes is high in the blood, water is drawn into the blood by osmosis to dilute the electrolytes, reducing their concentration.

Electrolytes and Nerve Conduction and Muscle Contraction Sodium and potassium are important for the conduction of nerve impulses (see Table 10.1). Nerve impulses are created by a change in the electrical charge across cell membranes. In the extracellular fluid, sodium is the most abundant positively charged electrolyte, and chloride is the principal negatively charged ion. Potassium is the principal positively charged ion inside cells, where it is 30 times more concentrated than outside the cell. An electrical charge, or membrane potential, exists across cell membranes because the number of negative ions just inside the cell membrane is greater than the number outside. Stimuli, such as neurotransmitters, change the cell membrane's permeability to sodium, allowing it to rush into the cells. This reverses, or depolarizes, the charge of the cell membrane at that location, and an electrical current is generated. The nerve impulse travels as an electrical current. Once the nerve impulse passes, the original membrane potential is rapidly restored by another change in cell membrane permeability; then the original distribution of sodium and

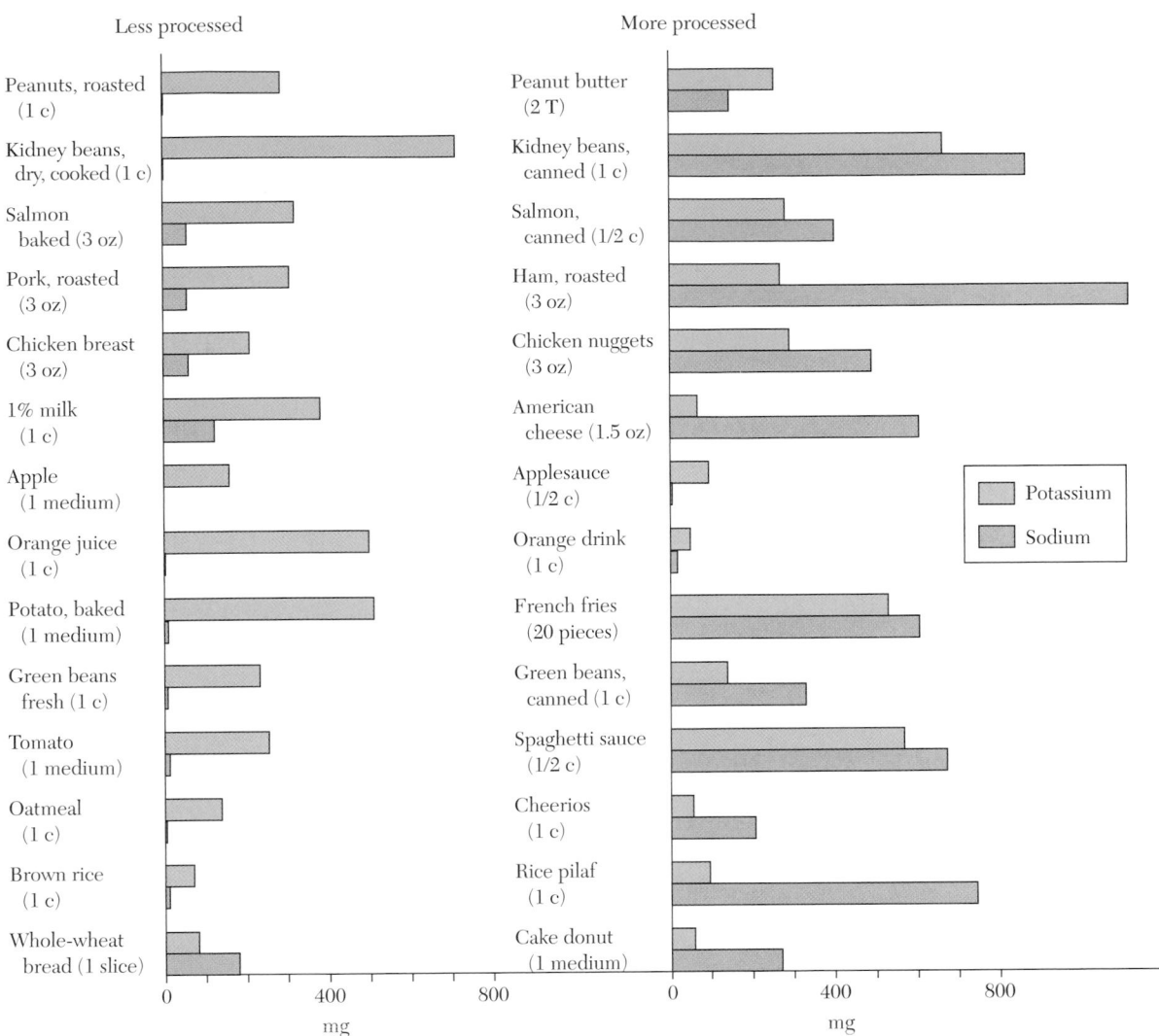

Figure 10.14
Less processed foods tend to be low in sodium and good sources of potassium. More processed foods are generally higher in sodium and may also be lower in potassium.

potassium ions across the cell membrane is restored by a sodium-potassium pump in the cell membrane (the sodium-potassium ATPase). A similar mechanism causes the depolarization of the muscle cell membranes, leading to muscle contraction.

Regulation of Electrolyte Balance Despite large variations in dietary intake, homeostatic mechanisms regulate the concentrations of these electrolytes within a narrow range. For example, in northern China, sodium chloride intake is greater than 13.9 grams per day; in the Kalahari Desert, it is less than 1.7 grams per day; and in an Indian population in Brazil, consumption may be less than 0.06 gram of salt per day. However, blood levels of sodium are not significantly different among these groups.

Sodium and chloride homeostasis is regulated to some extent by the intake of both water and salt. When salt intake is high, thirst is stimulated to increase water intake. When salt intake is very low, a salt appetite causes the individual to seek out the mineral. These mechanisms help ensure that appropriate proportions of salt and water are taken in. The kidneys, however, are the primary regulator of sodium, chloride, and potassium balance in the body. Excretion of these electrolytes in the urine is decreased when intake is low and increased when intake is high. Because water follows sodium by osmosis, the ability of the kidneys to conserve sodium provides a mechanism to conserve body water.

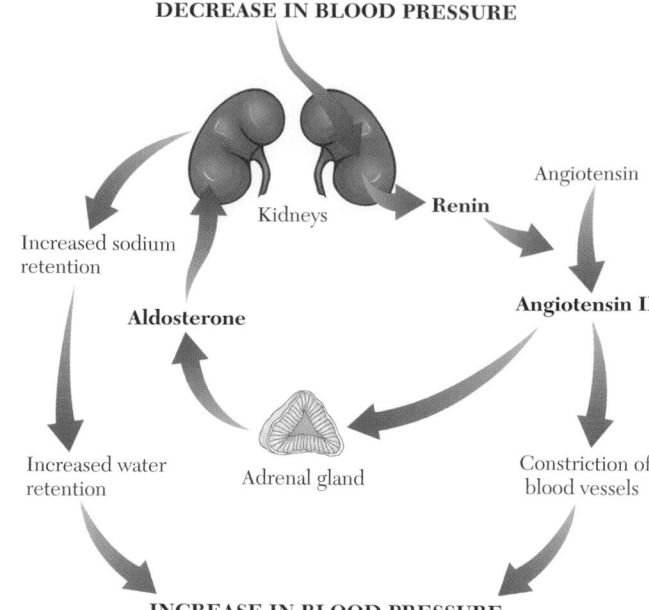

Figure 10.15
When blood pressure decreases, a series of events returns blood pressure to normal by constricting blood vessels and increasing sodium and water retention by the kidney.

Renin An enzyme produced by the kidney that aids in the conversion of angiotensin to its active form, angiotensin II.

Angiotensin II A compound that causes blood vessel walls to constrict and stimulates the release of the hormone aldosterone.

Aldosterone A hormone that increases sodium reabsorption and therefore enhances water retention by the kidney.

Sodium is the primary determinant of extracellular fluid volume. When the concentration of sodium in the blood increases, water follows, causing an increase in blood volume. Changes in blood volume can change blood pressure. Changes in blood pressure trigger the production and release of proteins and hormones that affect the amount of sodium, and hence water, retained by the kidneys. For example, when blood pressure decreases, the kidneys release the enzyme **renin**, beginning a series of events leading to the production of **angiotensin II** (Figure 10.15). Angiotensin II increases blood pressure both by causing the blood vessel walls to constrict and by stimulating the release of the hormone **aldosterone**, which acts on the kidneys to increase sodium reabsorption. Water follows the reabsorbed sodium, resulting in an increase in blood volume and, consequently, blood pressure. The increase in blood pressure then inhibits the release of renin and aldosterone so that blood pressure does not continue to rise.

As with sodium and chloride, the kidneys regulate potassium excretion to maintain a relatively constant amount of potassium in the body. If blood levels begin to rise, mechanisms are activated to stimulate the cellular uptake of potassium. This short-term regulation prevents the amount of potassium in the extracellular fluid from getting lethally high. The long-term regulation of potassium balance depends on aldosterone release, which causes the kidney to excrete potassium and retain sodium.

Electrolytes: How Much Do We Need?

Although DRI values have not yet been established for the electrolytes, the National Research Council has estimated minimum requirements. The estimated minimum for sodium is 500 mg per day for healthy adults.[5] The Daily Value on food labels recommends consuming no more than 2400 mg of sodium per day. This is below the typical intake in the United States of about 3600 mg per day of sodium. The estimated minimum requirement for chloride is 750 mg per day for adults. The Daily Value used on food labels is 3400 mg. The recommended minimum intake for potassium is 1600 to 2000 mg per day to maintain normal body stores and fluid concentrations. The Daily Value recommends at least 3500 mg per day of potassium for adults. Potassium intakes vary greatly depending on food selection. Diets containing few fruits and vegetables provide only about 2000 mg of potassium per day, and those high in fruits and vegetables provide 8000 to 11,000 mg.[6]

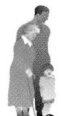

Pregnancy slightly increases sodium needs because the extracellular fluid volume increases. Pregnant women are advised to follow the recommendation for the general population for sodium intake (see Chapter 14).[7] At one time, a dietary salt restriction was common during pregnancy to prevent a syndrome known as pregnancy-induced hypertension. The cause of pregnancy-induced hypertension is not known, but salt restriction is no longer recommended. During lactation, sodium needs are increased to replace the amount secreted in milk. This is equal to about 135 mg per day. In infants, sodium needs are estimated from the amount consumed in human milk, which contains more chloride than sodium. This same chloride-to-sodium ratio has been recommended for infant formulas.

Potassium is needed to build new cells, so its requirement increases during times of growth. In pregnancy, extra potassium is needed to build new tissue. During lactation, the increased need is to replace losses in milk. In children, potassium is needed for growth; required amounts can be met by following the recommendations of the Food Guide Pyramid.

Electrolyte Deficiency and Toxicity

Deficiencies of sodium and chloride are rare in healthy individuals. Although the taste for salt that triggers your desire to plunge into a bag of salty chips is a learned preference rather than a response to physiological need, humans with very low salt intakes do have a true physiological drive to consume salt (Figure 10.16). Conditions that cause sodium and chloride depletion include heavy and persistent sweating, chronic diarrhea or vomiting, and kidney disease. A sodium or chloride imbalance can cause disturbances in acid-base and electrolyte balance.

Toxicities are also rare in healthy individuals. Excessive sodium intake has been related to hypertension in salt-sensitive individuals, but for individuals without salt-sensitive hypertension no toxic level of sodium intake has been documented as long as water needs are met and the kidneys are functioning properly. However, a high sodium intake increases calcium excretion and has been related to an increased risk of osteoporosis.[8]

Symptomatic potassium deficiency is also uncommon. It occurs as a result of vomiting, diarrhea, increased urinary losses, and excessive sweating. Individuals at risk include those with eating disorders who may vomit frequently or abuse laxatives, those consuming very-low-energy diets, and those taking diuretic medications, known as thiazide diuretics, to treat hypertension. Generally, potassium supplements are prescribed along with or incorporated into medications that cause potassium loss. Potassium deficiency results in poor appetite, muscle cramps, confusion, apathy, constipation, and, eventually, an irregular heartbeat.

Potassium toxicity from the diet is rare because urinary excretion is proportional to intake when kidney function is normal. If supplements are consumed in excess or kidney function is compromised, blood levels of potassium can increase and can eventually cause death due to an irregular heartbeat.

Hypertension

Electrolytes in the body are carefully regulated and, in turn, regulate fluid volume. As the extracellular fluid volume increases, blood pressure increases. A certain level of blood pressure is necessary to ensure that blood is delivered to all tissues. A healthy blood pressure is 120/80 mm of mercury or less. However, an increase in blood volume or a narrowing of the blood vessels can cause high blood pressure, or hypertension, generally defined as a blood pressure of 140/90 mm of mercury or greater. This is the level that is associated with increased risk of cardiovascular diseases such as atherosclerosis, heart attack, and stroke.[9] It also increases the risks for kidney disease and early death. It is estimated that 20% of adult Americans have a blood pressure in this range[8] (Figure 10.17).

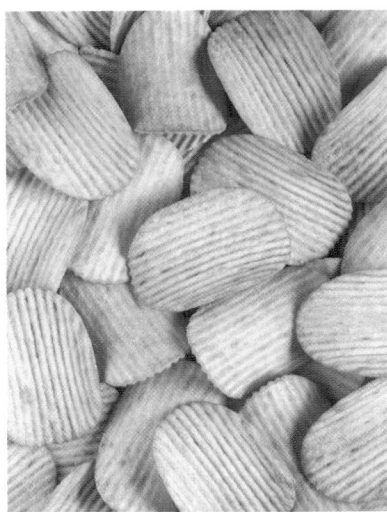

Figure 10.16

Our taste for salty chips is a learned preference. (© PhotoDisc, Inc.)

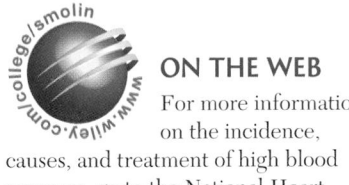

ON THE WEB

For more information on the incidence, causes, and treatment of high blood pressure, go to the National Heart, Lung, and Blood Institute at
www.nhlbi.nih.gov/siteindex

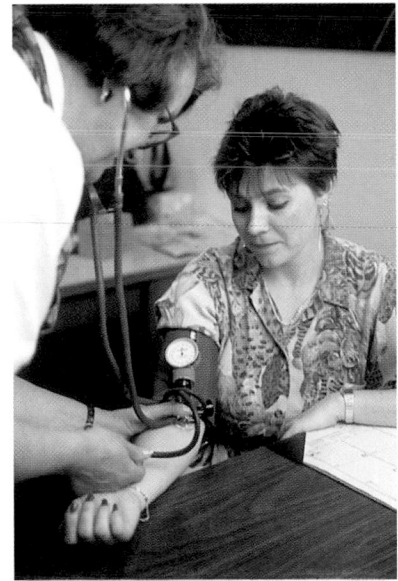

Figure 10.17

Hypertension has been called the silent killer because it has no outward symptoms but can lead to atherosclerosis, heart attack, stroke, kidney disease, and early death. Everyone should have their blood pressure monitored regularly since high blood pressure has no obvious symptoms. (Charles D. Winters)

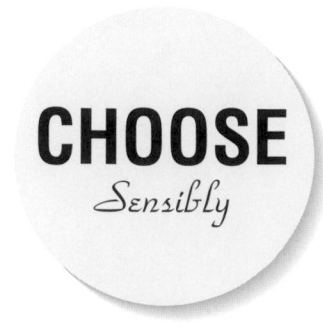

CHOOSE
Sensibly

Choose and prepare foods
with less salt

Figure 10.18
The Dietary Guidelines for Americans,
2000, recommends that Americans
"Choose and prepare foods with less
salt."

Causes of Hypertension Most people with high blood pressure have essential hypertension—hypertension with no obvious external cause. It is a complex disorder, most likely resulting from disturbances in one or more of the mechanisms that control body fluid and electrolyte balance. High blood pressure that occurs as a result of other disorders is referred to as secondary hypertension. There is a genetic predisposition to hypertension, so a family history of high blood pressure increases one's risk of developing this disorder. It is more common in African Americans, Puerto Ricans, and Cuban and Mexican Americans than in non-Hispanic whites. The increased incidence among African Americans is reflected in their 80% higher rate of death from stroke, 50% higher rate of death from heart disease, and 320% greater rate of hypertension-related kidney failure compared to Caucasians.[10] The risk of hypertension increases with age and is higher in those with diabetes or obesity, particularly when the excess body fat is visceral. Weight loss can prevent or delay the onset of hypertension in obese individuals. A lack of physical activity, heavy alcohol consumption, and stress can increase blood pressure.[11] Blood pressure is also affected by diet.

Minerals and Blood Pressure Diets high in salt are associated with a higher incidence of hypertension, whereas diets high in potassium, calcium, and magnesium are associated with a lower incidence of hypertension. A dietary pattern that incorporates a moderate sodium intake and larger amounts of these other nutrients has a greater impact than that of any single nutrient.[12]

Sodium and Salt The Intersalt study, which examined the incidence of hypertension in different populations, found that in populations consuming less than 4.5 grams of salt per day, average blood pressure was low and hypertension was rare or absent. In populations consuming 5.8 grams of salt or more per day, blood pressure increased with sodium intake.[13] As a result of epidemiological studies such as this one, a restriction of dietary sodium was commonly prescribed to reduce blood pressure in all hypertensive individuals. In addition, to decrease the incidence of hypertension in the population as a whole, moderate sodium intake is recommended by the Dietary Guidelines for Americans (Figure 10.18).

Whether the intake of sodium or salt affects blood pressure in all individuals is controversial.[14] Some research suggests that the impact of sodium intake on blood pressure depends on whether or not the individual is salt sensitive. In salt-sensitive individuals, a reduction in salt intake will cause a decrease in blood pressure. Of individuals with hypertension, about half are salt sensitive—that is, their hypertension is aggravated by a high-salt diet. In the other half, dietary salt does not affect blood pressure.[15] In individuals who are salt sensitive, sodium has been shown to have little effect on blood pressure unless it is consumed with chloride as salt.[16] However, data from a recent trial has questioned the theory of salt-sensitivity. In this trial, the lower the amount of sodium in the diet the lower the blood pressure. An intake of 2400 mg of sodium (the amount recommended by the Dietary Guidelines) reduced blood pressure in those with and without hypertension, and even more significant reductions were seen when sodium intake was reduced to 1500 mg of sodium per day.[12]

Potassium, Calcium, and Magnesium Epidemiology has shown that dietary patterns with high intakes of fiber and the minerals potassium, magnesium, and calcium are associated with lower blood pressure. For example, populations and individuals consuming vegetarian diets, which are high in these nutrients, generally have lower blood pressure than nonvegetarians.[17]

Primitive cultures worldwide and vegetarians in industrialized countries whose diets are high in potassium have a low incidence of hypertension, whereas groups that have low potassium intakes have a high incidence of hypertension.[18]

The risk of stroke, which is associated with hypertension, was found to be lower in men who consumed about 4.3 grams of potassium per day compared to those consuming 2.4 grams per day.[19] Because populations that have high intakes of sodium generally have low intakes of potassium, it is difficult to tell if the hypertension associated with a high-sodium diet is due to the high sodium or the low potassium. The fact that a high dietary sodium intake increases the excretion of potassium suggests that low levels of potassium in the body affect hypertension. Potassium supplements have been shown to decrease blood pressure.[20] Since excessive potassium intakes can cause an irregular heartbeat, potassium supplements are not recommended unless supervised by a physician. Increasing consumption of potassium-rich foods such as bananas, oranges, and potatoes is a safer way to increase potassium intake.

Epidemiology also supports a role for calcium and magnesium in regulating blood pressure. Numerous studies have found that individuals with low calcium intakes are more likely to have hypertension.[21] Calcium supplementation has been shown to lower blood pressure slightly in individuals with hypertension, and some analyses have also shown an effect in those with normal blood pressure.[22,23] Low dietary magnesium intake has also been associated with hypertension.[24,25]

The Total Dietary Pattern: The DASH Diet The results of the wide variety of studies on mineral intake and hypertension have been equivocal. This may be because the impact of each individual nutrient is small and a significant effect is seen only when several components of the diet are modified simultaneously. The Dietary Approaches to Stop Hypertension (DASH) trial examined the effect of dietary patterns on blood pressure and demonstrated that dietary pattern has a greater impact on blood pressure than individual nutrient intake.[26] Three diets were used, all containing 3000 mg of sodium per day, an amount somewhat greater than the Daily Value of 2400 mg per day. The first, a control diet, was a typical American dietary pattern—low in potassium, magnesium, calcium, and fiber, and high in fat and protein. One of the experimental diets was high in fruits and vegetables, providing 8 to 10 servings per day, making it higher in potassium, magnesium, calcium and fiber, but otherwise similar to the control diet. The other experimental diet was not only high in fruits and vegetables but also contained lowfat dairy products, whole grains, and lean meat, fish, and poultry, making it higher in potassium, magnesium, calcium, and fiber, and lower in fat, saturated fat, and cholesterol than the control diet. Both experimental diets lowered blood pressure in individuals both with hypertension and normal blood pressure. However, the effect was most dramatic in the diet that emphasized fruits and vegetables as well as lowfat dairy products, whole grains, and lean meats—a dietary pattern that has become known as the DASH Diet.[26] The reduction in blood pressure occurred after only two weeks of consuming the diet and persisted throughout the trial. Reductions were similar to that with drug therapy or diets that restrict sodium to very low levels of 1100 to 1800 mg per day.[27]

The DASH trial did not explore the effect of sodium on blood pressure, but a second trial called DASH-Sodium compared the effect of the DASH diet to a control diet at three different levels of sodium intake.[12] The high sodium diet provided 3300 mg sodium/day, slightly less than the average American intake; the intermediate diet provided 2400 mg sodium/day, the current government recommendation, and the low sodium diet provided 1500 mg sodium/day. Reducing sodium intake reduced blood pressure for both the DASH and control diets. The combination of the DASH diet and the lowest sodium intake reduced blood pressure more than either the DASH diet or low sodium alone.

The results of the DASH and DASH-Sodium trials demonstrate that changing the dietary pattern can lower blood pressure. In addition, the DASH dietary pattern may also reduce cancer risk, prevent osteoporosis, and protect against heart disease (see *Critical Thinking*: A Diet for Health).

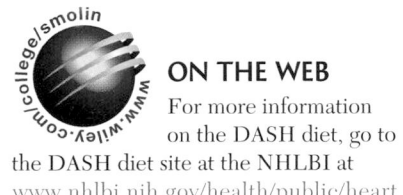

ON THE WEB
For more information on the DASH diet, go to the DASH diet site at the NHLBI at www.nhlbi.nih.gov/health/public/heart

CRITICAL THINKING

A Diet for Health

Rashamel is a 43-year-old father of three children. His father died of a stroke at the age of 54 as a result of undiagnosed and untreated high blood pressure. Rashamel wants to live to see his grandchildren, so he exercises as often as he can, about three times a week, quit smoking, and watches his diet and weight. Despite these efforts, at his recent physical his blood pressure was elevated to 144/92. Rather than start him on medication immediately, his doctor suggested a dietary approach first and referred him to a dietitian. A 24-hour recall reveals that Rashamel is maintaining a normal body weight of 175 pounds by consuming about 2500 kcal per day. After evaluating his current diet, the dietitian recommends he follow the DASH diet to reduce his blood pressure. The modified diet shown here illustrates the dietitian's recommendations.

▼

Current Diet		Modified Diet	
Breakfast		**Breakfast**	
Orange juice	¾ cup	Orange juice	¾ cup
1% lowfat milk	1 cup	1% lowfat milk	1 cup
Wheaties w/ 1 tsp sugar	1 cup	Wheaties w/1 tsp sugar	1 cup
		Banana	1 medium
Whole wheat bread w/ jelly	1 slice	Whole wheat bread w/jelly	2 slices
Margarine	1 tsp	Margarine	1 tsp
Lunch		**Lunch**	
Tuna salad	¾ cup	Tuna salad	¾ cup
Wheat bread	2 slices	Wheat bread	2 slices
		Carrot sticks	½ cup
		Bell pepper strips	½ cup
Chips	1 oz	Fruit cocktail (light syrup)	½ cup
Cola	1 can	1% lowfat milk	1 cup
Dinner		**Dinner**	
Baked chicken	3 oz	Chicken stir fry	3 oz
		Almonds	10
		Broccoli	½ cup
		Mushrooms	½ cup
Rice	1 cup	Rice	1½ cup
Salad	1 cup	Salad	1 cup
Light salad dressing	1 Tbsp	Light salad dressing	1 Tbsp
Dinner roll	1	Dinner roll	1
Margarine	2 tsp	Margarine	2 tsp
Cantaloupe	½ cup	Cantaloupe	½ cup
Iced tea (sweetened)	12 oz	1% lowfat milk	1 cup
Snacks		**Snacks**	
Cookies	2 large	Frozen yogurt	½ cup
Dried apricots	5	Dried apricots	5
Milky Way candy bar	1	Graham crackers	2
Cola	1 can		

How does the modified diet compare to the recommendations of the Food Guide Pyramid? to Rashamel's current diet?

▼

Answer:

How do these changes affect the sodium and potassium content of Rashamel's diet?

▼

His original diet was not high in sodium, containing about 2500 mg, which is slightly above the Daily Value of 2400 mg. The changes in his diet reduce his sodium slightly but increase his potassium intake from 2870 mg to 5000 mg. The amount of magnesium is also increased slightly.

Rashamel's wife Yuka is 42 years old. Although she is not concerned about her blood pressure, Yuka is concerned about osteoporosis because her mother was recently hospitalized with a hip fracture. She wants to make sure she is consuming adequate calcium. She is mildly lactose intolerant.

If she consumed the modified diet, would it meet her AI for calcium?

▼

Yes, her AI is 1000 mg, and the modified diet contains 1320 mg of calcium. Because of her lactose intolerance Yuka does not drink much milk. She can tolerate a small amount on her morning cereal and can consume yogurt and cheese in moderate amounts. If the milk consumed at lunch and dinner is eliminated from her diet, she would not meet the AI.

What changes would increase the amount of calcium from low lactose sources?

▼

To increase calcium, Yuka could substitute canned salmon for tuna in the salad at lunch. She could also include more tofu in her diet—a food she ate frequently while growing up in Japan. Including a serving of miso soup with tofu, or using tofu instead of chicken in the stir fry at dinner would increase calcium by about 130 mg. She can also replace the milk with small amounts of yogurt and lowfat cheese. She might also consider taking a calcium supplement.

Yuka only weighs 110 pounds and requires about 1800 kcal to maintain her body weight.

How could this diet be changed to reduce the energy content without reducing the calcium?

▼

Answer:

Table 10.2 *Suggestions for Keeping Blood Pressure in a Healthy Range*

- Choose and prepare foods with less salt.
- Aim for a healthy weight: Blood pressure increases with increases in body weight and decreases when excess weight is reduced.
- Increase physical activity: It helps lower blood pressure, reduce risk of other chronic diseases, and manage weight.
- Eat fruits and vegetables: They are naturally low in salt and kcalories. They are also rich in potassium, which may help decrease blood pressure.
- If you drink alcoholic beverages, do so in moderation. Excessive alcohol consumption has been associated with high blood pressure.

USDA, DHHS. Dietary Guidelines for Americans, 2000.

Choosing a Diet to Prevent Hypertension and Stay Healthy Reducing the incidence of hypertension in the United States is an important public health goal (Table 10.2). Both the Dietary Guidelines and the Daily Values recommend a reduction in sodium consumption. In addition, the Dietary Guidelines encourages the consumption of fresh fruits, vegetables, grains, meats, and dairy products, a dietary pattern that may provide more health benefits than just lowering blood pressure.[28]

Selecting a DASH Diet A diet that promotes healthy blood pressure provides plenty of potassium, calcium, and magnesium; is moderate in sodium chloride; and maintains a healthy weight. This DASH diet pattern can be achieved by using the Food Guide Pyramid as a guide and aiming toward the high end of the recommended number of servings of vegetables, fruits, dairy products, and grains. Dry beans and nuts should be frequent choices from the Meat, Poultry, Fish, Dry Beans, Eggs, & Nuts Group. Nutrient-dense choices from each group will ensure that the energy content of the diet does not exceed needs. Table 10.3 gives the number of servings recommended for several different energy levels. The risk of hypertension is minimized by combining this dietary pattern with the suggestions for reducing sodium intake given below.

Moderate Sodium Intake A diet that is moderate in sodium limits the use of salt added in cooking and at the table as well as that consumed in processed foods (Table 10.4). Food labels can be helpful in identifying high-sodium foods. All the sodium-containing additives are itemized in the ingredient list, and the total sodium content

Table 10.3 *Serving Recommendations for the DASH Diet*

Food Group	Number of Servings*			
Kcalorie level	1600	2000	2600	3100
Grains	6–7	7–8	10–11	12–13
Vegetables	3–4	4–5	5–6	6–7
Fruits	3–4	4–5	5–6	6–7
Lowfat dairy	2–3	2–3	3–4	3–4
Meats, fish, poultry	1–2	1–2	2	2–3
Beans, nuts, and seeds	1/3	1/2	2/3	3/4
Limit fats and sweets				

*Serving sizes correspond to the serving sizes recommended by the Food Guide Pyramid

Table 10.4   *Tips for Reducing Your Sodium Intake*

1. Reduce the salt in your diet gradually so that you learn to enjoy the unsalted flavors in foods.
2. When shopping:
   - Use food labels to select foods low in sodium.
   - Choose unprocessed foods—they have less sodium than processed foods.
   - Choose fresh or frozen vegetables rather than canned.
3. When cooking:
   - Prepare meals from scratch so you control the amount of salt added.
   - Do not add salt to the water when cooking rice, pasta, and cereals.
   - Flavor foods with ingredients such as lemon juice, onion or garlic powder (not salt), pepper, curry, dill, basil, oregano, or thyme rather than salt.
4. When eating:
   - Limit use of salt at the table.
   - Limit salted snack foods like potato chips, salted nuts, salted popcorn, and crackers, and replace them with fresh fruits and vegetables.
   - Limit cured, salted, or smoked meats such as bologna, corned beef, hot dogs, and smoked turkey to a few servings a week or less. Substitute sliced roasted turkey, chicken, or beef.
   - Limit salty or smoked fish such as sardines, anchovies, or smoked salmon (lox).
   - Limit foods prepared in salt brine such as pickles, olives, and sauerkraut.
   - Cut down on cheeses, especially processed cheeses.
   - Limit the amounts of soy sauce, Worcestershire sauce, barbecue sauce, ketchup, and mustard you add to food.
5. When eating out:
   - Choose foods without sauces, or ask for them to be served on the side.
   - Ask that food be prepared without added salt.

per serving is included in the Nutrition Facts section. Food labels also list the sodium content of a serving as a percent of the Daily Value, 2400 mg. The Nutrition Facts on the label in Figure 10.19 shows that a serving of spaghetti sauce contains 250 mg, or 10% of the sodium that should be included in the daily diet. Additional information can be obtained from descriptors relating to the salt or sodium content of a product (Table 10.5). Drug facts labels on over-the-counter medications can help identify those that contain large amounts of sodium.

Table 10.5   *Salt and Sodium Content Descriptors on Food Labels*

Descriptor	Definition
Sodium-free	Contains less than 5 mg of sodium per serving.
Salt-free	Must meet criterion for "sodium-free."
Very low sodium	Contains 35 mg or less of sodium per serving.
Low Sodium	Contains 140 mg or less of sodium per serving.
Reduced or less sodium	Contains at least 25% less sodium per serving than a reference food.
Light in sodium	Contains at least 50% less sodium per serving than the average reference amount for same food with no sodium reduction.
No salt added, without added salt, and unsalted	No salt added during processing, and the food it resembles and for which it substitutes is normally processed with salt. (If the food is not "sodium-free," the statement "not a sodium-free food" or "not for control of sodium in the diet" must appear on the same panel as the Nutrition Facts panel.)
Lightly salted	Contains at least 50% less sodium per serving than a reference amount. (If the food is not "low in sodium," the statement "not a low-sodium food" must appear on the same panel as the "Nutrition Facts" panel).

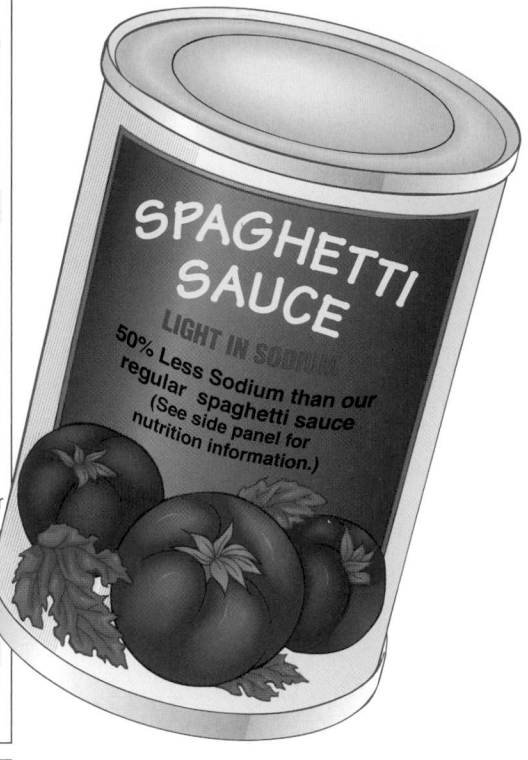

Nutrition Facts
Serving Size 1/2 cup (125g)
Servings Per Container about 3½

Amount Per Serving		
Calories 50	Calories from Fat 10	
		%Daily Value**
Total Fat 1g		**2%**
Saturated Fat 0g		**0%**
Cholesterol 0mg		**0%**
Sodium 250mg		**10%**
Potassium 530mg		**15%**
Total Carbohydrate 9g		**3%**
Dietary Fiber 1g		**4%**
Sugars 7g		
Protein 2g		
Vitamin A 10%	•	Vitamin C 25%
Calcium 2%	•	Iron 10%

*Percent Daily Values are based on a 2,000
calorie diet. Your daily values may be higher
or lower depending on your calorie needs.

	Calories:	2,000	2,500
Total Fat	Less than	65g	80g
Sat Fat	Less than	20g	25g
Cholesterol	Less than	300mg	300mg
Sodium	Less than	2,400mg	2,400mg
Potassium		3,500mg	3,500mg
Total Carbohydrate		300g	375g
Dietary Fiber		25g	30g

Light Spaghetti Sauce, 250 milligrams
(mg) per serving
Regular Spaghetti Sauce, 500mg per
serving

Figure 10.19
Food labels help determine how much
sodium a food contributes to the diet.

• MINERALS INVOLVED IN BONE HEALTH

Bone is composed of a protein framework that is hardened by deposits of minerals. There are two types of bone: cortical or compact bone, which forms the sturdy, dense outer surface layer, and trabecular or spongy bone, which forms an inner spongy lattice that supports the cortical shell (Figure 10.20). Healthy bone requires adequate dietary protein and vitamin C to maintain collagen—the most abundant protein in the bone-matrix—and a sufficient supply of minerals to ensure solidity. The mineral deposits of bone consist primarily of calcium and phosphorus but also include magnesium, fluoride, and other trace minerals (see Chapter 11). Adequate vitamin D (discussed in Chapter 9) is necessary to maintain appropriate levels of calcium and phosphorus.

Bone: A Living Tissue

Bone is a living, metabolically active tissue that is constantly being broken down and reformed in a process called **bone remodeling**. Bone is formed by cells called osteoblasts and broken down or resorbed by cells called osteoclasts. During bone formation the activity of the bone-building osteoblasts exceeds that of the osteoclasts. When bone is being broken down, the osteoclasts resorb bone more rapidly than the osteoblasts can rebuild it.

Most bone is formed early in life. In the growing bones of children, bone formation occurs more rapidly than breakdown. Even after growth stops, bone mass continues to increase into young adulthood when **peak bone mass** is achieved, somewhere

Bone remodeling The process whereby bone is continuously broken down and reformed to allow for growth and maintenance.

Peak bone mass The maximum bone density attained at any time in life, usually occurring in young adulthood.

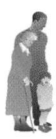

between the ages of 16 and 30.[29] In healthy adults, bone breakdown and formation are in balance, so bone mass remains constant. After about age 35 to 45, the amount of bone broken down begins to exceed that which is formed. Although both types of bone are lost with age, the loss of spongy trabecular bone begins earlier than does cortical bone loss. [30] If enough bone is lost, the skeleton is weakened and fractures occur easily. This is known as **osteoporosis**, a condition which generally has no symptoms until the fifth or sixth decade of life.

Osteoporosis

Osteoporosis is caused by a loss in both the protein matrix and the mineral deposits of bone, resulting in a decrease in the total amount of bone (Figure 10.21). In the United States, about 28 million people have osteoporosis or are at risk due to low bone mass, and 80% of them are women.[31,32] Osteoporosis leads to 1.5 million fractures annually, which account for $10 to $15 billion per year in medical cost.[31] The causes of osteoporosis are not fully understood, but the risk depends on the level of peak bone mass and the rate at which bone is lost.

Peak bone mass and the rate of bone loss are affected by age, genetics, gender, and lifestyle. The risk of osteoporosis increases progressively with age. Genetic factors are believed to account for as much as 70% of the variation in bone density, and osteoporosis risk.[33] Genetic differences between racial groups lead to differences in the risk of osteoporosis. For example, the incidence of osteoporosis in African American women is half that of Caucasian women despite similar environmental risk factors. The reason for the lower risk in African American women is that they begin menopause with higher bone density and have lower rates of bone loss after **menopause**.[34] Risk is greater in women than men because men have a higher peak bone mass and because bone loss is accelerated for about 5 years after menopause. This **postmenopausal bone loss** is related to a drop in levels of the hormone estrogen that occurs around menopause. Declining estrogen affects bone cells and decreases intestinal calcium absorption. During this period, women lose a disproportionate amount of trabecular bone. After the postmenopausal period, women continue to lose bone but more slowly. This **age-related bone loss**, which also occurs in men, involves the loss of both the compact cortical bone and the spongy trabecular bone. Osteoporosis-related fractures occur in one out of every two women over age 50 and in about one in every eight men over 50[38] (Figure 10.22).

Lifestyle factors that affect bone mass include smoking, alcohol consumption, exercise, and diet. Smoking and alcohol consumption can decrease bone mass, whereas weight-bearing exercise, such as walking and jogging, increase bone mass. Having more body fat decreases the risk of osteoporosis because adipose tissue produces estrogen, which helps maintain bone mass and enhances calcium absorption. A greater body weight also increases the amount of weight-bearing exercise that the individual gets in day-to-day activities, which increases bone mass. Although calcium is the most significant dietary mineral affecting osteoporosis risk, other minerals including sodium, phosphorus, magnesium, and several trace minerals affect bone mass and bone health by their effects on calcium absorption, urinary calcium losses, as well as bone physiology.

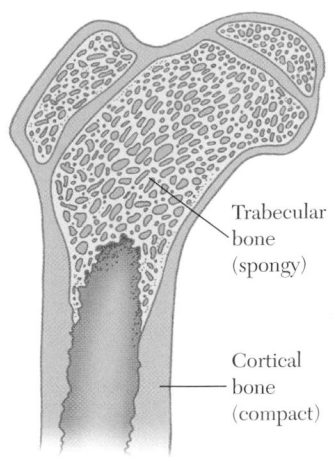

Figure 10.20
The compact bone that forms the outer layer of bone is called cortical bone and the spongy interior is called trabecular bone.

Osteoporosis A bone disorder characterized by a reduction in bone mass, increased bone fragility, and an increased risk of fractures.

Menopause The physiological changes that mark the end of a woman's capacity to bear children.

Postmenopausal bone loss The accelerated bone loss that occurs in women for about five years after estrogen production decreases.

Age-related bone loss The bone loss that occurs in both men and women as they age.

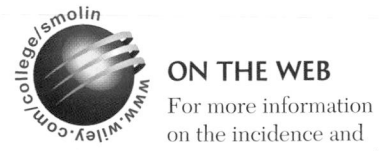

ON THE WEB
For more information on the incidence and risks of osteoporosis, go to the National Institutes of Health Osteoporosis and Related Bone Disease National Resource Center at
www.osteo.org/

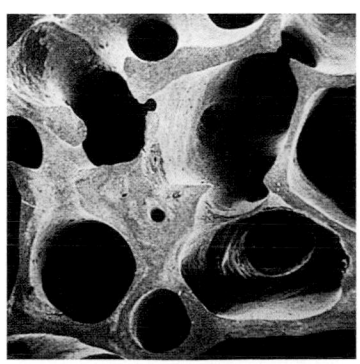
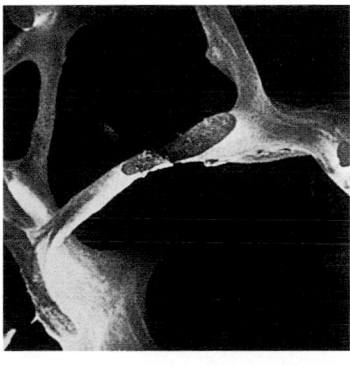

Figure 10.21
Osteoporosis causes a decrease in bone density and increases the risk of fractures. Normal bone (*left*). Bone weakened by osteoporosis (*right*). (Courtesy of Wyeth-Ayerst Laboratories)

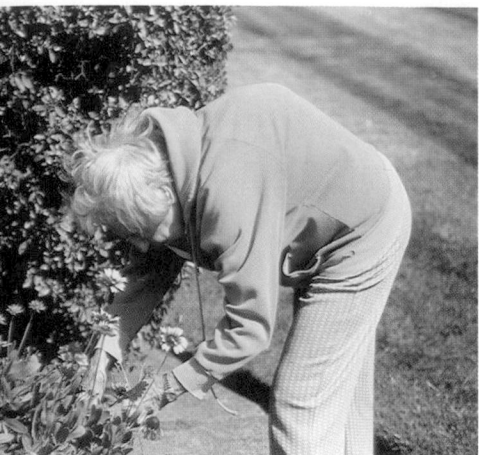

Figure 10.22

The bone loss due to osteoporosis can cause a stooped posture and a decrease in stature. (© Larry Mulvehill/Science Source/Photo Researchers, Inc.)

Calcium

Calcium is the most abundant mineral in the body. It accounts for 1 to 2% of adult body weight. Over 99% of the calcium in the body is found in the solid mineral deposit in bones and teeth.[36] The remaining 1% is present in intracellular fluid, blood, and other extracellular fluids, where it plays vital roles in nerve transmission, muscle contraction, blood pressure regulation, and the release of hormones.

Calcium in the Diet The main source of calcium in the North American diet is dairy products such as milk, cheese, and yogurt. Fish, such as sardines, that are consumed in their entirety, including the bones, are also a good source, as are legumes and some green vegetables such as broccoli, Chinese cabbage, and kale (Figure 10.23). Grains are only a moderate source of calcium, but because they are consumed in such large quantities they make a significant contribution to dietary calcium intake.

Some of the calcium in the diet is added to foods during food processing. Baked goods such as breads, rolls, and crackers, to which nonfat dry milk powder has been added, provide calcium. Tortillas that are treated with lime water (calcium hydroxide) provide calcium. Tofu is a good source when calcium is used in its processing. In addition, there are products on the market, such as orange juice and breakfast cereals, that are fortified with calcium.

Calcium in the Digestive Tract Calcium is absorbed by both active transport and passive diffusion. Active transport depends on the active form of vitamin D and accounts for most absorption when intakes are low to moderate. When vitamin D is deficient, absorption decreases dramatically. At high intakes, passive transport becomes more important. As calcium intake increases, the percentage that is absorbed declines.

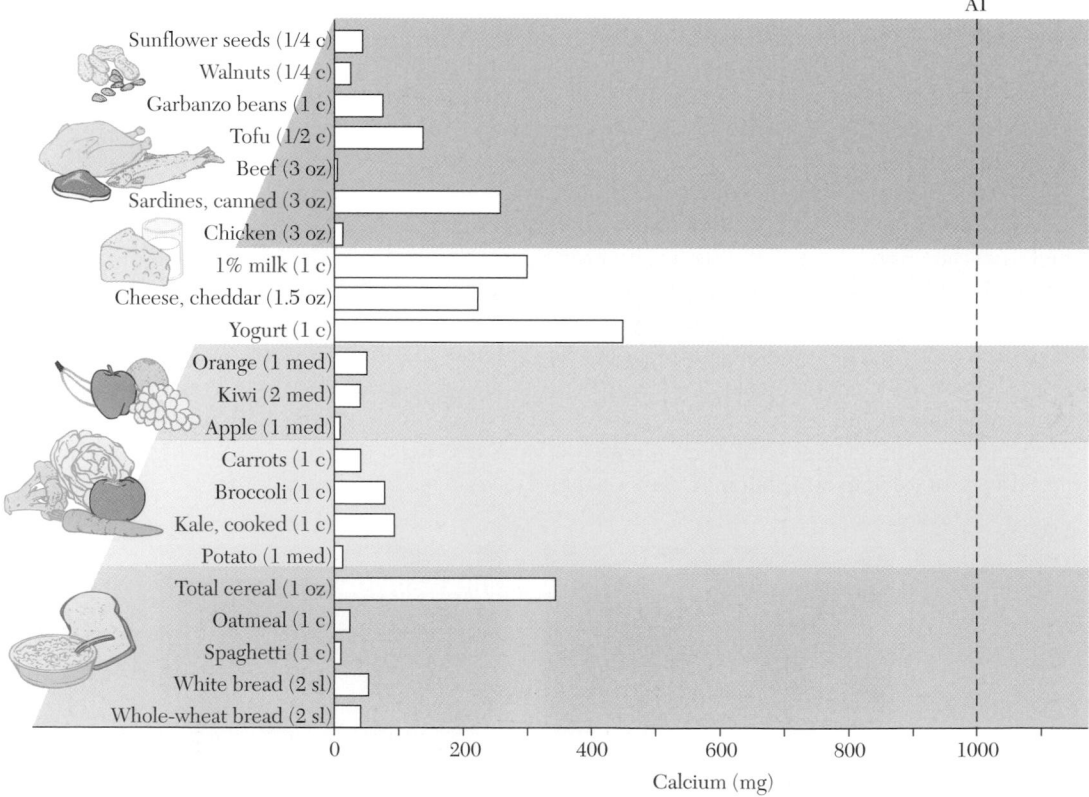

Figure 10.23

Calcium content of selections from each group of the Food Guide Pyramid. The dashed line represents the AI for men and women 19 to 50 years of age.

The bioavailability of calcium is affected by a number of other dietary factors, including the presence of lactose, which enhances calcium absorption, and tannins, fiber, phytates, and oxalates, which decrease calcium absorption. For example, spinach is a high-calcium vegetable but only about 5% of the calcium is absorbed;[37] the rest is bound by oxalates and excreted in the feces. Chocolate also contains oxalates, but chocolate milk is still a good source of calcium because the amount of oxalates from the chocolate is small. When calcium intake is low, dietary components that alter absorption may affect calcium status, but when calcium intake is adequate, these factors have little effect.[38]

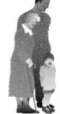

The efficiency of calcium absorption varies with life stage. During infancy, about 60% of calcium consumed is absorbed. In young adults absorption is about 25%. In older adults absorption declines due to a decrease in blood levels of the active form of vitamin D. An additional decrease in calcium absorption occurs in women after menopause due to the decrease in estrogen. During pregnancy, when calcium need is high, elevated estrogen helps increase calcium absorption.

Calcium in the Body Calcium is important in the maintenance of bones and teeth (see Table 10.1), where it is primarily found with phosphorus as solid mineral crystals known as **hydroxyapatite**. It also plays extremely important roles in cell communication and the regulation of body processes. Calcium helps regulate enzymes and is necessary in blood clotting. It is involved in transmitting chemical and electrical signals in nerves and muscles. It is necessary for the release of neurotransmitters, which allow nerve impulses to pass from one nerve to another and from nerves to other tissues. Inside the muscle cells, calcium allows the two muscle proteins, actin and myosin, to interact to cause muscle contraction. Calcium also plays a role in blood pressure regulation, possibly by controlling the contraction of muscles in the blood vessel walls and signaling the secretion of substances that regulate blood pressure.[21]

The roles of calcium are so vital to survival that powerful regulatory mechanisms ensure that constant intracellular and extracellular concentrations are maintained. Slight changes in blood calcium levels trigger responses that quickly raise or lower them back to normal levels. This homeostasis is maintained by the hormones **parathyroid hormone (PTH)**, which raises blood calcium, and **calcitonin**, which lowers blood calcium (Figure 10.24). If the level of blood calcium falls too low,

Hydroxyapitite A crystalline compound composed of calcium and phosphorus that is deposited in the protein matrix of bone to give it strength and rigidity.

Parathyroid hormone (PTH) A hormone secreted by the parathyroid gland that increases blood calcium levels.

Calcitonin A hormone secreted by the thyroid gland that reduces blood calcium levels.

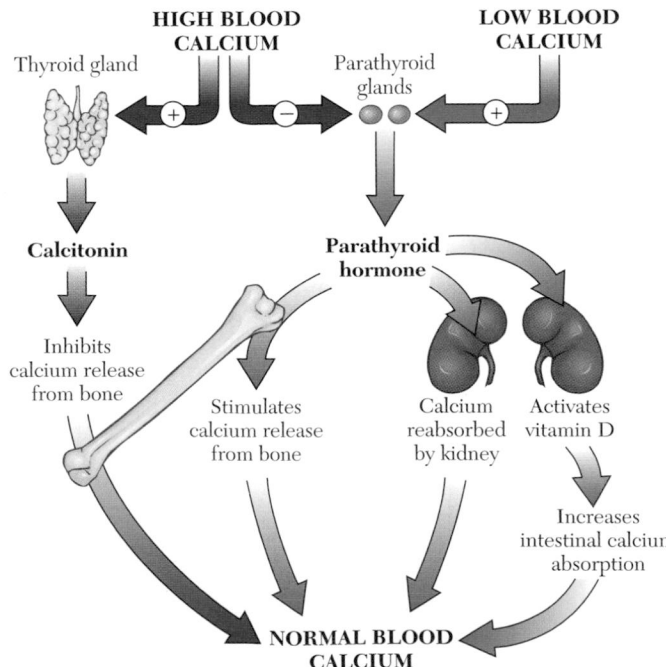

Figure 10.24
Levels of calcium in the blood are very tightly regulated by parathyroid hormone and calcitonin.

parathyroid hormone is released, stimulating the release of calcium from bone, reducing calcium excretion by the kidney, and activating vitamin D. Activated vitamin D increases the amount of calcium absorbed from the gastrointestinal tract and, with parathyroid hormone, stimulates calcium release from the bone. The overall effect is to rapidly increase blood calcium levels. If blood calcium levels become too high, the secretion of parathyroid hormone is shut off and calcitonin is secreted. Calcitonin acts primarily on bone to inhibit the release of calcium, resulting in a decrease in blood calcium levels.

How Much Calcium Do We Need? Ideally, calcium intake should be adequate to maintain bone and prevent fractures from osteoporosis later in life. However, it has not been possible to determine how much is needed at each life stage to prevent osteoporosis in older adults. Therefore, DRI values for calcium intakes have been set at the amount that allows maximum calcium retention. Increasing dietary calcium above this level will not increase the amount of calcium retained in the body. Adults may continue to lose bone mass at this intake level due to other causes such as loss of estrogen, smoking, and a sedentary lifestyle, but this loss is not due to inadequate calcium intake.

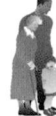

    Rather than an RDA, an AI has been determined for calcium because it was not possible to precisely estimate the dietary intake needed for maximum retention. The AI for adults age 19 through 50 years is 1000 mg per day.[36] Since absorption decreases with age, the AI for men and women age 51 and older is increased to 1200 mg per day. Postmenopausal bone loss cannot be prevented by increasing calcium intake, so the AI is not higher in women. For adolescents the AI is higher than for adults—1300 mg per day for boys and girls age 9 through 18. In children and adolescents the AI is set at a level that will support bone growth.

    Infants thrive on the amount of calcium they obtain from human milk. For infants, an AI is set based on the mean intake of infants fed principally with human milk. Because calcium is not as well absorbed from infant formulas, formula-fed infants require more. There is no specific AI for formula-fed infants, but formulas are higher in calcium than breast milk to compensate for the reduced absorption.

    The AI for calcium during pregnancy is not increased above nonpregnant levels. This is because there is an increase in maternal calcium absorption during pregnancy that helps to supply the calcium needed for the fetal skeleton. In addition, since there is no correlation between the number of pregnancies and bone mineral density, the maternal skeleton does not appear to be used as a supply of calcium for the fetus. However, during lactation, calcium is secreted in milk, and the source of this calcium does appear to be the maternal skeleton.[39] This bone resorption occurs regardless of calcium intake.[40] Since the loss of maternal skeleton is not prevented by increasing dietary calcium, and since the calcium lost appears to be regained following weaning, the AI is not increased during lactation.

Calcium Deficiency Bone acts as a calcium reservoir inside the body. When calcium intake is not adequate, normal blood levels are maintained by resorbing calcium from bone. This provides a steady supply of calcium to maintain its roles in cell communication and regulation. However, over time a deficient calcium intake contributes to oseteoporosis.

Calcium and Osteoporosis Low calcium intake during the years of bone formation results in a lower peak bone mass. Low intake after peak bone mass has been achieved increases the rate of bone loss and, along with it, the risk of osteoporosis.

    A low calcium intake is the most significant dietary factor contributing to osteoporosis, but intake alone does not predict the risk of osteoporosis. Genetics as well as other dietary and lifestyle factors also affect calcium status and bone mass. Diets high in phytates, oxalates, and tannins reduce calcium absorption, as does low vitamin D status. Some studies have demonstrated a connection between sodium chloride intake and calcium loss in the urine, but the impact of sodium on osteoporosis is still controversial.[41] Adequate protein is necessary for bone health but increasing protein intake increases urinary calcium losses. Despite this, high protein intakes are generally not associated with a higher risk of osteoporosis. This is because diets higher in protein are typically higher in calcium and bone mass depends more on the ratio of calcium to protein than the amount of protein alone. High levels of protein therefore do not have a negative effect on bone mass when calcium intake is adequate.[42] Higher intakes of zinc, magnesium, potassium, fiber, and vitamin C, nutrients that are plentiful in fruits and vegetable, are associated with greater bone mass.[43]

Preventing and Treating Osteoporosis   The best treatment for osteoporosis is to prevent it by achieving a high peak bone mass. Maximizing calcium deposition into bone is especially important during childhood and adolescence. Individuals with the highest peak bone mass after adolescence have a protective advantage over bone loss later in life.[31]

The risk of osteoporosis can be minimized by following appropriate dietary and lifestyle patterns throughout life. A diet rich in fruits and vegetables that is adequate in calcium and vitamin D and not excessive in phosphorus, protein, or sodium will reduce risk. Maintaining an active lifestyle that includes weight-bearing exercise and limiting smoking and alcohol consumption will help to further improve bone density. Once osteoporosis has occurred, it is difficult to restore lost bone.

Individuals who do not meet their calcium needs with diet alone can benefit from calcium supplementation. However, because high calcium intake can interfere with the absorption of other minerals, supplements should be taken with care. In young individuals who do not meet their calcium needs with food, supplemental calcium can increase peak bone mass. In postmenopausal women, calcium supplements have been found to be helpful in reducing bone loss but are not effective at increasing bone mass.[44] The effect of calcium supplements in decreasing calcium losses in postmenopausal women is greatest after the first five years of menopause and has more of an effect on cortical than on trabecular bone loss.[36] Benefits increase when calcium supplementation is combined with other therapies. For example, treatment with calcium and vitamin D has been shown to prevent bone loss, increase bone density, and decrease the frequency of bone fractures.[45] Replacing the estrogen lost in menopause—known as hormone replacement therapy—also has been shown to reduce bone loss and restore some lost bone, and the effectiveness of this therapy is enhanced by taking calcium supplements.[46]

Other treatments for osteoporosis include the hormone calcitonin and drugs known as bisphosphonates. Calcitonin injections or nasal spray can reduce bone resorption, and its effects are enhanced by calcium supplementation.[47] Bisphosphonates act by inhibiting bone resorption and have been shown to prevent postmenopausal bone loss and increase bone mineral density in patients with osteoporosis.[48] Exercise can also be helpful in treating osteoporosis. Minerals other than calcium that have been used to prevent and treat bone loss include magnesium, fluoride, and boron, but results with these have been equivocal (see *Off the Label*: Getting Enough Calcium?).

Calcium Toxicity   Adverse effects associated with high calcium consumption focus on intake from supplements. Too much calcium from supplements may cause kidney stone formation and kidney insufficiency, and may interfere with the absorption of other minerals. Calcium interacts with iron, zinc, magnesium, and phosphorus. Although calcium supplements inhibit iron absorption, there is no evidence that the long-term use of calcium supplements with meals affects iron status.[49] High intakes of calcium from supplements have also been found to reduce zinc absorption and thereby increase zinc needs in the diet.[50] There is no evidence of depletion of phosphorus or magnesium associated with calcium intake. A UL of 2500 mg per day has been set for adults age 19 to 70 years.

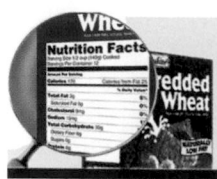

Off the Label
Getting Enough Calcium

Most people in the United States do not consume the recommended amount of calcium in their diets. The recommended calcium intake for adults is 1000 mg per day—the amount in a little more than three cups of milk. Do you get enough?

Milk is not the only food that provides calcium. Other dairy products, fish with bones, leafy green vegetables, and many fortified foods are good sources of calcium. Food labels can help you find good sources of calcium because the Nutrition Facts label must list the % Daily Value for calcium. To calculate the milligrams of calcium in a food, multiply the %Daily Value by 1000 (the Daily Value for calcium). For example, if the label on a box of fortified breakfast cereal indicates that a serving provides 25% of the Daily Value for calcium, a serving contains 250 mg of calcium (25% × 1000 mg = 250 mg calcium). If you eat more than one serving of the size indicated on the label, adjust your calcium calculation appropriately. Food labels may also use descriptors about their calcium content (see table), and foods that are a good source of calcium can carry a health claim about the association between calcium intake and the risk of osteoporosis. This information can help you judge whether your food choices make a significant contribution to your calcium intake.

Although you can meet your calcium needs with a carefully planned diet, many people choose to use supplements to ensure that they get enough calcium on a daily basis. Multivitamin and mineral supplements typically contain only a small portion of the Daily Value for calcium. So, if you want to get a significant amount of your calcium from a supplement, choose one that contains a calcium compound alone. The Supplement Facts label can help you determine how much of what form of calcium is in a supplement. The calcium in calcium carbonate is absorbed as well as the calcium from milk and the other forms, including calcium citrate, calcium gluconate, calcium lactate, calcium citrate-malate, and calcium phosphate are absorbed as well as calcium from a mixed diet.[1] Calcium preparations such as bone meal, powdered bone, dolomite (limestone), and oyster shell should be avoided because they may contain enough lead to be dangerous if consumed routinely.[2] And if supplements containing vitamin D are used, monitor the amount of vitamin D consumed because it is toxic in large doses. Some calcium supplements are also over-the-counter antacids. For instance, Tums, which contains calcium carbonate, is a safe, effective calcium supplement. However, antacids that contain aluminum and magnesium may negatively affect calcium status. These minerals bind phosphorus, preventing its absorption. As a result, phosphorus is released from bone to maintain blood levels, and in the process, calcium is also released and excreted in the urine.

How often and with what you take your calcium supplement are also important. Calcium absorption is lower when a large amount (400 mg or more) is taken in a single dose, so a lower dose supplement taken twice a day may provide more calcium than a single large dose.[3] And calcium absorption from food and supplements can be affected by other dietary factors. Acidic foods, lactose, and fat, which prolongs transit time, increase calcium absorption, whereas oxalate, phytates, and fiber inhibit calcium absorption.

Whether you are getting your calcium from high-calcium foods or supplements, check the label to make sure what you are choosing is the best way to meet your calcium needs.

[1]Mortensen, L., and Charles, P. Bioavailability of calcium supplements and the effect of vitamin D: comparisons between milk, calcium carbonate, and calcium carbonate plus vitamin D. *Am. J. Clin. Nutr.* 63:354–357, 1996.

[2]Bourgoin, B. P., Evans, D. R., Cornett, J. R., et al. Lead content in 70 brands of dietary calcium supplements. *Am. J. Public Health* 83:1155–1160, 1993.

[3]Heaney, R. P., Weaver, C. M., and Fitzsimmons, M. L. Influence of calcium load on absorption fraction. *J. Bone Miner. Res.* 5:1135–1138, 1990.

Nutrient Content Descriptors Related to Calcium

Descriptor	Definition
High-calcium, rich in calcium, excellent source of calcium	Contains 200 mg of calcium or more per serving
Good source of calcium	Contains 100 mg to 190 mg calcium per serving
More or added calcium	Contains at least 100 mg more per serving than reference food

Meeting Calcium Needs Americans typically do not consume enough calcium. It is estimated that only 25% of boys and 10% of girls ages 9 to 17 meet the recommendation of 1300 mg of calcium per day and only 50 to 60% of adults meet the recommendation of 1000 to 1200 mg per day.[31] Adequate calcium intake can be achieved by following the Food Guide Pyramid recommendation of 2 to 3 servings of milk, yogurt, or cheese daily plus 3 to 5 servings of vegetables a day. Ice cream, puddings, and soups made with milk are also good calcium sources. Sources of calcium that are low in lactose include dark-green leafy vegetables such as kale, broccoli, and mustard greens; soy products processed with calcium; and fish consumed with the bones. Fortified foods such as breakfast cereals and juice products also provide calcium.

Phosphorus

Phosphorus makes up about 1% of the adult body by weight, and 85% of this is found as a structural component of bones.[46] The phosphorus in soft tissues has both structural and regulatory roles. In nature, phosphorus is most often found in combination with oxygen as phosphate.

Phosphorus in the Diet Phosphorus is more widely distributed in the diet than calcium. Like calcium, it is found in dairy products such as milk, yogurt, and cheese, but meat, cereals, bran, eggs, nuts, and fish are also good sources (Figure 10.25). Food additives used in baked goods, cheese, processed meats, and soft drinks also provide phosphorus.

Phosphorus in the Digestive Tract Phosphorus is more readily absorbed than calcium. There is no evidence that the efficiency of absorption is affected by the amount in the diet. Vitamin D does aid phosphorus absorption via an active mechanism, but most absorption occurs by a mechanism that does not depend on vitamin D. Therefore, when vitamin D is deficient, phosphorus can still be absorbed, but its absorption is reduced.

Phosphorus in the Body Phosphorus is an important component of a number of molecules with structural and regulatory roles. The phosphorus and calcium in hydroxyapatite form the structure of bones. Phosphorus is a component of phospholipids, which form the structure of cell membranes. It is a major constituent of DNA and RNA. Phosphorus is also involved in regulating enzyme activity because the addition of a phosphate can activate or deactivate certain enzymes. The high-energy bonds of ATP are formed between phosphate groups. Phosphorus is also part of the phosphate **buffer** system that helps regulate pH in the cytoplasm of all cells so that chemical reactions can proceed normally.

Blood levels of phosphorus are not as strictly controlled as those of calcium, but levels are maintained in a ratio with calcium that allows bone mineralization. When

Buffer A substance that reacts with an acid or base to prevent changes in pH.

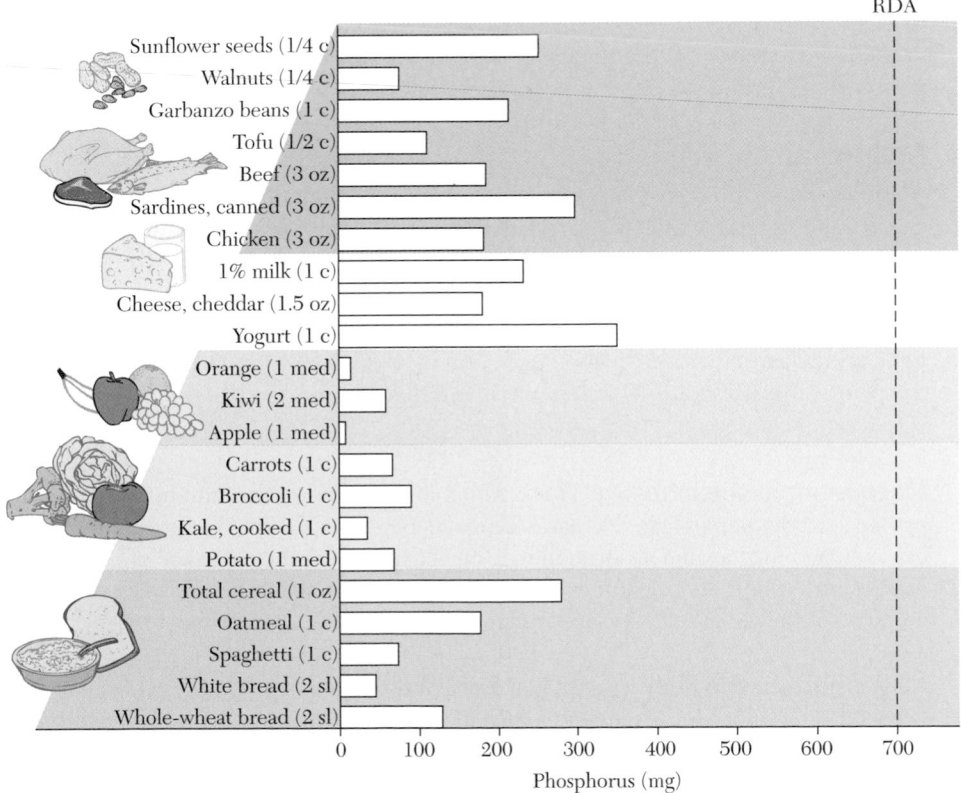

Figure 10.25
Phosphorus content of selections from each group of the Food Guide Pyramid. The dashed line represents the RDA for adults.

blood levels of phosphorus are low, the active form of vitamin D is synthesized. This increases the absorption of both phosphorus and calcium from the intestine and increases their release from bone. When phosphorus intake is high, more is lost in the urine so plasma levels rise only slightly. A rise in serum phosphorus indirectly stimulates parathyroid hormone release, causing phosphorus excretion and calcium retention by the kidney as well as calcium release from bone. When parathyroid hormone is not secreted (such as when calcium levels rise), phosphorus is retained by the kidney and calcium is excreted.

How Much Phosphorus Do We Need? For men and women 19 to 50 years of age the RDA for phosphorus is set at 700 mg.[36] This is the amount needed to maintain normal blood phosphorus levels. Because neither absorption nor urinary losses change significantly with age, the RDA is the same for older adults.

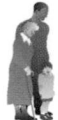

For growing children and adolescents, the RDA is based on the phosphorus intake necessary to meet the needs for bone and soft tissue growth. There is no evidence that phosphorus requirements are increased during pregnancy; intestinal absorption increases by about 10%, which is sufficient to provide the additional phosphorus needed by the mother and fetus. The RDA is not increased during lactation because the phosphorus in milk is provided by an increase in bone resorption and a decrease in urinary excretion that are independent of dietary intake of either phosphorus or calcium.

Phosphorus and Health Phosphorus deficiency can lead to bone loss, weakness, and loss of appetite. However, because phosphorus is so widely distributed in food, dietary deficiencies are rare. Marginal phosphorus deficiencies are most common in premature infants, vegans, alcoholics, and the elderly. Marginal phosphorus status may be caused by losses due to chronic diarrhea and over-use of aluminum-containing antacids, which prevent phosphorus absorption.

Toxicity from high phosphorus intake is rare in healthy adults, but excessive intakes can lead to bone resorption. The increased use of phosphorus-containing food additives has caused concern about its impact on bone health.[51] However, a study that monitored bone resorption found that it did not increase when phosphorus intake was doubled from 800 to 1600 mg per day.[52] Levels of phosphorus intake typical in the United States are not believed to affect bone health as long as calcium intake is adequate.[36] Based on the upper level of normal serum phosphate, a UL for phosphorus of 4.0 grams per day has been set for adults 19 to 70.

Magnesium

There are approximately 25 grams of magnesium in the adult human body. Magnesium is a mineral that affects the metabolism of calcium, sodium, and potassium.

Magnesium in the Diet Magnesium is found in leafy greens such as spinach and kale because it is a component of chlorophyll. The germ and bran of whole grains, nuts, seeds, and bananas are also good sources, but other fruits, fish, meat, and milk are poor sources (Figure 10.26). In areas with hard water, the water supply may provide a significant amount of magnesium.

Magnesium in the Digestive Tract About 50% of the magnesium in the diet is absorbed, and the percentage decreases as intake increases. The active form of vitamin D can enhance magnesium absorption to a small extent, and the presence of phytate decreases absorption. As calcium in the diet increases, the absorption of magnesium decreases, so the use of calcium supplements can reduce the absorption of magnesium.

Magnesium in the Body About 50 to 60% of the magnesium in the body is in bone where it is essential for the maintenance of structure. Magnesium is also involved in regulating calcium homeostasis and is needed for the action of vitamin D and many hormones including parathyroid hormone.[53]

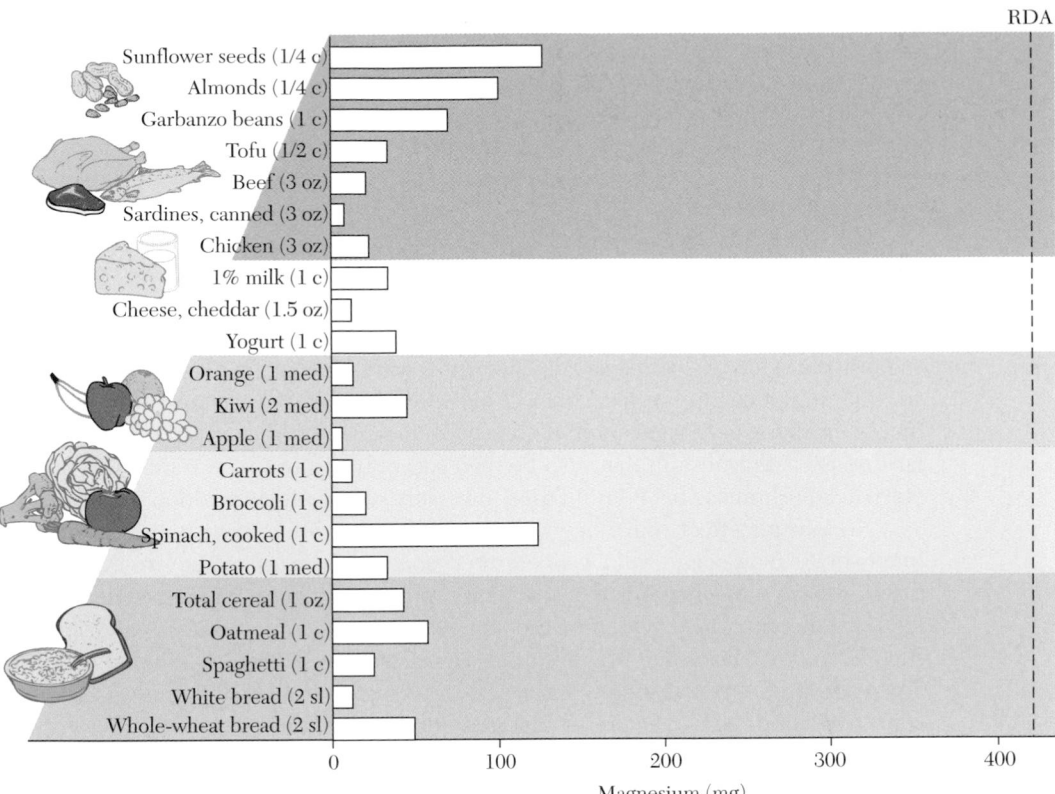

Figure 10.26

Magnesium content of selections from each food group of the Food Guide Pyramid. The dashed line represents the RDA for adult men age 31 and older.

Magnesium is a cofactor for over 300 enzymes. It is necessary for the generation of energy from carbohydrate, lipid, and protein (see Table 10.1). In some of these reactions it is involved indirectly as a stabilizer of ATP, and in others, directly as an enzyme activator. Magnesium is needed for the activity of sodium-potassium ATPase, responsible for active transport of sodium and potassium across membranes. It is therefore essential for maintenance of electrical potentials across cell membranes and proper functioning of the nerves and muscles, including those in the heart. It is important for DNA and RNA synthesis and for almost every step in protein synthesis. Therefore, magnesium is particularly important for dividing growing cells.

Blood levels of magnesium are closely regulated by the kidney. When magnesium intake is low, excretion in the urine is decreased. As intake increases, urinary excretion increases to maintain normal blood levels. This efficient regulation permits homeostasis over a wide range of dietary intakes.

How Much Magnesium Do We Need? The RDA for magnesium is 400 mg per day for young men and 310 mg per day for young women.[36] This is based on the maintenance of total body magnesium balance over time. The RDA is slightly higher for men and women age 31 and older.

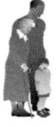

The requirement for pregnancy is increased by 35 mg per day to account for the addition of lean body mass. No increase is provided for lactation because magnesium is released when bone is resorbed and urinary excretion is decreased. An AI is set for infants based on the magnesium content of human milk. A serving of whole-grain breakfast cereal, spinach, or legumes contains about 100 mg of magnesium.

Magnesium and Health Magnesium deficiency is rare in the general population. However, it does occur in those with alcoholism, malnutrition, kidney disease, and gastrointestinal disease, as well as in those who use diuretics that increase magnesium loss in the urine. Deficiency symptoms include nausea, muscle weakness and cramping, irritability, mental derangement, and changes in blood pressure and heartbeat. Low blood magnesium levels affect levels of blood calcium and potassium; therefore some of these symptoms may be due to alterations in the levels of these other minerals.

Low intakes of magnesium have been associated with a number of chronic diseases. Oral magnesium supplements given to postmenopausal women with osteoporosis caused an increase in bone density and a decrease in fracture rate, suggesting that low magnesium status is related to osteoporosis.[53] Epidemiological evidence suggests that humans with good magnesium status are at a lower risk of atherosclerosis, and supplements improve blood lipid levels.[54] Areas with hard water, which is high in calcium and magnesium, tend to have lower rates of death from cardiovascular disease.[55] Magnesium may also be involved in blood pressure regulation, and dietary magnesium has been found to be inversely correlated with blood pressure.[24]

No adverse effects have been observed from ingestion of magnesium in foods, but toxicity may occur from concentrated sources such as magnesium-containing drugs and supplements. Toxicity has been reported in elderly patients with impaired kidney function who frequently use magnesium-containing laxatives and antacids such as milk of magnesia. Magnesium toxicity is characterized by nausea, vomiting, low blood pressure, and other cardiovascular changes. The UL for adults and adolescents over nine years of age is 350 mg of nonfood magnesium.

• SULFUR

Sulfur in the diet comes from organic molecules such as the sulfur-containing amino acids in proteins and the sulfur-containing vitamins. It is also found in some inorganic food preservatives such as sulfur dioxide, sodium sulfite, and sodium and potassium bisulfite, which are used as antioxidants. In the body, the sulfur-containing amino acids methionine and cysteine are needed for protein synthesis. Cysteine is also part of the compound glutathione, which is important in detoxifying drugs and protecting cells from oxidative damage. The vitamins thiamin and biotin, essential for energy production, contain sulfur. Sulfur-containing ions are important in regulating acid-base balance.

There is no recommended intake for sulfur, and no deficiencies are known when protein needs are met (see Table 10.1).

• APPLICATIONS •

1. Use one day of the food record you kept in Chapter 2 to see how your diet compares to the DASH diet.
   a. Compare the number of servings from each of the food groups to the recommended servings for your energy intake as shown in Table 10.3.
   b. Modify your diet to meet DASH guidelines.
   c. What difficulties or inconveniences do you see with following this dietary pattern?
   d. What other dietary or lifestyle changes might you make if you are at high risk of hypertension?
2. Keep a log of all the fluids you consume in one day.
   a. Calculate your fluid intake by totaling the volume of water, beverages, and foods that are liquid at room temperature, such as soup and ice cream, that you consumed.

   b. How does your intake on this day compare with your estimated requirement?
3. a. Using food labels, estimate the amount of sodium you consume from processed foods each day.
   b. Make a list of processed foods you commonly eat that contain more than 10% of the Daily Value for sodium (2400 mg) per serving.
4. Using the food record you kept in Chapter 2, calculate your average calcium intake.
   a. How does your intake compare with the AI for calcium for someone of your age and sex?
   b. If your calcium intake is below the AI, modify your diet to increase your calcium consumption without significantly increasing your energy intake.

SUMMARY

1. Water is an essential nutrient that constitutes about 60% of the adult human body. It is consumed in beverages and food, and a small amount is produced by metabolism. Fluid intake is stimulated by the sensation of thirst, which occurs in response to a decrease in body water.

2. Body water is distributed between intracellular and extracellular compartments. The amount in each compartment depends largely on the concentration of solutes. Since water will diffuse by osmosis from a compartment with a lower concentration of solutes to one with a higher concentration, the body regulates the distribution of water by adjusting the concentration of electrolytes and other solutes in each compartment.

3. Water helps to transport other nutrients and waste products within the body and to excrete wastes from the body. It also helps to protect the body, regulate body temperature, and lubricate areas such as the eyes and the joints. Its polar structure allows it to function as a solvent for the molecules involved in metabolism.

4. Water is lost from the body in urine and feces and through evaporation from the skin and lungs. The kidney is the primary regulator of water output. If water intake is low, antidiuretic hormone will cause the kidney to conserve water. If water intake is high, more water will be excreted in the urine. The amount of water required by the body, about 1 ml per kcalorie of intake, may vary depending on environmental conditions and activity level. Dehydration can occur if water intake is too low or output is excessive.

5. Minerals are elements needed by the body to regulate chemical reactions and provide structure. They come from plant and animal sources, and their bioavailability is affected by interactions with other minerals, vitamins, and other dietary components such as fiber, phytates, oxylates, and tannins. For some minerals, bioavailability is affected by body need.

6. The minerals sodium, chloride, and potassium are electrolytes important in the maintenance of fluid balance and the formation of membrane potentials. The North American diet is abundant in sodium and chloride from processed foods and table salt but generally low in potassium, which is high in unprocessed foods such as fresh fruits and vegetables.

7. Electrolyte and fluid homeostasis is regulated primarily by the kidneys. A decrease in blood pressure or blood volume signals the release of the enzyme renin, which helps form angiotensin II. Angiotensin II causes blood vessels to constrict and the hormone aldosterone to be released. Aldosterone causes the kidneys to reabsorb sodium and hence water, thereby increasing blood volume. Failure of these regulatory mechanisms may be a cause of hypertension.

8. Hypertension is common in the United States. A diet high in sodium increases blood pressure in some, if not all individuals. Other nutrients, including potassium, magnesium, and calcium, also affect blood pressure.

9. To reduce the risk of hypertension, public health recommendations suggest a moderate intake of salt and sodium, adequate dietary potassium, weight loss in overweight individuals, limited alcohol consumption, and increased exercise. The adoption of the DASH diet—a dietary pattern high in fruits, vegetables, low-fat dairy products, whole grains, and lean meat, fish, and poultry—is also recommended. This diet is rich in potassium, magnesium, calcium, and fiber, and low in fat, saturated fat, and cholesterol.

10. Bone is a living tissue that is constantly being broken down and reformed in a process known as bone remodeling. Early in life, bone formation occurs more rapidly than bone breakdown to allow bone growth and an increase in bone mass. Peak bone mass occurs in young adulthood. With age, bone breakdown begins to outpace formation, causing a decrease in bone mass; this is accelerated in women for about 5 years after menopause.

11. Osteoporosis is a condition in which loss of bone mass increases the risk of bone fractures. The risk of osteoporosis is related to the level of peak bone mass and the rate of bone loss. These are affected by race and gender as well as diet and exercise.

12. Most of the calcium and phosphorus in the body is in bone as hydroxyapatite. Calcium not found in bone is essential for nerve transmission, muscle contraction, blood clotting, and blood pressure regulation. Blood levels of calcium are regulated by parathyroid hormone and calcitonin. Parathyroid hormone stimulates the release of calcium from bone, decreases calcium excretion by the kidney, and activates vitamin D to increase the amount of calcium absorbed from the gastrointestinal tract and released from bone. Calcitonin blocks calcium release from bone.

13. The AI for calcium ranges from 1000 to 1200 mg per day for adults and is 1300 mg per day in adolescents. Sources of calcium in the American diet include dairy products, fish consumed with bones, and leafy green vegetables.

14. In addition to its structural role in bones and teeth, phosphorus is part of a buffer system that helps prevent changes in pH. It is an essential component of phospholipids, ATP, and DNA. Good sources of phosphorus include dairy products, meats, and grains. The RDA is 700 mg per day.

15. Magnesium is important for bone health, and it is needed as a cofactor for numerous reactions throughout the body. In reactions involved in energy production it acts as an enzyme activator and stabilizer of ATP. It is also needed to maintain membrane potentials; thus it is essential for nerve and muscle conductivity. Homeostasis is regulated by the kidney. Deficiency is rare, and the best dietary sources are whole grains and green vegetables.

16. Sulfur is needed in the diet as preformed organic molecules such as the amino acids methionine and cysteine, which are needed to synthesize proteins and glutathione, and the vitamins thiamin and biotin, needed for energy metabolism. Sulfur is also part of a buffer system that regulates acid-base balance. A dietary deficiency is unknown in the absence of protein malnutrition.

REVIEW QUESTIONS

1. How is the amount of water in the body regulated?

2. Describe the functions of water in the body.

3. What is the recommended water intake for adults?

4. List three factors that increase water needs.

5. How do sodium, potassium, and chloride function in the body?

6. What types of foods contribute the most sodium to the North American diet?

7. What types of foods are good sources of potassium?

8. What is the relationship between dietary sodium and blood pressure?

9. What is the DASH diet, and how does it affect blood pressure?

10. What is the major source of calcium in the North American diet?

11. How are blood calcium levels regulated?

12. How is calcium intake related to the risk of osteoporosis?

13. What factors other than calcium are related to the risk of osteoporosis?

14. What is the function of phosphorus in the body?

15. Name some food sources of phosphorous.

16. What is the function of magnesium in the body?

17. Where is sulfur found in the body?

REFERENCES

1. Askew, E. W. Nutrition and performance in hot, cold, and high altitude environments. In *Nutrition in Exercise and Sport*, 3rd ed. Wolinsky, I., ed. Boca Raton, FL: CRC Press, 1998, 597–619.
2. Sheng, H-P. Body fluids and water balance, In *Biochemical and Physiological Aspects of Human Nutrition*, Stipanuk, M., ed, Philadelphia, PA: W. B. Saunders, 2000, 843–865.
3. Armstrong, L. E. and Epstein, Y. Fluid-electrolyte balance during labor and exercise: Concepts and misconceptions. *Int. J. Sport Nutr.* 9:1–12, 1999.
4. Oppliger, R. A., Case, H. S., Horswill, C. A., et al. American College of Sports Medicine position statement: Weight loss in wrestlers. *Med. Sci. Sports Exerc.* 28:ix–xii, 1996.
5. National Research Council, Food and Nutrition Board. *Recommended Dietary Allowances*, 10th ed. Washington, D.C.: National Academy Press, 1989.
6. National Research Council. *Diet and Health: Implications for Reducing Chronic Disease Risk*. Washington, D.C.: National Academy Press, 1989.
7. Committee on Nutritional Status During Pregnancy and Lactation, National Academy of Sciences. *Nutrition During Pregnancy*. Washington, D.C.: National Academy Press, 1990.
8. Antonios, T. F., and MacGregor, G. A. Salt intake: Potential deleterious effects excluding blood pressure. *J. Hum. Hypertens.* 9:511–515, 1995.
9. Brown, M. J. and Haydock, S. Pathoeatiology, epidemiology and diagnosis of hypertension. *Drugs* 59: 1s–12s, 2000.
10. Sixth Report of the Joint National Committee on Prevention, Detection, Evaluation, and Treatment of High Blood Pressure. *Arch. Intern. Med.* 157:2413–2446, 1997.
11. American Heart Association. Factors That Contribute to High Blood Pressure. Available online at www.americanheart.org/presenter.jhtml?identifier=4650/ Accessed April 18, 2002.
12. Greenland, P. Beating High Blood Pressure with Low-Sodium DASH. *N. Engl. J. Med.* 344:53–55, 2001.
13. Carvalho, J. J., Baruzzi, R. G., Howard, P. F., et al. Blood pressure in four remote populations in the Intersalt study. *Hypertension* 14:238–246, 1989.
14. Graudal, N. A., Galloe, A. M., and Garrod, P. Effects of sodium restriction on blood pressure, renin, aldosterone, catecholamines, cholesterols, and triglyceride: A meta-analysis. *JAMA*, 279:1383–1391, 1998.
15. Luft, L. C., and Weinberger, M. H. Heterogeneous responses to changes in dietary salt intake: the salt sensitivity paradigm. *Am. J. Clin. Nutr.* 65(Suppl.):612S–617S, 1997.
16. Kotchen, T. A., and Kotchen, J. M. Dietary sodium and blood pressure: interactions with other nutrients. *Am. J. Clin. Nutr.* 65(Suppl.): 708S–711S, 1997.
17. Vogt, T. M., Appel, L. J., Obarzanwk, E., et al. Dietary Approaches to Stop Hypertension: Rationale, design and methods. DASH Collaborative Group, *J. Am. Diet. Assoc.* 99: s12–s18, 1999.
18. Young, D. B., Lin, H., and McCabe, R. D. Potassium's cardiovascular protective mechanisms. *Am. J. Physiol.* 268:R825–R837, 1995.
19. Ascherio, A. Rimm, E. B., Hernan, M.A., et al. Intake of potassium, magnesium, calcium, and fiber and risk of stroke among U.S. men. *Circulation* 98:1198–1204, 1998.
20. Whelton, P. K., He, J., Cutler, J. A., et al. Effects of oral potassium on blood pressure: Meta-analysis of randomized controlled clinical trials. *JAMA* 227:1624–1632, 1997.
21. Hamet, P. The evaluation of the scientific evidence for a relationship between calcium and hypertension. *J. Nutr.* 125(Suppl.):311S–400S, 1995.
22. Allender, P. S., Cutler, J. A., Follmann, D., et al. Dietary calcium and blood pressure: A meta-analysis of randomized clinical trials. *Ann. Intern. Med.* 124:825–831, 1996.
23. Dwyer, J. H., Dwyer, K. M., Scribner, R. A., et al. Dietary calcium, calcium supplementation, and blood pressure in African American adolescents. *Am. J. Clin. Nutr.* 68:648–655, 1998.
24. Singh, R. B., Niaz, M. A., Moshiri, M., et al. Magnesium status and risk of coronary artery disease in rural and urban populations with variable magnesium consumption. *Magnes. Res.* 10:205–213, 1997.
25. Ma, J., Folsom, A. R., Melnick, S. L., et al. Associations of serum and dietary magnesium with cardiovascular disease, hypertension, diabetes, insulin, and carotid arterial wall thickness: The ARIC study. Atherosclerosis Risk in Community Study. *J. Clin. Epidemiol.* 48:927–940, 1995.
26. Appel, L. J., Moore, T. J., Obarzanek, E., et al. A clinical trial of the effects of dietary patterns on blood pressure. *N. Engl. J. Med.* 336:1117–1124, 1997.
27. Zemel, M. B. Dietary pattern and hypertension: The DASH diet. *Nutr. Rev.* 55:303–305, 1997.
28. Kaplan, N. M. The dietary guidelines for sodium. *Am. J. Clin. Nutr.* 71: 1020–1026, 2000.
29. Teegarden, D., Lyle, R. M., McCabe, G. P., et al. Diet and bone mineral measure in young women. *Am. J. Clin. Nutr.* 68:749–754, 1998.
30. Groff, J. L., Gropper, S. S., and Hunt, S. M. *Advanced Nutrition and Human Metabolism*, 2nd ed. St. Paul, Minn.: 1995. West Publishing Company.
31. National Institutes of Health. Consensus Development Conference Statement. Osteoporosis Prevention, Diagnosis and Therapy, March 27–29, 2000. Available online at odp.od.nih.gov/consensus.cons/111/111_intro.htm/Accessed April 18, 2002.
32. Osteoporosis Overview. Osteoporosis and Related Bone Diseases National Resource Center. Available online at www.osteo.org/osteo.html/ Accessed April 18, 2002.
33. Eisman, J. A. Genetics of osteoporosis. *Endocr. Rev.* 20:788–804, 1999.
34. Bohannon, A. D. Osteoporosis and African American women. *J. Womens Health Gend. Based Med.* 8:609–615, 1999.
35. National Institutes of Health. Consensus Development Conference Statement: Osteoporosis Prevention, Diagnosis, and Therapy, march 27–29, 2000. Available online at odp.odnihgov/consensus/cons/111/111_intro.htm/Accessed Jan. 17, 2001.
36. Institute of Medicine, Food and Nutrition Board. *Dietary Reference Intakes for Calcium, Phosphorus, Magnesium, Vitamin D, and Fluoride*. Washington, D.C.: National Academy Press, 1997.
37. Heaney, R. P., Weaver, C. M., and Recker, R. R. Calcium absorption from spinach. *Am. J. Clin. Nutr.* 47:707–709, 1988.
38. Bronner, F., and Pansu, D. Nutritional aspects of calcium absorption. *J. Nutr.* 129:9–12, 1999.

39. Affinito, P., Tommaselli, G. A., DiCarlo, C., et al. Changes in bone mineral density and calcium metabolism in breast-feeding women: A one year follow-up study. *J. Clin. Endocrinol. Metab.* 81:2314–2318, 1996.

40. Cross, N. A., Hillman, L. S., Allen, S. H., and Krasue, G. F. Changes in bone mineral density and markers of bone remodeling during lactation and postweaning in women consuming high amounts of calcium. *J. Bone Miner. Res.* 10:1312–1320, 1995.

41. Burger, H., Grobbee, D. E., and Drueke, T. Osteoporosis and salt intake. *Nutr. Metab. Cardiovasc. Dis.* 10:46–53, 2000.

42. Heaney, R. P. Excess dietary protein may not adversely affect bone. *J. Nutr.* 128:1054–1057, 1998.

43. New, S. A., Robins, S. P., Campbell, M. K., et al. Dietary influences on bone mass and bone metabolism: Further evidence of a positive link between fruit and vegetable consumption and bone health. *Am. J. Clin. Nutr.* 71:142–151, 2000.

44. Riggs, B. L., O'Fallon, W. M., Muhs, J., et al. Long-term effects of calcium supplementation on serum parathyroid hormone level, bone turnover, and bone loss in elderly women. *J. Bone Miner. Res.* 13:168–174, 1998.

45. Reid, I. R. The roles of calcium and vitamin D in the prevention of osteoporosis. *Endocrinol. Metab. Clin. North Am.* 27:389–398, 1998.

46. Devine, A., Dick, I. M., Heal, S. J., et al. A 4-year follow-up study of the effects of calcium supplementation on bone density in elderly postmenopausal women. *Osteoporos. Int.* 7:23–28, 1997.

47. Nieves, J. W., Komar, L., Cosman, F., and Lindasya, R. Calcium potentiates the effect of estogen and calcitonin on bone mass: Review and analysis. *Am. J. Clin. Nutr.* 67:18–24, 1998.

48. Wimalawansa, S. J. A four-year randomized controlled trial of hormone replacement and bisphosphonate, alone or in combination, in women with postmenopausal osteoporosis. *Am. J. Med.* 104:219–226, 1998.

49. Minihane, A. M., and Fairweather-Tait, S. J. Effect of calcium supplementation on daily nonheme-iron absorption and long-term iron status. *Am. J. Clin. Nutr.* 68:96–102, 1998.

50. Wood, R. J., and Zheng, J. J. High dietary calcium intakes reduce zinc absorption and balance in humans. *Am. J. Clin. Nutr.* 65:1803–1809, 1997.

51. Calvo, M. S., and Park, Y. K. Changing phosphorus content of the U.S. diet: Potential for adverse effect on bone. *J. Nutr.* 126:1168S–1180S, 1996.

52. Bizik, B. K., Ding, W., and Cerklewski, F. L. Evidence that bone resorption of young men is not increased by high dietary phosphorus obtained from milk and cheese. *Nutr. Res.* 16:1143–1146, 1996.

53. Sojka, J. E., and Weaver, C. M. Magnesium supplementation and osteoporosis. *Nutr. Rev.* 53:71–74, 1995.

54. Dreosti, I. E. Magnesium status and health. *Nutr. Rev.* 53:S23–S27, 1995.

55. Rubenowitz, E., Axelsson, G., and Rylander, R. Magnesium in drinking water and death from myocardial infarction. *Am. J. Epidemiol.* 143:456–462, 1996.

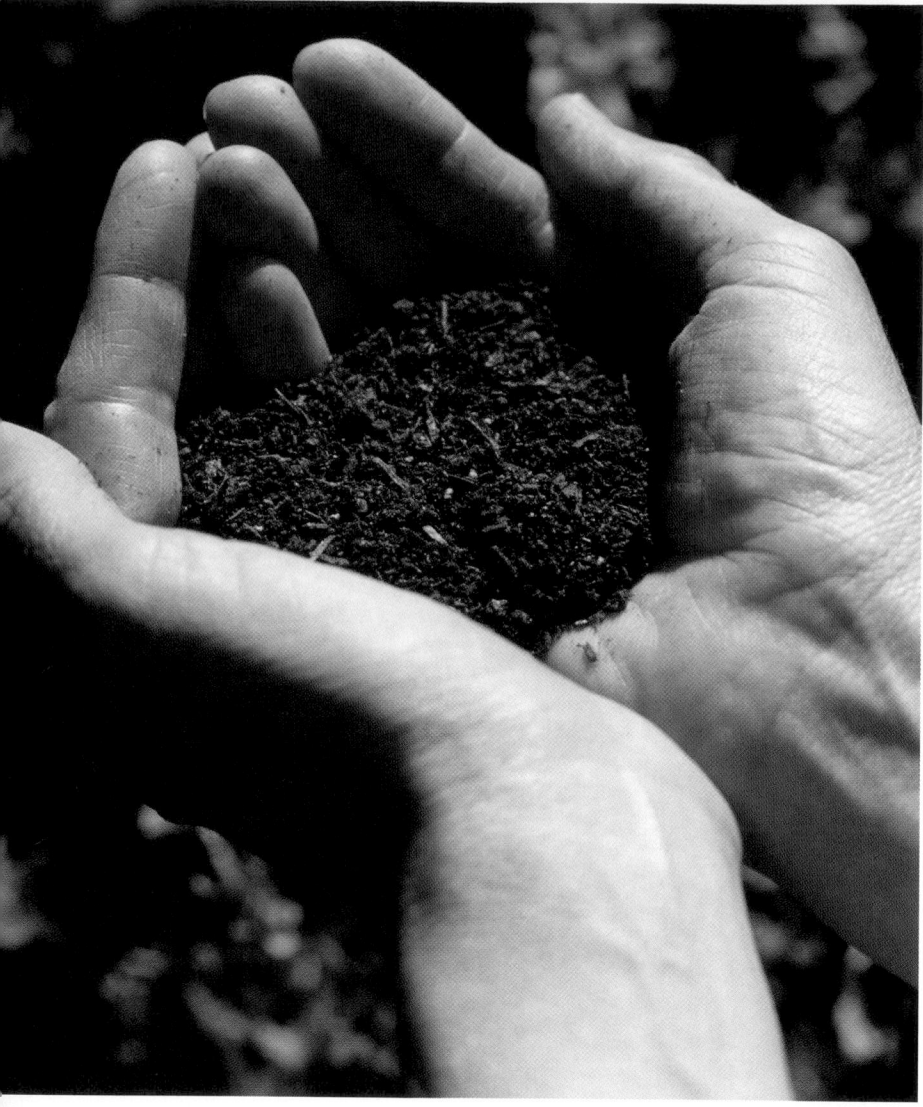

Chapter 11

The Trace Minerals: Our Elemental Needs

Chapter Outline

TRACE ELEMENT FUNCTIONS

IRON (FE)

ZINC (ZN)

COPPER (CU)

MANGANESE (MN)

SELENIUM (SE)

IODINE (I)

CHROMIUM (CR)

FLUORIDE (F)

MOLYBDENUM (MO)

OTHER TRACE ELEMENTS

(© Nancy R. Cohen/Photo Disc, Inc.)

Chapter Concepts

✔ Trace elements are required in the diet in small amounts but have important functions in regulating body processes.

✔ Iron is a component of the oxygen transport protein hemoglobin. Iron deficiency anemia is the most common nutritional deficiency worldwide, but too much iron can be toxic.

✔ Copper is needed to transport iron; therefore, a deficiency can cause anemia. Copper is also involved in the synthesis of connective tissue, lipid metabolism, and antioxidant protection.

✔ Zinc is a cofactor for many enzymes and also affects protein synthesis through gene expression. It is needed for tissue growth and repair, sexual development, and immune function.

✔ Manganese is a component of the antioxidant enzyme superoxide dismutase.

✔ Selenium is an essential part of the antioxidant enzyme glutathione peroxidase.

✔ Iodine is essential for the synthesis of the thyroid hormones, which regulate basal metabolic rate and other body functions.

✔ Chromium is needed for insulin to transport glucose into cells.

✔ Fluoride is important for healthy bones and teeth. An adequate intake reduces dental caries.

✔ Molybdenum is needed for the activity of several enzymes involved in uric acid production.

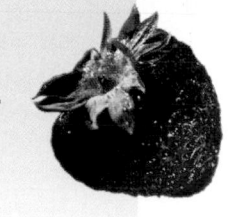

Can taking a supplement of one mineral cause a deficiency of another?

Are iron supplements dangerous?

Can taking chromium supplements change body composition?

Trace elements are the most recently recognized of the essential nutrients. By definition, trace elements are minerals that are required by the body in an amount of 100 mg or less per day or that are present in the body in an amount of 0.01% or less of body weight. The methods traditionally used to establish the essentiality of nutrients and to determine their requirements have not been effective for studying many of the trace elements. The requirements for some of these elements are so small and interactions among the elements and other dietary components so great that isolated deficiencies of trace elements have not always been possible to create, even in the laboratory. This has caused researchers to focus not only on the needs for individual nutrients, but on the importance of balanced interactions of nutrients within the total diet.

Determining the health impact of trace mineral deficiencies involves a mixture of addressing old challenges and exploring new frontiers. Deficiencies of iron and iodine have been public health concerns for generations. It is estimated that more than 2 billion people worldwide suffer from iron deficiency, including 8.5 million women, adolescent girls, and children in the United States.[1,2] Iodine deficiency, although virtually eradicated in the United States, is a major health problem in developing countries. While eliminating these deficiencies is a continuing challenge, new concerns have arisen about marginal deficiencies of some of the trace elements. For example, is impaired immune function due to a mild zinc deficiency a widespread public health problem or a rare condition? Does a marginal selenium deficiency increase cancer risk? Does a low chromium intake contribute to diabetes? There are no good ways to diagnose these marginal deficiencies, and there is still much to learn about the breadth of function of these trace elements.

• TRACE ELEMENT FUNCTIONS

As with the major minerals, some of the trace elements have complementary functions while others have separate unique functions. For example, a number of trace elements interact with oxygen—some by assuring it is delivered to cells and some by preventing oxidative damage. Minerals can also catalyze the formation of dangerous free radicals. To prevent this, the body stores, transports, and uses these minerals in forms that are bound to proteins and therefore unable to cause free radical formation. A number of enzymes that contain trace elements are able to destroy reactive oxygen molecules and protect cells from oxidative damage. Iron, copper, zinc, manganese, and selenium all serve as components of these antioxidant enzyme systems. In addition to these parallel roles, each trace element has additional unique functions. Iodine is a component of thyroid hormones, which help regulate metabolic rate. Chromium is important for allowing glucose to enter cells, and fluoride strengthens tooth enamel. Whether a mineral's role is unique or complements another, optimum function depends on adequate levels of all other nutrients.

• IRON (FE)

Iron was identified as a major constituent of blood in the 18th century. By 1832, iron tablets were used to treat young women in whom "coloring matter" was lacking in the blood. Today we know that the red color in blood is due to the iron-containing protein **hemoglobin** and that a deficiency of iron decreases hemoglobin production. Despite the fact that iron is one of the best understood of the trace elements, iron deficiency remains the most common nutritional deficiency in North America and worldwide.[1,2]

Hemoglobin An iron-containing protein in red blood cells that binds oxygen and transports it through the bloodstream to cells.

Iron in the Diet

Iron in the diet comes from both plant and animal sources. Much of the iron in animal products is **heme iron**—iron that is part of a chemical complex found in proteins, such as **myoglobin** in muscle and hemoglobin in blood. Meat, poultry, and fish are good sources of heme iron. Heme iron accounts for about 10 to 15% of the dietary iron in industrialized countries.[3]

Leafy green vegetables, legumes, and whole and enriched grains are good sources of **nonheme iron** (see Figure 11.1). Another source of nonheme iron in the diet is iron cooking utensils, from which iron leaches into food. Leaching is enhanced by acidic foods. For example, spaghetti sauce cooked in a glass pan contains

Heme iron A readily absorbed form of iron found in animal products that is chemically associated with proteins such as hemoglobin and myoglobin.

Myoglobin An iron-containing protein in muscle cells that binds oxygen.

Nonheme iron A poorly absorbed form of iron found in both plant and animal foods that is not part of the iron complex found in hemoglobin and myoglobin.

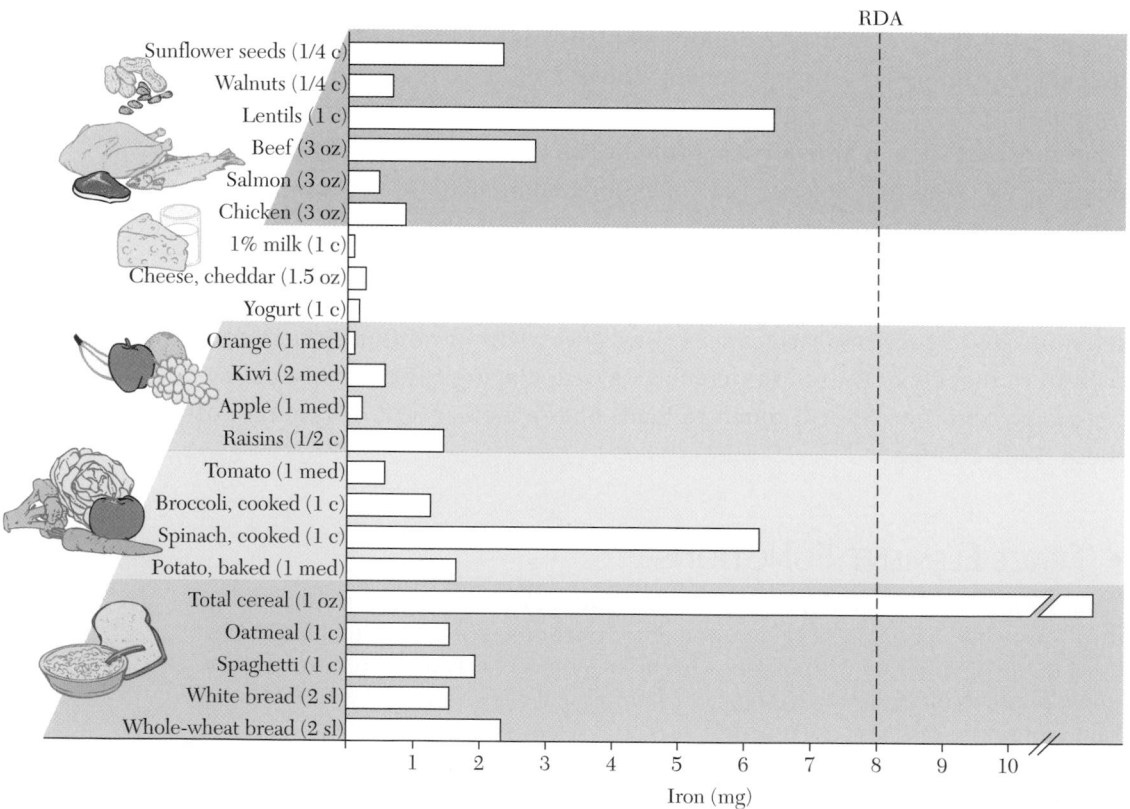

Figure 11.1

Iron content of selections from each group of the Food Guide Pyramid. The dashed line represents the RDA for adult men and postmenopausal women. Both plant and animal foods are good sources of iron, but the form in animal foods is more readily absorbed.

about 3 mg of iron, but the same sauce cooked in an iron skillet may contain more than 80 mg, depending on how long it is cooked.

Iron in the Gastrointestinal Tract

Heme iron is absorbed more than twice as efficiently as nonheme iron, and absorption is not affected by meal composition. The bioavailability of nonheme iron is affected by meal composition. Some dietary components enhance absorption, while others inhibit it. The presence of acids such as ascorbic acid (vitamin C), citric acid, lactic acid, and others enhance iron absorption by helping to keep iron in the ferrous (Fe^{2+}) form, which is better absorbed than the ferric (Fe^{3+}) form. The best studied of these acids is vitamin C, which enhances the absorption of iron for two reasons: First, as an acid, it keeps iron in its more absorbable form; and second, it forms a complex with iron that remains soluble and bioavailable, preventing iron from forming unabsorbable complexes in the gastrointestinal tract.[4] To have this effect, the vitamin C must be consumed in the same meal as the iron; it can then enhance nonheme iron absorption up to sixfold.[3] Consuming meats such as beef, fish, or poultry that are sources of heme iron also increases the absorption of nonheme iron. For example, a small amount of hamburger in a pot of chili will enhance the body's absorption of iron from the beans.

Dietary factors that interfere with the absorption of nonheme iron include fiber, phytates found in cereals, tannins found in tea, and oxalates found in some leafy greens such as spinach. These prevent absorption by binding iron in the gastrointestinal tract. The presence of other minerals may also decrease iron absorption. For instance, calcium supplements decrease iron absorption, particularly when both are consumed at the same meal.[5]

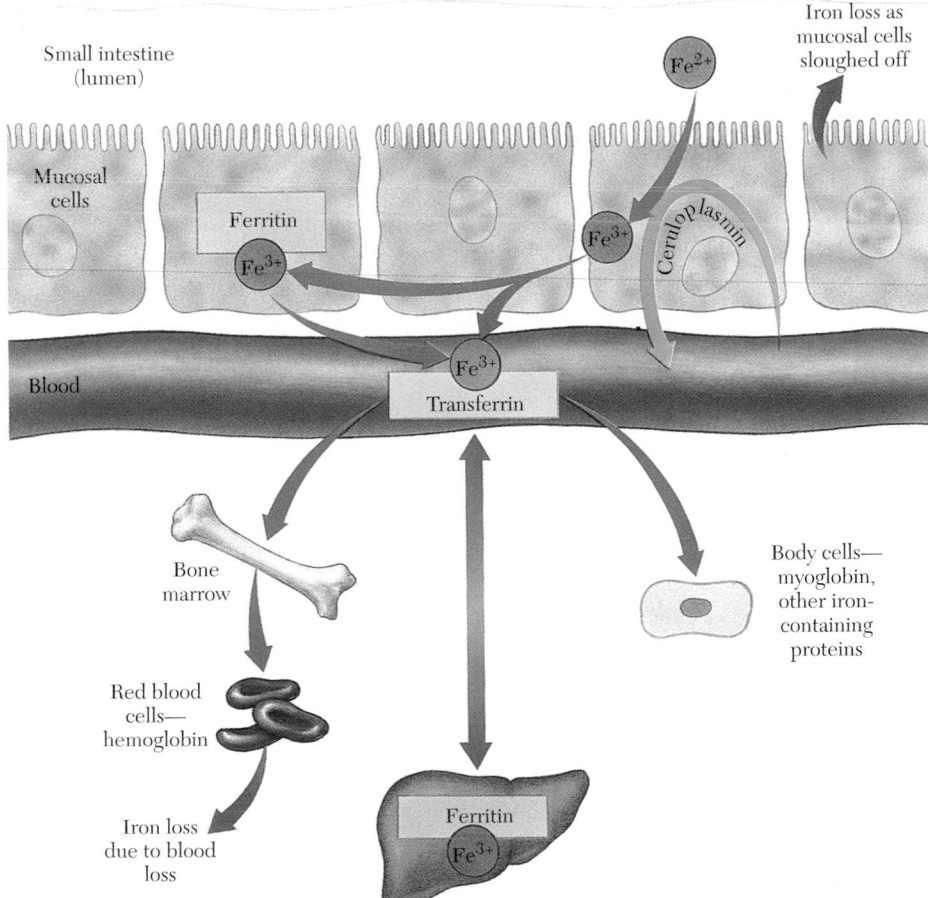

Figure 11.2

Ferrous iron (Fe^{2+}) is absorbed and converted to ferric iron (Fe^{3+}) by ceruloplasmin. The excess remains in mucosal cells bound to ferritin and is excreted when the cells die. Iron is transported in the blood bound to transferrin. It is delivered to bone, where it is needed to synthesize hemoglobin for red blood cells, and to other body cells, where it is used to synthesize myoglobin and other iron-containing proteins. When red blood cells die, the iron is released for reuse. Excess iron is stored primarily in the liver, bound to ferritin.

Ferritin The major iron storage protein.

Transferrin An iron transport protein in the blood.

Ceruloplasmin A copper-containing protein that converts iron to the ferric form, which can bind to iron storage and iron transport proteins.

Iron in the Body

The amount of iron in the body is controlled primarily at the intestine. Iron that has entered the mucosal cells of the small intestine can be bound to the iron storage protein **ferritin** or the iron transport protein **transferrin**. The copper-containing protein **ceruloplasmin** is needed to convert iron to the form that binds to either transferrin or ferritin. Iron that remains bound to ferritin is excreted in the feces when mucosal cells die and are sloughed off into the intestinal lumen (Figure 11.2). Iron that is picked up by transferrin is transported in the blood to the liver, bones, and other body tissues. The amount of iron transported from the mucosal cells to the rest of the body depends on need.

Before iron can enter cells for use, the iron-transferrin complex in the blood must bind to proteins on the cell membrane called transferrin receptors. When iron is in short supply, the number of transferrin receptors increases and less of the iron storage protein ferritin is made, reducing iron storage and allowing more iron to be transported into the cells. When iron is plentiful, more ferritin is made to increase storage capacity and the number of transferrin receptors decreases, so the capacity to pick up iron from the mucosal cells and transport it into body cells is reduced. More iron is then left in the mucosal cells and lost when they die.

Iron that is absorbed in excess of immediate needs can be stored in the protein ferritin primarily in the liver, spleen, and bone marrow. Levels of ferritin in the blood can be used to estimate iron stores. When ferritin concentrations in the liver become high, some is converted to an insoluble storage protein called hemosiderin. Iron can be mobilized from body stores as needed, and deficiency signs will appear only after stores are depleted.

Iron is not readily excreted. Even when red blood cells die, the iron in their hemoglobin is not lost from the body. The cells are removed from the blood by cells in the liver, spleen, and bone marrow and degraded; the iron is then attached to transferrin for transport back to body tissues including the bone where it can be incorporated into new red blood cells. Most iron loss even in healthy individuals occurs through blood loss, including that lost during menstruation and the small amounts lost from the gastrointestinal tract. Some iron is also lost through the shedding of cells from the intestine, skin, and urinary tract.[4]

Iron in the body is essential for the delivery of oxygen to cells. It is a component of two oxygen-carrying proteins, hemoglobin and myoglobin. Most of the iron in the body is part of hemoglobin. Hemoglobin in red blood cells transports oxygen to body cells and carries carbon dioxide away from cells for elimination by the lungs. Myoglobin is found in the muscle, where it enhances the amount of oxygen available for use in muscle contraction. Iron is also essential for energy production as a part of several proteins involved in the citric acid cycle and the electron transport chain. Iron-containing proteins are involved in drug metabolism and the immune system. Iron is also part of the enzyme catalase, which protects the cell from oxidative damage by destroying hydrogen peroxide before it can form free radicals.

Table 11.1 *Dietary Reference Intake Values for Iron*

Gender/ Life Stage	Recommended Intake
Infants	
0–6 months	0.27 mg°
7–12 months	11 mg
Children	
1–3 years	7 mg
4–8 years	10 mg
Males	
9–13	8 mg
14–18	11 mg
≥ 19	8 mg
Females	
9–13	8 mg
14–18	15 mg
19–50	18 mg
≥ 51	8 mg
Females taking oral contraceptives	
14–18	11.4 mg
19–50	10.9 mg
Pregnancy	27 mg
Lactation	
≤ 18	10 mg
19–50	9 mg
Vegetarians	
Men ≥ 19	14 mg
Menstruating women	33 mg
Adolescent girls	26 mg

°This value is an AI; all other values are RDAs.

How Much Iron Do We Need?

The RDA for iron is based on the amount needed to maintain normal function but only minimal iron stores. The RDA is set at 8 mg per day for adult men age 19 and older and for postmenopausal women.[6] The RDA for menstruating women is increased to 18 mg per day to compensate for the iron lost in menstruation. Other specific recommendations have been made for each gender and life-stage group by considering the percentage of dietary iron absorbed, iron losses from the body, and conditions that increase needs, such as growth and pregnancy (Table 11.1). For example, a separate RDA category was created for vegetarians because iron is poorly absorbed from plant sources.

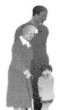

Iron Deficiency

When iron is deficient, hemoglobin cannot be produced. When not enough hemoglobin is available, the red blood cells that are formed are small and pale and unable to deliver adequate oxygen to the tissues. This is known as **iron deficiency anemia** (Figure 11.3). Iron deficiency is the most common nutritional deficiency in the United States, affecting 7.8 million adolescent girls and women of childbearing age and 700,000 children aged one to two years.[2] It is estimated that about 10% of women of childbearing age have insufficient iron stores and 3 to 5% have iron deficiency anemia. Among children aged one to three years, 9% are iron deficient and 3% have iron deficiency anemia.[2] Among low-income and minority women and children, the incidence is even greater. Only about one-fourth of adolescent girls and women of childbearing age meet the RDA for iron through their diet.[2]

Symptoms of iron deficiency anemia include fatigue, weakness, headache, decreased work capacity, an inability to maintain body temperature in a cold environment, changes in behavior, decreased resistance to infection, impaired development in infants, and an increased risk of lead poisoning in young children. One strange symptom thought to be related to iron deficiency is **pica**. This is a compulsion to eat nonfood items such as clay, ice, paste, laundry starch, paint chips, and ashes. Pica can lead to the consumption of substances containing toxic minerals, such as lead-based paints, and it can introduce substances into the diet that inhibit mineral absorption (see Chapter 14).

Women of reproductive age are at risk for iron deficiency anemia because of iron loss due to menstruation. The need for iron is also increased during pregnancy because of the increase in maternal blood volume and the growth of other maternal tissues and the fetus. Iron deficiency is common among pregnant women even in industrialized countries and can lead to premature delivery and greater risk to the mother.[7] Iron deficiency is common in infants and children because their rapid growth increases iron needs. Because the iron in human milk is more available than that in infant formula, the American Academy of Pediatrics recommends that infants

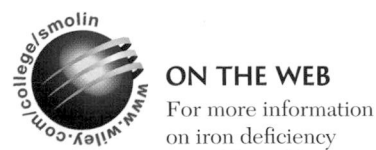

ON THE WEB

For more information on iron deficiency anemia, go to the World Health Organization website at

www.who.int

Iron deficiency anemia A condition that occurs when the oxygen-carrying capacity of the blood is decreased because there is insufficient iron to make hemoglobin. It is diagnosed in adults when hemoglobin concentration is less than 11 grams per 100 ml of blood.

Pica The compulsive ingestion of nonfood substances such as clay, laundry starch, and paint chips.

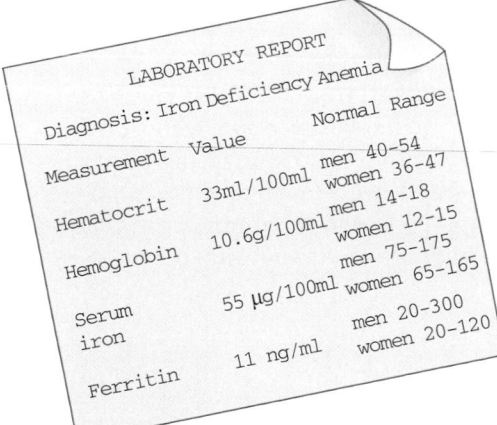

LABORATORY REPORT

Diagnosis: Iron Deficiency Anemia

Measurement	Value	Normal Range
Hematocrit	33ml/100ml	men 40–54 women 36–47
Hemoglobin	10.6g/100ml	men 14–18 women 12–15
Serum iron	55 μg/100ml	men 75–175 women 65–165
Ferritin	11 ng/ml	men 20–300 women 20–120

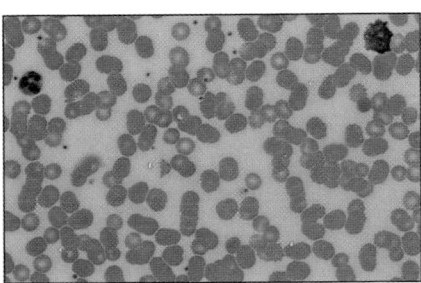

(a)

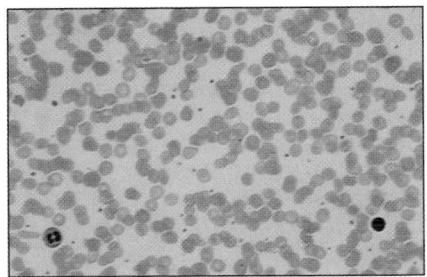

(b)

Figure 11.3

Iron deficiency anemia is diagnosed when levels of red blood cells or proteins containing iron are low. It causes the red blood cells to become small and pale. (*a*) Normal red blood cells. (*b*) Iron deficiency anemia. (*a*, © B & B Photos/Custom Medical Stock Photo; *b*, © Custom Medical Stock Photo)

who are not fed human milk should be fed iron-fortified formula.[8] Toddlers with finicky eating habits should be monitored to ensure they are consuming adequate iron from foods such as meats, leafy green vegetables, and fortified cereals (see Chapters 14 and 15).

Adolescents are also at risk for iron deficiency anemia. In adolescent boys, rapid growth and an increase in muscle mass and blood volume increase iron need. In adolescent girls, iron needs are increased because weight gain is almost as great as in boys and iron losses are increased by the onset of menstruation (see Chapter 15).

Athletes are another group susceptible to iron deficiency. This may be due to a low iron intake, as well as increased losses due to prolonged training. Based on the amount lost, the EAR may be 30 to 70% higher for athletes than for the general population[6] (see Chapter 13 and *Critical Thinking:* Increasing Iron Intake).

Iron Toxicity

Iron toxicity can be acute, resulting from ingestion of a single large dose at one time, or chronic, due to the accumulation of iron in the body over time (referred to as iron overload). Iron overload can result from the chronic consumption of large but nontoxic doses of iron over a long period, but generally occurs only in individuals with hereditary abnormalities in iron absorption (the most common cause), diseases requiring frequent blood transfusions, or conditions in which red blood cell synthesis is abnormal.[9] A UL has been set at 45 mg per day from all sources.

Acute Toxicity   Iron is toxic in large amounts. Even a single large dose can be life-threatening. Iron toxicity from supplements is one of the most common forms of poisoning among children under age six. Iron poisoning may cause damage to the intestinal lining, abnormalities in body pH, shock, and liver failure. Iron supplement overdose is the leading cause of liver transplants in children. To protect children from accidental poisoning from iron-containing drugs and supplements, these products display a warning on the label (Figure 11.4). In addition, since most cases of serious iron poisoning have occurred with products containing 30 mg or more per dose, these products are packaged in individual doses to make consumption of many pills difficult for a young child.[10]

Chronically Elevated Iron Stores   Iron stores that are above normal but below toxic levels have been hypothesized to be associated with a greater risk of both heart disease and cancer. The relationship between iron and heart disease was originally suggested because heart disease occurs less frequently in premenopausal women, who lose iron monthly, than in postmenopausal women and men. Elevated levels of the iron storage protein ferritin are associated with an increased risk of heart attacks.[11]

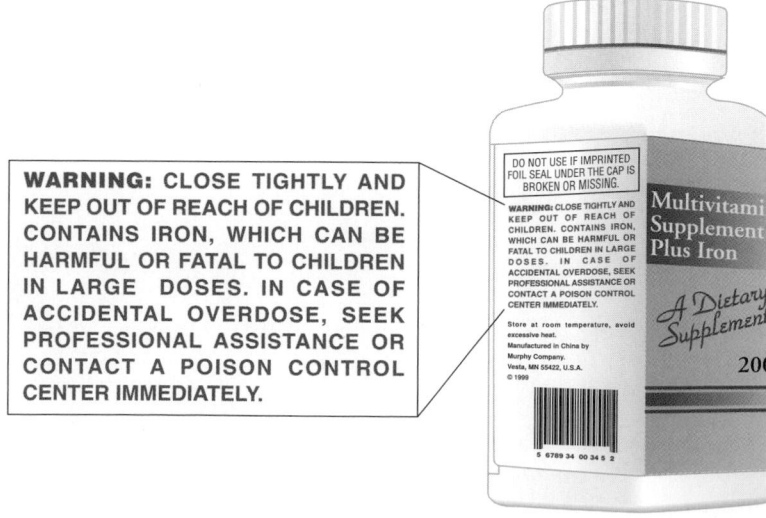

Figure 11.4
Labels on iron-containing supplements and medications must carry a toxicity warning.

Iron is hypothesized to increase the formation of oxidized LDL cholesterol, which then leads to atherosclerosis. Excess iron is suggested to increase cancer incidence by boosting the formation of free radicals, suppressing the activity of the immune system, and promoting cancer cell multiplication. However, there is not sufficient evidence to support a cause-and-effect relationship between iron and heart disease[12] or cancer.[9]

Hemochromatosis The most common cause of chronic iron overload is the genetic disorder **hemochromatosis**, which is a condition that allows increased iron absorption. Hemochromatosis afflicts about 1.5 million Americans. It is the most common inherited disease in Caucasian populations in North America, Australia, and Europe, occurring in about 1 in 300 individuals.[13] Although more frequent in Caucasian populations, it is also seen in African Americans and Hispanics. The accumulation of excess iron that occurs in hemochromatosis causes oxidative changes resulting in heart and liver damage, diabetes, and certain types of cancer. Iron deposits also darken the skin. To have these symptoms, an individual must inherit the hemochromatosis gene from both parents. The one in ten people who inherit the gene from only a single parent don't have these serious symptoms but do absorb iron better than people who do not have the gene at all.

The public health impact of hemochromatosis is potentially significant. The availability of red meat and the prevalence of iron-fortified foods in the American diet virtually assures that individuals with two genes for hemochromatosis will eventually accumulate damaging levels of iron. If individuals with hemochromatosis can be identified, treatment is simple: regular blood withdrawal. This will prevent the complications of iron overload, but to be effective it must be initiated before organs are damaged. Therefore, genetic screening to identify and treat young healthy individuals is essential in preventing complications.[14]

Hemochromatosis An inherited condition that results in increased iron absorption.

Meeting Iron Needs: Consider the Total Diet

To meet iron needs, both the amount and the bioavailability of iron from the diet should be considered. The best sources of iron are red meats and organ meats such as liver and kidney. Good vegetable sources are leafy greens such as spinach and kale, although the nonheme iron in plants is less well absorbed than the heme iron in animal sources (Figure 11.5). Iron absorption can be enhanced by including meat, fish, poultry, and foods rich in vitamin C in meals containing iron, while decreasing the consumption of dairy products, which are high in calcium, at these meals.[5]

Because iron is a nutrient at risk for deficiency in the American diet, the iron content of packaged foods must be listed on food labels. It is given as a percent of the Daily Value for iron, which is 18 mg for adults. Therefore, if your breakfast cereal provides 10% of the Daily Value for iron, it contains about 1.8 mg of iron per serving.

Although diet is the ideal way to meet iron needs, supplements are often recommended for groups at risk for deficiency such as small children, women of childbearing age, and pregnant women. Iron is commonly available as an individual supplement or as part of multivitamin and mineral supplements. These contain nonheme iron. As with nonheme iron in the diet, to enhance the absorption of iron in a supplement, it should be consumed with foods containing vitamin C, such as orange juice; taken with a meal containing meat, fish, or poultry; and not taken with dairy products or substances that bind iron. Iron from supplements that contain the ferrous form (Fe^{2+}) of iron, such as ferrous sulfate, is more readily absorbed than iron from those with the ferric form (Fe^{3+}). Iron supplements should not be taken at the same meal as calcium supplements. Large intakes of iron from supplements can interfere with the absorption of zinc and copper (Table 11.2). Iron-containing supplements should be taken only as suggested on the label and stored out of the reach of children or others who may consume them in excess.

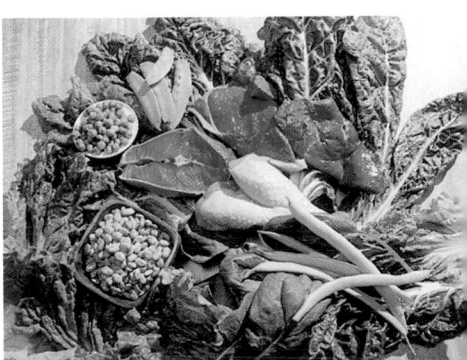

Figure 11.5
Iron in our diets comes from both animal and plant sources. (© Tony Freeman/PhotoEdit)

Table 11.2 *A Summary of the Trace Elements*

Mineral	Sources	Recommended Intake for Young Adults*†	Major Functions	Deficiency Diseases and Symptoms	Groups at Risk	Toxicity	Tolerable Upper Intake Levels (UL)†
Iron	Red meats, leafy greens, dried fruits, whole and enriched grains	8–18 mg	Part of hemoglobin, which delivers oxygen to cells, myoglobin, which binds oxygen in muscle, and electron carriers in the electron transport chain	Iron deficiency anemia, weakness, lethargy	Infants and preschool children, adolescents, women of childbearing age, pregnant women, athletes	Liver damage	45 mg
Zinc	Meat, seafood, milk, whole grains, eggs	8–11 mg	Regulates protein synthesis; functions in growth, development, wound healing, immunity, and superoxide dismutase SOD	Poor growth and development, dermatitis, decreased immune function	Vegetarians, low-income children, elderly	Decreased copper absorption	40 mg
Copper	Organ meats, nuts and seeds, whole grains, seafood	900 μg	Functions in proteins in iron and lipid metabolism, (SOD), nerve and immune function, collagen synthesis	Anemia, poor growth, bone abnormalities	Those who over-supplement zinc	Vomiting	10 mg
Manganese	Nuts, legumes, whole grains, tea	1.8–2.3 mg°	Functions in carbohydrate and lipid metabolism, SOD	Growth retardation	None	Nerve damage	11 mg
Selenium	Organ meats, eggs, and seafood	55 μg	Antioxidant as part of glutathione peroxidase, spares vitamin E, synthesis of thyroid hormones	Muscle pain and weakness, Keshan disease	Populations in areas with low-selenium soil	Nausea, diarrhea, vomiting, fatigue, hair changes	400 μg
Iodine	Iodized salt, saltwater fish, and seafood	150 μg	Needed for synthesis of thyroid hormones	Goiter, cretinism, mental retardation, growth and developmental abnormalities	Populations living where soil is iodine deficient and iodized salt is not used	Enlarged thyroid	1110 μg
Chromium	Liver, brewer's yeast, nuts, grains	25–35 μg°	Glucose tolerance	Impaired glucose metabolism	Malnourished children	None reported	ND
Fluoride	Fluoridated water, tea, fish, toothpaste	3–4 mg°	Strengthens tooth enamel, enhances remineralization of tooth enamel, reduces bacterial acid production	Increased risk of dental caries	Populations in areas with unfluoridated water	Mottled teeth, kidney damage, abnormal bones	10 mg
Molybdenum	Milk, organ meats, grains, legumes	45 μg	Cofactor for many enzymes	Unknown in humans	None	Arthritis and joint inflammation	2 mg

°Values with an asterisk (°) represent Adequate Intakes (AI). All other values are Recommended Dietary Allowances (RDA).

†Recommended intakes for all age groups and stages of life are given on the inside cover and UL values are in Appendix G.

ND = Insufficient evidence to determine a UL.

CRITICAL THINKING

Increasing Iron Intake

Odelia is a twenty-three-year-old college sophomore. She has been feeling tired and run down all semester. She recently read an article about iron deficiency in young women and became concerned about her iron status. She decides to go to the health center where she has blood drawn. Her lab values, shown in Figure 11.3, indicate that she has iron deficiency anemia.

A review of her typical diet shows that Odelia's iron intake is less than the recommended amount. She decides to try to increase the amount of iron she gets from her diet before considering iron supplements. Odelia is originally from Ghana. She enjoys many native foods and consumes a primarily vegetarian diet. At home in Ghana her mother prepared meals in iron cookware. Since moving to the United States, Odelia has used stainless steel cookware, and she believes that this may have contributed to her anemia.

Typical Diet

Food	Amount	Iron (mg)
Breakfast		
Grits with	1 cup	0.5
butter	1 tsp	0
Plantain	1	0.9
Whole wheat toast	1 slice	1.2
Apple juice	3/4 cup	0.7
Tea with	1 cup	0
sugar	1 tsp	0
Lunch		
Apple	1 medium	0.2
Cornbread with	1 piece	1.5
butter	1 tsp	0
Yogurt	1 cup	0.2
Tomato	1 medium	0.5
Tea with	1 cup	0
sugar	1 tsp	0
Dinner		
Rice	1 cup	2.4
Peanuts	1/3 cup	0.9
Kale	1 cup	1.2
Yams	1 cup	1.1
Apple juice	3/4 cup	0.7
Tea with	1 cup	0
sugar	1 tsp	0
Total		**12.0**

What dietary factors could contribute to Odelia's poor iron status?

▼

1. The RDA for a young female vegetarian is _____.
Her total iron intake is marginal at 12 mg per day .

2. The iron in her diet comes from plant sources. This might contribute to her deficiency because _____.

3. The diet is low in vitamin C-rich foods. This may contribute to her deficiency because _____.

4. The switch to stainless steel cookware may have reduced her iron intake because _____.

How could Odelia's breakfast and lunch be modified to increase her iron intake?
▼

Odelia is a vegetarian, so her iron sources are limited to plant foods, which are generally lower in iron and contain only the less-well-absorbed nonheme form of iron. There are, however, good plant sources of naturally occurring iron as well as sources fortified with iron. For instance, switching from the half cup of grits, containing about 0.5 mg of iron, to a fortified cereal will greatly increase her intake. Adding 2 tablespoons of raisins to the hot cereal contributes another 0.4 mg. Another good vegetarian source of iron is beans. A bowl of chili with beans at lunch will add 8 mg of iron.

What modifications could Odelia make to increase the iron content of her dinner?
▼

Answer:

Does Odelia's diet meet the recommendations of the Food Guide Pyramid for vegetarians? Are there other nutrient deficiencies for which she may be at risk?
▼

Answer:

• ZINC (ZN)

The essentiality of zinc in the human diet was first recognized about 30 years ago, when a syndrome of growth depression and delayed sexual development, seen in Iranian and Egyptian men consuming diets based on vegetable protein, was alleviated by supplemental zinc.[15] Although the diet was not low in zinc, it was high in grains containing phytates, which interfered with zinc absorption, causing a deficiency.

Zinc in the Diet

Zinc is found in foods from both plant and animal sources. Zinc from animal sources is better absorbed than that from plants, because the zinc in plant foods is often bound by phytates. Zinc is abundant in red meat, liver, eggs, dairy products, vegetables, and some seafood (Figure 11.6). Whole grains are a good source, but refined grains are not because zinc is lost in milling and not added back in enrichment. Grain products leavened with yeast provide more zinc than unleavened products because the yeast leavening of breads reduces the phytate content.[16]

Zinc in the Gastrointestinal Tract

The amount of zinc in the body is regulated in part by the amount that is absorbed. Zinc entering the mucosal cells of the intestine may be used by the mucosal cell itself,

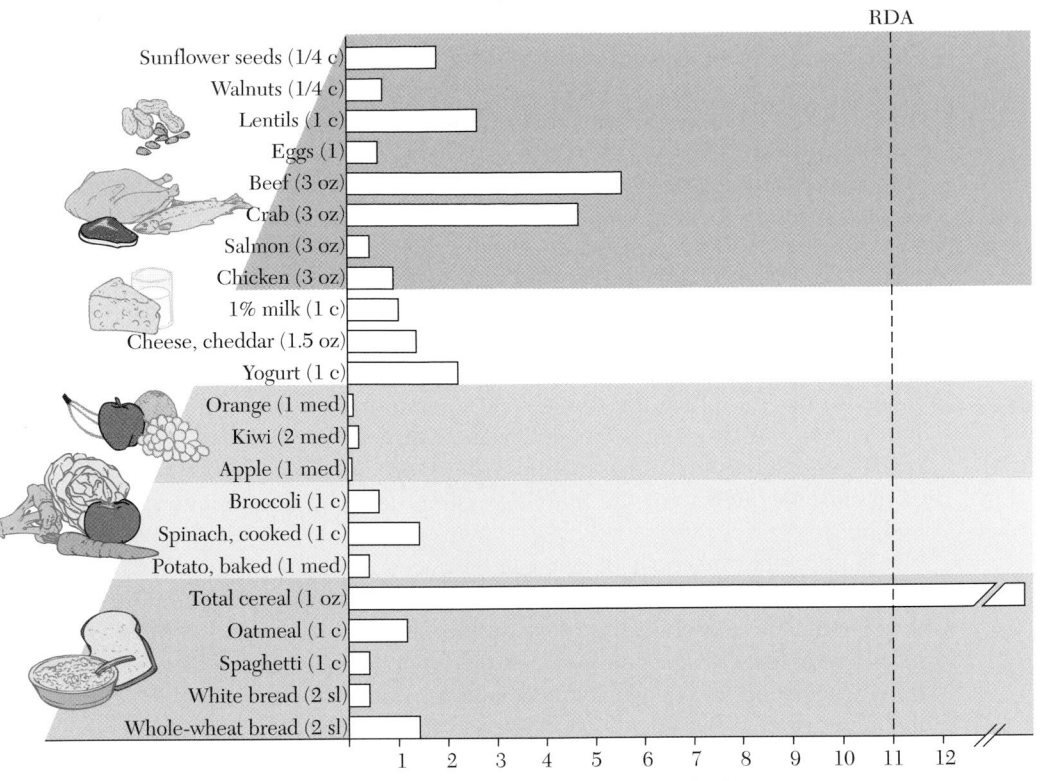

Figure 11.6
Zinc content of selections from each group of the Food Guide Pyramid. The dashed line represents the RDA for adult men. Meat, seafood, and dairy products as well as fortified foods are good sources of zinc.

pass through the cell into the blood, or be bound by the protein metallothionein, which helps regulate the amount of zinc that reaches body tissues. Zinc in the mucosal cell stimulates the synthesis of **metallothionein**, and when zinc intake is high more metallothionein is made. Zinc bound to metallothionein is not easily transported out of the muscosal cell and is lost when the cells die (Figure 11.7). Conversely, when zinc intake is low, metallothionein synthesis is not stimulated, so concentrations drop and zinc is readily transferred from the mucosal cells to the blood. Since metallothionein does not completely prevent zinc transfer, high intakes can override this regulatory mechanism.

Metallothionein A protein that binds zinc and copper in intestinal cells and limits their absorption into the blood.

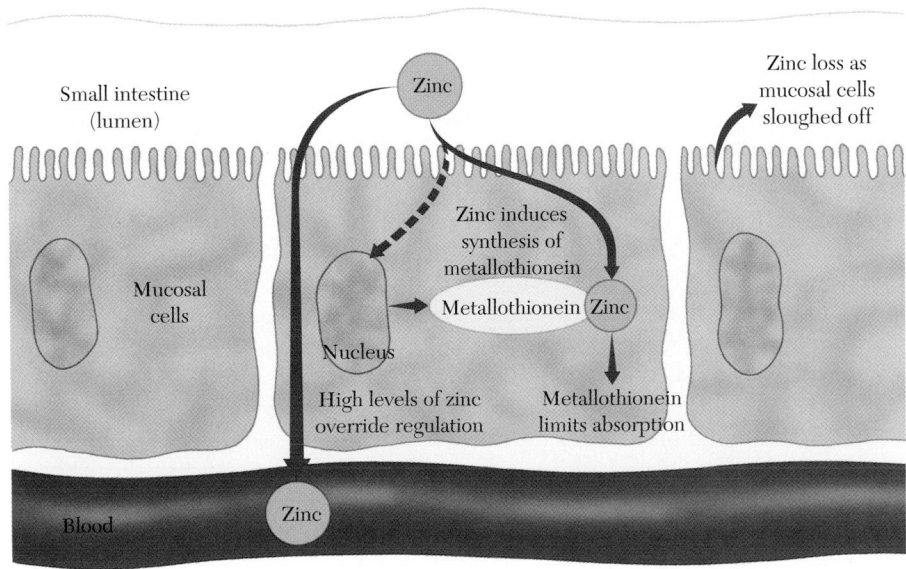

Figure 11.7
Zinc absorption is regulated by the protein metallothionein in intestinal mucosal cells.

Zinc in the Body

Once zinc has been absorbed, homeostasis can be maintained to some extent by regulating excretion. Zinc is secreted in pancreatic and intestinal juices, which enter the lumen of the intestine. When zinc levels are low, the zinc that enters the gastrointestinal tract can be reabsorbed and recycled. When levels are high, it is not reabsorbed and is therefore eliminated in the feces.

Zinc is the most abundant intracellular trace element. It is found in the cytosol, in cellular organelles, and in the nucleus. Zinc is involved in the functioning of nearly 100 different enzymes, including a form of **superoxide dismutase (SOD)**, which is vital for protecting cells from free radical damage. Zinc is also needed by enzymes that function in the synthesis of DNA and RNA, in carbohydrate metabolism, in acid-base balance, and in a reaction that is necessary for folate absorption. Zinc also plays a role in the storage and release of insulin, the mobilization of vitamin A from the liver, and the stabilization of cell membranes. It influences hormonal regulation of cell division and is therefore needed for the growth and repair of tissues, the activity of the immune system, and the development of sex organs and bone.

Some of the functions of zinc can be traced to its role in gene expression. For example, zinc stimulates the production of metallothionein by binding to a regulatory factor and activating the transcription of the gene for this protein. Zinc also plays a structural role in proteins essential for gene expression. Zinc-containing proteins are needed for the activity of vitamin A, vitamin D, and a number of hormones including thyroid hormones, estrogen, and testosterone. Without zinc, these nutrients and hormones cannot bind to DNA to increase or decrease gene expression and, hence, the synthesis of certain proteins.

Superoxide dismutase (SOD) An enzyme that protects the cell from oxidative damage by neutralizing superoxide free radicals. One form of the enzyme requires zinc and copper for activity, and another form requires manganese.

How Much Zinc Do We Need?

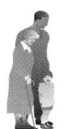

The RDA for zinc is 11 mg per day for adult men and 8 mg per day for adult women.[6] This is based on the amount of zinc needed to replace daily losses from the body.

During pregnancy, the recommendation for zinc is increased to account for the zinc that accumulates in maternal and fetal tissues. During lactation, the RDA is increased to compensate for zinc secreted in breast milk. For infants from newborn to six months of age, an AI has been established based on the zinc intake of breast-fed infants. RDAs have been established for older infants, children, and adolescents based on the amount of zinc lost from the body, the amount needed for growth, and the absorption of zinc from the diet. Although the RDA for older adults is the same as that for younger adults, the elderly population may be at risk for zinc deficiency because of low intakes.

Zinc Deficiency

The symptoms of zinc deficiency, which include poor growth and development, skin rashes, and impaired immune function, reflect its importance in protein synthesis and gene expression. Because it is needed for the proper functioning of vitamins A and D and the activity of numerous enzymes, deficiency symptoms can resemble deficiencies of other essential nutrients.

One of the main concerns with even moderate zinc deficiency is altered immune defenses. The impact of zinc deficiency on immune function is rapid and extensive, causing a decrease in the number and function of immune cells in the blood. The drop in immune function can lead to an increased incidence of infections.

Zinc deficiency has been seen in individuals with a genetic defect in zinc absorption and metabolism called acrodermatitis enteropathica, in those fed TPN solutions lacking zinc, and in those consuming low-protein, high-phytate diets. It may also occur in a number of disease states including kidney disease, sickle cell anemia, alcoholism, cancer, and AIDS.

The risk of zinc deficiency is greater in areas of the world where the diet is high in phytate, fiber, tannins, and oxalates, especially in the elderly, low-income children,

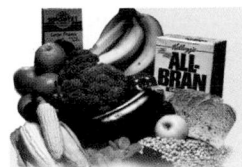

Off the Shelf

Will Zinc Cure the Common Cold?

Despite advances in modern medical science, the common cold remains as common as ever. Adults in the United States develop two to four colds per year, and children get six to eight.[1] Colds make you feel miserable and decrease productivity—and are responsible for 15 million sick days each year.

It is likely that man has been trying to cure the common cold for as long as viruses have been causing coughs and sneezes. Your great grandmother may have had little to offer but a bowl of chicken soup, or maybe some honey with lemon, for your cough. Today there are a multitude of over-the-counter medications to relieve symptoms. They will lower your fever, clear your nose, and suppress your cough, but they won't make your cold go away. Since folk remedies and pharmaceuticals are unable to cure the common cold and people are unwilling to take time out of their busy lifestyles to rest and drink plenty of fluids, many have turned to dietary supplements that promise to make colds go away. Vitamin C has been promoted as a cold cure for many years. And although it can't cure a cold, there is some evidence that it reduces a cold's duration and symptoms (see Chapter 8).

A more recent addition to the list of cold remedies is the zinc lozenge, which promises to reduce the duration and severity of the common cold. It has been suggested that zinc in lozenge form works when it comes in contact with the mucous membranes in the throat.[1] The zinc in a mineral supplement will not have any effect because this zinc goes to your stomach and doesn't contact the mucosal surfaces affected by cold viruses. The results of double-blind placebo-controlled clinical trials that have been completed to assess the efficacy of zinc lozenges have been inconsistent. When zinc gluconate and zinc acetate lozenges were compared to a placebo in individuals with natural colds and those with experimental colds, zinc was found to have little effect on the duration or severity of the colds.[2] A review of seven studies found only two that suggested zinc lozenges reduced the severity and duration of cold symptoms.[3] In addition, a recent meta analysis (a method that combines data from all available trials) found that the evidence for the effectiveness of zinc lozenges in reducing the duration of the common cold is still lacking.[4]

Should you take zinc lozenges? The evidence supporting their benefits is weak, but anything that shows promise in making the sniffles go away faster is irresistible to many. If you try zinc lozenges, try cautiously. Too much zinc can suppress the immune system, lower HDL cholesterol levels, and impair copper absorption. Zinc lozenges each contain about 11 to 14 mg of elemental zinc. Taking four of these in a day will exceed the UL of 40 mg per day.

[1]Novick, S. G., Godfrey, J. C., Pollack, R. L., and Wilder, H. R. Zinc-induced suppression of inflammation in the respiratory tract caused by infection with human rhinovirus and other irritants. *Med. Hypotheses* 49:347–357, 1997.

[2]Turner, R. B., and Cetnarowski, W. E. Effect of treatment with zinc gluconate or zinc acetate on experimental and natural colds. *Clin. Infect. Dis.* 31:1202–1208, 2000.

[3]Marshall, I. Zinc for the common cold, Cochrane Database Syst. Rev:CD001364, 2000.

[4]Jackson, J. L., Lesho, E., and Peterson, C. Zinc and the common cold: A meta-analysis revisited. *J. Nutr.* 130(Suppl):1512S–1515S, 2000.

and vegetarians—particularly female vegans. Groups likely to be at risk of deficiency in the United States include children from 1 to 3 years of age, adolescent females, and adults 71 years of age and older.[17] Symptomatic zinc deficiency is relatively uncommon in North America, but in developing countries it has important health and developmental consequences. Supplements have been shown to reduce the incidence of diarrhea and infections in children in developing nations.[18]

Zinc Toxicity and Supplements

Zinc can be toxic when consumed in excess of recommendations. A single dose of 1 to 2 g can cause gastrointestinal irritation, vomiting, loss of appetite, diarrhea, abdominal cramps, and headaches. This has occurred with consumption of foods and beverages contaminated with zinc that has leached from galvanized containers. Intakes in the range of 50 to 300 mg per day have been shown to decrease rather than enhance immune function and to reduce HDL cholesterol, the type of cholesterol that has a protective effect against heart disease.[19] Supplements providing 50 mg per day of zinc have been shown to interfere with the absorption of copper.[20] When high zinc intake inhibits copper absorption, it leads to a reduction in the activity of the copper-dependent enzyme copper-zinc superoxide dismutase in red blood cells. A UL has been set at 40 mg per day from all sources based on the adverse effect of excess zinc on copper metabolism.

Zinc is often marketed as a supplement to improve immune function, enhance fertility and sexual performance, and cure the common cold (see *Off the Shelf*: Will

Zinc Cure the Common Cold?). For individuals consuming adequate zinc, there is no evidence that extra is beneficial. In individuals with a mild zinc deficiency, supplementation may result in improved wound healing, immunity, and appetite; in children it can result in improved growth and learning. In healthy older adults, supplements of zinc have been shown to improve the immune response (see Chapter 16).[21] Over-supplementation may result in toxicity and can also contribute to copper deficiency.

• COPPER (CU)

The ability of copper to treat certain types of anemia helped establish the essentiality of copper in human nutrition.[22] Further understanding of the impact of copper deficiency in humans came from studying individuals who were inadvertently fed intravenous (TPN) solutions deficient in copper and those with a rare genetic disease in which there is a defect in copper utilization.

Copper in the Diet

The richest dietary sources of copper are organ meats such as liver and kidney. Seafood, nuts and seeds, whole grain breads and cereals, and chocolate are also good sources (Figure 11.8). As with many other trace elements, soil content affects the amount of copper in plant foods.

Copper in the Gastrointestinal Tract

About 30 to 40% of the copper in a typical diet is absorbed.[23] The absorption of copper is affected by the presence of other minerals and vitamins in the diet. The zinc content of the diet can have a major impact on copper absorption. When zinc intake is high, it stimulates the synthesis of the protein metallothionein in the mucosal cells. Metallothionein helps regulate zinc absorption; however, metallothionein preferentially binds copper rather than zinc. Therefore, when metallothionein is synthesized, it binds copper, preventing it from being moved out of mucosal cells into the blood.[20] The antagonism between copper and zinc is so great that phytates, which inhibit zinc absorption, actually increase the absorption and utilization of copper. Copper absorption is also reduced by high intakes of iron, manganese, and molybdenum. Other factors that affect copper absorption include vitamin C and large doses of antacids, which inhibit copper absorption and, over the long term, can cause copper deficiency.

Copper in the Body

Once absorbed, copper binds to albumin, a protein in the blood, and travels to the liver, where it binds to the protein ceruloplasmin for delivery to other tissues. Copper can be removed from the body by secretion in the bile and subsequent elimination in the feces.

Copper functions in a number of important proteins and enzymes that are involved in iron and lipid metabolism, connective tissue synthesis, maintenance of heart muscle, and function of the immune and central nervous systems.[6] The copper-containing protein ceruloplasmin converts iron into a form that can bind to transferrin for transport. Copper is also an essential component of a form of the antioxidant enzyme superoxide dismutase (SOD). Copper plays a role in cholesterol and glucose metabolism, and elevated blood cholesterol levels have been reported in copper deficiency. It is also needed for the synthesis of the neurotransmitters norepinephrine and dopamine, and several blood-clotting factors. It may be involved in the synthesis of myelin, which is necessary for transmission of nerve signals.

How Much Copper Do We Need?

The RDA for copper for adults is 900 μg per day. This recommendation is based on the amount of copper needed to maintain normal blood levels of copper and cerulo-

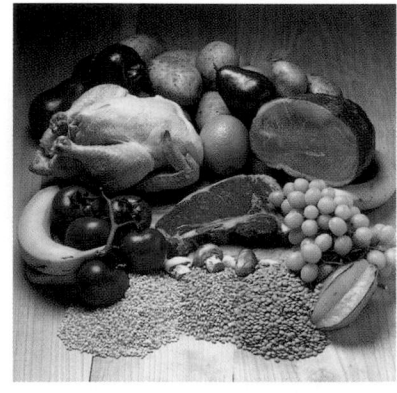

Figure 11.8
These foods are good sources of copper. (Charles D. Winters)

plasmin. During pregnancy, the RDA is increased to 1000 μg per day. The RDA for lactation is 1300 μg per day. The amount of copper in the North American diet is slightly above the RDA.

Copper Deficiency

Severe copper deficiency is relatively rare, occurring most often in preterm infants. Marginal copper deficiency may be more prevalent but has been difficult to diagnose.[24] The most common manifestation of copper deficiency is anemia. This is due primarily to the fact that the copper-containing protein ceruloplasmin is needed for iron transport. In copper deficiency, even if iron is sufficient in the diet, iron cannot be transported out of the intestinal mucosa. Copper deficiency causes skeletal abnormalities similar to those seen in vitamin C deficiency. This is because the enzyme needed for the cross-linking of connective tissue requires copper.[25] Copper deficiency has also been associated with impaired growth, degeneration of the heart muscle, degeneration of the nervous system, and changes in hair color and structure. Because of copper's role in the development and maintenance of the immune system, a diet low in copper decreases the immune response and increases the incidence of infection.[26]

Copper Toxicity

Copper toxicity from dietary sources is extremely rare but has occurred as a result of drinking from contaminated water supplies or consuming acidic foods or beverages stored in copper containers. Excessive copper intake causes abdominal pain, vomiting, and diarrhea. These effects may occur with copper intakes of 4.8 mg per day in some individuals, but there is evidence that people can adapt to higher exposures without experiencing symptoms. High doses of copper have also been shown to cause liver damage. The UL has been set at 10 mg of copper per day. This is consistent with the safe upper level of intake of 10 mg/day in women and 12 mg/day in men proposed by the World Health Organization.[27]

• MANGANESE (MN)

The best dietary sources of manganese are whole grains and nuts (Figure 11.9). Fruits and vegetables are fair sources; meat, dairy products and refined grains are poor sources.

Manganese homeostasis is maintained by regulating both absorption and excretion. Manganese absorption increases when intake is low and decreases when intake is high. Manganese is eliminated by secretion into the intestinal tract in bile. It is a constituent of some enzymes and an activator of others. Manganese-requiring enzymes are involved in amino acid, carbohydrate, and cholesterol metabolism; cartilage formation; urea synthesis; and antioxidant protection as a component of SOD.

How Much Manganese Do We Need?

There was not sufficient evidence to set an RDA for manganese; the AI is 2.3 mg/day for men and 1.8 mg/day for women based on the amounts consumed in the healthy population. Recommended intakes are higher during pregnancy and lactation.[6]

Manganese and Health

Manganese deficiency in animals results in growth retardation, reproductive problems, congenital malformations in the offspring, and abnormalities in brain function, bone formation, glucose regulation, and lipid metabolism.

Although a naturally occurring manganese deficiency has never been reported in humans, a man participating in a study of vitamin K was inadvertently fed a diet deficient in manganese for six months. He lost weight, his black hair turned a red color, and he developed dermatitis and low blood cholesterol. Manganese deficiency

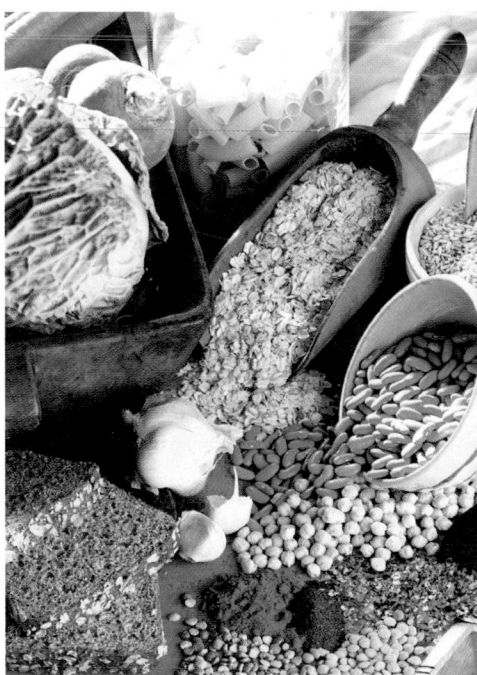

Figure 11.9

Legumes, nuts, and whole grains are high in manganese. (Rita Maas/The Image Bank)

was further studied in young male volunteers fed a manganese-deficient diet for 39 days. These men developed dermatitis and had altered blood levels of cholesterol, calcium, and phosphorus.[28]

Toxic levels of manganese result in damage to the nervous system. In humans, toxicity has been reported in manganese mine workers exposed to high concentrations of inhaled manganese dust. The UL is 11 mg per day from all sources.

• SELENIUM (SE)

Although selenium was discovered about 180 years ago, its essential role in human nutrition was not recognized until the 1970s. Selenium is necessary for the activity of an important antioxidant enzyme.

Selenium in the Diet

Seafood, kidney, liver, and eggs are excellent sources of selenium (Figure 11.10). Fruits, vegetables, and drinking water are generally poor sources. Grains and seeds can be good sources depending on the selenium content of the soil where they were grown. For example, wheat grown in Kansas has a different selenium content from wheat grown in Michigan. Soil selenium content can have a significant impact on the selenium intake of populations consuming primarily locally grown food.

Selenium in the Body

Glutathione peroxidase A selenium-containing enzyme that protects cells from oxidative damage by neutralizing peroxides.

Once selenium is absorbed, homeostasis is maintained by regulating its excretion in the urine. Selenium is an essential part of the enzyme **glutathione peroxidase**. Glutathione peroxidase neutralizes peroxides so they no longer form free radicals, which cause oxidative damage. By reducing free radical formation, selenium can spare some

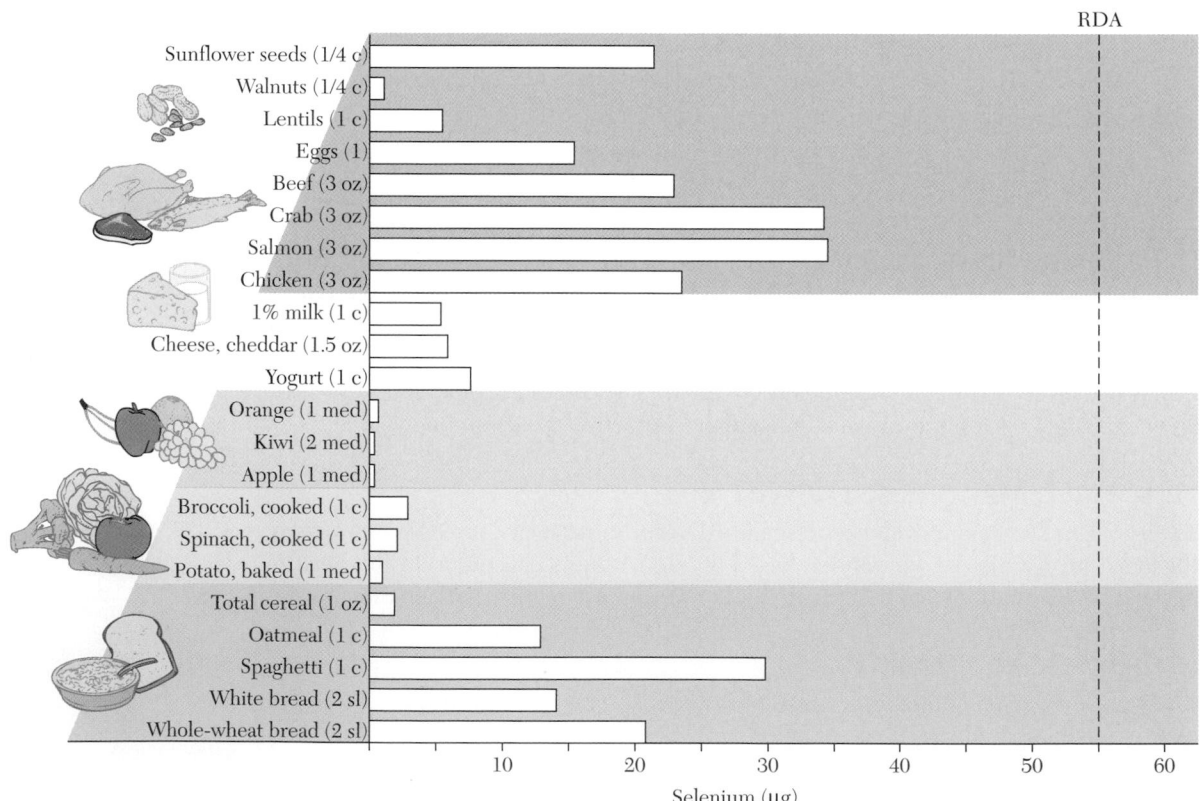

Figure 11.10

Selenium content of selections from each group of the Food Guide Pyramid. The dashed line represents the RDA for adults. Both plant and animal foods are good sources of selenium.

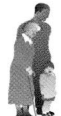

of the requirement for vitamin E, because vitamin E is used to stop the action of free radicals once they are produced (Figure 11.11). Selenium is also needed for the synthesis of the thyroid hormones, which regulate basal metabolic rate.

How Much Selenium Do We Need?

The RDA for selenium for adults is 55 μg per day. This is based on the amount needed to maximize the activity of the enzyme glutathione peroxidase in the blood. The estimated average intake of selenium in the United States meets or nearly meets this recommendation for all age groups.

An increase in selenium intake is recommended during pregnancy and lactation. The AI for infants is based on the amount contained in breast milk.

Selenium Deficiency

Symptoms of selenium deficiency include muscular discomfort and weakness. A form of heart disease called Keshan disease may also occur with selenium deficiency. Selenium supplements relieve most of the symptoms of Keshan disease and reduce its incidence, but selenium deficiency is not the only cause of this disease. It is hypothesized to be due to several interacting factors which include selenium deficiency, other nutritional factors, and an infectious agent.[29] Selenium deficiency is not likely to be a problem when the diet includes foods grown in many different locations.

Selenium and Cancer

Observations of an increased incidence of certain human cancers in regions where selenium intake is low as well as animal studies demonstrating that a high selenium intake reduces the incidence of cancer led to the hypothesis that selenium protects against cancer. Interest in the role of selenium in cancer prevention intensified when an intervention trial that provided supplements of 200 μg per day to skin cancer patients found that, although skin cancer recurrence was not reduced, total cancer incidence, cancer mortality, and cases of lung, prostate, and colon cancer all decreased in the selenium-supplemented group.[30] The mechanism of cancer protection is believed to be selenium's ability to turn on the self-destruct mechanism in cancer cells and therefore eliminate cancers before they spread.[31]

Selenium Toxicity and Supplements

In a region of China with very high selenium in the soil, an intake of 5 mg per day resulted in fingernail changes and hair loss. Selenium toxicity has also been reported in the United States because of a manufacturing error that created mineral supplements containing a dose of 27 mg of selenium per day. The individuals who used these supplements had symptoms which included nausea, diarrhea, abdominal pain, fingernail and hair changes, nervous system abnormalities, fatigue, and irritability.[28] Adverse effects such as hair and fingernail loss and gastrointestinal upset have been reported at much lower levels. The UL for adults is 400 μg/day from diet and supplements.

Selenium supplements are marketed with claims that they will protect against environmental pollutants, prevent cancer and heart disease, slow the aging process, and improve immune function. Although selenium does play a role in these processes, supplements of selenium have not been shown to be of additional benefit in the general population.

• IODINE (I)

Iodine is needed for the synthesis of thyroid hormones. In the early 1900s, iodine deficiency was common in the central United States and Canada, but it has virtually disappeared due to the addition of iodine to table salt. Iodine deficiency, however, remains a world health problem.

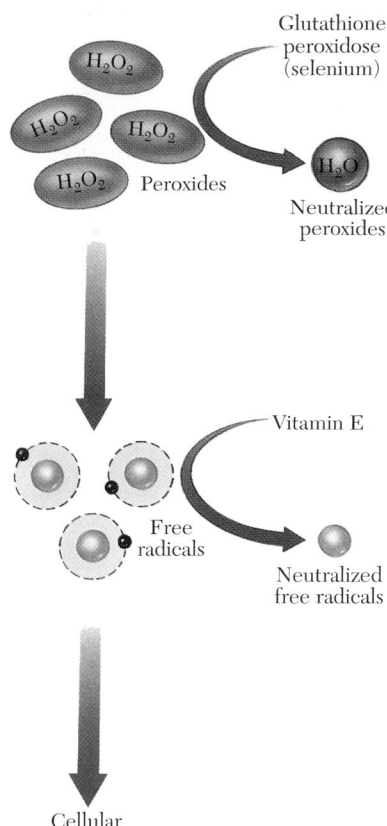

Figure 11.11

Selenium is a part of the enzyme glutathione peroxidase, which neutralizes peroxides before they form free radicals. This can spare some of the need for vitamin E.

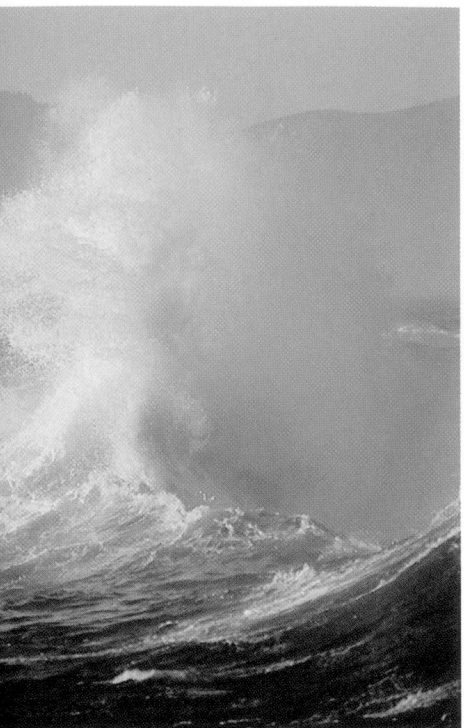

Figure 11.12

Most of the iodine in our diet comes from the sea. (© Darrell Gulin/Stone)

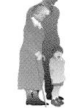

Goiter An enlargement of the thyroid gland caused by a deficiency of iodine.

Iodine in the Diet

Most of the iodine in our diets comes from the sea. There are high concentrations of iodine in seawater and seafood (Figure 11.12). Plants grown close to the sea are high in iodine. The amount of iodine in plants grown inland depends on the iodine content of the soil.

Iodine in our diet also comes from contaminants and additives in foods. Dairy products may contain iodine because of the iodine-containing additives used in cattle feed and the use of iodine-containing disinfectants on cows, milking machines, and storage tanks. Iodine-containing sterilizing agents are also used in fast-food restaurants, and iodine is used in dough conditioners and some food colorings. Most of the iodine in the North American diet comes from salt fortified with iodine, referred to as iodized salt. It is commonplace in the United States, and only iodized salt is sold in Canada. Iodized salt should not be confused with sea salt, which is a poor source of iodine because the iodine is lost in the drying process.

Iodine in the Body

Iodine is an essential component of the thyroid hormones and, along with selenium, is essential for the synthesis of thyroid hormones. Thyroid hormones regulate basal metabolic rate, growth and development, and promote protein synthesis. If blood levels of the thyroid hormones drop, thyroid-stimulating hormone is released. This hormone signals the thyroid gland in the neck to take up iodine and synthesize thyroid hormones. When the supply of iodine is adequate, thyroid hormones can be made and their presence turns off the synthesis of thyroid-stimulating hormone (Figure 11.13).

How Much Iodine Do We Need?

The RDA for iodine in adult men and women is 150 μg per day. This is based on the amount needed to maintain normal iodine levels in the thyroid gland. Since the iodinization of salt, the intake of iodine in North America has met or exceeded the RDA.

Iodine needs are increased during pregnancy and lactation. The recommended intake for infants is based on the amount obtained from breast milk.

Iodine Deficiency

Iodine deficiency reduces the production of thyroid hormones. Metabolic rate slows with insufficient thyroid hormones, causing fatigue and weight gain. The most obvious outward sign of deficiency is an enlarged thyroid gland called a **goiter** (Figure

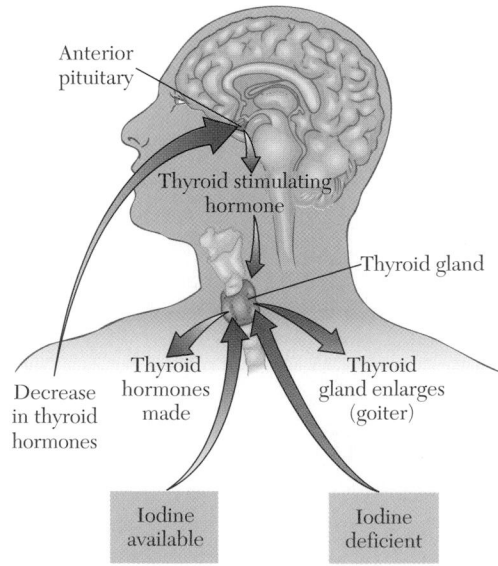

Figure 11.13

When thyroid hormone levels drop too low, thyroid-stimulating hormone stimulates the thyroid gland to take up iodine and synthesize more hormones. If iodine is not available, the stimulation continues and the thyroid enlarges, forming a goiter.

11.14). A goiter forms when reduced thyroid hormone levels cause thyroid-stimulating hormone to be released, stimulating the thyroid gland to make more thyroid hormones. Because iodine is unavailable, the hormones cannot be made and the stimulation continues causing the thyroid gland to enlarge. In milder cases of goiter, treatment with iodine causes the thyroid gland to return to normal size, but this result is not consistent in more severe cases.

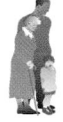

A number of other iodine deficiency disorders occur because of the effect of iodine on growth and development. If iodine is deficient during pregnancy, it increases the risk of stillbirth and spontaneous abortion. Deficiency also can cause a condition called **cretinism** in the offspring. Cretinism is characterized by symptoms such as mental retardation, deaf mutism, and growth failure. Iodine deficiency during childhood and adolescence can also result in goiter and impaired mental function.

The risk of iodine deficiency is increased by consuming **goitrogens**, substances in food that interfere with the utilization of iodine or with thyroid function. Goitrogens are found in turnips, rutabaga, cabbage, and cassava. Most are destroyed in cooking or are present in foods that do not play an important role in human diets. However, in African countries where cassava is a dietary staple, high goitrogen intake may play a role in the development of iodine deficiency disorders.[32]

Iodine Fortification

Since it was first used in Switzerland in the 1920s, iodized salt has been the major means of combating iodine deficiency (see *Off the Label*: Should You Choose Iodized Salt?). Because of the fortification of table salt with iodine, cretinism and goiter are now rare in North America, but worldwide, 600 million people have goiter and 1.5 billion people are at risk for iodine deficiency.[33] At the recommendation of the United Nations Joint Committee on Health Policy, salt iodinization is now being applied in most countries with an iodine deficiency disease problem of public health significance.[34] For groups who do not have access to iodized salt or who will not use it, other forms of iodine supplementation, such as injections or oral doses of iodized oil, may be effective for control of iodine deficiency.[35]

Iodine Toxicity

Acute toxicity can occur with very large doses of iodine. Intakes between 200 and 500 μg per kilogram of body weight have caused death in laboratory animals.[28] Chronically high intakes of iodine can cause an enlargement of the thyroid gland that resembles goiter. The UL for adults is 1100 μg of iodine per day from all sources. Goiter from excessive iodine can also occur if iodine intake changes drastically. For example, in a population with a marginal intake, a large increase in intake due to supplementation can cause thyroid enlargement even at levels that would not be toxic in a healthy population.

• CHROMIUM (CR)

Chromium is essential for insulin to function normally. Currently it is recognized by many as the popular supplement chromium picolinate, promoted to increase lean body mass.

Chromium in the Diet

Dietary sources of chromium include liver, brewer's yeast, nuts, and whole grains. Milk, vegetables, and fruit are poor sources. Refined carbohydrates such as white breads, pasta, and white rice are also poor sources because chromium is lost in milling and not added back in the enrichment process. Chromium intake can be increased by cooking in stainless steel cookware because chromium leaches from the steel into the food.

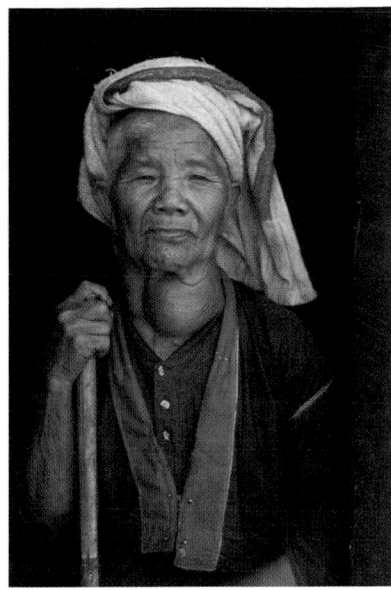

Figure 11.14
Iodine deficiency causes enlargement of the thyroid gland, a condition called goiter. (© Alison Wright/Corbis)

Cretinism A condition resulting from poor maternal iodine intake during pregnancy that causes stunted growth and poor mental development in offspring.

Goitrogens Substances that interfere with the utilization of iodine or the function of the thyroid gland.

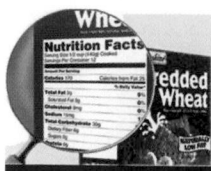

Off the Label
Should You Choose Iodized Salt?

When selecting a box of salt for the kitchen cupboard, you can choose one that just says "salt" or one that is labeled "iodized salt." Iodized salt is salt to which the trace element iodine has been added. Which should you choose?

Iodine is an essential nutrient. The amount we consume in our diet depends as much on where foods are grown as on which foods we choose. Foods produced in regions where the soil is rich in iodine are better sources of iodine than foods produced in regions where the soil is iodine-poor. The iodine content of plants grown in iodine-deficient soil may be 100 times less than those grown in iodine-rich soil.[1] When the earth was formed, all soils were high in iodine, but today iodine is most plentiful in areas close to the sea. Mountainous areas and river valleys have little iodine left in the soil because it has been washed out by glaciers, snow, rain, and flood waters. The iodine washed from the soil has accumulated in the oceans, where it is present as iodide ions. When these ions come in contact with sunlight, they are oxidized to form iodine, which can escape into the air. Every year approximately 400,000 tons of iodine escapes into the atmosphere from the ocean surface. The iodine in the atmosphere is returned to the soil in rain, but the return is slow and the amounts returned to the soil are small. In areas where the forces of nature have resulted in iodine-deficient soil, the iodine deposited from rain will be washed away again by these same forces. Therefore, iodine-deficient soil will remain deficient.

Iodine-depleted soil is not new to the planet's ecology. Its effect on human health has become a part of history in many areas of the world. In Europe the presence of iodine deficiency was recorded by classical art, which portrayed even the wealthy with goiter and cretinism. Leonardo da Vinci is said to have been more knowledgeable about goiter than medical professors of his time.[2] A century ago goiter was endemic in the central regions of North America. And in parts of

Asia today, iodine deficiency is a major public health problem.

In the United States, Switzerland, and some other European countries, iodine deficiency was virtually eliminated in the early part of the 20th century by the iodinization of salt. And today, developing nations, where iodine deficiency is still a public health problem, have experimented with iodized salt[3,4] as well as iodine-fortified fish sauce, sugar, and drinking water as ways to add iodine to the diet.[5,6]

Why fortify salt? Salt was selected as the vehicle for added iodine because it is a food item consistently consumed by the majority of the population at risk. People did not need to change their eating habits to include the fortified product in their diet. The iodine also could be added to salt uniformly, inexpensively, and in a form that was well utilized by the body. It could be added in amounts that would eliminate deficiency when typical quantities of salt were consumed by the population, but would not cause toxicity in those consuming larger amounts of iodized salt or in those who already meet their iodine needs from other sources.

For about 50 years the average intake of iodine in the United States has exceeded the RDA, and iodine deficiency has been rare.[7] The typical diet includes iodine from iodized salt as well as from foods from across the country and around the world. However, recent data from NHANES III has shown a significant reduction in the average American iodine intake. The average intake is still considered sufficient, but the drop has increased the number of people who are at risk of deficiency. There are many factors that may have contributed to the decrease in iodine intake.[8] Egg yolks are rich in iodine, but egg consumption has declined due to concerns about dietary cholesterol intake. The amount of salt added in the home may also have declined due to recommendations regarding blood pressure. And, most of the salt in the American diet comes from processed foods, which contain noniodized salt. There have also been

changes in the amounts of iodine-containing additives and contaminants in foods. The dairy industry has made an effort to reduce the iodine content of milk and the baking industry has replaced some of the iodine-containing dough conditioners with bromine salts, thus reducing the iodine content of commercially manufactured breads. Despite this decrease, most people get plenty of iodine, especially if they live on the coast or buy food in a supermarket. However, for those who eat little seafood, live inland where the soil is deficient in iodine, and consume primarily foods grown locally, choosing salt labeled "iodized" will ensure their iodine needs are met.

[1] Hertzel, B. S., and Clugston, G. A. Iodine. In *Modern Nutrition in Health and Disease*, 9th ed. Shils, M. E., Olson, J. A., Shike, M., and Ross, A. C. Baltimore: Williams & Wilkins, 1999, 253–264.

[2] Underwood, B. A. Micronutrient malnutrition: is it being eliminated? *Nutr. Today* 33:121–129, 1998.

[3] Melse-Boonstra, A., Rozendaal, M., Rexwinkel, H., et al. Determination of discretionary salt intake in rural Guatemala and Benin to determine the iodine fortification of salt required to control iodine deficiency disorders: studies using lithium-labeled salt. *Am. J. Clin. Nutr.* 68:636–641, 1998.

[4] Ranganathan, S., and Reddy, V. Human requirements of iodine and safe use of iodized salt. *Indian J. Med. Res.* 102:227–232, 1995.

[5] Eltom, M., Elnagar, B., Sulieman, E. A., et al. The use of sugar as a vehicle for iodine fortification in endemic iodine deficiency. *Int. J. Food Sci. Nutr.* 46:281–289, 1995.

[6] Saowakhontha, S., Sanchaisuriya, P., Pongpaew, P., et al. Compliance of population groups of iodine fortification in endemic areas of goiter in northeast Thailand. *J. Med. Assoc. Thai.* 77:449–454, 1994.

[7] Hollowell, J. G., Staehling, N. W., Hannon, W. H., et al. Iodine nutrition in the United States. Trends and public health implications: Iodine excretion data from National Health and Nutrition Examination Surveys I and III (1971–1974 and 1988–1994). *J. Clin. Endocrinol. Metab.* 83:3401–3408, 1998.

[8] Lee, K., Bradley, R., Dwyer, J., and Lee, S. L. Too much versus too little: The implications of current iodine intake in the United States. *Nutr. Rev.* 57:177–181, 1999.

Chromium in the Body

When carbohydrate is consumed, insulin is released and binds to receptors in cell membranes. This binding triggers the uptake of glucose by cells, an increase in protein and lipid synthesis, and other effects. Chromium is part of a small peptide that stabilizes the bound insulin and amplifies its effect.[36] When chromium is deficient, it takes more insulin to produce the same effect.

How Much Chromium Do We Need?

Based on the amount of chromium in a balanced diet, an AI has been set at 35 μg/day for men and 25 μg/day for women. The AI is increased during pregnancy and lactation. The AI for older adults is slightly lower because energy intake decreases with age.

Chromium Deficiency

Overt chromium deficiency is not a problem in the U.S. population. Deficiencies have been reported in patients receiving long-term TPN not containing chromium and in malnourished children. Deficiency symptoms include impaired glucose tolerance with diabetes-like symptoms, such as elevated blood glucose levels and increased insulin levels. There is some evidence that chromium deficiency may play a role in the development of type 2 diabetes, but its role is not clear.[37] Chromium deficiency may also cause elevated blood cholesterol and triglyceride levels, but the role of chromium in lipid metabolism is not fully understood.[38]

Chromium Toxicity and Supplements

Despite widespread use of chromium supplements among athletes, no dietary toxicity has been reported in humans. Chromium supplementation of 200 to 1000 μg per day has been shown to have beneficial effects on blood glucose, insulin, and cholesterol levels in individuals with type 2 diabetes.[39] Chromium supplements, particularly as chromium picolinate, are also marketed to reduce body fat and increase lean body tissue (Figure 11.15). This appeals to individuals wanting to lose weight as well as to athletes trying to build muscle. Because chromium is needed for insulin action and insulin promotes protein synthesis, it is likely that adequate chromium is necessary to increase lean body mass. However, most recent studies on the effects of chromium picolinate or other chromium supplements in healthy human subjects have found no beneficial effects on muscle strength, body composition, weight loss, or other aspects of health.[40]

Controlled trials have reported no dietary toxicity in humans.[41] Despite the apparent safety of chromium supplements, a few concerns have been raised. Two cases of renal failure have been associated with chromium picolinate supplements, but both of these individuals were taking other drugs known to cause renal toxicity, so it is unclear that the effect was due to the chromium supplement.[41] The safety of chromium picolinate has also been questioned because of studies in cell culture that suggest it may cause DNA damage.[42] This effect is specific to the picolinate form of chromium and may be due to the ability of this form to generate DNA-damaging free radicals.[43] Human studies using the standard supplemental doses of chromium picolinate have not detected an increase in DNA damage, but more work is needed to completely rule out any risk.[44] Despite these concerns, the DRI committee concluded that there was insufficient data to establish a UL for chromium.

• FLUORIDE (F)

The importance of fluoride for dental health has been recognized since the 1930s, when an association between the fluoride content of drinking water and the prevalence of dental caries was noted (Figure 11.16).

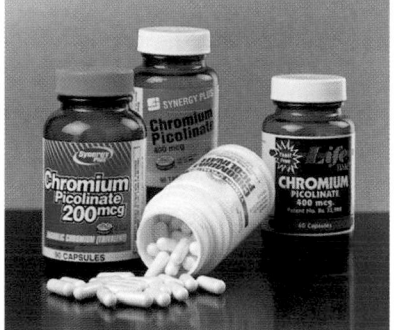

Figure 11.15

Chromium supplements are marketed to increase lean body mass and decrease body fat. (George Semple)

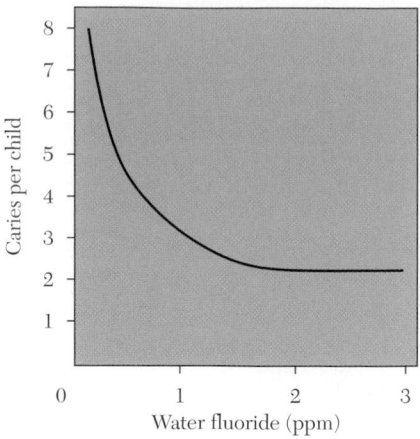

Figure 11.16

This graph illustrates the effect of water fluoridation level on dental caries in children 12 to 14 years of age. (Food and Nutrition Board, Institute of Medicine. *Dietary Reference Intakes for Calcium, Phosphorus, Magnesium, Vitamin D and Fluoride.* Washington, D.C.: National Academy Press, 1997)

Fluoride in the Diet

Fluoride is present in small amounts in almost all soil, water, plants, and animals. The richest dietary sources of fluoride are fluoridated water, tea, and marine fish consumed with their bones. Tea contributes significantly to total fluoride intake in countries that consume large amounts of the beverage. Brewed tea contains 1 to 6 mg of fluoride per liter depending on the amount of dry tea used, the brewing time, and the fluoride content of the water.[45] In the United States, most of the fluoride in the diet comes from toothpaste and from fluoride added to the water supply—usually 0.7 to 1.2 mg per liter (Water companies often report fluoride levels in parts per million [ppm], 1 mg/liter = 1 ppm). Because food readily absorbs the fluoride in cooking water, the fluoride content of food can be significantly increased when it is handled and prepared using fluoridated water. Cooking utensils also affect food fluoride content. Foods cooked with Teflon utensils can pick up fluoride from the Teflon, whereas aluminum cookware can decrease fluoride content. Fluoride is absorbed into the body in proportion to its content in the diet.

Fluoride in the Body

Fluoride has a high affinity for calcium and so is usually associated with calcified tissues such as bones and teeth. In teeth, fluoride is incorporated into the enamel crystals, where it forms the compound fluorhydroxyapatite, which is more resistant to acid than the hydroxyapatite crystals it replaces.

How Much Fluoride Do We Need?

Epidemiology has confirmed the effectiveness of fluoridated water in reducing dental cavities.[46] The criterion used to establish an AI for fluoride was the estimated intake shown to reduce the occurrence of dental caries maximally without causing unwanted side effects. The AI for fluoride from all sources is set at 0.05 mg per kg per day for everyone 6 months of age and older because it protects against dental caries with no adverse effects.[45] Thus, for children age 4 through 8 years, the AI is set at 1.1 mg per day using a reference weight of 22 kg. For adult men age 19 and older, the AI is 3.8 mg per day based on a weight of 76 kg, for women, it is 3.1 mg per day based on a weight of 61 kg. The AI is not increased in pregnancy or lactation.

Breast milk is low in fluoride, and ready-made infant formulas are prepared with unfluoridated water. Unless infant formula is prepared at home with fluoridated water, it contains little fluoride. The American Academy of Pediatrics suggests a supplement of 0.25 mg per day for children 6 months to 3 years of age, 0.5 mg per day for ages 3 to 6 years, and 1.0 mg per day for ages 6 to 16 who are receiving less than 0.3 mg per liter of fluoride in the water supply.[47] These supplements are available by prescription for children living in areas with low water fluoride concentrations. Swallowed toothpaste is estimated to contribute about 0.6 mg per day of fluoride in young children.[45]

Fluoride and Health

Adequate dietary fluoride is important for bone and dental health. Fluoride has its greatest effect on dental caries prevention early in life, during maximum tooth development up to the age of 13, but it has been shown to have some effect in adults.[48] In addition to making tooth enamel more acid resistant, fluoride protects teeth in other ways. Fluoride in saliva reduces cavities by reducing acid produced by bacteria, inhibiting the dissolution of tooth enamel by acid, and increasing enamel remineralization after acid exposure.[49] Fluoride seems to stimulate new bone formation and has therefore been suggested to strengthen bones in adults with osteoporosis. Slow-release fluoride supplements have been shown to increase bone mass and prevent new fractures.[50]

Fluoridated Water The fluoridation of public drinking water to prevent dental caries began in Grand Rapids, Michigan, in 1945. Today, over half of the U.S. population lives in communities with fluoridated drinking water.[46] Some people believe that water fluoridation represents a public health hazard and increases the risk of cancer. These beliefs are not supported by scientific facts. Based on epidemiological data and available evidence related to the adverse effects of fluoride, the small amounts consumed in drinking water do not pose a risk for health problems such as cancer, kidney failure, or bone disease.[51]

Fluoride Toxicity Fluoride can cause adverse effects in high doses. Fluoride intakes of 2 to 8 mg per day can cause mottled teeth in children (Figure 11.17). A recent increase in the prevalence of this condition in the United States has occurred due to the chronic ingestion of toothpaste containing fluoride. In adults doses of 20 to 80 mg per day can result in changes in bone health that can be crippling, as well as changes in kidney function and possibly nerve and muscle function. Death was reported with an intake of 5 to 10 grams per day. Due to concern over excess fluoride intake, a new warning is now required on fluoride-containing toothpastes. The label must state, "If you accidentally swallow more than used for brushing, seek professional help or contact a poison control center immediately."

The UL for fluoride is set at 0.1 mg per kg per day for infants and children less than 9 years of age, and at 10 mg per day for people ages 9 through 70.[45]

ON THE WEB
For more information on fluoride and dental caries, go to the American Dental Association Oral Health Topics at www.ada.org/public/topics

• MOLYBDENUM (MO)

Like many other trace elements, molybdenum is needed to activate enzymes. The molybdenum content of food varies with the molybdenum content of the soil where the food is produced. The most reliable sources include milk, milk products, organ meats, breads, cereals, and legumes.

Molybdenum is readily absorbed from foods. The amount in the body is regulated by excretion in the urine and bile. Molybdenum is a cofactor for enzymes necessary for the metabolism of sulfur-containing amino acids and nitrogen-containing compounds present in DNA and RNA, the production of uric acid, and the oxidation and detoxification of various other compounds.

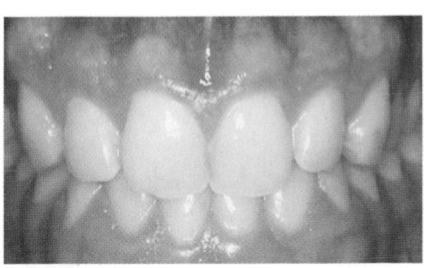
(a)

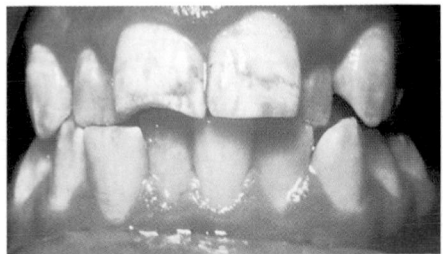
(b)

Figure 11.17
Too much dietary fluoride causes the teeth to appear mottled (enamel fluorosis). (*a*) Normal teeth. (*b*) Teeth showing enamel fluorosis. (*a*, © Edward H. Gill/Custom Medical Stock Photo; *b*, © NIH/Custom Medical Stock Photo)

Although molybdenum deficiency in humans has been reported as a result of long-term TPN, a naturally occurring deficiency has never been reported. Deficiency has been induced in laboratory animals by feeding them high doses of the element tungsten, which inhibits molybdenum absorption. The resulting deficiency caused growth retardation, decreased food intake, impaired reproduction, and decreased life expectancy.

Based on the results of molybdenum balance studies, an RDA has been set at 45 μg per day for adults. The RDA is increased for pregnancy and lactation. An AI has been set for infants based on the amount of molybdenum in breast milk.

There are few data on adverse effects of high intakes of molybdenum in humans. A UL of 2000 μg per day was set based on impaired growth and reproduction in animals.[6]

• OTHER TRACE ELEMENTS

Many other trace elements are found in minute amounts in the human body. Some of these may be essential for human health, and others may be present only as a result of environmental exposure. There is sufficient evidence of a role for arsenic, boron, nickel, silicon, and vanadium in human health for these to have been reviewed by the DRI committee.[6] There was not sufficient data to establish an AI or an RDA for any of these elements, but ULs have been set for boron, nickel, and vanadium. Other trace elements that play a physiological role include aluminum, bromine, cadmium, germanium, lead, lithium, rubidium, and tin. The specific functions of these have not been defined, and they have not been evaluated by the DRI committee. All the minerals, both those known to be essential and those that are still being assessed for their role in human health, can be obtained by choosing a variety of foods from each of the groups of the Food Guide Pyramid.

• APPLICATIONS •

1. Using the three-day food intake record you kept in Chapter 2:
   a. Calculate your average daily intake of iron.
   b. How does your iron intake compare with the recommendation for someone of your age and sex?
   c. If your intake is low, suggest modifications to your diet to meet the RDA for iron for someone your age and sex.
   d. If your diet already meets the recommendations for iron, make a list of foods you like that are good sources of iron.
   e. Identify the major food sources of iron in your diet and indicate whether they contribute heme iron.

2. Using your food record, calculate your zinc intake.
   a. If you eliminated meat from your diet, would you meet the RDA for zinc?
   b. What foods could you substitute for meat that are good sources of zinc?

3. Using the Internet, search for information on a supplement discussed in this chapter—for instance, zinc lozenges or chromium picolinate.
   a. How does the information compare to the discussion in the text?
   b. Who provided the information? Does it promote the sale of a product?
   c. Is the information supported by scientific studies?

SUMMARY

1. The amount of iron that is absorbed from the diet depends on the type of iron, other dietary components, and the body's need for the element. Much of the iron in animal-based food products is heme iron, an easily absorbable form. Nonheme iron, which is not well absorbed, comes from both animal and plant sources. If iron stores are low, more iron is transported from the intestinal mucosa to body cells. When body stores are adequate, less iron is transported from the mucosa.

2. Iron functions as part of hemoglobin, which transports oxygen in the blood, and myoglobin, which enhances the amount of oxygen available during muscle contraction. When iron is deficient, adequate hemoglobin cannot be made, resulting in iron deficiency anemia—the most common nutritional deficiency worldwide. Iron is also a component of many enzymes, including some in the electron transport chain and the antioxidant enzyme catalase.

3. Iron can be toxic. Ingestion of a single large dose can be fatal. The accumulation of iron in the body over time causes heart and liver damage and contributes to diabetes and certain types of cancer. The most common cause of chronic iron overload is hemochromatosis, a genetic disorder in which too much iron is absorbed.

4. Zinc is needed for the activity of many enzymes, including a form of the antioxidant enzyme superoxide dismutase. Many of the functions of zinc are believed to be related to its role in gene expression. Zinc is needed for tissue growth and repair, development of sex organs and bone, proper immune function, storage and release of insulin, mobilization of vitamin A from the liver, and stabilization of cell membranes. Good sources of zinc include red meats, eggs, dairy products, and whole grains. Zinc deficiency results in poor growth, delayed sexual maturation, skin changes, hair loss, skeletal abnormalities, and depressed immunity.

5. Zinc absorption is regulated by metallothionein, a protein that binds zinc in the mucosal cells and limits how much can enter the blood. Since copper binds the same protein, an excess of zinc can stimulate metallothionein synthesis and trap copper in the mucosal cells, causing a copper deficiency.

6. Copper functions in a number of important proteins that affect iron and lipid metabolism, synthesis of connective tissue, and antioxidant protection. The copper-containing protein ceruloplasmin is needed for iron transport. The richest sources of copper in the diet are organ meats. A copper deficiency can cause anemia and bone abnormalities.

7. Manganese is necessary for the activity of some enzymes, including a form of the antioxidant enzyme superoxide dismutase. Manganese is involved in carbohydrate and lipid metabolism and brain function. Good dietary sources include whole grains and nuts.

8. Selenium protects against oxidative damage as an essential part of the enzyme glutathione peroxidase. Glutathione peroxidase destroys peroxides before they can form free radicals. Adequate dietary selenium reduces the need for vitamin E. Dietary sources include seafood, eggs, organ meats, and plant foods grown in selenium-rich soils. Severe selenium deficiency is rare except in regions with very low soil selenium content and limited diets. In China, selenium deficiency is associated with a heart condition known as Keshan disease. Low selenium intake has been linked to increased cancer risk.

9. Iodine is an essential component of thyroid hormones, which control basal metabolic rate, growth, and development. The best sources of iodine in the diet are seafood, foods grown near the sea, and iodized salt.

10. When iodine is deficient, continued release of thyroid-stimulating hormone causes the thyroid gland to enlarge, forming a goiter. Iodine deficiency during pregnancy causes a condition in the offspring known as cretinism, which is characterized by growth failure and mental retardation. Iodine deficiency during childhood and adolescence can impair mental function. Although iodine deficiency is a world health problem, it has been virtually eliminated in North America through the use of iodized salt.

11. Chromium is needed for normal insulin action and glucose utilization. It is found in liver, brewer's yeast, nuts, and whole grains.

12. Fluoride is necessary for the maintenance of bones and teeth. Adequate dietary fluoride helps prevent dental caries. Most of the fluoride in the diet in the United States comes from fluoridated drinking water and toothpaste.

13. Molybdenum is a cofactor for enzymes involved in the metabolism of the amino acids methionine and cysteine and nitrogen-containing compounds such as DNA and RNA.

14. There is evidence that boron, arsenic, nickel, silicon, and vanadium may be essential in humans as well as animals. They may be necessary in small amounts but can be toxic if consumed in excess.

REVIEW QUESTIONS

1. Why does iron deficiency cause red blood cells to be small and pale?

2. List three life stage groups at risk for iron deficiency anemia.

3. List several good sources of iron in the diet and indicate if they contain heme iron.

4. Discuss three factors that affect iron absorption.

5. What is hemochromatosis?

6. How does zinc affect the synthesis of proteins?

7. Why does excess zinc cause a deficiency of copper?

8. Explain why a deficiency of copper can contribute to anemia.

9. What is the role of selenium in the body?

10. Why does selenium decrease the need for vitamin E?

11. What is a goiter and what causes it?

12. What is the role of chromium in the body?

13. How does fluoride function in dental health?

REFERENCES

1. Underwood, B. A. Micronutrient malnutrition: Is it being eliminated? *Nutr. Today* 33:121–129, 1998.
2. Centers for Disease Control and Prevention. Recommendations to prevent and control iron deficiency in the United States. *Morb. Mortal. Wkly. Rep.* 47:1–29, 1998. Available online at *www.cdc.gov/mmwr/preview/mmwrhtml/00051880.htm* Accessed April 18, 2002.
3. Lynch, S. R. Interaction of iron with other nutrients. *Nutr. Rev.* 55:102–110, 1997.
4. Bothwell, T. H. Overview and mechanisms of iron regulation. *Nutr. Rev.* 53:237–245, 1995.
5. Whiting, S. J. The inhibitory effect of dietary calcium on iron bioavailability: a cause for concern? *Nutr. Rev.* 53:77–80, 1995.
6. Food and Nutrition Board, Institute of Medicine. *Dietary Reference Intakes: Vitamin A, Vitamin K, Arsenic, Boron, Chromium, Copper, Iodine, Iron, Manganese, Molybdenum, Nickel, Silicon, Vanadium, and Zinc.* Washington, D.C.: National Academy Press, 2001.
7. Allen, L. H. Pregnancy and iron deficiency: unresolved issues. *Nutr. Rev.* 55:91–101, 1997.
8. AAP (American Academy of Pediatrics). Iron fortification of infant formulas. *Pediatr.* 104:119–123, 1999.

9. Guthrie, J. F., and Schwenk, N. E. Current issues related to iron status: Implications for nutrition education and policy. *USDA, Family Economics and Nutrition Review* 9:2–19, 1996.

10. Iron-containing supplements and drugs: label warning statements and unit-dose packaging requirements. *Federal Register*, January 1997.

11. Klipstein-Grobusch, K., Koster, J. F., Grobbee, D. E., et al. Serum ferritin and the risk of myocardial infarction in the elderly: The Rotterdam Study. *Am. J. Clin. Nutr.* 69:1231–1236, 1999.

12. Clarkson, P. M., and Haymes, E. M. Exercise and mineral status of athletes: calcium, magnesium, phosphorus, and iron. *Med. Sci. Sports Exerc.* 27:831–843, 1995.

13. Halliday, J. W. Hemochromatosis and iron needs. *Nutr. Rev.* 56(II):S30–S37, 1998.

14. Edwards, C. Q., Griffin, L. M., Ajioka, R. S., and Kushner, J. P. Screening for hemochromatosis: phenotype versus genotype. *Semin. Hematol.* 35:72–76, 1998.

15. Prasad, A. S. Discovery of human zinc deficiency and studies in an experimental human model. *Am. J. Clin. Nutr.* 53:403–412, 1991.

16. King, J. C., and Keen, C. L. Zinc. *In Modern Nutrition in Health and Disease*, 9th ed. Shils, M. E., Olson, J. A., Shike, M., and Ross A. C., eds. Baltimore: Williams & Wilkins, 1999, 223–239.

17. Briefel, R. R., Bialostosky, K., Kennedy-Stephenson, J., et al. Zinc intake of the U.S. population: Findings from the Third National Health and Nutrition Examination Survey, 1988–1994. *J. Nutr.* 130:1367S–1373S, 2000.

18. Fraker, P. J., King, L. E., Laakko, T., and Vollmer, T. L. The dynamic link between the integrity of the immune system and zinc status. *J. Nutr.* 130: 1399S–1406S, 2000.

19. Sandstead, H. H. Requirements and toxicity of essential trace elements, illustrated by zinc and copper. *Am. J. Clin. Nutr.* 61(suppl):621S–624S, 1995.

20. Turnlund, J. R. Copper. *In Modern Nutrition in Health and Disease*, 9th ed. Shils, M. E., Olson, J. A., Shike, M., and Ross, A. C., eds. Baltimore: Williams & Wilkins, 1999, 241–252.

21. Bogden, J. D. Studies on micronutrient supplements and immunity in older people. *Nutr. Rev.* 53:S59–S65, 1995.

22. Mills, E. S. The treatment of idiopathic (hypochromic) anemia with iron and copper. *Can. Med. Assoc.* J. 22:175–178, 1930.

23. Wapnir, R. A. Copper absorption and bioavailability. *Am. J. Clin. Nutr.* 67(suppl):1054S–1060S, 1998.

24. Milne, D. B. Copper intake and assessment of copper status. *Am. J. Clin. Nutr.* 67(suppl):1041S–1045S, 1998.

25. Uauy, R., Olivares, M., and Gonzales, M. Essentiality of copper in humans. *Am. J. Clin. Nutr.* 67(Suppl.):952S–959S, 1998.

26. Percival, S. S. Copper and immunity. *Am. J. Clin. Nutr.* 67(Suppl.):1064S–1068S, 1998.

27. World Health Organization. Copper. In *Trace Elements in Human Nutrition and Health*. Geneva: World Health Organization, 1996, 123–143.

28. National Research Council, Food and Nutrition Board. *Recommended Dietary Allowances*, 10th ed. Washington, D.C.: National Academy Press, 1989.

29. Levander, O. A., and Beck, M. A. Interacting nutritional and infectious etiologies of Keshan disease: insights from coxsackie virus B–induced myocarditis in mice deficient in selenium or vitamin E. *Biol. Trace Elem. Res.* 56:5–21, 1997.

30. Clark, L. C., Combs, G. F. Jr., Turnbull, B. W., et al. Effect of selenium supplementation for cancer prevention in patients with carcinoma of the skin. *JAMA* 276:1957–1968, 1996.

31. Harrison, P. R., Lanfear, J., Wu, L., et al. Chemopreventive and growth inhibitory effects of selenium. *Biomed. Environ. Sci.* 10:235–245, 1997.

32. Rao, P. S., and Lakshmy, R. Role of goitrogens in iodine deficiency disorders and brain development. *Indian J. Med. Res.* 102:223–226, 1995.

33. Underwood, B. A. From research to global reality: the micronutrient story. *J. Nutr.* 128:145–151, 1998.

34. van der Haar, F. The challenge of the global elimination of iodine deficiency disorders. *Eur. J. Clin. Nutr.* 51(Suppl.):S3–S8, 1997.

35. Furnee, C. A. Prevention and control of iodine deficiency: a review of a study on the effectiveness of oral iodized oil in Malawi. *Eur. J. Clin. Nutr.* 51(Suppl.):S9–S10, 1998.

36. Vincent, J. B. The biochemistry of chromium. *J. Nutr.* 130:715–718, 2000.

37. Anderson, R. A. Chromium as an essential nutrient for humans. *Regul. Toxicol. Pharmacol.* 26:S35–S41, 1997.

38. Anderson, R. A. Recent advances in the clinical and biochemical manifestations of chromium deficiency in human and animal nutrition. *J. Trace Elem. Exp. Med.* 11:241–250, 1998.

39. Anderson, R. A., Cheng, N., Bryden, N. A., et al. Elevated intakes of supplemental chromium improve glucose and insulin variables in individuals with type 2 diabetes. *Diabetes* 46:1786–1791, 1997.

40. Lukaski, H. C. Chromium as a supplement. *Ann. Rev. Nutr.* 19:279–301, 1999.

41. Jeejeebhoy, K. N. The role of chromium in nutrition and therapeutics and as a potential toxin. *Nutr. Rev.* 57:329–335, 1999.

42. Stearns, D. M., Wise, J. P. Sr., Patierno, S. R., and Wetterhahn, K. E. Chromium (III) picolinate produces chromosome damage in Chinese hamster ovary cells. *FASEB J.* 9:1643–1648, 1995.

43. Speetjens, J. K., Collins, R. A., Vincent, J. B., and Woski, S. A. The nutritional supplement chromium (III) tris(picolinate) cleaves DNA. *Chem. Res. Toxicol.* 12:483–487, 1999.

44. Kato, I., Vogelman, J. H., Dilman, V., et al. Effect of supplementation with chromium picolinate on antibody titers to 5-hydroxymethyl uracil. *Eur. J. Epidemiol.* 14:621–626, 1998.

45. Institute of Medicine, Food and Nutrition Board. *Dietary Reference Intakes for Calcium, Phosphorus, Magnesium, Vitamin D, and Fluoride*. Washington, D.C.: National Academy Press, 1997.

46. Horowitz, H. S. The effectiveness of community water fluoridation in the United States. *J. Pub. Hlth. Dent.* 56:253–258, 1996.

47. ADA (American Dental Association Council on Dental Therapeutics). New fluoride guidelines proposed. *J. Am. Dent. Assoc.* 125:366, 1994.

48. American Dental Association. Fluoridation facts. Available online at www.ada.org/consumer/fluoride/facts/ff-menu.html/ Accessed April 7, 2002.

49. Marquis, R. E. Antimicrobial actions of fluoride for oral bacteria. *Can. J. Microbiol.* 41:955–964, 1995.

50. Pak, C. Y., Sakhaec, K., and Zerwekh, J. E. Sustained-release sodium fluoride in the management of established menopausal osteoporosis. *Am. J. Med. Sci.* 313:23–32, 1997.

51. National Research Council. *The Health Effects of Ingested Fluoride. Report of the Subcommittee on the Health Effects of Ingested Fluoride.* Committee on Toxicology, Board of Environmental Studies and Toxicology, Commission on Life Sciences. Washington, D.C.: National Academy Press, August 16, 1993.

Meeting Our Needs: Food, Fortified Food, and Supplements

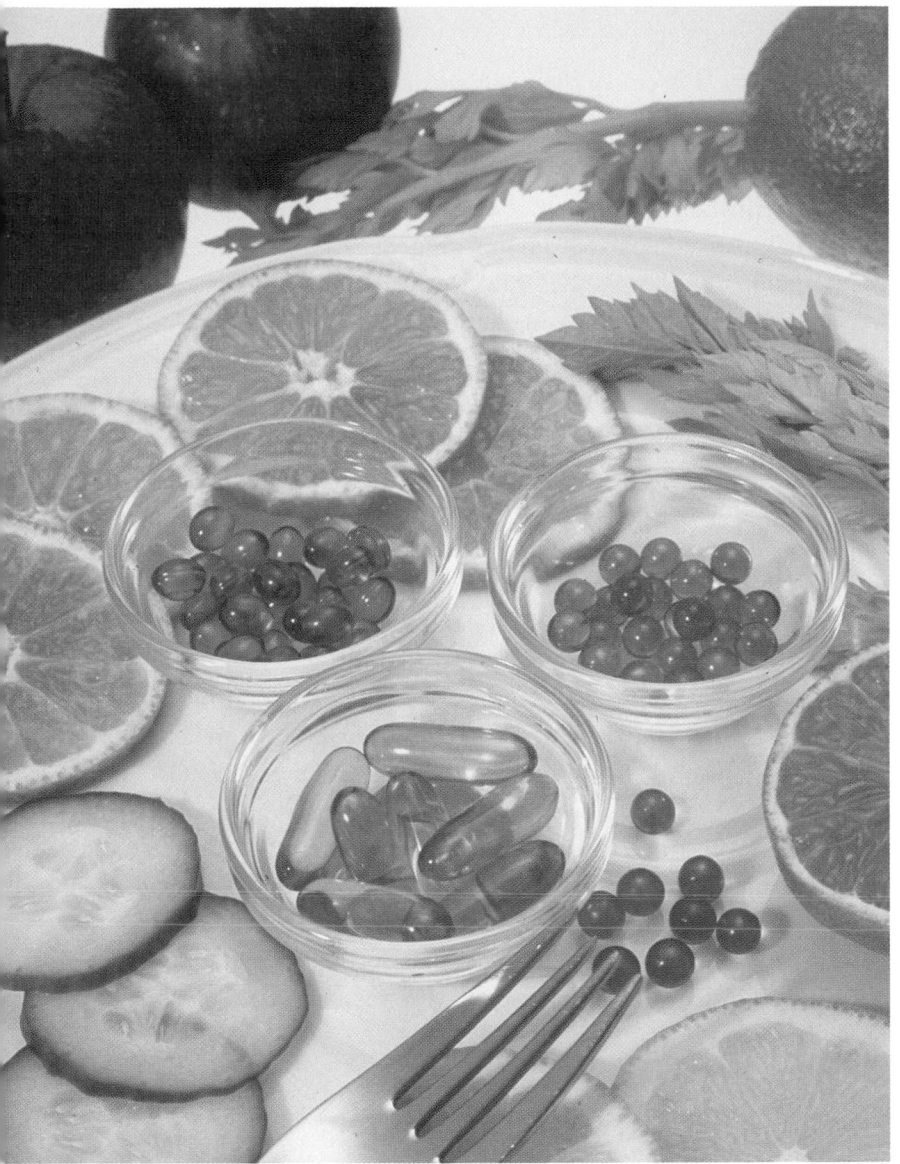

(© Anthony Johnson/The Image Bank)

Chapter Concepts

✔ A well-chosen diet can provide all of the nutrients needed by most healthy people.

✔ Food processing, storage, and preparation can cause nutrient loss.

✔ In the United States, many foods are fortified with added nutrients.

✔ Food contains substances that provide health benefits beyond their nutrient content.

✔ When the diet cannot provide for all nutrient needs, nutrient supplements are available.

✔ Although there are no mandatory standards for the manufacture of dietary supplements, the FDA regulates their labeling and monitors them for safety.

✔ Supplemental sources of vitamins and minerals are recommended for nutritionally vulnerable groups.

✔ Many substances that are not nutrients are available as supplements.

✔ Dietary supplements must be chosen carefully to assure that needs are met without the risk of toxicity.

Can a well-planned diet meet your nutrient needs?

Does the government set standards for the manufacture of dietary supplements?

Can you assume herbs are safe because they are natural?

All that nutrition scientists have learned about nutrient structures, functions, and interactions helps us understand our nutrient needs—but it doesn't always help us meet them. Choosing a diet that contains too little or too much energy or nutrients can lead to debilitating deficiency diseases, cause toxic reactions, and in some cases increase the risk of chronic disease. Meeting needs requires that we choose the right combination of foods in the proper proportions from the foods that are available to us. The fact that many people do not or cannot consume a nutritionally adequate diet has led to the proliferation of nutrient-fortified foods and dietary supplements.

Americans drink milk fortified with vitamin A and vitamin D, eat bread enriched with B vitamins and iron, and cook with salt containing added iodine. They can choose a breakfast cereal that provides 100% of the Recommended Dietary Allowance (RDA) for a host of vitamins, orange juice fortified with calcium, and a cornucopia of supplement pills. Americans consume these supplemental nutrients not only to ensure that their nutrient needs are met but also to prevent birth defects and protect themselves from diseases such as cardiovascular disease, cancer, and osteoporosis. The concept of nutrients as a defense against disease has fueled enthusiasm for fortified foods and dietary supplements.

The many options for meeting nutrient needs has made selecting a healthy diet harder than ever. Because we do not yet know all there is to know about essential nutrients and other biologically active components in foods and supplements, consumers must be aware of the importance of wise food choices and the risks of oversupplementation.

• MEETING YOUR NUTRIENT NEEDS

In order to maintain health and allow for growth and reproduction, individuals must consume sufficient amounts of energy and all the essential nutrients. These needs can be met by a diet that includes a variety of wholesome foods. However, the exact requirement for each nutrient does not need to be consumed every day in order to meet needs. It is the total diet, consisting of the average intake consumed over a period of days or weeks, that is important.

There are many factors that affect how difficult it is for an individual to meet their nutrient needs. Gender, life stage, and health status affect nutrient requirements. It is more difficult to meet needs at some stages of life than at others. For example, pregnant women need more protein and iron than nonpregnant women, and elderly individuals may have more difficulty obtaining adequate vitamin B$_{12}$ than younger people because the absorption of this vitamin may decrease with age. In the developed world the food supply is plentiful and varied, but food choices and food preparation methods can affect what proportion of nutrient needs are met each day. In areas where food availability and variety are limited, it is difficult to meet nutrient needs even when foods are chosen and prepared wisely (see Chapter 18).

There are some circumstances under which it is difficult to meet needs without supplemental sources of nutrients. This fact has been recognized by the nutrient intake recommendations of the Dietary Reference Intakes (DRI) and addressed by government food fortification programs. It has also motivated the manufacturers of dietary supplements to offer a huge variety of supplement options.

Despite the appeal of supplements, consumers should not rely heavily on these to meet their needs. Epidemiological research has shown that supplements do not provide all the benefits that foods do. Studies show that people who eat more fruits and vegetables have a lower incidence of a host of chronic diseases. These same benefits are not duplicated by taking supplements of nutrients found in these foods. In addition to nutrients, foods contain phytochemicals and other substances that are not nutrients but that have health-promoting properties. Scientists have not yet identified all the substances contained in foods, nor have they determined all of their effects on human health. What is clear is that a wholesome, varied diet is important for optimal health (Figure 12.1).

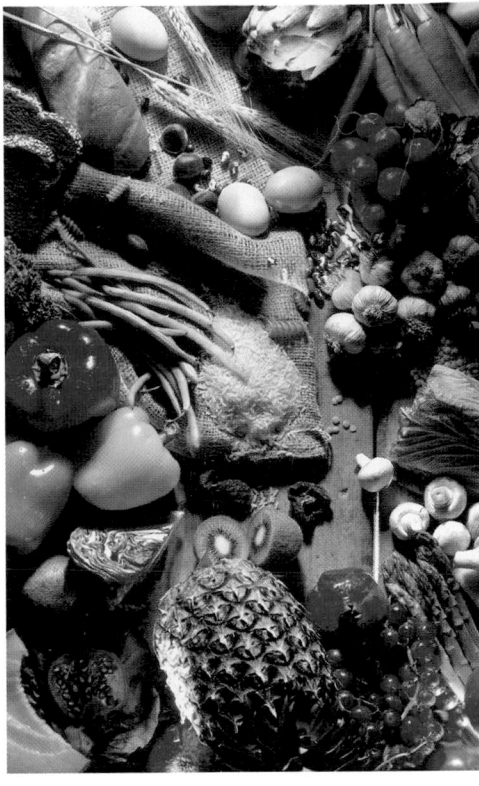

Figure 12.1
A well-chosen varied diet can provide all of our nutrient needs. (© Rick Lance/ Phototake)

• GETTING IT ALL FROM FOOD

A healthy diet includes a wide variety of foods. Many of these should be less processed choices such as fresh fruits and vegetables and whole grains; these are good sources of a multitude of nutrients and other health-promoting substances. Some choices may also be foods fortified with nutrients.

Choosing Wisely

Each food choice we make provides some nutrients, but none provides them all. Grains are good sources of iron and zinc and most of the B vitamins, including folate; leafy green vegetables provide iron, calcium, magnesium, vitamin A, folate, vitamin E, and vitamin K; fruits provide potassium, vitamin A, and vitamin C; meat provides iron, zinc, thiamin, vitamins B_6 and B_{12}; milk contains calcium, phosphorus, riboflavin, vitamin A, and vitamin D; and oils contain vitamin E (Figure 12.2). The recommendations of the Food Guide Pyramid are a good place to start when

Figure 12.2
Each food group of the Food Guide Pyramid provides sources of vitamins and minerals, but no one group can meet all micronutrient needs.

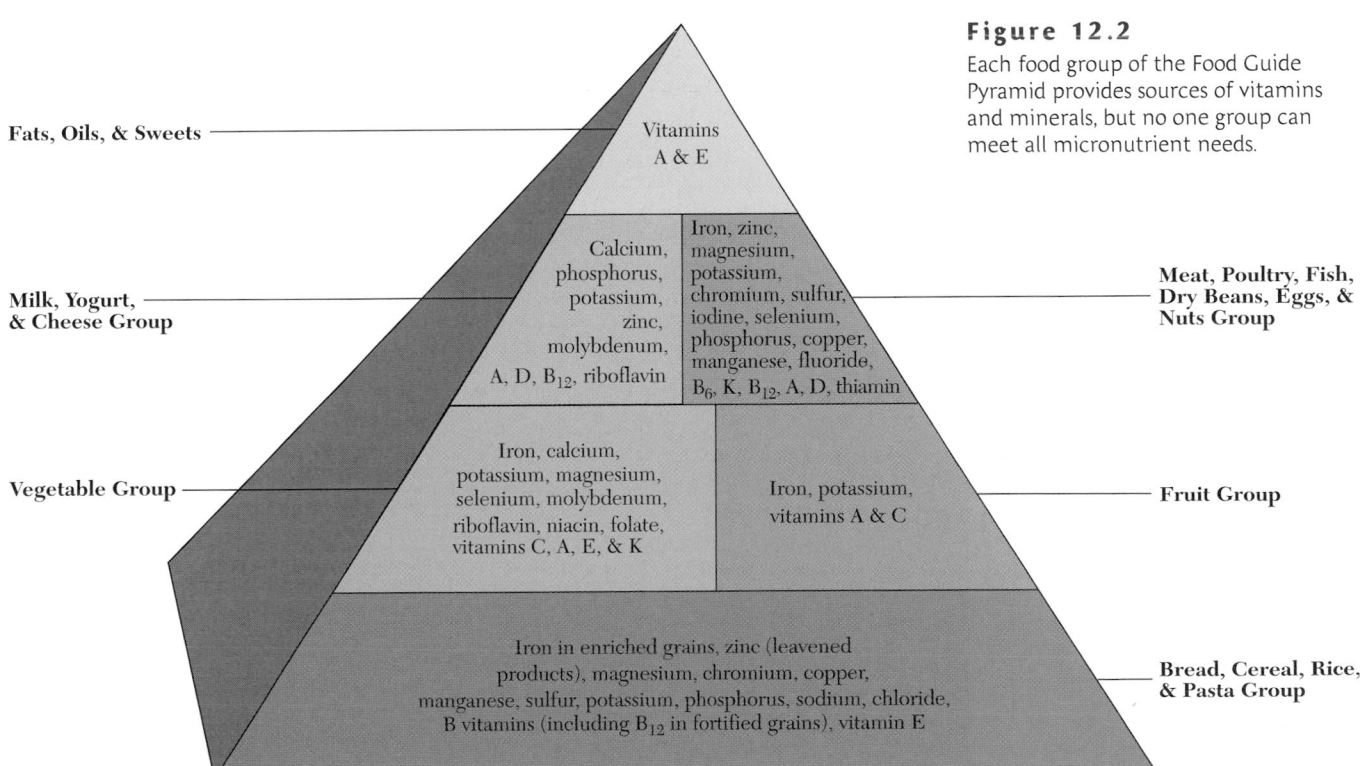

Fats, Oils, & Sweets — Vitamins A & E

Milk, Yogurt, & Cheese Group — Calcium, phosphorus, potassium, zinc, molybdenum, A, D, B_{12}, riboflavin

Meat, Poultry, Fish, Dry Beans, Eggs, & Nuts Group — Iron, zinc, magnesium, potassium, chromium, sulfur, iodine, selenium, phosphorus, copper, manganese, fluoride, B_6, K, B_{12}, A, D, thiamin

Vegetable Group — Iron, calcium, potassium, magnesium, selenium, molybdenum, riboflavin, niacin, folate, vitamins C, A, E, & K

Fruit Group — Iron, potassium, vitamins A & C

Bread, Cereal, Rice, & Pasta Group — Iron in enriched grains, zinc (leavened products), magnesium, chromium, copper, manganese, sulfur, potassium, phosphorus, sodium, chloride, B vitamins (including B_{12} in fortified grains), vitamin E

choosing a balanced diet. However, not all choices from each food group provide the same nutrients. Only a diet that contains a variety of nutrient-dense choices from within each group and has been handled carefully to avoid nutrient losses will meet nutrient needs.

Choices from within Food Guide Pyramid Groups When making selections from each group of the Food Guide Pyramid, variety and nutrient density are both important considerations (see Chapter 2, Table 2.1). Variety is important because different choices from within each food group provide different amounts and types of nutrients. For example, corn and kale are both in the vegetable group of the Food Guide Pyramid, but they provide very different nutrients. Corn is a good source of carbohydrate and fiber but contains almost no vitamin A; kale is high in β-carotene (a vitamin A precursor) as well as folate, calcium, and vitamin C. If your three vegetable servings each day are all corn, you will be missing out on vitamin A and other nutrients that you would have consumed in a more varied diet. Choosing a varied diet is also important because nutrients and other food components interact. Interactions may be positive, enhancing nutrient utilization, or negative, inhibiting nutrient use. Variety averages out these interactions. In addition, foods may contain toxic substances such as pesticides, fertilizers, and natural toxins. Different foods contain different amounts of different substances, so a variety of foods ensures you will not get too much of any harmful substance.

The amount of essential nutrients in a food relative to the energy provided, or nutrient density, is another important factor in choosing foods. For instance, you can get 50% of your RDA for thiamin and niacin from a Big Mac or from a turkey sandwich. Choosing the turkey sandwich, which is more nutrient dense (the Big Mac contains over 500 kcalories, whereas the turkey sandwich contains about 300 kcalories), allows you to eat more of other foods, which contain other nutrients, without exceeding your energy requirements.

Minimize Nutrient Losses Heat, light, air, and the passage of time all cause the loss of nutrients from foods (Table 12.1). Therefore, it is important to consider how the foods you are choosing have been handled; food transport, storage, processing, and preparation can all affect nutrient content. For example, fresh-picked vegetables may seem like a more nutritious choice than frozen or canned vegetables even though they are often less available. However, if the "fresh vegetable" has actually

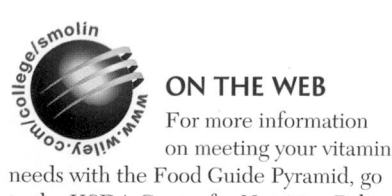

ON THE WEB
For more information on meeting your vitamin needs with the Food Guide Pyramid, go to the USDA Center for Nutrition Policy and Promotion at
www.usda.gov/cnpp/
or the National Cancer Institute's 5-a-day program at
www.5aday.gov/

Table 12.1 *Vitamin Losses in Handling*

Vitamin	Causes of Loss
Thiamin	Heat, air, and neutral or low-acid conditions
Riboflavin	Light, especially in moist and low-acid environments. Also destroyed by heat. When it is dry or in a food, it is more stable.
Niacin	Stable
Biotin	Heat
Pantothenic acid	Heat and low- or high-acid conditions
Vitamin B$_6$	Heat and light
Folate	Heat, air, light, and acid conditions
Vitamin B$_{12}$	Oxygen and light
Vitamin C	Light, heat, contact with iron or copper cooking utensils. More stable in the presence of acid than in neutral or low-acid conditions, so citrus fruits maintain their vitamin C content longer than other sources. One of the most easily destroyed vitamins.
Vitamin A and β-carotene	Oxygen, light, and acid. Fairly stable in cooking
Vitamin D	Oxygen, light, heat, and low-acid conditions
Vitamin E	High-temperature frying, light, air, and freezing
Vitamin K	Light and low- or high-acid conditions

Table 12.2 *Minimizing Nutrient Losses*

Food Storage

- Store canned and fresh foods in a cool location.
- Keep refrigerated fresh produce tightly wrapped to retain moisture and decrease exposure to air.
- For long storage, freezing is best. To retain flavor and to stop enzyme activity that destroys vitamins, fresh vegetables should be boiled briefly before freezing.

Food Preparation

- Cut or cook vegetables just before serving. This minimizes the time they are exposed to air, heat, or light.
- Cut vegetables in large pieces. The smaller the pieces into which they are cut, the greater the surface area exposed—and the greater the nutrient losses.
- Do not soak vegetables before cooking—this causes loss of water-soluble B vitamins and vitamin C.
- Do not wash rice before cooking because the water-soluble vitamins added in enrichment will be washed away.
- Do not thaw or wash frozen vegetables before cooking.

Cooking

- Do not overcook vegetables—they should remain slightly crisp.
- Minimize exposure to water and cooking times by trying steaming, pressure cooking, microwaving, roasting, grilling, stir-frying, or baking.

been a week in transport and another week in the refrigerator, frozen vegetables may actually supply more vitamins. Manufacturers of frozen vegetables often freeze their produce in the fields where they are grown, thereby preserving most of the nutrients. The processing and heating of canned foods reduces their nutrient content. However, because canned foods keep for a long time, do not require refrigeration, and are often less expensive than fresh or frozen, they provide an available, affordable source of nutrients that may be the best choice in some situations.

Exposure to oxygen, light, and heat can destroy vitamins, but appropriate food storage, preparation, and cooking can minimize losses (Table 12.2). To reduce losses, store food away from heat and light and begin preparation as close to serving time as possible. Cooking time and temperature as well as cooking method can also affect nutrient loss; the higher the temperature and the longer the heat is applied, the greater the loss. Pressure cookers and microwaves can reduce cooking times, thereby reducing nutrient losses. Because water-soluble vitamins can be washed away, cooking techniques that do not bring food into direct contact with water, such as steaming, or that use dry heat such as roasting, grilling, stir-frying, or baking, are best (Figure 12.3). If foods are cooked in water, some of the vitamins can be retrieved by using the cooking water to make soups and sauces.

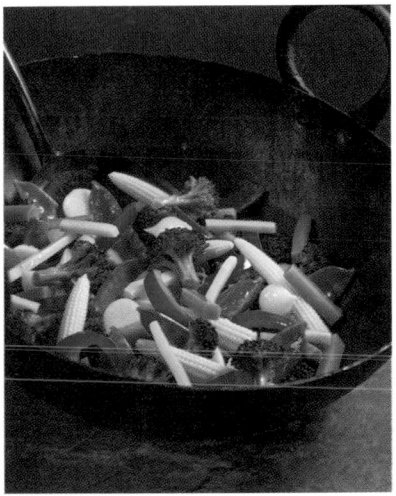

Figure 12.3
Cooking methods that do not use water, such as stir-frying, minimize nutrient losses.   (© Dennis Gottlieb/Foodpix)

Fortified foods Foods to which one or more nutrients have been added.

Fortified Foods

Fortified foods are foods to which one or more nutrients have been added. The added nutrients may or may not have been present in the original food. Fortified foods can be used to increase the intake of nutrients that are deficient in the diet without relying on consumers to make the recommended choices or to take nutrient supplements. Fortification is an effective way to increase nutrient intake and reduce deficiency diseases in a population. Recently, fortification has become a marketing tool for food manufactures.

Fortification: An Historical Perspective The fortification of foods in the United States has a long history. One of the earliest successful fortification efforts was the fortification of salt with iodine. This program was initiated in 1924 to prevent goiter, cretinism, and other iodine deficiency disorders. In the early 1930s vitamin D was added to cow's milk to enhance calcium absorption and prevent rickets. In 1938 voluntary enrichment of flours and breads with thiamin, niacin, riboflavin, and iron was motivated by the widespread deficiency of these nutrients in the diet. In 1943 enrichment of grains with these nutrients became mandatory. This enrichment program required the addition of many but not all of the nutrients lost in the milling of grain for the purpose of restoring them to the same or a higher level than originally present. Thiamin was added to prevent beriberi, niacin to prevent pellagra, riboflavin because it is needed for proper functioning of vitamin B$_6$ and niacin, and iron was added to prevent iron deficiency anemia. Other fortification programs have been implemented to enhance the quality of certain foods. For example, vitamin A is added to lowfat and nonfat cow's milk because vitamin A is lost when the fat is removed from whole milk. Margarine is fortified with vitamin A because it is often used instead of butter, which naturally contains vitamin A. The most recent fortification program in the Untied States, begun in 1998, is the fortification of grain products with folic acid to reduce the incidence of neural tube birth defects. Fortification programs are used throughout the world to increase the intake of nutrients likely to be deficient in the diet of local populations (see Chapter 18, Nutrification).

Fortification to Improve the Public Health Government-supported fortification programs are developed to improve public health. Both what foods are to be fortified and how much of the nutrient or nutrients should be added are carefully considered. Dietary staples are typically selected for fortification because they are consistently consumed by the majority of the population. The level of fortification chosen must be high enough to benefit those who need to increase their intake but not so high as to increase the risk of excessive intakes in others. For example, the level of folic acid used in fortification was determined by evaluating the average grain consumption by various groups in the United States and then choosing a fortification level that would benefit the majority of the population but not be toxic to any one subgroup of the population. The level of folic acid currently added to grain products is not high enough for women of childbearing age to meet the recommendation of 400 µg from these products alone because if it was high enough to satisfy this need it would have also been high enough to mask vitamin B$_{12}$ deficiency.

Fortified Foods in the Marketplace Fortification today extends beyond government-mandated programs. Manufacturers are now choosing to fortify their products with nutrients that are of concern to the population. For example, because many people know their diets are low in calcium, a variety of cereals and juices are fortified with calcium. Because more is viewed as better, cereals are available with 100% of the Daily Values for vitamins, and because herbs are thought to be helpful, fruit punch may come with ginseng and St. John's Wort. This voluntary fortification can be beneficial, but it can also result in toxicities and nutrient imbalances.

The purpose of consuming fortified foods is to meet nutrient needs. However, with the plethora of products currently available, exceeding the Tolerable Upper Intake Levels (ULs) is a potential problem. For example, almost all breakfast cereals contain a complement of B vitamins as well as iron and calcium (Figure 12.4). When these are consumed in addition to a multivitamin, it would be easy to exceed the UL for some nutrients. For example, teens who take a multivitamin supplement and consume three cups of breakfast cereal each morning are exceeding the RDA for many nutrients. National food survey data indicates that 20 to 30% of young children may exceed the UL for folic acid because of the frequent use of fortified breakfast cereals and supplements in addition to fortified grain products.[1] And extensive fortification in the breakfast cereal industry has made it difficult for those who must limit iron intake to find breakfast cereals that are not fortified with iron.

To meet nutrient needs but not risk nutrient excesses, consumers must be aware of what has been added to the foods they are choosing and consider all the sources of nutrients: foods, fortified foods, and supplements.

Functional Foods

Food provides an unlimited variety of tastes, textures, smells, and nutrient combinations. In addition to nutrients and gastronomic delight, food contains factors that af-

Fortified Breakfast Cereal

Nutrition Facts
Serving Size 1 Cup (50g/1.8 oz.)
Servings per Container About 10

Amount Per Serving	Cereal	Cereal with 1/2 Cup Vitamins A&D Fat Free Milk
Calories	180	220
Calories from Fat	5	5

	% Daily Value**	
Total Fat 0.5g*	**1%**	**1%**
Saturated Fat 0g	0%	0%
Cholesterol 0mg	**0%**	**0%**
Sodium 280mg	**12%**	**14%**
Potassium 100mg	**3%**	**9%**
Total Carbohydrate 43g	**14%**	**16%**
Dietary Fiber 2g	9%	9%
Sugars 15g		
Other Carbohydrate 26g		
Protein 3g		

Vitamin A	15%	20%
Vitamin C	25%	25%
Calcium	0%	15%
Iron	100%	100%
Vitamin D	10%	25%
Vitamin E	100%	100%
Thiamin	100%	100%
Riboflavin	100%	110%
Niacin	100%	100%
Vitamin B$_6$	100%	100%
Folic Acid	100%	100%
Vitamin B$_{12}$	100%	110%
Pantothenate	100%	100%
Phosphorus	10%	20%
Magnesium	8%	10%
Zinc	100%	100%
Copper	4%	6%

*Amount in cereal. One half cup of fat free milk contributes an additional 40 calories, 65mg sodium, 6g total carbohydrate (6g sugars), and 4g protein.

**Percent Daily Values are based on a 2,000 calorie diet. Your daily values may be higher or lower depending on your calorie needs.

		Calories	2,000	2,500
Total Fat	Less than		65g	80g
Sat. Fat	Less than		20g	25g
Cholesterol	Less than		300mg	300mg
Sodium	Less than		2,400mg	2,400mg
Potassium			3,500mg	3,500mg
Total Carbohydrate			300g	375g
Dietary Fiber			25g	30g

Calories per gram: Fat 9 • Carbohydrate 4 • Protein 4

Figure 12.4

The amount and variety of nutrients added to fortified breakfast cereals is almost as great as that contained in multivitamin supplements.

fect absorption and nutrient utilization and offer disease protection. Foods that provide health benefits beyond basic nutrition have been termed **functional foods**. The substances in foods that provide health benefits include both **zoochemicals**, health-promoting compounds found in animal foods, and **phytochemicals,** health-promoting compounds found in plant foods (Figure 12.5). Although these terms are relatively new, interest in the therapeutic properties of foods is not new. Early medicine relied on many food prescriptions to treat disorders, and Eastern cultures have long used foods for their medicinal benefits. Until recently most of this was based on cultural beliefs and tradition rather than scientific evidence. During the last decade, however, many studies have examined the relationships among the consumption of specific foods, typical dietary patterns, and health. Most of this research has focused on phytochemicals.

Aren't All Foods Functional? In the broadest interpretation of the definition, almost any food can be considered a functional food. The simplest functional foods are unmodified whole foods that naturally contain substances that provide a health benefit beyond that provided by the nutrients they contain. Many fruits and vegetables fit into this category. For instance, broccoli and other **cruciferous** vegetables have been associated with a decreased cancer risk in epidemiological studies. Further research has shown that these vegetables contain a number of phytochemicals that have anticancer properties. There are also animal products that can be considered functional foods. For example, fish is functional; consumption of a diet high in fish has been related to a reduced risk of heart attacks.[2] The omega-3 fatty acids in fish are believed to play a role. Other functional foods are manufactured or fortified to contain specific health-promoting properties or substances. For example, some margarines contain added plant sterols (Benecol® and Take Control®) to help lower blood cholesterol. These modified foods have also been called designer foods or nutraceuticals[3] (see page 346, *Off the Shelf:* Are They Foods? Should You Choose Them?).

Labeling Functional Foods Although labels generally do not use the term "functional food," food and supplement labels can be helpful in determining the health-related functions that foods provide. Health claims on food labels are one source of this information. Functional foods that contain nutrients or other substances that have been demonstrated by careful research to affect a disease or health-related condition may carry a health claim on their labels (see Chapter 2). For example, oats contain a soluble fiber that helps lower cholesterol. The evidence supporting this effect was strong enough for the FDA to permit foods containing oats to claim that it helps reduce blood cholesterol. Other foods may contain substances that have been associated with health benefits, but the evidence is not strong enough for a health claim to have been approved. Foods and substances sold as dietary supplements may

Functional foods Foods that provide a health benefit beyond that provided by the nutrients they contain.

Zoochemicals Substances found in animal foods (*zoo* means animal) that are not essential nutrients but may have health-promoting properties.

Phytochemicals Substances found in plant foods (*phyto* means plant) that are not essential nutrients but may have health-promoting properties.

Cruciferous A group of vegetables (also called crucifers) named for the cross shape of their four-petal flowers. They include broccoli, Brussels sprouts, cabbage, cauliflower, kale, kohlrabi, mustard greens, rutabagas, and turnips. Their consumption is linked with lower rates of cancer.

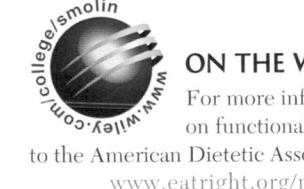

ON THE WEB
For more information on functional foods go to the American Dietetic Association at www.eatright.org/nfs/ and look for the nutrition fact sheet on vitamins, minerals, and functional foods.

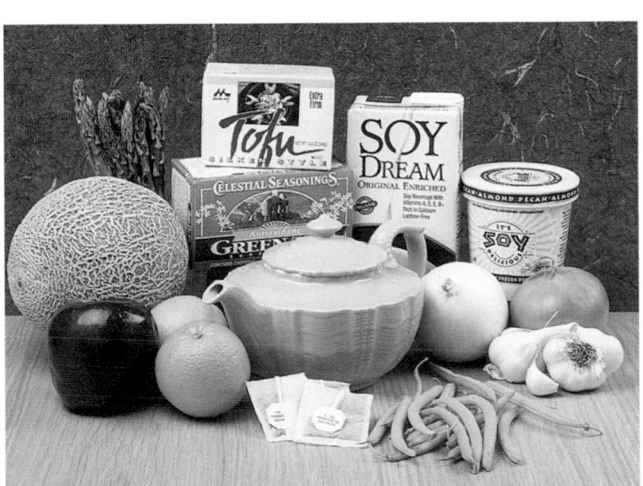

Figure 12.5
These plant products contain phytochemicals that have health-promoting properties. As Hippocrates wrote—"Let food be thy medicine and medicine be thy food." (George Semple)

also include structure/function claims on the label (see pp. 344–345, *Off the Label: Labeling Dietary Supplements*). Table 12.3 lists some examples of foods that can be considered functional foods.

Phytochemicals

The term "phytochemical" literally means plant chemical—phyto is derived from the Greek word for plant. The term refers to the hundreds, perhaps thousands, of biologically active nonnutritive chemicals found in plants. In plants, phytochemicals serve as protection. For example, compounds in onions and garlic serve as natural pesticides, protecting plants from insects. We ingest hundreds of plant chemicals in our diet. Most have no effect on health, some promote health, and others can be toxic. For instance, chemicals in some wild mushrooms can cause symptoms ranging from stomach upset, dizziness, and hallucinations to liver and kidney failure, coma, and death. However, we generally use the term "phytochemical" to refer to those substances found in plants that have health-promoting properties.

Food, Phytochemicals, and Health Phytochemicals that have health-promoting properties have been recognized because of epidemiological observations that identified relationships between diets high in certain plant foods and a reduction in chronic disease. Further evaluation of these foods has led researchers to specific phytochemicals that may be responsible for the health benefits. Foods such as garlic, soybeans, cruciferous vegetables, legumes, onions, citrus fruits, tomatoes, whole grains, and a variety of herbs have been found to be excellent sources of these health-promoting compounds.[4] The phytochemicals found in these foods include allium compounds, isoflavones, saponins, indoles, isothiocyanates, dithiolthione, ellagic acid, polyacetylenes, flavonoids, carotenoids, phytates, lignans, glucarates, phthalides, and terpenoids.[5]

Most phytochemicals are found in more than one type of plant food, and many have multiple actions within the body. Carotenoids, flavonoids, and saponins act as antioxidants.[6] Phytoestrogens have structures similar to hormones and act by blocking or mimicking hormone function. Phytosterols and saponins bind to other molecules, such as cholesterol, and alter their metabolism. Sulfides and isothiocyanates

Table 12.3 *Examples of Functional Foods*

Functional Food	Key Component	Potential Benefit
Whole-grain products	Fiber	Reduced risk of cancer and heart disease
Oatmeal	β-glucan soluble fibers	Reduced blood cholesterol
Lowfat products	Reduced fat content	Reduced risk of cancer and heart disease
Grape juice	Phenols	Improved cardiovascular health
Tea	Tannins, catechins	Reduced cancer and heart disease risk
Fish	Omega-3 fatty acids	Reduced heart disease risk
Soy	Phytoestrogens, soy protein	Reduced risk of cancer and heart disease, reduced menopause symptoms
Garlic	Organic sulfur compounds	Reduced risk of cancer and heart disease
Foods containing sugar alcohols	Sugar alcohols	Reduced risk of tooth decay
Cereal fortified with folic acid	Folic acid	Reduced risk of neural tube defects
Juice fortified with calcium	Calcium	Reduced risk of osteoporosis
Modified margarine	Plant sterols, plant stanol esters	Reduced blood cholesterol
Juices and soups with herbal additives	Echinacea, St. John's wort	Enhanced immune function, improved mood

Table 12.4 *Examples of Phytochemicals*

Phytochemical Name or Class	Biological Activities and Possible Effects	Food Sources
Carotenoids (α-carotene, β-carotene, β-cryptoxanthin, lutein, lycopene, zeaxanthin)	Vitamin A precursors (some), antioxidants; increase cell-cell communication; decrease risk of macular degeneration (some)	Yellow-orange-colored fruits and vegetables (apricots, carrots, cantaloupe, tomatoes, sweet potatoes), broccoli, leafy greens such as spinach, dairy products, eggs, margarine
Flavonoids (quercetin, kaempferol, myricetin), flavones (apigenin), flavonols (catechins)	Decrease capillary fragility and permeability; block carcinogens and slow growth of cancer cells	Fruits, vegetables, berries, citrus fruits, onions, margarine, purple grapes, tea, red wine
Phytoestrogens (isoflavones such as genistein, biochanin A, and daidzein; lignins)	Metabolized to estrogen-like compounds in the GI tract; induce cancer cell death; slow the growth of cancer cells; reduce the risk of cancers of the breast, ovaries, colon, and prostate; inhibit cholesterol synthesis; may reduce risk of osteoporosis	Isoflavones are in soybeans and soy-based foods Lignins are in flax, rye, some berries, and vegetables
Phytosterols (beta-sitosterol, stigmasterol, and campesterol)	Decrease cholesterol absorption from the GI tract; decrease proliferation of colonic cells	Vegetable oils, nuts, seeds, cereals, legumes
Saponins (soyasaponins, soyasapogenols)	Bind bile acids and cholesterol in the GI tract to reduce absorption; toxic to tumor cells; antioxidant	Soybeans, modified margarines
Glucosinolates (glucobrassicin), Isothiocyanates (sulphorophane), Indoles (indole-3-carbinol)	Increase the activity of enzymes that deactivate carcinogens; alter estrogen metabolism; affect the regulation of gene expression	Cruciferous vegetables (broccoli, Brussels sprouts, cabbage), horseradish, mustard greens
Sulfides and thiols (dithiolthiones and allium compounds such as diallyl sulfides, allyl methyl trisulfides)	Increase the activity of enzymes that deactivate carcinogens; decrease conversion of nitrates to nitrites in the intestine; may lower cholesterol, blood clotting, and blood pressure	Sulfides are in onions, garlic, leeks, scallions Dithiolthiones are in cruciferous vegetables
Inositol phosphates (phytate, inositol, pentaphosphate)	Bind metal ions and prevent them from generating free radicals; protect against cancer	Cereals, soybeans, soy-based foods, cereal grains, nuts and seeds (especially abundant in sesame seeds and soybeans)
Phenolic acids (caffeic and ferulic acids, ellagic acid)	Anticancer properties; prevent the formation of carcinogens in the stomach	Blueberries, cherries, apples, oranges, pears, potatoes Ellagic acid is in berries and nuts
Protease inhibitors	Bind to trypsin and chymotrypsin; decrease growth of cancer cells; inhibit malignant changes in cells; inhibit hormone binding; may aid DNA repair, which can slow cancer cell division and help return a cell to its normal state; prevent tumors from releasing proteases that destroy neighboring cells	Soybeans, other legumes, cereals, vegetables
Tannins	Antioxidants; may inhibit activation of carcinogens and cancer promotion	Grapes, tea, lentils, red and white wine, black-eyed peas
Capsaicin	Modulates blood clotting	Hot peppers
Coumarin (phenolic)	Promotes functions of enzymes that protect against cancer	Citrus fruits
Curcumin (phenolic)	Inhibits enzymes that activate carcinogens; anti-inflammatory and antioxidant properties	Turmeric, mustard
Monoterpene (limonene)	Triggers production of enzymes to detoxify carcinogens; inhibits cancer promotion and cell proliferation; affects blood clotting and cholesterol levels	Citrus fruit peels and oils, garlic

stimulate the activity of enzymes that help deactivate carcinogens. Other phytochemicals are health-promoting due to their ability to inhibit carcinogens, alter the way in which cells communicate, affect DNA repair mechanisms, or influence other cell processes that may affect cancer development.[5,7] Some classes of phytochemicals, their mechanism of action, and food sources are given in Table 12.4 and a few of the better studied phytochemcials are discussed here.

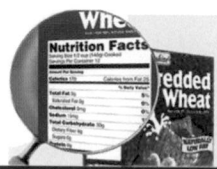

Off the Label
Labeling Dietary Supplements

Thousands of types of dietary supplements are available in today's market. Some provide a combination of essential nutrients in amounts close to the recommendations, some provide large doses of single nutrients, and others provide chemicals and herbs not known to be dietary essentials. Many are designed to supply nutrients that may be lacking in a typical diet, while others are formulated for purposes such as enhancing athletic performance, promoting weight loss, alleviating colds, and even extending life. They come in many forms; pills, tablets, liquids, and powders. Despite the enormous variety of supplements, they all must meet the definition of a dietary supplement and follow the regulations for labeling and advertising established by the Dietary Supplement Health and Education Act of 1994.

In order to help consumers wade through the thousands of choices, products sold as supplements must display a standard label. Each product must include the words "dietary supplement" on the label and carry a "Supplement Facts" panel similar to the "Nutrition Facts" panel found on food labels. The Supplement Facts panel lists the recommended serving size and the name and quantity of each ingredient per serving. The source of the ingredient may be given with its name in the "Supplement Facts" panel or in the ingredient list below the panel. The nutrients for which Daily Values have been established are listed first followed by other dietary ingredients for which no Daily Values have been established (see figure on opposite page).[1]

The types of health claims that can be made on supplement labels are also regulated. Three types of claims are allowed: nutrient content claims, health claims, and nutrition support claims.[2] Nutrient content claims describe the level of a nutrient in a supplement. For example, a supplement containing at least 20% of the Daily Value (12 mg) of vitamin C per serving can state that it is an "excellent source of vitamin C." The terms "high potency" and "antioxidant" are also types of nutrient content claims that can only be used when the supplement meets certain criteria. When describing an individual vitamin or mineral, high potency means that a serving provides 100% or more of the Daily Value. For multinutrient products, high potency means that a serving provides more than 100% of the Daily Value for two-thirds of the vitamins and minerals present. A supplement may use the term "antioxidant" if it is "a good source of" or "high in" a nutrient for which there is an established Daily Value and for which there is scientific evidence of its function as an antioxidant. For example, a supplement containing 60 mg of vitamin C could be labeled as an antioxidant supplement.

Health claims point out a link between a supplement and a disease or health-related condition. Health claims must be approved by the FDA before they are permitted on the labels of dietary supplements, whereas nutrition support claims do not require FDA approval. Nutrition support claims describe the relationship between a nutrient and a deficiency disease that can result if the nutrient is lacking in the diet. For example, a vitamin C supplement could state that "vitamin C prevents scurvy." Nutrition support claims can also include structure-function claims. These refer to the effect of a supplement on maintaining the normal structure or function of the body. These may not directly or indirectly refer to a disease or health-related condition. For example, a calcium supplement might say that "calcium builds strong bones." The ginseng supplement shown here claims that ginseng improves performance by stating that "when you need to perform your best, take ginseng."

Carotenoids Carotenoids are a group of more than 600 yellow, orange, and red compounds found in living organisms. Carotenoids have antioxidant properties,[8] and some also have vitamin A activity. The most prevalent carotenoids in the North American diet include β-carotene, α-carotene, β-cryptoxanthin, lycopene, lutein, and zeaxanthin. The major sources of carotenoids in the diet are fruits and vegetables. Because of this, blood carotenoid levels are a good indicator for fruit and vegetable intake.

The intake of carotenoid-containing fruits and vegetables has been associated with a reduced risk of certain cancers, cardiovascular disease, and age-related eye diseases such as cataracts and macular degeneration.[9] The antioxidant properties of carotenoids are believed to be responsible for some of these effects. β-carotene is the best known carotenoid, but it may be a less effective antioxidant than others. Lycopene, the carotenoid that gives tomatoes their color, is a more potent antioxidant than other dietary carotenoids.[10] The carotenoids lutein and zeaxanthin are most strongly associated with reduced risk of macular degeneration, the leading cause of blindness in older adults. Some carotenoids may also promote oxidative damage depending on the particular carotenoid as well as the amount of oxygen present, the

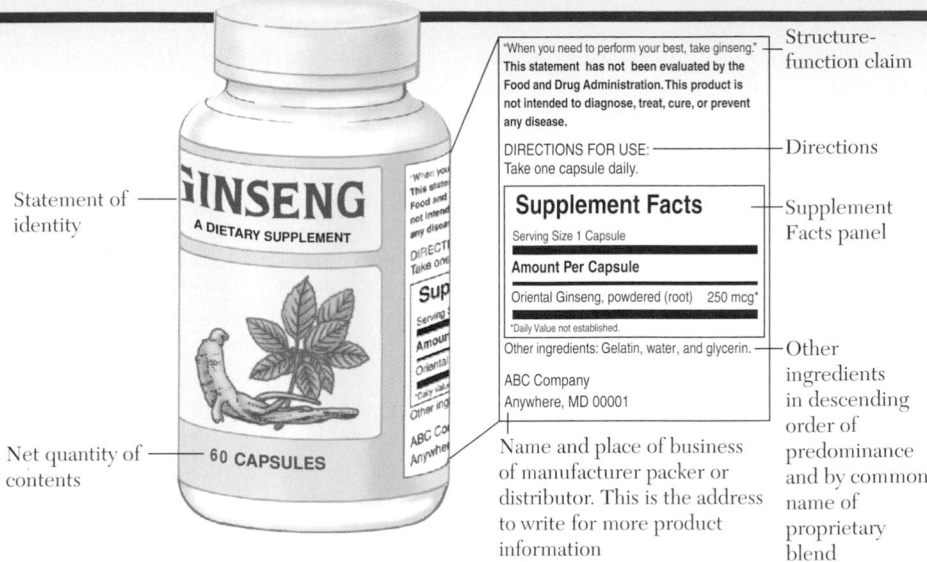

Statement of identity

Net quantity of contents

60 CAPSULES

"When you need to perform your best, take ginseng." This statement has not been evaluated by the Food and Drug Administration. This product is not intended to diagnose, treat, cure, or prevent any disease.

DIRECTIONS FOR USE: Take one capsule daily.

Supplement Facts

Serving Size 1 Capsule

Amount Per Capsule

Oriental Ginseng, powdered (root)   250 mcg*

*Daily Value not established.

Other ingredients: Gelatin, water, and glycerin.

ABC Company
Anywhere, MD 00001

Structure-function claim

Directions

Supplement Facts panel

Other ingredients in descending order of predominance and by common name of proprietary blend

Name and place of business of manufacturer packer or distributor. This is the address to write for more product information

Structure-function claims are based on the manufacturer's review and interpretation of the scientific literature and must not be untrue or misleading. Each label bearing a structure-function claim must carry the disclaimer that "This statement has not been evaluated by the Food and Drug Administration. This product is not intended to diagnose, treat, cure, or prevent any disease."

Although the Dietary Supplement Health and Education Act limits the claims manufacturers can use on labels, products may still be promoted by using information in the form of articles, book chapters, and scientific abstracts that are displayed separately from the products. This information must not be false or misleading or promote a particular brand of supplement, and it must be presented in a balanced fashion.

Supplement labels provide important information about the contents of dietary supplements. However, they are not a reliable guide for supplement use. Before purchasing a supplement, con-

sumers should know what they are purchasing and why. When consuming supplements, consumers should follow dosage recommendations and, when available, use the ULs established by the DRIs to avoid toxicities.

[1] New FDA labeling rules for dietary supplements. *FDA Consumer* 32:2, Jan./Feb., 1998.

[2] Kurtzweil, P. An FDA guide to dietary supplements. *FDA Consumer* 32:28–35, Sept./Oct., 1998.

amount of the carotenoid, and interactions with other antioxidants. Some studies show that when β-carotene is added to a vitamin E-deficient diet, it acts as a pro-oxidant.[11] But in the presence of vitamin E, β-carotene acts as an antioxidant. One explanation for the increase in the incidence of lung cancer among smokers supplemented with β-carotene is that pro-oxidant activity prevails over antioxidant activity.

Flavonoids Flavonoids are found in fruits, vegetables, wine, grape juice, and tea. One of the most abundant types of flavonoids is the anthocyanins, which give the blue and red colors to blueberries, raspberries, and red cabbage (Figure 12.6). These compounds are strong antioxidants that protect against cancer and cardiovascular disease. The pigments that give the pale yellow color to potatoes, onions, and orange rinds are also flavonoids. Citrus fruits contain about 60 flavonoids that inhibit blood clotting and have antioxidant, anti-inflammatory, and anticancer properties.[5]

Phytoestrogens Phytoestrogens are believed to interrupt cancer development and affect health by interfering with the action of the hormone estrogen. Phytoestrogens include isoflavones and lignins. These compounds are modified by the microflora in

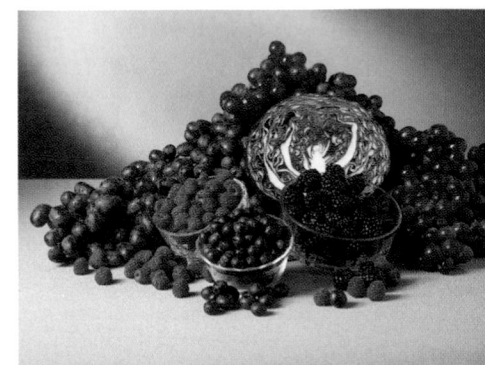

Figure 12.6
Phytochemicals called anthocyanins give the red and purple colors to these foods. (Andy Washnik)

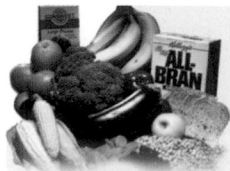

Off the Shelf
Are They Foods? Should You Choose Them?

An energy bar that contains soy protein and 23 vitamins and minerals; a canned soft drink with 100% of the Daily Value for B vitamins plus Echinacea; a fruit juice designed for women with 600% of the Daily Value for thiamin, riboflavin, vitamin B_6, and vitamin B_{12} along with guarana and Dong Quai; bottled water with 100% of the Daily Value for vitamin C—are these foods?

As food manufacturers cash in on the concept that "health sells," the line between what is a supplement and what is a food has become blurred. Claims that a product provides nutrients or other substances that will promote health, reduce disease risk, or enhance athletic performance do sell products. But do these products provide the benefits they claim, and are these benefits ones you need? Should they be part of your diet? As with dietary supplements, it is important to know what you are choosing and to consider the risks and benefits of the product before you consume it.

One of the first things to consider when selecting a fortified product is what nutrients it provides. These products must all carry either a Nutrition Facts or Supplement Facts label. If you are looking for a way to ensure that you get enough vitamins, you may choose a breakfast cereal or beverage that provides close to 100% of your vitamin needs. These products can provide this insurance when taken as an alternative to a multivitamin pill. Some nutrients may even be better absorbed when they are included with food than when consumed in a pill. For example, powdered breakfast drinks that are mixed with milk often provide extra calcium. Since the lactose in milk enhances calcium absorption, this product may provide more absorbable calcium than a supplement taken with a glass of water. The advantages may be less clear for other products. Some advertise that they provide benefits from added nutri-

ents, phytochemicals, or herbs but a close look at the label reveals that the amounts of these substances added is almost insignificant.

If the product provides nutrients or other substances you want to add to your diet, it is then important to see if it also contains things you don't want to supplement. For example, an energy bar with added soy may help you increase your intake of soy protein. But if it also includes more energy, fat, and added vitamins than you want, you may do better getting your soy protein from tofu. Likewise, fortified fruit juice may seem like a good way to get your vitamins, but if the juice also includes one or more herbs that you don't want, a glass of orange juice with a vitamin pill might be a better choice.

Finally, what are the risks of the product? When you consider this food as a part of your total diet, are you exceeding the recommended intakes for any nutrients? We are used to consuming foods in amounts that satisfy our sensory desires, fill our stomachs, and quench our thirst. In contrast, we dole out vitamin pills in accordance with the recommended dose. Too much of a supplement can be toxic, but it is almost impossible to consume harmful amounts of nutrients in unfortified foods. However, when the food resembles a supplement, we may consume it with the abandon of a food but be exposed to the risks of a supplement. For example, adults need to consume about eight cups of fluid per day. Drinking eight cups of water a day is healthy and safe. But if that water is fortified with vitamin C, niacin, vitamin E, and vitamins B_6 and B_{12} the risk of toxicity increases with every glass. If it is a hot day and you drink an extra bottle you may be consuming these nutrients well in excess of your needs and be increasing your risk of a toxic dose. What if these products also contain herbs? Is it an herb that you have researched and determined will be a

healthy addition to your diet (see Table 12.6: Considerations for Choosing a Dietary Supplement and *Off the Shelf:* Are You Choosing an Herbal Benefit or an Herbal Risk?) There are no Daily Values or ULs for herbs, so you may not be able to tell if you are getting a dose that is too low to have any effect or perhaps high enough to cause an adverse effect.

There are a variety of products on the market—promoted to enhance your health and nutrition—that lie somewhere between foods and supplements. These products may have enticing claims, but their contents should be carefully considered before adding them to your diet on a regular basis. Do you really need water that is fortified with vitamins? Are the benefits worth the extra cost? Does the juice with St. John's wort provide any benefit? Or does it pose a risk? Consumers today enjoy a great variety of choices, but they need to choose wisely to be sure they are getting health benefits, not health risks.

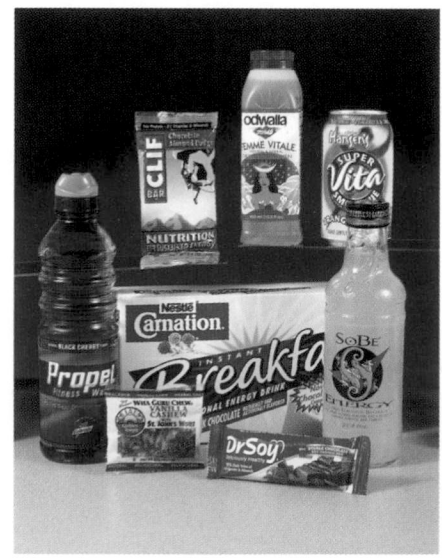

(Andy Washnik)

the intestines to form compounds that are structurally similar to estrogen. They are suspected of blocking estrogen function by tying up estrogen receptors on cells. Isoflavones, the best known of which is genistein, are found in soybeans and are believed to protect against some types of cancers.[12] Research also indicates that isoflavones may protect against osteoporosis, but more research is needed before firm conclusions can be drawn.[13] They are also hypothesized to decrease hot flashes and other symptoms of menopause, although studies have shown this effect to be minimal[14] (see Chapter 6, *Off the Shelf:* Soy Protein for Your Health?). Flax seed is rich in lignins. Lignin metabolites are structurally similar to estrogen and have been shown to inhibit the growth of estrogen-stimulated breast cancer.[5]

Phytochemicals That Mimic Cholesterol Phytosterols and saponins are classes of phytochemicals that have structures resembling cholesterol. They decrease cholesterol absorption from the gastrointestinal tract and therefore lower blood cholesterol—a major risk factor for cardiovascular disease. Phytosterols, such as β-sitosterol, are added to some margarines to help lower cholesterol.

Sulfur-Containing Phytochemicals Isothiocyanates, dithiolthiones, and sulfides all contain sulfur. These classes of phytochemicals stimulate the activity of enzymes that detoxify carcinogens. Cruciferous vegetables such as broccoli, cauliflower, Brussels sprouts, and cabbage are particularly good sources of isothiocyanates and dithiolthiones. Sulforaphane, an isothiocyanate found in high concentrations in broccoli, is particularly effective at boosting the activity of enzyme systems that detoxify carcinogens and has been shown to protect animals from breast cancer.[15] Sulfides include the allium compounds found in garlic, onions, leeks, chives, and shallots. Allium compounds also act by boosting the activity of cancer-destroying enzyme systems. In addition, these compounds prevent bacteria in the gut from converting nitrates into nitrites that can form carcinogens.

How Much Should You Consume? The concept that dietary recommendations should be made for substances in foods that are not essential nutrients is relatively new. Choline, which has not yet been determined to be a dietary essential for everyone, was discussed along with the DRIs for B vitamins, and carotenoids were considered along with the antioxidant nutrients. No recommendations were given for dietary carotenoid consumption and no specific recommendations currently exist for the amounts of other phytochemicals that should be consumed in the diet. A set of DRIs that will consider phytochemical intake has been proposed.

Even though there are no quantitative recommendations for phytochemical intake, following recommendations for a healthy diet will provide a diet high in phytochemicals. The concept of choosing a varied diet that will meet nutrient needs and provide a generous supply of phytochemicals is emphasized in many public health recommendations. The Dietary Guidelines' "Build a Healthy Base" tells consumers to use the Food Guide Pyramid to guide food choices and emphasizes the consumption of a variety of grain products, vegetables, and fruits (Figure 12.7). The "Five A Day" program recommends consuming at least five fruit and vegetable servings daily. Nonetheless, recent surveys of the typical American diet suggest that although our fruit and vegetable intake has increased, only 24% of those surveyed met their recommended intake for fruit and for vegetables.[16] White potatoes represented a disproportionately large share of our total vegetable intake, while phytochemical- and nutrient-rich dark green and deep yellow vegetables account for a disproportionately small share.[17] Table 12.5 includes some suggestions for increasing the intake of foods that provide a variety of phytochemicals.

The effect of food preparation on phytochemicals varies. Most phytochemicals are heat stable and so are not destroyed by cooking or lost in cooking water. Cooking may even increase the availability of some phytochemicals such as the carotenoids in broccoli.[5]

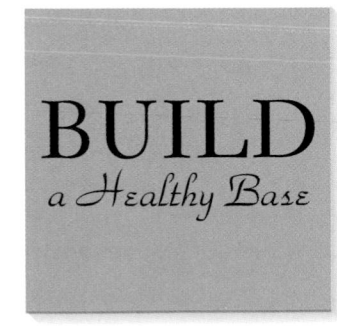

BUILD
a Healthy Base

- Let the Pyramid guide your food choices.
- Choose a variety of grains daily, especially whole grains.
- Choose a variety of fruits and vegetables daily.

Figure 12.7
Three of the recommendations of the Build a Healthy Base tier of the Dietary Guidelines emphasize variety, balance, and the consumption of grains, fruits, and vegetables.

Table 12.5   *Suggestions for Increasing Fruit, Vegetable, and Grain Intake*

Try a new fruit or vegetable each week.

Eat fruits and vegetables for snacks.

Put fruit on your cereal in the morning or vegetables in your eggs.

Try dried fruit instead of candy.

Drink fruit or vegetable juices instead of soft drinks.

Try baked fruit for dessert.

Double your typical serving of vegetables.

Increase your use of herbs and spices such as garlic, basil, turmeric, parsley, oregano, and hot peppers.

Eat a vegetarian dinner at least once a week.

Add vegetables to your favorite entrees such as spaghetti sauces and casseroles.

CRITICAL THINKING

Supplemental Choices

Hazel has her third cold of the winter. She is tired of being sick! She decides that she needs to improve her diet. In the grocery store she looks for foods that have the highest nutrient content. When she describes her concern at a local health food store, the clerk recommends several supplements to keep her healthy. These include a vitamin C supplement, a stress formula B vitamin supplement called B_{50}, and another supplement called Prevention Plus. When she gets home with her new health food program, her friend who is a nutrition student questions whether Hazel needs all of these products.

What are Hazel's nutrient needs?

▼

Hazel is a generally healthy 22-year-old. Her Body Mass Index (BMI) is in the healthy range. She exercises a couple of days each week. Therefore, Hazel's needs should be met by the recommendations for someone of her age and sex.

How healthy is Hazel's typical diet?

▼

Hazel tries to eat well. Comparing her diet to the Food Guide Pyramid, she finds that she meets all of the serving recommendations except for dairy products and fruits.

Using information from each product's Supplement Facts label, Hazel compiles a list of the amounts and % Daily Values of each ingredient in her supplements.

▼

Supplement	Ingredient	Dose	% DV/ dose	Frequency	Total amount (% DV)
Vitamin C	Vitamin C	500 mg	833%	3/day	1500 mg (2500%)
B50	Thiamin	50 mg	3333%	3/day	150 mg (10,000%)
	Niacin	50 mg	250%		150 mg (750%)
	Vitamin B6	60 mg	2500%		180 mg (7500%)
	Riboflavin	50 mg	2941%		150 mg (8823%)
	Biotin	50 μg	16.66%		150 μg (50%)
	Pantothenic Acid	50 mg	500%		150 mg (1500%)
	Folic Acid	50 μg	12.5%		150 μg (38%)
	Vitamin B12	50 μg	833%		150 μg (2500%)
Prevention Plus	Vitamin C	1000 mg	1667%	1/day	1000 mg (1667%)
	Zinc	15 mg	100%		15 mg (100%)

Will Hazel's intake exceed the UL for any nutrients if she takes these products?

▼

- Vitamin C: Her total intake from all of these at the recommended frequency would be 2500 mg per day, which exceeds the UL of 2000 mg/day.
- Niacin: Three tablets of B50 provides 150 mg daily. This is well in excess of the UL of 35 mg.
- Vitamin B_6: Three tablets of B50 a day provide 180 mg and will exceed the UL of 100 mg.
- In addition, although there are no ULs for the other B vitamins, her intake for many is well above 100% of the Daily Value.

What about fortified foods?

▼

In searching for nutritious foods, Hazel selected a highly fortified breakfast cereal. A look at the label reveals that if she eats this cereal every day she will be consuming an additional 20 mg of niacin and 2 mg of vitamin B_6 as well as at least another 50% of the Daily Value for the other B vitamins. This will further increase her risk of an adverse effect from excess intakes.

What would you recommend to Hazel?

▼

Answer:

• DIETARY SUPPLEMENTS

About half of the adults in the United States use some kind of dietary supplement.[18] They are available from the shelves of health food stores, grocery stores, and drug stores, as well as through mail-order catalogs, TV advertisements, and the Internet. Of the supplements sold, about 40% are vitamin supplements, 8% are mineral supplements, and the remaining are herbal and botanical supplements, sports supplements, and other specialty products.[19] If food provides all the nutrients we need as well as phytochemicals, why then are dietary supplements such big sellers? People take supplements to energize themselves, to protect themselves from disease, to cure their illnesses, to enhance what they get in food, and simply to ensure against deficiencies. Although dietary supplements may be beneficial to some individuals under some circumstances, they can also carry risks. Concentrated doses of vitamins and minerals can result in toxicity, and supplements of other substances, such as herbs, may have side effects that outweigh any benefits they may provide. Dietary supplements are easily obtained without a prescription. If they are used to treat illnesses that require medical attention, they may delay conventional therapy causing additional harm. The following sections discuss some of the risks and benefits of a variety of supplements; many others are discussed in relation to specific nutrients and life stages in other chapters of this book.

Regulation of Dietary Supplements

Dietary supplements are regulated by the Dietary Supplement Health and Education Act of 1994. As defined by this law, a dietary supplement includes any product intended for ingestion as a supplement to the diet and may contain one or more of

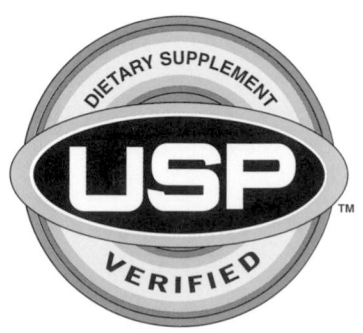

Figure 12.8
This DSVP mark indicates that the supplement has been manufactured according to quality, purity, and potency standards set by the US Pharmacopoeia (USP) Convention.

the following ingredients: vitamins; minerals; herbs, botanicals, or other plant-derived substances; amino acids; enzymes; concentrates; and extracts. In the following discussion, dietary supplements are divided into those that provide vitamins and minerals and those that contain primarily nonvitamin/nonmineral substances. There are also many products that contain a combination of nutrients and substances not determined to be nutrients.

Labels and Safety According to the Dietary Supplement Health and Education Act, products intended for ingestion as supplements must include the words "dietary supplement" on the label and carry a standardized label similar to food labels. Information that may be contained in advertising and package inserts and literature is also regulated. However, these products do not need to be approved by the FDA for safety and effectiveness before they are marketed. According to the Dietary Supplement Health and Education Act, the manufacturer is responsible for ensuring that a supplement is safe before it is sold. The FDA is only involved if a problem is reported once the product has been marketed. The FDA has the authority to remove a product from the market if it can prove that the product carries significant risk.

Manufacturing Standards Because there are no mandatory standards in manufacturing, the amount of an ingredient in a dietary supplement and how well it is absorbed by the body may vary from dose to dose. To address this problem, the United States Pharmacopoeia (USP) Convention, which sets the standards for drug manufacture, has developed the USP Dietary Supplement Verification Program (DSVP).[20] This program evaluates and confirms the contents of dietary supplements, manufacturing processes, and compliance with standards of purity. A dietary supplement company that wishes to participate in the program must submit its products to the USP, which then inspects manufacturing facilities, reviews manufacturing procedures, analyzes samples of the product, and evaluates the manufacturer's quality control systems. Products that have been reviewed and meet USP criteria can use the DSVP verification mark on the label or the statement "made to US Pharmacopoeia (USP) quality, purity, and potency standards" (Figure 12.8). Consumers can be assured that products that have been USP verified contain the ingredients as listed on the label, meet requirements for limits on contaminants, and comply with good manufacturing practices. Once a product has been verified by the USP, it will be routinely surveyed to ensure that it continues to meet USP criteria.

Vitamin and Mineral Supplements

Eating a variety of foods is the best way to meet nutrient needs, and most healthy adults who consume a reasonably good diet do not need supplements. In fact, an argument against the use of supplements is that it gives people a false sense of security, causing them to pay less attention to the nutrient content of the foods they choose.

Many people take supplements because they are concerned that their diets don't provide adequate amounts of vitamins and minerals. These concerns are justified for some nutrients but not for others. Analysis of the current U.S. diet has shown that average intakes of thiamin, riboflavin, niacin, and vitamin C meet or exceed recommendations. However, the average calcium intake in the American diet is only 700–800 mg per day—well below the recommended intake for any group over the age of 8 years. Unfortunately, oftentimes it is people who already eat the most healthful diets who are most likely to take supplements.[21]

Some individuals cannot meet all their nutrient requirements with food, either because they have increased needs or excess losses. Groups for whom vitamin and mineral supplements are typically recommended include dieters, vegans, pregnant women and women of childbearing age, older adults, individuals suffering from chronic disease, and others who are nutritionally vulnerable because of the use of cigarettes or alcohol (Figure 12.9).

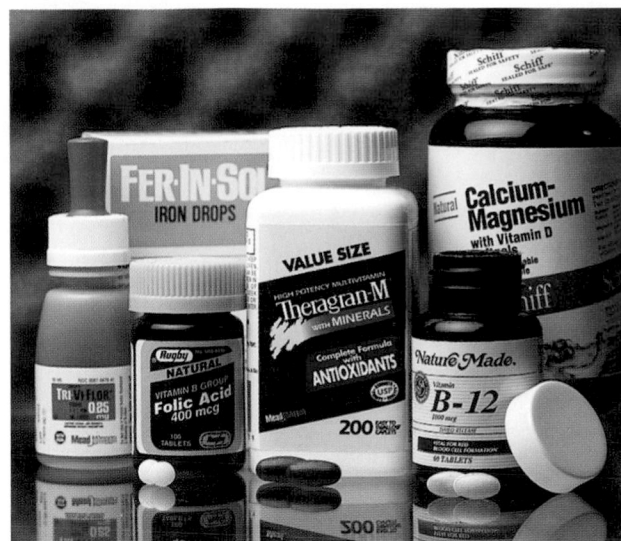

Figure 12.9
Many vitamin and mineral supplements are targeted to groups with increased needs for certain nutrients. (George Semple)

Dieters Individuals dieting to lose weight restrict their energy intake and consequently reduce their intake of micronutrients. It is difficult to consume the recommended amounts of all vitamins and minerals if energy intake is less than 1200 kcalories per day, no matter how well planned the diet is. Therefore, it is important to supplement diets that contain fewer than 1200 kcalories with a multivitamin-mineral supplement that meets the DRI recommendations (see Chapter 7).

Vegans Vegan diets must be supplemented with vitamin B_{12} in order to meet needs. Although vegetarian diets are generally high in micronutrients, a vegan diet, which excludes all animal food products, will be deficient in vitamin B_{12}. Vegans need to obtain vitamin B_{12} from fortified foods or from supplements (see Chapters 6 and 8).

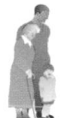

Young Women Women of childbearing age whether or not they are pregnant may need supplements to meet their micronutrient needs. Research demonstrating that the risk of bearing children with neural tube defects is reduced by folic acid supplementation has led to the recommendation that women capable of becoming pregnant obtain 400 μg of synthetic folic acid daily from either fortified foods or supplements in addition to consuming food folate from a varied diet (see Chapter 8). Once a woman becomes pregnant, the need for folate remains high and iron requirements increase. Although a well-planned diet can meet the needs of pregnant women, supplements of iron and folate are recommended, and multivitamin and mineral supplements are usually prescribed (Figure 12.10).

Older Adults Micronutrient supplements may also benefit older adults because the capacity to absorb or utilize vitamins may decrease with aging. For example, 10 to 30% of individuals over 50 have a condition called atrophic gastritis, which reduces the ability to absorb vitamin B_{12} bound in food. Foods fortified with B_{12} or supplements are therefore recommended for this age group (see Chapters 8 and 16). Meeting the AI for vitamin D and calcium may also be difficult for older adults. The AI for vitamin D is 10 μg for those 51 to 70 and increases to 15 μg for those over 70 years of age. The AI for calcium is 1200 mg for those 51 and over. Dietary assessment can identify those who are able to meet the recommended levels of calcium and vitamin D from dietary sources (and from sunlight), and those who would benefit from supplements and fortified foods.

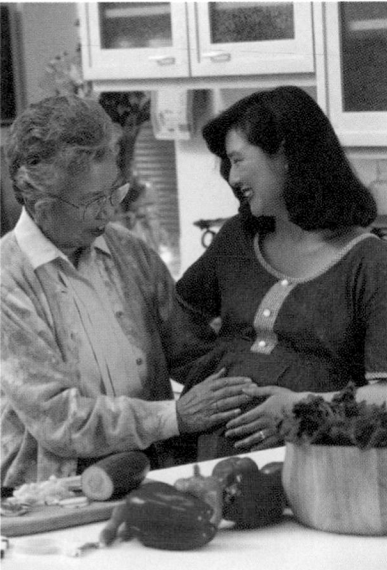

Figure 12.10
Pregnant women and older adults are life-stage groups that may benefit from micronutrient supplements. (Larry Dale Gordon/The Image Bank)

Chronic Disease Individuals with chronic diseases that affect nutrient utilization, or those taking certain medications, may require vitamin and mineral supplements. For instance, individuals with pernicious anemia require injections of vitamin B_{12} or mega doses of oral supplements to meet their needs. Individuals who take certain blood pressure medications (thiazide diuretics) may require supplemental potassium (see Chapter 10). Individuals who routinely take medications should discuss nutrient–drug interactions and the need for specific vitamin and mineral supplementation with their doctor or pharmacist (see Chapter 16).

There are also some chronic diseases that are treated with nutrient supplements. In these cases, the supplements are really being used as drugs and not nutrients. For example, high doses of the nicotinic acid form of niacin can be used to lower LDL cholesterol levels. Large doses of vitamin B_6, folic acid, and vitamin B_{12} can be used to lower homocysteine levels in individuals with inherited abnormalities in homocysteine metabolism. Likewise, supplements of carnitine and some amino acids are required by people with metabolic disorders that limit the body's ability to supply them. When dietary supplements are used to treat a disease, it should be done under a physician's supervision.

Smokers and Drinkers The use of cigarettes and alcohol also affects vitamin requirements. Heavy cigarette smokers, for instance, require more vitamin C to maintain the blood concentrations of vitamin C found in nonsmokers. The DRIs recommend an additional 35 mg per day of vitamin C for those who smoke cigarettes.[22] Alcohol consumption affects nutrient needs because it inhibits the absorption of thiamin, niacin, vitamin B_6, and folate and may affect their metabolism (see Chapters 15 and 16).

Nonvitamin/Nonmineral Supplements

The use of dietary supplements that contain substances that are not classified as either vitamins or minerals has increased dramatically (Figure 12.11). Depending on how the surveys were conducted, the percent of adults who are using nonvitamin/nonmineral supplements is now somewhere between 20 and 68%.[23] Some of these supplements contain nutrients, such as amino acids and carbohydrates. Some contain compounds that are found in the body but are not considered essential in the diet, and others include nonnutrient compounds found in plants (see *Off the Shelf: Are You Choosing an Herbal Benefit or an Herbal Risk?*). A brief discussion of some of these supplements is included below, and others are discussed throughout the text.

Macronutrients as Supplements Protein and amino acid supplements are often taken to increase muscle mass. Although amino acids are needed to synthesize muscle tissue, muscle growth is stimulated by exercise, not by supplements. Some amino acids are also taken for specific reasons. For example, some weight loss products contain arginine and ornithine, which are purported to increase fat loss. Carbohydrates are frequently supplemented in products designed for athletes as is discussed in Chapter 13. In addition, fiber is found in products designed to increase satiety and promote weight loss or to reduce blood cholesterol levels. Fatty acids are supplemented for a variety of reasons. For example, supplements of omega-3 fatty acids from fish oils are used to lower the risk of heart disease, and supplements of flax seed oil are taken to reduce breast cancer risk.[5] There is valid scientific evidence to back up the claims made for some of these products, but many do not provide enough of the nutrient to have the advertised effect.

Compounds Found in the Body Some of the ingredients in supplements are substances that are found in the body or that are their precursors or metabolites. These are not dietary essentials because they are synthesized in the body in sufficient quantities to meet needs, and no deficiency symptoms occur when they are absent from the diet. However, some consumers take these supplements because they believe that body levels may not be sufficient for optimal health. Substances that fit into this category include enzymes, hormones, and vitamin-like substances that function in metabolism. The risks of each need to be considered individually.

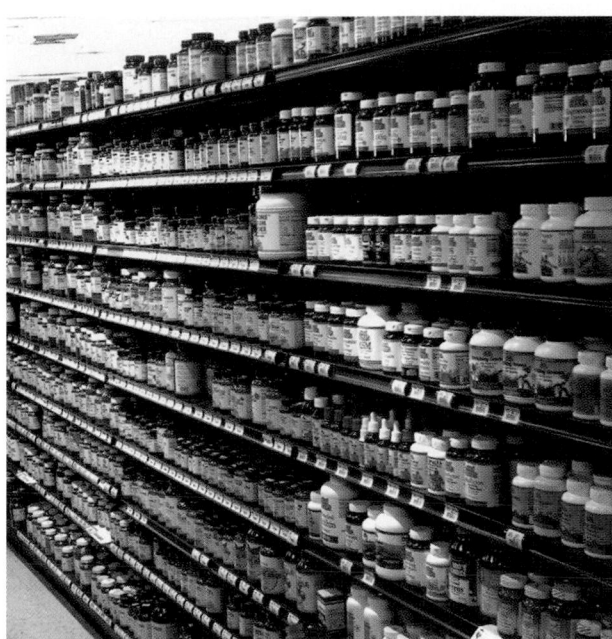

Figure 12.11
There are thousands of different types of dietary supplements available on the shelves of health food stores, drug stores, and grocery stores. (Tom Carter/PhotoEdit)

Enzymes and Hormones Supplements of enzymes and hormones frequently do not reach the target organs they are supposed to affect. Enzymes, which are proteins, and protein hormones are broken down into amino acids in the GI tract before they reach cells inside the body and therefore have little effect on body function (see Chapter 6). However, lipid hormones may be absorbed and reach the bloodstream intact, thereby affecting function. For example, DHEA and melatonin are taken in the hope that boosting the levels of these hormones will delay aging (see Chapter 16). Anabolic steroids are hormones taken by athletes to increase muscle mass; however, they are illegal and have dangerous side effects (see Chapter 13, *Off the Shelf:* Ergogenic Hormones: Anything for an Edge).

Structural and Regulatory Molecules Glucosamine and chondroitin sulfate provide substances needed for the formation of healthy joints and are sold to alleviate the pain and progression of arthritis (see Chapter 16: *Off the Shelf:* Arthritis Remedies).[24] Inositol is a component of phospholipids in cell membranes where it plays a role in relaying messages to the inside of the cell. Inositol can be synthesized from glucose. There is no evidence that it is essential in the human diet, but it may have some clinical value in treating diseases such as diabetes and kidney failure.[25] Para-aminobenzoic acid (PABA) is a part of the folate molecule but has no vitamin activity on its own and cannot be used by humans to synthesize folate. It is purported to be beneficial in disorders of the skin and connective tissue and even to darken graying hair; however, none of these effects have been backed-up by research. Topical PABA is used as a sunblock, but there is no evidence that oral PABA offers protection from the sun or anything else, and in large doses it may cause liver damage.

Carnitine is needed to transport fatty acids into the mitochondria where they are broken down to generate ATP (see Chapters 5 and 13). It is taken by athletes in the hopes that it will enhance the use of fat as an energy source, spare glycogen, and hence increase endurance. Most studies show no increase in endurance with carnitine use. Creatine is also frequently taken by athletes. It is a precursor of creatine phosphate, a molecule that provides a quick source of ATP in the muscle. Supplements have been shown to increase creatine phosphate levels in the muscle and to enhance strength, performance, and recovery from high intensity exercise, but not to benefit endurance (see Chapter 13, Table 13.4). SAMe, chemically known as S-adenosyl-methionine, is present in the body normally as an intermediate in the

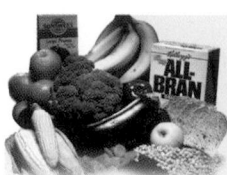

Off the Shelf

Are You Choosing an Herbal Benefit or an Herbal Risk?

The popularity of herbal supplements is on the rise. They are taken to cure a variety of ailments such as colds, arthritis, depression, and menopausal symptoms as well as to slow aging, improve memory, and enhance well being. Because they are "natural"—herbs are often viewed as harmless. Natural, however, is no guarantee of safety. Why are herbs so popular? How can you tell whether you are choosing an herbal risk or an herbal benefit?

Herbal supplements are readily available and relatively inexpensive. They can be purchased without a trip to the doctor or a prescription. Although consumers who want to manage their own health may view this as beneficial, it can also cause problems. When a drug is prescribed by a physician, we assume that it will have a beneficial effect on our ailment, that each dose will contain the same amount of drug, that the physician or pharmacist has considered other medications we are taking and other medical conditions that may alter the effectiveness of the drug, and that the drug itself will not cause a severe side effect. These assumptions cannot be made with herbs. Some herbs may be toxic either alone or in combination with other drugs and herbs being consumed. Some may contain bacteria or other contaminants. And it is difficult to know what dose of an herb you are taking. Even those pressed and packaged into pills may not provide the same dose in each pill. For example, a study of ephedra-containing dietary supplements, a product taken for weight loss, found that the ephedra content of pills often differed by 20% or more from label claims and was inconsistent between two lots of some products.[1] Also, because consumers decide what to treat, herbal remedies can be used inappropriately or can be used instead of necessary medical intervention.

Consumers who choose to use herbal remedies should research the product they plan to take and analyze the potential benefits and risks of the product for them. The suggestions for judging nutrient claims discussed in Chapter 1 of this text can be helpful in analyzing herbs. For example, a consumer considering taking echinacea, an herbal immune enhancer often taken to prevent or treat cold symptoms, would want to think about whether the claims made for the herb make sense. The claim that it may help prevent or reduce cold symptoms is reasonable. Then the consumer would consider the source of the claim? Much of the information available on echinacea is anecdotal—that is, it comes from personal testimonies but there is some good research in humans that supports the claim that this herb enhances the immune response. The cost is also an important consideration. A bottle of echinacea capsules costs about $5.00—similar to the cost of other over-the-counter cold medications. Then the consumer would want to check out the product's safety record, particularly for people of similar life stage and with similar health conditions as themselves. Research has shown echinacea to be relatively nontoxic in healthy adults. However, individuals with the disease lupus, in which the immune system attacks body tissues, should not take this supplement because echinacea can worsen symptoms of the disease. So for most people, the risks of echinacea are small and the benefits may be real. However, this is not true for all herbal products.

For some herbs, the risks outweigh the benefits. Serious side effects from excessive doses or unusual combinations of herbs and medications are not uncommon. For example, herbs such as comfrey and chamomile, which are consumed in tea, can be toxic in high doses. The use of herbal supplements also may be inappropriate at certain times. For example, St. John's wort can prolong and intensify the effects of narcotic drugs and anesthetic agents, so it should not be taken before surgery.[2] It is recommended that herbal products not be used for 2 to 3 weeks prior to surgery.

Some guidelines to follow if you are considering taking herbs or herbal supplements are listed below:

- If you are ill or taking medications, consult your physician before taking herbs.
- Do not take herbs if you are pregnant.
- Do not give herbs to children.
- Do not assume herbal products are safe.
- Do not take herbs with known toxicities.
- Read label ingredients and the list of precautions.
- Start with low doses, and stop taking any product that causes side effects.
- Do not take combinations of herbs.
- Do not use herbs for long periods.

The accompanying table lists some of the suggested benefits and potential risks associated with popular herbal supplements.

---

[1] Gurley, B. J., Gardner, S. F., and Hubbard, M. A. Content versus label claims in ephedra-containing dietary supplements. *Am. J. Health Syst. Pharm.* 57:963–969, 2000.

[2] Jones, D. M., and Weintraub, P. S. Anesthesiologists warn: If you're taking herbal products, tell your doctor before surgery. Available online at www.asahq.org/PublicEducation/herbal.html Accessed May 25, 2000.

Potential Benefits and Side Effects of Common Herbal Ingredients

Product	Suggested Benefit	Side Effects
Astralagus (Huang ch')	Immune stimulant	Low blood pressure, dizziness, fatigue
Cat's Claw (uña de gato)	Relieves arthritis and indigestion, immune stimulant	Should not be taken by individuals with thrombocytopenia (a blood disorder)
Chamomile[a]	Aids indigestion, promotes relaxation	Allergy possible
Chaparral[b,c∘]	Cancer cure, acne treatment, antioxidant	Liver damage, possibly irreversible
Comfrey (borage, coltsfoot)[b,c∘]	As a poultice for wounds and sore joints; as a tea for digestive disorders	Do not take orally, even as a tea; obstruction of blood flow to liver resulting in liver failure and possibly death
Dong Quai[a]	Increases energy	May cause birth defects
Echinacea (purple cone flower, snake root, Indian head)[b,d]	Topically for wound healing, internally as an immune stimulant, cold remedy	Allergy possible, adverse effects in pregnant women and people with autoimmune disorders
Ephedra (Ma Huang, Chinese ephedra, epitonin)[b,c∘]	Relieves cold symptoms, weight loss	High blood pressure, irregular heartbeat, heart attack, stroke, death
Ginger[a]	Relieves motion sickness and nausea	Irregular heartbeat with large doses
Ginkgo biloba[b] (maiden hair, kew tree, Pak ko)	Improved memory and mental function, improved circulation	GI distress, headache, allergic skin reactions
Ginseng[b]	Enhanced immunity, improved sexual function	High blood pressure
Germander[c]	Weight loss, increased energy	Liver disease, possibly death
Kombochu tea[b] (mushroom tea, kvass tea, kwassan, kargasck)	General well-being	GI upset, liver damage, possibly death
Lobelia[b,c∘] (Indian Tobacco)	Relaxation respiratory remedy	Breathing problems, rapid heartbeat, low blood pressure, convulsions, coma, death
Milk thistle[a]	Protects against liver disease	May decrease effectiveness of some medications
Saw palmetto[b]	Improves urinary flow with enlarged prostate	Stomach upset
St. John's wort[b] (hypericum)	Promotes mental well-being	Contains similar ingredients as the antidepressant drug fluoxetine (Prozac) and should not be used by people taking antidepressants
Stephania[b,c∘] (magnolia)	Weight loss	Kidney damage, including kidney failure resulting in transplant or dialysis
Valerian[b]	Mild sedative	GI upset, headache, restlessness
Willow bark[b,c∘]	Pain and fever relief	Reye's syndrome, allergies
Wormwood[c∘]	Relieves digestive ailments	Numbness or paralysis of legs, delirium, paralysis
Yohimbe[b]	Aphrodisiac	Tremors, anxiety, high blood pressure, rapid heart beat, psychosis, paralysis

∘Has been shown to have serious side effects and should be avoided.

[a]Mayo Clinic. Blurbs on Herbs. Available online at www.mayohealth.org/mayo/9703/htm/herb_sb.htm Accessed May 15, 2000.
[b]Mayo Clinic. Herbs can have many health effects—some beneficial, some dangerous. Available online at www.mayohealth.olrg/mayo/0707/htm/me_6sb.htm Accessed Apr. 1, 2000.
[c]Kurtzweil, P. An FDA guide to dietary supplements. *FDA Consumer* 32:28–35, Sept./Oct., 1998.
[d]Bartels, C. L., and Miller, S. J. Herbal and related remedies, *NCP* 13:5–14, 1998.

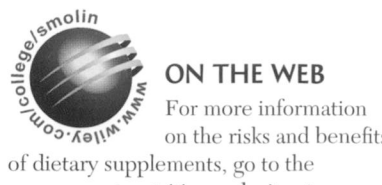

metabolism of methionine. SAMe is claimed to be effective for treating such diverse conditions as depression, arthritis, and liver disease. Although there is preliminary evidence that SAMe may be somewhat beneficial in individuals with depression and arthritis, the results of large, well-controlled studies are not yet available and the risks of taking this supplement have not been adequately assessed.[26]

Coenzymes Lipoic acid is a coenzyme needed for the conversion of pyruvate into acetyl-CoA and for a reaction of the citric acid cycle. Although essential to energy production, lipoic acid can be synthesized in adequate amounts by human cells. Ubiquinone, or coenzyme Q, is important for the production of energy from carbohydrate, fat, and protein because it is one of the electron carriers in the electron transport chain. As its name implies, it is present ubiquitously, in animals, plants, and microorganisms, and it is synthesized in the human body. Supplements of ubiquinone have been reported to improve reproductive performance in rats fed a diet deficient in vitamin E, but there is no evidence that it is needed in the diet of healthy humans.

Herbs, Botanicals, and Other Plant-Derived Substances Technically an herb is a non-woody seed-producing plant that dies at the end of the growing season. However, the term herb is generally used to refer to any botanical or plant-derived substance. Throughout human history herbs have been used as medicine. This herbal or phyto medicine is an ancient art based in folklore and tradition. Herbal products available today, such as Dong Quai, Indian Tobacco, and St. John's wort, borrow from the traditional medicine of many cultures. These herbal supplements are offered to improve general well being as well as for their specific medicinal functions. The physiological effects of some of these are rooted in tradition and anecdote. For others, scientific research has determined that the plant has an effect on human physiology. Supplements that are currently popular include garlic, ginseng, gingko biloba, St. John's wort, and echinacea, as well as a variety of phytochemicals.

Garlic has been used medicinally for centuries, and recent research has shown that it may lower blood cholesterol (see Chapter 5, *Off the Shelf:* Are Supplements a Safe Way to Reduce Blood Cholesterol?). Garlic supplements allow consumers to increase garlic intake without eating this odiferous food at every meal; some preparations contain a deodorized form. Ginseng has been used in Asia for centuries for its energizing, stress-reducing, and aphrodisiac properties. High doses may cause nervousness and heart palpitations. Gingko biloba, also called "maiden hair," is an herb that has been used to enhance memory and to treat a variety of circulatory ailments. Consumption of the leaves may cause side effects such as headaches, gastrointestinal upset, and dizziness. Consumption of other parts of the plant can cause allergic skin reactions. St. John's wort is an herb taken to promote mental well-being. Analysis reveals that it contains low doses of the chemical found in the antidepressant drug fluoxetine (Prozac). Individuals taking antidepressant drugs should not take St. John's wort. Petals of the echinacea plant were used by Native Americans as a treatment for colds, flu, and infections. Today, it is a popular herbal cold remedy. Studies have documented that it is an immune system stimulant. Although side effects have not been reported, allergies are possible[27] (Figure 12.12).

As already discussed, plants contain hundreds of phytochemicals. Some companies try to bottle the health-promoting properties of phytochemicals by extracting them and pressing them into pills or capsules. Popular phytochemical supplements include carotenoids, such as β-carotene and lutein, and flavonoids, such as rutin, hesperidin, and pycnogonol. Lutein is a carotenoid found in leafy green vegetables that does not have vitamin A activity. It is absorbed into the body and, along with another carotenoid, zeaxanthin, makes up the pigment in the macula of the eye. Diets high in lutein have been associated with a reduced incidence of age-related eye disorders, such as macular degeneration. Even though the same effect has not been demonstrated with supplements, lutein supplements are often taken to promote healthy vision.[28] As discussed above, flavonoids and bioflavonoids are antioxidants. Supplements containing them are advertised as cures for arthritis, heart disease,

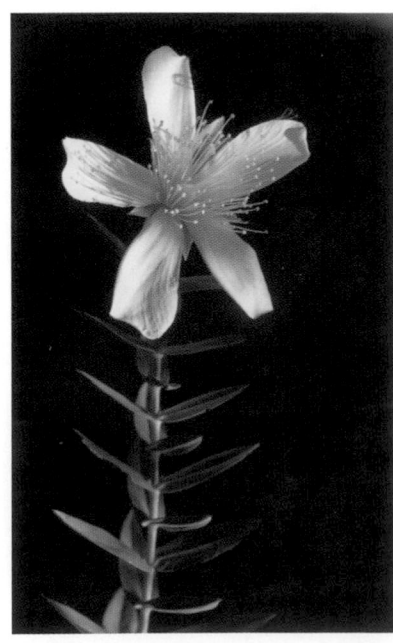

Figure 12.12

Just because herbs such as this St. John's wort are natural doesn't mean they are safe for everyone at any dose. (Bryan Knox/Corbis Images)

high blood pressure, and colds. Although the foods containing these phytochemicals have been shown to have health promoting properties, supplements have not been shown to have the same health effects.

• DO YOU NEED SUPPLEMENTAL NUTRIENTS?

How can you be sure that you are meeting your needs with food or if you should take a supplement? Our diets contain some foods that are naturally high in nutrients, some processed foods from which nutrients have been lost, and many foods fortified with nutrients. Some of these were carefully selected for fortification at a level designed to avoid potential deficiencies and toxicities. Others are somewhat randomly fortified depending on the most current craze in the nutrition marketplace. The only way to determine if you need to supplement your intake is to have a complete nutritional assessment that analyzes both your individual nutrient needs and your typical dietary intake. Although there is little evidence that the average person benefits from a low-dose multivitamin or multivitamin-mineral supplement that does not exceed 100% of the RDA, there is also little evidence of harm.

Toxicity Concerns

Just as there is a minimum amount of a vitamin necessary to prevent deficiency, so is there a maximum level above which symptoms of toxicity are likely to occur. For years it was thought that only the fat-soluble vitamins could build up to toxic levels in the body and that excesses of water-soluble vitamins were merely excreted in the urine and could not reach toxic levels. However, as use of nutrient supplements became more popular, reports of toxicities of water-soluble vitamins, such as niacin and vitamin B_6, began to appear. If the popularity of fortified foods and supplements continues, toxicity symptoms are likely to become more common.

The level at which a nutrient becomes toxic is not always clear. Although the DRIs include an upper limit standard (UL), there is often too little information available to set a UL. The Food and Nutrition Board was unable to set a UL for many of the nutrients reviewed thus far because studies on the adverse effects of high doses of these nutrients were unavailable or inadequate. If no UL is available, extra caution should be taken when consuming levels above the recommended amount.

Other than ULs, there is little information available to consumers regarding supplement toxicities. Vitamin suppliers tell consumers the benefits but are less likely to reveal risks, particularly for subgroups in the population. For example, β-carotene supplements are widely available and do not carry a warning that they may increase the risk of lung cancer among smokers. Excess folic acid can be dangerous for those with marginal vitamin B_{12} intake because the supplemental folic acid can mask the symptoms used to diagnose the B_{12} deficiency. Iron can be a more serious toxicity concern in those with the inherited condition hemochromatosis, in which regulation of iron absorption is abnormal.

If You Choose to Supplement

If you choose to take a dietary supplement, whether to ensure an adequate nutrient intake, prevent disease, or optimize health, products must be chosen with care to assure that nutrient needs are met and the possibility of toxicity is minimal. But choosing a supplement can be confusing. The FDA estimates that there are 29,000 different products available as dietary supplements.[19] Some claim to have special formulations designed to alleviate stress or maximize antioxidant protection. Others target the needs of women, men, athletes, or seniors. Some claim to be all natural, others add herbal ingredients that promise everything from a better memory to a reduced risk of cancer. They entice you with terms like "mega," "advanced formula," "high potency," and "ultra." Are these really better than a plain old multivitamin/mineral supplement?

When considering a supplement, the Supplement Facts panel is helpful in determining how much of each nutrient or other substance is in a daily dose (Table 12.6). It is easy to see if any nutrients are present in amounts that exceed 100% of the Daily Value. Although the Daily Values are not the same as specific RDA values, for most nutrients they are close and represent safe and adequate amounts. The nutrients most likely to be present in amounts greater than 100% of the Daily Value are the B vitamins. These are inexpensive and many, but not all, are safe in higher doses. For any nutrients that are present at more than 100% of the Daily Value, you can check to see if the amount exceeds the UL (see Appendix G). Taking any nutrient in amounts that exceed this value significantly increases the risk of potentially serious toxicity symptoms.

If the amounts are safe, the label can then be reviewed to be sure that the product provides all the nutrients you need to satisfy your individual concerns. Does it provide minerals as well as vitamins? If you want to increase your calcium intake, does it provide the amount of calcium you want? If you are anemic, does it provide iron? Does it provide enough vitamin B_{12} to meet your needs if you are over 50 or eat a vegan diet? If you are a woman of childbearing age, you might want to ensure that you get 400 μg of folic acid from your supplement. Special formulas for men, seniors, or women may not necessarily provide what you need even if you fit into the group they target. These claims are not regulated so it is up to the company to decide what each special group needs. Make sure to consider your medical condition and medications you are taking that may interact with supplements. For example, individuals taking anticoagulant medications should not take supplements containing vitamin E. People who tend to get kidney stones should avoid vitamin C supplements. Those with iron storage disorders should not take iron supplements. Check with your physician, dietitian, or pharmacist to help identify these interactions.

Another concern with choosing a supplement is nonvitamin/nonmineral ingredients. Even standard brands of multivitamin supplements are now offering formulations with added herbal ingredients. Know the health risks and benefits of these before you take them. There are no Daily Values for herbs, carotenoids, flavonoids, isoflavones, and other phytochemicals, so it is difficult to assess whether the amount in a supplement is high or low. A supplement that has a complete assortment of vitamins and minerals does not have much room for large amounts of other ingredients. Often the amounts of these substances added to multivitamin/mineral supplements are too small to be significant. In addition, the presence of these ingredients or a label term such as "natural" may increase the cost more than the ingredients contained in the formula.

Finally, once you select a product, store it safely and use it properly. Check the expiration date. Some vitamins will degrade over time, so make sure you will be using

---

Table 12.6 *Considerations for Choosing a Dietary Supplement*

- Why do you want a supplement? If you are taking it for insurance, does it provide both vitamins and minerals? If you want to supplement specific nutrients, are they contained in the product?

- Does it contain potentially toxic levels of any nutrient? Check the % DV. For any nutrients that exceed 100%, check to see if they exceed the UL (see Appendix G).

- Does it contain any nonvitamin/nonmineral ingredients? If so, have any been shown to be toxic to someone like you?

- Do you have a medical condition that recommends against certain nutrients or other ingredients? Are you a smoker? (Smoking increases the need for vitamin C, but also increases the risks associated with taking β-carotene.)

- Are you taking prescription medication with which an ingredient in the supplement may interact? Check with your physician, dietitian, or pharmacist to help identify these interactions.

- How much does it cost? Just as more isn't always better, more expensive is not always better either. Compare costs and ingredients before you buy.

the supplement before it has expired. Follow the serving recommendations. If the label says 2 tablets provide 100% of the Daily Value, you don't need to take 4 tablets a day. More is not always better when it comes to supplements. If you suffer a harmful effect or illness that you think is related to the use of a supplement, seek medical attention and report the incident to FDA MedWatch by calling 1–800-FDA-1088 or going into the MedWatch Web site.

• APPLICATIONS •

1. Use the Internet to identify several supplements on the market that contain phytochemicals.
   a. What health promises are made about these supplements?
   b. Do they contain a single compound or are they an extract of a whole plant containing multiple compounds?
   c. What are the advantages and disadvantages of these supplements? Would you recommend them to a friend? Why or why not?

2. Do a survey of 10 people.
   a. Record all of the dietary supplements they take including the number of doses taken per day as well as the reason they chose to take each supplement.
   b. Tabulate the total amount of each vitamin, mineral, or other component.
   c. Are there any nutrients consumed in excess of the recommendation (RDA or AI)?
   d. Are any consumed in excess of the UL?
   e. Do you think these supplements will fulfill the expectations of the consumers? Why or why not?

3. Make a table listing the micronutrient content of three varieties of breakfast cereal.
   a. Is the amount of iron the same in each? What is the range of % Daily Values of iron?
   b. Is the amount of folic acid the same in each? What is the range of % Daily Values of folic acid?
   c. Find a cereal that would be safe to consume if you suffered from iron overload.

SUMMARY

1. A wholesome varied diet is important for optimal health. Dietary supplements and fortified foods may be needed by some groups to meet nutrient needs.

2. Our needs for vitamins and minerals can be met by a carefully selected diet that follows the recommendations of the Food Guide Pyramid. Balance the diet by choosing foods from all food groups. From within each group choose a variety of nutrient dense foods.

3. Fortified foods provide supplemental nutrients—some foods are fortified with nutrients according government guidelines to promote public health. Others are fortified according to manufacturers' perceptions of what will sell in the marketplace.

4. Foods that contain substances that provide physiological benefits beyond that of simply meeting nutrient needs are termed functional foods. Health-promoting substances in plant foods are called phytochemicals; those in animal foods are zoochemicals.

5. Phytochemicals have been associated with reductions in the risk of cancer and other degenerative diseases. Some act as antioxidants, some affect the activity of enzymes or hormones, and others work by other mechanisms. A diet rich in plant foods is rich in phytochemicals.

6. About half the adult population in the United States takes some type of dietary supplement. Dietary supplements may contain vitamins; minerals; herbs, botanicals, or other plant-derived substances; amino acids; enzymes; concentrates or extracts. The FDA regulates dietary supplements, but since they are not classified as drugs, regulations are not strict.

7. Vitamin and mineral supplements are recommended for some groups of individuals such as dieters, vegetarians, pregnant women and women of childbearing age, older adults, and nutritionally vulnerable groups.

8. Many substances that are not nutrients are available as supplements. Some dietary supplements contain compounds that are already present in the body but are not essential in the diet. Others contain plant extracts and herbs. These products may have beneficial physiological actions, but they can also have dangerous side effects.

9. Supplemental sources of nutrients—either from fortified foods or supplements—must be used carefully to avoid toxicity. When choosing a dietary supplement, it is important to carefully consider both the potential risks and benefits of the product.

REVIEW QUESTIONS

1. Can everyone meet all their nutrient needs with foods? Why or why not?

2. Why is it important for the diet to include a variety of foods from each group of the Food Guide Pyramid?

3. Explain how and why the nutrient content of fresh raw green beans, fresh cooked green beans, cooked frozen green beans, and canned green beans might differ.

4. Who determines which nutrients are added to fortified foods?

5. Define functional foods and give an example.

6. What are phytochemicals?

7. List three types of phytochemicals and their suggested health benefits.

8. What are zoochemicals?

9. How can you ensure that your diet is plentiful in phytochemicals?

10. List three groups for whom micronutrient supplements may be beneficial?

11. What types of ingredients can be included in dietary supplements?

12. Can the label on a dietary supplement tell you if the dose of an herbal ingredient is safe? Why or why not?

REFERENCES

1. Lewis, C. J., Crane, N. T., Wilson, D. B., and Yetley, E. A. Estimated folate intakes: data updated to reflect food fortification, increase bioavailability, and dietary supplement use. *Am. J. Clin. Nutr.* 70:198–207, 1999.

2. American Dietetic Association. Omega-3s: Something Fishy. Available online at www.eatright.com/erm/erm060299.html/ Accessed March 26, 2002.

3. American Dietetic Association. Position of the American Dietetic Association: Functional Foods. *J. Am. Diet. Assoc.* 99:1278–1285, 1999.

4. Fund, W. C. R. *Food, Nutrition, and the Prevention of Cancer: A Global Perspective.* Washington, D.C.: American Institute for Cancer Research, 1997.

5. Craig, W. J. Phytochemicals: guardians of our health. *J. Am. Diet. Assoc.* 97:199–204, 1997.

6. Beecher, G. R. Phytonutrients' role in metabolism: Effects on resistance to degenerative processes. *Nutr. Rev.* 57(II):S3–S6, 1999.

7. Steinmetz, K. A., and Potter, J. D. Vegetables, fruit, and cancer prevention: a review. *J. Am. Diet. Assoc.* 96:1027–1039, 1996.

8. Pryor, W. A., Stahl, W., and Rock, C. L. Beta carotene: From biochemistry to clinical trials. *Nutr. Rev.* 58(I): 39–53, 2000.

9. Cooper, D. A., Eldridge, A. L., and Peters, J. P. Dietary carotenoids and certain cancers, heart disease, and age-related macular degeneration: a review of recent research. *Nutr. Rev.* 57:201–214, 2000.

10. Miller, N., Sampson, J., Candeias, L. P., et al. Antioxidant activities of carotenes and xanthophylls. *FEBS Lett.* 384:240–246, 1996.

11. Palozza, P. Prooxidant actions of carotenoids in biologic systems. *Nutr. Rev.* 56:257–265, 1998.

12. Messina, M., Gardner, C., and Barnes, S. Gaining insight into the health effects of soy but a long way still to go: commentary on the fourth international symposium on the role of soy in preventing and treating chronic disease. *J. Nutr.* 132:547S–551S, 2002.

13. Messina, M., and Messina, V. Soyfoods, soybean isoflavones, and bone health: A brief overview. *J. Ren. Nutr.* 1:63–68, 2000.

14. Vincent, A., and Fitzpatrick, L. A. Soy isoflavones: Are they useful in menopause? *Mayo Clin. Proc.* 75:1174–1184, 2000.

15. Fehey, J. W., Zhang, Y., and Talalay, P. Broccoli sprouts: An exceptionally rich source of inducers of enzymes that protect against carcinogens. *Proc. Natl. Acad. Sci. USA* 94:10367–10372, 1997.

16. Cleveland, L. E., Cook, A. J., Wilson, J. W., et al. Pyramid Servings Data Results from the USDA's CSFII, ARS Food Surveys Research Group. Available online at www.barc.usda.gov/bhnrc/foodsurvey/home/htm/Accessed March 13, 2002.

17. Krebs-Smith, A. M., and Kantor, L. S. Choose a variety of fruits and vegetables daily: Understanding the complexities. *J. Nutr.* 131:487S–501S, 2001.

18. American Dietetic Association. American's Food and Nutrition Attitudes and Behaviors—Nutrition and You: Trends 2000. Available online at www.eatright.org/pr/2000/010300a.html/ Accessed March 26, 2002.

19. Sarubin, A. *The Health Professional's Guide to Popular Dietary Supplements.* Chicago, IL: American Dietetic Association; 2000.

20. USP Dietary Supplement Verification Program. Available online at www.usp-dsvp.org. Accessed June 11, 2002.

21. American Dietetic Association. Position of the American Dietetic Association: Food fortification and dietary supplements. *J. Am. Diet. Assoc.* 101:115–125, 2001.

22. Food and Nutrition Board. Institute of Medicine. *Dietary Reference Intakes for Vitamin C, Vitamin E, Selenium, and Carotenoids.* Washington, D.C.: National Academy Press, 2000.

23. Radimer, K. L., Subar, A. F., and Thompson, F. E. Nonvitamin, nonmineral dietary supplements: Issues and findings from NHANES III. *J. Am. Diet. Assoc.* 100:447–454, 2000.

24. Kelly, G. S. The role of glucosamine sulfate and chondriotin sulfates in the treatment of degenerative joint disease. *Altern. Med. Rev.* 3:27–39, 1998.

25. Aukema, H. M., and Holub, B. J. Inositol and pyroloquinoline quinone. In *Modern Nutrition in Health and Disease*, 8th ed. Shils, M. E., Olson, J. A., and Shike, M., eds. Philadelphia: Lea & Febiger, 1994. 449–458.

26. Ramos, L. Beyond the headlines: SAMe as a supplement. *J. Am. Diet. Assoc.* 100: 414, 2000.

27. Bartels, C. L., and Miller, S. L. Herbal and related remedies. *NCP* 13:3–18, 1998.

28. Mares-Perlman, J. A., and Erdman, J. W. Can lutein protect against chronic disease. *Symposium. J. Nutr.* 132: 517s–540s, 2002.

Fueling Fitness: Nutrition and Exercise

Chapter **13**

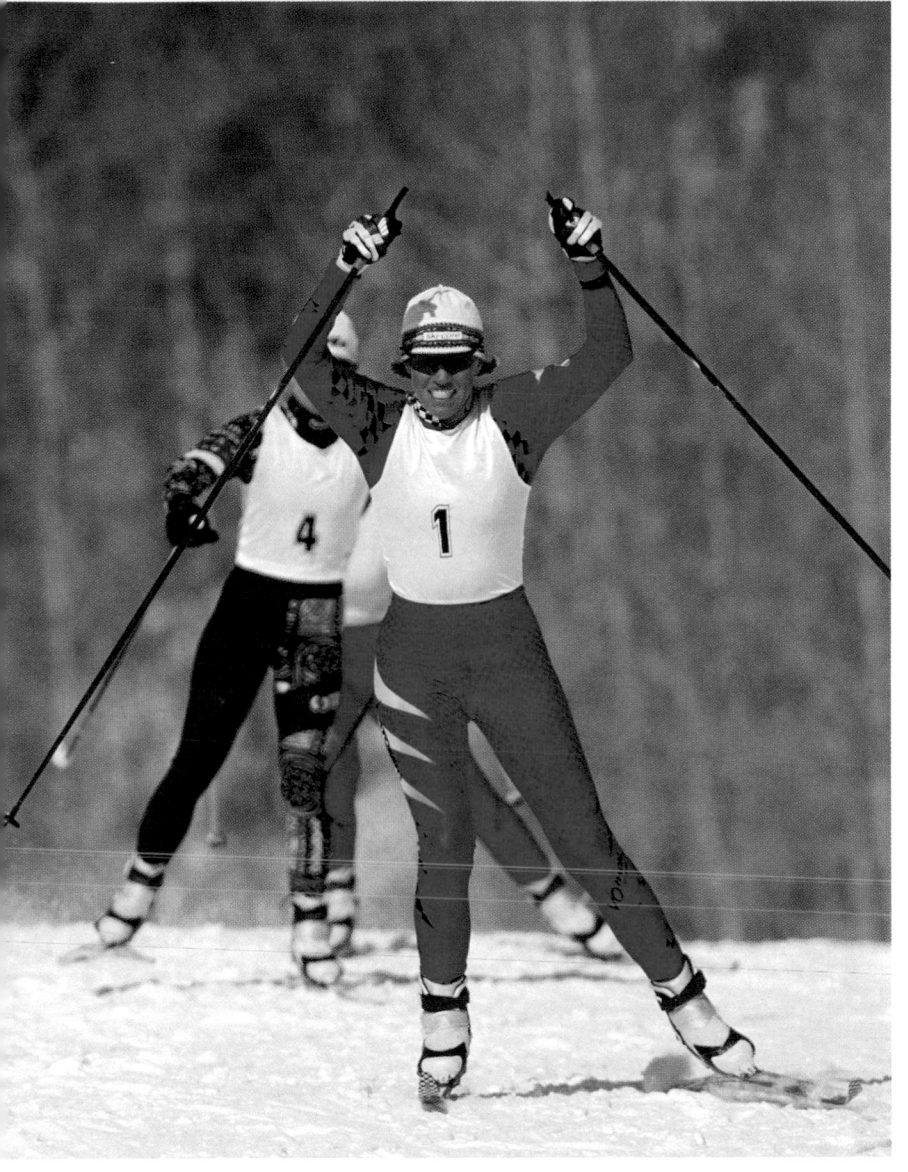

(© Nathan Bilow/Allsport)

Chapter Concepts

✔ Regular exercise can improve fitness and overall health and reduce the risk of chronic disease.

✔ An active lifestyle should include aerobic activities as well as those that improve flexibility and strength.

✔ Activity requires energy generated from the breakdown of carbohydrate, fat, and protein. The availability of oxygen affects which nutrients can be used to produce ATP and how much is produced.

✔ Diets for physically active individuals should provide adequate energy and the same proportions of carbohydrate, fat, and protein that are recommended for the general population.

✔ Sufficient water is essential during all types of exercise to transport nutrients, eliminate wastes, and cool the body.

✔ Nutrient intake before, during, and after competition may affect athletic performance.

✔ The popularity of performance-enhancing (ergogenic) supplements continues to increase among athletes. Before they are used, the risks should be weighed against the benefits.

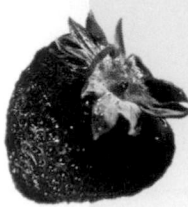

Just a Taste

How much exercise is enough?

Does exercise increase protein needs?

Can dietary supplements enhance athletic performance?

Good nutrition and adequate physical activity are both important throughout life. The amount of exercise an individual gets influences one's nutritional status and overall health. In turn, diet and nutritional status can influence exercise performance.

Although many of us think of exercise as running marathons and competing in the Olympic Games, even moderate exercise can improve health and fitness. For some, fitness means being able to easily walk around the block, mow the lawn, or play with their children. For more seasoned athletes, fitness means optimal performance of strenuous exercise. For everyone, fitness reduces the risk of chronic diseases such as cardiovascular disease and obesity. Whether your goal is maintaining your health or competing in athletic events, nutrition provides a launching pad from which physical fitness can be improved. The right mixture of the energy-yielding nutrients—carbohydrate, fat, and protein—along with adequate micronutrients and water enhances the performance of the body "machine."

• FITNESS IN YOUR LIFE

Fitness The ability to perform routine physical activity without undue fatigue.

Exercise improves **fitness**. You don't need to run 10-kilometer races or swim the English Channel to be physically fit. Even a small amount of exercise is better than none, and, within reason, more exercise is better than less. Whether you are 16 or 60, fitness through regular exercise can improve your overall health.

The Many Faces of Fitness

Being fit means maintaining cardiorespiratory endurance, muscle strength and endurance, flexibility, and a healthy body composition. These parameters of fitness are important for athletes but also extend to every aspect and task of daily life.

Cardiorespiratory system The circulatory and respiratory systems, which together deliver oxygen and nutrients to cells.

Aerobic exercise Endurance exercise such as jogging, swimming, or cycling that increases heart rate and requires oxygen in metabolism.

Cardiorespiratory Endurance Cardiorespiratory endurance determines how long you can continue a task, whether it is climbing stairs, raking leaves, or running a race. It requires muscle strength but also involves the cardiovascular and respiratory systems, referred to jointly as the **cardiorespiratory system**. Endurance is increased by **aerobic exercise**, the type of exercise that increases the heart rate and uses oxygen. To be aerobic, an activity should be performed at an intensity low enough to allow you to carry on a conversation but high enough that you cannot sing while exercising. Aerobic activities include walking, dancing, jogging, cross-country skiing, cycling, and swimming.

Stroke volume The volume of blood pumped by each beat of the heart.

Resting heart rate The number of times that the heart beats per minute while a person is at rest.

Regular aerobic exercise strengthens heart muscle and increases **stroke volume**, which is the amount of blood pumped with each beat of the heart. This in turn decreases **resting heart rate**, which is the rate at which the heart must beat to supply blood to the tissues at rest. Resting heart rate can be measured by counting the number of pulses, or heartbeats, per minute while at rest (Figure 13.1). The more fit someone is, the lower their resting heart rate and pulse and the more activity they can perform before reaching **maximum heart rate**. Maximum heart rate is the maximum number of beats per minute that the heart can attain. It is dependent on age and can be estimated by subtracting one's age from 220. Aerobic exercise should be performed at a heart rate of 60 to 90% of maximum heart rate. For example, a 40-year-old individual would have a maximum heart rate of 180 beats per minute and should exercise at a pace that keeps the heart rate between 108 and 162 beats per minute (Figure 13.2).

Aerobic exercise also increases **maximal oxygen consumption**, or **VO$_2$ max**, which is the maximum amount of oxygen that can be consumed by the body's cells during exercise. VO$_2$ max is dependent on the ability of the cardiorespiratory system to deliver oxygen to the cells and the ability of the cells to use oxygen to produce energy. The greater the VO$_2$ max, the more intense activity a person can perform before a lack of oxygen affects performance. VO$_2$ max can be determined in an exercise laboratory by measuring oxygen uptake during exercise.

To perform this measurement, an individual runs on a treadmill while the air he or she breathes is measured. Oxygen consumption or uptake is calculated by subtracting the amount of oxygen exhaled from the amount of oxygen inhaled. The workload is then increased by increasing the speed and/or grade of the treadmill until the individual can no longer continue (Figure 13.3). The amount of oxygen consumed at the highest workload achieved is the VO$_2$ max. A trained athlete will have a greater VO$_2$ max than an untrained individual.

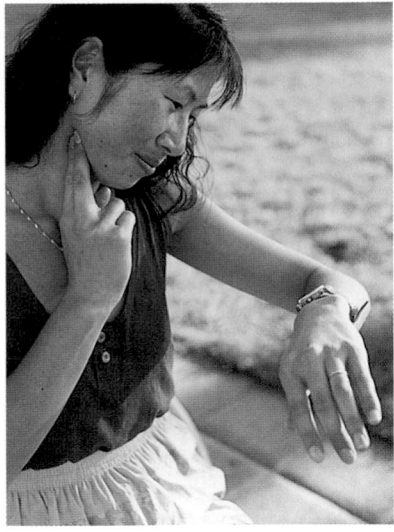

Figure 13.1

Heart rate can be estimated by feeling the pulse at the side of the neck just below the jaw bone. A pulse is caused by the heart beating and forcing blood through the arteries. The number of pulses per minute equals heart rate. (© Michael Newman/PhotoEdit)

Maximum heart rate The maximum number of beats per minute that the heart can attain. It declines with age and can be estimated by subtracting age in years from 220.

Maximal oxygen consumption or VO$_2$ max The maximum amount of oxygen that can be consumed by the tissues during exercise.

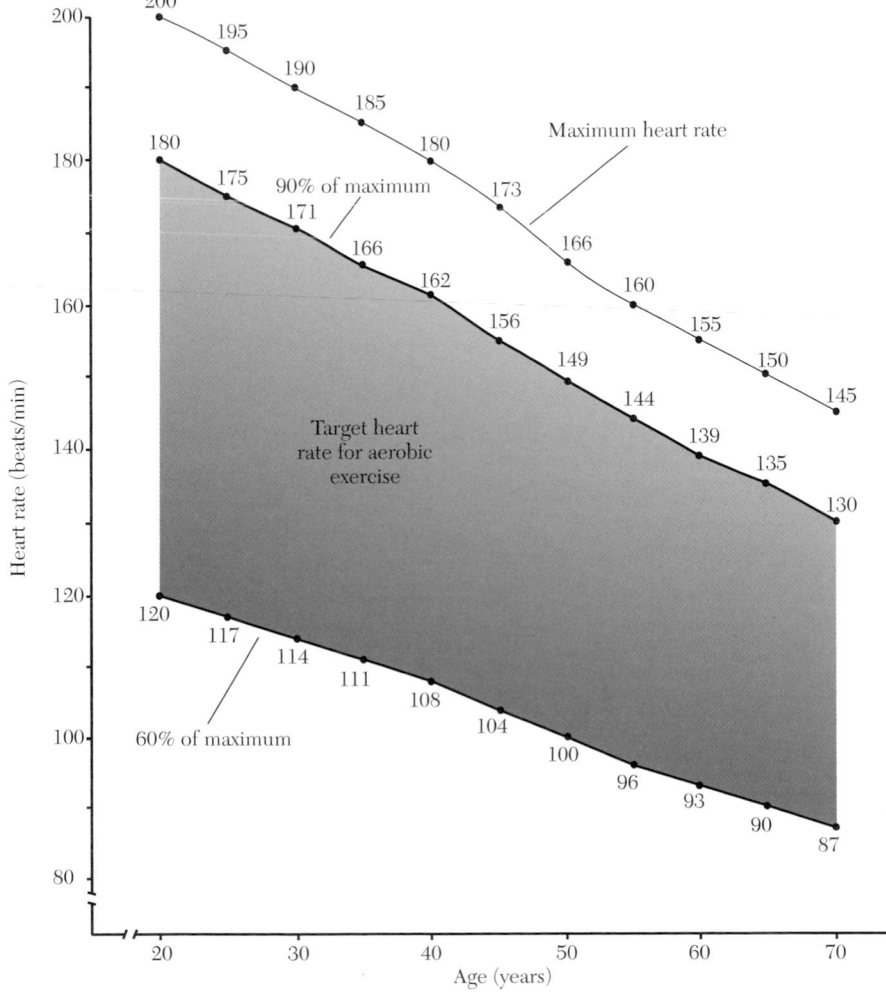

Figure 13.2

The orange area represents the target heart rate for aerobic exercise—between 60 and 90% of maximum heart rate. Exercise performed at this level will benefit cardiovascular health. (Adapted from McArdle, W. D., Katch, F. I., and Katch, V. L. *Exercise Physiology: Energy, Nutrition, and Human Performance*, 3rd ed. Philadelphia: Lea & Febiger, 1991.)

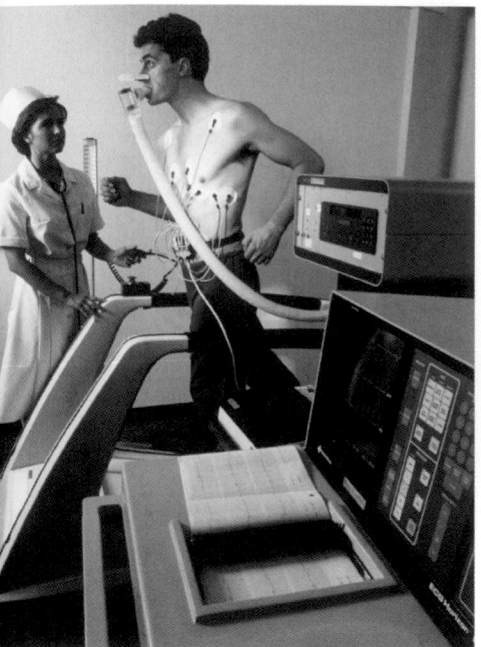

Figure 13.3
Maximal oxygen consumption can be estimated by measuring oxygen uptake while running to exhaustion on a treadmill. (© Julian Calder/Stone)

Endorphins Compounds that act as natural euphorics and reduce the perception of pain under certain stressful conditions.

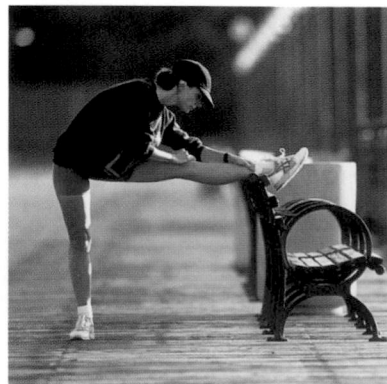

Figure 13.4
Stretching muscles to increase and maintain flexibility is an important component of any exercise regimen. (© David Madison/Stone)

Muscle Strength and Endurance Muscle strength and endurance enhance the ability to perform tasks such as pushing or lifting. In daily life, this could mean lifting a bag of groceries, unscrewing the lid of a jar, or shoveling snow from your driveway. Muscle strength and endurance are increased by repeatedly using muscles in activities that require moving against a resisting force. This type of exercise is called strength-training or resistance-training exercise and includes activities such as weight lifting.

Flexibility Flexibility determines range of motion—how far one can bend and stretch muscles and ligaments. If flexibility is poor, you cannot easily bend to tie your shoes or stretch to remove packages from the car. Regularly moving the limbs, neck, and torso through their full ranges of motion helps increase and maintain flexibility (Figure 13.4).

Body Composition Individuals who are physically fit have a greater proportion of lean body tissue than unfit individuals of the same body weight. In general, women have more stored body fat than men. For adult women, the desirable percent of body fat is 20 to 30% of total weight; in adult men, the desirable percent is about 12 to 20%.[1] The proportions of lean and fat tissue that are associated with optimal fitness also depend on individual goals. For example, a competitive athlete such as a runner or a weight lifter may need a higher percentage of lean tissue than a nonathlete to be considered fit. With aging, lean body mass decreases in both men and women, and there is an increase in the percentage of body fat even if body weight remains the same. Some of this change may be prevented by physical activity (see Chapter 16).

The Health Benefits of Exercise

In addition to making the tasks of everyday life easier, maintaining fitness through regular activity offers many health benefits. A regular exercise program makes it easier to maintain a healthy body weight; helps maintain muscles, bones, and joints; and reduces the risk of osteoporosis. It can also help to prevent or delay the onset of cardiovascular disease, hypertension, diabetes, and colon cancer. It can prevent depression and improve mood, sleep patterns, and overall outlook on life. Exercise stimulates the release of chemicals called **endorphins**, which are thought to be natural tranquilizers that play a role in triggering what athletes describe as an "exercise high." In addition to causing this state of exercise euphoria, endorphins are thought to aid in relaxation; improve mood, pain tolerance, and appetite control; and reduce anxiety.

Weight Management The more energy one expends, the more food one can consume while maintaining a healthy weight. Exercise makes weight management easier because it increases energy needs. During exercise, energy expenditure can rise well above the resting rate and some of this increase persists for many hours after activity slows.[2] Exercise can also boost energy expenditure through its effect on body composition. Exercise increases lean tissue mass and because, even at rest, lean tissue uses more energy than fat tissue, this increases basal energy needs. The combination of increased energy output during exercise, the rise in expenditure that persists after exercise, and the increase in basal needs can have a major impact on total energy expenditure. Besides increasing energy needs, exercise also promotes the loss of body fat and slows the loss of lean tissue that occurs with energy restriction. This makes exercise an essential component of any weight-reduction program.

Cardiovascular Disease Exercise reduces the risk of cardiovascular disease.[3] Aerobic exercise strengthens the heart muscle, thereby reducing resting heart rate and decreasing the heart's workload. Exercise may also lower blood pressure and increase HDL cholesterol levels in the blood, both of which reduce the risk of cardiovascular disease.[4]

Diabetes People with excess body fat are more likely to develop diabetes. By keeping body fat within the normal range, aerobic exercise can decrease one's risk of developing diabetes. Physical activity that includes both aerobic exercise and strength training is also important in the treatment of type 2 diabetes because it can increase the sensitivity of tissues to insulin.[5] Exercise can reduce or eliminate the need for medication to maintain normal blood glucose levels. People with diabetes should develop exercise programs with the help of physicians and dietitians, because exercise can affect dietary and medication needs.

Osteoporosis and Joint Disorders Exercise reduces the risk of osteoporosis. One of the causes of bone loss, like muscle loss, is lack of use; therefore, weight-bearing exercise such as walking, running, and aerobic dance can increase peak bone mass and prevent bone loss (see Chapter 10). Exercise can also benefit individuals with arthritis because the strength and flexibility promoted by exercise help arthritic joints move more easily.

Cancer Individuals who exercise regularly may be reducing their cancer risk. There is some evidence that exercise reduces breast cancer risk, but it is not clear whether risk reduction is related to exercise intensity, duration, or the age at which the exercise is performed.[6] The evidence that exercise reduces colon cancer risk is stronger; active individuals are less likely to develop colon cancer than their sedentary counterparts.[7] When evaluating the impact of exercise on cancer risk, diet and other lifestyle factors also must be carefully considered. It is possible that some of the effect is due to the fact that people who exercise regularly are more likely to have healthier overall diets and lifestyles.

Exercise Recommendations

Most adult Americans do not exercise regularly; 25% get no physical activity at all during their leisure time.[8] Because exercise reduces the incidence of chronic disease, public health guidelines recommend an increase in activity level[9,10] (Figure 13.5). The most recent recommendations, made by the DRIs, advise Americans to engage in 60 minutes of moderate exercise every day.[2] This is an increase from previous recommendations of 30 minutes of moderate exercise on most days of the week. The recommendation was changed because this higher level of activity is associated with maintaining weight in the healthy BMI range and maximizing the other health benefits of exercise.

What Is Moderate Activity? The DRIs define moderate activity as the equivalent of walking or jogging at a rate of 3 to 4 mph, cycling leisurely, or swimming slowly. Sixty minutes of moderate exercise each day, in addition to the activities of daily living, is considered an "active" physical activity level (see Chapter 7, Table 7.4). An "active" level can be achieved with less than 60 minutes of exercise if the exercise is more intense, for example, jogging at 6 mph or greater or swimming at a moderate to fast pace. Individuals who perform moderate exercise for more than 2.5 hours per day or more intense exercise for more than 1 hour per day are categorized as "very active." This higher activity level increases energy needs but does not necessarily enhance other health benefits. Individuals who perform no exercise other than the activities of daily living are considered "sedentary," and those who perform less than an hour of moderate activity fit into the "low active" category. This amount of exercise is not enough to promote the maintenance of a healthy body weight or fully reduce chronic disease risk.

Components of a Good Exercise Regimen A well-planned exercise regimen includes aerobic exercise, which raises heart rate and therefore improves cardiorespiratory fitness; stretching, which promotes and maintains flexibility; and strength training, which increases the strength and endurance of specific muscles. Each exercise session should begin with a warm-up, such as mild stretching and easy jogging, to increase blood flow to the muscles, and end with a cool-down period, such as walking or stretching, to help prevent muscle cramps and slowly reduce heart rate.

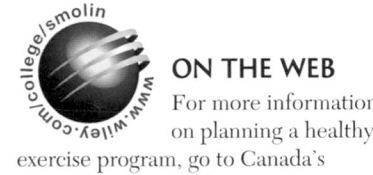

ON THE WEB
For more information on planning a healthy exercise program, go to Canada's physical activity guide at
www.hc-sc.gc.ca/hppb/paguide/
the Washington Coalition for Promoting Physical Activity at
www.beactive.org/
or
www.healthfinder.gov/

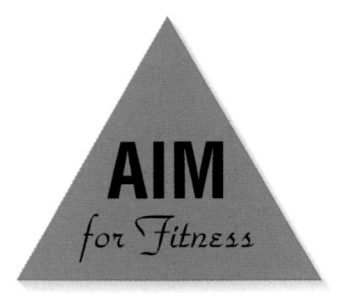

▲ Be physically active each day

Figure 13.5
The Dietary Guidelines, 2000, recommends that Americans "Be physically active each day."

Aerobic exercise, such as walking, bicycling, skating, swimming, or jogging, should be performed for 30 to 60 minutes (depending on intensity) most days of the week. For optimal benefit, aerobic activity should be performed at a level that raises the heart rate to 60 to 90% of its maximum (see Figure 13.2). For a sedentary individual beginning an exercise program, mild exercise such as walking can raise the heart rate into this range. As fitness improves, exercisers must perform more intense activity to raise their heart rates to this level.

To improve and maintain flexibility, stretching exercises should be done at least three days a week. Muscles should be stretched to a position of mild discomfort and held for 10 to 30 seconds. Each stretch should be repeated three to five times.

Strength training, such as weight lifting, should be done two to three days a week at the start of an exercise program, and two days a week after the desired strength has been achieved. Each session should include a minimum of 8 to 10 exercises that train the major muscle groups. Each exercise should be repeated 8 to 12 times. The weights should be heavy enough to cause the muscle to be near exhaustion after the 8 to 12 repetitions. Increasing the amount of weight lifted will increase muscle strength, whereas increasing the number of repetitions will improve endurance.

A good way to maintain or improve fitness is to use the Activity Pyramid shown in Figure 13.6.[11] The base of the pyramid includes suggestions on how to increase

The Activity Pyramid

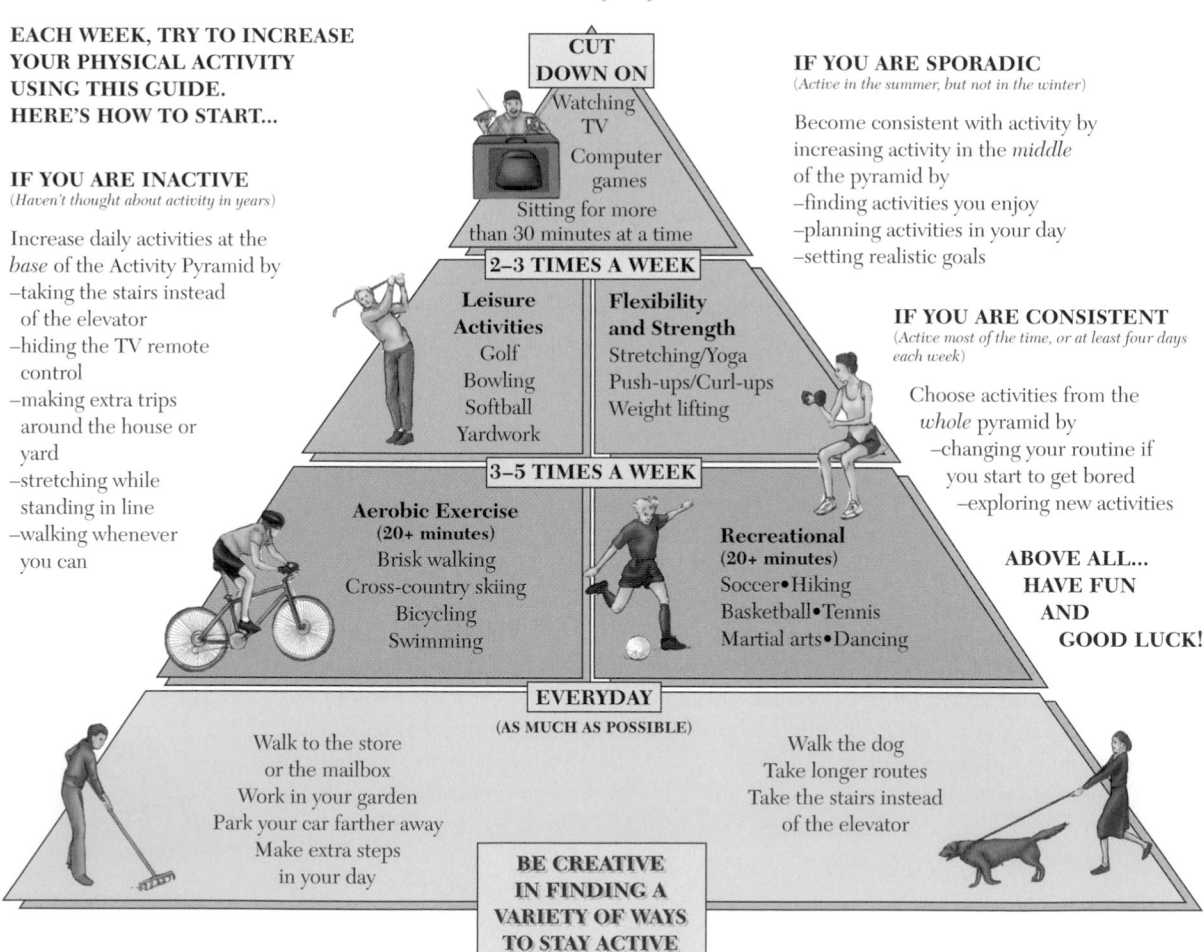

EACH WEEK, TRY TO INCREASE YOUR PHYSICAL ACTIVITY USING THIS GUIDE. HERE'S HOW TO START...

IF YOU ARE INACTIVE
(*Haven't thought about activity in years*)

Increase daily activities at the *base* of the Activity Pyramid by
–taking the stairs instead of the elevator
–hiding the TV remote control
–making extra trips around the house or yard
–stretching while standing in line
–walking whenever you can

CUT DOWN ON
Watching TV
Computer games
Sitting for more than 30 minutes at a time

2–3 TIMES A WEEK

Leisure Activities
Golf
Bowling
Softball
Yardwork

Flexibility and Strength
Stretching/Yoga
Push-ups/Curl-ups
Weight lifting

3–5 TIMES A WEEK

Aerobic Exercise (20+ minutes)
Brisk walking
Cross-country skiing
Bicycling
Swimming

Recreational (20+ minutes)
Soccer•Hiking
Basketball•Tennis
Martial arts•Dancing

EVERYDAY
(AS MUCH AS POSSIBLE)

Walk to the store or the mailbox
Work in your garden
Park your car farther away
Make extra steps in your day

Walk the dog
Take longer routes
Take the stairs instead of the elevator

BE CREATIVE IN FINDING A VARIETY OF WAYS TO STAY ACTIVE

IF YOU ARE SPORADIC
(*Active in the summer, but not in the winter*)

Become consistent with activity by increasing activity in the *middle* of the pyramid by
–finding activities you enjoy
–planning activities in your day
–setting realistic goals

IF YOU ARE CONSISTENT
(*Active most of the time, or at least four days each week*)

Choose activities from the *whole* pyramid by
–changing your routine if you start to get bored
–exploring new activities

ABOVE ALL... HAVE FUN AND GOOD LUCK!

Figure 13.6
The Activity Pyramid. A pyramid shape can be used to build an active lifestyle. At the base are activities of daily living. Layered over this base are aerobic exercise, recreational activities, and strength and flexibility exercises. At the very top are sitting activities that should be less frequent.

the amount of activity in your daily life. At the next level of the pyramid are aerobic exercises, such as walking and swimming, that focus on improving heart and lung function. The third level of the pyramid includes exercises to build flexibility and strength, such as golf or yoga. As with the Food Guide Pyramid, the narrow tip of the Activity Pyramid focuses on things that should be limited, such as watching TV and playing computer games.

Exercise Recommendations for Children Children and adolescents should spend at least 60 minutes per day in developmentally appropriate exercise.[2,9] Activity for young children should be intermittent, with periods of moderate to vigorous activity lasting 10 to 15 minutes or more along with periods of rest and recovery. To promote this amount of exercise, a variety of enjoyable activities should be stressed and competition de-emphasized (Figure 13.7). Modern lifestyles, however, do not promote activity in children; television, computers, and video games are often chosen over physical activity. Studies have found that children who watch four or more hours of television per day have more body fat and a greater body mass index than those who spend fewer than two hours watching TV.[12] Children who learn to enjoy physical activity are more likely to be active adults who maintain a healthy body weight and have a lower risk of cardiovascular disease, diabetes, osteoporosis, and certain types of cancer. Learning by example is always best. Children who have physically active parents are the leanest and the fittest.

Getting Started Almost everyone can participate in some form of exercise, no matter where they live, how old they are, or what physical limitations they have. Exercise classes are taught in nursing homes. Heart patients, amputees, the blind, and those confined to wheelchairs compete in athletic events. You are never too old to exercise, and it is never too late to start.

Changing Behavior Incorporating exercise into day-to-day life may require a behavior change, and changing behavior is not easy. The first step in beginning an exercise program is to recognize the reasons for not exercising and identify ways to overcome them. Many people avoid exercise because they do not enjoy it, feel they have to join an expensive health club, have little motivation to do it alone, or find it inconvenient and uncomfortable. Finding a type of exercise that is enjoyable, a time that is realistic and convenient, and a place that is appropriate and safe are important first steps in adopting an exercise program. Riding your bike to class or work rather than driving or taking the bus, taking a walk on your lunch break, and enjoying a game of catch or tag with your children are all effective ways to increase your everyday activity level. The goal is to gradually make lifestyle changes that increase physical activity. Behavioral strategies such as those listed in Table 13.1 may help promote regular exercise (see *Critical Thinking*: Incorporating Exercise Sensibly).

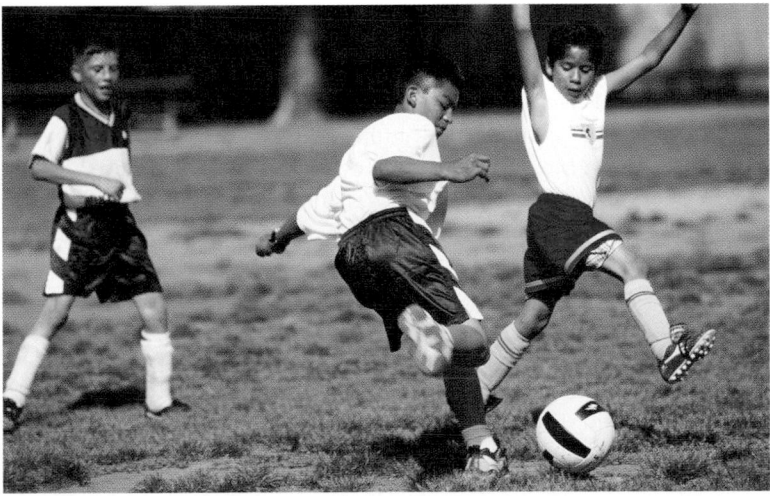

Figure 13.7
Children who participate in and enjoy exercise are more likely to have active lifestyles as adults. (© Carl Schneider/ FPG International)

Table 13.1 *Suggestions for Beginning and Maintaining an Exercise Program*

- Start slowly—Instead of planning to run 3 miles a day, plan to start with a nightly walk around the block.
- Make it fun—Choose activities you enjoy and find a partner with whom to exercise.
- Set specific attainable goals—"I will walk for 20 minutes after dinner 3 days a week."
- Make it convenient—Plan to walk early in the morning, during your lunch hour at work, or after dinner.
- Include a warm-up and a cool-down period—Warming up helps prepare muscles, ligaments, and tendons for the upcoming activity and mobilizes fuel supplies needed for activity. A cool-down helps to prevent muscle cramps.
- Challenge your strength or endurance once or twice a week and do moderate workouts on other days.
- Don't overdo it. Some days you may do more and others less, include some rest each week.
- Record your progress—Keep a record of your activity so you can track your progress and keep yourself motivated.
- Listen to your body—Symptoms such as lightheadedness or chest pain or pressure require immediate attention. Paying attention to more minor aches and pains allows you to stop before an injury occurs.
- Reward yourself—Plan to reward yourself when you succeed at your goal: a new book, a movie.

Exercising Safely Safety should be a concern in planning any exercise regimen. Before beginning, everyone should check with their physician to be sure that their plans are safe considering their medical history. Then the location and environment for exercise can be considered. Busy work schedules often force people to exercise in the dark early-morning or evening hours. Exercisers who use the street for walking or jogging should wear light-colored, reflective clothing so they can be seen by motorists. Exercising with a partner is safer and more enjoyable.

Weather conditions can be a health concern. Physical activity produces heat, which normally is dissipated to the environment, partly by the evaporation of sweat. When the environmental temperature is high, heat is not efficiently transferred to the environment, and when humidity is high, sweat evaporates slowly, making it difficult to cool the body. Thus, exercise should be reduced or curtailed in hot and humid conditions. Cold environments can also pose problems for the outdoor exerciser. In general, cold does not impair exercise capacity, but the numbing of exposed flesh and the bulk of extra clothing can cause problems for joggers and bicyclists. Because exercise produces heat, clothing must allow for evaporation of sweat while providing protection from the cold. For swimmers, cold water can cause performance to deteriorate.

Balancing Exercise Frequency, Intensity, and Duration The combination of exercise frequency, duration, and intensity that is needed to achieve a desired fitness level depends on the needs, goals, and abilities of the exerciser. For example, a short intense workout may suit the needs of some individuals, while others prefer a longer workout at a lower intensity. Some may choose to exercise for a longer period once during the day, while others may spread their exercise throughout the day in shorter bouts of 15-minute duration. Also, what is best for a middle-aged man trying to reduce his risk of chronic disease is different from what is best for an 18-year-old college basketball player, and different still from what is best for an octogenarian trying to continue living independently. Young healthy athletes may require very intense activity to obtain a training effect. Older adults and those who have not previously been active can increase their fitness by exercising at a lower intensity if the duration and frequency of exercise are increased.

Don't Overdo It To improve muscle strength and cardiorespiratory fitness, the body must be stressed and respond to the stress by increasing muscle size and strength. Initially, training can cause fatigue and weakness, but during rest the body rebuilds to become stronger. If not enough rest occurs between exercise sessions, there is no time to regenerate so fitness and performance do not improve. In athletes, excessive training can lead to **overtraining syndrome**, which involves emotional, behavioral, and physical symptoms that persist for weeks to months. It is caused by repeatedly training without sufficient rest to allow for recovery. The most common symptom of overtraining syndrome is fatigue that limits workouts and is felt even at rest. Some athletes experience a decrease in appetite and weight loss as well as muscle soreness, increased frequency of viral illnesses, and increased incidence of injuries. They may become moody, easily irritated, depressed, have altered sleep patterns, or lose their competitive desire and enthusiasm. Overtraining syndrome occurs only in serious athletes who are training extensively, but rest is essential for anyone working to increase fitness.

Overtraining Syndrome A collection of emotional, behavioral, and physical symptoms that occurs when training without sufficient rest persists for weeks to months.

CRITICAL THINKING

Incorporating Exercise Sensibly

Nicole recently turned 45 years old. Her promise to herself was to get back in shape. She is 5 feet 4 inches tall and weighs 140 pounds. Although her body mass index is still within the healthy range, she is about 5 pounds above her usual weight. Currently Nicole exercises about once a month and then suffers from a few days of sore muscles. When the family goes on outings, she finds that she tires long before her husband and children. She would like to lose a few pounds, but more importantly she would like to increase her strength and endurance.

Before beginning her exercise program she checks with her physician, who agrees that she should increase her exercise and recommends that she do stretching and strength-training exercises as well as aerobic activities that keep her heart rate between 60 and 90% of her maximum.

What is 60 to 90% of Nicole's maximum heart rate?

▼

Maximum heart rate = 220 − age = 220 − 45 = 175 beats per minute

60% of maximum = 175 × 0.6 = 105 beats per minute

90% of maximum = 175 × 0.9 = 158 beats per minute

She should exercise at a heart rate of at least 105 but no more than 158 beats per minute.

Nicole's fitness plan

Nicole decides she will exercise for 90 minutes a day, 5 days a week. Her plan is to join a gym and stretch and lift weights for 30 minutes, followed by an hour of aerobic exercise outdoors, either jogging or riding a bicycle in the park.

After three days on her new schedule, a rainy day keeps Nicole indoors. She realizes that her family is angry and feels abandoned. She hasn't been able to do an hour of aerobics without exceeding her maximum heart rate. She is tired, sore, and ready to give up and accept the fact that she is never going to get back in shape.

Where did she go wrong?

▼

It is unrealistic to go from exercising one day a month to five days a week. It is unnecessary to lift weights five days a week to gain muscle strength, and Nicole can reach 60 to 90% of her maximum heart rate by walking quickly. A more achievable goal might be to start with a stretching routine at home, a 20-minute walk at a moderate rate three days a week, and two weight-lifting sessions per week. As her strength and endurance improve, she can increase the frequency, intensity, and duration of her exercise. Nicole needs to find a time for her exercise program that will fit into her daily routine. She also needs to set alternative plans for bad weather and allow time for a warmup before her work out and a cool-down after she is finished.

Nicole's new fitness plan

She continues her gym membership but only goes to lift weights two evenings a week, when her husband can watch the children. As a treat afterwards she relaxes in the whirlpool before returning home. She shares her story with a friend at work, and they decide to walk during their lunch hour three days a week. As her fitness improves, she adds walks in the morning before her family gets up and is able to walk faster, keeping her heart rate between 60 and 90% of maximum.

How has this change in activity affected Nicole's energy needs?

▼

Before her activity change, Nicole's physical activity level was in the sedentary category. Her estimated energy requirement (EER) can be calculated using the equations on the inside cover of this text.

For an adult woman:

$$EER = 354 - (6.91 \times age\ in\ yrs) + PA\,[(9.36 \times weight\ in\ kg) + (726 \times height\ in\ m)]$$

$$Age = 45\ yrs,\ PA = 1.0,\ weight = 63.6\ kg,\ height = 1.63\ meters$$

$$EER = 354 - (6.91 \times 45) + 1.0[(9.36 \times 63.6) + (726 \times 1.63)]$$
$$= 1822\ kcalories/day$$

Nicole now walks for 45 minutes 3 days a week. At the gym twice a week, she does 30 minutes of weight lifting and light calisthenics. On average she therefore engages in a little over 3 hours of moderate physical activity per week, or about 30 minutes per day. This increases her physical activity level from the sedentary to the low active category and increases her EER as follows:

$$EER = 354 - (6.91 \times age\ in\ yrs) + PA[(9.36 \times weight\ in\ kg) + (726 \times height\ in\ m)]$$

$$Age = 45\ yrs,\ PA = 1.12,\ weight = 63.6\ kg,\ height = 1.63\ meters$$

$$EER = 354 - (6.91 \times 45) + 1.12\,[(9.36 \times 63.6) + (726 \times 1.63)\,]$$
$$= 2035\ kcalories/day$$

As Nicole's fitness level improves, she finds she has more energy and can increase her other activities. Within a few months, she finds she is getting the recommended 60 minutes per day of moderate activity putting her in the active category.

What is Nicole's EER now that she is in the active physical activity category?

▼

Answer:

• FUELING ACTIVITY

Just as an automobile engine runs on energy from gasoline, the body machine runs on energy from the carbohydrate, fat, and protein in food and body stores. These fuels are needed whether you are writing a letter, walking around the block, or running a marathon. But the amount of each of these nutrients that is used depends on the type of activity that is performed, how long it is performed, and the physical conditioning of the exerciser.

Energy for Activity

Carbohydrate, fat, and protein are the fuel sources for the body. But before they can be used to fuel activity, their energy must be converted into the high-energy compound ATP. ATP is the immediate source of energy for all body functions. In a resting muscle, there is enough stored ATP to sustain activity for a few seconds. As the ATP in muscle is used, enzymes break down another high-energy compound, called **creatine phosphate**, to replenish the ATP supply. As with ATP, the amount of creatine phosphate stored in the muscle at any time is small. During the first 10 to 15 seconds of exercise, the muscles use energy from the ATP and creatine phosphate that is stored there. But activity of longer duration requires that the body replenish ATP from the metabolism of the energy-yielding nutrients (Figure 13.8).

Creatine phosphate A compound found in muscle that can be broken down quickly to make ATP.

Converting Fuels to Energy

Carbohydrate, fat, and protein all can be used to produce ATP when oxygen is available. When no oxygen is available, only carbohydrate can be used, and although it produces ATP rapidly, it is not used efficiently. The availability of oxygen in muscle cells is determined both by how quickly the heart can pump blood from the lungs—where it picks up oxygen—to the muscle cells, and by the amount of hemoglobin in the blood, which determines how much oxygen the blood can carry.

Anaerobic metabolism or **anaerobic glycolysis** Metabolism in the absence of oxygen. In glycolysis, two molecules of ATP are produced from each molecule of glucose. Glucose is metabolized in this way when the blood cannot deliver oxygen to the tissues quickly enough.

Producing Energy from Carbohydrate The carbohydrate fuel used for exercise is glucose. It can be used as a fuel source whether or not oxygen is available at the cells. The glucose used to power muscle activity may come from glycogen inside the muscle or from glucose delivered via the bloodstream. The glucose delivered in the blood comes from that released by the liver or absorbed from the diet.

Lactic acid A compound produced from the breakdown of glucose in the absence of oxygen.

The first step of glucose metabolism does not require oxygen and is referred to as **anaerobic metabolism** or **anaerobic glycolysis**. It breaks down glucose to form the three-carbon compound pyruvate, releases electrons, and produces two molecules of ATP. When oxygen is unavailable, the metabolism of carbohydrate stops and the pyruvate and released electrons combine to form **lactic acid**. When oxygen is available, the pyruvate and electrons proceed through **aerobic metabolism**, producing carbon dioxide, water, and more ATP. Aerobic metabolism includes the con-

Aerobic metabolism Metabolism in the presence of oxygen. In aerobic metabolism, the conversion of pyruvate to acetyl CoA, the citric acid cycle, and the electron transport chain break down carbohydrates, fatty acids, and amino acids into carbon dioxide and water to produce ATP.

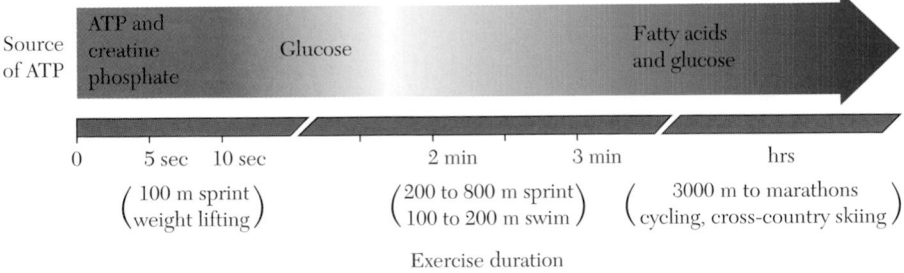

Figure 13.8

When exercise begins, ATP and creatine phosphate stored in the muscle provide ATP for muscle contraction. As creatine phosphate stores become depleted, anaerobic glycolysis, which breaks down glucose from the blood or from muscle glycogen, becomes the predominant source of ATP. After about 3 minutes, aerobic metabolism, which uses fatty acids and glucose to produce ATP, begins to predominate.

version of pyruvate to acetyl-CoA; the citric acid cycle, which breaks down acetyl-CoA, producing some ATP and releasing electrons; and the electron transport chain, which passes electrons down a chain of molecules to oxygen, releasing energy to make ATP. Aerobic metabolism produces ATP more efficiently than anaerobic metabolism. The same molecule of glucose that produces two molecules of ATP in anaerobic glycolysis can produce about 36 to 38 molecules of ATP when metabolized aerobically (Figure 13.9).

Producing Energy from Fat Fatty acids from the diet and from body stores can be used for fuel, but oxygen must be present. Stored fat accounts for 90% of stored energy in a typical adult. It provides a lightweight, energy-dense fuel supply.

During exercise, triglycerides in adipose tissue and in muscle fibers are broken down into fatty acids and glycerol. Fatty acids from adipose tissue are released into the blood and are then taken up by the muscle cells. Inside the muscle cell, fatty acids from triglycerides within the muscle and those delivered by the blood must be transported into the mitochondria to produce ATP. Inside the mitochondria, fatty acids are broken into two-carbon units to form acetyl-CoA. Acetyl-CoA is metabolized via the citric acid cycle and electron transport chain to produce ATP, carbon dioxide, and water (see Figure 13.9).

The rate at which fatty acids can be used by the muscle depends on how quickly they can be delivered to mitochondria in the muscle cells. To enter the mitochondria, fatty acids must be activated with the help of **carnitine**, a molecule produced in the body from the amino acids lysine and methionine. Carnitine supplements are marketed to athletes with the promise that they will enhance the utilization of fat

Carnitine A molecule synthesized in the body that is needed to transport fatty acids and some amino acids into the mitochondria for metabolism. Supplements of carnitine are marketed to athletes to enhance performance.

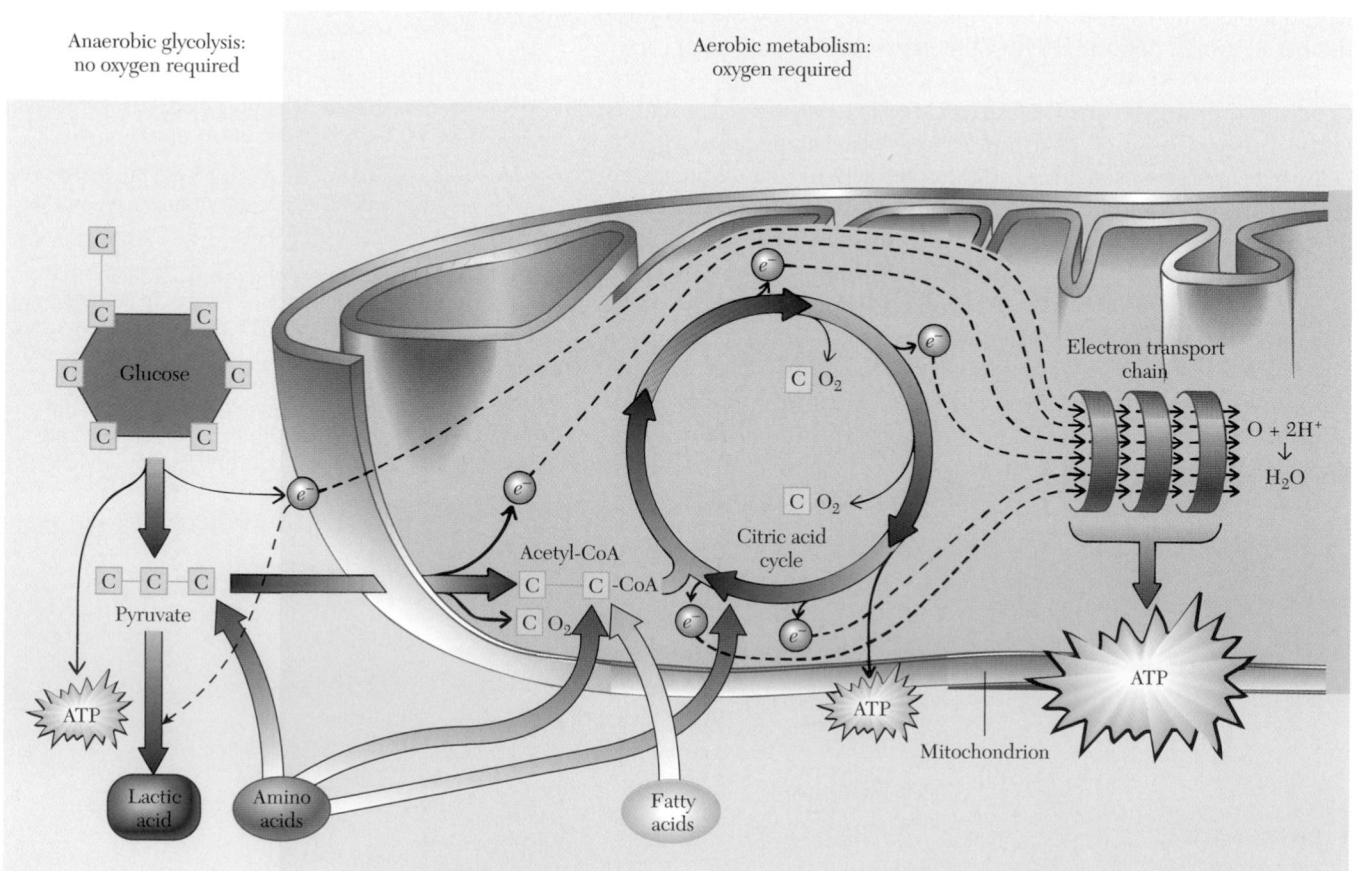

Figure 13.9

In the absence of oxygen, ATP is produced by the anaerobic glycolysis of glucose. When oxygen is present, ATP is produced by aerobic metabolism of glucose, fatty acids, and amino acids.

during exercise. This would spare carbohydrate and thereby allow athletes to exercise for a longer time before exhaustion. Carnitine is made by the cells, so it does not need to be supplied in the diet to ensure the efficient use of fatty acids. Studies that examined the effect of carnitine supplements found that they did not affect the utilization of fat as fuel during exercise or improve exercise endurance.[13]

Producing Energy from Protein Protein can be broken down into amino acids which can also be used to produce ATP when oxygen is available. For most exercise, protein contributes only a small percentage of the energy used. It becomes an important source of energy only when exercise continues for many hours. Endurance exercise increases the use of amino acids both as an energy source and for glucose production via gluconeogenesis to maintain blood glucose levels.

Which Fuels Are Used?

The intensity and duration of exercise and the conditioning of the exerciser can affect the contributions that carbohydrate and fat make as fuels for energy production. Fuel utilization in turn affects how long exercise can continue before **fatigue** sets in.

Exercise Intensity and Duration While at rest, the cardiorespiratory system is able to deliver adequate blood, and, consequently, oxygen, to the muscles to allow aerobic metabolism of fatty acids. During exercise, however, the delivery of oxygen to tissues can become limiting, causing the muscle cells to rely at least partially on the anaerobic metabolism of glucose. Generally, the more intense the exercise, the more the muscles rely on glucose to provide energy (Figure 13.10). Thus, with low-intensity exercise, the cardiorespiratory system can deliver enough oxygen to muscles to allow aerobic metabolism to predominate, so fatty acids and some glucose are used as fuel. When intensity reaches the VO_2 max, most energy is derived from anaerobic metabolism of glucose.

Fatigue The inability to continue an activity at an optimal level.

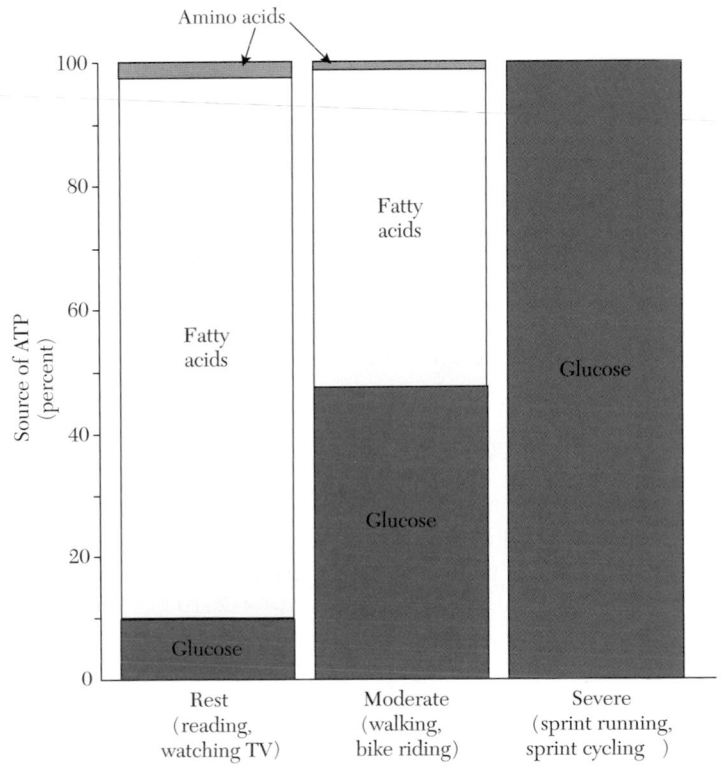

Figure 13.10

As exercise intensity increases, the proportion of energy supplied by carbohydrate increases. During exercise the total amount of energy expended is greater than at rest. (Adapted from Horton, E. S. Effects of low-energy diets on work performance. *Am. J. Clin. Nutr.* 35:1228–1233, 1982.)

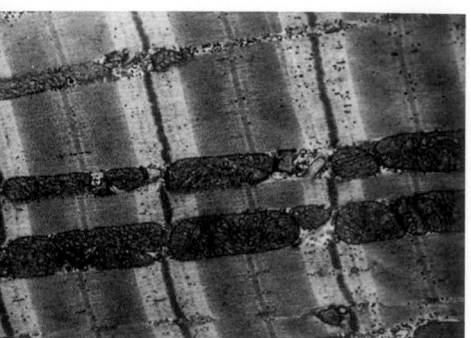

Figure 13.11
Mitochondria are the site of aerobic metabolism. In trained athletes, the number of mitochondria in muscle cells increases. (Don W. Fawcett/ Visuals Unlimited)

ATP production via anaerobic metabolism is rapid, but it is not efficient. When glucose is metabolized anaerobically, muscle glycogen is used 18 times faster than when the glucose is fully oxidized by aerobic metabolism. Because the amount of stored glycogen available to produce glucose during exercise is limited, intense exercise cannot be continued for long periods of time before glycogen is depleted and the athlete becomes fatigued. Lower-intensity exercise can continue for longer periods because aerobic metabolism predominates after the first few minutes of exercise. Aerobic metabolism is more efficient and uses both glucose and fatty acids for energy. However, even aerobic metabolism uses some glucose, so if exercise continues long enough, glycogen stores will eventually be depleted.

Exercise fatigue occurs because of the depletion of liver and muscle glycogen and the accumulation of lactic acid. When athletes run out of glycogen, they experience a feeling of overwhelming fatigue that is sometimes referred to as "hitting the wall" or "bonking." During intense exercise that relies on anaerobic metabolism, fatigue occurs quickly because of rapid glycogen depletion and also because pyruvate is converted to lactic acid (see Figure 13.9). The accumulation of lactic acid changes the acidity of the muscle, reducing its ability to contract. Lactic acid also inhibits the mobilization of fat from adipose tissue, forcing the muscle to rely more on glycogen, thus depleting it even faster. When exercise stops and oxygen is available again, lactic acid can be either carried away by the blood to other tissues to be broken down or metabolized aerobically in the muscle. After intense exercise, a mild cool-down, such as walking, may allow enough blood flow to the muscle to remove built-up lactic acid and prevent cramping.

The Conditioning of the Exerciser Training with repeated bouts of aerobic exercise causes physiological changes that increase the amount of oxygen that can be delivered to and used by the muscle cells. The heart becomes larger and stronger so that the stroke volume is increased. The number of capillary blood vessels in the muscles increases so that blood is delivered to muscles more efficiently. And the total blood volume and number of red blood cells expands, increasing the amount of hemoglobin so more oxygen can be transported to the cells. Training also causes changes at the cellular level that affect the ability of cells to use different types of fuel to produce ATP. There is an increase in the ability to store glycogen, and there is an increase in the number and size of muscle-cell mitochondria (Figure 13.11). Because aerobic metabolism occurs in the mitochondria, this increases the cell's capacity to burn fatty acids to produce ATP. The use of fatty acids spares glycogen, which delays the onset of fatigue. Because trained athletes store more glycogen and use it more slowly, they can sustain aerobic exercise for longer periods at higher intensities than can untrained individuals. A conditioned athlete can also exercise at a higher percentage of her VO_2 max before lactic acid begins to accumulate.

Living and working at high altitudes, where the atmosphere contains less oxygen, also causes adaptations that improve the capacity of the cardiorespiratory system to deliver oxygen. Therefore, endurance athletes often train at high altitudes to enhance their aerobic capacity.

• EXERCISING GOOD NUTRITION

Adequate nutrition is essential to performance whether you are a marathon runner or a mall walker. For every exerciser, diet must provide sufficient energy from the appropriate sources to fuel activity, protein to maintain muscle mass, micronutrients to allow utilization of the energy-yielding nutrients, and water to transport nutrients and cool the body.

Energy Needs

The amount of energy needed for an activity depends on the duration and frequency of the activity, as well as the characteristics of the exerciser, and even his location. For a casual exerciser, the energy needed for activity may increase energy expenditure by a few hundred kcalories a day. For an endurance athlete, such as a marathon runner, the energy needed for training may increase expenditure by 2000 to 3000 kcalories per day. Some athletes require 6000 kcalories a day to maintain body weight. In general, the more intense the activity, the more energy it requires (see Table 13.2 and Appendix K). For example, riding a bicycle involves less work than running the same distance and therefore requires less energy. The more time spent exercising, the more energy it requires. Riding a bicycle for 60 minutes requires six times the energy needed to ride for 10 minutes. The body weight of the exerciser is another factor in determining energy needs. Moving a heavier body requires more energy than moving a lighter one. Therefore, it requires less energy for a 120-pound woman to walk for 5 minutes than it does for a 250-pound woman.

There are also some special considerations that affect the energy needs for activity. For example, because of the buoyancy of adipose tissue, the energy required for

Table 13.2 *Energy Expended for Activity*

Activity	Energy (kcal/hr)						
Body Weight (kg) (lb)	50 110	57 125	64 140	70 155	77 170	84 185	91 200
Aerobics (moderate)							
Male	455	480	506	531	556	582	607
Female	394	413	433	453	472	492	511
Biking (12 mph)							
Male	380	401	422	443	464	486	507
Female	329	345	361	378	394	410	427
Bowling (recreational)							
Male	121	128	135	142	148	155	162
Female	105	110	115	121	126	131	136
Dancing (recreational)							
Male	364	384	405	425	445	465	486
Female	315	331	346	362	378	393	409
Gardening (moderate)							
Male	303	320	337	354	371	388	405
Female	263	276	289	302	315	328	341
Golf (walking w/bag)							
Male	425	448	472	496	519	543	567
Female	368	386	404	422	441	459	477
Jumping rope (moderate)							
Male	595	628	661	694	727	760	793
Female	515	540	566	591	617	642	668
Running (10 min/mi)							
Male	619	653	688	722	757	791	826
Female	536	562	589	615	642	669	695
Sitting at ease							
Male	73	77	81	85	89	93	97
Female	63	66	69	72	76	79	82
Swimming (moderate)							
Male	364	384	405	425	445	465	486
Female	315	331	346	362	378	393	409
Walking (15 min/mi)							
Male	257	271	285	300	314	328	342
Female	222	233	244	255	266	277	288
Weight lifting							
Male	340	359	378	397	415	434	453
Female	294	309	323	338	352	367	382

Source: ESHA Research, Salem, Ore.

an overfat individual to swim may be less than his lean counterpart. But if a lean individual and an obese individual were in the weightlessness of space, it would require no more energy for one to leap across the room than for the other. There are also special circumstances that affect the amount of energy an individual needs for daily activity. A paraplegic in a wheelchair may have lower energy needs because many of the major muscles in the body are always inactive. At the other extreme, a person with the form of cerebral palsy that causes uncontrolled muscle movements may have higher energy needs because the muscles never stop moving.

Weight Loss and Weight Gain

Body weight and composition can affect exercise performance. Athletes involved in activities where small, light bodies offer an advantage—for instance, ballet, gymnastics, and certain running events—may restrict energy intake to maintain a low body weight. While a slightly leaner physique may be beneficial, dieting to maintain an unrealistically low weight may threaten health and performance. An athlete who needs to lose weight should do so in advance of the competitive season to prevent the restricted diet from affecting performance. The general guidelines for healthy weight loss should be followed—reduce energy intake, increase activity, and change the behaviors that led to weight gain (see Chapter 7). To preserve lean body mass and enhance fat loss, weight loss should be at a rate of about 1/2 to 2 pounds per week. This can be accomplished by reducing total energy intake by 200 to 500 kcalories per day and increasing exercise.

In adolescents, athletic activities combined with weight loss may affect the maturation process and increase the risks of developing anorexia or bulimia.[14] Female ballerinas and gymnasts who maintain extremely low levels of body fat often have delayed menses and delayed sexual maturation. Sporadic diets that severely restrict fluid and energy intake are sometimes used by athletes in sports such as wrestling to fit into a specific weight class. Such dietary practices may be detrimental to health and performance (see discussion of fluid needs in the following section).[15]

In sports such as football in which being large is advantageous, an increase in body weight may be desirable. To gain weight, 500 to 1000 extra kcalories per day should be consumed.[16] Strength training should accompany weight gain to promote an increase in lean tissue.

Carbohydrate, Fat, and Protein Needs

The source of dietary energy is often as important as the amount of energy. In general, the diets of physically active individuals should contain the same proportion of carbohydrate, fat, and protein as is recommended to the general public—about 45 to 65% of total energy as carbohydrate, 20 to 35% of energy as fat, and 10 to 35% of energy as protein.[16]

Carbohydrate Carbohydrate is needed to maintain blood glucose levels during exercise and to replace glycogen stores after exercise. The amount recommended for athletes depends on the total energy expenditure, type of sport, gender, and environmental conditions but ranges from 6 to 10 grams per kilogram of body weight per day.[16] Most of the carbohydrate in the diet should be complex carbohydrates from whole grains and starchy vegetables, with some naturally occurring simple sugars from fruit and milk. These foods provide vitamins, minerals, phytochemicals, and fiber as well as energy.

Fat Dietary fat supplies fat-soluble vitamins and essential fatty acids as well as an important source of energy. Body stores of fat provide enough energy to support the needs of even the longest endurance events. For physically active individuals, diets providing 20 to 25% of energy as fat have been recommended to allow adequate carbohydrate intake and facilitate weight management where necessary.[16] No performance benefits have been associated with diets containing less than 15% fat. Excess dietary fat is unnecessary and excess energy consumed as fat, carbohydrate, or protein can cause an increase in body fat.

Protein Protein is essential to maintain muscle mass and strength. But eating extra protein does not produce bigger muscles. Muscle growth is stimulated by exercise, not by increasing protein intake (Figure 13.12). Supplements of synthetic anabolic steroids are often used by athletes to increase muscle mass; however, these are illegal and have dangerous side effects (see *Off the Shelf*: Ergogenic Hormones: Anything for an Edge).

A diet that contains the RDA for protein (0.8 g/kg) provides adequate protein for most active individuals. Competitive athletes participating in endurance and strength sports may require more protein. In endurance events such as marathons, protein is used for energy and to maintain blood glucose so these athletes may benefit from 1.2 to 1.4 grams of protein per kilogram per day. Strength athletes who require amino acids to synthesize new muscle proteins may benefit from 1.4 to 1.8 grams per kilogram per day.[17] This amount, however, is not much more than the amount contained in the typical American athlete's diet. For example, an 85-kg man consuming 3000 kcalories, 18% of which is from protein, would be consuming 135 g, or 1.6 g of protein per kg body weight.

Protein supplements are often marketed with the promise of enhancing muscle growth or improving performance. There are hundreds of protein powders and bars available. Although certain types of exercise do increase protein needs, the protein provided by expensive supplements will not meet an athlete's needs any better than the protein found in a balanced diet.

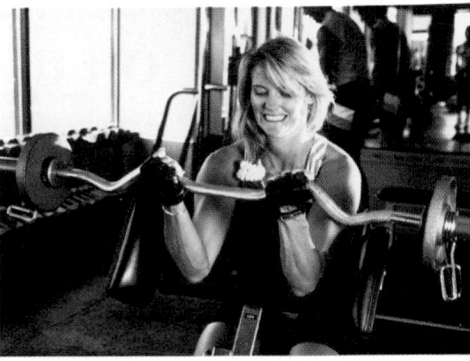

Figure 13.12
Building muscle requires time and hard work. It is accomplished by increasing resistance exercise, not by simply increasing protein intake.
(© Alan Becker/The Image Bank)

Vitamin and Mineral Needs

Adequate vitamin and mineral intake is essential to optimal performance. In addition, the need for some micronutrients may be increased by exercise. However, most athletes who consume a balanced diet that meets energy needs also meet their micronutrient needs. For example, B vitamins are involved in energy production and are required for red blood cell synthesis, protein synthesis, and tissue repair and maintenance. These processes are increased during exercise, therefore exercise may increase the need for B vitamins.[18] However, because energy expenditure is increased, a diet that provides enough food to meet energy needs will most likely provide sufficient B vitamins. Athletes who consume lowfat diets or restrict their intake of energy or specific food groups may be at risk for micronutrient deficiencies. Iron and calcium are of particular concern.

Iron For most individuals, exercise does not increase iron needs. However, in athletes, particularly female athletes, a reduction in the amount of stored iron is common. If this situation progresses to anemia, it can impair exercise performance as well as reduce immune function and affect other physiologic processes.[19]

Poor iron status may be caused by inadequate iron intake, increased iron needs, increased iron losses, or a redistribution of iron due to exercise training. Dietary iron intake may be limited in athletes who are attempting to keep body weight low, or in those who consume a vegetarian diet and therefore do not eat meat—an excellent source of readily absorbable heme iron. Iron needs may be increased in athletes because exercise stimulates the production of red blood cells, so more iron is needed for hemoglobin synthesis. Iron is also needed for the synthesis of muscle myoglobin and the iron-containing proteins needed for ATP production in the mitochondria. An increase in iron losses with prolonged training, possibly because of increased fecal, urinary, and sweat losses, also contributes to increased iron needs in athletes.[16] Iron balance may also be affected by the breaking of red blood cells from impact in events such as running (foot-strike hemolysis) or by the contraction of large muscles. How-

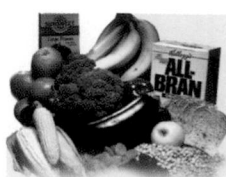

Off the Shelf
Ergogenic Hormones: Anything for an Edge

"Citius, altius, fortius"—faster, higher, stronger—the Olympic motto. For as long as there have been competitions, athletes have yearned for something—anything—that would give them the competitive edge. Everything from desiccated liver to bee pollen and shark cartilage has been used as an ergogenic aid. The majority of these potential performance boosters have turned out to offer more of a psychological edge than a physiological one. However, when athletes from Eastern European nations began to dominate international strength events, the athletic community became aware of the muscle-building effects of large doses of anabolic steroids. Finally, an effective ergogenic aid had been found. Since then, anabolic steroids have been determined to be dangerous, and their use is now illegal. They are regulated as controlled substances under the 1988 Anti-Drug Abuse Act and the Anabolic Steroids Act of 1990. However, the effectiveness of these hormones in building muscle and improving performance has led athletes to experiment with these and other hormones in the endless search for a competitive edge.

Anabolic Steroids The term "anabolic steroid" refers to steroid hormones that accelerate protein synthesis and growth. The anabolic steroids used by athletes are synthetic versions of the human steroid hormone testosterone. Natural testosterone stimulates and maintains the male sexual organs and promotes the development of bones and muscles and the growth of skin and hair. The synthetic testosterone used by athletes has a greater effect on muscle development and bone, skin, and hair than it does on sexual organs. When synthetic testosterone is taken in conjunction with exercise and an adequate diet, muscle mass increases. However, these drugs also make the body think testosterone is being produced, and therefore the body reduces its production of natural testosterone. Without natural testosterone, the sexual organs are not maintained; this leads to testicular shrinkage and a decrease in sperm production. In adolescents, the use of synthetic testosterone causes bone growth to stop and height to be stunted. Anabolic steroid use may also cause oily skin and acne, water retention in the tissues, yellowing of the eyes and skin, coronary artery disease, liver disease, and sometimes death. Users may have psychological and behavioral side effects such as violent outbursts and depression, possibly leading to suicide. The dangers of steroid use are increased by the fact that they are illegal, so their manufacturing and distribution procedures are not regulated. Users can never be sure of the potency and purity of what they are taking.

Steroid Precursors Steroid precursors are compounds that can be converted into steroid hormones in the body. These include androstenedione, androstenediol, DHEA, norandrostenediol, and norandrostenedione. Steroid precursors can be sold legally as dietary supplements.

The best known of the steroid precursors is androstenedione, often refered to as "andro." It is a precursor to testosterone that is marketed as an alternative to anabolic steroids to increase levels of testosterone. Andro has been used for years by bodybuilders, but it was launched to public prominence when professional baseball player Mark McGwire announced his use of it during the 1998 major league baseball season when he hit 70 home runs to break the league's single-season home-run record. McGwire has subsequently stopped using andro, and it has been banned by the International Olympic Committee, the National Collegiate Athletic Association, and all major international sports federations except major league baseball.

Despite andro's popularity, few studies had until recently examined whether it actually increases blood testosterone or produces anabolic effects. Recent studies have not conclusively answered these questions. One study found no difference between the increase in muscle strength, muscle mass, and lean body mass and the decrease in fat mass that occurred in subjects taking andro and subjects in a control group not taking the supplement after 8

---

ever, this rarely causes anemia because the breaking of red blood cells stimulates the production of new ones.[20]

Some athletes experience a condition known as sports anemia, which is a temporary decrease in hemoglobin concentration that occurs during exercise training. This is an adaptation to training that does not seem to impair delivery of oxygen to tissues. It occurs when blood volume expands to increase oxygen delivery, but the synthesis of red blood cells lags behind the increase in plasma volume.

Calcium Calcium is needed to maintain blood calcium levels and promote and maintain bone density, which in turn reduces the risk of osteoporosis. In general, exercise—particularly weight-bearing exercise—increases bone density, thereby reducing the risk of osteoporosis. However, in female athletes with extremely low body weight and fat, calcium status can be at risk.

Female athletes who strive to reduce body weight and fat to improve performance, achieve an ideal body image, and meet goals set by coaches, trainers, or par-

weeks of resistance training.[1] In addition to failing to demonstrate anabolic effects, this study found that andro caused a decrease in HDL cholesterol, suggesting that it may increase the risk of heart disease. In a second study, a similar dose of andro was found to raise testosterone levels, but the researchers did not measure muscle strength or mass.[2] Another study found that andro had no anabolic effect on muscle protein metabolism.[3]

As with any dietary supplement, the fact that andro is available over the counter does not guarantee its safety. Scientists still do not know how much androstenedione is absorbed, where it acts, or how much is converted to testosterone. It is not known whether androstenedione will cause testicular shrinkage, liver disease, and heart disease like anabolic steroids. In addition, the purity of what is sold commercially is unknown, unregulated, and probably quite variable.

Peptide Hormones Peptide hormones now compete with anabolic steroids on the black market of alleged tissue-building performance-enhancing drugs. The ability of manufacturers to produce peptide hormones through genetic engineering has increased their availability not only to individuals with conditions that require these hormones, but also to athletes.

Human growth hormone is a peptide hormone that is produced naturally by the pituitary gland. It is important for tissue building during growth in children. Growth hormone produced by genetic engineering is used to treat children who are small due to growth hormone deficiency. Growth hormone levels decline with age and may account for some of the decrease in fat-free mass that occurs with age. In adults, growth hormone maintains lean tissue, stimulates fat breakdown, increases the number of red blood cells, and boosts heart function. This hormone is appealing to athletes because it increases muscle protein synthesis. But despite these physiological effects, the ergogenic benefits of growth hormone among athletes remain unproven.[4] Increases in muscle strength obtained from resistance training were not improved by growth hormone. Growth hormone did cause a greater increase in fat-free mass, but there was no increase in incorporation of amino acids into muscle, suggesting that the increase was likely due to fluid retention or accumulation of connective tissue.[5] Prolonged use of growth hormone can cause heart dysfunction and high blood pressure as well as excessive growth of some body parts, such as hands, feet, and facial features. Growth hormone is on the World Anti-Doping Association's list of banned substances.

Another peptide hormone that is popular among endurance athletes is erythropoietin, known as EPO. Natural erythropoietin is produced by the kidneys and stimulates stem cells in the bone marrow to differentiate into red blood cells. Genetically engineered EPO is used to treat anemia due to kidney disease, chemotherapy, HIV infection, and blood loss. It can enhance the performance of endurance athletes by increasing the ability to transport oxygen to the muscles. It therefore increases VO_2 max and aerobic performance and spares glycogen. However, too much EPO can cause production of too many red blood cells, which can lead to excessive blood clotting, heart attacks, and strokes. The International Olympic Committee banned EPO in 1990 after it was linked to the death of more than a dozen cyclists.[6]

[1]King, D. S., Sharp, R. L., Vukovich, M. D., et al. Effect of oral androstenedione on serum testosterone and adaptations to resistance training in young men: a randomized controlled trial. *JAMA* 28:2020–2028, 1999.

[2]Leder, B. Z., Longcope, C., Catlin, D. H., et al. Oral androstenedione administration and serum testosterone concentrations in young men. *JAMA* 283:779–782, 2000.

[3]Rasmussen, B. B., Volpi, E., Gore, D. C., and Wolfe, R. R. Androstenedione does not stimulate muscle protein anabolism in young healthy men. *J. Clin. Endocrinol. Metab.* 85:55–59, 2000.

[4]Jenkins, P. J. Growth hormone and exercise. *Clin. Endocrinol.* 50:683–689, 2000.

[5]Frisch, H. Growth hormone and body composition in athletes. *J. Endorcinol. Invest.* 22(Suppl):106–109, 1999.

[6]Ritter, S. K. Faster, higher, stronger. *Chem. Engineering News* 77:42–52, 1999.

---

ents are at risk for a syndrome of interrelated disorders referred to as the **female athlete triad**. This syndrome includes disordered eating, **amenorrhea**, and osteoporosis (Figure 13.13). The extreme energy restriction that occurs in eating disorders can create a physiological condition similar to starvation and contribute to menstrual abnormalities. High levels of exercise can also affect the menstrual cycle by increasing energy demands or causing hormonal changes.[21] When combined, energy restriction and excessive exercise can contribute to amenorrhea—the delayed onset or absence of menses in women. Amenorrhea results in low estrogen levels and interferes with calcium balance, consequently causing reductions in bone mass and bone-mineral density. Low estrogen levels reduce calcium absorption and, when combined with poor calcium intake (common in female athletes and females in general), lead to premature bone loss, failure to reach maximal peak bone mass, and an increased risk of stress fractures. Neither adequate dietary calcium nor the increase in bone mass caused by weight-bearing exercise can compensate for bone loss due to low estrogen levels. If menses resume, bone loss can at least be partially reversed, but whether these athletes are at greater risk of osteoporosis later in life is not known.[22]

Female athlete triad The combination of disordered eating, amenorrhea, and osteoporosis that occurs in some female athletes, particularly those involved in sports in which low body weight and appearance are important.

Amenorrhea Delayed onset of menstruation or the absence of three or more consecutive menstrual cycles.

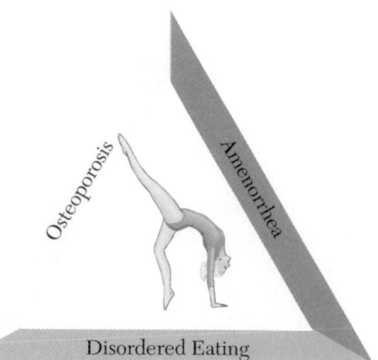

Figure 13.13

The female athlete triad includes disordered eating, amenorrhea, and osteoporosis. Women with these conditions typically have low body fat and may experience multiple or recurrent stress fractures. This syndrome is more common in women who are perfectionists, highly competitive, and have a low self-esteem.

Fluid Needs

Water is needed to regulate body temperature and to transport both oxygen and nutrients to the muscles and waste products away from the muscles. Failure to consume adequate fluids to replace water lost through the lungs and in sweat can be critical to even the most casual exerciser.

Water and the Regulation of Body Temperature During exercise, heat production increases as exercise intensity increases. If heat cannot be lost from the body, body temperature rises and exercise performance as well as health may be jeopardized. The ability to dissipate the heat generated during exercise is affected by the hydration status of the exerciser as well as by environmental conditions. At rest in a temperate environment, an individual loses about 1.2 liters (about 4.5 cups) of water per day, or 50 ml per hour, through evaporation from the skin and lungs. Exercise in a hot environment can increase this more than tenfold. Adequate fluids should be consumed before, during, and after exercise. Since thirst is not a reliable indicator of fluid needs, it is important for anyone exercising to schedule regular fluid breaks. Strenuous exercise should be avoided if the weather is too hot or too humid.

Consequences of Inadequate Hydration Inadequate body water leads to thermal distress, which includes dehydration, heat cramps, heat exhaustion, and heat stroke. Dehydration occurs when water loss is great enough for blood volume to decrease, thereby reducing the ability to deliver oxygen and nutrients to exercising muscles. Even mild dehydration—a body water loss of 1% of body weight—can impair exercise performance (Figure 13.14). Heat cramps are involuntary cramps and spasms in the muscles involved in exercise. They occur when water and salt have been lost during extended exercise and are caused by an imbalance of the electrolytes sodium and potassium at the muscle cell membranes. Heat exhaustion occurs when fluid loss causes blood volume to decrease so much that it is not possible to both cool the skin and deliver oxygen to active muscles. It is characterized by a rapid weak pulse, low blood pressure, fainting, profuse sweating, and disorientation. Heat stroke, the most serious form of thermal distress, occurs when the temperature regulatory center of the brain fails. Heat stroke is characterized by elevated body temperature, hot dry skin, extreme confusion, and unconsciousness. It requires immediate medical attention.

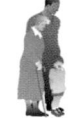

Children are at a greater risk for dehydration and thermal distress because they produce more heat, are less able to transfer heat from muscles to the skin, take longer to acclimatize to heat, and sweat less than adults. To reduce risks, children should rest periodically in the shade, consume fluids frequently, and limit the intensity and duration of activities on hot days. Also, children lose more heat in cold environments than adults because they have a greater surface area per unit of body weight. Therefore, they are more prone to **hypothermia**.

Hypothermia A condition in which body temperature drops below normal. Hypothermia depresses the central nervous system, resulting in the inability to shiver, sleepiness, and eventually coma.

Weight Loss through Dehydration Athletes involved in sports with weight classes, such as wrestling and boxing, sometimes go to unhealthy extremes to keep body weight down so they can compete in lower weight classes (competing at the

Figure 13.14

As the level of dehydration increases, exercise performance declines. (Adapted from Saltin, B., and Castill, D. I. Fluid and electrolyte balance during prolonged exercise. In *Exercise, Nutrition, and Energy Metabolism.* Horton, E. S., and Tergung, R. I., eds. New York: Macmillan, 1988.)

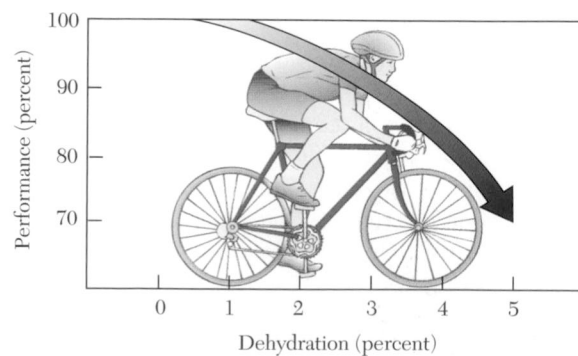

high end of a weight class is thought to give an advantage over smaller opponents).[15] Frequently, this rapid weight loss is accomplished by dehydration, through such practices as vigorous exercise, fluid restriction, wearing vapor-impermeable suits, and using hot environments such as saunas and steam rooms. More extreme measures include vomiting and the use of diuretics and laxatives. These practices can be dangerous and even fatal. They may reduce performance and can adversely affect heart and kidney function, temperature regulation, and electrolyte balance.[23]

Fluid Intake for Exercise Anyone exercising should consume extra fluids. Typically, however, exercising individuals ingest amounts of fluids that are equal to only about one- to two-thirds of the amount lost in sweat.[24]

How Much to Consume? To ensure adequate hydration, exercisers should drink generous amounts of fluid in the 24 hours before the exercise session and about 2 cups of fluid 2 hours before exercise. On warm days, athletes should consume an additional 1 to 2 cups about 30 to 60 minutes before exercising.[25] During exercise, whether casual or competitive, exercisers should try and drink enough water to prevent weight loss (Figure 13.15). Drinking at least 3 to 6 ounces of fluid every 10 to 15 minutes should maintain adequate hydration. Typically athletes do not consume enough fluids during exercise to balance fluid losses. To restore lost water after exercise, each pound of weight lost should be replaced with 16 to 24 ounces (1 to 1.5 pounds) of fluid (Table 13.3).

What to Consume? For most exercisers, water is the best fluid to drink.[25] Alcohol and beverages containing caffeine, such as colas, iced tea, and coffee should be avoided. They act as diuretics and therefore reduce body fluids rather than increase them. For exercise lasting longer than 60 minutes, beverages containing a small amount of carbohydrate are recommended. For extreme events lasting 8 hours or more, fluids with carbohydrate and electrolytes are needed.

Exercise depletes body carbohydrate stores. Consuming carbohydrate in a beverage helps to maintain blood glucose levels, therefore providing a source of glucose for the muscle and delaying fatigue. Beverages containing 4 to 8 grams of carbohydrate per 100 ml of fluid are best. This is the amount of carbohydrate found in popular sports beverages such as Gatorade and Powerade (see *Off the Label*: Sports Beverages and Bars: What Are You Really Getting?). Although not necessary, these beverages are also suitable for exercise lasting less than an hour. As the amount of carbohydrate in the beverage increases, the rate at which the solution leaves the stomach decreases. Therefore, beverages containing larger amounts of carbohydrate, such as fruit juices and soft drinks, are not recommended unless they are diluted with an equal volume of water.

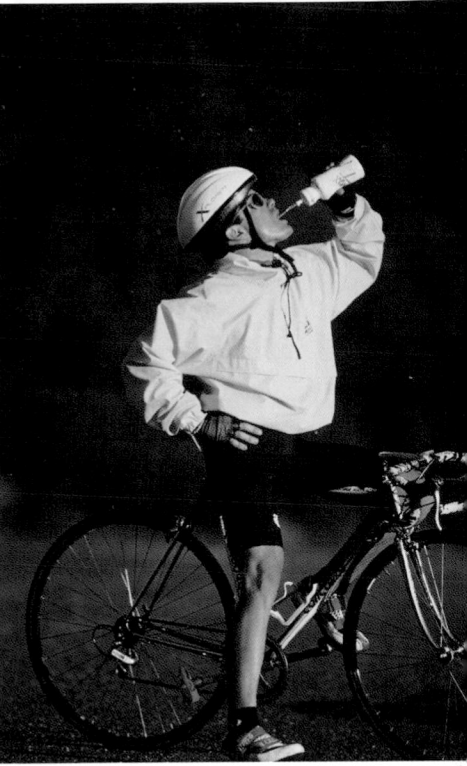

Figure 13.15
Fluids should be consumed before, during, and after exercise. (© Karl Weatherly/Corbis)

Table 13.3 *Recommended Fluid Intake for Exercise*

Before Exercise

Begin exercise well hydrated by consuming generous amounts of fluid in the 24 hours before exercise.

Consume about 2 cups of fluid 2 hours before exercise.

During Exercise

Consume at least 3 to 6 ounces of fluid every 15 minutes.

For exercise lasting less than 60 minutes, water is the best fluid.

For exercise lasting longer than 60 minutes, consuming a fluid containing about 6% carbohydrate may improve endurance.

For exercise lasting longer than 8 hours, a fluid containing carbohydrate and electrolytes may be beneficial.

After Exercise

Begin fluid replacement immediately after exercise.

Consume 16 to 24 ounces of fluid for each pound of weight lost.

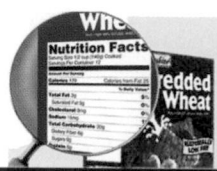

Off the Label
Sports Beverages and Bars: What Are You Really Getting?

Exceed, Gatorade, Power Burst, Power Bar. . . . Beverages and bars claim to provide you with that extra boost that makes your workout more satisfying or your performance more competitive. They are marketed to people at all levels of activity, from strollers to professional athletes. Can they enhance your exercise program? Their benefits depend on what your individual needs are and why you want to consume them. Read labels carefully to be sure your ergogenic snack won't slow you down.

Sports Beverages Fluids before, during, and after exercise are important to prevent dehydration, and sports drinks claim to be the fluid you need for exercise. A glance at the label finds that sports drinks are really water, sugar, and salt. Most of what exercisers lose in sweat is water—so the best beverage to replace it is water. Because small amounts of minerals, including sodium, are also lost in sweat, many sports drinks are marketed with the promise of replacing these lost electrolytes. However, during everyday workouts and most athletic events only small amounts are lost in sweat, and these are easily replaced from foods eaten during the next meal. Although electrolyte replacement is physiologically unnecessary even for events lasting as long as a marathon, the amount of sodium in the typical sports drink is not harmful. In addition, the sodium may improve the taste and therefore increase the amount of fluid

consumed as well as increase the rate of fluid absorption.[1]

The sugar in sports drinks is included to help maintain blood glucose. For moderate exercise such as a 20-minute jog, 40 minutes at the gym, or a brisk walk through the park, glucose-containing beverages offer no advantage over a water bottle filled at the drinking fountain. And they may be counterproductive if the goal of exercise is losing weight. A typical sports drink contains about 50 kcalories per cup, so drinking a 16-ounce bottle at the gym will replace about half of the 200 kcalories expended during your 40-minute ride on the stationary bicycle.

For exercise of longer duration (60 minutes or more), consuming glucose does help to maintain blood glucose and has been shown to increase endurance. To be effective, the drink should contain 10 to 20 grams of glucose in an 8-ounce serving. Less than this may not enhance performance, and more may delay stomach emptying and cause abdominal cramps. The ingredient list shows you the source of the carbohydrate. Most provide glucose, but some beverages contain short chains of glucose molecules called glucose polymers. These leave the stomach more quickly than the same amount of glucose but have not been shown to offer any additional performance benefit.[2]

Other sports beverages use fructose instead of glucose, but studies have shown that there is no advantage over glucose in terms of stomach emptying or perfor-

mance, and fructose is more likely to cause gastric distress. If fructose is tolerated, fruit juice diluted with an equal volume of water will provide the same amount of carbohydrate as a sports drink at about half the cost.

For most activities, sports drinks provide no performance or health advantages over plain water, but if a flavored beverage is consumed more readily than plain water, their use may provide the benefit of enhanced fluid intake.

Sports Bars Another type of "sports food" is the sports bar. There are many different types that vary in composition and in the promises they make. Some are high in carbohydrate and are advertised to optimize performance. Others are higher in protein and are advertised to build lean muscle, reduce body fat, increase strength, and speed recovery. All are marketed as a snack that can be eaten before, during, or after exercise.

If you are choosing a sports bar as a precompetition meal, read the label and choose one that provides about 300 kcalories—60 to 70% of kcalories as carbohydrate, 10 to 25% of kcalories as fat, and 10 to 20% of kcalories as protein. Use the total kcalories and grams of total carbohydrate, total fat, and protein to calculate the percent of energy from each (see figure). A bar that meets these recommendations can also be eaten during an activity to prevent hunger and maintain blood glucose. Bars that are lower in carbohydrate and higher

Small amounts of minerals, including sodium and chloride, are lost in sweat, but sweat consists mostly of water. Therefore, for most activities, replacing electrolytes is not a primary concern. The amounts of sodium and other minerals lost in sweat during exercise lasting even as long as 5 hours are not enough to affect health or performance and can easily be replaced by food eaten after the exercise has stopped. Only in extremely long events lasting 8 hours or more, such as ultramarathons or Ironman triathalons, are there significant losses of sodium and other minerals in the sweat. If, during one of these endurance events, an athlete were to drink water without electrolytes, the water would dilute the sodium remaining in the blood. When the blood is diluted, it signals the brain to stop the thirst sensation and stimulates the production of urine by the kidneys, increasing water loss and resulting in dehydration. The consumption of fluids containing electrolytes will prevent blood from becoming too diluted. It is recommended that these ultraendurance athletes include 0.5 to 0.7

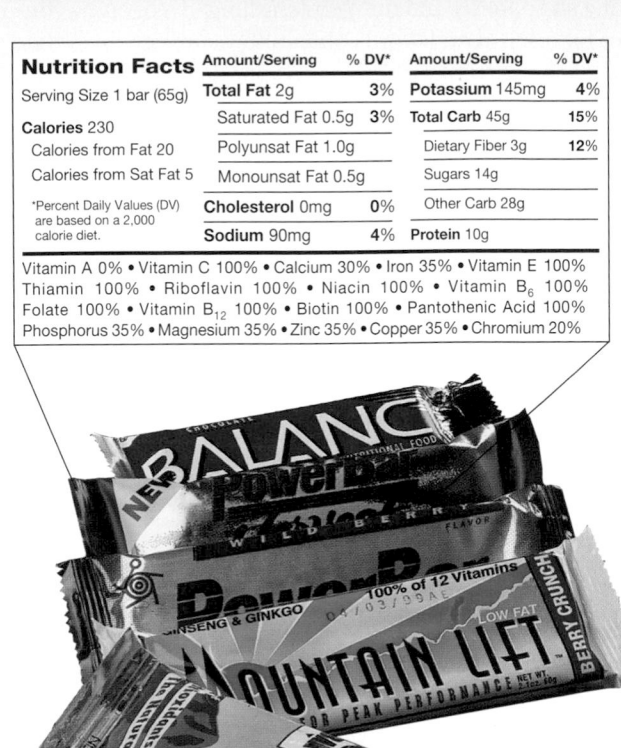

Nutrition Facts	Amount/Serving	% DV*	Amount/Serving	% DV*
Serving Size 1 bar (65g)	Total Fat 2g	3%	Potassium 145mg	4%
Calories 230	Saturated Fat 0.5g	3%	Total Carb 45g	15%
Calories from Fat 20	Polyunsat Fat 1.0g		Dietary Fiber 3g	12%
Calories from Sat Fat 5	Monounsat Fat 0.5g		Sugars 14g	
*Percent Daily Values (DV) are based on a 2,000 calorie diet.	Cholesterol 0mg	0%	Other Carb 28g	
	Sodium 90mg	4%	Protein 10g	

Vitamin A 0% • Vitamin C 100% • Calcium 30% • Iron 35% • Vitamin E 100%
Thiamin 100% • Riboflavin 100% • Niacin 100% • Vitamin B_6 100%
Folate 100% • Vitamin B_{12} 100% • Biotin 100% • Pantothenic Acid 100%
Phosphorus 35% • Magnesium 35% • Zinc 35% • Copper 35% • Chromium 20%

(George Semple)

in protein or fat may not significantly increase blood glucose and will take longer to digest, possibly causing stomach upset. Such a bar is fine for a snack during the day but is not the best choice immediately before or during exercise.

Although sports bars look and often taste like candy bars, comparing the labels will show that most are lower in fat than candy bars; provide more fiber; and contain vitamin C, vitamin E, calcium, iron, magnesium, copper, zinc, and a host of B vitamins. The percent Daily Value of many of these vitamins and minerals may not be included in the Nutrition Facts portion of the label, but the nutrients added will appear in the ingredient list. Whether sports bars are eaten before, during, or after an activity, they are just one part of the total diet and should not take the place of the whole grains, fresh vegetables and fruits, dairy products, and meats or meat substitutes that make up a healthy diet.

The greatest advantage of sports bars is convenience. They are pre-portioned, ready to eat, and transportable. If having a compact, individually wrapped bar that will fit in a pocket or bicycle pack means the difference between consuming this food or no snack at all, they can be beneficial. They provide carbohydrate, protein, fat, and many micronutrients, but they don't provide fluid. If you choose to use these bars, eat them with plenty of water. Sports beverages and sports bars may also provide a psychological edge if the consumer believes they will enhance performance.

[1]Senay, L. C. Water and electrolytes during physical activity. In *Nutrition in Exercise and Sport*, 3rd ed. Wolinski, I., ed. Boca Raton, Fla.: CRC Press, 1998. 257–276.

[2]Puhl, S. M., and Buskirk, E. R. Nutrient beverages for exercise and sport. In *Nutrition in Exercise and Sport*, 3rd ed. Wolinski, I., ed. Boca Raton, Fla.: CRC Press, 1998. 277–314.

gram of sodium per liter (1.2 to 1.8 g of sodium chloride per liter) in their rehydration drinks.[16] Consuming salt alone in pill form is unnecessary and dangerous because the salt will draw water away from the tissues and may cause dehydration, nausea, and vomiting. Therefore, the common belief that salt pills are necessary to replace the sodium lost in sweat and prevent dehydration is a misconception.

• FOOD AND DRINK FOR SPORT

For most of us, a trip to the gym requires no special nutritional planning beyond that needed to consume a balanced diet and plenty of water. For competitive athletes, however, foods eaten in preparation for competition may give or take away the extra seconds that can mean victory or defeat. Thus far, no magic pill that maximizes performance has been discovered, but there are a number of sound sports nutrition recommendations.

Glycogen Supercompensation: Maximizing Glycogen Stores

Glycogen supercompensation or **carbohydrate loading** A regimen of diet and exercise training designed to maximize muscle glycogen stores before an athletic event.

Larger glycogen stores allow exercise to continue for longer periods. Glycogen depletion is not an issue for most exercisers, but it is a problem for endurance athletes. One way to maximize glycogen stores before an event is to follow a regimen of **glycogen supercompensation** or **carbohydrate loading**. This involves depleting glycogen stores by exercising strenuously and then replenishing glycogen by consuming a high-carbohydrate diet for a few days before competition, during which time only light exercise is performed. The current practice is to taper down exercise during the six days before competition while progressively increasing the carbohydrate content of the diet to about 550 grams, or 70% of energy, during the three days before competition.[26] Since consuming this much carbohydrate can be difficult, there are a number of high-carbohydrate beverages available which contain 50 to 60 grams of carbohydrate in 8 fluid ounces. These should not be confused with sports drinks designed to be consumed during competition, which contain only about 10 to 20 grams of carbohydrate in 8 fluid ounces. A glycogen supercompensation regimen will increase glycogen stores 20 to 40% above the level that would be achieved on a typical diet.[27]

Although glycogen supercompensation is beneficial to endurance athletes, it will provide no benefit and even has some disadvantages for those exercising for periods less than 90 minutes. For every gram of glycogen in the muscle, 3 grams of water are also deposited. This water will cause a 2- to 7-pound weight gain and may cause some muscle stiffness. As glycogen is used, the water is released. This can be an advantage when exercising in hot weather, but the extra weight is a disadvantage for those competing in events of short duration.

Meals for Exercise

The goal of meals eaten before exercise is to maximize glycogen stores and provide adequate hydration while minimizing any digestion, hunger, and gastric distress. The wrong meal can hinder performance more than the right one can enhance it. The goal for meals after exercise is to replenish fluid, electrolyte, and glycogen losses.

The Pre-exercise Meal Meals before athleteic events should ensure that liver glycogen stores are full. Muscle glycogen is depleted by exercise, but liver glycogen is used to supply blood glucose and is depleted even during rest if no food is ingested. A high-carbohydrate meal eaten 2 to 4 hours before the event will fill liver glycogen stores. The meal should be high in carbohydrate (60 to 70%), low in fat (10 to 25%), and moderate in protein (10 to 20%), and provide about 300 kcalories—for example, a cup of pasta with tomato sauce and a slice of bread, or a turkey sandwich and a cup of juice. High-fiber foods should be avoided to prevent feeling bloated during competition. Spicy foods that could cause heartburn, and large amounts of simple sugars that could cause diarrhea, should also be avoided unless the athlete is accustomed to eating these foods.

In addition to providing nutritional clout, a meal that includes "lucky" foods may provide some athletes with an added psychological advantage. Some athletes find that in addition to a precompetition meal, a small high-carbohydrate snack or beverage consumed shortly before an event may enhance endurance.[27] Because foods affect people differently, athletes should test the effect of these meals and snacks during training, not during competition.

During Exercise For short-term activities food consumption is not necessary, but fluid consumption is important during all exercise. As discussed with fluid needs, consuming carbohydrate during intense exercise lasting more than an hour helps maintain blood glucose and enhance performance. Carbohydrate intake should begin shortly after exercise commences and should include glucose or a combination of glucose and fructose.[16] Fructose alone is not as effective and may cause diarrhea. Some athletes may prefer to obtain this carbohydrate in sports drinks but consuming a solid food snack with water is also effective.

Postexercise Meals When exercise ends, the body must shift from the catabolic state of breaking down glycogen, triglycerides, and muscle proteins for fuel to the anabolic state of restoring muscle and liver glycogen, depositing lipids, and synthesizing muscle proteins. The first priority for all exercisers is to replace fluid losses. For serious athletes, appropriate postexercise intake can replenish muscle and liver glycogen within 24 hours of the athletic event. To maximize glycogen replacement, a high-carbohydrate meal or drink should be consumed as soon as possible after the competition and again every 2 hours for 6 hours after the event. Ideally the meals should provide about 0.7 to 1.5 grams of carbohydrate per kg of body weight, which is about 50 to 100 grams of carbohydrate for a 70-kg (150 pound) person—the equivalent of two pancakes with syrup and a glass of fruit punch.[26] Approximately 600 grams of carbohydrate, or about 8 to 10 g per kg, should be consumed during the 24 hours after exercise. The consumption of fructose compared to glucose induces less muscle glycogen synthesis and more liver glycogen synthesis. This type of program to restore glycogen is critical for athletes who must perform again the following day, but is not necessary if the athlete has one or more days to replace glycogen stores before the next intense exercise.

• ERGOGENIC AIDS: DO SUPPLEMENTS ENHANCE ATHLETIC PERFORMANCE?

Athletes use a variety of **ergogenic aids** to enhance their performance. Anything designed to enhance performance can be considered an ergogenic aid; running shoes are mechanical aids; psychotherapy is a psychological aid; drugs are pharmacological aids. Many dietary supplements are also used as ergogenic aids (Figure 13.16). Although many of these supplements are expensive and most have not been shown to improve performance, athletes are vulnerable to their enticements. When considering the use of an ergogenic supplement, an athlete should first weigh the health risks against potential benefits; dietary supplements do not have to be proven safe or effective before they can be sold (see Chapter 12) (Table 13.4).

Ergogenic aids Anything designed to increase work or improve performance.

Vitamin Supplements

Many of the promises made about the benefits of vitamin supplements to athletes are extrapolated from their biochemical functions. For example, B vitamin supplements are promoted to enhance energy production because of their roles in muscle energy metabolism. Vitamins B_6, B_{12}, and folic acid are promoted for aerobic exercise because they are involved in the transport of oxygen to exercising muscle.

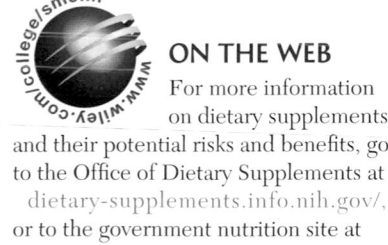

ON THE WEB

For more information on dietary supplements and their potential risks and benefits, go to the Office of Dietary Supplements at dietary-supplements.info.nih.gov/, or to the government nutrition site at www.nutrition.gov/

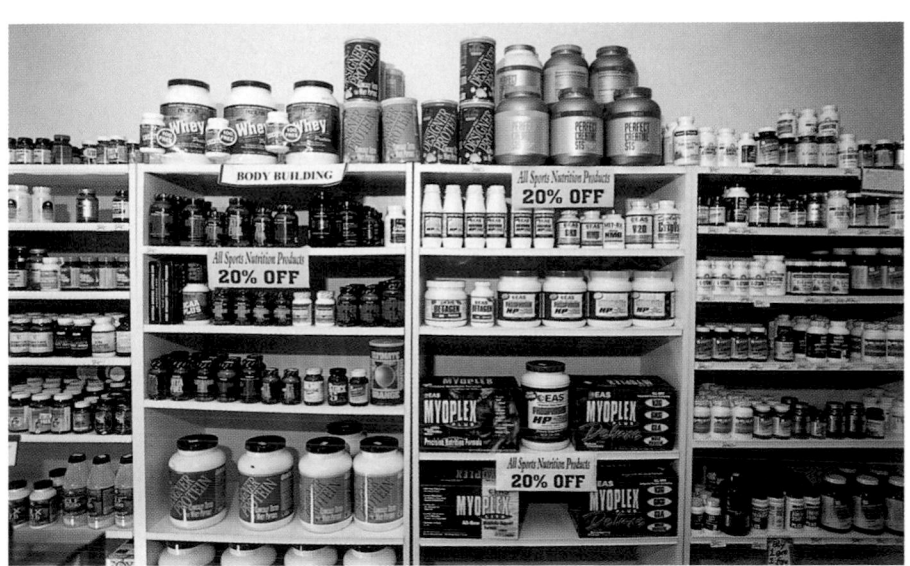

Figure 13.16

Many types of supplements are marketed to athletes as ergogenic aids. (George Semple)

Table 13.4 *Claims, Effectiveness, and Risks of Popular Ergogenic Aids*

Ergogenic Aid	Claim	Effectiveness	Risk
Androstenedione	Converted to testosterone, which increases muscle growth and strength.	No long-term human studies on safety or ergogenic effects.	May have risks similar to illegal steroids
Arginine, ornithine, and lysine	Causes the release of growth hormone, which stimulates muscle development and decreases body fat.	No increase in lean body mass observed with supplementation.	Reduced absorption of other amino acids. Diarrhea at high doses.
Bee pollen	Causes faster recovery from training workouts, which enables a higher level of training.	No evidence that it improves training level.	Allergic reactions.
Bicarbonate (sodium bicarbonate, baking soda)	Helps buffer lactic acid produced during exercise, thereby delaying fatigue.	Increases blood pH and may enhance performance and strength in intense anaerobic activities.	Bloating, diarrhea, and high blood pH
Branched chain amino acids (leucine, isoleucine, and valine)	Improves endurance and prevents fatigue.	Evidence of an effect is equivocal.	No toxicity reported.
Caffeine	Increases the release of fatty acids from adipose tissue, spares glycogen, and enhances endurance.	Increases endurance in some individuals.	Dehydration, nervousness, anxiety, insomnia, digestive discomfort, abnormal heartbeat
Carnitine	Enhances the utilization of fatty acids and spares glycogen.	No increase in fatty acid utilization or improvement in exercise performance found.	D, L-Carnitine and D carnitine forms can be toxic.
Chromium (chromium picolinate)	Increases lean body mass, decreases body fat, delays fatigue.	No effect on protein or lipid metabolism unless a chromium deficiency exists.	No toxicity reported in humans.
Creatine (creatine monohydrate)	Increases energy production and speeds recovery after high-intensity exercise	Increases muscle creatine and creatine phosphate synthesis after exercise, and enhances strength, performance, and recovery from high-intensity exercise.	Stomach pain.
DHEA (dehydro-epiandrosterone)	Builds muscles, burns fat, and delays chronic diseases associated with aging.	No proven benefits.	Acne, oily skin, facial hair, voice deepening, hair loss, mood changes, liver damage, and stimulation of existing cancers.
Ephedra (Chinese ephedra, Ma Huang)	Increases time to exhaustion, inhibits hunger, and stimulates energy expenditure and fat breakdown.	Causes selective fat breakdown with weight loss and increases time to exhaustion especially when taken with caffeine.	Dizziness, headache, gastrointestinal distress, irregular heartbeat, heart palpitations, heart attack, stroke, seizure, psychosis, and death.
Ginseng (*P. Ginseng* or Chinese ginseng)	Enhances performance	May improve muscle strength and aerobic capacity.	May increase the effects and side effects of other stimulants such as caffeine.
Glutamine	Increases muscle glycogen deposition following intense exercise, enhances immune function, and prevents the adverse effects of overtraining	Little evidence that it increases immune function, prevents the symptoms of overtraining, or increases glycogen synthesis.	No evidence of toxicity.
HMB (β-hydroxy β-methyl butyrate)	Increases ability to build muscle and burn fat in response to exercise.	Some evidence of an increase in lean body mass and strength.	No toxicity in animals, but little information in humans.
Medium-chain triglycerides (MCT)	Provides energy without promoting fat deposition; reduces muscle protein breakdown	No evidence of a benefit in humans.	None known.
Vanadium (vanadyl sulfate)	Aids insulin action; allows more rapid and intense muscle pumping for bodybuilders.	No evidence to support a benefit for bodybuilders.	Reduces insulin production.

These vitamins are indeed needed for energy metabolism, and a deficiency of one or more of these would interfere with energy production and impair athletic performance, but supplements aren't generally necessary. Because athletes must consume more food to meet energy needs, more vitamins are consumed as well, so a reasonably well-planned diet based on grains, vegetables, and fruits and including some meat and milk will provide enough of all the B vitamins to meet an athlete's needs.

The claims that athletes should consume supplements of vitamin E, vitamin C, and β carotene are based on their antioxidant functions. Exercise increases oxidative processes, and therefore increases the production of free radicals, which have been associated with fatigue during exercise.[28] It has been suggested that antioxidant supplements delay fatigue, but research examining the effect of exercise on the need for antioxidants is equivocal. There is no clear consensus on whether supplementation of antioxidant nutrients is beneficial.[18] As long as athletes do not consume antioxidant supplements in amounts that exceed the Tolerable Upper Intake Levels (ULs), there is little risk associated with their use; however, a diet that includes plenty of fruits and vegetables will ensure adequate intakes of these nutrients as well as provide other antioxidants.

Mineral Supplements

Some of the minerals advertised as endurance enhancers include chromium, vanadium, selenium, zinc, and iron.

Chromium supplements, as chromium picolinate, claim to increase lean body mass and decrease body fat. Chromium is needed for insulin action and insulin promotes protein synthesis. Therefore, adequate chromium status is likely to be important for lean tissue synthesis. The picolinate form is believed to be absorbed better than other forms of chromium. Studies in humans have not consistently demonstrated an effect of supplemental chromium picolinate on muscle strength, body composition, body weight, or other aspects of health.[29] Because no adverse effects have been associated with chromium intake from food or supplements, no UL has been established.[20] The safety of the picolinate form has been questioned because of studies in cell culture that suggest it may cause DNA damage.[30] Although human studies using the standard supplemental dose of chromium picolinate have not detected an increase in DNA damage, more work is needed to completely rule out any risk.[31]

Vanadium, usually as vanadyl sulfate, is another mineral marketed for its ability to assist the action of insulin. Vanadium supplements promise to increase lean body mass, but there is no evidence that they have an anabolic effect, and toxicity is a concern.[32] A UL of 1.8 mg per day of elemental vanadium has been set for adults age 19 and older. Selenium is marketed for its antioxidant properties and zinc for its role in protein synthesis and tissue repair, but neither of these supplements has been found to improve athletic performance in individuals with adequate mineral status. Iron is also marketed as an ergogenic mineral because it is needed for hemoglobin synthesis. If an iron deficiency exists, as it frequently does in female athletes, supplements can be of benefit.

Amino Acid Supplements

Amino acid supplements are also promoted to athletes. Supplements of some single amino acids affect hormone levels and muscle physiology, but their effect on exercise performance is unclear. Glycine supplements are promoted because glycine is a precursor to creatine, but it does not provide the ergogenic effects that creatine supplements do (see next section). The amino acids ornithine, arginine, and lysine are marketed with the promise that they will stimulate the release of growth hormone and, in turn, enhance the growth of muscles. Large doses of these amino acids have been shown to stimulate growth hormone release, but in the amounts typically supplemented, serum growth hormone levels are not increased and there is no effect on muscle growth or strength in weight lifters.[32]

Glutamine supplements promise to increase muscle glycogen deposition following intense exercise, to enhance immune function, and to prevent the adverse effects of overtraining such as fatigue and increased incidence of certain infections. Glutamine supplementation has not been found to increase glycogen synthesis.[33] Glutamine is important for immune system cells, and decreases in plasma glutamine have been reported following prolonged exercise; however, the effects of glutamine supplementation on immune function or the symptoms of overtraining are inconsistent.[32]

The branched-chain amino acids (leucine, isoleucine, and valine) are the predominant amino acids used for fuel during exercise. Supplements of these are promoted to improve performance in endurance athletes. Studies examining the effect of branched-chain amino acids on endurance performance have found that they do not enhance performance.[34]

There is little evidence to support the use of amino acid supplements by athletes, and in general these supplements are not recommended. High doses of individual amino acids may interfere with the absorption of other amino acids from the diet (see Chapter 6). In addition, there have been several reports of illness caused by contaminants in the supplements. Like any dietary supplement, amino acid supplements should be taken with caution and the risks weighed against potential benefits.

Other Ergogenic Aids

Substances that are not nutrients are also marketed as ergogenic aids. Creatine, bicarbonate, and caffeine are not nutrients but may have an ergogenic effect for some types of activity. Many herbal preparations, such as ginseng and ephedra, may have ergogenic effects, but in the case of ephedra, the risk of serious side effects is great. Many other supplements that are sold to enhance performance, such as bee pollen, wheat germ oil, brewer's yeast, ginseng, royal jelly, DNA, and RNA, have not been found to be ergogenic.

Creatine Creatine is a nitrogen-containing compound found in the body, primarily in muscle, where it is used to make creatine phosphate. It is synthesized by the kidney, liver, pancreas, and other tissues and is consumed in the diet in meat and milk. The more creatine in the diet, the greater the muscle creatine stores. Creatine supplements have been shown to increase levels of both creatine and creatine phosphate in muscle (Figure 13.17).[35] Higher levels of these provide muscles with more quick energy for activity, delay fatigue, prevent the accumulation of lactic acid, and allow creatine phosphate to be regenerated more quickly after exercise.[36] These effects make creatine supplementation beneficial for exercise that requires explosive bursts of energy, such as sprinting and weight lifting, but do not enhance performance in long-term endurance activities such as marathons. Creatine supplements have also been found to increase body mass mostly through lean tissue. This increase is believed to be due to water retention related to creatine uptake in the muscle. An increase in muscle mass and strength may also occur in response to the greater amount and intensity of training that may be achieved.[35]

A number of studies have suggested that creatine supplements are safe, but controlled toxicology studies have not been done and the safety and efficacy of the long-term use of high-dose supplements is unknown.[37] Product purity is also a concern. Because large doses of 5 to 30 g (1 to 6 teaspoons) are needed to be effective, even a minor contaminant might be consumed in significant amounts. Ingestion of creatine before or during exercise is not recommended, and the FDA has advised consumers to consult a physician before using creatine.

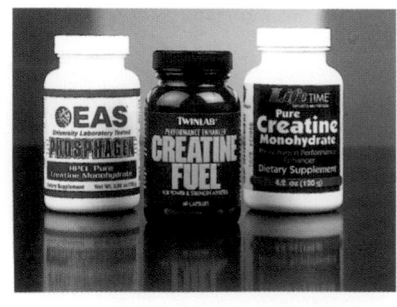

Figure 13.17
Creatine supplements are marketed to athletes to delay fatigue and increase muscle mass. (George Semple)

Bicarbonate Bicarbonate ions act as a buffer in the body, so supplements have been hypothesized to neutralize lactic acid and thus delay fatigue and allow improved performance. Taking bicarbonate before exercise has been found to improve performance and delay exhaustion in sports such as sprint cycling, which involve intense exercise lasting only 1 to 7 minutes, but it is of no benefit for lower-intensity aerobic exercise.[32]

Caffeine Some athletes may try to enhance endurance by consuming caffeine before an event. Caffeine has been shown to enhance performance during prolonged moderate-intensity endurance exercise and short-term intense exercise.[38] This is hypothesized to occur because caffeine enhances the release of fatty acids, and when fatty acids are used as a fuel source, glycogen is spared, delaying the onset of fatigue. Athletes who are unaccustomed to caffeine respond better than those who routinely consume it. In some athletes caffeine may impair performance by increasing water loss in the urine or by causing gastrointestinal upset. Regardless of its effectiveness, athletes should know that excess caffeine is illegal. The International Olympic Committee prohibits athletes from competing when urine caffeine levels are 12 μg per ml or greater. For urine caffeine to reach this level, an individual would need to drink 6 to 8 cups of coffee within about a 2-hour period. Caffeine is also found in pill form in products such as NoDoz, which contains about 100 mg of caffeine per tablet—about the same amount as that in a cup of coffee (Table 13.5).

Herbal Supplements Most herbs that are used as ergogenic aids are poorly researched, so the evidence for their benefits is only anecdotal. Ginseng and ephedra are the best studied of the herbal ergogens.[39]

Ginseng is promoted to increase endurance. Human clinical trials of Chinese ginseng (*P. ginseng*) have shown that when taken in appropriate doses for long enough by individuals engaged in physical activity of sufficient intensity, it may increase muscle strength and aerobic capacity.[39] The benefits may be greater for untrained or older subjects. Ginseng supplements are generally considered safe based on over 2000 years of use with few reported side effects. Side effects may, however, occur in some individuals, and it has been shown to increase the effects and side effects of other stimulants such as caffeine.[39]

Ephedrine, also called ephedra, Chinese ephedra, or Ma Huang, is also taken to improve performance. Unlike other herbal supplements, the active ingredient, ephedrine, is well characterized; ephedrine is used in many over-the-counter and prescription antihistamine, decongestant, and appetite suppressant products. Ephedrine is a stimulant that mimics the effects of epinephrine. Large doses of ephedrine, about 25 mg, have not been shown to improve athletic performance and when combined with large amounts of caffeine (> 100 mg), have been associated with serious side effects including nervousness, headaches, nausea, hypertension, cardiac arrhythmias, and even death. Lower doses of ephedrine combined with moderate amounts of caffeine have been shown to increase the time to exhaustion in exercise and to promote a

Table 13.5 *The Caffeine Content of Commonly Consumed Foods and Medications*

Food or Medication	Amount	Caffeine (mg)
Coffee, regular	1 cup (240 ml)	139
Coffee, decaffeinated	1 cup	3
Tea, brewed	1 cup	45
Pepsi	12 oz (1 can)	37
Diet Pepsi	12 oz (1 can)	50
Mountain Dew	12 oz (1 can)	54
Hot chocolate	1 cup	7
Brownie	1	14
Chocolate bar	1 oz	15
NoDoz	1 tablet	100
Excedrin	1 tablet	65
Empirin, Anacin	1 tablet	32

reduction in body fat during weight loss. The use of ephedrine, whether herbal or synthetic, has been banned from amateur sporting events.[39]

Other Supplements Bee pollen is a mixture of the pollen of flowering plants, plant nectar, and bee saliva. It contains no extraordinary factors and has not been shown to have any performance-enhancing effects. In addition, ingesting or inhaling bee pollen can be hazardous to individuals allergic to various plant pollens.[40] Brewer's yeast is a source of B vitamins and some minerals but has not been demonstrated to have any ergogenic properties. Likewise, there is no evidence to support claims that wheat germ oil will aid endurance. As an oil, it is high in fat, but it is no better as an energy source than any other fat. Royal jelly is a substance produced by worker bees to feed to the queen bee. While it helps the queen bee grow to twice the size of worker bees and to live 40 times longer, royal jelly does not appear to enhance athletic capacity in humans. Finally, DNA and RNA are marketed to aid in tissue regeneration. In the body, they carry genetic information and are needed to synthesize proteins, but DNA and RNA are not required in the diet, and supplements do not help replace damaged cells (see *Critical Thinking*: An Ergogenic Boost?).

CRITICAL THINKING

An Ergogenic Boost?

Andrew is on the college track team. He would like to improve his performance and decides to experiment with some ergogenic aids. Based on the articles and advertisements he's read in sports magazines, he selects creatine to improve his sprint times and chromium to increase his lean body mass. But before he begins taking these, he wants to explore their risks and benefits.

The ads and articles about these supplements make the following claims:

> Creatine will increase muscle creatine phosphate levels to provide quick energy and speed recovery after exercise.

> Chromium will increase lean body tissue and enhance fat loss.

Do the claims made for these products make sense?
▼

Creatine is a precursor for creatine phosphate, which is a source of ATP for short-term exercise. Therefore, the claim that it will increase creatine phosphate levels and provide more energy for sprint types of activity seems logical.

Chromium is a mineral that is needed for insulin to perform its functions. Insulin is needed for many essential roles, including getting glucose into cells, turning on protein synthesis, and stimulating the synthesis of fat. The claim that it will increase lean tissue makes some sense metabolically, but Andrew is not sure why taking chromium would enhance only the protein-building aspect of insulin's function.

Is there evidence that these supplements work?
▼

The advertisements show photographs of sprinters and body builders and quote their testimonials on the effectiveness of these products. Andrew is not convinced by this type of anecdotal evidence, so he makes a trip to the library to explore the scientific literature.

Where should Andrew look for more information?

▼

In order to find sound scientific studies he should look for articles in well-respected peer-reviewed journals in the field of nutrition and sports, such as the *International Journal of Sport Nutrition*, and *Medicine and Science in Sports and Exercise*. He should then focus on studies that include athletes involved in the types of activities he performs. He can also look at the government nutrition site at www.nutrition.gov for links to information on dietary supplements.

Do these supplements live up to their promoters' promises?

▼

Andrew finds several articles on creatine and chromium. The studies of creatine involve exercise that requires bursts of activity such as sprinting and weight lifting and demonstrate enhanced performance when compared to a placebo. For chromium, the studies are contradictory. One shows an increase in the amount of weight gained and a decrease in body fat in college weight trainers, while another study finds no significant effects.

What are the risks of taking creatine and chromium?

▼

No deleterious effects of creatine have been reported in healthy humans, but Andrew could not find any well-controlled studies on the long-term effects of this supplement. Because the doses of creatine are large (1 to 6 teaspoons), Andrew is concerned about the purity of the products. He decides to select one that displays the USP verification mark on the label (see Chapter 12).

Chromium is an essential mineral, but the muscle building effects of chromium are still questionable. The doses in supplements are about 200 μg per day. Although the evidence for chromium toxicity was not substantial enough to establish a UL, one study found that the picolinate form of chromium caused DNA damage in cells grown in the laboratory. Andrew decides that he will wait for more research to be done before he takes chromium picolinate as an ergogenic aid. Because he eats a balanced diet and takes a multivitamin and mineral supplement that contains chromium, he concludes that he is getting adequate chromium. He is still considering creatine but is unsure whether it will offer more benefits than risks.

What would you recommend Andrew do?

▼

Answer:

• APPLICATIONS •

1. Keep a log of your activity for one day.
   a. Note the number of hours you spend in (1) activities of daily living, (2) moderate intensity activity, and (3) vigorous activity (see Chapter 7).
   b. What is your physical activity level? (Use Table 7.4.)
   c. What is your estimated energy expenditure (EER)? (Use Table 7.2.)
   d. If you increased your exercise enough to move to the "active" physical activity level, what would your new EER be?
   (If you are already active, what would your EER be in the "very active" level?)
   e. Make a list of foods that you could add to your diet to balance the added expenditure of this increase in activity.

2. Taking into consideration your typical weekly schedule of activities and events, design a reasonable exercise program for yourself using the Activity Pyramid. Include the types of activities, the times during the week you will be involved in each activity, and the length of time you will engage in each

activity. Choose activities you enjoy and schedule them for reasonable lengths of time and at reasonable frequencies.

a. What everyday changes have you made that will increase the energy expended in day-to-day activities?

b. Which activities are aerobic, which improve flexibility, and which are for strength training?

c. Can each of these activities be performed year-round? Suggest alternative activities and locations for inclement weather.

3. Do a risk-benefit analysis of an ergogenic aid (a quick way to do this is to use the Internet to collect information). List the risks and benefits and then write a conclusion as to why you would or would not take this substance.

SUMMARY

1. Fitness, which is the ability to perform routine physical activity without undue fatigue, is defined by an individual's cardiorespiratory endurance, muscle strength and endurance, flexibility, and body composition.

2. Regular exercise improves fitness in individuals of all ages and can reduce the risk of chronic diseases such as obesity, heart disease, diabetes, and osteoporosis. Exercise can also delay some of the changes in body composition and metabolism that occur with age.

3. A well-designed fitness program involves aerobic exercise, stretching, and strength training. To maintain a healthy body weight and maximize health, 60 minutes per day of moderate exercise should be performed in addition to the activities of daily living. One way to create a more active lifestyle is to choose enjoyable activities and follow the recommendations of the Activity Pyramid.

4. Activity is fueled by ATP generated from carbohydrate, fat, and protein. When oxygen is limited, anaerobic glycolysis produces ATP from carbohydrate. When oxygen is plentiful, aerobic metabolism generates ATP. Aerobic metabolism is more efficient than anaerobic glycolysis and can utilize carbohydrate, fatty acids, and amino acids as energy sources.

5. The availability of oxygen and the proportion of carbohydrate and fat used as fuel for a given activity depend on the intensity and duration of the activity and the conditioning of the exerciser. For short-term, high-intensity activity, ATP is generated primarily from the anaerobic metabolism of glucose from muscle glycogen stores. For lower-intensity exercise of longer duration, aerobic metabolism predominates, and both glucose and fatty acids become important fuel sources. Protein becomes an important source of energy only when exercise continues for many hours. Training improves oxygen delivery and utilization, allowing aerobic exercise to be sustained for longer periods at higher intensity.

6. The diet of an active individual should provide sufficient energy to fuel activity. In general, it should contain about 45 to 65% of total energy as carbohydrate from whole grains, fruits, vegetables, and milk to ensure that glycogen stores are replenished after daily exercise; 20 to 35% of energy as fat; and about 10 to 35% of energy as protein.

7. Adequate fluid intake before exercise ensures that athletes begin exercise well hydrated. Fluid intake during and after exercise must replace water lost in sweat and from evaporation through the lungs. Water is needed to ensure that the body can be cooled and that nutrients and oxygen can be delivered to body tissues. If water intake is inadequate, dehydration can lead to a decline in exercise performance and thermal distress may occur. Plain water is the best fluid to consume for most exercise. During exercise lasting longer than 60 minutes, athletes might benefit from fluids containing glucose. Electrolyte replacement is not harmful but is only necessary during ultraendurance activities lasting more than 8 hours.

8. Sufficient micronutrients are needed to generate ATP from macronutrients, to maintain and repair tissues, and to transport oxygen and wastes to and from the cells. Some athletes are at risk for deficiencies of iron and calcium.

9. Competitive endurance athletes may utilize glycogen supercompensation regimens to maximize glycogen stores before an event.

10. Meals eaten before competition should provide about 300 kcalories; should be high in carbohydrate, low in fat, moderate in protein, and low in fiber; and should satisfy the psychological needs of the athlete. Postcompetition meals should replace lost fluids and electrolytes and begin restoring muscle and liver glycogen.

11. Many types of ergogenic aids are marketed to improve athletic performance. Some are beneficial for certain types of activity, but many offer little or no benefit. An individual risk-benefit analysis should be used to determine if a supplement is appropriate for you.

REVIEW QUESTIONS

1. List the health benefits of fitness.

2. What is aerobic exercise?

3. What is strength training?

4. How does aerobic exercise affect resting heart rate?

5. How much exercise is enough?

6. What is maximal oxygen consumption and how is it affected by aerobic exercise?

7. What fuels are used to produce ATP in anaerobic metabolism?

8. Which is more efficient, aerobic or anaerobic metabolism?

9. What factors affect the availability of oxygen and the type of fuel used during exercise?

10. What fuels are used in exercise of long duration such as marathon running?

11. What are the recommendations for fluid intake before, during, and after exercise?

12. How does exercise affect protein needs?

13. What is glycogen supercompensation or carbohydrate loading?

14. Can ergogenic aids enhance exercise performance? How? Are they safe?

REFERENCES

1. Abernathy, R. P., and Black, D. R. Healthy body weights: An alternative perspective. *Am. J. Clin. Nutr.* 63 (Suppl.):448S–451S, 1996.

2. Institute of Medicine, Food and Nutrition Board. *Dietary Reference Intakes for Energy, Carbohydrates, Fiber, Fat, Protein and Amino Acids.* Washington, D.C.: National Academy Press, 2002.

3. Haennel, R. G., and Lemire, F. Physical activity to prevent cardiovascular disease. How much is enough? *Can. Fam. Physican* 48:65–71, 2002.

4. American College of Sports Medicine. American College of Sports Medicine Position Stand: Exercise and physical activity for older adults. *Med. Sci. Sports Exerc.* 30:992–1008, 1998.

5. Albright, A., Franz, M., Hornsby, G. et al. American College of Sports Medicine Position Stand. Exercise and type 2 diabetes. *Med. Sci. Sports Exerc.* 32:1345–1360, 2000.

6. Gammon, M. D., John, E. M., and Britton, J. A. Recreational and occupational physical activities and risk of breast cancer. *J. Natl. Cancer Inst.* 90:100—117, 1998.

7. Colditz, G. A., Cannuscio, C. C., and Frazier, A. L. Physical activity and reduced risk of colon cancer: Implications for prevention. *Cancer Causes Control* 8:649–667, 1997.

8. U.S. Department of Health and Human Services. *Physical Activity and Health: A Report of the Surgeon General.* Centers for Disease Control and Prevention, 1996.

9. U.S. Department of Agriculture, U.S. Department of Health and Human Services. *Nutrition and Your Health: Dietary Guidelines for Americans*, 5th ed. Home and Garden Bulletin No. 232. Hyattsville, Md.: U.S. Government Printing Office, 2000.

10. Healthy People 2010. Available online at www.health.gov/healthy people/ Accessed May 6, 2002.

11. Exploring the Activity Pyramid, Institute for Research and Education. Healthsystem Minnesota. Available online at www.hsmnet.com/HSM/ BHC/IRE/HEC/EXPLORE.HTM/ Accessed January 10, 2000.

12. Andersen, R. E., Crespo, C. J., Bartlett, S. J., et al. Relationship of physical activity and television watching with body weight and level of fatness among children: Results from the Third National Health and Nutrition Examination Survey. *JAMA* 279:938–942, 1998.

13. Brass, E. P. Supplemental carnitine and exercise. *Am. J. Clin. Nutr.* 72(Suppl.):618S–623S, 2000.

14. Beals, K. A., and Manore, M. M. Nutritional status of female athletes with subclinical eating disorders. *J. Am. Diet. Assoc.* 98:419–425, 1998.

15. Oppliger, R. A., Case, H. S., Horswill, C. A., et al. American College of Sports Medicine Position Statement: Weight-loss in wrestlers. *Med. Sci. Sports Exerc.* 28:ix–xii, 1996.

16. Nutrition and athletic performance—Position of the American Dietetic Association, Dietitians of Canada, and the American College of Sports Medicine. *J. Am. Diet Assoc.* 100:1543–1556, 2000.

17. Paul, G. L., Gautsch, T. A., and Layman, D. K. Amino acid and protein metabolism during exercise and recovery. In *Nutrition in Exercise and Sport*, 3rd ed. Wolinski, I., ed. Boca Raton, Fla.: CRC Press, 1998. 125–158.

18. Manore, M. M. The effect of physical activity on thiamin, riboflavin, and vitamin B6 requirements. *Am. J. Clin. Nutr.* 72(Suppl.):598S–606S, 2000.

19. Beard, J., and Tobin, B. Iron status and exercise. *Am. J. Clin. Nutr.* 72(Suppl.):594S–597S, 2000.

20. Food and Nutrition Board, Institute of Medicine. *Dietary Reference Intakes: Vitamin A, Vitamin K, Arsenic, Boron, Chromium, Copper, Iodine, Iron, Manganese, Molybdenum, Nickel, Silicon, Vanadium, and Zinc.* Washington, D.C.: National Academy Press, 2001.

21. Otis, C. L., Drinkwater, B. L., Johnson, M., et al. American College of Sports Medicine position stand on female athlete triad. *Med. Sci. Sports Exerc.* 29:i–ix, 1997.

22. Bennell, K. L., Malcolm, S. A., Wark, J. D., and Brukner, P. D. Skeletal effects of menstrual disturbances in athletes. *Scand. J. Med. Sci. Sports* 7:261–273, 1997.

23. Remick, D., Chancellor, K., Pederson, J., et al. Hyperthermia and dehydration-related deaths associated with intentional rapid weight loss in three collegiate wrestlers—North Carolina, Wisconsin, and Michigan, November–December, 1997. *MMWR* 47:105–108, 1998. Available online at www.cdc.gov/epo/mmwr/mmwr_wk.html/ Accessed February 5, 2001.

24. Senay, L. C. Water and electrolytes during physical activity. In *Nutrition in Exercise and Sport*, 3rd ed. Wolinski, I., ed. Boca Raton, Fla.: CRC Press, 1998. 257–276.

25. American College of Sports Medicine. Position stand on exercise and fluid replacement. *Med. Sci. Sports. Exerc.* 28:i–vii, 1996.

26. Wilkinson, J. G., and Lieberman, M. Carbohydrate metabolism in sport and exercise. In *Nutrition in Exercise and Sport*, 3rd ed. Wolinski, I., ed. Boca Raton, Fla.: CRC Press, 1998. 63-99.

27. Coyle, E. F. Substrate utilization during exercise in active people. *Am. J. Clin. Nutr.* 61(Suppl.):968S–979S, 1995.

28. Dekkers, J. C., van Doornen, L. J. P., and Kemper, H. C. G. The role of antioxidant vitamins and enzymes in the prevention of exercise-induced muscle damage. *Sports Med.* 21:213–238, 1996.

29. Lukaski, H. C. Chromium as a supplement. *Ann. Rev. Nutr.* 19:279–301, 1999.

30. Stearns, D. M., Wise, J. P., Patierno, S. R., and Wetterhahn, K. E. Chromium (III) picolinate produces damage in Chinese hamster ovary cells. *FASEB J.* 9:1643:1643–1648, 1995.

31. Kato, I., Vogelman, J. H., Dilman, V., et al. Effect of supplementation with chromium picolinate on antibody titers to 5-hydroxymethyl uracil. *Eur. J. Epidemiol.* 14:621–626, 1998.

32. Williams, M. H. Facts and fallacies of purported ergogenic amino acid supplements. *Clin. Sports Med.* 18:633–649, 1999.

33. van Hall, G., Saris, W. H., van de Schoor, P. A., and Wagenmakers, A. J. The effect of free glutamine and peptide ingestion on the rate of muscle glycogen resynthesis in man. *Int. J. Sports Med.* 21:25–30, 2000.

34. Davis, J. M., Welsh, R. S., De Volve, K. L., and Alderson, N. A. Effects of branched-chain amino acids and carbohydrate on fatigue during intermittent, high-intensity running. *Int. J. Sports Med.* 20:309–314, 1999.

35. Terjung, R. L., Clarkson, P., Eichner, E. R., et al. American College of Sports Medicine roundtable: The physiological and health effects of oral creatine supplementation. *Med. Sci. Sports Exerc.* 32:706–717, 2000.

36. Feldman, E. B. Creatine: a dietary supplement and ergogenic aid. *Nutr. Rev.* 57:45–50, 1999.

37. Poortmans, J. R., Francaux, M. Adverse effects of creatine supplementation: Fact or fiction? *Sports Med.* 30:155–170, 2000.

38. Spriet, L. L. Caffeine and performance. *Int. J. Sport Nutr.* 5(Suppl.):84S–99S, 1995.

39. Bucci, L. R. Selected herbals and human exercise performance. *Am. J. Clin. Nutr.* 72: 624S–636S, 2000.

40. Bauer, L., Kohlich, A., Hirschwehr, R., et al. Food allergy: Pollen or bee products? *J. Allergy Clin. Immunol.* 97:65–73, 1996.

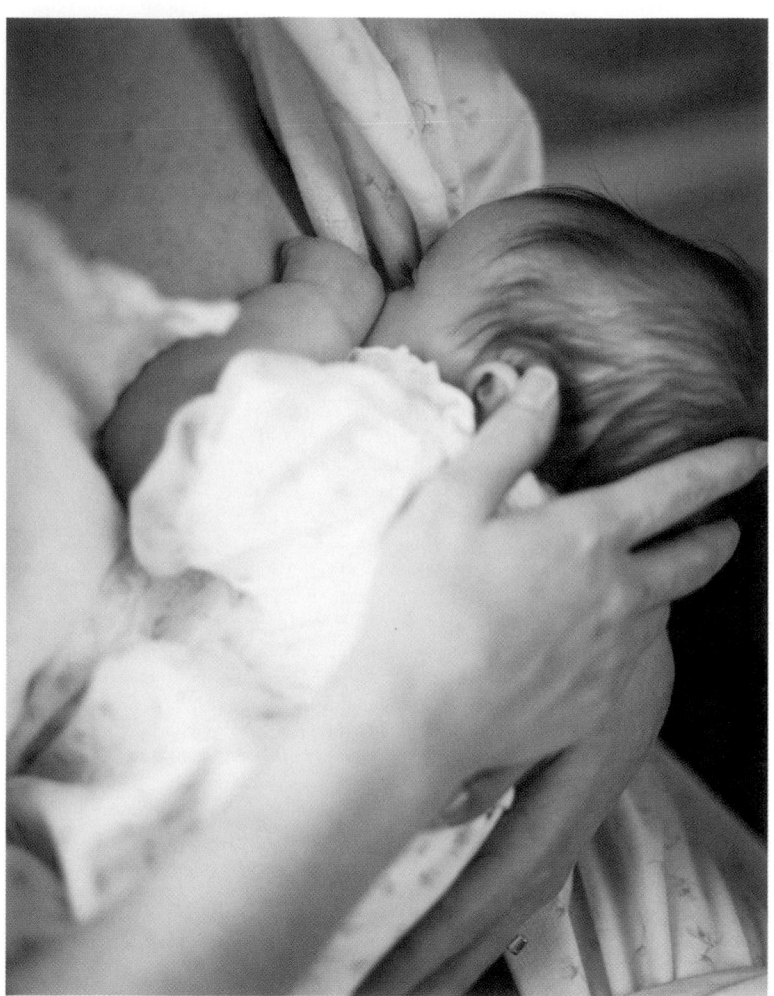

(© Anderson Ross/PhotoDisc, Inc.)

Chapter Outline

Chapter Concepts

✔ A woman's nutrient intake during pregnancy must meet her needs and those of the fetus.

✔ In order to support pregnancy and prepare for lactation, a pregnant woman's body undergoes many changes.

✔ Energy, protein, water, vitamin, and mineral needs increase during pregnancy.

✔ Adequate weight gain during pregnancy is essential to the health of the mother and unborn baby.

✔ The age, health, lifestyle, and nutritional status of the mother can affect her developing child.

✔ Lactation increases the mother's nutrient needs.

✔ A newborn infant's energy and protein needs are higher per unit of body weight than at any other time of life.

✔ An infant's growth rate is the best measure of the adequacy of his diet.

✔ Breast feeding is the ideal way to nourish most infants.

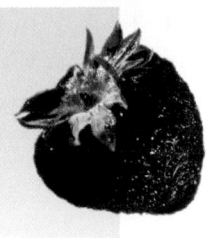

Just a Taste

Do pregnant women need vitamin and mineral supplements?

Should overweight women gain weight during pregnancy?

Is breast feeding the best option for all newborn infants and their mothers?

For a single cell to develop into a complete human being, it must multiply and differentiate to form the specific shapes and specialized tissues of a human infant. This development requires a safe environment to which oxygen and nutrients are provided in the right amounts and at the right times and from which waste products are removed. The mother's uterus provides this environment, and the nutrients and waste products are transported by her blood supply. Therefore, the mother's health and nutritional status are crucial to a successful pregnancy outcome.

To help ensure the health of her baby, a woman must start her pregnancy in good nutritional health, and during pregnancy her diet must be carefully planned to supply the nutrients needed to maintain her health, support the physiological changes in her body, and provide for the rapid growth and development of her unborn baby. A deficiency or excess of nutrients, as well as the use of alcohol, drugs, and cigarettes, may cause birth defects, premature births, and low birth weights. Although good nutrition cannot always prevent these problems, adequate nutrition and consistent prenatal care can reduce the number of babies born disabled, too soon, or too small.

After delivery, the newborn must continue to receive adequate nutrition. Breast-fed infants depend on nutrients from the mother to meet their needs. Lactation has high nutrient demands, and the composition of breast milk can be affected by maternal intake, so a nursing woman's diet must be selected carefully. Formula-fed infants rely on the nutrients in infant formulas to meet their needs.

• THE PHYSIOLOGY OF PREGNANCY

Pregnancy, from **conception** to birth, usually lasts 40 weeks, or about nine months in humans. During pregnancy, a single cell grows and develops into an infant that is ready for life outside the womb. Many physiological changes take place in the mother to support her developing offspring and prepare her for **lactation**.

Prenatal Growth and Development

Reproduction requires the **fertilization** of an egg, or ovum, from the mother by a sperm from the father. Fertilization, which occurs in the **fallopian tube** or **oviduct**, produces a single-celled **zygote**. The zygote travels down the mother's fallopian tube into the uterus. Along the way the zygote divides many times to form a ball of smaller cells. In the uterus it attaches to the uterine lining in a process known as **implantation**. Once implantation has occurred, two new organs, the **amniotic sac** and **placenta**, form to protect and nourish the developing offspring (Figure 14.1). The amniotic sac is a fluid-filled membrane that surrounds the unborn baby and protects it from the bumps and bruises of the outside world. The placenta provides a network of blood vessels that allow nutrients and oxygen to be transferred from mother to baby and waste products to be transferred from the baby to the mother's blood for elimination. It is formed when the implanted ball of cells develops branch-

Conception The union of sperm and egg (ovum) that results in pregnancy.

Lactation Milk production and secretion.

Fertilization The union of sperm and egg (ovum).

Fallopian tubes or **oviducts** Narrow ducts leading from the ovaries to the uterus

Zygote The cell produced by the union of sperm and ovum during fertilization.

Implantation The process by which the developing ball of cells embeds in the uterine lining.

Amniotic sac A membrane surrounding the fetus that contains the amniotic fluid.

Placenta An organ produced from both maternal and embryonic tissues. It secretes hormones, transfers nutrients and oxygen from the mother's blood to the fetus, and removes wastes.

395

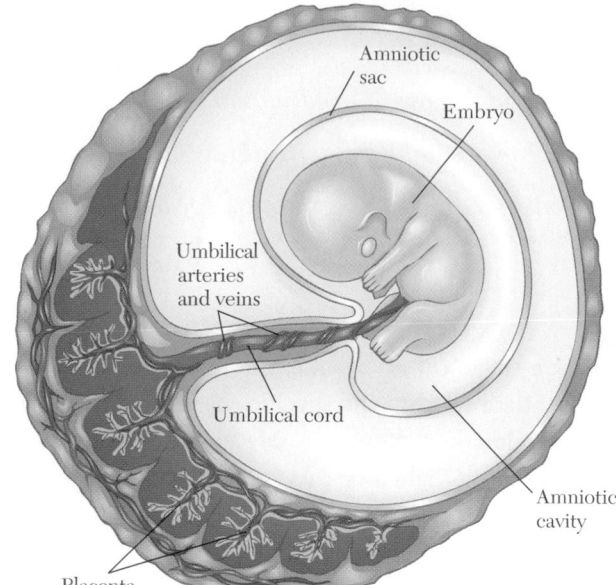

Figure 14.1
During pregnancy, the amniotic sac protects the fetus, and the placenta allows nutrients and wastes to be transferred between mother and baby.

Embryo The developing human from two to eight weeks after fertilization. All organ systems are formed during this time.

Fetus The developing human from the ninth week to birth. Growth and refinement of structures occur during this time.

Spontaneous abortion or **miscarriage** Interruption of pregnancy prior to the seventh month.

like projections that grow into the lining of the uterus, allowing blood vessels that supply the developing baby to lie in close proximity to maternal blood. The placenta also secretes hormones necessary to maintain pregnancy.

As these structures develop, the ball of cells continues to grow. The cells differentiate to form the multitude of specialized cell types that make up the body, and arrange themselves in the proper shapes and locations to form body organs and structures. About two weeks after fertilization, the developing offspring is known as an **embryo**. The embryonic stage of development lasts until the eighth week after fertilization, when rudimentary organ systems have been formed. The embryo at this point is approximately 3 cm long (a little more than an inch) and has a beating heart. All major external and internal structures have been formed. Beginning at the ninth week of development and continuing until birth, the developing offspring is known as a **fetus** (Figure 14.2). During the fetal period of development, structures that appeared during the embryonic period continue to grow and mature. Anything that interferes with development can result in birth defects. If the defect is severe, it may result in a **spontaneous abortion** or **miscarriage**.

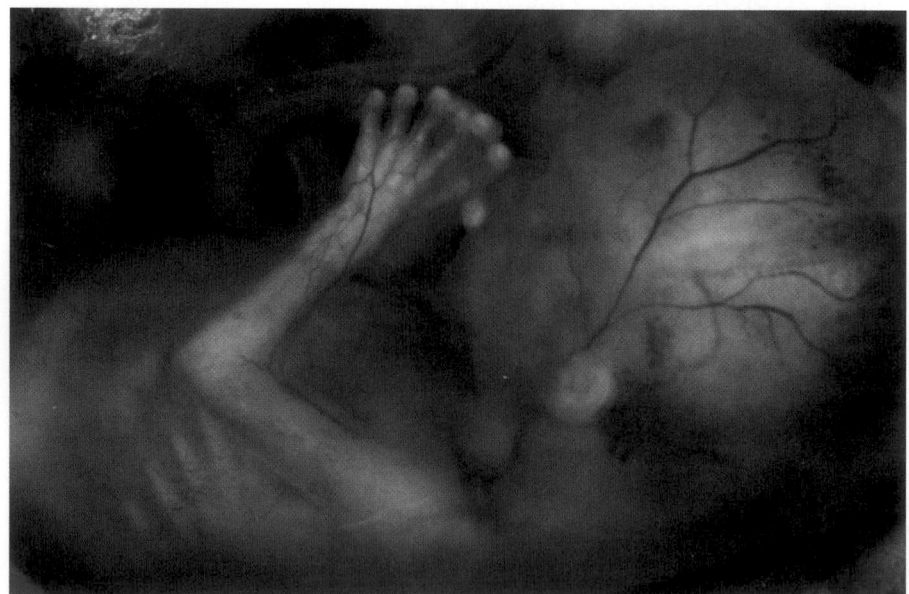

Figure 14.2
At 16 weeks, the fetus is about 16 cm (6.4 inches) long. (Custom Medical Stock Photo)

The fetal period usually ends after 40 weeks of **gestation** with the birth of an infant weighing about 3 to 4 kilograms (6.6 to 8.8 lb).[1] Infants who are born on time but have failed to grow well in the uterus are said to be **small-for-gestational-age**. Those born before 37 weeks of gestation are said to be **preterm** or **premature**.

Whether born too soon or just too small, **low birth weight** infants (those weighing less than 2.5 kg [5.5 lb] at birth) and **very low birth weight** infants (those weighing less than 1.5 kg [3.3 lb]), are at increased risk for illness and early death.[2] They often require special care and a special diet in order to successfully continue to grow and develop. Survival improves with increasing gestational age and birth weight. Today, with advances in medical and nutritional care, infants born as early as 25 weeks of gestation and those weighing as little as 1 kg (2.2 lb) can survive.

Changes in the Mother

A woman's body undergoes many changes during pregnancy to develop and maintain the systems necessary to support the growing fetus. Her blood volume increases by 50%, and her heart, lungs, and kidneys work harder to deliver nutrients and oxygen and remove wastes. The placenta develops, and the hormones produced by it orchestrate other changes: They promote uterine growth; they relax muscles and ligaments to accommodate the growing fetus and allow for childbirth; they promote breast development; and they increase fat deposition to provide the energy stores that will be needed during late pregnancy and lactation. These changes all result in weight gain and can affect the type and level of physical activity that is safe. In some cases they can also cause uncomfortable or dangerous side effects.

Weight Gain During Pregnancy Adequate weight gain during pregnancy is essential to the health of both mother and fetus. Typically the weight of the infant at birth is about 25% of the total pregnancy weight gain. Changes in maternal tissues account for the rest of the weight gained during pregnancy. This includes increases in the size of the uterus and breasts, in the volume of blood and extracellular fluid, and in fat stores (Figure 14.3).

Gestation The time between conception and birth, which lasts about nine months (or about 40 weeks) in humans.

Small-for-gestational-age An infant born at term weighing less than 2.5 kg (5.5 lb).

Preterm or **premature** An infant born before 37 weeks of gestation.

Low birth weight A birthweight less than 2.5 kg (5.5 lb).

Very low birth weight A birthweight less than 1.5 kg (3.3 lb).

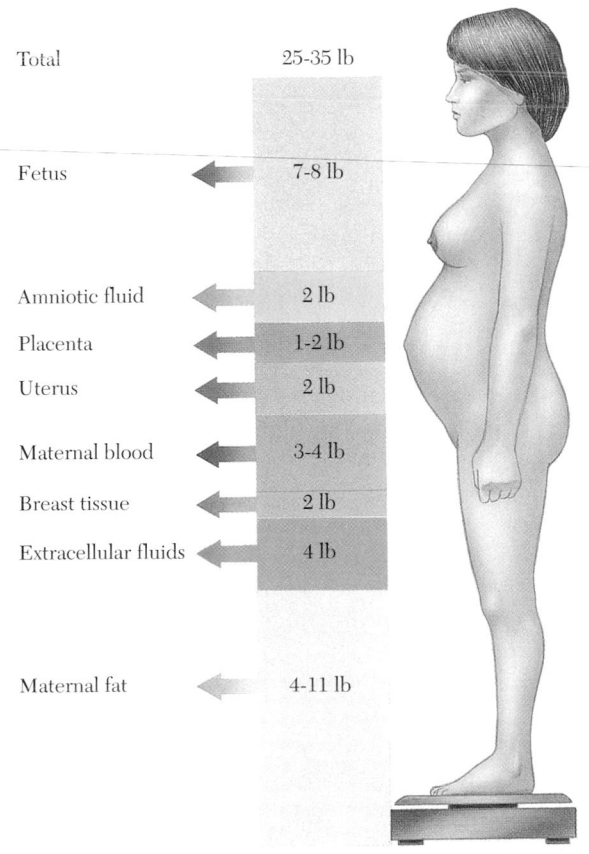

Total	25-35 lb
Fetus	7-8 lb
Amniotic fluid	2 lb
Placenta	1-2 lb
Uterus	2 lb
Maternal blood	3-4 lb
Breast tissue	2 lb
Extracellular fluids	4 lb
Maternal fat	4-11 lb

Figure 14.3

The weight gained by the mother during pregnancy includes increases in the weight of her tissues as well as the weight of the fetus, placenta, and amniotic fluid.

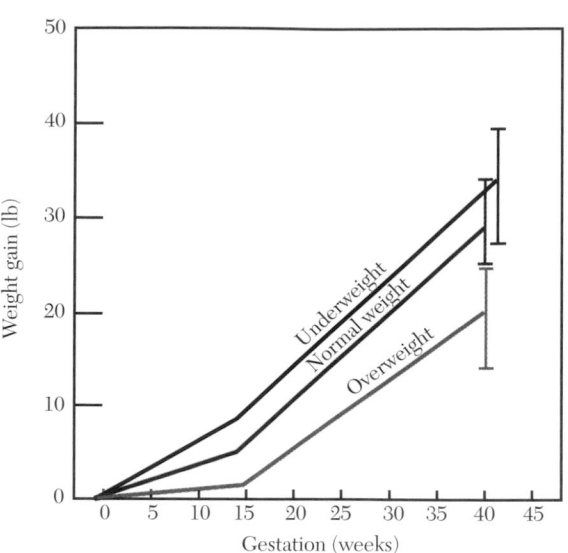

Figure 14.4
The same pattern of weight gain is recommended for women who are normal weight, underweight, or overweight at the start of pregnancy, but the recommendations for total weight gain are different. (Adapted from Committee on Nutritional Status During Pregnancy and Lactation. *Nutrition During Pregnancy.* Washington, D.C.: National Academy Press, 1990.)

Trimester A term used to describe each third, or three-month period, of a pregnancy.

Cesarean section The surgical removal of the fetus from the uterus.

Large-for-gestational-age An infant weighing greater than 4 kg (8.8 lb) at birth.

The recommended weight gain during pregnancy is 25 to 35 pounds (11.4 to 15.9 kg) for healthy, normal-weight women. The rate of weight gain is as important as the total weight gain. Little gain is expected in the first three months, or **trimester**, of pregnancy—usually about 2 to 4 pounds (0.9 to 1.8 kg). In the second and third trimesters, when the fetus grows from less than a pound to 6 to 8 pounds, the recommended maternal weight gain is about 1 pound (0.45 kg) per week. Women who are underweight or overweight at conception should also gain weight at a slow, steady rate (Figure 14.4). Weight gains of up to 40 pounds (18 kg) are recommended for women who begin pregnancy underweight. Overweight women should gain less, only about 15 to 25 pounds (6.8 to 11.4 kg) over the course of pregnancy.

Gaining too much or too little weight as well as being underweight or overweight can affect the health of both mother and child.[1] Being underweight by 10% or more at the onset of pregnancy or gaining too little weight during pregnancy increases the risk of producing a low birth weight baby. Excess weight, whether present before conception or gained during pregnancy, can also compromise the outcome of the pregnancy. The mother's risks for high blood pressure, gestational diabetes, difficult delivery, and **cesarean section** are increased by excess weight, as is the risk of having a **large-for-gestational-age** baby. Dieting during pregnancy is not advised even for obese women. If possible, excess weight should be lost before the pregnancy begins or, alternatively, after the child is born and weaned.

Some women are concerned that weight gained during pregnancy will be permanent, but most lose all but about 2 pounds within a year of delivery. Approximately 10 pounds are lost at birth from the weight of the baby, amniotic fluid, and placenta. In the week after delivery, another 5 pounds of fluid are typically lost. Once this initial fluid and tissue weight is lost, further weight loss requires that energy intake be less than energy output. After the mother has recovered from delivery, a balanced low-energy diet combined with moderate exercise will promote weight loss and the return of muscle tone.

Physical Activity During Pregnancy For healthy, well-nourished women, carefully chosen moderate exercise is recommended during pregnancy. Physical activity during pregnancy improves overall fitness, reduces stress, prevents excess weight gain, prevents low back pain, improves digestion, reduces constipation, prevents gestational diabetes, improves mood and body image, and speeds recovery from childbirth. Too much exercise that is too intense has the potential to harm the fetus by reducing the amount of oxygen and nutrients it receives or by increasing body temperature. Therefore, guidelines have been developed to minimize the risks and maximize the benefits of exercise during pregnancy (Table 14.1). However, all

Table 14.1 *Guidelines for Physical Activity During Pregnancy*

Obtain medical permission before beginning an exercise program.

If inactive before pregnancy, increase activity very gradually.

Regular exercise (at least three times per week) is preferable to intermittent activity.

Stop exercising when fatigued and do not exercise to exhaustion.

Choose non-weight-bearing activities such as swimming that have minimal risk of falls or abdominal injury.

Avoid strenuous exertion during the first trimester; at other times, strenuous exercise should not be continued for more than 15 minutes.

After the first trimester avoid exercise that is performed lying on one's back.

Avoid exercising in hot or humid environments.

Drink plenty of liquids before, during, and after exercise.

Prepregnancy exercise routines should be resumed gradually after the birth of the child.

Modified from Dewey, K. G., and McCrory, M. A. Effects of dieting and physical activity on pregnancy and lactation. *Am. J. Clin. Nutr.* 59 (Suppl.):446S–453S, 1994; and American College of Obstetricians and Gynecologists. *Exercise During Pregnancy and the Postpartum Period (Technical Bulletin #189).* Washington, D.C.: ACOG, 1994.

pregnant women should check with their physicians before engaging in any exercise program.

Women who were physically active before their pregnancy can continue their exercise programs, but women who begin an exercise program after becoming pregnant should start slowly, with low-intensity, low-impact activities such as walking.[3] During pregnancy, the risk of injury is greater because women weigh more and carry that weight in the front of their bodies where it can interfere with balance and place stress on the bones, joints, and muscles. Activities that have a risk of abdominal trauma, falls, or joint stress, such as contact and racquet sports, should be avoided.[4] Exercise in the water is recommended because the body's buoyancy in water compensates for the changes in weight distribution (Figure 14.5). To ensure adequate delivery of oxygen and nutrients to the fetus, intense exercise should be limited during pregnancy. To prevent overheating, plenty of fluids should be consumed, and exercise should be carried out in a well-ventilated environment.

Discomforts of Pregnancy

The physiological changes that occur during pregnancy can cause uncomfortable side effects for the mother. Some are caused by changes in fluid distribution, others by hormonal changes that affect the digestive tract. Most of these problems are minor, but in some cases they may endanger the mother and the fetus.

Edema During pregnancy, blood volume expands to nourish the fetus, but this expansion may also cause the accumulation of extracellular fluid in the tissues, known as **edema**. Edema is characterized by swelling, particularly in the feet and ankles (Figure 14.6). Restriction of dietary sodium below the amount recommended for the general population is not recommended, nor is fluid restriction. Edema can be uncomfortable but does not increase medical risks unless it is accompanied by a rise in blood pressure.

Morning Sickness **Morning sickness** is a syndrome of nausea and vomiting that occurs during pregnancy. The term "morning sickness" is somewhat of a misnomer because symptoms can occur anytime during the day or night. It is thought to be related to the hormonal changes of pregnancy and may be alleviated to some extent by eating small frequent snacks of dry starchy foods, such as plain crackers or bread. In most women symptoms decrease significantly after the first trimester, but in some cases the symptoms last for the entire pregnancy and, in severe cases, may require intravenous nutrition to assure that needs are met.

Edema Swelling due to the buildup of extracellular fluid in the tissues.

Morning sickness Nausea and vomiting that affects many women during the first few months of pregnancy and in some women can continue throughout the pregnancy.

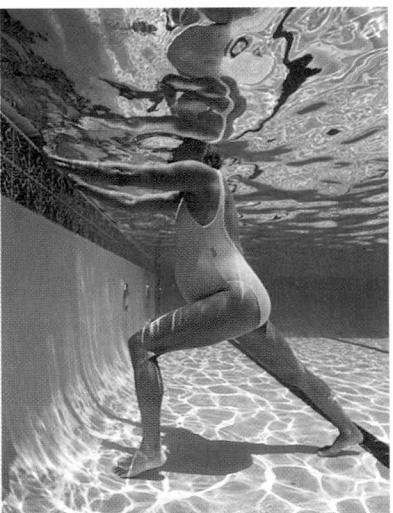

Figure 14.5
During pregnancy, exercising in the water can reduce stress on joints and help keep the body cool. (© Tracy Frankel/The Image Bank)

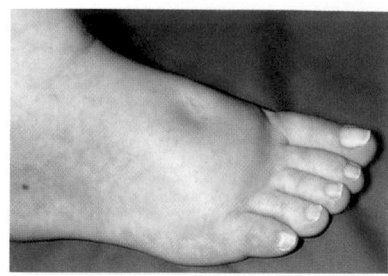

Figure 14.6
Edema in feet and ankles is a common complication of pregnancy. Elevating the feet will help reduce swelling. (© Dr. P. Marazzi/Science Photo Library/Photo Researchers, Inc.)

Heartburn Heartburn is another common digestive complaint during pregnancy because the hormones produced to relax the muscles of the uterus also relax the muscles of the gastrointestinal tract. This involuntary relaxation of the lower esophageal sphincter allows the acidic stomach contents to back up into the esophagus, causing irritation. The problem gets more severe as pregnancy progresses because the growing baby crowds the stomach. The fuller the stomach, the more likely that its contents will back up into the esophagus. Therefore, heartburn can be reduced by consuming many small meals throughout the day rather than a few large meals. Because high-fat foods, such as fried foods, rich sauces, and desserts, leave the stomach slowly, a lowfat diet of grains, fruits, vegetables, plain meats, and lowfat dairy products is less likely to cause heartburn. Because a reclining position makes it easier for acidic juices to flow into the esophagus, remaining upright after eating also reduces heartburn. Avoiding substances that are known to cause heartburn, such as caffeine and peppermint, can also be helpful.

Constipation Constipation is a frequent complaint during pregnancy. The pregnancy-related hormones that cause muscles to relax also decrease intestinal motility and slow transit time. Constipation becomes more of a problem late in pregnancy when the weight of the uterus puts pressure on the gastrointestinal tract. Maintaining a moderate level of physical activity and consuming at least one-half gallon of water and other fluids per day, as well as high-fiber foods such as whole grains, vegetables, and fruits, are recommended to prevent constipation. Hemorrhoids are also more common during pregnancy, as a result of both constipation and physiological changes in blood flow.

Gestational Diabetes

Gestational diabetes A consistently elevated blood glucose level that develops during pregnancy and returns to normal after delivery.

Consistently elevated blood glucose level during pregnancy is known as **gestational diabetes**. It occurs in 2 to 6% of all pregnancies and is most common in obese women.[5] This form of diabetes usually disappears when the pregnancy is completed, although the mother remains at higher risk for developing type 2 diabetes (see Chapter 4).

High levels of glucose in the mother's blood can adversely affect the fetus. Glucose in the mother's blood passes freely across the placenta, so high maternal blood sugar provides extra energy to the fetus. This extra energy can produce a baby who is large for gestational age and consequently at increased risk of complications. As with other types of diabetes, the treatment of gestational diabetes involves consuming a carefully planned diet, moderate daily exercise, and in some cases, medication.

Pregnancy-Induced Hypertension

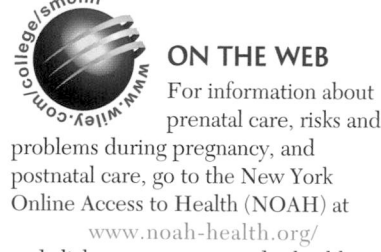

ON THE WEB
For information about prenatal care, risks and problems during pregnancy, and postnatal care, go to the New York Online Access to Health (NOAH) at www.noah-health.org/ and click on pregnancy under health topics.

Pregnancy-induced hypertension A spectrum of conditions involving elevated blood pressure during pregnancy. **Preeclampsia** is characterized by an increase in body weight, elevated blood pressure, protein in the urine, and edema. It can progress to **eclampsia**, which can be life threatening to mother and fetus.

Pregnancy-induced hypertension is a spectrum of conditions involving elevated blood pressure that occurs in about 6 to 8% of pregnancies. It is a major risk factor for maternal and fetal illness and death; it accounts for nearly 15% of pregnancy-related maternal deaths in the United States.[6] It is more common in mothers under 20 or over 35 years of age, those in low-income groups, and women with chronic hypertension or kidney disease.

The mildest form of pregnancy-induced hypertension is **gestational hypertension**, which is an abnormal rise in blood pressure that occurs after the twentieth week of pregnancy. **Preeclampsia** is a form that causes an increase in blood pressure, excretion of protein in the urine, and edema. Its onset is often signaled by a weight gain of several pounds within a few days. It can progress to a more severe form, **eclampsia**, in which life-threatening seizures occur.

The cause of pregnancy-induced hypertension is not known, but research suggests that low calcium intake may be involved. Evidence is not strong enough to support routine supplementation of all pregnant women, but pregnant teens, individuals with inadequate calcium intake, and women known to be at risk of developing pregnancy-induced hypertension may benefit from additional dietary calcium.[7–9]

Treatment includes bed rest and careful medical attention. Dietary sodium intake should be moderate, but sodium restriction is not a cure. The condition usually resolves after delivery.

• THE NUTRITIONAL NEEDS OF PREGNANCY

Nutrition is important before pregnancy to support conception and maximize the likelihood of a healthy pregnancy. During pregnancy maternal intake must provide all the nutrients needed for the growth and development of the fetus while continuing to meet the mother's needs. Because the increased need for energy is proportionately smaller than the increased need for protein, vitamins, and minerals, a well-balanced, nutrient-dense diet is required.

The Importance of Nutrition Before Pregnancy

A woman's nutritional status before she becomes pregnant may affect her ability to conceive and successfully complete a pregnancy. Starvation diets, anorexia nervosa, and excessive athletic activity, such as marathon running, can interfere with ovulation and therefore make conception less likely. Obesity can alter hormone levels and decrease fertility. Deficiencies or excesses of nutrients can also affect pregnancy outcome. For instance, a deficiency of folate or an excess of vitamin A early in pregnancy can cause birth defects.

Nutritional status can be affected by some birth control methods, and these can therefore have an impact on a subsequent pregnancy. For example, oral contraceptives are associated with reduced blood levels of vitamins B_6 and B_{12}.[9] If conception occurs soon after oral contraceptive use stops, these levels will not have time to return to normal before pregnancy begins. The use of drugs—whether over-the-counter, prescribed, or illicit—can also affect both fertility and pregnancy outcome. A woman who is considering pregnancy should discuss her plans with her physician in order to determine the risks associated with any medication she is taking.

Energy and Macronutrient Needs During Pregnancy

Energy needs increase during pregnancy to deposit and maintain the new fetal and maternal tissues. The EER for pregnancy is calculated as the sum of the total energy expenditure for nonpregnant women, the increase in energy expenditure due to pregnancy, and the energy deposited in tissues.[4] During the first trimester, total energy expenditure changes little, so the EER is not increased above nonpregnant levels. During the second and third trimesters, an additional 340 and 452 kcalories per day, respectively, is recommended (Figure 14.7). Although the RDA for carbohydrate and the AI for linoleic acid and alpha-linolenic are increased during pregnancy, the macronutrient distribution of the diet should be about the same as that recommended for the general population.

Protein Needs Protein needs are also increased during pregnancy (see Figure 14.7). Protein is needed for the structure of all new cells in both the mother and the fetus. An increase of 25 grams of protein per day above the RDA for nonpregnant women or 1.1 g/kg/d is recommended for the second and third trimesters of pregnancy to provide for the increase in maternal blood volume; the development of the placenta, breasts, uterus, and uterine muscles; and the development and growth of all fetal structures. For a woman weighing 136 pounds (62 kg), this increases protein needs to about 75 grams per day.

Fluid Needs The need for water is increased during pregnancy because of the increase in blood volume, the production of amniotic fluid, and the needs of the fetus. This requires the consumption of only an extra ounce per day. Adequate fluid consumption, about 2 liters per day, throughout pregnancy is also important in preventing constipation.

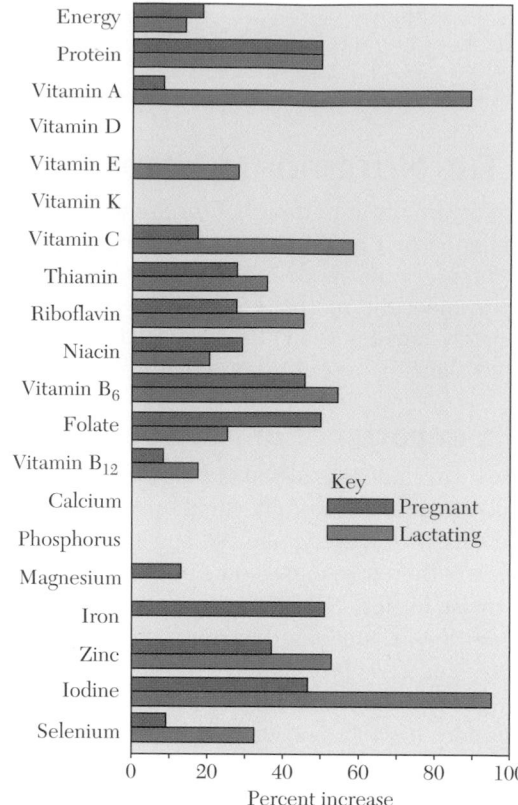

Figure 14.7
This graph illustrates the percentage increase in recommended nutrient intakes for a 25-year-old woman during the third trimester of pregnancy and lactation. The RDA for iron during lactation is equal to half the RDA for nonpregnant, nonlactating women.

Micronutrient Needs During Pregnancy

The need for many vitamins and minerals is increased during pregnancy. Due to growth in maternal and fetal tissues as well as increased energy utilization, the requirements for the B vitamins, such as thiamin, niacin, and riboflavin, increase. To meet the needs for increased protein synthesis in fetal and maternal tissues, the requirements for vitamin B_6 and zinc increase. The needs for calcium, vitamin D, and vitamin C increase to provide for the growth and development of bone and connective tissue. To form new maternal and fetal cells the needs for folate, vitamin B_{12}, zinc, and iron are increased.

Calcium The fetus retains about 30 grams of calcium over the course of gestation. Most of the calcium is deposited in the last trimester when the fetal skeleton is growing most rapidly and the teeth are forming. The increased need for calcium does not increase maternal bone resorption, and studies have found no correlation between the number of pregnancies a woman has had and the density of her bones. There is an increase in the absorption of calcium from the diet during pregnancy,[10] which may be due in part to an increase in estrogen and an increase in the concentration of active vitamin D in the blood.[11] Therefore, the AI for calcium for pregnant women age 19 and older—1000 mg a day—is not increased above nonpregnant needs. This AI can be met by consuming 3 to 4 servings of milk or other dairy products daily. Women who are lactose intolerant can meet their calcium needs with yogurt, cheese, reduced-lactose milk, calcium-rich vegetables, and calcium-fortified foods.

Vitamin D Adequate vitamin D is essential to ensure efficient calcium absorption, but the recommended intake for vitamin D is not increased above nonpregnant levels. When pregnant women receive regular exposure to sunlight, vitamin D supplements are unnecessary. If exposure to sunlight is limited and sufficient vitamin D is not consumed in the diet, supplements should be considered. Most prenatal supplements provide 10 μg of vitamin D, which is twice the AI but well below the UL for pregnancy of 50 μg.[10] Inadequate vitamin D may be a particular problem in African American women because their calcium intake is often low due to lactose intolerance and their darker pigmentation reduces the synthesis of vitamin D in the skin.

Vitamin C   Vitamin C is important for bone and connective tissue formation because it is needed for the synthesis of collagen, which gives structure to skin, tendons, and the protein matrix of bones. Vitamin C deficiency during pregnancy increases the risk for premature birth and eclampsia. The RDA is increased by 10 mg per day during pregnancy. The requirement for vitamin C can easily be met with foods such as citrus fruit, and supplements are generally not necessary.

Folate   Folate is needed for the synthesis of DNA and thus for cell division. During pregnancy, cells multiply to form the placenta, expand maternal blood, and allow for fetal growth. Adequate folate intake is crucial even before conception because rapid cell division occurs in the first days and weeks of pregnancy.

Folate is believed to be essential for proper formation of the **neural tube**, which is the portion of the embryo that develops into the brain and spinal cord. During development, neural tissue forms a groove; the groove closes when the sides fold together to form a tube (Figure 14.8). This neural tube closure occurs between 21 and 28 days of development. If it does not occur normally, the infant will be born with a neural tube defect, such as spina bifida, a defect in which the neural tube does not close completely (see Chapter 8). It has been hypothesized that folate might overcome a deficit in the production of DNA or protein at a critical time in neural tube closure, or that it selectively increases the spontaneous abortion rate of affected fetuses.[13]

Because the neural tube closes so early in development, often before a woman even knows she is pregnant, the DRIs recommend that women capable of becoming pregnant consume 400 μg daily of synthetic folic acid from fortified foods, supplements, or a combination of the two, in addition to consuming a varied diet rich in natural sources of folate (see Chapter 8, *Critical Thinking: Four Hundred of Fortified Folate*).

Folate continues to be important even after the neural tube closes. Inadequate folate intake is associated with premature and low birth weight births and fetal growth retardation.[14] In the mother, it can result in megaloblastic anemia—the type of anemia in which blood cells do not mature properly (see Chapter 8). The RDA for pregnancy is set at 600 μg of dietary folate equivalents per day. Natural sources of folate include orange juice, legumes, leafy green vegetables, and organ meats. Fortified sources include breads, cereals, and other grain products. Folic acid supplements can also be used to meet this goal. Most prenatal supplements contain 400 μg of folic acid.

Vitamin B$_{12}$ Vitamin B$_{12}$ is essential for the regeneration of active forms of folate, so a deficiency of vitamin B$_{12}$ can also result in megaloblastic anemia. Vitamin B$_{12}$ is transferred from the mother to the fetus during pregnancy. Based on the amount transferred and the increased efficiency of B$_{12}$ absorption that occurs during pregnancy, the RDA for pregnancy is set at 2.6 μg per day.[9] This amount is easily met by a diet containing animal products. Vegans must consume foods fortified with vitamin B$_{12}$ or take vitamin B$_{12}$ supplements to meet the needs of mother and fetus.

Zinc   Zinc is involved in the synthesis and function of DNA and RNA and the synthesis of proteins. It is therefore extremely important for growth and development. Zinc deficiency during pregnancy is associated with an increased risk of fetal malformations, prematurity, and low birth weight.[15] Because zinc absorption is inhibited by high iron intakes, iron supplements may compromise zinc status if the diet is low in zinc. The RDA is 11 mg per day for pregnant women 19 years of age and older.[16]

Neural tube A portion of the embryo that develops into the brain and spinal cord.

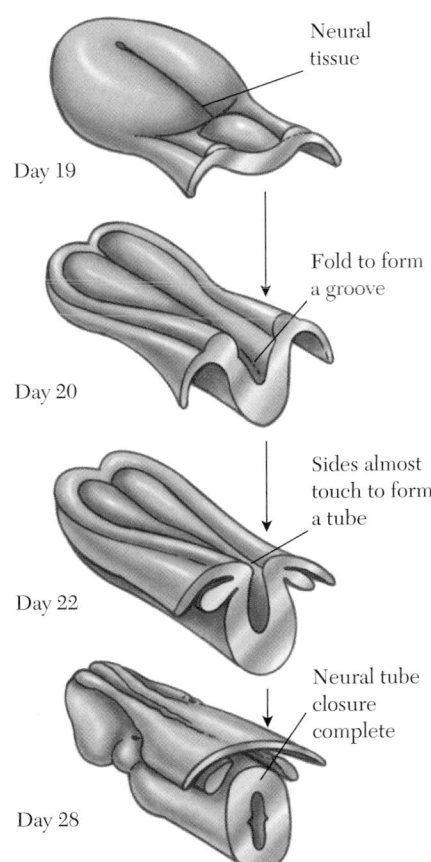

Neural tissue

Day 19

Fold to form a groove

Day 20

Sides almost touch to form a tube

Day 22

Neural tube closure complete

Day 28

Figure 14.8
During embryonic development, a flat plate of neural tissue forms a groove and then the edges fold up and join to form the neural tube, which will become the brain and spinal cord.

Iron Iron deficiency anemia is common during pregnancy. It has been associated with an increased risk of low birth weight and preterm delivery.[17] Because low iron stores are so common among women of childbearing age, many women start pregnancy with diminished iron stores and quickly become deficient. This occurs despite the fact that iron absorption is increased during pregnancy and iron losses are decreased due to the cessation of menstruation.

Iron needs are high during pregnancy to provide for the synthesis of hemoglobin and other iron-containing proteins in both maternal and fetal tissues. The fetus draws iron from the mother to ensure adequate fetal hemoglobin production, mostly during the last trimester. Babies born prematurely may not have had time to accumulate sufficient iron, but babies born at term usually have adequate iron stores even if the mother is deficient.

The RDA for iron during pregnancy is 27 mg per day compared with 18 mg for nonpregnant women.[16] It takes an exceptionally well-planned diet to meet iron needs during pregnancy. Red meats, leafy green vegetables, and fortified cereals are good sources of iron. Foods that enhance iron absorption, such as citrus fruit or meat, should also be included in the diet. Iron supplements are often recommended during the second and third trimesters (see *Critical Thinking*: Nutrient Needs for a Successful Pregnancy).

Meeting Nutrient Needs During Pregnancy

The energy and protein needs of pregnancy can be met by following the Food Guide Pyramid recommendations for pregnant women (Figure 14.9). The additional servings recommended from the Bread, Cereal, Rice, & Pasta Group and

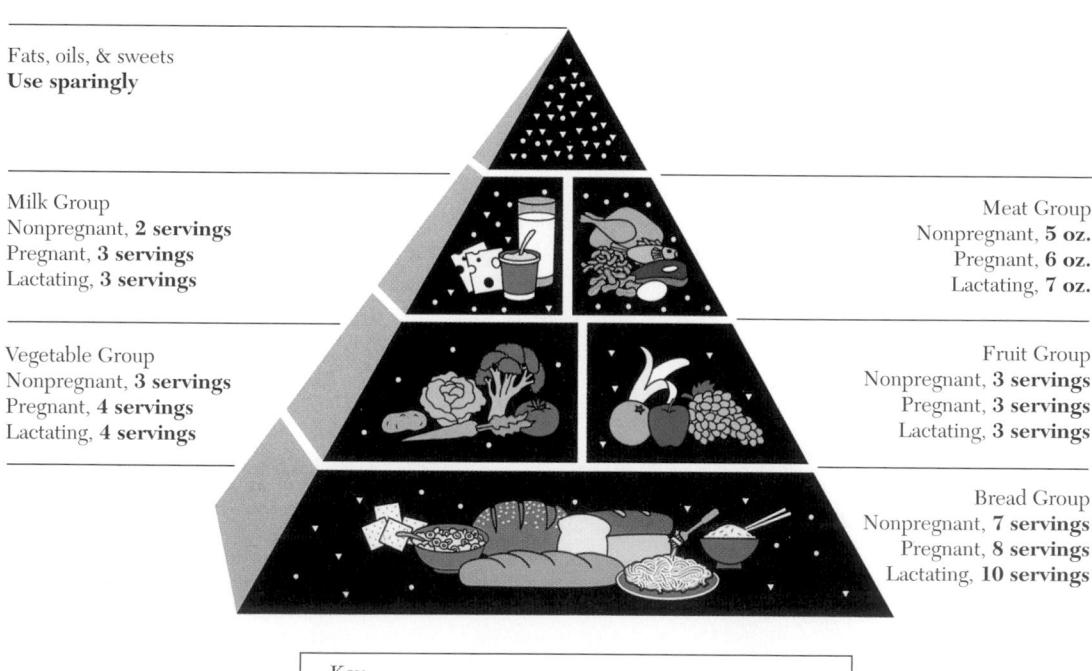

Food Guide Pyramid
A Guide to Daily Food Choices

Fats, oils, & sweets
Use sparingly

Milk Group
Nonpregnant, **2 servings**
Pregnant, **3 servings**
Lactating, **3 servings**

Meat Group
Nonpregnant, **5 oz.**
Pregnant, **6 oz.**
Lactating, **7 oz.**

Vegetable Group
Nonpregnant, **3 servings**
Pregnant, **4 servings**
Lactating, **4 servings**

Fruit Group
Nonpregnant, **3 servings**
Pregnant, **3 servings**
Lactating, **3 servings**

Bread Group
Nonpregnant, **7 servings**
Pregnant, **8 servings**
Lactating, **10 servings**

Key
○ Fat (naturally occurring and added)   ▽ Sugars (added)
These symbols show fats, oils, and added sugars in foods.

USDA, 1992

Figure 14.9

The recommendations of the Food Guide Pyramid can be applied during pregnancy and lactation. Shown here are the recommended servings for a 25-year-old woman before pregnancy and during pregnancy and lactation. (U.S. Department of Agriculture, Home and Garden Bulletin No. 252, 1992.)

the Vegetable Group provide energy, protein, micronutrients, and fiber, particularly if whole grains are chosen. The extra serving of milk that is recommended provides energy, protein, calcium, vitamin D, and riboflavin. The additional one ounce of meat provides energy, protein, vitamin B_6, vitamin B_{12}, iron, and zinc. These recommendations can be met by adding a snack such as a sandwich, an apple, and a glass of milk.

Food Cravings and Aversions Most women change their diets during pregnancy. Some changes are made in an effort to improve nutrition to ensure a healthy infant, but other changes are based on cravings, aversions, or cultural or family traditions. Foods that are commonly craved include sweets and dairy products. Common aversions include coffee and other caffeinated drinks, highly seasoned foods, or fried foods.[18] It has been suggested that hormonal or physiological changes during pregnancy—in particular, changes in taste and smell—may be the cause of such cravings and aversions.

An unusual type of food craving that is more common in pregnancy is **pica**. This is an abnormal craving for and ingestion of nonfood substances having little or no nutritional value. Commonly consumed substances include clay, laundry starch, ice and freezer frost, baking soda, cornstarch, and ashes. Pica during pregnancy is potentially dangerous. The consumption of large amounts of nonfood substances may cause micronutrient deficiencies by reducing the intake of nutrient-dense foods and by reducing nutrient absorption from food. The substances consumed could also cause intestinal obstruction or perforation and could contain toxins or parasites.

Anemia and pregnancy-induced hypertension are more common in mothers who practice pica, but it is not clear if pica is a result of these conditions or a cause. In newborns, anemia and low birth weight are often related to pica in the mother. Because of the association of these conditions with micronutrient intake, it was once thought that pica was an attempt to meet micronutrient needs. It is now believed that pica may be more related to cultural factors than the need for micronutrients.

Pica An abnormal craving for and ingestion of unusual food and nonfood substances.

Are Vitamin and Mineral Supplements Necessary? A healthy diet is essential to satisfy all of the nutrient requirements of pregnancy; even when a prenatal supplement is taken, a woman's diet must be carefully planned.[1] Supplements that are generally recommended include folic acid before and during pregnancy, and iron during the second and third trimesters.[1] A multivitamin and mineral supplement may also be necessary in those whose food choices are limited, such as vegetarians, or in those whose needs are very high, such as pregnant teenagers. (see *Off the Shelf*: Prenatal Supplements).

CRITICAL THINKING

Nutrient Needs for a Successful Pregnancy

Chevon is four months pregnant. From the start—before she tried to conceive—she has been careful about her nutritional health. She took care to consume plenty of both fortified grain products to obtain enough folic acid and foods that are naturally high in folate. Now that she is entering her second trimester, her doctor is concerned about her intake of iron and other nutrients and has prescribed a prenatal supplement. Chevon follows his advice and takes the supplement, but she is curious about whether her diet meets the nutrient needs of pregnancy without supplements. She records her intake for a typical day:

Food	Food Guide Pyramid Group
Breakfast	
1 cup corn flakes	1 grain
with 1 cup reduced-fat milk	1 milk
3/4 cup orange juice	1 fruit
1 cup decaffeinated coffee	
with sugar and cream	fats, oils, and sweets
Lunch	
Tuna sandwich	
3 oz tuna	1 meat
2 tsp mayonnaise	fats, oils, and sweets
2 slices white bread	2 grain
20 french fries	2 vegetable
1 can orange soda	fats, oils, and sweets
3 chocolate chip cookies	1 grain
1 apple	1 fruit
Dinner	
3 oz chicken leg	1 meat
1/2 cup peas	1 vegetable
1 piece corn bread	2 grain
1 tsp margarine	fats, oils, and sweets
1 cup lettuce and tomato salad	1 vegetable
1 Tbsp dressing	fats, oils, and sweets
1 cup reduced-fat milk	1 milk

Her current diet meets the recommendations of the Food Guide Pyramid for a nonpregnant woman, but during her pregnancy, she will also need as much as 450 extra kcalories per day. To obtain this extra energy she should add a serving of vegetables, a serving of milk, an ounce of meat, and a serving of grain products.

What nutrients are provided by these additions?
▼

An added serving of whole grains will add iron, zinc, fiber, and B vitamins. The extra serving of vegetables will add folate, fiber, and vitamin C or A. The extra serving of dairy products will add protein, riboflavin, vitamin D, and calcium. Even though the recommendation for calcium intake is not increased during pregnancy, most young women do not meet calcium needs, and three servings from this group provide about 1000 mg, the AI for young adults. The extra meat adds protein, and if it is from red meat, it provides an excellent source of absorbable iron and zinc as well as vitamins B_{12} and B_6.

Chevon is overweight. Should she still add these foods to her diet?
▼

Answer:

How could her original diet be improved to increase nutrient density?
▼

Answer:

**Does Chevon's diet meet the iron needs of pregnancy
without supplements?**

▼

Answer:

• NUTRITION AND THE RISKS OF PREGNANCY

Most of the four million women who give birth every year in the United States are healthy during pregnancy and produce healthy babies. However, childbearing is not without risks. In the United States, 300 to 500 women die yearly as a result of childbirth. Eleven percent of babies are born too soon, 7.4% are low birth weight, and 7.2 out of each 1000 born alive die within the first year of life.[19] The reasons for poor pregnancy outcome vary. Some women are at increased risk because of their age and preexisting health problems; others have limited access to health care, lack a supportive home environment, or lack the money and facilities to acquire nutritious foods. Others are at risk because they smoke, drink alcohol, or use drugs.

Maternal Health Status

The health of the mother affects the outcome of pregnancy. Women who begin pregnancy with chronic diseases such as diabetes, hypertension, and PKU must manage their health carefully to assure a healthy pregnancy. Maternal age and reproductive history can also have an impact on nutritional status, maternal health, and pregnancy outcome.

The Pregnant Teenager Although the rate of teen pregnancy has been decreasing over the past decade, from 62.1 babies per 1000 teens in 1991, to 48.5 per thousand in 2001, it remains a major public health problem.[20] Pregnant teenagers face economic, social, and medical problems as well as nutritional problems.

Pregnancy places a nutritional strain on a woman's body at any age, and this stress is compounded when the mother herself is still growing. Adolescent girls continue to grow and mature physically for about 4 to 7 years after menstruation begins. Therefore, the risk of pregnancy is greater during this time than it is in women who have stopped growing. To better address the nutritional goals of the pregnant teenager, the Dietary Reference Intakes include an age category within pregnancy that focuses on the needs of pregnant teens.

Consuming a diet that meets the needs for a teenage mother's growth as well as the needs of pregnancy can be difficult. For example, pregnant teens typically consume a diet that contains less calcium, iron, zinc, magnesium, vitamin D, folate, and vitamin B_6 than is recommended. Teenagers are at greater risk of pregnancy-induced hypertension and are more likely to deliver preterm and low birth weight babies. Socioeconomic and demographic factors also contribute to poor pregnancy outcomes in teenage girls. The pregnant teenager needs early medical intervention and nutritional counseling to produce a healthy baby.

The Older Mom The nutritional requirements for older women during pregnancy are no different than for women in their 20s, but pregnancy after the age of 35 does carry additional risks because older women are more likely to start pregnancy with medical conditions such as cardiovascular disease, kidney disorders, obesity, and diabetes.[21] During pregnancy, they also are more likely to develop gestational diabetes, pregnancy-induced hypertension, and other complications. They also have a higher incidence of low birth weight deliveries and of chromosomal abnormalities, especially

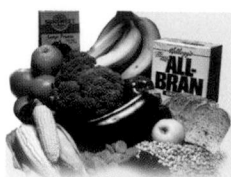

Off the Shelf
Prenatal Supplements

Most pregnant women leave their first prenatal doctor's visit with a prescription for a prenatal vitamin and mineral supplement. Yet public health agencies only recommend routine supplementation of iron and folate.[1,2] The supplements prescribed by physicians contain iron and folate, but they also contain about 15 other vitamins and minerals. Should women take these supplements?

There is nothing wrong with taking a multivitamin and mineral supplement during pregnancy as long as the recommended dosage is not exceeded. The concern of public health agencies is that individuals taking supplements may ignore other components of their diet, thinking that the supplement will meet all their needs. Even when a prenatal supplement is taken, a woman's diet must be carefully planned to satisfy all of the requirements of pregnancy.

Prenatal vitamin and mineral supplements supply many nutrients at levels that meet or slightly exceed the recommended intake for pregnancy, but some are present in amounts that do not meet the needs of pregnancy, and others are missing altogether. For example, the tablet shown in the table contains only 200 mg of calcium, which is only 20% of the AI for a pregnant woman age 19 or older.[3] The reason it does not contain more is that the tablet would have to be very large to provide the recommendation of 1000 mg. To meet her needs a pregnant woman would need to consume this tablet plus the amount of calcium in about three glasses of milk. For similar reasons, the tablet doesn't meet the recommendation for magnesium. Even if all the calcium and magnesium needed for pregnancy could be packed into a little pill, it still would not provide an adequate diet. Prenatal supplements do not contain the

Nutrients Commonly Contained in a Prenatal Supplement

Nutrient	Amount per Tablet	Recommendations for Pregnancy
Vitamin A (μg)	800	770
Vitamin D (μg)	10	5°
Vitamin E (mg α-tocopherol)	11–15	15
Vitamin C (mg)	80–120	85
Folate (μg DFE)	680–1700	600
Thiamin (mg)	1.5	1.4
Riboflavin (mg)	1.6–3.0	1.4
Niacin (mg)	17–20	18
Vitamin B_6 (mg)	2.6–10	1.9
Vitamin B_{12} (μg)	2.5–12	2.6
Biotin (μg)	30	30°
Pantothenic acid (mg)	7	6°
Calcium (mg)	200	1000°
Iron (mg)	60–65	27
Magnesium (mg)	100	350
Copper (mg)	2–3	1.0
Zinc (mg)	25	11

Values given are for a pregnant woman 19 to 30 years of age during her third trimester. Unless indicated, values represent Dietary Reference Intake RDA values.

°Adequate Intake (AI).

protein needed for tissue synthesis or the complex carbohydrates needed for energy. They lack fiber, which helps prevent constipation, and they do not contain fluid for expanding tissues and blood volume and maintaining normal bowel function. They are also lacking in food components such as the phytochemicals that are supplied by a diet rich in whole grains, fruits, and vegetables.

Prenatal supplements are not absolutely necessary to meet the nutrient needs of pregnancy, but a very carefully planned diet is necessary to provide all the substances needed to produce a healthy baby. If a prenatal supplement is taken, it must be part of a healthy diet.

[1]Committee on Nutritional Status During Pregnancy and Lactation, National Academy of Science. *Nutrition During Pregnancy.* Washington, D.C.: National Academy Press, 1990.

[2]Institute of Medicine, Food and Nutrition Board. *Dietary Reference Intakes for Thiamin, Riboflavin, Niacin, Vitamin B-6, Folate, Vitamin B-12, Pantothenic Acid, Biotin, and Choline.* Washington, D.C.: National Academy Press, 1998.

[3]Institute of Medicine, Food and Nutrition Board. *Dietary Reference Intakes for Calcium, Phosphorus, Magnesium, Vitamin D, and Fluoride.* Washington, D.C.: National Academy Press, 1997.

Down syndrome A disorder caused by extra genetic material that results in distinctive facial characteristics, mental retardation, and other abnormalities.

Down syndrome. Today, careful medical monitoring throughout pregnancy is reducing the risks to older mothers and their babies (Figure 14.10).

Reproductive History Frequent pregnancies, with little time between, increase the risk for malnutrition because the mother may not have replenished nutrient stores depleted in the first pregnancy when she becomes pregnant again. A short interval between pregnancies also increases the risk of preterm and low birth weight

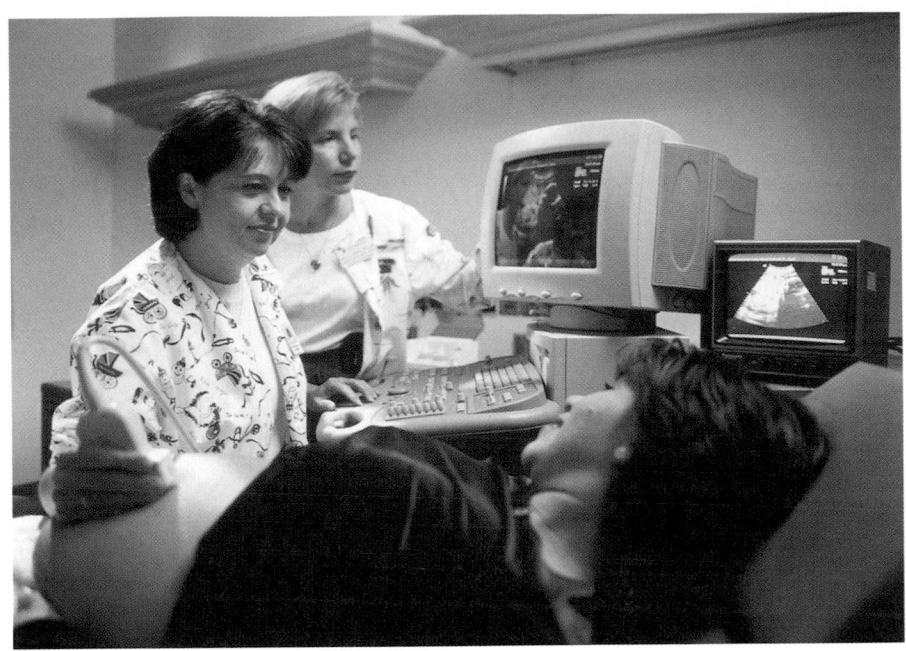

Figure 14.10
Prenatal care with careful medical monitoring can help older women have uncomplicated pregnancies and produce healthy babies. (Stewart Cohen/Stone)

infants. Women with a history of poor pregnancy outcome are also at increased risk. For example, a woman who has had a number of miscarriages is more likely to have another, and a woman who has had one child with a birth defect has an increased risk for defects in subsequent children.

Socioeconomic Factors

One of the greatest risk factors for poor pregnancy outcome is low-income level. Poverty limits access to food, education, and health care.[22] Low-income women have a higher incidence of low birth weight and preterm infants. Low-income women are unlikely to receive any care until late in pregnancy. One federally funded program that addresses the nutritional needs of pregnant women is the Special Supplemental Nutrition Program for Women, Infants, and Children (WIC). WIC has been shown to reduce health-care costs by providing preventative care to low-income pregnant women through nutrition education and food vouchers.[23] This program provides services to pregnant women, to nonlactating women for 6 months after birth, to lactating women for 12 months after birth, and to infants and children up to 5 years of age, but it does not address the need for good nutrition for women planning a pregnancy.

Substances That Affect Pregnancy Outcome

Many substances can affect the health of the embryo and fetus during pregnancy. Some of these are environmental toxins, some are consumed in the diet, and others are the result of maternal behaviors such as smoking and drug use (Figure 14.11).

The Embryo and Fetus Are Particularly Vulnerable The rapidly dividing cells of the embryo and fetus are sensitive to many substances that might normally be a part of a woman's daily routine. Any chemical, biological, or physical agent that causes birth defects is called a **teratogen**. The placenta prevents some teratogens from passing from the mother's blood to the embryonic or fetal blood, but it cannot prevent the passage of all hazardous substances.

The developing embryo and fetus are particularly vulnerable to assault when cells are dividing, differentiating, and moving to form body structures and organs. During these critical periods of development, anything that interferes with development causes irreversible damage. Because each organ system develops at a different rate and time, the period when a nutritional, chemical, or other insult occurs deter-

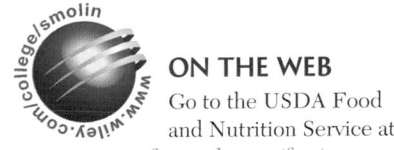

ON THE WEB
Go to the USDA Food and Nutrition Service at
www.fns.usda.gov/fns/
for information about programs such as WIC that are designed to improve the nutrition of women and children.

Teratogen A substance that can cause birth defects.

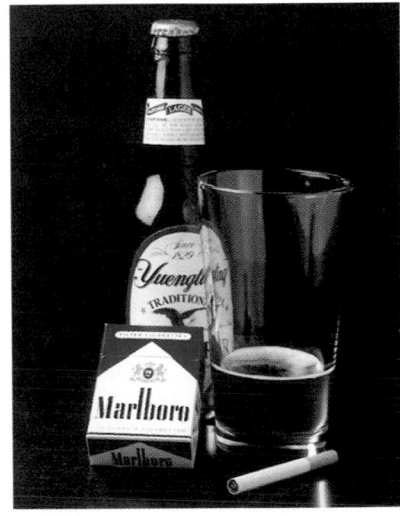

Figure 14.11
Women who smoke, drink alcohol, or use illicit drugs during pregnancy put their babies at risk. (George Semple)

mines which organ system is primarily affected. Because the majority of cell differentiation occurs during the embryonic period, this is the time when exposure to teratogens can do the most damage, but vital body organs can still be affected during the fetal period (Figure 14.12). Severe damage to an embryo or fetus usually results in a spontaneous abortion.

Nutrients as Teratogens Deficiencies or excesses of some nutrients can have teratogenic effects. As discussed previously, inadequate folate intake may affect neural tube development. Excess vitamin D can cause mental retardation. Too much preformed vitamin A is of particular concern because the risk of abnormalities in the offspring increases even when maternal intake is not extremely high. A UL of 3000 μg/day has been established for pregnant women, ages 19 to 50 years. Supplements consumed during pregnancy should therefore contain beta-carotene, which is not teratogenic.

Alcohol Alcohol is a teratogen that impairs fetal growth and development. It is a toxin that reduces blood flow to the placenta, thereby decreasing the delivery of oxygen and nutrients to the fetus. The use of alcohol can also impair maternal nutritional status, further increasing the risk to the embryo or fetus. Alcohol can cause learning and developmental disabilities and behavioral abnormalities referred to as **alcohol-related birth defects** or **fetal alcohol effects**. Alcohol-related birth defects are the leading cause of preventable birth defects and mental retardation.[24] They occur in 1 out of every 1000 live births in the United States and in 43 of every 1000 babies born to heavy drinkers.

More severe alcohol-related damage during pregnancy is called **fetal alcohol syndrome**. Fetal alcohol syndrome is a pattern of facial deformities, growth retardation, and permanent brain damage that causes problems throughout the child's life-

Alcohol-related birth defects or **fetal alcohol effects** A spectrum of abnormalities such as learning and developmental disabilities and behavioral abnormalities in a child due to maternal alcohol consumption during pregnancy.

Fetal alcohol syndrome A characteristic group of physical and mental abnormalities in an infant resulting from maternal alcohol consumption during pregnancy.

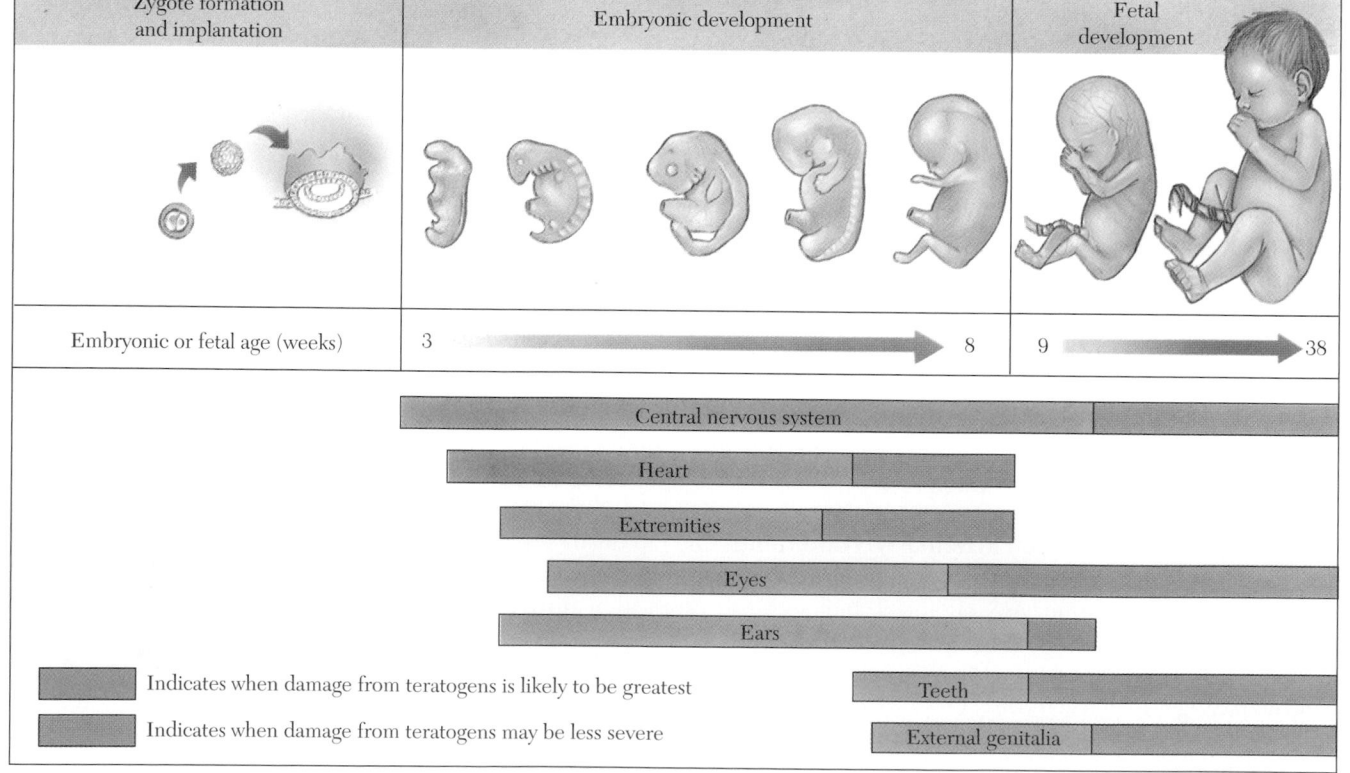

Figure 14.12

The critical periods of development are different for different body systems. (Adapted from Moore, K., and Persaud, T. *The Developing Human*, 5th ed. Philadelphia: W. B. Saunders Company, 1993.)

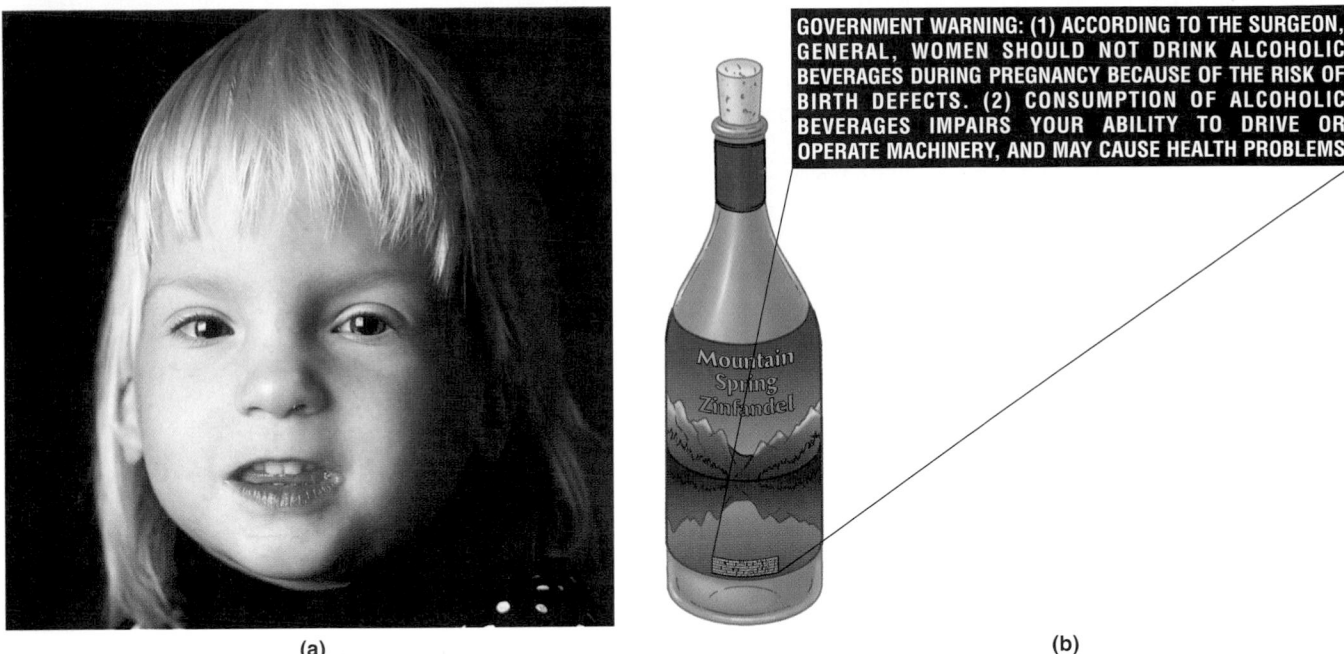

GOVERNMENT WARNING: (1) ACCORDING TO THE SURGEON, GENERAL, WOMEN SHOULD NOT DRINK ALCOHOLIC BEVERAGES DURING PREGNANCY BECAUSE OF THE RISK OF BIRTH DEFECTS. (2) CONSUMPTION OF ALCOHOLIC BEVERAGES IMPAIRS YOUR ABILITY TO DRIVE OR OPERATE MACHINERY, AND MAY CAUSE HEALTH PROBLEMS

(a) (b)

Figure 14.13

(a) Children with fetal alcohol syndrome have common facial characteristics, including a low nasal bridge, a short nose, distinct eyelids, and a thin upper lip. (b) Alcoholic beverage packages include a warning against alcohol consumption during pregnancy. (a, © George Steinmetz)

time. The head circumference is small, the cheekbones are poorly developed, the nose is short with a low nasal bridge between the eyes, the area under the nose is flat, and the upper lip is thin (Figure 14.13a). Growth retardation either during gestation or after birth is common. Newborns with the syndrome may be shaky and irritable, with poor muscle tone and alcohol withdrawal symptoms. Other problems include heart and urinary tract defects, impaired vision and hearing, and delayed language development. Mental retardation is the most common and most serious effect.

Because alcohol consumption in each trimester has been associated with abnormalities, and because there is no level of alcohol consumption that is known to be safe during pregnancy, complete abstinence from alcohol during pregnancy is recommended, and warning labels to this effect appear on containers of beer, wine, and hard liquor (see Figure 14.13b).

Cigarettes Exposure to cigarette smoke affects the baby before birth and throughout life.[25] Compounds in tobacco smoke bind to hemoglobin and reduce oxygen delivery to fetal tissues. In addition, the nicotine absorbed from cigarette smoke constricts arteries and limits blood flow, reducing both oxygen and nutrient delivery to the fetus. Low birth weight babies are common among smokers; it is estimated that 20% of all such births could be prevented if women stopped smoking while pregnant. The risks of miscarriage, stillbirth, and premature birth are also increased in mothers who smoke.[26] The risk of **sudden infant death syndrome (SIDS,** or **crib death)** and respiratory problems are increased in children exposed to cigarette smoke both in the uterus and after birth.[27] The effects of maternal smoking follow children throughout life.

Caffeine Caffeine is a natural component of coffee, tea, and chocolate and is added to some soft drinks and medications (see Table 13.6). Caffeine has not been found to be a teratogen in humans, but consumption of more than 300 mg of caffeine per day by the mother during pregnancy has been associated with small reductions in birth weight and an increase in the risk for spontaneous abortion.[28] A typical cup of American coffee contains about 140 mg of caffeine, so this amount would be equivalent to about $2\frac{1}{2}$ cups of coffee per day.

Sudden infant death syndrome (SIDS) or **crib death** The unexplained death of an infant, usually during sleep.

Illicit Drug Abuse Substance abuse during pregnancy is a national health issue. Exposure to cocaine, opiates, or amphetamines has been shown to affect infant behavior and impact learning and attention span during childhood.[29]

Cocaine increases the risk of complications to the mother and creates problems for the infant before, during, and after delivery. Cocaine use during pregnancy is associated with a high rate of miscarriages, intrauterine growth retardation, premature labor and delivery, low birth weight infants, birth defects, and sudden infant death syndrome.[30] This drug easily crosses the placenta and causes damage by constricting blood vessels, thereby reducing the flow of oxygen and nutrients to the rapidly dividing fetal cells.[31] At birth, cocaine-exposed babies are small and overly excitable. They have a small head circumference, which is associated with lower IQ scores. Cocaine also affects brain chemistry by altering the action of neurotransmitters. This may cause the impulsiveness and moodiness characteristic of some cocaine-exposed children. Some of these babies also have physical deformities.

Marijuana also crosses the placenta and enters fetal blood. Thus far, results of studies on the effect of marijuana use on pregnancy outcome have been conflicting—some show no negative effects, while others show that these infants are shaky and easily startled.[32]

• LACTATION

The nutrient requirements of pregnancy include those needed to prepare for lactation. After childbirth, the breast-feeding mother's nutrient intake must support milk production and can influence the nutrient composition of her milk.

The Physiology of Lactation

During pregnancy, changes occur in the breasts to prepare for milk production, and body fat is deposited to ensure that energy is available for lactation. After birth, the suckling of the infant causes the release of the pituitary hormone prolactin, which stimulates milk production. The more the infant suckles, the more milk is produced. The release of milk from the milk-producing glands and its movement through the ducts and storage sinuses is referred to as **let-down** (Figure 14.14). The let-down of milk is

Let-down A hormonal reflex triggered by the infant's suckling that causes milk to be released from the milk glands and flow through the duct system to the nipple.

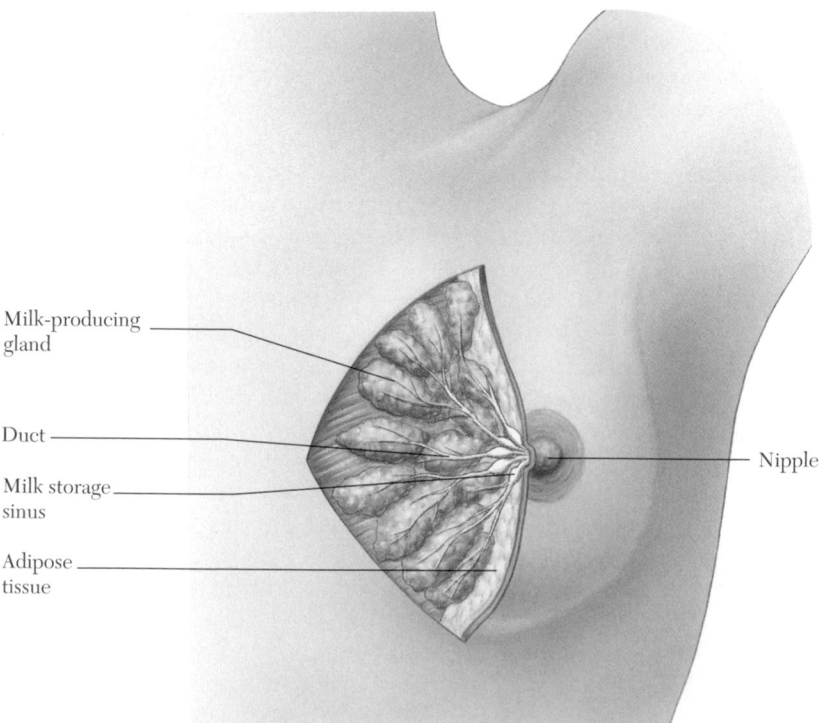

Milk-producing gland

Duct

Milk storage sinus

Adipose tissue

Nipple

Figure 14.14

During lactation, milk travels from the milk-producing glands through the ducts to milk storage sinuses and then to the nipple.

caused by oxytocin, another hormone produced by the pituitary gland. Oxytocin release is also stimulated by the suckling of the infant, but as nursing becomes more automatic, oxytocin release and the let-down of milk may occur in response to the sight or sound of an infant. It can be inhibited by nervous tension, fatigue, or embarrassment. The let-down response is essential for successful breast feeding and makes suckling easier for the child. If let-down is slow, the child can become frustrated and difficult to feed.

Maternal Nutrient Needs During Lactation

The need for many nutrients is even greater during lactation than during pregnancy. This is because the mother is still providing for all of the nutrient needs of the infant, who is growing faster and is more active than the fetus. The newborn also has greater energy and nutrient needs for processes such as body temperature regulation and digestion that were partially or completely managed by the mother when the fetus was still in the womb. Meeting the needs of lactation requires a varied nutrient-dense diet that follows the Food Guide Pyramid recommendations for lactating women (see Figure 14.9). Most lactating women can meet all their needs without supplements.

Energy and Macronutrient Needs During Lactation During the first six months of lactation, approximately 600 to 900 ml, or 2.5 to 3.75 cups, of milk is produced daily. The amount is increased or decreased depending on the amount that the infant consumes.

Energy Human milk contains about 160 kcalories per cup (240 ml). Providing an infant with 750 ml of milk would require approximately 500 kcalories from the mother. Much of this must come from the diet, but some can be met from mobilization of maternal fat stores. The EER for lactation is estimated by adding the total energy expenditure of nonlactating women and the energy in milk and then subtracting the energy supplied by maternal fat stores.[4] This is equal to an additional 330 kcalories per day during the first 6 months of lactation, and 400 kcalories per day during the second 6 months (see Figure 14.7).

Many women are concerned about losing weight after pregnancy. It is normal to lose weight during the first six months after delivery. Some studies report that breast feeding does not affect the amount of weight lost, whereas others suggest it does so initially or if breast feeding continues for at least six months.[33] Beginning one month after birth, most lactating women lose 0.5 to 1 kilogram (1 to 2 lb) per month for 6 months. Some women will lose more, and others may maintain or even gain weight regardless of whether or not they breast feed. Rapid weight loss is not recommended during lactation because it can decrease milk production; regular exercise may speed weight loss and does not impair milk production.

Protein, Carbohydrate and Fat To ensure adequate protein for milk production, the RDA for lactation is increased by 25 grams/day. The RDA for carbohydrate and the AIs for linoleic and alpha-linolenic acids are also higher during lactation (see inside cover).[4]

Water To avoid dehydration and ensure adequate milk production, fluid intake should be increased by about 1 liter per day. This can be done by consuming an extra glass of milk, juice, or water at every meal and whenever the infant nurses. When fluid intake is low, the mother's urine will become more concentrated to conserve water for milk production.

Micronutrient Needs During Lactation The recommended intakes for several vitamins and minerals are increased during lactation to meet the metabolic needs of synthesizing milk and to replace the nutrients secreted in the milk itself (see Figure 14.7). Maternal intake of some vitamins including C, B_6, B_{12}, A, and D can affect milk composition. When maternal intake is low, the amounts in milk are decreased. The recommended intakes of vitamin B_6, B_{12}, other B vitamins, and vitamins A, C, and E are increased above nonlactating levels.

For other nutrients, including calcium and folate, levels in the milk are maintained at the expense of maternal stores. Much of the calcium secreted in human milk comes from an increase in maternal bone resorption. However, the AI for calcium is not increased above nonlactating levels because the loss of calcium from maternal bones is not prevented by increases in dietary calcium. Calcium supplements during lactation also do not affect the concentration of calcium in the milk or maternal bone mineral changes.[34] Although lactation is associated with maternal bone loss, the calcium lost is replaced after weaning.[35] Folate needs are increased above nonpregnant levels to account for the amount needed to replace folate secreted in milk plus the amount needed by nonlactating women to maintain folate status.[16] Iron needs are not increased during lactation because little iron is lost in milk, and, in most women, losses are decreased because menstruation is absent. The RDA for lactation is 9 mg/day, half that of nonlactating women.

• NUTRITION FOR THE INFANT

When a child is born and the umbilical cord is cut, he or she suddenly becomes actively involved in obtaining nutrients rather than being passively fed through the placenta (Figure 14.15). Nutrient needs are high to support growth, development, and activity. Suckling from either the breast or bottle must satisfy all nutrient needs.

Nutrient Needs of the Newborn

During the first few months after birth, growth is more rapid than at any other time of life. Many of the infant's organ systems and metabolic processes are still developing. Since infants' digestive abilities are limited and they have no teeth, a special type of diet is required.

Energy and Macronutrient Needs   Intakes in infants must supply enough energy for their rapid growth. EERs for infants are calculated from total energy expenditure plus the energy deposited in tissues due to growth (see inside cover).[4] Differences in growth rates are reflected in the separate EER prediction equations for infants 0 to 3 months, 4 to 6 months, and 7 to 12 months.

Fat   Healthy infants consume about 55% of their energy as fat during the first 6 months of life, and 40% during the second 6 months. This energy-dense diet allows the infant's small stomach to hold enough food to meet energy needs. An AI for total fat has been set at 31 g/day for infants from birth to 6 months of age and at 30 g/day for infants 7 to 12 months of age. A sufficient supply of the long chain polyunsaturated fatty acids docosahexaenoic acid (an omega-3 fatty acid) and arachidonic acid (an omega-6 fatty acid) are important for nervous system development. These fatty acids are constituents of cell membranes and are incorporated into the retina of the eye and brain tissue. Infants can synthesize docosahexaenoic acid and arachidonic acid from their precursors, alpha-linolenic acid and linoleic acid, respectively, but the rate of conversion may not be optimal.[36] AIs for infants have been set for total omega-3 and total omega-6 fatty acids based on the amounts of these types of fatty acids in human milk.[4]

Carbohydrate   Carbohydrate is a major contributor to energy intake in the infant. The source of carbohydrate in breast-fed infants and most bottle-fed infants is lactose. About 39% of the energy in breast milk is from lactose. As the infant grows and solid foods are introduced into the diet, the percentage of kcalories from carbohydrate in the diet increases and the percent from fat decreases.

Protein   The infant's protein requirement per unit of body weight is very high compared with the adult requirement: The AI is 1.52 grams per kilogram from birth to

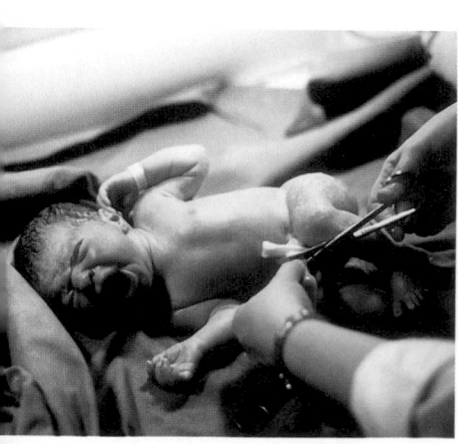

Figure 14.15

At birth the umbilical cord is cut and the child must obtain nutrients orally. (© Jerry Cooke/Photo Researchers, Inc.)

six months of age, compared with 0.8 gram per kilogram for an adult. The ideal protein source for newborns is human milk. Infant formulas are designed to mimic this amino acid pattern. A diet too high in protein may lead to dehydration because the excretion of metabolic wastes produced when excess protein is consumed increases water loss.

Water The fluid requirements of infants are also very high compared with those of adults. Infant kidneys are poorly developed and unable to reabsorb much of the water that is filtered out of the blood. Therefore, infants lose proportionately more water in their urine than adults. Infants also lose proportionately more water through evaporation than do adults because they have a large surface area compared with their total body weight. These factors, in addition to the fact that infants cannot tell us they are thirsty, puts them at risk for dehydration. It is recommended that infants consume 150 ml of water per kilogram of body weight. Usually the amount of water in breast milk or formula is enough to meet needs. Hot weather, fever, diarrhea, and vomiting increase water loss, and therefore require that additional water be given.

In the developing world, diarrhea is the most common cause of infant death, and in the United States it kills one child each day. The cause of the diarrhea is usually a bacterial or viral infection; the cause of death is dehydration. The fluid intake of infants with diarrhea should be monitored carefully, and a pediatrician should be contacted. Mixtures of sugar, water, and electrolytes are available to replace lost fluids.

Micronutrients There are several vitamins and minerals that may be limited in the unsupplemented infant diet. These include iron, vitamin D, vitamin K, fluoride, and vitamin B_{12}.

Iron is the nutrient most commonly deficient in infants who are consuming adequate energy and protein. Iron deficiency is usually not a problem during the first 4 to 6 months of life because infants have iron stores at birth and the iron in human milk, though not particularly abundant, is very well absorbed. The AI for iron from birth to 6 months is only 0.27 mg/day. After 4 to 6 months, iron stores are depleted but iron needs remain high. The RDA for 7 to 12 months is 11 mg/day. The diets of breast-fed infants should contain other sources of iron, such as iron-fortified rice cereal. Formula-fed infants should be fed iron-fortified formula.

Newborns are also potentially at risk for vitamin D deficiency. Breast milk is relatively low in vitamin D, so breast-fed infants who do not receive adequate exposure to sunlight, such as those living in cold climates, may not obtain adequate vitamin D. An AI of 5 μg of vitamin D has been set for infants 0 to 12 months of age. This may be provided as a supplement for breast-fed infants. Infant formulas contain 10 μg of vitamin D per liter of formula. To synthesize adequate vitamin D, about 15 minutes per day of sun exposure, with only the face exposed, is needed for light-skinned babies; a longer time is required for darker-skinned babies.

Vitamin K, important in blood clotting, is another nutrient for which newborns are at risk of deficiency. Little of this vitamin crosses the placenta from mother to fetus, and because the gut is sterile at birth, no microbial vitamin K synthesis occurs. Breast milk is also low in vitamin K, so breast-fed infants are at risk of hemorrhage due to vitamin K deficiency. Most newborns receive a vitamin K injection at birth to prevent the possibility of hemorrhage. This provides them with enough vitamin K to last until their intestines are colonized with the bacteria that synthesize it.

Fluoride is important in the development of teeth, even before they erupt. Breast milk is low in fluoride, and formula manufacturers use unfluoridated water in preparing liquid formula. Therefore, breast-fed infants, infants fed premixed formula, and those fed formula mixed with low-fluoride water are often supplemented beginning at six months of age. In areas where the drinking water is fluoridated, infants fed formula reconstituted with tap water should not be given fluoride supplements.

Vitamin B_{12} may be deficient in the breast milk of vegan mothers. Therefore, infants of vegan mothers should be supplemented with vitamin B_{12}.

How Much Is Enough: Assessing Infant Growth

Although nutrient needs for infants are fairly well defined, it is difficult to calculate an infant's actual nutrient intake. The best indicator of adequate nourishment is normal growth. Most healthy infants follow standard patterns of growth, so an infant's growth can be monitored by comparing length, weight, and head circumference to standards for infants of the same age[37] (see Appendix B).

Growth charts plot typical growth patterns of infants, children, and adolescents in the United States (Figure 14.16). An infant's pattern of growth can be monitored and compared with that of other infants of the same age. The resulting ranking, or percentile, indicates where the infant's growth falls in relation to population standards. For example, if a newborn boy is at the 20th percentile for weight, it means that 19% of newborn boys weigh less and 80% weigh more. Children usually continue at the same percentiles as they grow. For instance, a child who is at the 50th percentile for height and 25th percentile for weight should continue to follow ap-

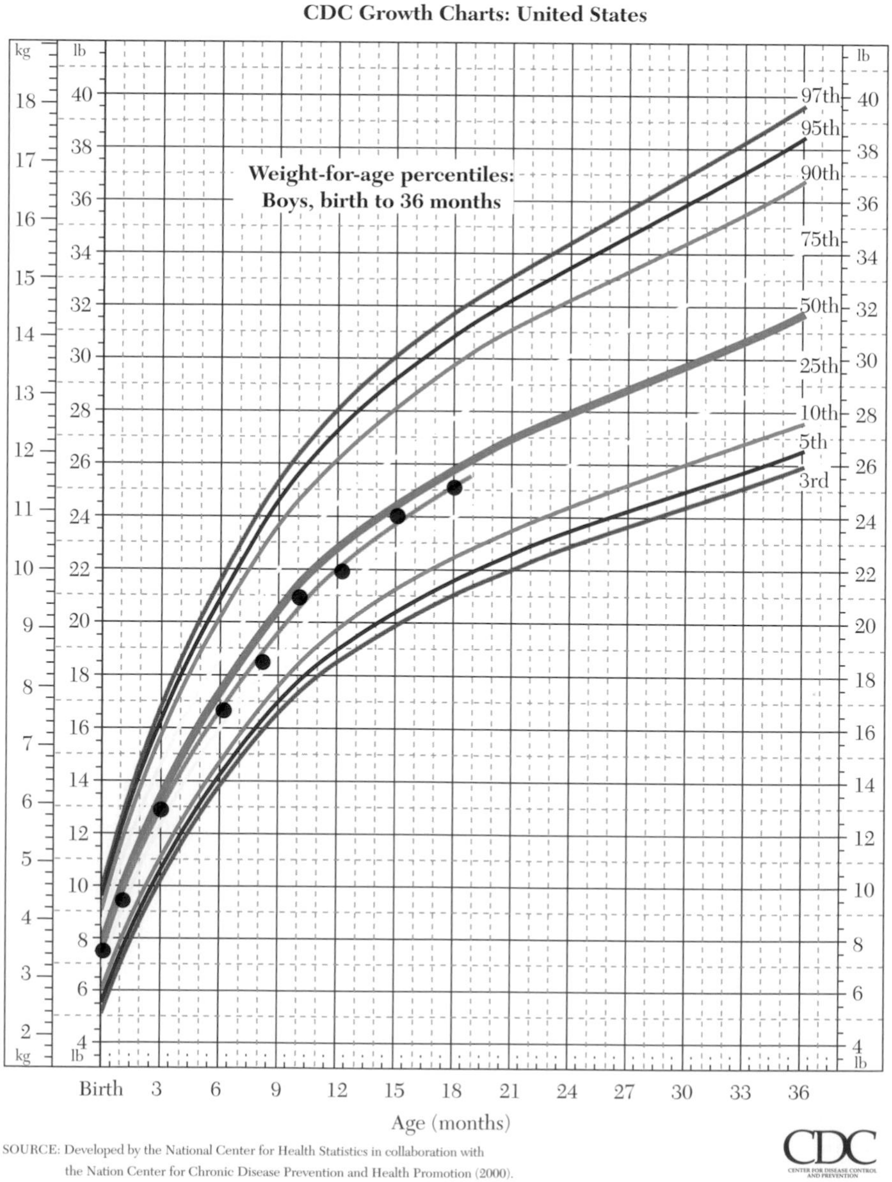

CDC Growth Charts: United States

Figure 14.16

Growth charts, such as this one, which shows weight-for-age percentiles for boys from birth to 36 months of age, demonstrate typical patterns of growth. The blue line follows the pattern of growth for an infant whose birth weight was at the 40th percentile and continued to grow along this curve.

SOURCE: Developed by the National Center for Health Statistics in collaboration with the Nation Center for Chronic Disease Prevention and Health Promotion (2000).

proximately these height and weight curves. A dramatic deviation from the pattern could indicate overnutrition or undernutrition.

Whether an infant is 6 pounds or 8 pounds at birth, the rate of growth should be approximately the same—rapid initially and slowing slightly as the infant approaches one year of age. A rule of thumb is that an infant's birth weight should double by four months and triple by one year of age. In the first year of life, most infants increase their length by 50%. Breast-fed and bottle-fed infants have similar growth for the first three to four months, but then bottle-fed infants grow at a faster rate. Small infants and premature infants often follow a pattern parallel to but below the growth curve for a period of time and then experience catch-up growth that brings them onto the growth curve in a place compatible with their genetic growth potential. Slight fluctuations in growth rate are normal, but a consistent pattern of not following the growth curve or a sudden change in growth pattern is cause for concern.

A rapid increase in weight without an increase in height may be an indicator that the infant is being overfed. Growth that is slower than the predicted pattern indicates **failure to thrive**. This is a catch-all term for any type of growth failure in a young child. The cause may be a congenital condition, the presence of disease, poor nutrition, neglect, abuse, or psychosocial problems. The treatment is usually an individualized plan that includes adequate nutrition and careful monitoring by physicians, dietitians, and other health-care professionals. Just as there are critical periods in fetal life, there are critical periods for growth and development during infancy when undernutrition can permanently affect development.

Failure to thrive The inability of a child's growth to keep up with normal growth curves.

Feeding the Newborn

Newborns have small stomachs, can consume only liquids, and have high nutrient requirements. They should be fed on demand throughout the day and night, about eight times daily. The ideal food for the newborn is breast milk, but infant formula can also meet a newborn's needs. Solid food should not be introduced into the diet until the child is at least 4 to 6 months of age. Introducing solid food before 4 months is not recommended because the infant's feeding abilities and gastrointestinal tract are not mature enough to handle foods other than breast milk or formula.

A relatively common problem in infants is **colic**. Colic involves daily periods of inconsolable crying that cannot be stopped by holding, feeding, or changing the infant. Colic usually begins at a few weeks of age and continues through the first two to three months. It occurs in both breast- and bottle-fed infants. Although its cause is unknown, it is hypothesized that colic is related to intestinal gas caused by milk intolerance, improper feeding practices, or immaturity of the central nervous system.

Colic Inconsolable crying that is believed to be due to pain from gas buildup in the gastrointestinal tract or immaturity of the central nervous system.

Meeting Nutrient Needs with Breast Feeding Breast milk is designed specifically for the human newborn, it requires no special preparation, and the amount available varies with demand. Thus, breast feeding is the preferred form of infant nutrition and is usually the recommended choice for feeding the newborn of a healthy, well-nourished mother.[38]

Advantages to Mother and Child Breast feeding has nutritional, immunological, physiological, and psychological benefits for both mother and child. Breast milk provides protection against infection early in life by passing immune factors from the mother to the infant. Breast-fed babies have fewer allergies, ear infections, respiratory illnesses, and urinary tract infections than formula-fed babies, and have fewer problems with constipation and diarrhea. There is also evidence that breast feeding protects against sudden infant death syndrome, diabetes, and chronic digestive diseases.[39] The strong suckling required by breast feeding aids in the development of facial muscles, which help in speech development and the correct formation of teeth. Breast-fed babies are also less likely to be overfed, because the amount of milk consumed cannot be monitored visually. In bottle feeding, it is often tempting to encourage the baby to finish the entire bottle whether or not he is hungry. For the mother, breast feeding has the advantage of providing a readily available and inexpensive source of nourishment for her infant. It requires no preparation or bottles and nipples that must be washed. It is more ecological because it doesn't require energy for manufacture or generate waste from discarded packaging. Physiologically, breast feeding causes contractions that help the mother's uterus return to size more quickly and may promote weight loss in some women, especially when continued for more than 6 months.[40] Women who breast feed may have a lower risk of developing osteoporosis and breast and ovarian cancer. Lactation also inhibits ovulation, lengthening the time between pregnancies; however, it does not reliably prevent ovulation and so cannot be effectively used for birth control. Oral contraceptives can be used immediately postpartum, but those containing only progestin are preferable because they do not affect milk volume or composition. Oral contraceptives containing estrogen may decrease milk volume. Psychologically, breast feeding can be a relaxing, emotionally enjoyable interaction for both mother and infant (Table 14.2).

Table 14.2 *Risks and Benefits of Breast and Bottle Feeding*

Risk/Benefit	Breast Feeding	Bottle Feeding
Nutrients	Ideal food for human babies. Composition changes as they eat and grow.	Modeled after human milk, but certain components cannot be duplicated. Composition does not change with time. Must be prepared carefully to supply the correct nutrient mix and ratio of nutrients to fluid.
Amount	Underfeeding can be a problem in newborns if the mother is not well versed in breast feeding and the signs of dehydration in the infant.	Overfeeding is a risk because of the desire of caregivers to have the baby empty the bottle.
Immunity	Immune factors are transferred from mother to infant.	There are no immune factors in formula.
Allergies	Allergies to breast milk are very rare and the risk of food allergies is reduced.	There are a variety of choices if the infant is allergic to one type of formula.
Risk from mother	Certain contaminants such as environmental pollutants, medications, illicit drugs, and disease-causing organisms such as HIV can pass from mother to baby.	None.
Environmental contamination	Breast milk is sterile, but pumped milk can become contaminated if stored improperly.	Bacterial contamination is a risk if formula is prepared under unsanitary conditions or stored improperly.
Ease for caregivers	No equipment to wash, always available, but may require more time from the mother.	Requires more preparation and washing, but other family members can share responsibility for feeding.
Ease for baby	Suckling is harder for the baby but aids in development of teeth and facial muscles needed for speech. Pumped breast milk can be easily consumed by weak or sick infants.	Easier for baby, which is especially important for weak or sick infants.
Benefit to mother	Promotes uterine contractions which help the uterus return to prepregnancy size. May promote loss of weight and body fat if continued for more than six months. May reduce risk of breast cancer.	May allow more sleep.
Cost	Cheaper, but the mother must be well nourished.	More expensive than nursing and includes cost of formula as well as equipment and energy used in preparation.

How Long Should Breast Feeding Continue? Physiologically, lactation can continue as long as suckling is maintained. Breast feeding alone is sufficient to support optimal growth for about six months, and the American Academy of Pediatrics recommends breast milk along with supplemental feeding of solids for the first year of life—and longer—as mutually desired by mother and child.[39] As part of its Integrated Management of Childhood Illness Program, the World Health Organization recommends that infants in developing nations be breast fed for two years.[41] After 12 months, the baby no longer needs breast milk to meet nutrient needs. As the infant obtains more and more of its energy from solid foods, milk production decreases due to reduced demand by the infant. However, breast feeding beyond 12 months continues to provide nutrition, comfort, and an emotional bond between mother and child.

How Much Is Enough? A strong, healthy baby will be able to suckle shortly after birth. Within a week, milk production and breast feeding are usually fully established (Figure 14.17). Infants should be fed on demand every 1.5 to 3 hours. A feeding should last approximately 8 to 12 minutes at each breast. Although it is difficult to measure the amount of milk an infant takes from the breast, a well-fed newborn should urinate enough to soak six to eight diapers a day and gain about $\frac{1}{3}$ to $\frac{1}{2}$ pound per week.

Practical Aspects of Breast Feeding Breast feeding does not always come naturally to mother or infant and can require practice and patience. Effective suckling by the infant and relaxation of the mother are essential to successful breast feeding. Some foods and other substances in the mother's diet, such as garlic or spicy foods, contain chemicals or flavors that pass into breast milk and cause adverse reactions in some babies. These reactions seem to be individual to the mother and child. As long as a food does not affect the infant's response to feeding, it can be included in the mother's diet. Caffeine in the mother's diet can make the infant jittery and excitable, so large amounts should be avoided while breast feeding. Alcohol, which is harmful for infants, passes into breast milk. It is most concentrated an hour to an hour and a half after consumption and is cleared from the milk at about the same rate it disappears from the bloodstream. Therefore, occasional limited alcohol consumption while breast feeding is probably not harmful if intake is timed to minimize the amount present in milk when the infant is fed.

Breast feeding does not mean that a mother must be available for every feeding. Milk may be pumped from the breast and stored for later feedings. If prescription drugs are taken by the mother for only a short time, a breast pump may be used to maintain milk production and the milk discarded, until the medication is no longer needed (Figure 14.18). Since pumped milk is exposed to pumps and bottles, care must be taken to avoid contamination. If pumped milk is not immediately fed to the baby, it should be refrigerated. It can be kept refrigerated for 24 to 48 hours, but if it will not be used within that period, it should be frozen in a clean container. Warming breast milk in a microwave is not recommended, because this destroys some of its immune properties and it may result in dangerously hot portions of the milk. The best way to warm milk is by running warm water over the bottle.

Composition of Human Milk The nutrient composition of breast milk is specifically designed for the human infant and changes as the infant develops. The first fluid that is produced by the breast after delivery is called **colostrum**. Not actually milk, colostrum is a yellowish fluid that is higher in water, protein, immune factors, minerals, and some vitamins than milk. It is produced for up to a week after delivery. While colostrum is produced, it may seem that the newborn is not receiving enough to eat; however, supplemental bottle feedings are not necessary. The nutrients in colostrum meet infant needs until mature milk production begins. During the first few months of life, the immune factors provided first by colostrum, and later by mature milk, compensate for the infant's immature immune system. Colostrum also has

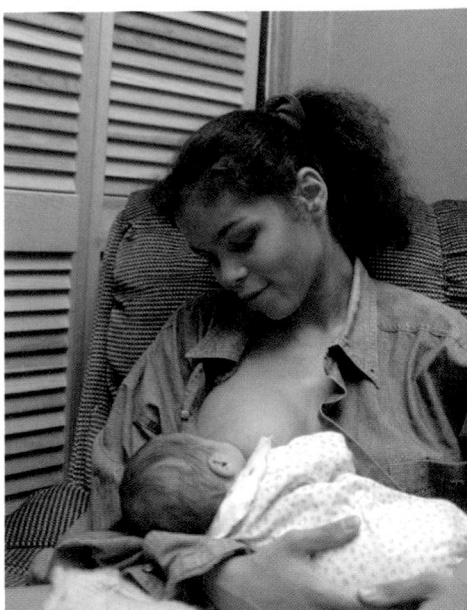

Figure 14.17
By the time the infant is a week old, mother and child have usually adjusted to breast feeding. (© Richard Lord/ The Image Works.)

Colostrum The first milk, which is secreted in late pregnancy and up to a week after birth. It is rich in protein and immune factors.

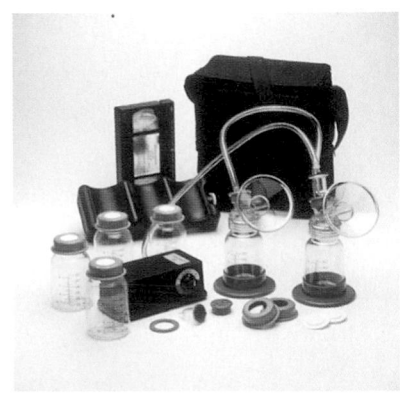

Figure 14.18
Breast pumps can be used to pump milk for bottle feedings. This relieves the mother from responsibility for all feedings. (Bailey Medical Engineering)

beneficial effects on the gastrointestinal tract, acting as a laxative that helps the baby excrete the thick, mucousy stool produced during life in the womb.

The composition of mature human milk changes over time, meeting the nutrient needs of the child for up to the first year of life. Mature human milk contains about 160 kcalories per cup (240 ml) and is a good source of protein, fat, magnesium, and calcium. When compared with cow's milk, it is very different in both appearance and composition. Human milk looks thin and watery and has less protein and minerals than cow's milk. Lactalbumin, the predominant protein in human milk, forms a soft, easily digested curd in the infant's stomach. The amino acids methionine and phenylalanine, which are difficult for the infant to metabolize, are present in lower amounts in human milk proteins than in cow's milk proteins. Human milk is also a good source of taurine, an amino acid needed for bile salt formation and eye and brain function.

The fat in human milk is more easily digested than that in cow's milk. Human milk is higher in cholesterol and the essential fatty acid linoleic acid. It is also higher in arachidonic and docohexaenoic fatty acids, which are essential for normal brain development, eyesight, and growth.[42] The fat content of breast milk changes throughout a feeding, gradually increasing during the nursing session. Thus, for the baby to attain satiety and obtain adequate energy, it is important for nursing to continue long enough for the infant to obtain the higher-fat milk.

Lactose is the primary carbohydrate in human milk. It is digested slowly, so it stimulates the growth of acid-producing bacteria. It also promotes the absorption of calcium and other minerals and provides a source of galactose for nervous system development.

Human milk is low in iron, but the iron present is easily absorbed. About 50% of the iron in human milk is absorbed, compared with only 2 to 30% from many other foods.

Human milk also contains a number of other substances that protect the infant from disease. Antibody proteins and immune system cells pass from the mother into her milk to provide the infant immune protection. A number of enzymes and other proteins prevent the growth of harmful microorganisms. Several carbohydrates have been identified that protect against disease-causing organisms, including viruses that cause diarrhea. One substance favors the growth of the beneficial bacterium *Lactobacillus bifidus* in the infant's colon, which inhibits the growth of disease-causing organisms.

Meeting Nutrient Needs with Bottle Feeding   A hundred years ago a baby who could not be breast fed had little chance of survival. Today infants who cannot breast feed can still thrive. There are many commercially available infant formulas modeled after the nutrient content of breast milk. Unmodified cow's milk should never be fed to infants; its higher protein and mineral content taxes the kidneys and predisposes the infant to dehydration. Young infants may also become anemic if fed cow's milk because it contains little absorbable iron and can lead to iron loss by causing small amounts of gastrointestinal bleeding.

When Is Bottle Feeding Best?   There are some situations when breast feeding is not the best choice. An infant who is small or weak may not have the strength to receive adequate nutrition from breast feeding. In this case, formula, which provides almost the same nutrients as breast milk, can be used, or pumped breast milk can be offered to the infant in a bottle.

Bottle feeding reduces the transmission of drugs and disease via breast milk. Hepatitis and HIV infection, which causes AIDS, can be transmitted to the infant in breast milk, but common illnesses such as colds, flu, and skin infections should not interfere with breast feeding.[43] In the United States, women who are infected with HIV are advised not to breast feed, but in developing nations, the risk of malnutrition associated with not breast feeding outweighs the risk of passing this infection on to the infant. Women who are taking medications should check with their physician as to whether it is safe to breast feed. Because alcohol and drugs such as cocaine and marijuana can be passed to the baby in breast milk, alcoholic and drug-addicted mothers are counseled not to breast feed. Nicotine from cigarette smoke is also rapidly transferred from maternal blood to milk, and heavy smoking may decrease the supply of milk.

How Much Is Enough? As with breast-fed infants, formula-fed infants should be fed on demand every few hours. Newborns have small stomachs, so at each feeding they may consume only a few ounces of formula. As the infant grows, the amount consumed at each feeding will increase to 4 to 8 ounces. Caregivers should respond to cues from the infant that hunger is satisfied, even if a bottle of formula is not finished. Encouraging infants to finish every bottle can result in overfeeding and excess weight gain. As with breast-fed infants, adequate intake can be judged from the amount of urine produced and the amount of weight gained.

Practical Aspects of Bottle Feeding Infant formula must be prepared carefully in order to avoid mixing errors and contamination. If the proper measurements are not used in preparing formula, the child can receive an excess or deficiency of nutrients and an improper ratio of nutrients to fluids. If the water and all the equipment used in preparing formula are not clean or if the prepared formula is left unrefrigerated, food-borne illness may result. Because sanitation is often a problem in developing nations, infections that lead to diarrhea and dehydration occur more commonly in formula-fed than in breast-fed infants. Commercially prepared formulas are sterile and powdered formulas contain no harmful microorganisms. To avoid introducing harmful microorganisms, the water used to mix powdered formula should be boiled for one to two minutes and allowed to cool before mixing. Hands should be washed before preparing formula, and bottles and nipples should be washed in a dishwasher or placed in a pan of boiling water for 5 minutes. Formula should be prepared immediately before a feeding, and any excess should be discarded. Opened cans of ready-to-feed and liquid concentrate formula should be covered and refrigerated and used within the time indicated on the can. Formula may be fed either warm or cold, but the temperature should be consistent.

The position of the child is important during feeding. The infant's head should be higher than the stomach, and the bottle should be tilted so that there is no air in the nipple (Figure 14.19). If the hole in the nipple is too large, the infant may feel full before receiving adequate nutrition. If the hole is too small, the infant may tire before nutrient needs are met. Just as breast-fed infants alternate breasts, bottle-fed infants should be held alternately between the left and right arms to promote equal development of the head and neck muscles.

Infants should never be put to bed with a bottle of formula. At night, while the child sleeps, the flow of saliva is decreased and the sugary formula liquid is allowed to remain in contact with the teeth for many hours. This causes the rapid and serious decay of the upper teeth referred to as **nursing bottle syndrome**. Usually, the lower teeth are protected by the tongue and are unaffected (Figure 14.20).

Formula Choices Infant formulas can never duplicate the living cells, active hormones, enzymes, and immune system molecules in human milk, but formulas today try to replicate human milk as closely as possible in order to match the growth, nutrient absorption, and other parameters obtained with breast feeding. Formula is available in ready-to-feed, liquid concentrate, or powdered forms (see *Off the Shelf*: Choosing an Infant Formula).

There are also special formulas available for infants with conditions, such as allergies, prematurity, and genetic abnormalities, that alter dietary needs. For infants who cannot tolerate human or cow's milk, soy protein formulas are available. And for those who cannot tolerate soy protein, formulas made from predigested proteins, called protein hydrolysates, are an option.

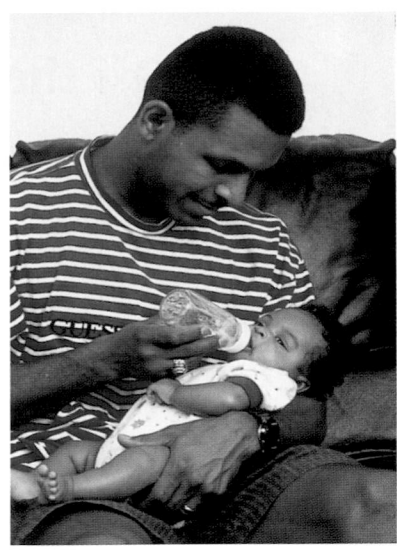

Figure 14.19
During bottle feeding, the position of the baby and the bottle are both important. (© Erika Stone/Photo Researchers, Inc.)

Nursing bottle syndrome Extreme tooth decay in the upper teeth resulting from putting a child to bed with a bottle containing milk or other sweetened liquids.

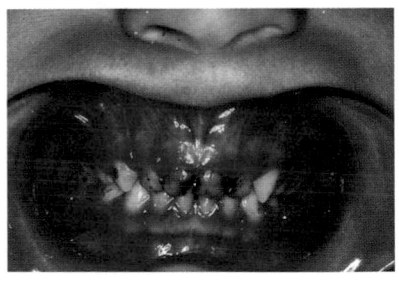

Figure 14.20
Nursing bottle syndrome causes rapid decay of the upper front teeth. (K. L. Boyd, D.D.S./Custom Medical Stock Photo)

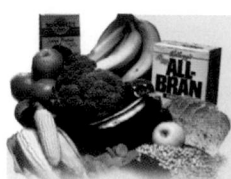

Off the Shelf

Choosing an Infant Formula

Which infant formula is best? Infants are often formula-fed from birth, and most are formula-fed after a few months of breast feeding. Selecting an infant formula can be confusing. Is cow's milk formula better than a soy-based formula? Is one safer or more nutritious than the other? Is a less expensive formula likely to be missing certain nutrients? Is premixed formula better than powdered?

The safety and nutrient content of commercially prepared infant formulas do not need to be considerations in choosing a formula because they are regulated by the FDA. The FDA guidelines for the amounts of nutrients in formulas are based on the composition of human milk and follow the recommendations by the American Academy of Pediatrics Committee on Nutrition.[1] Strict quality control regulations require that each batch of formula be tested for stability and analyzed to ensure it contains the appropriate amounts of required nutrients.

Cow's milk is the standard base for infant formula. If cow's milk formula is not well tolerated by an infant, hydrolyzed cow's milk and soy-based formula are available. Cow's milk hydrolysates are usually recommended over soy formula because they provide higher quality protein and the calcium they contain is better ab-

sorbed. Soy-based formulas are necessary for infants who cannot tolerate the protein in cow's milk and for those who are lactose intolerant, because soy formula contains sucrose or corn syrup instead of lactose.

Formulas are marketed in three basic forms: ready-to-feed, liquid concentrates, and powdered. Ready-to-feed formulas require no preparation and are available in sizes ranging from 4-ounce bottles to 32-ounce containers. Liquid concentrates are prepared for use by mixing equal amounts of the concentrate and water. Powdered formulas are prepared by mixing 1 tablespoon of powder for every 2 ounces of water. When properly prepared, all of these provide the needed nutrients in an appropriate concentration. Problems arise when formulas are mixed incorrectly or when the water used to prepare them is contaminated. Incorrect mixing can result from a lack of understanding, poor measuring techniques, the addition of extra water to make the formula last longer, or the belief that a more concentrated formula will make the baby grow better. Even correctly mixed formula is a health hazard if the water used to mix it contains contaminants such as lead or disease-causing microorganisms. Water for formula should come from a safe source and be boiled before use.

Since the composition and safety of infant formulas are regulated, the major

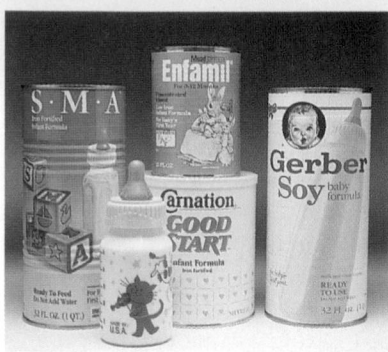

(Charles D. Winters)

considerations when choosing a formula are cost, ease of transport, and convenience of preparation. Ready-to-feed formulas are easiest to use but may cost more and are heavier and bulkier to carry home from the store. Liquid concentrates are a good compromise because they provide more formula for less weight and are easy to mix. Powders are the least expensive and the easiest to transport home in a grocery bag but require more measuring and mixing. Since all of these products are nutritionally comparable, this choice depends on the needs of the caregivers.

[1]Stehlin, I. B. Infant formula: Second best but good enough. *FDA Consumer*, 29:17–20, June 1996.

Premature infants have special needs because they do not have fully developed organ systems or metabolic pathways. If they are too small or weak to nurse or take a bottle, pumped breast milk or formula can be fed through a tube. Some nutrients that are produced in the bodies of full-term infants are essential in the diets of premature infants. For example, preterm infants are less able to synthesize the amino acids tyrosine and cysteine and the fatty acid docosahexaenoic acid. These and other substances, such as taurine and carnitine, are needed in higher amounts by premature babies. The energy, protein, and micronutrient requirements of preterm infants are also higher due to their rapid growth and development. Preterm infant formulas are available to meet the needs of premature babies.

Genetic abnormalities that prevent the normal metabolism of specific nutrients may alter dietary needs. For instance, infants with the genetic disease phenylketonuria (PKU) lack an enzyme needed to metabolize the amino acid phenylalanine (see Chapter 6). If a child with PKU is fed breast milk or a formula that contains phenylalanine, the by-products of phenylalanine metabolism accumulate and can cause brain damage. This can be prevented by feeding infants with PKU a special formula that provides only enough phenylalanine to meet the need for protein synthesis. Because this special diet must be started as soon as possible, infants born in the United States and Canada are tested for PKU at birth.

• APPLICATIONS •

1. Assume that one day of the food record you kept in Chapter 2 is the record of a 25-year-old pregnant woman.
   a. Does this diet meet her energy and protein needs? If not, what foods would you add to the diet to meet the needs of pregnancy?
   b. Does this diet meet the iron and calcium needs of a 25-year-old pregnant woman? List three foods that are good sources of each.
   c. Does this diet meet the folate needs of a 25-year-old pregnant woman? What foods could you add to a diet that is low in folate to meet needs without supplements? What foods in this diet are fortified with folic acid?

2. For each of the following nutrients, describe any differences between the needs of nonpregnant, pregnant, and lactating women. Explain why the requirements for pregnancy and lactation do or do not differ from those for the nonpregnant state.
   a. Energy
   b. Protein
   c. Calcium
   d. Iron
   e. Folate

3. Use the Internet to find out about the WIC program in your area.
   a. Would it be easy for you to use this program if you were a pregnant or lactating woman or had a young child?
   b. What income levels does it serve?

SUMMARY

1. Pregnancy begins with the fertilization of an egg by a sperm, producing a zygote. About three weeks after fertilization, the embryonic period of development begins. The embryo grows, and the cells differentiate and move to form the organs and structures of the body. At nine weeks, the fetal period of development begins. It continues until birth, about 40 weeks after fertilization.

2. During pregnancy, maternal physiology changes to support the pregnancy and prepare for lactation. The amniotic sac and the placenta develop; maternal blood volume increases; the uterus and supporting muscles expand; body fat is deposited; the heart, lungs, and kidneys work harder; the breasts enlarge; and total body weight increases.

3. Recommended weight gain during pregnancy is 25 to 35 pounds for normal-weight women. If too little weight is gained, the infant may be small at birth and at increased risk for illness and death. Too much weight gain can place both mother and baby at risk, but weight loss should never be attempted during pregnancy. Normal-weight, underweight, and overweight mothers should gain weight at a steady rate during pregnancy.

4. During healthy pregnancies, a carefully planned program of moderate-intensity exercise can be beneficial and safe.

5. The hormones that direct changes in maternal physiology and the growth and development of the fetus sometimes cause unwanted side effects. Digestive system discomforts that are common in pregnancy include morning sickness, heartburn, constipation, and hemorrhoids. Changes in glucose utilization can cause gestational diabetes. An elevation in blood pressure, called pregnancy-induced hypertension, can cause edema, weight gain, and protein in the urine (preeclampsia), and in severe cases can be life threatening (eclampsia).

6. Nutritional status is important before, during, and after pregnancy. Poor nutrition before pregnancy can decrease fertility or lead to a poor pregnancy outcome. During pregnancy the requirements for energy, protein, water, vitamins, and minerals increase. The B vitamins are needed to support increased energy and protein metabolism; calcium, vitamin D, and vitamin C are needed for bone and connective tissue growth; protein, folate, vitamin B_{12}, and zinc are needed for cell replication; and iron is needed for red blood cell synthesis.

7. Because the embryo and fetus are rapidly developing and growing, they are susceptible to damage from poor nutrition and physical, chemical, or other environmental teratogens.

8. Factors that increase the risks of pregnancy include poor maternal health status; age that is under 20 or over 35 years; a short interval between pregnancies; a history of poor reproductive outcomes; poverty; and behaviors such as smoking, alcohol use, and drug use.

9. During lactation the need for protein, fluid, and many vitamins and minerals is even greater than during pregnancy.

10. Newborns grow more rapidly and require more energy and protein per kilogram of body weight than at any other time in life. Fat and fluid needs are also proportionately higher than in adults. A diet that meets energy, protein, and fat needs may not necessarily meet the need for iron, fluoride, and vitamins D and K.

11. Breast milk is the ideal food for new babies. It is designed specifically for the human newborn; is always available; requires no special equipment, mixing, or sterilization; and provides immune protection. If breast feeding is not chosen, there are many infant formulas on the market that are patterned after human milk and provide adequate nutrition to the baby.

12. Infant formulas are the best option when the mother is ill or is taking prescription or illicit drugs, or when the infant has special nutritional needs. The major disadvantages of bottle feeding are the potential for bacterial contamination, overfeeding, and the possibility of errors in mixing formula.

REVIEW QUESTIONS

1. List three physiological changes that occur in the mother's body during pregnancy.

2. How do the requirements for energy and protein change during pregnancy?

3. Why does the mother's recommended intake for iron increase during pregnancy?

4. How much weight should a woman gain during pregnancy?

5. How do the recommendations for weight gain differ for overweight and underweight women?

6. What kind of exercise is safe during pregnancy?

7. Are vegetarian diets safe for pregnant women? Why or why not?

8. How does alcohol consumed by a woman during pregnancy affect the child?

9. How does maternal age affect nutrient requirements during pregnancy?

10. How do maternal energy and protein requirements change during lactation?

11. What are the advantages of breast feeding?

12. When is bottle feeding a better choice?

REFERENCES

1. Committee on Nutritional Status during Pregnancy and Lactation, National Academy of Sciences. *Nutrition during Pregnancy*. Washington, D.C.: National Academy Press, 1990.

2. Bryson, S. R., Theriot, L., Ryan, N. J., et al. Primary follow-up care in a multidisciplinary setting enhances catch-up growth of very-low-birth-weight infants. *J. Am. Diet. Assoc.* 97:386–390, 1997.

3. American College of Sports Medicine. *ACSM's Guidelines for Exercise Testing and Prescription*, 5th ed. Baltimore: Williams & Wilkins, 1995.

4. Institute of Medicine, Food and Nutrition Board. *Dietary Reference Intakes for Energy, Carbohydrates, Fiber, Fat, Protein and Amino Acids*. Washington, D.C.: National Academy Press, 2002.

5. Sullivan, B. A., Henderson, S. T., and Davis, J. M. Gestational diabetes. *J. Am. Pharm. Assoc.* (Wash) 38:364–371, 1998.

6. Report of the National High Blood Pressure Education Program Working Group on High Blood Pressure in Pregnancy. *Am. J. Obstet. Gynecol.* 183:S1–S22, 2000.

7. Ritchie, L. D., and King, J. C. Dietary calcium and pregnancy-induced hypertension: Is there a relation? *Am. J. Clin. Nutr.* 71(Suppl.):1371S–1374S, 2000.

8. Villar, J., and Belizán, J. M. Same nutrient, different hypothesis: disparities in trials of calcium supplementation during pregnancy. *Am. J. Clin. Nutr.* 71(Suppl.):1375S–1379S, 2000.

9. Food and Nutrition Board, Institute of Medicine. *Dietary Reference Intakes for Thiamin, Riboflavin, Niacin, Vitamin B-6, Folate, Vitamin B-12, Pantothenic Acid, Biotin, and Choline*. Washington, D.C.: National Academy Press, 1998.

10. Food and Nutrition Board, Institute of Medicine. *Dietary Reference Intakes for Calcium, Phosphorus, Magnesium, Vitamin D, and Fluoride*. Washington, D.C.: National Academy Press, 1997.

11. Ritchie, L. D., Frung, E. B., Halloran, B. P., et al. A longitudinal study of calcium homeostasis during human pregnancy and lactation and after resumption of menses. *Am. J. Clin. Nutr.* 67:693–701, 1998.

12. Food and Nutrition Board, Institute of Medicine. *Dietary Reference Intakes for Vitamin C, Vitamin E, Selenium, and Carotenoids*. Washington, D.C.: National Academy Press, 2000.

13. Hook, E. B., and Czeizel, A. E. Can terathanasia explain the protective effect of folic-acid supplementation on birth defects? *Lancet* 350:513–515, 1997.

14. Scholl, T. O., and Johnson, W. G. Folic acid: influence on the outcome of pregnancy. *Am. J. Clin. Nutr.* 71(Suppl.):1295S–1303S, 2000.

15. King, J. C. Determinants of maternal zinc status during pregnancy. *Am. J. Clin. Nutr.* 71(Suppl.):1334S–1343S, 2000.

16. Food and Nutrition Board, Institute of Medicine. *Dietary Reference Intakes for Vitamin A, Vitamin K, Arsenic, Boron, Chromium, Copper, Iodine, Iron, Manganese, Molybdenum, Nickel, Silicon, Vanadium, and Zinc*. Washington, D.C.: National Academy Press, 2001.

17. Allen, L. H. Anemia and iron deficiency: Effects on pregnancy outcome. *Am. J. Clin. Nutr.* 71(Suppl.):1280S–1284S, 2000.

18. Mitchell, M. K. *Nutrition Across the Life Span*. Philadelphia: W. B. Saunders, 1997.

19. Centers for Disease Control and Prevention. Available online at www.cdc.gov/ Accessed February 8, 2001.

20. Women Are Having More Children, New Report Shows Teen Births Continue to Decline. *National Center for Health Statistics*. Available online at www.cdc.gov/nchs/releases/02news/womenbirths.htm/ Accessed April 30, 2002.

21. Prysak, M., and Kisly, A. Age greater than thirty-four years is an independent pregnancy risk factor in nulliparous women. *J. Perinatol.* 17:296–300, 1997.

22. Kramer, M. S., Seguin, L., Lydon, J., and Goulet, L. Socio-economic disparities in pregnancy outcome: Why do the poor fare so poorly? *Paediatr. Perinat. Epidemiol.* 14:194–210, 2000.

23. Owen, A. L., and Owen, G. M. Twenty years of WIC: A review of some effects of the program. *J. Am. Diet. Assoc.* 97:777–782, 1997.

24. Appelbaum, M. G. Fetal alcohol syndrome: the nurse practitioner's perspective. *Nurse Pract.* 2:27–33, 1996.

25. Kendrick, J. S., and Merritt, R. K. Women and smoking: an update for the 1990s. *Am. J. Obstet. Gynecol.* 175:528–535, 1996.

26. DiFranza, J. R., and Lew, R. A. Effect of maternal smoking on pregnancy complications and sudden infant death syndrome. *J. Fam. Pract.* 40:385–394, 1995.

27. Klonoff-Cohen, H. S., Edelstein, S. L., Lefkowitz, E. S., et al. The effect of passive smoking and tobacco exposure through breast milk on sudden infant death syndrome. *JAMA* 273:795–798, 1995.

28. Hinds, T. S., West, W., Knight, E. M., and Hartland, B. F. The effect of caffeine on pregnancy outcome variables. *Nutr. Rev.* 54:203–207, 1996.

29. Wagner, C. L., Katikaneni, L. D., Cox, T. H., and Ryan, R. M. The impact of prenatal drug exposure on the neonate. *Obstet. Gynecol. Clin. North Am.* 25:169–194, 1998.

30. Fox, C. H. Cocaine use in pregnancy. *J. Am. Board Fam. Pract.* 7:225–228, 1994.

31. Plessinger, M. A., and Woods, J. R., Jr. Maternal, placental, and fetal pathophysiology of cocaine exposure during pregnancy. *Clin. Obstet. Gynecol.* 36:267–278, 1994.

32. Lee, M. J. Marijuana and tobacco use in pregnancy. *Obstet. Gynecol. Clin. North Am.* 25:65–83, 1998.

33. Haiek L. N., Kramer M. S., Ciampi A., and Tirado R. Postpartum weight loss and infant feeding. *J Am Board Fam Pract.* 14:85–94, 2001.

34. Prentice, A. Calcium requirements of breast-feeding mothers. *Nutr. Rev.* 56:124–130, 1998.

35. Krebs, N. F., Reidinger, C. J., Robertson, A. D., and Brenner, M. Bone mineral density changes during lactation: Maternal dietary and biochemical correlates. *Am. J. Clin. Nutr.* 65:1738–1746, 1997.

36. Bendich, A., and Brock, P. E. Rationale for the inclusion of long chain polyunsaturated fatty acids and for concomitant increase in

vitamin E in infant formulas. *Int. J. Vitam. Nutr. Res.* 67:213–231, 1997.

37. U.S. Department of Health and Human Services, Centers for Disease Control and Prevention, National Center for Health Statistics CDC growth charts: United States, Advance Data, No. 314, June 8, 2000 (revised). Available online at www.cdc.gov/growthcharts/ Accessed February 8, 2001.

38. American Dietetic Association. Position paper on promotion of breast-feeding. *J. Am. Diet. Assoc.* 97:662–666, 1997.

39. American Academy of Pediatrics, Working Group on Breast-Feeding. Breast-feeding and the use of human milk. *Pediatrics* 100:1035–1039, 1997.

40. Kelsey, J. J. Hormonal contraception and lactation. *J. Hum. Lact.* 12:315–318, 1996.

41. WHO Fact Sheet No. 178: Reducing mortality from major childhood killer diseases. September 1997. Available online at www.who.int/inf-fs/en/fact178.html Accessed August 1, 2002.

42. Williams, R. D. Breast-feeding best bet for babies. *FDA Consumer* 28:19–23, October 1995.

43. Golding, J. Unnatural constituents of breast milk—medication, lifestyle, pollutants, viruses. *Early Hum. Dev.* 29 (Suppl.):S29–S43, 1997.

15 The Growing Years: Infancy to Adolescence

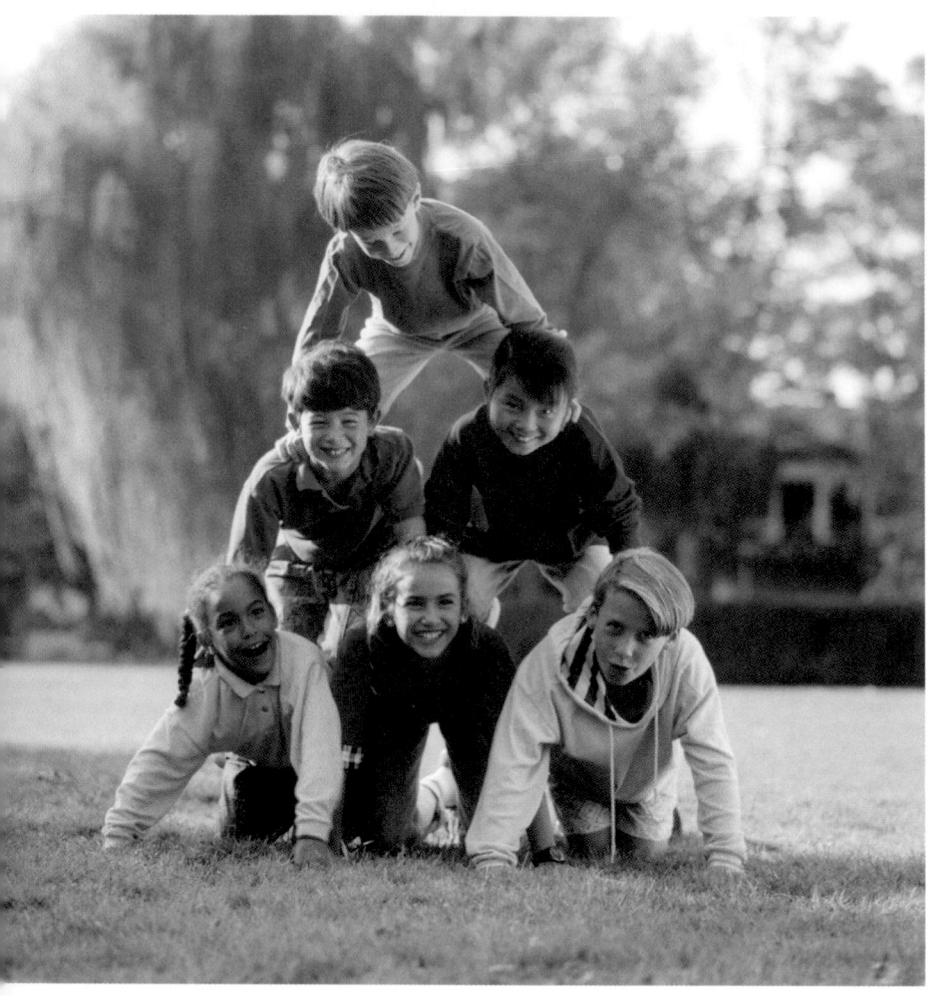

(© Richard Hutchings/PhotoEdit)

Chapter Outline

STARTING RIGHT: HEALTHY EATING FOR LIFE
Teaching Nutritious Eating Habits
Providing for Optimal Growth and Development
Reducing the Risk of Chronic Disease

NOURISHING THE INFANT: INTRODUCING SOLID FOOD
Meeting the Infant's Nutrient Needs
Food Allergies
Food Intolerances

NOURISHING TODDLERS AND YOUNG CHILDREN
Children's Nutrient Needs
Meeting Children's Nutrient Needs
Nutrition-Related Problems in Children
Influences from the Outside World

ADOLESCENCE: TRANSITION TO ADULTHOOD
The Changing Body: Sexual Maturation
Adolescent Nutrient Needs
Meeting Adolescent Nutrient Needs
A Changing World: Influences on Adolescent Nutrition

Chapter Concepts

✔ The eating patterns learned in childhood can affect health over the course of a lifetime.

✔ Normal growth is the best indication of adequate nutrient intake in children and teens.

✔ Nutrient intake in childhood can affect the risk of developing chronic disease later in life.

✔ After 4 to 6 months of age, solid foods can gradually be introduced into the infant's diet.

✔ Nutrient intakes for children must meet the needs for growth as well as for maintenance and activity.

✔ Nutrient intake in children and adolescents is influenced by their environment and their peers.

✔ Nutrient requirements of males and females change with sexual maturation.

✔ Alcohol consumption can affect nutritional status, judgment, and health.

Just a Taste

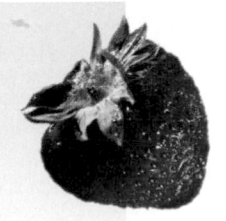

Do parents' eating habits affect those of their children?

Are high blood cholesterol and high blood pressure concerns in children?

Can fast food and sweetened cereals be part of a healthy diet?

Nutrient intake during childhood helps shape the adult that the child will become. Thus, in the words of William Wordsworth, "the child is father of the man." Nutrition can affect the ability to achieve maximum growth potential as well as the propensity for developing chronic disease later in life. Eating habits developed during childhood and adolescence may last a lifetime.

Many physical changes occur between infancy and adulthood. During this period of rapid growth from birth to about 18 years of age, the diet must supply the nutrients needed for growth and development as well as for maintenance and activity. Many factors other than nutrient needs determine which foods a child consumes. From the start, which foods are offered is a major determinant of what is consumed, but individual taste always plays a role in food choices. As the child grows, influences from the outside world increase. When a child is enrolled in day-care or preschool programs, parents may no longer be in control of—or even aware of—what the child is eating. When the child is in school, carefully packed lunches may be discarded or traded for more appealing foods. During adolescence, physiological changes dictate nutritional needs but peer pressure may dictate food choices.

• STARTING RIGHT: HEALTHY EATING FOR LIFE

Good nutrition early in life is key to health in later years. What children eat depends on what they have learned to eat as well as their personal preferences. A well-balanced eating pattern allows children to meet their nutrient needs for growth and development and to prevent or delay the onset of the chronic diseases that plague American adults.

Teaching Nutritious Eating Habits

The development of nutritious eating habits starts with caregivers offering a balanced and varied diet adequate in energy and essential nutrients and appropriate to the child's developmental needs. The caregiver is responsible for deciding what foods should be offered to the child, when they should be offered, and where they should be eaten. The child must then decide whether to eat, what foods to eat, and how much to consume.

Providing Nutritious Food Because children learn by imitation, caregivers should demonstrate healthy eating habits. If role models eat a diet high in fat and low in fruits and vegetables, children will follow suit. When children enter day care, preschool, or school, teachers, staff, and friends also influence their eating behavior.

What and When to Offer? Meals for children should be planned according to the groups and serving recommendations of the Food Guide Pyramid. Food choices should be developmentally appropriate. Young children have small stomachs and high energy needs, so frequent meals and snacks are necessary. A meal or snack

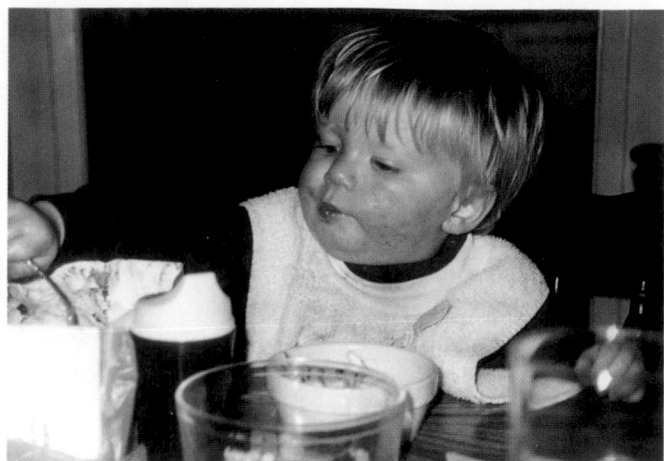

Figure 15.1
Caregivers should offer a variety of healthy food choices and allow children to select what they will eat and how much. (Mary Grosvenor)

should be offered every 2 to 3 hours and, because children thrive on routines and feel secure in knowing what to expect, a consistent pattern should be maintained from day to day. The texture of foods should also be appropriate to the child's developmental age. Foods that may cause choking should be avoided. Vegetables should be cooked until soft for easy chewing. Food should not be too hot or too spicy. As children grow, choices should change to meet their developmental abilities.

No matter how erratic children's food intake may be, caregivers should offer a variety of appropriate healthy food choices at each meal and let their children select what and how much they will eat (Figure 15.1). To increase the likelihood that a new food will be accepted, it should be introduced at the beginning of a meal when the child is hungry. If a new food becomes associated with a bad experience, such as burning the mouth, the child will be unlikely to try it again.

Breakfast: Nutrition for Learning Does it really matter at what time during the day nutrients are consumed? Children and teens who are not particularly hungry first thing in the morning will gladly go off with an empty stomach. Whether the child is in preschool or high school, this may be detrimental to both school performance and total nutrient intake.[1] Breakfast provides dietary energy for the morning. Without breakfast, the brain must rely on glucose from body stores for fuel. Studies have found that children who eat breakfast perform better on achievement tests and have fewer behavior problems in school.[2] Breakfast also makes a significant contribution to total daily nutrient intake. One study found that children who eat breakfast are more likely to meet their nutritional needs than children who skip breakfast.[3]

A good breakfast should meet a quarter to a third of the day's nutrient needs. For example, toast, a bowl of oatmeal with milk and raisins, and a glass of orange juice provides about 450 kcalories as well as B vitamins; vitamins C, A, and D; and calcium and iron. Though not every child will eat this good breakfast, even children who do not like breakfast may be willing to consume a slice of toast with peanut butter or a bowl of interestingly shaped colored cereal. Even the most sugary cereal has some redeeming features. For example, while 40% of the energy in Cap'n Crunch is from simple sugars, it provides 20% or more of the Daily Value for thiamin, riboflavin, niacin, vitamin B_6, folate, vitamin B_{12}, pantothenic acid, and iron. When 1/2 cup of reduced-fat milk is added to the cereal, it also provides 15% of the Daily Value for calcium. Children who eat ready-to-eat cereals, sugared or not, have a higher overall intake of vitamins and minerals than children who do not.[1] Although a bowl of oatmeal is preferable to a breakfast of Cookie Crisp, sugared cereals can make an important contribution to children's diets.

Children who cannot or will not eat breakfast before they leave the house can take a snack to be eaten on the way to school or during recess if they get hungry before lunch. Fruit, yogurt, a bag of dry cereal, or half a sandwich is certainly a better alterna-

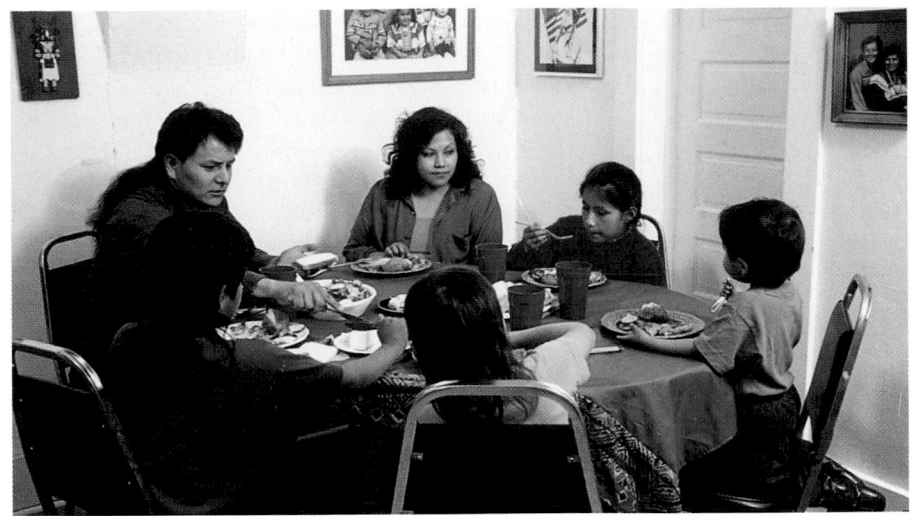

Figure 15.2
Companionship and conversation at meals help create a positive eating environment. (© Lawrence Migdale/Photo Researchers, Inc.)

tive than a candy bar from a vending machine. Having breakfast at school is also an option. The National School Breakfast Program is available in about half the nation's schools and serves more than seven million children. Children participating in the National School Breakfast Program have higher achievement test scores than eligible nonparticipants.[2] The breakfasts served must provide at least 25% of the 1989 RDA for certain nutrients and furnish at least 1 serving of milk; 1 serving of fruit, juice, or vegetables; and either 2 servings of bread, 2 servings of meat, or 1 serving of each. Meals are provided free or at a reduced cost for families who meet income guidelines.

A Positive Eating Environment To develop sound eating habits children need companionship, conversation, and a pleasant location at mealtimes. They eat better with company—caregivers should sit with children and eat what they eat (Figure 15.2).[3] Children need time to finish eating. Slow eaters are unlikely to finish eating if they are abandoned by siblings who run off to play and adults who leave to wash dishes.

To make mealtime a nutritious, educational, and enjoyable experience, it should not be a battle zone.[3] Threats and bribes are counterproductive and can create a problem where none had previously existed. Food is not a reward or a punishment: It is simply nutrition. If caregivers follow these guidelines, it is then up to the child to decide whether to eat at all, what to choose from the offered foods, and how much to eat.

Providing for Optimal Growth and Development

The ultimate size (height and weight) that a child will attain is affected by genetic, environmental, and lifestyle factors. A child whose parents are 5 feet tall may not have the genetic potential to grow to 6 feet, but when adequately nourished, most children follow standard patterns of growth. A normal growth pattern is the best indicator of adequate nourishment.

Growth is most rapid in the first year of life, when an infant's length increases by 50%, or about 10 inches. In the second year of life, children generally grow about 5 inches; in the third year, 4 inches; and thereafter, about 2 to 3 inches per year. During adolescence, there is a period of growth that is almost as rapid as that of infancy.

Children's growth can be monitored by comparing their pattern of growth to standard patterns using growth charts (see Appendix B).[4] To account for the variability among ethnic groups and breast-fed and bottle-fed babies, the growth charts were developed using data from all segments of the U.S. population. For infants, charts are available to monitor weight-for-age, length-for-age, and head-circumference-for-age. For children and adolescents age 2 to 20 years, these charts as well as one for BMI-for-age are available. The BMI-for-age growth chart is the recommended method for identifying children and adolescents who are over- and underweight.

Growth occurs in spurts and plateaus, but overall growth patterns are predictable. If a child's overall pattern of growth changes, his dietary intake should be evaluated to determine the reason for the sudden change. There are critical periods in childhood when malnutrition can cause lasting damage for which adequate nutrition later on may not be able to compensate. For example, malnutrition can have a profound effect on children's physical, emotional, and cognitive development.[5]

If sufficient energy is not consumed weight will decrease and if the deficiency continues, growth in height will slow or stop. A child who falls below the fifth percentile of the BMI-for-age distribution is considered underweight and should be evaluated to determine the cause of his or her low body weight. Nutritional intervention can help increase body weight. Offering children small frequent nutrient-dense meals and snacks can increase energy intake. Underweight adolescents can increase their weight by combining muscle-building exercises with increases in energy intake.

A drastic increase in body weight may be due to an energy intake that exceeds output. Research has found that overweight children and adolescents are more likely than their normal-weight counterparts to be overweight as adults.[6] As with adults, excess body weight in childhood and adolescence increases the risk of chronic disease. A child is considered overweight when BMI falls at or above the 95th percentile and is at risk of being overweight when BMI is greater than or equal to the 85th percentile and less than the 95th percentile (Figure 15.3).

CDC Growth Charts: United States

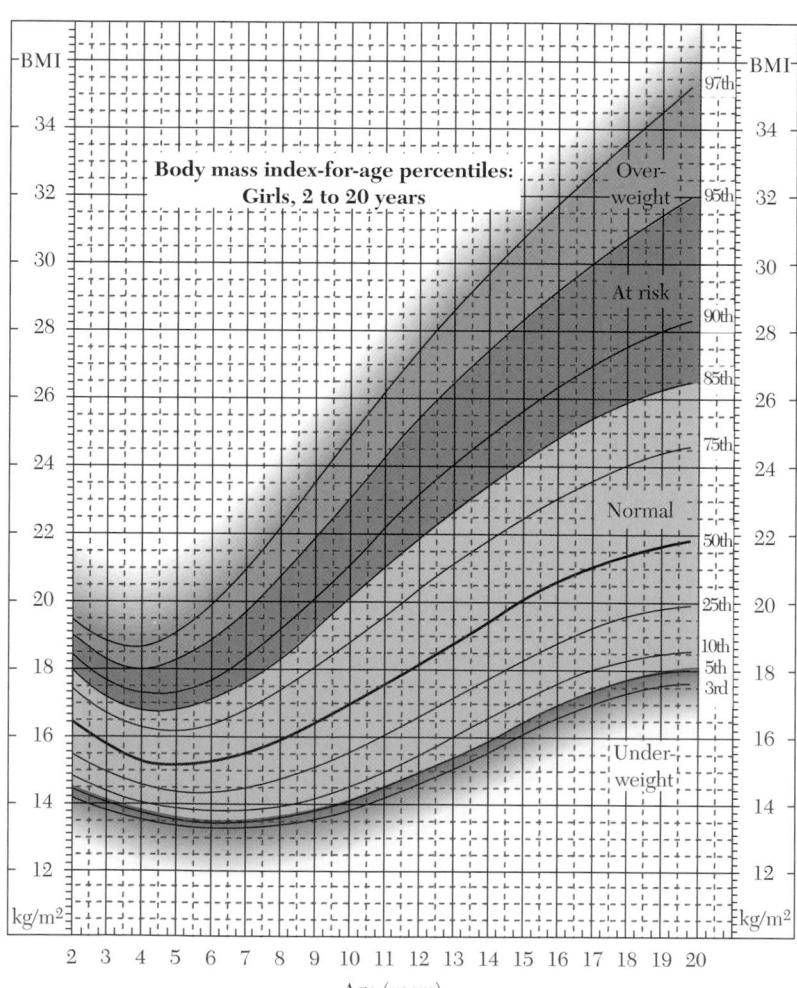

Figure 15.3

Growth charts are helpful for monitoring a child's pattern of growth. This example illustrates body mass index-for-age percentiles for girls ages 2 to 20. Body mass index (BMI) can be used beginning at two years of age, when an accurate stature can be obtained. BMI is predictive of body fat and has been recommended to screen for underweight and overweight children, ages two years and older. The colored areas represent BMI values that are associated with underweight, normal weight, at risk of overweight, and overweight.

SOURCE: Developed by the National Center for Health Statistics in collaboration with the Nation Center for Chronic Disease Prevention and Health Promotion (2000).

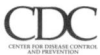

Reducing the Risk of Chronic Disease

The diets of children and adolescents can affect their health and longevity. Nutrient deficiencies can affect growth and nutritional excesses can result in childhood obesity and an increased risk for chronic disease later in life. Most children and adolescents in the United States consume more saturated fat and sodium than is recommended. They consume a dietary pattern that is low in fruits and vegetables and high in sweet and salty processed foods (Figure 15.4).

Obesity Overweight and obesity are major problems in children in the United States.[5] It is estimated that more than 13% of American children ages 6 to 19 are overweight.

Heredity and environment and lifestyle play a role in childhood obesity. Obese parents are more likely to have obese offspring not only because they pass on a genetic tendency to be overweight but because their children may learn poor eating and exercise habits. If sound nutrition and exercise habits are developed early and are followed throughout life, obesity can be avoided despite a genetic predisposition.

As with adult obesity, childhood obesity increases the risks of chronic disease. Obese children may have high blood cholesterol and glucose levels and elevated blood pressure. These risk factors may increase the chances that they will develop heart disease, hypertension, and diabetes. In addition to its health impact, obesity's psychosocial impact is great for children. Obese children in the United States are less well accepted by their peers than normal-weight children and are frequently ridiculed and teased. They often have a poor self-image and low self-esteem.

The goal in treating overweight children is to allow them to grow into their current weight. As long as the rate of weight gain is slowed, a child at the 95th percentile for weight at age 7 can be at the 90th percentile by age 9 and at the 75th percentile by age 11. This requires that the child's behavior be modified to reduce energy intake to a moderate level and to increase activity (see *Critical Thinking:* At Risk for Malnutrition).

Changing Behavior As with adults, weight gain in children is related to patterns of eating and exercise. Any permanent change in weight requires a permanent change in lifestyle. Changing eating patterns and activity is key to developing and maintaining a healthy weight. Because children, like adults, may overeat for comfort, self-reward, or out of boredom, parent involvement in helping the child find other sources of gratification can be vital.

Reducing Intake Modifying a child's food consumption patterns can be difficult. Denying food may promote further overeating by making the child feel that there will not be enough to satisfy hunger. The child may then overeat whenever there is a chance. Thus, energy intake restrictions should be relatively mild, allowing adequate nutrition to continue growth in height with little weight gain. Healthy foods such as whole grains, fruits and vegetables, lean meats, and reduced-fat dairy products should be offered at meals and for snacks. Planning ahead can help manage eating at social events. For example, a teenage girl with a weight problem could plan how much she will eat at a pizza party and then increase her exercise to burn off the excess calories.

Increasing Activity Although energy intake among American children overall is not increasing, they are getting heavier, suggesting that a major contributor to the increase in body weight is lack of physical activity.[7] Watching television, playing video games, and surfing the Web have replaced neighborhood games of tag and soccer for many children.

Overweight children are less likely to be physically active than lean children. They may be embarrassed by their bodies and shy away from participating in group activities. Increases in physical activity need to be gradual in order to make exercise

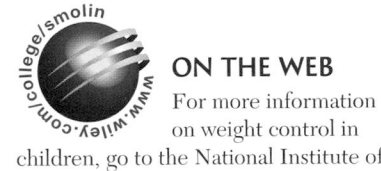

ON THE WEB
For more information on weight control in children, go to the National Institute of Diabetes and Digestive and Kidney Disorders at
www.niddk.nih.gov
and click on weight loss and control under health information.

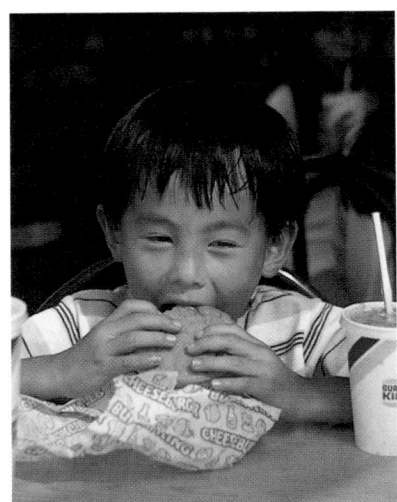

Figure 15.4
Many children in the United States consume a diet that is high in fat and low in fruits and vegetables. (© Arthur R. Hill/Visuals Unlimited)

a positive experience. A good way to start is to encourage activities such as games, walks after dinner, bike rides, hikes, swimming, and volleyball that can be enjoyed by the whole family. This sends a positive message to "be more active" rather than a negative message of "do not eat so much." Again, involvement of the whole family is key. Parents who are active, play with their children, watch their children compete or play, or take children to physical activity or sports events have more active children.

Activity Guidelines Whether or not a child is obese, he or she should be physically active. The Dietary Guidelines and the DRIs recommend that children be physically active for at least an hour per day.[8] Children have short attention spans, so their activities should be intermittent. Periods of moderate to vigorous activity lasting 10 to 15 minutes or more each day should be interspersed with periods of rest and recovery. Preadolescent children should be exposed to a variety of different types of activities that are of various levels of intensity (Figure 15.5). Learning to enjoy sports and exercise in childhood will set the stage for an active lifestyle in adulthood.

Type 2 Diabetes Until recently, type 2 diabetes was considered a disease that affected primarily adults over 40, but it is now on the rise among America's youth.[9] The typical picture of type 2 diabetes in this population is a child from age 10 to

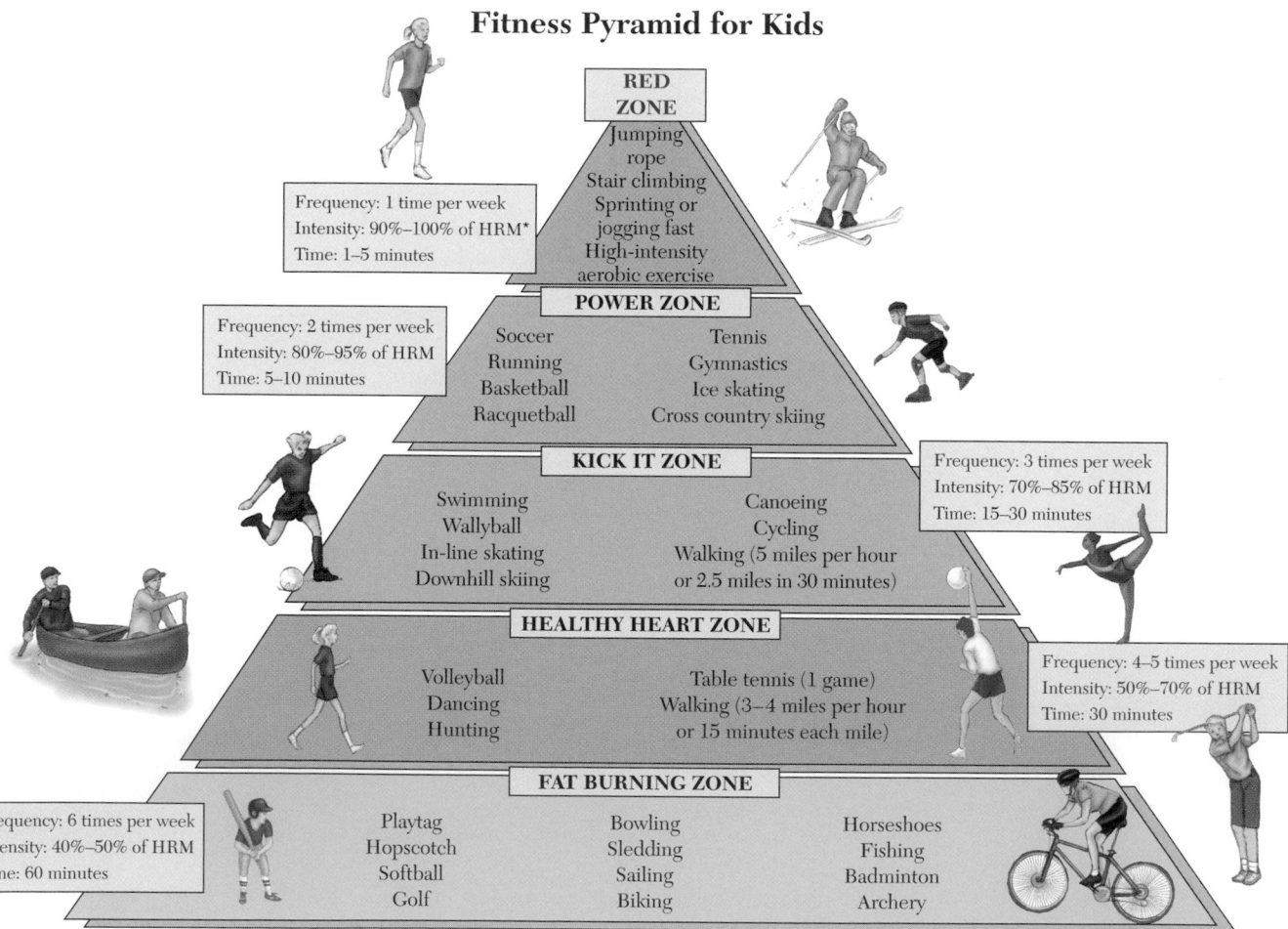

Fitness Pyramid for Kids

RED ZONE
Jumping rope
Stair climbing
Sprinting or jogging fast
High-intensity aerobic exercise

Frequency: 1 time per week
Intensity: 90%–100% of HRM*
Time: 1–5 minutes

POWER ZONE
Soccer
Running
Basketball
Racquetball
Tennis
Gymnastics
Ice skating
Cross country skiing

Frequency: 2 times per week
Intensity: 80%–95% of HRM
Time: 5–10 minutes

KICK IT ZONE
Swimming
Wallyball
In-line skating
Downhill skiing
Canoeing
Cycling
Walking (5 miles per hour or 2.5 miles in 30 minutes)

Frequency: 3 times per week
Intensity: 70%–85% of HRM
Time: 15–30 minutes

HEALTHY HEART ZONE
Volleyball
Dancing
Hunting
Table tennis (1 game)
Walking (3–4 miles per hour or 15 minutes each mile)

Frequency: 4–5 times per week
Intensity: 50%–70% of HRM
Time: 30 minutes

FAT BURNING ZONE
Playtag
Hopscotch
Softball
Golf
Bowling
Sledding
Sailing
Biking
Horseshoes
Fishing
Badminton
Archery

Frequency: 6 times per week
Intensity: 40%–50% of HRM
Time: 60 minutes

°HRM—Heart Rate Maximum

(Adapted from: American Dietetic Association. Position of the American Dietetic Association: Dietary guidance for healthy children ages 2 to 11 years. *J. Am. Diet. Assoc.* 99:93–101, 1999)

Figure 15.5
Children should enjoy participating in a variety of activities of varying intensity.

mid-puberty, overweight, with a family history of the disease. Little is known about this disease in children, but based on experience with adults, it is thought to be a progressive disease that increases in severity with time from diagnosis. The longer an individual has the disease, the greater the risk of complications that involve the circulatory system or nervous system and that can lead to blindness, kidney failure, heart disease, or amputations (see Chapter 4).[10]

The goal of treatment is to keep blood glucose levels in the normal range and treat related conditions such as hypertension and high blood lipid levels. The recommended treatment for children who have elevated blood glucose but are not symptomatic is education about the disease to promote a lifestyle change that includes a balanced diet moderate in energy and increased physical activity. However, due to the progressive nature of diabetes, most will eventually require drug treatment. Preventative measures that may delay or prevent the onset of type 2 diabetes include weight management and increased physical activity.

Blood Cholesterol and Heart Disease Children in the United States and Canada currently consume about 11% of their energy from saturated fat.[11] This exceeds the amounts recommended for a healthy diet and can lead to elevated blood cholesterol levels. The recommended level for blood cholesterol in children aged 2 to 18 is less than 170 mg per 100 ml. In the United States, many children have blood cholesterol levels higher than this. Elevated blood cholesterol levels during childhood and adolescence are associated with higher blood cholesterol and higher mortality rates from cardiovascular disease in adulthood.[12]

The American Academy of Pediatrics recommends blood cholesterol monitoring for high-risk children and teenagers. This includes those with parents or grandparents who developed heart disease before age 55, and those whose parents have cholesterol levels over 240 mg per 100 ml. To reduce the risk of developing high blood cholesterol levels and, subsequently, heart disease, the diets of children over the age of 3 should contain no more than 25 to 35% of energy from fat and be low in cholesterol, saturated fat, and *trans* fat.[8] Lowfat diets have been found to promote healthy blood lipid levels without interfering with growth.[13]

Hypertension Those who have blood pressure at the high end of normal as youngsters are more likely to develop high blood pressure as adults.[14] Blood pressure can be affected by the amount of body fat, activity level, and sodium intake, as well as by the total pattern of dietary intake, so attention should be paid to these nutritional and lifestyle factors in children. This is particularly important if there is a family history of hypertension.

CRITICAL THINKING

At Risk for Malnutrition

Bobby is eight years old and has a history of iron deficiency anemia. His parents have recently become concerned because all he wants to do is lie around and watch TV, and he is gaining weight. Previously he played active, imaginative games with his toys, enjoyed playing basketball with his friends, and was eager to go on hikes with the family. Since Bobby's parents are both overweight, they are concerned that he will also have a weight problem, so they take him to see their pediatrician.

The nurse weighs and measures Bobby and draws a blood sample to check for iron deficiency anemia. She compares Bobby's weight for height to last year's measurements. Last year he was at the 50th percentile, and he is now almost at the 75th.

The pediatrician reports that Bobby is anemic again and prescribes an iron supplement. She refers Bobby and his parents to a dietitian for dietary counseling on weight management as well as iron intake. The dietitian reviews Bobby's diet and exercise patterns. She learns that Bobby has been watching TV or playing video games for about 6 hours a day. Below are the results of a food frequency questionnaire that she recorded:

Food		Frequency	
		Servings/Day	Servings/Week
Milk and dairy products:	Regular fat	6	
	Reduced fat		
	Fat free		
Meat and eggs:	Red meat		1
	Chicken		2
	Fish		1
	Eggs		
Grains and cereals:	Whole grains	2	
	Refined grains	4	
Fruit and juices:	Citrus	1	
	Other	2	
Vegetables:	Dark green leafy		
	Other	1	
Added fats:		3	
Snack foods:	Chips, etc.	1	
	Candy	1	

What nutrients are likely to be excessive or deficient in this dietary pattern?
▼

Bobby's high intake of regular dairy products provides a good source of calcium but adds a lot of fat and saturated fat to his diet. His low intake of meats means that heme iron is low in the diet, and the lack of leafy green vegetables means his intake of nonheme iron from vegetables is low. His low intake of vegetables and whole grains means his fiber intake is low, and some vitamins and minerals may be low in the diet. The candy and chips add energy, fat, sugar, and/or salt with few other nutrients.

Why might excessive consumption of dairy products contribute to Bobby's anemia?
▼

Dairy products are an important source of protein, vitamins, and minerals, particularly calcium, but they are a poor source of iron. In addition, the high calcium they provide decreases absorption of iron consumed at the same meal.

Suggest some dietary changes that would increase Bobby's iron intake and absorption.
▼

Answer:

How can Bobby reduce the energy content of his diet?
▼

Because Bobby is well past the age when he needs a high-fat diet for growth and development and his weight is increasing more rapidly than his height, the dietitian recommends that he switch to lowfat milk and dairy products. The dietitian also suggests that the family make some changes in the types of food they have around the house so Bobby can have more low-kcalorie, nutrient-dense choices such as fruits and vegetables to snack on. The dietitian encourages the family to bake, broil, or grill their meat, trimming off excess fat. She also recommends the family work together to increase the amount of exercise they get.

Suggest some activities you enjoyed as a child that would help Bobby to increase his activity level.
▼

Answer:

• NOURISHING THE INFANT: INTRODUCING SOLID FOOD

Solid and semisolid foods can be gradually introduced into the infant's diet starting between the fourth and sixth months of life when the infant's feeding abilities and gastrointestinal tract are mature enough to handle foods other than breast milk or formula. Since the young infant takes milk by a licking motion of the tongue called suckling, which strokes or milks the liquid from the nipple, solid food placed in the mouth at an early age is usually pushed out as the tongue thrusts forward. By four to six months of age the early reflex to bring the tongue to the front of the mouth to suckle has diminished, and the tongue is held farther back in the mouth, allowing solid food to be accepted without being expelled. By this age, the infant also can hold the head up steadily and is able to sit, either with or without support. Internally, the digestive tract has developed, and enzymes are present for starch digestion. The kidneys are more mature and better able to concentrate urine. With all of these changes, the child is ready to begin a new approach to eating.

Meeting the Infant's Nutrient Needs

Until one year of age, most nutritional needs are still met by breast milk or formula. Even though some suggest that the addition of infant cereal to the bottle during the first few months will help the infant sleep through the night, studies have shown that there is no difference in sleeping patterns based on such feeding practices.

First Foods The most commonly recommended food to be fed first to a child is iron-fortified infant rice cereal mixed with formula or breast milk. Rice cereal is the recommended first food because it is easily digested and rarely causes allergic reactions. After rice has been successfully included in the diet, other grains can be introduced, with wheat cereal given last because it is most likely to cause an allergic reaction. To monitor for food allergies, it is important to introduce new foods one at a time. Each new food should be offered for a few days without the addition of any other new foods. If an allergic reaction occurs, it is most likely due to the newly introduced food. Foods that cause symptoms such as rashes, digestive upsets, or respiratory problems should be discontinued before any other new foods are added. After cereals are introduced, puréed vegetables or fruits can be tried; some suggest that vegetables be offered before fruits so that the child will learn to enjoy food that is not sweet before being introduced to sweet foods. Once teeth have erupted, foods with more texture can be added. For the 6- to 12-month-old child, small pieces of soft or ground fruits, vegetables, and meats are appropriate (Table 15.1).

Table 15.1   *Typical Meal Patterns for Infants*

Food	Serving Size	Servings per Day		
		4–6 Months	6–8 Months	9–12 Months
		(tongue able to stay in back of mouth and not push food out)	(can easily move hand to mouth)	(can use a cup and easily consume finger foods)
Formula or breast milk°	8 oz	4	4	4
Dry infant cereal	2 Tbsp	2	4	4
Vegetables	2–3 Tbsp	—	2	3
Fruits	2 Tbsp	—	2	4
Fruit juice	4 oz	—	—	1 (by cup)
Meats (or egg yolks)	1 Tbsp	—	2–4 (strained)	4–6 (chopped)
Finger foods		—	1†	4‡

°Includes that added to cereal.

†Dry toast, teething biscuits.

‡Table foods except "choking" foods (foods in shapes and sizes that are likely to cause choking, such as large pieces of meat, whole grapes, or hot dogs or carrots cut in circular slices.)

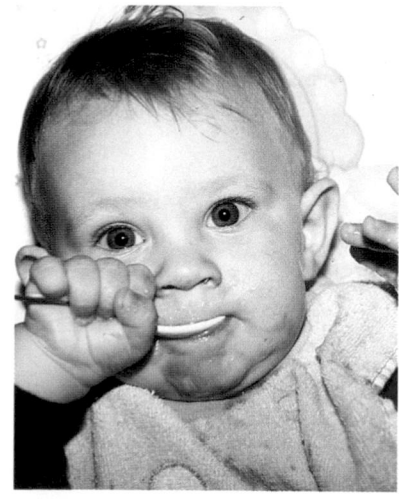

Figure 15.6
Self-feeding is important in infant development but is not a tidy process. (Gregory Smolin)

Allergen A substance, usually a protein, that stimulates an immune response.

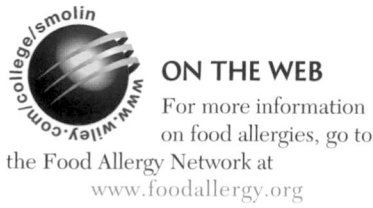

ON THE WEB
For more information on food allergies, go to the Food Allergy Network at www.foodallergy.org

Developmentally Appropriate Choices As the child becomes familiar with more variety, food choices should be made from each of the food groups in the Food Guide Pyramid. At one year of age, whole cow's milk should be offered and continued until two years of age, after which reduced fat milks can be used. To avoid choking, foods that can easily lodge in the throat, such as carrots, grapes, and hot dogs, should not be offered to infants or toddlers.

As children become more independent, they will want to feed themselves. Although this is not always a neat and clean process, it is important for development (Figure 15.6). By the age of eight or nine months, infants can hold a bottle and self-feed finger food such as crackers. By ten months, most infants can drink from a cup, so water and fruit juices can be offered. Juice should not be served in a bottle because it may contribute to nursing bottle syndrome. Excess quantities of apple and pear juice should be avoided; they contain sorbitol, a poorly absorbed sugar alcohol, that can cause diarrhea. Added sugars should be offered in moderation to ensure a nutrient-dense diet. Honey and corn syrup should not be served to children less than a year old because these foods may contain spores of *Clostridium botulinum*, the bacterium that causes botulism poisoning (see Chapter 17). Older children and adults are not at risk from botulism spores because the environment in a mature gastrointestinal tract prevents the bacterium from growing.

Food Allergies

True allergic reactions to food, or food allergies, are relatively rare, occurring in about 1.4% of young children.[15] They occur when incompletely digested proteins are absorbed from the intestine, enter the lymph and/or bloodstream, and cause a reaction involving the immune system. Exposure to an **allergen** for the first time causes the immune system to produce antibodies to that allergen. When the allergen is encountered again by eating the same food, allergy symptoms such as vomiting, diarrhea, asthma, hives, eczema, runny nose and swelling of tissues, hay fever, and general cramps and aches may result as the immune system battles the allergen. The symptoms may occur almost immediately or take up to 24 hours to appear, and can vary from mild to severe and life threatening. Foods that commonly cause allergies include wheat, peanuts, eggs, milk, nuts, seafood, soy products, and some meats.

Food allergies are common in infants because their digestive tracts are not fully mature. After about three months of age, the risk of developing food allergies is reduced because incompletely digested proteins are less likely to be absorbed. Many children who develop food allergies before the age of three will outgrow them. For example, of children allergic to eggs at one year of age, only 4% were still allergic by age five.[15] Allergies that appear after three years are more likely to be a problem for life.

Diagnosis Several laboratory methods are available to identify foods that are likely to cause an individual's allergic reaction, but they cannot determine the source of the problem with 100% reliability. The cause of a food allergy can be confirmed by using an **elimination diet** and **food challenge**. This involves removing all foods suspected of causing an allergic reaction from the diet. When a diet that causes no symptoms has been established, it is followed for two to four weeks. Then in the food challenge, small amounts of a food suspected of causing a reaction are reintroduced under a doctor's supervision. If no reaction to the food occurs, then increasing amounts are introduced until a normal portion is offered. If there is still no reaction, then the food can be ruled out as an allergen (see *Off the Shelf:* Peanut Allergy).

Elimination diet and **food challenge** A program that eliminates potential allergy-causing foods from an individual's diet and then systematically adds them back to identify any foods that cause an allergic reaction.

Prevention and Management Preventing the development of food allergies is not always possible. Breast feeding can reduce the risk of food allergies and is recommended for infants from families with a history of allergies. Infants who are breast fed are less likely to be exposed to foreign proteins that cause food allergies. In addition, their gut matures earlier and they are protected by antibodies and other components of human milk.[15] The benefits of breast feeding are increased if the mother avoids eating common allergy-causing foods such as peanuts, eggs, fish, and dairy products during lactation. To decrease the chances of developing allergies when solid foods are introduced, wheat, eggs, and fish should not be introduced until the child is 12 months of age, and peanuts should not be given until 36 months.[15]

The best way to manage a food allergy is to avoid consuming the offending food. The information on food labels can be helpful in identifying foods that contain allergy-causing ingredients (see Chapter 6, *Off the Label*: Identifying Protein Sources).

Food Intolerances

Adverse reactions to foods are also caused by **food intolerances.** Food intolerances do not involve antibody production by the immune system. Rather, they are caused by foods that are difficult or impossible to digest. Food intolerances can be caused by chemical components in foods, by toxins that occur naturally in foods, by substances added to foods during processing or preparation, or simply by large amounts of foods, such as onions or prunes, that cause local GI irritation.[15] Lactose intolerance is an example of a food intolerance caused by a reduced ability to digest milk sugar. It is not an allergy to milk proteins.

Food intolerance An adverse reaction to a food that does not involve antibody production by the immune system.

• NOURISHING TODDLERS AND YOUNG CHILDREN

Nourishing a growing child is not always an easy task. Foods offered must be appropriate for children's physical development as well as suit their developing tastes. Whether children are toddlers (ages one to three), or in early childhood (ages four through eight), they are becoming independent eaters.

Children's Nutrient Needs

As children grow, their nutrient requirements per unit of body weight decrease, but total needs increase because they gain weight and become more active. Recommended intakes are not different for boys and girls until about nine years of age, at

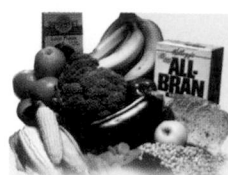

Off the Shelf
Peanut Allergy

Peanut-free schools. Peanut-free airline seats. Why all the attention to peanuts? People with lactose intolerance or allergies to seafood do not force these items from their neighbor's plates, so is it a violation of civil rights to force a school to eliminate peanut butter from the menu for the few children who have this allergy? Should we give up our bag of peanuts on the airplane because one passenger might be allergic to them? The answers to these questions are in the hands of the courts, but the rationale behind them is easily explained.

An allergy to peanuts is one of the most common food allergies. It is rarely outgrown, and life-threatening reactions occur from exposure to minuscule doses. Amounts of peanut protein as low as 100 μg can cause a reaction, whereas for other food allergies, up to a thousandfold more—50–100 mg of an allergen—must be eaten before a reaction occurs.[1] And individuals who are allergic to peanuts may be at risk even if the peanuts do not find their way into their mouths. A survey found that 66% of allergic individuals develop symptoms simply from contact with peanuts.[2] Some even experience reactions when peanut allergen is merely inhaled. Reactions to peanut exposure vary but often include difficulty breathing, skin reactions such as flushing and hives, and a drop in blood pressure. When an allergic individual has a reaction that includes respiratory symptoms, it must be treated immediately with an epinephrine injection and the person should be taken to a hospital emergency room for further treatment.

Because reactions occur with such low levels of peanut exposure, individuals with peanut allergy must avoid all contact with peanuts. This, however, may not be easy, especially for children. Peanut butter sandwiches are a staple of many children's diets, and a peanut butter–smeared finger or shirt could cause a reaction in an allergic friend. If the same knife that spread peanut butter is dipped into the jelly jar, the allergic child who is served only jelly crackers may suffer a peanut reaction.

Shopping for safe foods for someone with peanut allergy is challenging. Indi-

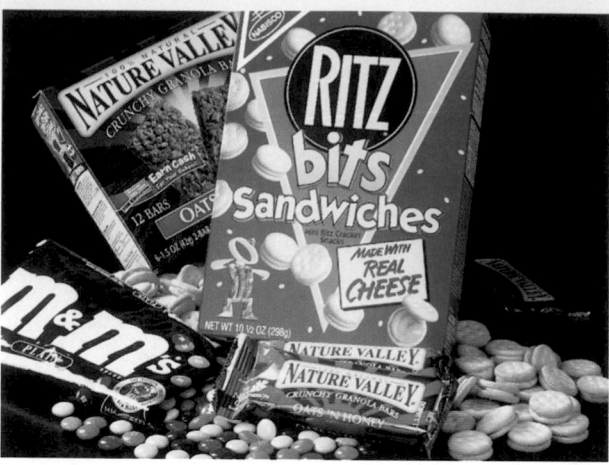

Parents of children with allergies must read labels carefully. These products all contain peanut products or indicate that they may have inadvertently become contaminated with peanuts during manufacture (George Semple).

viduals with peanut allergy or their caregivers need to rely on food labels to identify safe and unsafe choices. Peanuts, peanut butter, and peanut butter candy are obvious foods to avoid. Others are not so obvious; some foods, such as cookies and crackers, contain peanut flour and peanut oil. Crude peanut oil (less refined) was found to cause an allergic reaction in 10% of allergic subjects, whereas refined peanut oil did not cause a reaction in any of those studied.[3] Food labels, however, do not indicate which type of oil is used in a product.

Even foods manufactured in the same location as peanut-containing foods can pose a risk. For instance, cheese "sandwich" crackers seem like a safe snack, but a thorough reading of the ingredient list reveals the last ingredient on the list to be peanuts. This is because the cheese crackers were manufactured in the same processing facility as peanut butter sandwich crackers, so the label reflects the possibility of cross-contamination. Other products may list "peanut fragments" or state either that the product "may contain peanuts" or that it was manufactured in a facility that processes peanuts. This information protects both the company from legal action and the allergic individual

from inadvertently consuming peanut-containing products.

So should your school be peanut free? Serving peanut-free foods is challenging even for a mother trying to keep her own child safe, but it is nearly impossible for school cafeteria workers to be aware of all the ingredients in the food they serve. Even if allergic children bring all their own food from home, they are not necessarily safe if peanuts are being eaten all around them. So, will prohibition of peanuts prevent allergic reactions? Does it violate the rights of children who like peanut butter and jelly sandwiches? While this may be decided by the legal system, awareness of the problem may protect an allergic child.

[1]Hourihane, J. O., Kilburn, S. A., Nordlee, J. A., et al. An evaluation of the sensitivity of subjects with peanut allergy to very low doses of peanut protein: A randomized, double-blind, placebo-controlled food challenge study. *J. Allergy Clin. Immunol.* 100:596–600, 1997.

[2]Hourihane, J. O., Kilburn, S. A., Dean, P., and Warner, J. O. Clinical characteristics of peanut allergy. *Clin. Exp. Allergy* 27:634–639, 1997.

[3]Hourihane, J. O., Bedwani, S. J., Dean, T. P., and Warner, J. O. Randomized double blind crossover challenge study of allergenicity of peanut oils in subjects allergic to peanuts. *BMJ.* 314:1084–1088, 1997.

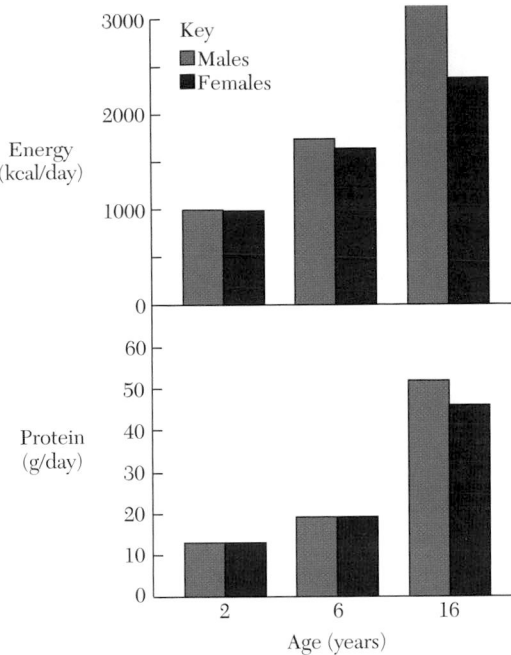

Figure 15.7

The total need for both energy and protein increases with age. Source: Institute of Medicine

which time sexual maturation causes differences in nutrient needs between the sexes. The Dietary Reference Intakes make nutrient recommendations that include two age groups for children; toddlers (ages 1 through 3) and early childhood (ages 4 through 8). Children 9 and older are included in the adolescent group.

Energy, Protein, and Water The total need for energy and protein increases as body size increases. The average 2-year-old needs about 1000 kcalories and 13 grams of protein per day. By age 6, that child will need about 1700 kcalories and 19 grams of protein per day (Figure 15.7).[16]

Fluid requirements increase in proportion to energy requirements. By one year of age, a child's kidneys have matured and the fluid lost through evaporation has decreased, so fluid requirements are similar to those of adults: 1 ml of fluid per kcalorie of energy consumed.

Fat Infants need a high fat diet (40–55% of energy intake) to support their rapid growth and development (see *Off the Label*: Labeling Food for Young Children). As children grow, the recommended intake for fat is reduced to provide adequate energy without increasing the risk of developing chronic disease (Figure 15-8). The acceptable range for fat intake is 30 to 40% of energy for children ages 1 to 3 years and 25 to 35% of energy for those 4 through 18 years of age. Specific AIs have been set for linoleic and α-linolenic acid at each life stage.[16]

Carbohydrate and Fiber Carbohydrate recommendations for children over age two are the same as those for adults: 45 to 65% of energy. Specific fiber recommendations have not been made for infants, but for children an AI has been established based on data that show an intake of 14 grams of fiber per 1000 kcalories reduces the risk of heart disease. Fiber supplements are not recommended for children, since high intakes can limit the amount of food and, consequently, the nutrients that a small child can consume. As in the adult diet, most of the carbohydrate in a child's diet should be from whole grains, fruits, and vegetables. Foods high in added sugars, such as cookies, candy, and soda, should be limited.

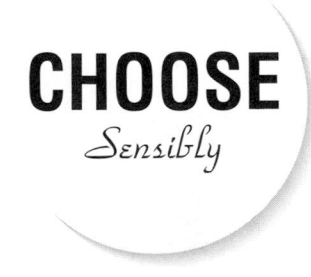

Choose a diet that is low in saturated fat and cholesterol and moderate in total fat

Figure 15.8

The Dietary Guidelines recommends that everyone over the age of two years consume a diet that is low in saturated fat and cholesterol and moderate in fat. (USDA, DHHS, 2000)

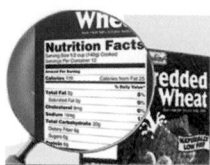

Off the Label
Labeling Food for Young Children

Children have different nutrient needs than adults. Therefore, the labels on foods designed for young children must follow different labeling rules.

Infancy and early childhood is a period of rapid growth and development, and dietary fat serves as an energy source, a carrier of fat-soluble vitamins, and a source of essential fatty acids. Thus, labels for foods intended for children under two are not permitted to list the amount of saturated fat, polyunsaturated fat, monounsaturated fat, cholesterol, kcalories from fat, and kcalories from saturated fat on the label out of concern that caregivers might restrict fats in the diets of young children.[1] Labels for foods for children under two are also not allowed to carry most of the claims about a food's nutrient content, such as whether it is lowfat and low-cholesterol, and they cannot carry the FDA-approved health claims about the relationship between a nutrient or food and a health concern.[1]

After the age of one, the amount of fat in the diet can safely be reduced.

Therefore, labels on foods designed for 2- to 4-year-olds must include information on the amount of cholesterol and saturated fat per serving and can voluntarily provide information on the number of kcalories from fat and saturated fat and the amount of polyunsaturated and monounsaturated fat per serving. The serving sizes listed are based on servings appropriate for small children.

Another difference between standard food labels and those for foods designed for children under age four is the absence of percent Daily Values for total fat, saturated fat, cholesterol, total carbohydrate, fiber, and sodium.[1] Daily Values for these nutrients have not been established for children under four; for this age group, the FDA has set Daily Values only for vitamins, minerals, and protein. Labels include the percent Daily Values for these nutrients when they are present in significant amounts.

A few nutrient and health claims are allowed on young children's foods. These include claims that describe the percentage

of vitamins or minerals in a food as they apply to the Daily Values for children under age 2, such as, "provides 50% of the Daily Value for vitamin C." Also, for children under 2, the descriptors "unsweetened" and "unsalted" are allowed. "No sugar added" and "sugar free" are approved only for use on dietary supplements for children.

The labels of foods intended for young children provide information needed to make wise food selections, but many of the foods consumed by young children do not have special labels because they are also adult foods. When selecting these foods, keep in mind that the needs of young children, especially for fat, are different than the needs of adults.

[1]Kurtzweil, P. Labeling rules for young children's foods. *FDA Consumer* 29:14–18, March 1995.

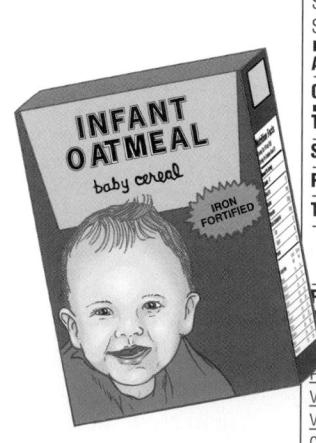

Nutrition Facts

Serving Size 1/4 cup (15g)
Servings Per Container About 30

Amount Per Serving

Calories 60

Total Fat		1g
Sodium		0mg
Potassium		50mg
Total Carbohydrate		10g
Fiber		1g
Sugars		0g
Protein		2g

Daily Value	Infants 0-1	Children 1-4
Protein	7%	6%
Vitamin A	0%	0%
Vitamin C	0%	0%
Calcium	15%	10%
Iron	45%	60%
Vitamin E	15%	8%
Thiamin	45%	30%
Riboflavin	45%	30%
Niacin	25%	20%
Phosphorus	15%	10%

Nutrition label for foods for children under age two.

Nutrition Facts

Serving Size 1 jar (140g)

Amount Per Serving

Calories 110	Calories from Fat 0

Total Fat	0g
Saturated Fat	0g
Cholesterol	0mg
Sodium	10mg
Total Carbohydrate	27g
Dietary Fiber	4g
Sugars	1
Protein	0g

% Daily Value		
Protein 0%	•	Vitamin A 6%
Vitamin C 45%	•	Calcium 2%
Iron 2%		

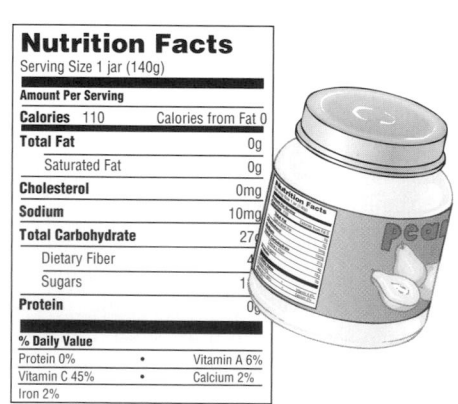

Nutrition label for foods for children ages two to four.

Micronutrient Needs As children grow, so do their vitamin and mineral requirements. Surveys indicate that the diets of children in the United States are likely to be deficient in vitamin A, vitamin C, vitamin E, calcium, iron, and zinc.[17]

Calcium Adequate calcium intake during childhood is essential for achieving maximum peak bone mass, which is important in preventing osteoporosis later in life (see Chapter 10). The AI for calcium for toddlers is 500 mg per day and for young children is 800 mg per day. Despite the importance of calcium for maximizing peak bone mass, calcium intake in school-age American children is declining, primarily due to a decrease in the consumption of dairy products, such as milk, yogurt, and cheese.[5]

Iron Iron deficiency anemia is one of the most prevalent forms of malnutrition in children. Although iron intake by American children has increased over the last 20 years, iron deficiency is still a public health problem.[18] Iron deficiency anemia can lower the child's resistance to illness and slow recovery time. It can affect learning ability, intellectual performance, stamina, and mood. Good sources of iron that are acceptable to small children include fortified grains and breakfast cereals, raisins, eggs, and lean meats. If anemia is diagnosed, iron supplements are usually prescribed until iron stores are repleted. These supplements should be kept out of the reach of children. Overdoses of iron-containing supplements are the leading cause of poisoning deaths among children under 6 years of age.[19] To help protect children, products containing iron include a warning about the hazards to children of ingesting large amounts of iron. Products containing 30 mg or more per dose are packed in individual doses to reduce the chances of consuming enough to cause toxicity.

Meeting Children's Nutrient Needs

Children over the age of two, like adults, need a varied diet based on whole grains, vegetables, and fruits, adequate in milk and other high-protein foods, and moderate in fat and sodium. Snacks should be as nutritious as meals.

Balance and Variety A healthy diet can be provided by following the recommendations of the Food Guide Pyramid, choosing the low end of the suggested range of servings, and modifying portion sizes. For instance, an adult serving of milk would be 1 cup, whereas a serving for a 2-year-old would be 4 ounces and for a 5-year-old it would be 6 ounces (see Table 15.2). A Food Guide Pyramid, designed to be appealing to young children, has been developed (Figure 15.9).

Creativity may be necessary to convince a young child to consume a varied diet. Substituting appropriate nutritious choices for refused foods can increase the variety of the diet. If vegetables are refused, they can be added to soups and casseroles. Fruit can be served on cereals or in milkshakes. Cheese can be included in recipes such as macaroni and cheese, cheese sauce, and pizza. Milk can be added to hot cereal, cream soups, puddings, and custards. And powdered milk can be used in baking. Meats can be added to spaghetti sauce, stews, casseroles, burritos, or pizza. Children often have periods known as food jags, when they will eat only certain foods and nothing else. For example, a child may refuse to eat anything other than peanut butter and jelly sandwiches for breakfast, lunch, and dinner. The general guideline is to continue to offer other foods along with those the child is focused on. What children will not touch at one meal, they may eat the next day or the next week.

Do Children Need Vitamin and Mineral Supplements? As with adults, children who consume a well-selected, varied diet can meet all their vitamin and mineral requirements with food. Occasional skipped meals and unfinished dinners are a normal part of most children's eating behavior. However, children with particularly erratic eating habits, those on regimens to manage obesity, those with limited food availability, and those who consume a vegan diet may benefit from supplements that

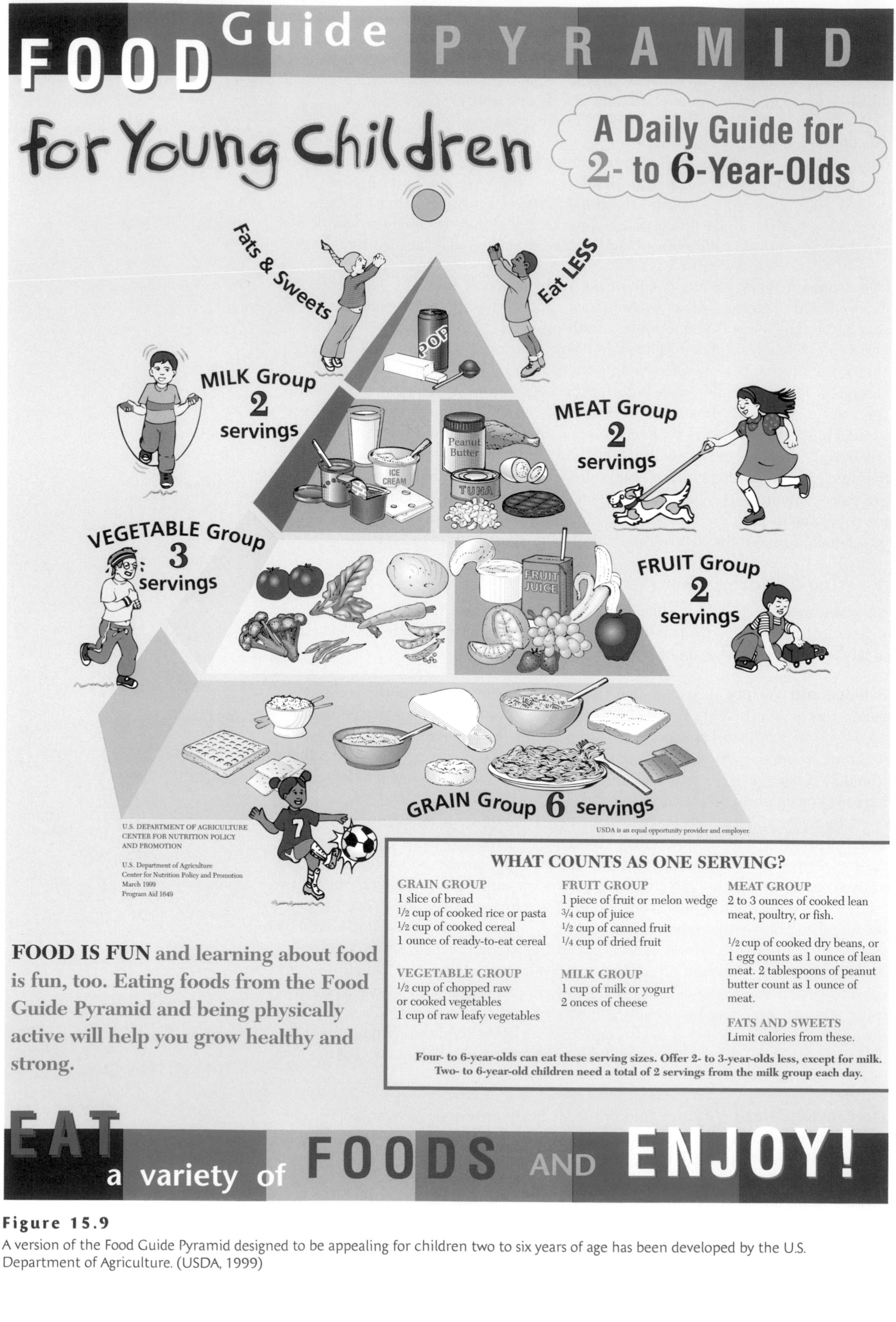

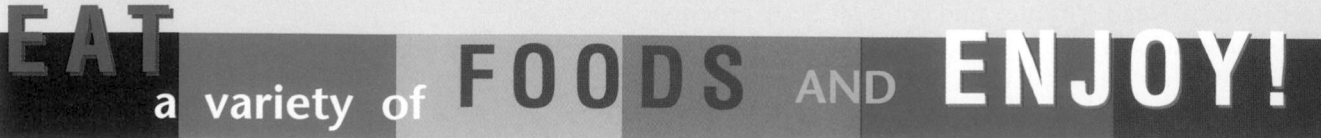

Figure 15.9

A version of the Food Guide Pyramid designed to be appealing for children two to six years of age has been developed by the U.S. Department of Agriculture. (USDA, 1999)

Table 15.2 A Typical Day's Food Intake for Three- and Eight-Year-Old Children

Three-Year-Old Child			Eight-Year-Old Child		
Food	Amount	Food Group	Food	Amount	Food Group
Breakfast					
Corn flakes	3 Tbsp	grain	Corn flakes	3/4 cup	grain
Milk, 2 %	1/2 cup	milk	Milk, 2%	3/4 cup	milk
Banana	3 Tbsp	fruit	Banana	half	fruit
Snack					
Peanut butter	1 Tbsp	meat			
Wheat crackers	3	grain			
Apple juice	1/2 cup	fruit			
Lunch					
Vegetable soup	1/4 cup	vegetable	Vegetable soup	1 cup	vegetable
Grilled tuna sandwich	half	grain, meat	Grilled tuna sandwich	1	grain, meat
Tomato	1/4	vegetable	Tomato	1/2	vegetable
Milk, 2%	1/2 cup	milk	Milk, 2%	3/4 cup	milk
Snack					
Hot cocoa	1/2 cup	milk	Hot cocoa	3/4 cup	milk
			Peanut butter and jelly sandwich	1	grain, meat
Cookie	1	grain	Cookies	2	grain
Snack					
Pretzels	2	grain	Pretzels	4	grain
Orange juice	1/2 cup	fruit	Orange juice	1/2 cup	fruit
Dinner					
Rice	3 Tbsp	grain	Rice	3/4 cup	grain
Chicken	1 drumstick	meat	Chicken	2 drumsticks	meat
Broccoli	1 floret	vegetable	Broccoli	3 florets	vegetable
Milk, 2%	1/2 cup	milk	Milk, 2%	3/4 cup	milk
Ice cream	1/2 cup	milk	Ice cream	3/4 cup	milk

provide no more than 100% of the Daily Values. If a children's supplement is offered, it should be monitored by caregivers and stored safely.

Nutrition-Related Problems in Children

In addition to nutrient deficiencies, a number of other problems related to food and nutrient intake can develop during childhood.

Dental Caries Carbohydrate-containing foods promote tooth decay. Decay occurs when there is prolonged contact between sugar and bacteria on the surface of the teeth. Because the primary teeth guide the growth of the permanent teeth, maintaining healthy primary teeth is just as important as preserving permanent ones. Preventing tooth decay involves limiting carbohydrate snacks, especially those that stick to teeth; brushing teeth frequently to remove sticky sweets; and consuming adequate fluoride (Figure 15.10). Children three years of age and over should be seen by a dentist regularly.

Hyperactivity Hyperactivity is a problem in 5 to 10% of school-age children, occurring more frequently in boys than in girls. This syndrome involves extreme physical activity, excitability, impulsiveness, distractibility, short attention span, and a low tolerance for frustration. Hyperactive children have more difficulty learning but usually are of normal or above-average intelligence. Hyperactivity is now considered part of a larger syndrome known as **attention deficit hyperactive disorder**.

Attention deficit hyperactivity disorder A condition that is characterized by a short attention span and a high level of activity, excitability, and distractibility.

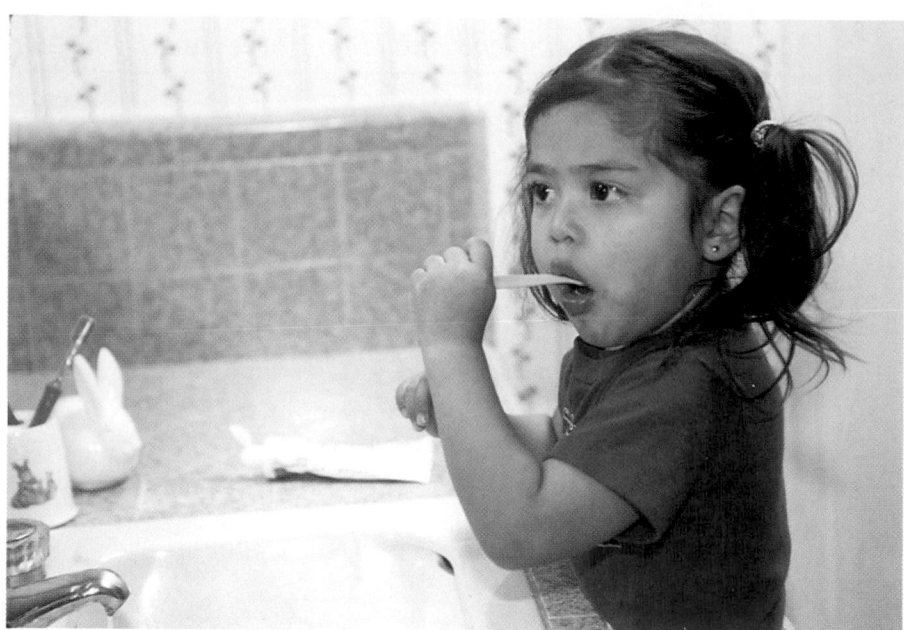

Figure 15.10
Frequent supervised toothbrushing by children can help prevent dental caries. (© David Young-Wolff/PhotoEdit)

One popular misconception is that hyperactivity is caused by a high sugar intake, but research on sugar intake and behavior has failed to support this hypothesis.[20] Hyperactive behavior that is observed after sugar consumption is likely the result of other circumstances in that child's life. For example, the excitement of a birthday party rather than the cake is most likely the cause of hyperactive behavior. Other situations that might cause hyperactivity include lack of sleep, overstimulation, the desire for more attention, or lack of physical activity.

Specific foods and food additives have also been implicated as a cause of hyperactivity. Numerous studies have been done to test the hypothesis that food sensitivities cause hyperactivity, but the results have been inconsistent.[21] Some children with this disorder seem to improve when particular foods or additives are eliminated, while others do not.

Another possible cause of hyperactive behavior in children is caffeine. Caffeine is a stimulant that can cause sleeplessness, restlessness, and irregular heartbeats. Beverages, food, and medicines containing caffeine are often a part of children's diets. For example, caffeinated beverages such as Coke and Mountain Dew are often included in children's fast-food meals.

Lead Toxicity Lead is an environmental contaminant that can be toxic, especially in children under six. Children are particularly susceptible because they absorb lead much more efficiently than do adults. It is estimated that children may absorb as much as 30 to 75% of ingested lead, whereas adults absorb only about 11%.[22] Once absorbed from the gastrointestinal tract, lead circulates in the bloodstream and then accumulates in the bones and, to a lesser extent, the brain, teeth, and kidneys. Lead disrupts the functioning of neurotransmitters and thus interferes with the functioning of the nervous system. Higher levels of lead can contribute to iron deficiency anemia, changes in kidney function, nervous system changes, and even seizures, coma, and death.[23] In young children, lead poisoning can cause learning disabilities and behavior problems.[24] In adults, lead poisoning can damage the reproductive organs and cause high blood pressure.[25] During pregnancy, lead toxicity can damage the fetal nervous system.

Lead is found naturally in the earth's crust, but over the years industrial activities have redistributed it in the environment. Lead is now found in soil contaminated with lead paint dust; it also enters drinking water from old corroded lead plumbing, lead solder on copper pipes, or brass faucets. It is found in polluted air, in leaded glass, and in glazes used on imported and antique pottery. These can contaminate

Table 15.3 *What You Can Do to Reduce Lead Exposure*

Reducing exposure from lead paint: If you live in a house built before 1978, it may contain lead paint or lead paint may have been sanded or scrapped off at some time.

- Wash floors and other surfaces weekly with warm water and detergent.
- Wipe soil off shoes before entering the house.
- Cover exposed soil in the yard with grass or mulch.

Reducing exposure from tap water: If your home has old plumbing, lead may be leaching into your tap water. More leaches into hot water than cold, and water that has been standing in the pipes has more lead.

- Use cold water for drinking and cooking.
- Allow water to run for 30 seconds before use.

Reducing exposure from food containers: Pottery glazes and lead crystal contain lead. The FDA limits the amount of lead allowed in ceramic foodware, but the lead content of pottery designed for ornamental use is not regulated.

- Look for engraved warnings such as "Not for Food Use—May Poison Food" and "For Decorative Purposes Only" to identify pottery that should not be used to serve food.
- Do not store acidic foods such as fruit juices or tomato juice in ceramic containers.
- Limit the use of antique or collectible housewares for food or beverages to special occasions.
- Use your lead crystal stemware to drink from, but do not store anything in lead crystal.
- Pregnant women should not routinely use lead crystal glasses.
- Infants should not be fed from crystal baby bottles.

For additional information: Contact the Centers for Disease Control and Prevention at 1-888-232-6789; the Environmental Protection Agency's Safe Drinking Water Hotline at 1-800-426-4791; the Consumer Product Safety Commission at 1-800-638-CPSC; the National Lead Information Center at 1-800-LEAD-FYI; or access Web sites for these agencies and organizations.

food and beverages. Because of the risks of lead toxicity from environmental contamination, lead is no longer used in house paint, gasoline, or solder. As a result, the number of children with elevated blood lead levels has decreased by 85% over the last 20 years.[26] Despite these gains, nearly a million children under six years of age have blood lead levels that are high enough to cause damage. For a number of reasons, the problem is greatest among children living in poverty. Their exposure is likely to be greater because they tend to live in older buildings where chipped paint and old plumbing may be contaminated with lead. In addition, children living in poverty are more likely to be malnourished, and malnutrition increases lead absorption because lead is better absorbed from an empty stomach and when other minerals such as calcium, zinc, and iron are deficient.

Children should have their blood lead levels tested.[26] The effects of lead poisoning are permanent, but if high levels are detected early, the lead can be removed with medical treatment (Table 15.3).

Eating Disorders Typically, eating disorders are thought of as a problem affecting teens and young women; however, such disorders are becoming more and more common in younger children. Eating disorders are usually not diagnosed until adolescence, but the excessive concern about weight and body image that characterizes these conditions may begin as early as the preschool years. These abnormal concerns can lead to battles over food and eating and to excessive finickiness, resulting in poor growth and abnormal development.

Influences from the Outside World

Forty years ago mothers had a greater impact on children's food choices because they were home to offer three meals a day. Today, the increase in the number of working mothers and single-parent households means children consume an increasing number of meals away from home—in day-care facilities, schools, and restaurant/fast-food establishments. Because of modern lifestyles, children make many of their own food choices, which are influenced by their home life, time spent away from home, and what they see on television.

Fast Food Isn't All Bad Children generally love fast food, and there is nothing wrong with an occasional fast-food meal. But these meals are typically lacking in milk, fruits, and vegetables. They are high in kcalories and fat and low in calcium, fiber, and vitamins A and C. To fit fast food into a healthy diet, more nutrient-dense fast-food choices need to be made and other meals and snacks throughout the day need to supply the missing nutrients. Many fast-food franchises now offer vegetables, salads, and milk. And some of the old standbys are not bad choices. A plain, single-patty hamburger provides a lot less fat and energy than one with two patties and a high-fat sauce. A chicken sandwich can be a lowfat choice if it is grilled or barbecued, not breaded and fried (see Appendix A). French fries are high in fat, but if they are combined with lowfat foods throughout the day, they can still be part of a healthy diet. A fast-food meal is only one part of the total diet. If the missing milk, fruits, and vegetables are consumed at other times during the day, the total diet can still be a healthy one.

Meals at Day Care or School Providing nutritious meals away from home is not always easy. A lunch taken to day care or school should contain foods that do not require refrigeration (even if a refrigerator is available, the child is likely to forget to put the lunch in it). Packing a lunch does not guarantee that it will be eaten, so caregivers should make sure the child likes what is sent; even the most carefully planned lunch is not nutritious if it is not eaten.

For children who buy their lunch at school, the National School Lunch Program provides low-cost meals designed to meet nutrient needs and promote healthy diets. The goals of this program are to improve the dietary intake and nutritional health of America's children, and to promote nutrition education by teaching children to make appropriate food choices.[27] Each lunch meal must provide one-third of the 1989 RDA for protein, vitamin A, vitamin C, iron, calcium, and energy and meet the Dietary Guidelines recommendations of no more than 30% of energy from fat and 10% from saturated fat. Within these guidelines, each school or school district can decide which foods to serve and how they are prepared. In addition to lunches, federal guidelines regulate foods sold in snack bars and vending machines that compete with school lunch programs. These must provide at least 5% of the RDA for one or more of the following: protein, vitamin A, vitamin C, niacin, riboflavin, calcium, and iron. An analysis of the foods students choose to eat from the meal offered found that students who participated in the school lunch program consumed one-third of the RDA for energy, protein, vitamin A, vitamin C, vitamin B_6, calcium, iron, and zinc and drank twice as much milk as students not participating in school lunch programs.

Television Reduces Activity and Influences Food Choices Many children today spend more time watching television than they do in any activity other than sleep.[28] Television affects nutritional status in a number of ways: It introduces children to foods they might otherwise not be exposed to, it promotes snacking, and it reduces physical activity (Figure 15.11).

Through advertising, television has a strong influence on the foods selected by young children. A review of commercials broadcast during children's programming found that over 60% were for food products—primarily sweetened breakfast cereals; sweets such as candy, cookies, doughnuts, and other desserts; snacks; and beverages—that are high in sugar, fat, or salt.[29] Television also promotes snacking behavior. Although snacks are an important part of a growing child's diet, many children snack on sweet and salty foods that are low in nutrient density while watching TV.

Perhaps the most important nutritional influence of television is that it reduces activity. Hours spent watching television are hours when physical activity is at a minimum. One study showed that children who watch four or more hours of TV per day had more

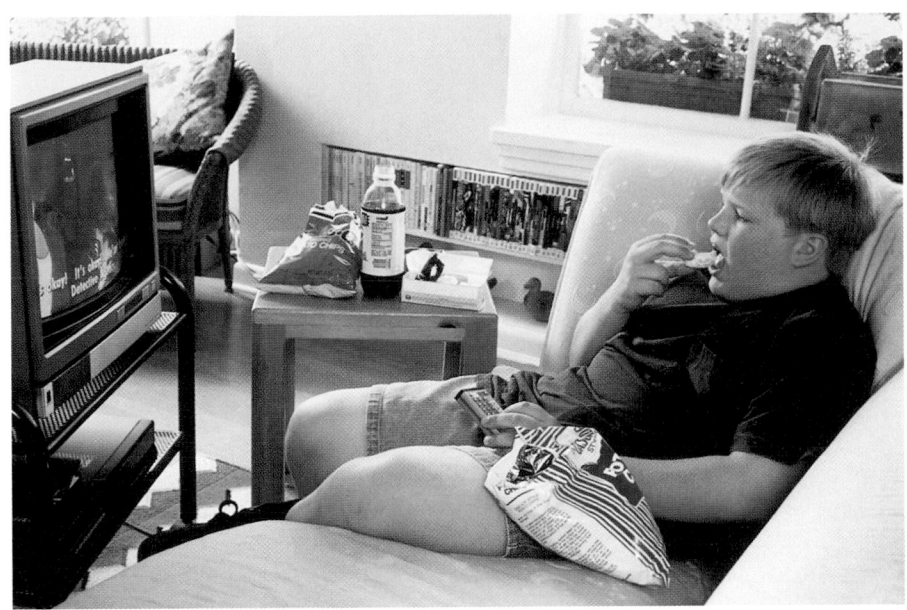

Figure 15.11
Television watching influences activity
level, snacking behavior, and the kinds
of foods children choose. (© Donna
Day/Stone)

body fat and a greater BMI than those who watch fewer than two hours a day.[30] In addition to television, children and adolescents today replace time spent at more physically demanding activities with time spent playing computer and video games.

• ADOLESCENCE: TRANSITION TO ADULTHOOD

Once a child has reached about 9 to 12 years of age, the physical changes associated with sexual maturation begin to occur. The maturation process creates differences between the nutrient requirements of males and females. As with children, the nutrient intake of adolescents is affected by psychosocial development and the environment in which they live. The DRIs begin recommendations for adolescent intake at age nine because the hormonal changes that mark the beginning of adolescence occur by this age in some girls, particularly in African Americans. The DRIs divide recommended intakes for adolescence into ages 9 through 13 and ages 14 through 18.[31]

The Changing Body: Sexual Maturation

During adolescence, organ systems develop and grow, body composition changes, and the growth rates and nutritional requirements of boys and girls diverge. This period of rapid change, which ends in sexual maturation, is called **puberty**. During adolescence, boys and girls grow about 11 inches and gain about 40% of their eventual skeletal mass.[32] From ages 10 to 17, girls gain about 53 pounds and boys about 70 pounds. During adolescence, there is an 18- to 24-month period of peak growth velocity, called the **adolescent growth spurt**. In girls, the growth spurt occurs between the ages of 10 and 13. In boys, it occurs between ages 12 and 15.

The hormonal changes that occur with sexual development orchestrate the type of growth that occurs and the change in body composition that results. During the growth spurt, boys tend to grow taller and heavier than girls and do so at a faster rate. Boys gain fat but also add so much lean mass as muscle and bone that their percentage of body fat actually decreases (Figure 15.12). In girls, **menarche**, the onset of menstruation, is typically followed by a deceleration in growth rate and an increase in fat deposition. By age 20, females have about twice as much adipose tissue as males and only about two-thirds as much lean tissue. These physiologic changes affect nutrient needs. Because there is a large individual variation in the age at which

Puberty A period in life characterized by rapid growth and physical changes that ends in the attainment of sexual maturity.

Adolescent growth spurt An 18- to 24-month period of peak growth velocity that begins at about ages 10 to 13 in girls and 12 to 15 in boys.

Menarche The onset of menstruation, which occurs normally between the ages of 10 and 15.

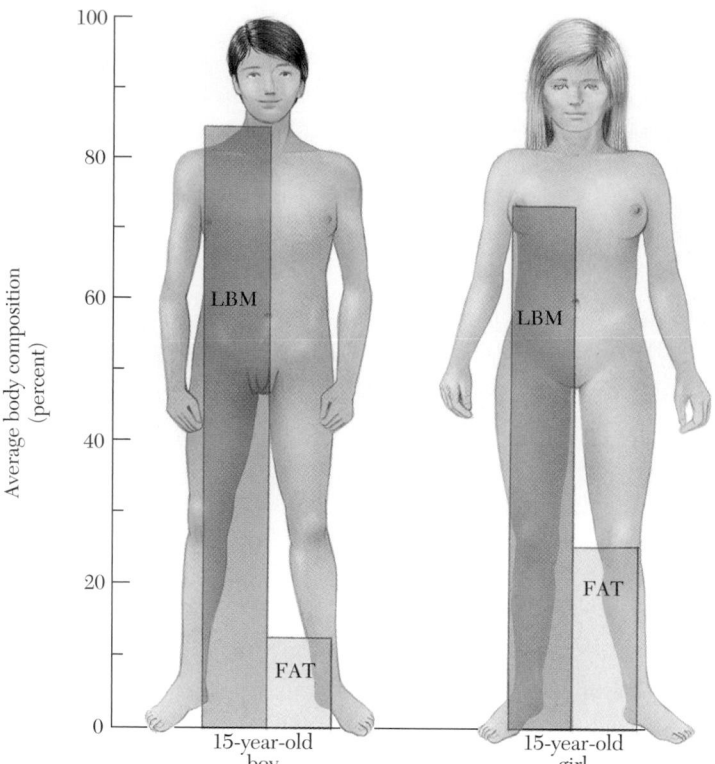

Figure 15.12
After puberty, males have a higher percentage of lean body mass and less body fat than females. (Adapted from Forbes, G. B., Body composition. In *Present Knowledge in Nutrition*, 6th ed. Brown, M. L. ed. Washington, D.C.: International Life Sciences Institute-Nutrition Foundation, 1990).

these growth changes occur, the stage of maturation is often a better indicator of nutritional requirements than actual chronological age.

Nutrition during childhood and adolescence can affect sexual development. Nutritional deficiencies can cause poor growth and delayed sexual maturation. Taller, heavier children usually enter puberty sooner than shorter, lighter ones.[33]

Adolescent Nutrient Needs

Total nutrient needs are greater during adolescence than at any other time of life. The best indicators of adequate intake are satiety and growth that follows the curve of the growth charts.

Energy and Macronutrients Energy requirements for boys exceed those for girls because boys have more muscle and a greater body size. Adolescent girls need 2100 to 2400 kcalories per day, and boys require about 2200 to 3150 kcalories per day (see Figure 15.7). Protein requirements for both groups reach the adult recommendation of 0.8 gram per kilogram by about age 19, but since boys are generally heavier, they require more total protein than girls. These higher requirements for males continue throughout life.

Vitamins The need for B vitamins involved in energy metabolism is much higher in adolescence than in childhood because of higher energy intakes. Riboflavin is frequently low in teen diets, especially in those of girls, possibly due to low milk intake. Vitamin B_6 is needed for protein synthesis; therefore, need is increased during the rapid growth of adolescence. Folate and vitamin B_{12} needs are increased because of the high rate of cell division for tissue growth. Vitamin B_{12} intake is typically adequate, but folate is a vitamin at risk for deficiency in the adolescent population.[34] The need for vitamin D increases with skeletal growth. The AI for vitamin D is set at 5 μg per day, but in active teens who engage in outdoor activities, much of the requirement is met by synthesis. Additional amounts of vitamins A, C, and E are needed to preserve the structure and function of the newly synthesized cells. These vitamins are generally adequate in the teen diet.

Iron Iron deficiency anemia is common in adolescence. Iron is needed to synthesize hemoglobin for the expansion of blood volume and myoglobin for the increase in muscle mass. Because blood volume expands at a faster rate in boys than in girls, boys require more iron for tissue synthesis than girls. However, the iron loss due to menstruation makes total needs greater in young women, yet their intake is typically less than the recommended amount. The RDA is set at 11 mg for boys and 15 mg for girls ages 14 to 18.[35] Good sources of iron acceptable to teens include fortified grains and breakfast cereals and lean red meats.

Calcium The adolescent growth spurt increases both the length and the mass of bones, and adequate calcium is essential to form healthy bone. Calcium retention varies with growth rate, with the fastest-growing adolescents retaining the most calcium. The AI for calcium during adolescence is 1300 mg per day for both sexes, but intake is typically below this in both adolescent boys and girls.[34] This may compromise the level of peak bone mass achieved, increasing the risk of developing osteoporosis later in life.

Foods common in the teen diet that are good sources of calcium include milk, yogurt and frozen yogurt, ice cream, and cheese added to hamburgers, nachos, and pizza. Although milk and cheese are the biggest source of calcium in teen diets, they can be high in saturated fat, so adolescents should be encouraged to consume reduced-fat dairy products and vegetable sources of calcium. Adolescent girls are likely to skimp on drinking milk, favoring low-kcalorie soft drinks. This may put them in double jeopardy, since diet soda does not supply calcium and some varieties are high in caffeine, which increases calcium excretion, and a form of phosphorus that increases calcium losses (Figure 15.13).[36]

Zinc During adolescence, the increase in protein synthesis required for the growth of skeletal muscle and the development of organs increases the need for zinc. The RDA is 11 mg for boys and 9 mg for girls ages 14 to 18. A long-term deficiency results in growth retardation and altered sexual development. Although severe zinc deficiency is rare in developed countries, even mild deficiency can cause poor growth, affect appetite and taste, impair immune response, and interfere with vitamin A metabolism. Since adolescents are growing rapidly and maturing sexually, adequate zinc is essential for, but not typically consumed by, this age group.[35] Good sources include meats and whole grains.

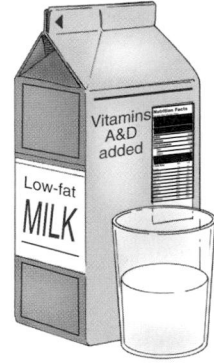
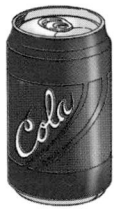

	Lowfat milk	Cola soft drink
Serving size	8 oz	12 oz
Energy (kcal)	102	150
Protein (g)	8	0
Calcium (mg)	300	0
Phosphorus (mg)	235	45
Riboflavin (mg)	0.4	0
Vitamin A (μg)	144	0
Vitamin D (μg)	2.5	0
Caffeine (mg)	0	40

Figure 15.13

An 8-ounce glass of milk is a good source of protein, calcium, riboflavin, vitamin A, and vitamin D. A serving of a carbonated beverage (12 fluid ounces) contains more energy, contributes few nutrients, and often contains caffeine.

Meeting Adolescent Nutrient Needs

Skipped meals and meals away from home are common among adolescents. No matter when foods are consumed throughout the day, an adolescent's diet should follow the recommendations of the Food Guide Pyramid—choosing at the high end of the range of serving recommendations. For example, a diet containing 3000 or more kcalories should contain 11 servings of grains. This may seem a staggering number, but it is not when spread over the course of a day. A large bowl of cereal and two slices of toast for breakfast is 4 servings; two tacos for lunch and crackers after school is 4 more servings; and a dinner of spaghetti and garlic bread can add another 3 or 4 servings. The diet should also provide 5 to 9 servings of fruits and vegetables. Unfortunately, fruits and vegetables are the food groups most likely to be lacking in the American diet: french fries, which are high in fat and salt, are the most frequently consumed vegetable. And many people never consume fruit. Sources of fruits and vegetables acceptable to teens include fruit juice, salads, and tomato sauce and vegetables on pizza and spaghetti.

Since the teen diet, especially that of teenage boys, is typically high in fat, saturated fat, cholesterol, and sodium, meals offered at home should be low in fat and sodium. Teens are no longer fed by their parents, but healthy choices, such as reduced-fat milk and dairy products, vegetables, and fruits, should be available at home (see *Critical Thinking*: Less Food May Not Mean Fewer Kcalories).

CRITICAL THINKING

Less Food May Not Mean Fewer Kcalories

Jenny is a busy 16-year-old high school junior. Until recently she hadn't paid much attention to her diet because she ate all her meals at home or at school. Now she has a part-time job and frequently eats dinner and snacks on her own. She notices that she has gained a few pounds and decides that she should change her diet.

Jenny's Original Diet			Jenny's New Diet		
Food	Energy (kcal)	Fat (g)	Food	Energy (kcal)	Fat (g)
Breakfast					
Corn flakes	97	0	Bagel	187	1
Lowfat milk	120	5			
Orange juice	112	0			
Toast	140	2.2			
Margarine	68	7.6			
Lunch					
Hamburger	260	10	Frozen yogurt	288	13
Apple	81	0.5			
Lowfat milk	120	5			
Corn chips	153	9.5			
Snack					
Slice of pizza	200	5	Double burger	576	32
Cola	185	0	French fries	315	16
			Vanilla shake	503	14
Dinner					
Ham and cheese sandwich	350	15	Candy bar	300	21
Potato chips	150	10	Potato chips	150	10
Cola	185	0			
Total	**2221**	**69.8**		**2319**	**107**

How has Jenny's intake changed?

▼

Although she eats less food, Jenny's new diet is actually higher in energy and fat, and lower in micronutrients. Her original diet provided 2221 kcalories, 28% of which was from fat, and met her micronutrient needs. Her new diet has more energy, contains about 42% fat, and does not supply the recommended amounts of vitamin A, folate, vitamin C, vitamin E, calcium, magnesium, zinc, or iron.

How could she modify her original diet to reduce her energy intake, provide the essential nutrients she needs, and still fit her busy schedule?

▼

Answer:

A Changing World: Influences on Adolescent Nutrition

Many psychosocial changes occur during adolescence. Teens are searching for their own identities and at the same time are afraid of some of the physical and social consequences of maturation. Social activities, peer pressure, and convenience are more important determinants of food intake and eating habits than is health. There is no sense of urgency about consuming a diet to reduce the risk of developing chronic disease. Nutrition concerns focus instead on environmental issues, appearance, weight loss or gain for appearance or athletic performance, or simply a full stomach. Factors outside the home, such as the use of drugs and alcohol, and other lifestyle choices that may have an impact on nutrition have more and more influence on what foods teens choose.

Vegetarian Diets Many teens today are turning to vegetarian eating. Some do it for health reasons or to lose weight, but most give up meat because they are concerned about animals and the environment. Although vegetarian diets can be a healthful alternative, foods must be carefully chosen to meet needs and avoid excesses. Meatless diets can be low in iron and zinc, and vegan diets, which contain no animal products, may put teens at risk of vitamin B_{12} deficiency and inadequate calcium intake. Although we think of vegetarian diets as healthy, they are not necessarily low in fat, particularly if high-fat dairy products are chosen. A slice of cheese pizza and a can of cola provides calcium but is high in fat and low in iron. However, when chosen carefully, a vegetarian diet can be low in saturated fat, and cholesterol and high in complex carbohydrate, fiber, and micronutrients. For example, a vegetarian lunch of a pita sandwich with hummus (chickpeas), tomatoes, and spinach, along with some dried fruit and a glass of reduced-fat milk, is low in fat and contains good sources of calcium and plant sources of iron.

Appearance and Body Image There is probably no other time in life when appearance is of more concern than during adolescence. The hormonal changes of puberty often cause acne, and many teens are unhappy with their bodies. Many girls want to lose weight even if they are not overweight. Many boys, on the other hand, want to gain weight to achieve a muscular, strong appearance.

Acne Acne, which is common in adolescence, is triggered by the hormonal changes that occur with the onset of puberty. At one time, acne was believed to be related to diet, and long lists of foods to avoid were doled out to teens with acne. Since then, restrictions on the intake of foods such as chocolate, french fries, and soft drinks have been found to have no effect on the severity of acne. Anxiety, lack of sleep, and hormonal fluctuations of the menstrual cycle are more likely to cause acne flare-ups than specific foods, but a well-balanced diet will ensure that the skin has all the nutrients needed to maintain its integrity. Medications are also available to treat acne. A prescription medication which is a derivative of vitamin A, called 13-*cis*-retinoic acid (Accutane), can be taken orally to treat a severe form of acne called cystic acne. Another prescription vitamin A derivative, called Retin-A, is used topically to treat acne. In addition to reducing acne, Retin-A tightens the skin and decreases wrinkles, making it a popular drug with older adults. Neither Accutane nor Retin-A should be used during pregnancy. Although these drugs are derivatives of vitamin A, vitamin A supplements cannot be substituted as a treatment for acne. In addition, large doses of vitamin A are toxic.

Body Weight Because of the importance of physical appearance during adolescence, being overweight can be particularly devastating. Obese adolescents may be discriminated against by adults as well as by their peers. This can lead to feelings of rejection, social isolation, and low self-esteem. The isolation of obese adolescents from teen society results in boredom, depression, inactivity, and withdrawal—all of which can cause an increase in eating and a decrease in energy output, worsening the problem (Figure 15.14). Adolescent weight-loss diets should be carefully planned to supply essential nutrients for growth without excess energy. Meals should be low in fat and high in whole grains, vegetables, and fruits. Breakfast and lunch should not be skipped because this may actually increase energy intake by increasing the amount of food consumed later in the day.

Eating Disorders Eating disorders such as bulimia and anorexia nervosa are more common in adolescence than at any other time in life (see Chapter 7). The pressure of taking on the responsibilities of adulthood, combined with pressure from peers and society to be thin, may contribute to this high incidence. Many individuals with eating disorders feel ineffectual in their lives and may be using food to achieve some measure of self-control. Disordered eating is often hidden by other eating patterns. For example, vegetarian adolescent females were twice as likely as nonvegetarians to report frequent dieting, four times as likely to report intentional vomiting, and eight times more likely to purge using laxatives.[37]

The Impact of Athletics Despite all the benefits of exercise, the nutrition misinformation that is common in school athletics can lead to serious health problems. Excessive use of dietary supplements, the use of anabolic steroids, inappropriate training diets, and fad diets can all cause problems (see Chapter 13).

Teen athletes may require more water, energy, protein, carbohydrate, and micronutrients than their less active peers, but supplements are rarely needed to meet these needs. Fluid should be consumed before, during, and after exercise to prevent dehydration. If the extra energy needs of teen athletes are met with whole grains, fresh fruits and vegetables, and dairy products, their protein, carbohydrate, and micronutrient needs will easily be met. An exception is iron, which may need to be supplemented, particularly in female athletes. The combination of poor iron intake, iron losses from menstruation and sweat, and increased needs for building new lean tissue puts many female athletes at risk for iron deficiency anemia.[38]

Some of the most dangerous practices associated with adolescent sports are those that attempt to control body weight. Some sports such as football demand that the athlete be large and heavy. In order to "bulk up," high school athletes may experiment with anabolic steroids, androstenedione, and creatine. Anabolic steroids are illegal, and although they do increase muscle mass, the risks far outweigh the benefits. Androstenedione is a testosterone precursor that is legally sold as a dietary supplement, but the long-term health effects of this supplement have not yet been determined. Creatine improves exercise performance in sports requiring short bursts of activity and has not been associated with serious side effects.[39] Nonetheless, the best

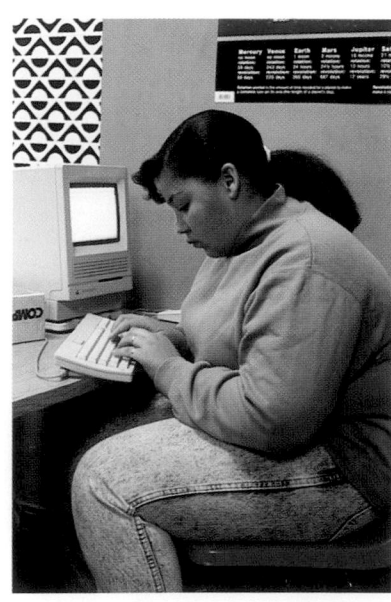

Figure 15.14

The prevalence of obesity is increasing among teens in the United States. (© Lawrence Migdale/Photo Researchers, Inc.)

and safest way for young athletes to increase muscle mass is the hard way: Lift weights and eat more.

Female athletes involved in sports that require lean, light bodies, such as gymnastics and ballet, are likely to abuse weight-loss diets. Sexual maturation, which causes an increase in body fat and changes in weight distribution, can be disturbing to young women involved in such sports. The combination of hard training and weight restriction can lead to a syndrome known as the female athlete triad that includes disordered eating, amenorrhea, and osteoporosis (see Chapter 13).[40]

Weight loss is also a concern for adolescents participating in sports such as wrestling that require athletes to fit into a specific weight class on the day of the event. In these athletes, dangerous methods of quick weight loss—such as severe energy intake restriction, water deprivation, vomiting, and diuretic and laxative abuse—are common practice. Low-energy diets can interfere with normal growth and may be too limited in variety to meet these athletes' needs for vitamins and minerals. Even more of a danger is the practice of restricting water intake and encouraging sweat loss to decrease body weight. This may achieve the temporary weight loss necessary to put the athlete in a lower weight class, but dehydration is dangerous and can impair athletic performance.[41]

Sexual Maturity As discussed earlier, sexual maturity in girls affects nutrition because it increases body fat and iron needs. The use of oral contraceptives and pregnancy during adolescence can also affect nutritional status.

Oral Contraceptive Use Oral contraceptive hormones may be prescribed to adolescent girls for a number of reasons and can affect nutrition because they affect nutrient metabolism. Oral contraceptives may cause a rise in fasting blood sugar and a tendency toward abnormal glucose tolerance in those with a family history of diabetes. They may also cause changes in body composition, including weight gain due to water retention and an increase in lean body mass. Oral contraceptives may reduce the need for iron by reducing menstrual flow and increasing iron absorption. Therefore, a special RDA for iron of 11.4 mg/day has been established for those taking oral contraceptives.[35] Blood levels of some B vitamins have been found to be low in oral contraceptive users, although it is not known whether these changes in blood levels reflect an increased need for these nutrients.[42,43]

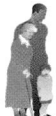

Teenage Pregnancy Because adolescent girls continue to grow and mature for several years after menstruation starts, the pregnant teenager must meet her own nutrient needs for growth and development as well as the needs of pregnancy. This puts the pregnant adolescent at nutritional risk. In order for the mother and fetus to remain healthy, special attention must be paid to all aspects of prenatal care, including nutrient intake (see Chapter 14). Due to the special nutrient needs of this group, the DRIs have included a life-stage group for pregnant girls age 18 or younger.

Alcohol Use Although it is illegal to sell alcohol to adolescents, alcoholic beverages are commonly available at teen social gatherings, and the peer pressure to consume them is strong. Alcohol is a drug that has short-term effects that occur soon after ingestion and long-term health consequences that are associated with overuse. It provides 7 kcalories per gram.

What Are the Immediate Effects of Alcohol Consumption? Alcohol is a small molecule that is rapidly and almost completely absorbed in the upper gastrointestinal tract. Some is absorbed directly from the stomach, so the effects of alcohol consumption are almost immediate, especially if it is consumed on an empty stomach. If there is food in the stomach when alcohol is consumed, less will be absorbed there because less is in contact with the stomach wall. Food also slows stomach emptying and therefore decreases the rate at which alcohol is absorbed in the small intestine. Some alcohol is metabolized by alcohol dehydrogenase in the stomach. Women tend

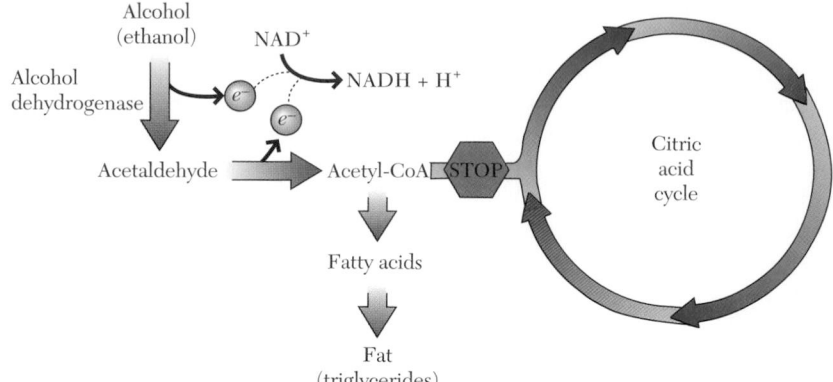

Figure 15.15
The breakdown of alcohol causes a buildup of NADH. This prevents acetyl-CoA from entering the citric acid cycle and diverts it for fat synthesis.

to have less of this stomach enzyme, which may be one reason women become intoxicated after consuming less alcohol than men.

Absorbed alcohol is metabolized in the liver. It is broken down by liver alcohol dehydrogenase to form acetaldehyde, which is then further degraded to form acetyl-CoA. As the alcohol molecule is broken down, electrons and hydrogen ions are released and picked up by NAD, producing NADH. The buildup of NADH inhibits acetyl-CoA from entering the citric acid cycle to produce ATP, so much of the acetyl-CoA generated is used to synthesize fatty acids (Figure 15.15).

The liver can break down about 0.5 oz of alcohol per hour, depending on body size, amount of previous drinking, food intake, and general health. When alcohol intake exceeds the ability of the liver to break it down, the excess circulates in the bloodstream until the liver enzymes can metabolize it. At the kidney, alcohol acts as a diuretic, increasing fluid excretion. Therefore, excessive alcohol intake can cause dehydration. At the brain, alcohol acts as a depressant. First it affects reasoning; if drinking continues, the vision and speech centers of the brain are affected. Next, large-muscle control becomes impaired, causing lack of coordination. Finally, the individual loses consciousness. If drinking were to continue, the anesthetic effects would suppress breathing and heart rate. It is possible for an individual to drink fast enough for alcohol levels to continue to rise after he or she has lost consciousness, resulting in death. This can occur with binge drinking, defined as frequently downing five or more drinks at a time. Binge drinking is a problem on college campuses, causing about 50 deaths and hundreds of cases of alcohol poisoning annually.[44]

Some alcohol is eliminated by the lungs. The amount lost through the lungs is predictable and reliable enough to be used to estimate blood alcohol level from a measure of breath alcohol. This is the basis of the Breathalyzer tests administered by the police to determine if an individual is driving under the influence of alcohol. The effects of alcohol on the central nervous system are what make driving while under the influence of alcohol so dangerous. Alcohol affects reaction time, eye-hand coordination, accuracy, and balance. Not only does alcohol impair one's ability to operate a motor vehicle, but it also impairs one's judgment in the decision to drive.

What Happens with Chronic Alcohol Use? One risk associated with regular alcohol consumption is the possibility of addiction. Alcohol addiction, like any other drug addiction, is a physiological problem that needs treatment. Alcoholism is believed to have a genetic component that makes some people more likely to become addicted, but environment also plays a significant role. Thus, someone with a genetic predisposition toward alcoholism whose peers do not consume alcohol is much less likely to become addicted.

Long-term excessive alcohol consumption has serious health implications. Alcohol either directly or indirectly affects every organ in the body and increases the risk of malnutrition and many chronic diseases. Alcohol contributes energy but few other nutrients and replaces more nutrient-dense energy sources in the diet. Alcohol dam-

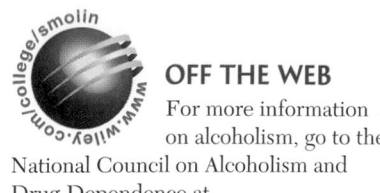

OFF THE WEB
For more information on alcoholism, go to the National Council on Alcoholism and Drug Dependence at
www.ncadd.org/
or the National Institute on Drug Abuse at
www.nida.nih.gov/

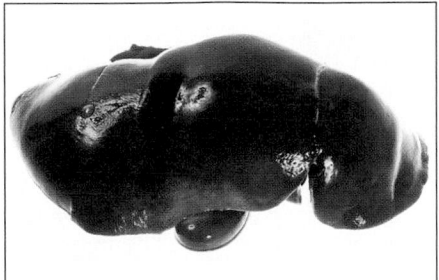 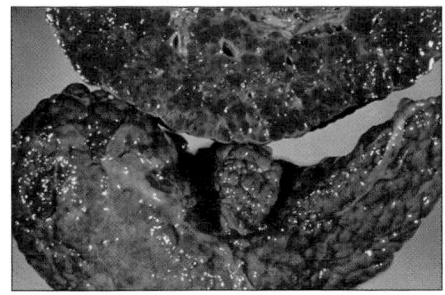

ages the lining of the small intestine, decreasing the absorption of several B vitamins and vitamin C. Thiamin deficiency is a particular concern with chronic alcohol consumption. Alcohol can also alter the storage, metabolism, and excretion of other vitamins and some minerals.

The most significant physiological effects of chronic alcohol consumption occur in the liver. Alcoholic liver disease progresses in a number of phases. The first phase is **fatty liver**, a condition that occurs when alcohol consumption increases the synthesis and deposition of fat in the liver. The second phase, **alcoholic hepatitis**, is an inflammation of the liver. Both of these conditions are reversible if alcohol consumption is stopped and good nutritional and health practices are followed. If alcohol consumption continues, **cirrhosis** may develop. This is an irreversible condition in which fibrous deposits scar the liver and interfere with its function. Since the liver is the primary site of many metabolic reactions, cirrhosis is often fatal (Figure 15.16). In addition to causing liver disease, heavy drinking is associated with hypertension, heart disease, and stroke.

Safe Drinking There are certain groups who should not drink, such as children, women who are pregnant or trying to conceive, alcoholics, individuals who plan to drive or engage in another activity that requires attention or skill, and individuals using prescription or over-the-counter medication (see Chapter 16, *Off the Shelf*: Alcohol: A Risk-Benefit Analysis). Excess alcohol consumption, whether occasional or chronic, is hazardous to health. Individuals who do drink should not drink in excess (Figure 15.17). When alcohol is consumed, it should be consumed slowly with meals, which slows absorption. It usually takes an hour to metabolize the alcohol in one drink (one drink is 0.5 oz distilled liquor, 12 oz beer, or 5 oz wine), so no more than one drink should be consumed every 1.5 hours. Sipping, not gulping, allows the liver time to break down what has already been consumed. Unfortunately, once alcohol has been consumed, the rate at which it is metabolized and eliminated from the body cannot be accelerated. Cold showers, brisk walks, and black coffee may wake you up, but they will not sober you up.

Fatty liver The accumulation of fat in the liver.
Alcoholic hepatitis Inflammation of the liver caused by alcohol consumption.
Cirrhosis Chronic liver disease characterized by the loss of functioning liver cells and the accumulation of fibrous connective tissue.

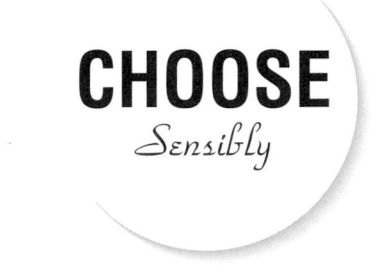

CHOOSE *Sensibly*

If you drink alcoholic beverages, do so in moderation

Figure 15.17
The Dietary Guidelines for Americans recommends that alcohol be consumed in moderation. (USDA, DHHS, 2000)

• APPLICATIONS •

1. Assume you had a Big Mac, fries, and a 16-ounce cola for lunch.
   a. How many servings from each food group of the Food Guide Pyramid does this represent?
   b. List the numbers of additional servings from each food group that you would need to satisfy the daily recommendations of the Food Guide Pyramid.
   c. Select foods from each group to complete your intake for the day.
   d. Do the foods you selected meet the selection recommendations of the Food Guide Pyramid and your energy needs?
2. The table gives height and weight measurements recorded for a girl from age six to age nine.
   a. Calculate her BMI and plot the values on a growth chart.
   b. What recommendations would you have about her weight?

Age	Height (in.)	Weight (lb)
6	45	44
7	48	53
8	50	77
9	52	97

3. Use the Internet or a diet analysis computer program to look up the nutrient composition of your favorite fast-food meal.
   a. What is the percent of kcalories from carbohydrate and fat in the meal?
   b. Compare the amount of energy, fat, protein, iron, calcium and vitamin A to the recommended intake for someone of your age, weight and lifestage.

SUMMARY

1. Good nutrition in childhood sets the stage for nutrition and health in the adult years. The diet must meet the needs for growth and development as well as reduce the risk of chronic disease later in life. Growth that follows standard patterns indicates adequate nutrition. Overweight children are likely to become overweight adults and develop elevated blood pressure, high blood cholesterol, and heart disease.

2. Introducing solid foods between four and six months of age adds iron and other nutrients to the diet and aids in muscle development. Newly introduced foods should be appropriate to the child's stage of development and offered one at a time to monitor for food allergies.

3. Food allergies are caused by the absorption of allergens, most of which are proteins. Food allergies involve antibody production by the immune system and are more common in infancy because the infant's immature gastrointestinal tract is likely to absorb whole proteins. Specific foods that cause allergies can be identified by an elimination diet and food challenge. Unlike food allergies, food intolerances do not involve the immune system.

4. Children like to have control over what they eat. In order to meet nutrient needs and develop nutritious habits, a variety of healthy foods should be offered at meals and snacks throughout the day.

5. Energy and protein needs per kilogram of body weight decrease as children grow, but total needs increase because of the increase in total body weight and activity level. The acceptable range of fat intake is higher for children than adults. Dietary carbohydrates should come primarily from whole grains, vegetables, fruits, and milk.

6. Low dietary intakes of vitamin A, vitamin C, calcium, iron, and zinc put some American children at risk of deficiencies. Meals away from home at school or fast-food restaurants are common and impact overall nutrient intake.

7. During adolescence, accelerated growth and sexual maturation have an impact on nutrient requirements. Body composition and the nutritional requirements of boys and girls diverge. Males gain more lean body tissue, while females have a greater increase in body fat.

8. During the adolescent growth spurt, total energy and protein requirements are higher than at any other time of life. Young men require more protein and energy than young women.

9. In adolescence, vitamin requirements increase to meet the needs of rapid growth. The minerals calcium, iron, and zinc are likely to be low in the adolescent diet. Iron deficiency anemia is common, especially in girls as they begin losing iron through menstruation.

10. The food intake of adolescents may be determined more by social activities, peer pressure, and participation in athletics than by nutrient needs. Since meals are frequently missed, healthy snacks should be included in the diet.

11. Psychosocial changes occurring during the adolescent years make physical appearance of great concern. Obesity can be psychologically and socially devastating. Eating disorders are more common in adolescence than at any other time. Adolescent athletes are susceptible to nutrition misinformation, and they may try dangerous practices such as using anabolic steroids to increase muscle mass or fad diets and fluid restriction to lose weight.

12. During the teen years, pregnancy, the use of oral contraceptives, and the consumption of alcohol may affect nutritional status.

13. Alcohol has short-term effects on the central nervous system, including the impairment of reasoning, judgment, and coordination, and eventually the loss of consciousness. Chronic alcohol use damages the liver and can cause malnutrition by decreasing nutrient intake and absorption and interfering with nutrient utilization.

REVIEW QUESTIONS

1. How does nutrient intake during childhood affect health later in life?

2. What is the best way to determine if a child is eating enough?

3. What impact does parents' weight have on a child's weight?

4. When should solid and semisolid foods be introduced into an infant's diet?

5. How should new foods be introduced to monitor for the development of food allergies?

6. What factors influence the maximum height a child will reach?

7. How do the recommendations for fat intake change as a child gets older?

8. Why is anemia a problem in young children? in teenage girls?

9. Why are snacks an important part of children's diets?

10. Why is breakfast important?

11. What nutritional problems can be signaled by sudden changes in weight patterns?

12. How can fast foods be incorporated into a healthy diet?

13. What is the adolescent growth spurt? How does it affect nutrient requirements?

14. Describe two physiological differences between males and females after puberty that affect their nutrient needs.

15. Why are teenagers particularly susceptible to eating disorders?

16. How can alcohol consumption affect nutritional status?

REFERENCES

1. Nicklas, T. A., O'Neil, C. E., and Berenson, G. S. Nutrient contribution of breakfast, secular trends, and the role of ready-to-eat cereals: A review of the data from the Bogalusa Heart Study. *Am. J. Clin. Nutr.* 67:757S–763S, 1998.

2. Kennedy, E., and David, C. USDA School Breakfast Program. *Am. J. Clin. Nutr.* 67:798S–803S, 1998.

3. Nahikian-Nelms, M. Influential factors of caregivers' behaviors at mealtime: a study of 24 child care providers. *J. Am. Diet. Assoc.* 97:505–509, 1997.

4. U.S. Department of Health and Human Services, Centers for Disease Control and Prevention, National Center for Health Statistics. CDC growth charts: United States. Advance Data, No. 314, June 8, 2000

(revised). Available online at www.cdc.gov/growthcharts/ Accessed August 28, 2000.

5. American Dietetic Association. Position of the American Dietetic Association: dietary guidance for healthy children aged 2 to 11 years. *J. Am. Diet. Assoc.* 99:93–101, 1999.

6. Daniels, S. R., Morrison, J. A., Sprecher, D. L., et al. Association of body fat distribution and cardiovascular risk factors in children and adolescents. *Circulation* 99:541–545, 1999.

7. Nutrition and Health Promotion Program, International Life Sciences Institute. A survey of parents and children about physical activity patterns. September–October 1996. Key findings Available online at www.ilsi.org/nhppress.html#2 Accessed July 31, 2002.

8. U.S. Department of Agriculture, U.S. Department of Health and Human Services. *Nutrition and Your Health: Dietary Guidelines for Americans*, 4th ed. Home and Garden Bulletin No. 232. Hyattsville, Md.: U.S. Government Printing Office, 2000.

9. American Diabetes Association. Type 2 diabetes in children and adolescents. *Diabetes Care* 23:381–386, 2000.

10. National Institute of Diabetes & Digestive & Kidney Diseases, National Institutes of Health, National Diabetes Information Clearinghouse. Fact Sheet on Diabetes Statistics. NIH Publication No. 98–3926, Nov. 1997; updated Feb. 1998. Available online at www.niddk.nih.gov/health/diabetes/pubs/dmstats/dmstats.htm/ Accessed November 27,2000.

11. McDowell, M. A., Briefel, R. R., Alaimo, K., et al. Energy and macronutrient intakes of persons 2 months and over in the United States. *Third National Health and Nutrition Examination Survey, Phase I, 1988–1991.* Advance data from Vital and Health Statistics: No. 255. Hyattsville, Md.: NCHS, 1994.

12. Berenson, G. S., Wattigney, W. A., Srinivasan, S. R., and Radhakrishnamurthy, B. Rationale to study the early natural history of heart disease: the Bogalusa Heart Study. *Am. J. Med. Sci.* 310(Suppl.):22S–28S, 1995.

13. Obarzanek E., Kimm, S. Y., Barton, B. A., et al. Long-term safety and efficacy of a cholesterol-lowering diet in children with elevated low-density lipoprotein cholesterol: Seven-year results of the Dietary Intervention Study in Children (DISC). *Pediatrics.* 107:256–264, 2001.

14. Bao, W., Threefoot, S. A., Srinivasan, S. R., and Berenson, G. S. Essential hypertension predicted by tracking of elevated blood pressure from childhood to adulthood: The Bogalusa Heart Study. *Am. J. Hypertens.* 8:657–661, 1995.

15. Chandra, R. K. Food hypersensitivities and allergic disease: A selective review. *Am. J. Clin. Nutr.* 66(Suppl.):526S–529S, 1997.

16. Institute of Medicine, Food and Nutrition Board. *Dietary Reference Intakes for Energy, Carbohydrate, Fiber, Fat, Protein and Amino Acids.* Washington, D.C.: National Academy Press, 2002.

17. Tippett, K. S., Mickle, S. J., Goldman, J. D., et al. Food and nutrient intake by individuals in the United States, 1 day 1989–1991. Nationwide Food Surveys Report No. 91–92, 1995.

18. Centers for Disease Control and Prevention. Recommendations to prevent and control iron deficiency in the United States. *MMWR Morb. Mortal. Wkly. Rep.* 47:1–29, 1998. Available online at www.cdc.gov/epo/mmwr/mmwr_mrr.html/ Accessed April 5, 2002.

19. Hingley, A. T. Preventing childhood poisoning. *FDA Consumer* 30:7–11, March 1996.

20. Wolraich, M. L., Wilson, D. B., and White, J. W. The effect of sugar on behavior or cognition in children: A meta analysis. *JAMA* 274:1617–1618, 1995.

21. Breakey, J. The role of diet and behavior in childhood. *J. Paediatr. Child Health* 33:190–194, 1997.

22. Farley, D. Dangers of lead still linger. *FDA Consumer* 32:16–21, January/February 1998.

23. Hammad, T. A., Sexton, M., and Langenberg, P. Relationship between blood lead and dietary iron intake in preschool children. *Annals Epidemiol.* 6:30–33, 1996.

24. Needleman, H. L., Reiss, J. A., Tobin, M. J., et al. Bone lead levels and delinquent behavior. *JAMA* 275:363–369, 1996.

25. Fackelmann, K. Hypertension's lead connection: Does low-level exposure to lead cause high blood pressure? *Sci. News* 149:382–383, 1996.

26. Update: blood lead levels—United States, 1991–1994. *MMWR, Morb. Mortal. Wkly. Rep.* 46:141–146, 1997.

27. U.S. Department of Agriculture. Nutrition Program Facts: National School Lunch Program: Qs and As on the National School Lunch Program. Available online at www.usda.gov/cnd/Lunch/default.htm Accessed August 1, 2002.

28. Gortmaker, S. I., Must, A., and Sobol, A. M. Television viewing as a cause for increasing obesity among children in the United States. *Arch. Pediatr. Adolesc. Med.* 150:356–360, 1996.

29. Sylvester, G. P., Achterberg, C., and Williams, J. Children's television and nutrition: friends or foes? *Nutrition Today* 30:6–15, February 1995.

30. Andersen, R. E., Crespo, C. J., Bartlett, S. J., et al. Relationship of physical activity and television watching with body weight and level of fatness among children: Results from the third National Health and Nutrition Examination Survey. *JAMA* 279:938–942, 1998.

31. Institute of Medicine, Food and Nutrition Board. *Dietary Reference Intakes for Calcium, Phosphorus, Magnesium, Vitamin D, and Fluoride.* Washington, D.C.: National Academy Press, 1997.

32. Mitchell, M. K. *Nutrition Across the Life Span*, Philadelphia: W. B. Saunders, 1997.

33. Slyper, A. H. Childhood obesity, adipose tissue distribution, and the pediatric practitioner. *Pediatrics* 102:e4, 1998.

34. USDA Agriculture Research Service. 1997 Results from USDA's 1994–1996 CSFII and 1994–1996 Diet and Health Knowledge Survey. ARS Food Surveys Research Group. Available online at www.bare.usda.gov/bhnrc/foodsurvey/home.htm Accessed July 23, 2002.

35. Institute of Medicine, Food and Nutrition Board. *Dietary Reference Intakes for Vitamin A, Vitamin K, Arsenic, Boron, Chromium, Copper, Iodine, Iron, Manganese, Molybdenum, Nickel, Silicon, Vanadium, and Zinc.* Washington, D.C.: National Academy Press, 2001.

36. Calvo, M. S., and Park, Y. K. Changing phosphorus content of the U.S. diet: Potential for adverse effect on bone. *J. Nutr.* 126:1168S–1180S, 1996.

37. Neumark-Sztainer, D., Story, M., Resnick, M. D., and Blum, R. W. Adolescent vegetarianism: A behavioral profile of a school-based population in Minnesota. *Arch. Pediatr. Adolesc. Med.* 151:833–838, 1997.

38. American Dietetic Association. Timely statement of the American Dietetic Association: nutrition guidance for adolescent athletes in organized sports. *J. Am. Diet. Assoc.* 96:611–612, 1996.

39. Terjung, R. L., Clarkson, P., Eichner, E. R., et al. American College of Sports Medicine roundtable: The physiological and health effects of oral creatine supplementation. *Med. Sci. Sports Exerc.* 32:706–717, 2000.

40. Beals, K. A., and Manore, M. M. Nutritional status of female athletes with subclinical eating disorders. *J. Am. Diet. Assoc.* 98:419–425, 1998.

41. Bazzarre, T. L. Nutrition and strength. In *Nutrition in Exercise and Sport*, 3rd ed. Wolinski, I., ed. Boca Raton, Fla.: CRC Press, 1998, 369–419.

42. Green,T. J., Houghton, L. A., Donovan,U., et al. Oral contraceptives did not affect biochemical folate indexes and homocysteine concentrations in adolescent females. *J. Am. Diet. Assoc.* 98:49–54, 1998.

43. Food and Nutrition Board, Institute of Medicine, *Dietary Reference Intakes for Thiamin, Riboflavin, Niacin, Vitamin B-6, Folate, Vitamin B-12, Pantothenic Acid, Biotin, and Choline.* Washington, D.C.: National Academy Press, 1998.

44. Wechsler H., Dowdall, G. W., Maenner, G., et al. Changes in binge drinking and related problems among American college students between 1993 and 1997. Results of the Harvard School of Public Health College Alcohol Study. *J. Am. Coll. Health* 47:57–68, 1998.

Chapter 16 Nutrition and Aging: The Adult Years

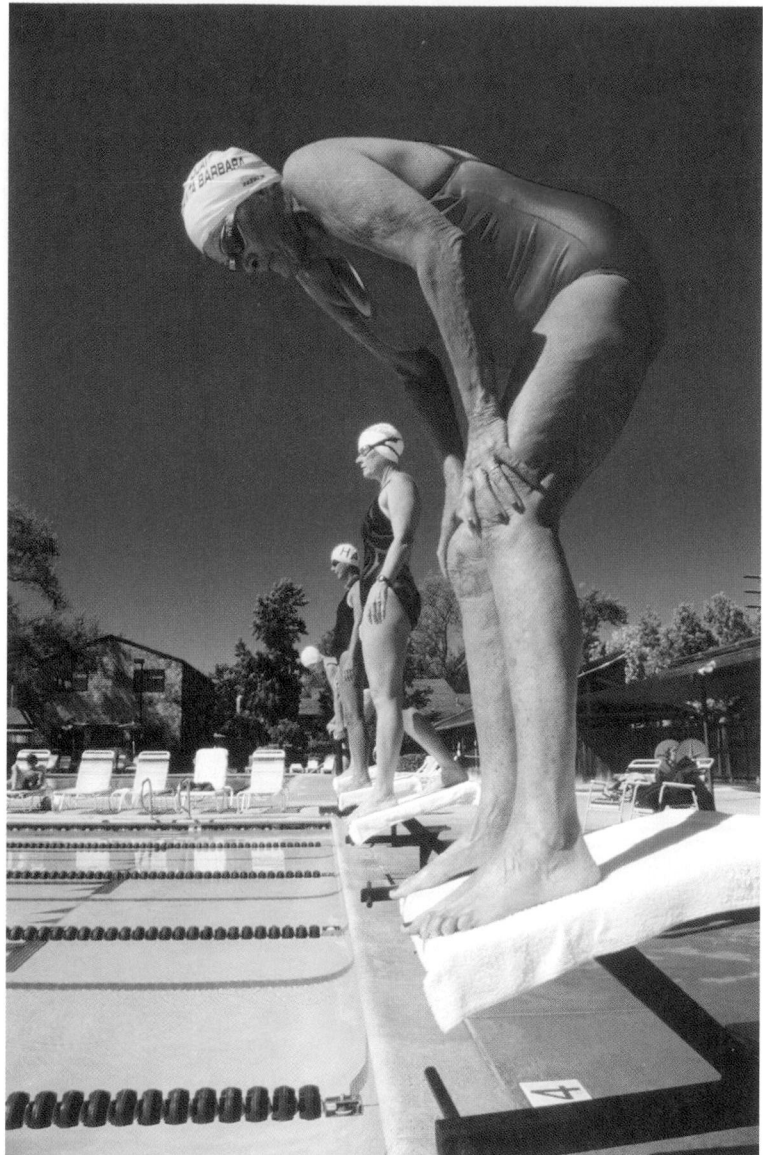

(© Joseph Sohm/ChromoSohm/Corbis Images)

Chapter Outline

WHAT IS AGING?
What Causes Aging?
How Long Can We Expect to Live
and Stay Healthy?

MALNUTRITION AND AGING

NUTRITION AND THE AGING PROCESS
Physiological Changes of Aging
Medical Consequences of Aging
Social and Economic Impact of Aging

NUTRITION FOR OLDER ADULTS
Can Nutrition Keep Us Young?
Nutrient Needs of Older Adults
Meeting the Nutrient Needs
of Older Adults

Chapter Concepts

✔ Aging is the accumulation of changes that occur over a lifetime.

✔ Americans are living longer than ever before; now the goal is to increase the number of healthy years.

✔ The risk of malnutrition increases with age.

✔ Many of the changes that occur with aging affect nutritional status.

✔ Aging increases the likelihood of disease and disability.

✔ Social and economic changes that occur with increasing age can also affect access to food and the risk of malnutrition.

✔ A healthy lifestyle can prevent or postpone some of the changes that occur with aging.

✔ Older adults need to consume nutrient-dense diets because their energy needs are decreased but their nutrient needs remain the same.

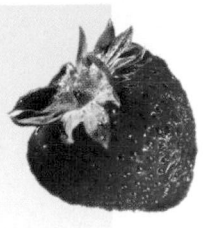

Just a Taste

Can consuming a healthy diet delay the changes that occur with aging?

Is malnutrition inevitable in the elderly?

Can antioxidant supplements slow aging?

We are all getting older in a society obsessed with youth. Youth symbolizes beauty, fitness, and health. Aging is symbolized by gray hair, wrinkled skin, weak bodies, and forgetful minds. Can the diet and lifestyle choices we make slow or prevent these changes?

When trying to stop the physiological clock, nutrition is not always the first place people turn. They cover gray hair with dyes and washes and soften and fade wrinkles with creams, cleansers, and plastic surgery. These methods result only in cosmetic changes that help people look younger. They do not help maintain vitality at a youthful level. On the other hand, a healthy lifestyle may not remove the crow's feet, but it can affect the health and vitality of one's later years.

Postponing the changes that occur with age is an important public health goal for the new millennium. Currently over 34 million Americans are over 65 years of age. It is estimated that this number will increase to about 70 million by the year 2030. Because the incidence of disease and disability increases with increasing age, this older population accounts for a large part of the public health budget. Thus, keeping older adults healthy is beneficial not only for those individuals but for the national health-care system as well.[1]

• WHAT IS AGING?

Biologically, aging is not something that begins at age 55, 65, or 75; it is a process that begins with conception and continues throughout life (Figure 16.1). It can be defined as the inevitable accumulation of changes with time that are associated with and responsible for an ever-increasing susceptibility to disease and death. When do we become "old"? Often the definition of "old" depends on who is defining the term. To a 5-year-old, anyone over age 15 seems old, but to a healthy 80-year-old, "old" may mean 90. Chronological age is not always the best indicator of health. A person who is chronologically 75 may have the vigor and health of someone only 55, or vice versa. There are 70-year-olds riding bicycles and others in wheelchairs; some are healthy, independent, and active, while others are chronically ill, dependent, and at high risk for malnutrition. Although universal to all living things, aging is a process we don't fully understand. We do know that our genetic makeup and the environment and lifestyle in which we spend our years affect how long we live and how long we remain healthy.

What Causes Aging?

As organisms become older, the number of cells they contain decreases and the function of the remaining cells declines. As tissues and organs lose cells, the ability of the organism to perform the physiological functions necessary to maintain homeostasis decreases; disease becomes increasingly common and the risk of malnutrition increases. This loss of cells and cell function occurs throughout life, but the effects

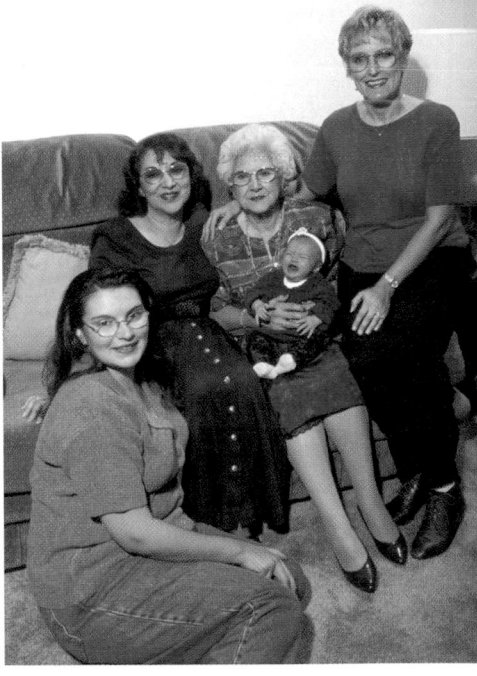

Figure 16.1
Aging is a process that occurs continuously in individuals of all ages. (© Tony Freeman/PhotoEdit)

459

Reserve capacity The amount of functional capacity that an organ has above and beyond what is needed to sustain life.

are not felt for many years because humans and other organisms begin life with extra functional capacity, or **reserve capacity**. Reserve capacity allows an organism to continue functioning normally despite a decrease in the number and function of cells. In young adults, the reserve capacity of organs is four to ten times that required to sustain life. As a person ages and reserve capacity decreases, the effects of aging become evident in all body systems.

There are two major hypotheses to explain why aging occurs. One favors the idea of a genetic clock and argues that the cell death associated with aging is a genetically programmed event. The other views the events of aging as the result of cellular wear and tear. The actual cause of the cell death associated with aging is probably some combination of both of these, and the rate at which cell death occurs and at which aging proceeds is determined by the interplay among genetics, environment, and lifestyle.

Programmed Cell Death One hypothesis about aging proposes that cell death is triggered when genes that disrupt cell function are activated.[2] This causes the selective, orderly death of individual cells or groups of cells and is referred to as **programmed cell death**. This hypothesis is supported by the fact that cells grown in the laboratory divide only a certain number of times before they die. Cells from older individuals will divide fewer times than those from younger individuals, and those from longer-lived species will divide more times than those from shorter-lived species. If cells in an organism stop reproducing and continue to die, the total number of cells will decline, resulting in a loss of organ function.

Programmed cell death The death of cells at specific predictable times.

Wear and Tear Another hypothesis suggests that aging is the result of an accumulation of cellular damage. This wear and tear may result from errors in DNA synthesis, increases in glucose levels, or damage caused by free radicals. Free radicals are reactive chemical substances that are generated from both normal metabolic processes and exposure to environmental factors. They cause oxidative damage to proteins, lipids, carbohydrates, and DNA, and may also indirectly harm cells by producing toxic products. For example, age spots—brown spots that appear on the skin with age—are caused by the oxidation of lipids, which produces a pigment called lipofuscin, or age pigment. The damage done to cells by free radicals is associated with aging and has been implicated in the development of a number of chronic diseases common among the aging, including cardiovascular disease and cancer.

Genetics, Environment, and Lifestyle The rate at which the changes associated with aging accumulate depends on genetics, environment, and lifestyle. Genes determine the efficiency with which cells are maintained and repaired. Individuals with less cellular repair capacity will lose cells and consequently age more quickly. Likewise, genes determine susceptibility to age-related diseases such as cardiovascular disease and cancer. However, individuals who inherit a low capacity to repair cellular damage may live long lives if they live in an environment with few factors that damage cells and if they eat well and exercise regularly. In contrast, individuals with exceptional cellular repair ability may accumulate cell damage rapidly if they smoke cigarettes, consume a diet high in fat and low in antioxidant nutrients, and live sedentary lives. No matter what individuals' genes predict about how long they will live, their actual **longevity** is also affected by lifestyle factors and the extent to which they are able to avoid accidents and disease (Figure 16.2).

Longevity The duration of an individual's life.

How Long Can We Expect to Live and Stay Healthy?

The maximum age to which any human can live—the **life span**—is about 100 to 120 years. Most individuals do not live that long. **Life expectancy**, the average length of time that a person can be expected to live, varies between and within populations. It

Life span The maximum age to which members of a species can live.
Life expectancy The average length of life for a population of individuals.

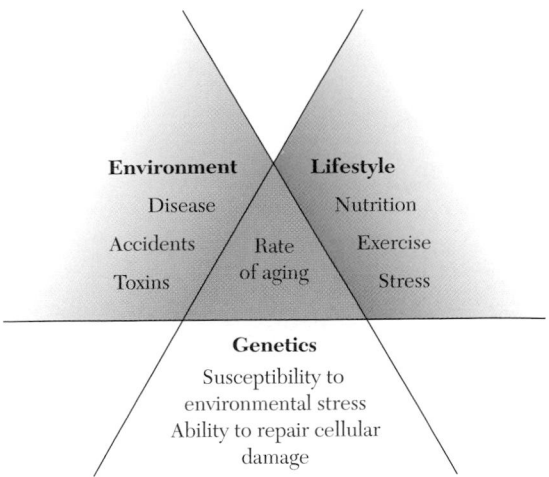

Figure 16.2

The rate at which individuals age is affected by their genetic makeup, the environment in which they live, and the lifestyle choices they make.

is affected by genetics, lifestyle, and environmental factors. In the United States in 1900, life expectancy was 50 years, but today, with advances in technology and improved nutrition and health care, the average is over 76 years.[3] Currently, 13% of the population is over 65 years of age and the number is increasing (Figure 16.3).

Even though average life expectancy in the United States has increased to over 76 years, the average healthy life span is only about 64 years. The last 12 years of life are often restricted by disease and disability, which become more and more common with advancing age.[5] The goal of successful aging is to increase not only life expectancy but the number of years of healthy life that an individual can expect. This is achieved by slowing the changes that accumulate over time and postponing the diseases of aging long enough to approach or reach the limits of life span before any symptoms appear. This is referred to as **compression of morbidity**. When applied to the population as a whole, this term means that people are healthier and living longer (Figure 16.4); applied to the individual, it means staying healthy until the limits of life span are reached. The fastest-growing segment of the population in industrialized nations is the individuals over the age of 85.[4] Keeping these individuals healthy by compression of morbidity benefits not only aging individuals but also the family members who must find the time and resources to care for them and the public health programs that attempt to meet their needs.

ON THE WEB

For public health data and statistical information on older adults, go to the National Center for Health Statistics at www.cdc.gov/nchs/.

Compression of morbidity The postponement of the onset of chronic disease such that disability occupies a smaller and smaller proportion of the life span.

• MALNUTRITION AND AGING

Aging increases the risk of malnutrition. Although the aging process itself is usually not a cause of malnutrition in healthy active adults, nutritional health can be compromised by conditions that become increasingly common with advancing age[6]

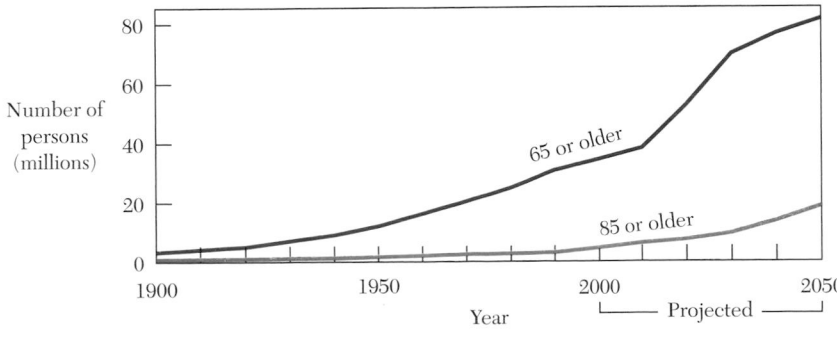

Figure 16.3

This graph illustrates the increase in the total number of persons age 65 and older and 85 and older. Data through 2050 are based on projections of the population and indicate that in the next few decades there will be almost 80 million people in the United States who are 65 or older. (*U.S. Census Bureau, Decennial Census Data and Population Projections.* Available online at www.agingstats.gov)

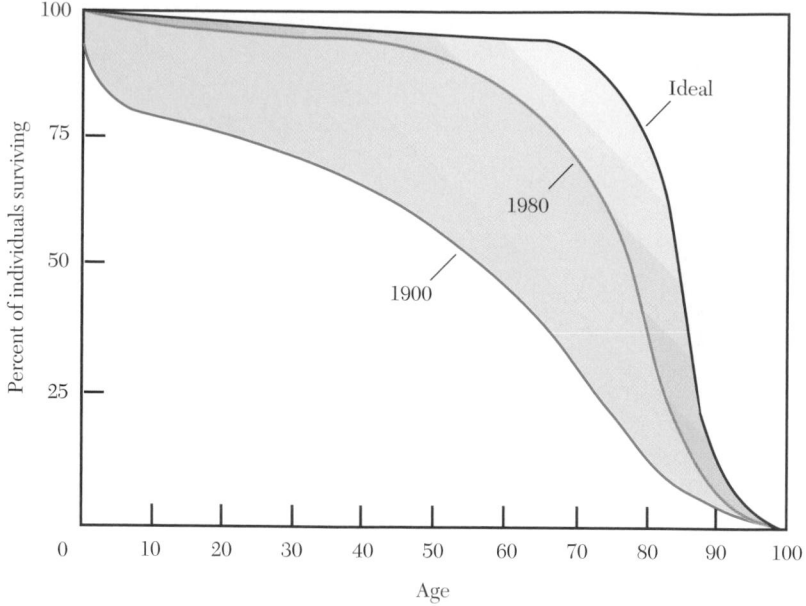

Figure 16.4
This graph illustrates the effect of compression of morbidity on survival in a population. The decline in deaths from infectious diseases between 1900 and 1980 allowed more people to survive into adulthood. Delaying the onset of chronic diseases will allow more people to remain healthy and survive into their seventies and eighties. (Adapted from Fries, J. F. Aging, natural death, and the compression of morbidity. *N. Engl. J. Med.* 303:130–135, 1980.)

Food insecurity An inability to acquire appropriate foods in a socially acceptable way.

(see Table 16.1). Any circumstance, whether physical, psychological, emotional, social, or economic, that interferes with the availability of or the ability to acquire desirable foods in socially acceptable ways can lead to **food insecurity**, and, subsequently, malnutrition. It is estimated that from 2.5 to 4.9 million older Americans experience food insecurity in any given six-month period.[7]

To address concerns over the nutritional health of the elderly, the federal Nutrition Screening Initiative was developed to promote screening for and intervention in nutrition-related problems in older adults.[8] This program is working to increase the awareness of nutritional problems in the elderly by involving practitioners and community organizations as well as relatives, friends, and others caring for the elderly in

Table 16.1 *Factors That Increase the Risk of Malnutrition Among the Elderly*

Reduced food intake due to:

Decreased appetite due to lack of exercise, depression, or social isolation

Changes in taste, smell, and vision

Dental problems

Limitations in mobility

Medications that restrict meal times or affect appetite

Lack of money to buy food

Lack of nutrition knowledge

Reduced nutrient absorption and utilization due to:

Gastrointestinal changes

Medications that affect absorption

Diseases such as diabetes, kidney disease, alcoholism, and gastrointestinal disease

Increased requirements due to:

Illness with fever or infection

Injury or surgery

Increased losses due to:

Medications that increase excretion of nutrients

Diseases such as gastrointestinal and kidney disease

Table 16.2   *DETERMINE: A Checklist of the Warning Signs of Malnutrition*

Disease	Any disease, illness, or condition that causes changes in eating can predispose one to malnutrition. Memory loss and depression can also interfere with nutrition if they affect food intake.
Eating poorly	Eating either too little or too much can lead to poor health.
Tooth loss/mouth pain	A healthy mouth, teeth, and gums are needed to eat.
Economic hardship	Having to or choosing to spend less than $25–$30 per person per week on food interferes with nutrition.
Reduced social support	Being with people on a daily basis has a positive effect on morale, well-being, and eating.
Multiple medicines	The more medicines one takes, the greater the chances of side effects such as weakness, drowsiness, diarrhea, changes in taste and appetite, nausea, and constipation.
Involuntary weight loss/gain	Unintentionally losing or gaining weight is a warning sign that should not be ignored. Being overweight or underweight also increases the risk of malnutrition.
Needs assistance in self-care	Difficulty walking, shopping, and cooking increases the risk of malnutrition.
Elder above age 80	The risks of frailty and health problems increase with increasing age.

evaluating the nutritional status of the aging population. This program developed the DETERMINE checklist (see Table 16.2) based on an acronym for the physiological, medical, and socio-economic situations that increase the risk of malnutrition among the elderly. The elderly themselves, family members, and caregivers can use this tool to identify when malnutrition is a potential problem.

• NUTRITION AND THE AGING PROCESS

The physiological changes that occur with age can affect nutritional status. These changes also increase the frequency of disease and the need to take medications, both of which can affect nutritional status. Likewise, there are social and economic changes that are common in aging and that increase the risk of food insecurity and, consequently, malnutrition (Figure 16.5).

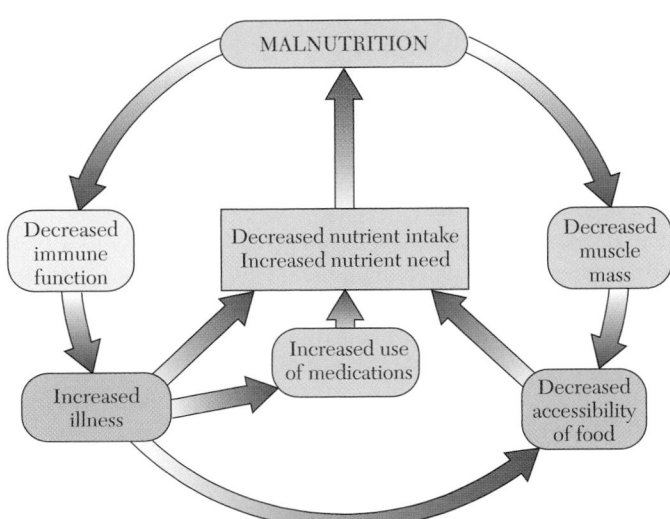

Figure 16.5
The causes and consequences of malnutrition are linked.

Physiological Changes of Aging

It is difficult to determine which of the changes that occur with aging are inevitable consequences of the aging process and which are the effect of disease states. But whether caused by disease or the inescapable loss of cells and cell function, the changes that occur in organs and organ systems can affect nutritional status by altering the appeal of food, digestion and absorption, nutritional requirements, and the ability to obtain food.

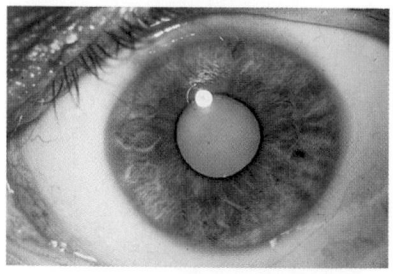

Figure 16.6
Cataracts cause the lens of the eye to become cloudy and impair vision. (© Science VU/Visuals Unlimited)

Sensory Changes Beginning around age 60, there is a progressive decline in the ability to taste and smell, which becomes more severe in persons over 70. The decline of these senses can contribute to impaired nutritional status by decreasing the appeal and enjoyment of food.[9] Some studies suggest that the decline in taste acuity is due to a reduction in the number of taste buds on the tongue; others suggest that it is the result of changes in sensitivity to specific flavors such as salty and sweet.[10] The sense of smell is important because odors provide important clues to food acceptability before food enters the mouth. Once in the mouth some molecules reach the nasal cavity where their odor is detected. It is the blending of the odor message from the nasal cavity and the taste message from the tongue that provides the overall food flavor. When the sense of smell is diminished, food is not as flavorful. Changes in taste and smell have been related to a greater intake of sweet foods among older adults.[10]

Vision also typically declines with age, making shopping for and preparation of food difficult. **Macular degeneration** is the most common cause of blindness in older Americans. The macula is a small area of the retina of the eye that distinguishes fine detail. With age, oxidative damage reduces the number of viable cells in the macula. As the macula degenerates, visual acuity declines, ultimately resulting in blindness. **Cataracts** are another common reason for declining sight. Of people who live to age 85, half will have cataracts that impair vision (Figure 16.6). Oxidative damage is believed to cause both macular degeneration and cataracts. Therefore, a diet high in foods containing antioxidant nutrients might slow or prevent these eye disorders.[11]

Macular degeneration Degeneration of a portion of the retina that results in a loss of visual detail and blindness.

Cataracts A disease of the eye that results in cloudy spots on the lens (and sometimes the cornea), which obscure vision.

Gastrointestinal Changes Aging causes changes in the gastrointestinal tract and its accessory organs that may alter the palatability as well as the digestion of food and the absorption of nutrients. One change is a decrease in the secretion of saliva into the mouth. Saliva mixes with food to allow it to be tasted and to provide lubrication for easy swallowing. A decrease in saliva causes dryness which decreases the taste of food and makes swallowing difficult. Saliva is also an important defense against tooth decay because it helps wash material away from the teeth and contains substances that kill bacteria. Thus a dry mouth increases the likelihood of tooth decay and **periodontal disease**. Loss of teeth and improperly fitting dentures also limit food choices and can contribute to poor nutrition in the elderly.

Periodontal disease A degeneration of the area surrounding the teeth, specifically the gum and supporting bone.

Aging may delay stomach emptying and cause changes in gastric secretions. Delayed stomach emptying can reduce hunger and, therefore, nutrient intake.[10] Reduced gastric secretions can affect the absorption of some nutrients. It is estimated that 10 to 30% of American adults over age 50 and 40% of those into their 80s have **atrophic gastritis**, an inflammation of the stomach lining accompanied by a decrease in the secretion of stomach acid.[12,13] When stomach acid is reduced, the enzymes that release vitamin B_{12} from food do not function properly and vitamin B_{12} in food cannot be absorbed. Absorption of iron, folate, calcium, and vitamin K may also be reduced.[13] Reduced stomach acid secretion also allows microbial overgrowth in the stomach and small intestine.[12,14] The increased populations of microbes in the gut further reduce B_{12} absorption by competing for available vitamin B_{12}.

Atrophic gastritis An inflammation of the stomach lining that causes a reduction in stomach acid and allows bacterial overgrowth.

With age there is also a reduction in digestive enzymes from the pancreas and small intestine, but there is enough reserve capacity that digestion and absorption are rarely significantly impaired. In the colon there are functional changes, including decreased motility and elasticity, weakened abdominal and pelvic muscles, and decreased sensory perception, which can lead to constipation. Low fiber and fluid intakes and lack of activity also contribute to constipation. Although constipation occurs in about the same frequency in all age groups,[15] it is estimated that 20 to 30% of individuals over age 65 are dependent on laxatives.[16] Maintaining regular exercise and consuming adequate fluid and fiber are safer ways to prevent constipation.

Age-related changes in other organs may affect nutrient metabolism. Most absorbed nutrients travel from the intestine to the liver for metabolism or storage. The liver has a greater regenerative capacity than most organs, but with age, there is a decrease in liver size and blood flow and an increase in fat accumulation, which eventually decrease the liver's ability to metabolize nutrients and break down drugs and alcohol. With age, the pancreas may become less responsive to blood glucose levels, and the body cells may become more resistant to insulin, resulting in diabetes. Changes in the heart and blood vessels reduce blood flow to the kidneys, making waste removal less efficient. The kidneys themselves become smaller and their ability to filter blood and to excrete the products of protein breakdown declines.[17] In some individuals blood urea levels may increase if protein intake is too high. The kidney's ability to concentrate urine also decreases with age, as does the sensation of thirst, increasing the risk of dehydration.

Changes in Body Composition and Weight Many people gain weight in their twenties, thirties, and forties, but after age 65, it is more common for people to lose weight. In addition to changes in body weight, aging is accompanied by an increase in body fat, especially in the abdomen, and a decrease in lean tissue, including a loss of muscle mass and strength and a decrease in bone mass (Figure 16.7).[18] Increases in body fat increase the risk of chronic disease, but the risks associated with excess body fat are lower for older adults than for younger ones.[19] The decline in muscle size and strength affects both the skeletal muscles needed to move the body and the heart and respiratory muscles needed to deliver oxygen to the tissues. Therefore, both strength and endurance are decreased, making the tasks of day-to-day life more difficult. The changes in muscle strength contribute not only to physical frailty, which is characterized by general weakness, impaired mobility and balance, and poor endurance, but also to the risk of falls and fractures. Loss of bone mass also increases the risk of fractures. In the oldest old, loss of muscle strength becomes the limiting factor determining whether they can continue to live independently. Some of the reduction in muscle strength and mass is due to changes in hormone levels

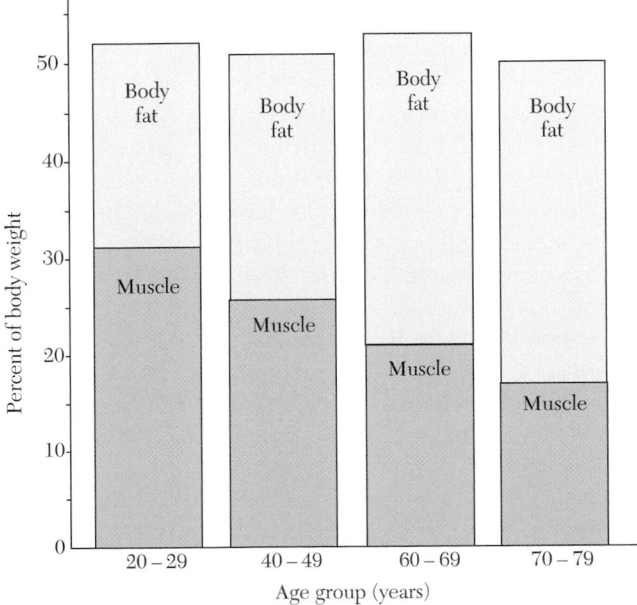

Figure 16.7

In most individuals, the proportion of muscle mass decreases and body fat increases with age. (Adapted from Cohen, S. H., et al. Compartmental body composition based on the body nitrogen, potassium, and calcium. *Am. J. Physiol.* 239:192–200, 1980.)

Figure 16.8

Magnetic resonance image of a thigh cross section from a 25-year-old man (*left*) and a 65-year-old man (*right*). The thighs are of similar size, but the thigh from the older man has a greater amount of fat (shown in white) around and through the muscle, indicating significant muscle loss. (S. A. Jubrias and K. E. Conley, University of Washington Medical Center)

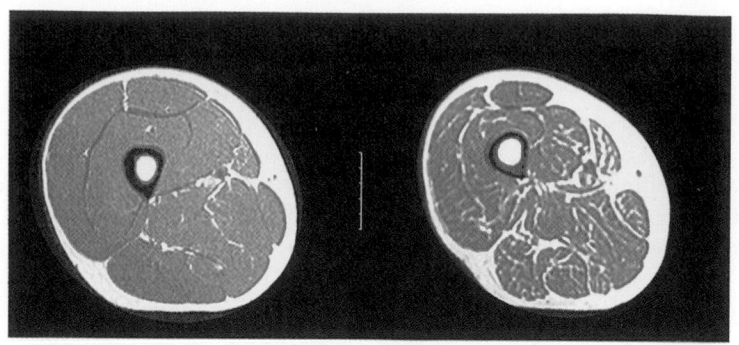

and in muscle protein synthesis, but a lack of exercise is also an important contributor (Figure 16.8).[20] Regular exercise can help maintain muscle mass, bone strength, and cardiorespiratory function and can increase energy needs.[21]

Stable body weight is a sign of good health. Extreme thinness or unintentional weight loss is a health risk, especially among older adults.[22] Although laboratory studies in animals have found that a diet deficient in energy can slow aging and extend life span,[23] this effect has not been demonstrated in humans.

Hormonal Changes Declining levels of some hormones are hypothesized to play a role in the aging process. Hormonal changes related to age can affect the ability to regulate blood glucose levels, body water, and body temperature and can cause changes in body composition. One of the most common hormone-related changes that occurs with aging is elevated blood glucose. This is due to both a decrease in the amount of insulin released by the pancreas and a decrease in insulin sensitivity at the tissues. This decreased insulin sensitivity is related to poor diet, inactivity, increased abdominal fat mass, and decreased lean mass. About 40% of individuals between the ages of 65 and 74 and 50% of those over 80 have diabetes, and about half of these cases are undiagnosed.[18] Another common hormonal change that occurs with age is a decline in levels of thyroid hormones. Changes in thyroid function are generally treated by administering hormones.

Many of the other hormonal changes, including decreases in growth hormone, DHEA (dehydroepiandosterone), melatonin, estrogen, and testosterone, are considered part of the normal physiology of aging. Some of these hormonal changes are partially responsible for the changes in body composition discussed above.

Growth hormone stimulates growth and protein synthesis; its levels gradually decline with age in both men and women and may be responsible for some of the decrease in lean body mass. Controlled studies, however, do not support a benefit to growth hormone replacement. When compared to a program of regular exercise, growth hormone injections did not produce any greater increases in muscle size or strength.[24] In addition, growth hormone administration has side effects including edema, carpal tunnel syndrome, and decreases in insulin sensitivity.

DHEA is a precursor to sex hormones such as testosterone, estrogen, and progesterone. Even though low levels of this hormone are not known to be the cause of age-associated disorders, DHEA supplements are available over-the-counter and promise to strengthen bones, muscles, and the immune system, and to prevent diabetes, obesity, heart disease, and cancer. Although some of these effects have been demonstrated when DHEA is administered to animals, beneficial effects of DHEA supplementation in humans have not been clearly established.[25] In addition, it is not clear whether the increases in sex hormones that may occur with DHEA administration create a risk of developing ovarian, prostate, or other types of cancer.[18]

Melatonin is a hormone that is secreted by the pineal gland. It is involved in regulating the body's cycles of sleep and wakefulness. A decline in melatonin is hypothesized to influence aging by affecting body rhythms and triggering genetically programmed aging at a cellular level.[26] Melatonin is also an antioxidant and may enhance immune function. It is available as a dietary supplement, but its effect on aging in humans has not been determined.

The most striking and rapidly occurring age-related hormonal change is **menopause**. Menopause normally occurs in women around the age of 50. During menopause, the cyclical release of the female hormones estrogen and progesterone slows and eventually stops, causing ovulation and menstruation to cease. The period of decline in estrogen is accompanied by changes in mood, skin, and body composition (an increase in body fat and a decrease in lean tissue). The reduction in estrogen decreases the risk of breast cancer but increases the risk of heart disease to a level more similar to that in men. Reduced estrogen also increases the risk of osteoporosis by increasing the rate of bone breakdown and decreasing calcium absorption from the intestine.

Menopause does not occur in men, but with age men do experience a gradual decrease in testosterone levels, which may contribute to the decrease in muscle mass and strength.

Menopause Physiological changes that mark the end of a woman's capacity to bear children.

Changes in Immune Function The ability of the immune system to fight disease declines with age. As it does, the incidence of infections, cancers, and autoimmune diseases increases, and the effectiveness of immunizations declines. Some of the decrease in immune function may be due to nutritional deficiencies. In turn, the increases in infections and chronic disease that occur can affect nutritional status.

The immune response depends on the ability of cells to differentiate, divide rapidly, and secrete immune factors, so nutrients that are involved in cell differentiation, division, and protein synthesis can influence the immune response. Supplements of β-carotene and several micronutrients, including zinc, vitamin E, and vitamin B_6, have been shown to improve immune response in both healthy and diseased elderly.[27,28] However, these individuals may have been deficient in these prior to supplementation.[27,28] High doses of some nutrients, including zinc, copper, and iron, depress immune function, so supplements should be taken with care.

Medical Consequences of Aging

With age there is an increase in the incidence of both acute and chronic illness. The reduction in reserve capacity and decline in immune function make infectious disease more frequent and more serious in the elderly. In addition, most older adults have at least one chronic medical condition.[1] The incidence of cardiovascular disease, diabetes, osteoporosis, hypertension, cancer, arthritis, and Alzheimer's disease all increase with age. Some of these diseases change nutrient requirements, some decrease the appeal of food, and some impair the ability to obtain and prepare an adequate diet by affecting mobility and mental status. All of these can cause food insecurity.

Conditions That Decrease Mobility More than half of the older population suffers from some form of physical disability, and the incidence increases with increasing age. Over 4.4 million older adults have difficulty carrying out the activities of daily life, including shopping, eating, and getting around the house.[1] These limitations affect the ability to maintain good nutritional health. Arthritis, a condition that causes pain upon movement, is the most common cause of disability in older individuals (see *Off the Shelf*: Arthritis Remedies). Osteoporosis and its associated fractures can also affect mobility. Some of the decrease in mobility that is due to disease and normal aging can be prevented by a healthy diet and lifestyle.

Conditions That Affect Mental Status Altered mental status can affect nutrition. Although many individuals maintain adequate nervous system function into old age, the incidence of dementia increases with age. **Dementia** refers to an impairment in memory, thinking, and/or judgment that is severe enough to cause personality changes and affect daily activities and relationships with others. Causes of dementia include multiple strokes, alcoholism, and Alzheimer's disease. Vitamin B_{12} status

Dementia A deterioration of mental state resulting in impaired memory, thinking, and/or judgment.

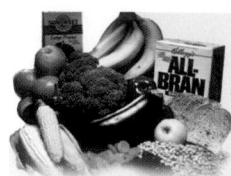

Off the Shelf
Arthritis Remedies

Osteoarthritis is a disease that affects over 33 million Americans.[1] It occurs when the connective tissue that prevents the bones in joints from rubbing together degenerates over time, causing pain. The goal for treatment is to control pain and slow or reverse the progression of the disease. Traditionally, arthritis has been treated with drugs that reduce inflammation, such as aspirin and ibuprofen, and with pain relievers such as acetaminophen. These drugs can reduce pain and inflammation but do not repair the tissue. They also have side effects if taken over long periods of time. Over the years, many alternative treatments—ranging from copper bracelets to special diets and dietary supplements—have been promoted, but none of these have been beneficial. Recently, however, the availability of supplements containing glucosamine and chondroitin sulfate has offered a new alternative for arthritis sufferers.

Glucosamine and chondroitin sulfate are not essential nutrients. They are molecules found in and around the cells of cartilage, the type of connective tissue that cushions our joints. They are made in the body and consumed in the diet in meat. In the body, glucosamine and chondroitin sulfate are needed for the synthesis of large molecules that bind water to form a porous, gel-like material that allows cartilage to resist crushing forces and cushion

the joints. It has been suggested that when consumed in the diet, glucosamine and chondroitin sulfate provide the raw materials needed to synthesize these large cushioning molecules. Glucosamine may also inhibit inflammation and increase the production of a compound that contributes to the lubricating and shock-absorbing properties of cartilage. Supplements of both glucosamine and chondroitin sulfate are said to reduce arthritis pain, stop cartilage degeneration, and possibly stimulate the repair of damaged joint cartilage.

Much of the research that has been done to test the effectiveness of these supplements indicates that they are safe and beneficial, but how beneficial is unclear. Some studies found large improvements while others found that the supplements had only small effects. The variation in effect is even more striking between individuals. Some people experienced more relief when taking glucosamine or chondroitin sulfate than they did with anti-inflammatory drugs, while others found that these supplements provided no benefits at all. A study that integrated results from many different trials concluded that these supplements had moderate to large effects on the symptoms of osteoarthritis.[2] The benefits occurred after the supplements had been taken for approximately 4 to 6 weeks and were sustained for 4 to 8 weeks after the supplements were discontinued.[3] Cur-

rently, the National Institutes of Health (NIH) is conducting a large trial in centers across the country to evaluate the effects of glucosamine and chondroitin sulfate, given separately and in combination, for reducing pain and improving function in patients with osteoarthritis of the knee.[4]

Should you try these to relieve your sore joints? The risks are low, and the benefits observed thus far make these supplements a promising treatment for an age-old disease. However, until these compounds are fully tested, the Arthritis Foundation and the American College of Rheumatology are urging patients with osteoarthritis to continue proven treatments and disease-management techniques and to inform their physicians if they are considering using these supplements.

[1]National Center for Health Statistics, Fast Stats A to Z, Arthritis. Available online at www.cdc.gov/nchs/fastats/arthrits.htm/ Accessed May 9, 2002.

[2]McAlindon, T. E., LaValley, M. P., Gulin, J. P., and Felson, D. T. Glucosamine and chondroitin for treatment of osteoarthritis: A systematic quality assessment and meta-analysis. *JAMA* 283:1469–1475, 2000.

[3]Hochberg, M. C., and Dougados, M. Pharmacological therapy of osteoarthritis. *Best Pract, Res. Clin. Rheumatol.* 15:583–593, 2001.

[4]Brief, A. A., Maurer, S. G., and Di Cesare, P. E. Use of glucosamine and chondroitin sulfate in the management of osteoarthritis. *J. Am. Acad. Orthop. Surg.* 9:71–78, 2001.

---

may also affect mental function in the elderly. With aging there is a decrease in blood vitamin B_{12} levels and a rise in metabolites indicative of poor B_{12} status. In most cases, vitamin B_{12} supplements do not improve neurological function; however, in some elderly patients with mild dementia and low blood levels of vitamin B_{12}, supplementation improved mental function.[29]

Over half of the cases of dementia in the elderly are due to **Alzheimer's disease**, a progressive, incurable loss of mental function. The brains of patients with Alzheimer's disease are characterized by the accumulation of an abnormal protein and a loss of certain types of nerve cells.[30] Its cause is unknown, but there does appear to be a genetic component in some cases. Many ineffective nutritional cures have been marketed for Alzheimer's disease. Supplements of choline and lecithin have been promoted to increase levels of the neurotransmitter acetylcholine, which is deficient in Alzheimer's patients. Antioxidant supplements have been suggested to prevent free radical damage. And when high aluminum levels were discovered in the brains of Alzheimer's patients, many people tried to reduce exposure by restricting the use of aluminum cookware and aluminum-containing deodorants. To date, neither nutritional supplements nor aluminum restriction has proved helpful in treating or preventing Alzheimer's disease.

Alzheimer's disease A disease that results in the relentless and irreversible loss of mental function.

Increased Use of Prescription and Over-the-Counter Medications Because health problems increase with increasing age, older adults are likely to take medications. Almost half of older Americans take multiple medications daily.[31] The use of prescription and over-the-counter medications can affect nutritional status. The more medications taken, the greater the chance of side effects such as increased or decreased appetite, changes in taste, constipation, weakness, drowsiness, diarrhea, and nausea. Illness related to incorrect doses or inappropriate combinations of medications is a significant health problem in the elderly (Figure 16.9). Both the effects of drugs on nutritional status and the effects of nutritional status on the effectiveness of the drugs must be considered.

Medications Can Affect Nutritional Status Medications can affect nutrition by altering appetite, nutrient absorption, metabolism, or excretion (Table 16.3). They have the greatest impact on individuals who must take medications for extended periods, those who take multiple medications, and those who already have marginal nutritional status.

Some medications directly affect the gastrointestinal tract. More than 250 drugs, including blood pressure medications, antidepressants, decongestants, and the pain reliever ibuprofen (found in Advil, Motrin, and Nuprin), can cause mouth dryness, which can decrease interest in eating by interfering with taste, chewing, and swallowing. Aspirin is a stomach irritant and can cause small amounts of painless bleeding in the gastrointestinal tract, resulting in iron loss. Digoxin, which is a heart

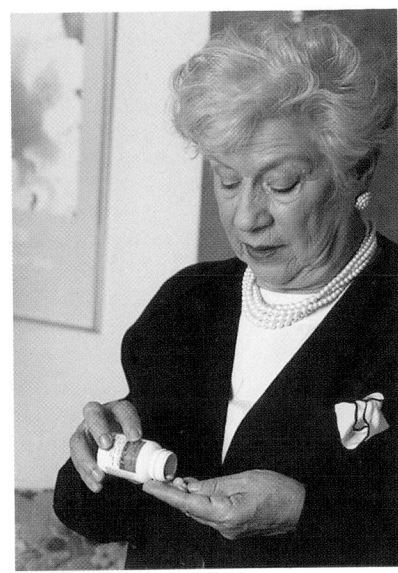

Figure 16.9

Many older adults take one or more medications every day. (© Michael Newman/PhotoEdit)

Table 16.3 *Commonly Used Drugs That May Cause Nutritional Deficiencies*

Drug Group	Drug	Potential Deficiency
Antacids	Sodium bicarbonate	Folate, phosphorus, calcium, copper
	Aluminum hydroxide	Phosphorus
Anticonvulsants	Phenytoin, phenobarbital, primidone	Vitamins D and K
	Valproic acid	Carnitine
Antibiotics	Tetracycline	Calcium
	Gentamicin	Potassium, magnesium
Antibacterial agents	Neomycin	Fat, nitrogen
	Boric acid	Riboflavin
	Trimethoprim	Folate
	Isoniazid	Vitamins B_6, D, and niacin
Anti-inflammatory agents	Sulfasalazine	Folate
	Prednisone	Calcium
	Aspirin	Vitamin C, folate, iron
Anticancer drugs	Colchine	Fat, vitamin B_{12}
	Methotrexate	Folate, calcium
Anticoagulant drugs	Warfarin	Vitamin K
Antihypertensive drugs	Hydralazine	Vitamin B_6
Diuretics	Thiazides	Potassium
	Furosemide	Potassium, calcium, magnesium
Hypocholesterolemic agents	Cholestyramine	Fat, fat-soluble vitamins, iron, folate, vitamin B_{12}
Laxatives	Mineral oil	Fat-soluble vitamins
	Phenolphthalein	Potassium, calcium
	Senna	Fat, calcium, vitamin B_6, folate, vitamin C
Tranquilizers	Chlorpromazine	Riboflavin

Adapted from Roe, D. A. *Diet and Drug Interactions*, New York: Van Nostrand Reinhold, 1989.

stimulant, can cause gastrointestinal upset, loss of appetite, and nausea. Narcotic pain medications such as codeine can lead to constipation, nausea, and vomiting.

Other drugs can decrease nutrient absorption. Cholestyramine (Questran), which is used to reduce blood cholesterol, can decrease the absorption of fat-soluble vitamins, vitamin B_{12}, iron, and folate. Antacids that contain aluminum or magnesium hydroxide (Rolaids or Maalox) combine with phosphorus in the gut to form compounds that cannot be absorbed; chronic use can result in loss of phosphorus from bone and possibly accelerate osteoporosis. Repeated use of stimulant laxatives can deplete calcium and potassium. Mineral oil laxatives prevent the absorption of fat-soluble vitamins. If it is not possible to prevent constipation by consuming a diet high in fiber and fluid, bulk-forming laxatives are a safer choice.

The metabolism of drugs can also affect nutritional status. For example, anticonvulsive drugs (used to prevent seizures) increase the liver's capacity to metabolize and eliminate vitamin D, therefore increasing the need for vitamin D.

Some drugs affect nutrient excretion. Diuretics, which are used to treat hypertension and edema, cause water loss, but some types (thiazides) also increase the excretion of potassium. People taking thiazide diuretics are advised to include several good sources of potassium in their diet each day or are prescribed supplements.

Food and Nutritional Status and Effectiveness of Medications Food components can either enhance or retard the absorption and metabolism of drugs. Some drugs, such as the pain medication Darvon, are absorbed better or faster if taken with food. Other drugs, such as aspirin and ibuprofen, should be taken with food because they are irritating to the gastrointestinal tract. Since food can delay how quickly drugs leave the stomach, some are best taken with just water. Other drugs interact with specific foods. For instance, the antibiotic tetracycline should not be taken with milk because it binds with calcium, making both unavailable.

Nutritional status can also affect drug metabolism. If nutritional status is poor, the body's ability to detoxify drugs may be altered. For example, in a malnourished individual, theophylline, used to treat asthma, is metabolized slowly, resulting in high blood levels of the drug, which can cause loss of appetite, nausea, and vomiting.

Specific nutrients can also affect the metabolism of drugs. High-protein diets enhance drug metabolism in general, and low-protein diets slow it. Vitamin K hinders the action of anticoagulants, taken to reduce the risk of blood clots. On the other hand, omega-3 fatty acids, such as those in fish oils, inhibit blood clotting and may intensify the effect of an anticoagulant drug and cause bleeding. It is safe to eat fish while taking anticoagulant drugs; however, the use of fish oil supplements is not recommended. Drugs can also interact with each other. For example, alcohol affects the metabolism of over a hundred medications. Drug interactions can exaggerate or, in some cases, diminish the effect of a medication. Individuals taking any medication should consult their doctor, pharmacist, or dietitian regarding how the drug could affect the action of other drugs they may be taking, how the drug could affect their nutrition, and how their nutrition could affect the action of the drug.

Alcohol Use Alcohol is a drug that, like other drugs, has risks as well as benefits. The risks posed by alcohol depend on the consumer and the amount consumed. Some people should not consume any alcohol. For instance, women who are pregnant or trying to conceive should not consume alcohol because it can damage the fetus. Children and adolescents should not consume alcohol because they are more likely to suffer its toxic effects—drunkenness and poisoning leading to seizures, coma, and death.[32] Individuals who plan to drive or operate machinery should not consume alcohol because it can impair coordination and reflexes. Alcoholics should avoid alcohol because they cannot restrict their drinking to moderate levels. Finally, individuals taking medications that can interact with alcohol should avoid alcohol.[33]

For some, moderate alcohol consumption (defined by the Dietary Guidelines as no more than one drink per day for women and two drinks per day for men) may have some benefits. Alcoholic beverages consumed before or with meals can stimulate appetite and improve mood. It can be relaxing, producing a euphoria that can enhance social interactions. Studies have shown that light drinking is associated with a reduction in mortality.[34] This is most likely due to the inverse relationship between heart disease and consumption of small amounts of alcohol.[35] This reduction in heart disease risk occurs mainly in men over 45 and women over 55.[33] Alcohol consumption increases HDL cholesterol level and may have an effect on the aggregation of platelets. These benefits are stronger when red wine is consumed, likely due to the phytochemicals (phenols) in red wine.[36] Wine consumption has been suggested as one reason for the French paradox: The fact that the French diet is higher in fat than the American diet but the French suffer from far less heart disease.

For everyone, the risks of *excess* alcohol consumption outweigh the benefits. Excess alcohol causes medical and social consequences that affect drinkers and their families. The abuse of alcohol contributes to domestic violence and leads to more than 100,000 deaths per year, including 20,000 from traffic accidents. The incidence of alcohol poisoning, especially among college students who binge drink, is on the rise.

Social and Economic Impact of Aging

There are a variety of social and economic changes that often accompany aging. These factors are all interrelated and affect nutritional status by decreasing the motivation to eat and the ability to acquire and enjoy food.

Income About 3.4 million elderly persons live below the poverty level.[1] The highest rates of poverty occur among the oldest of the old, minorities, women, persons living alone, and those with disabilities. Many older individuals, regardless of income level, must live on a fixed income when they retire from their jobs, making it difficult to afford health care, especially medications, and a healthy diet. Food is often the most flexible expense in one's budget, so limiting the types and amounts of foods consumed may be the only option available for older adults trying to meet expenses. Substandard housing and inadequate food preparation facilities can make the situation worse because food cannot easily be prepared and eaten at home.

Dependent Living Although many older adults continue to live independently in their own homes, the physical and psychological decline associated with aging causes some to eventually require assistance in living (Figure 16.10). Poor eyesight and other physical restrictions can limit the ability to drive a car. Without help, many

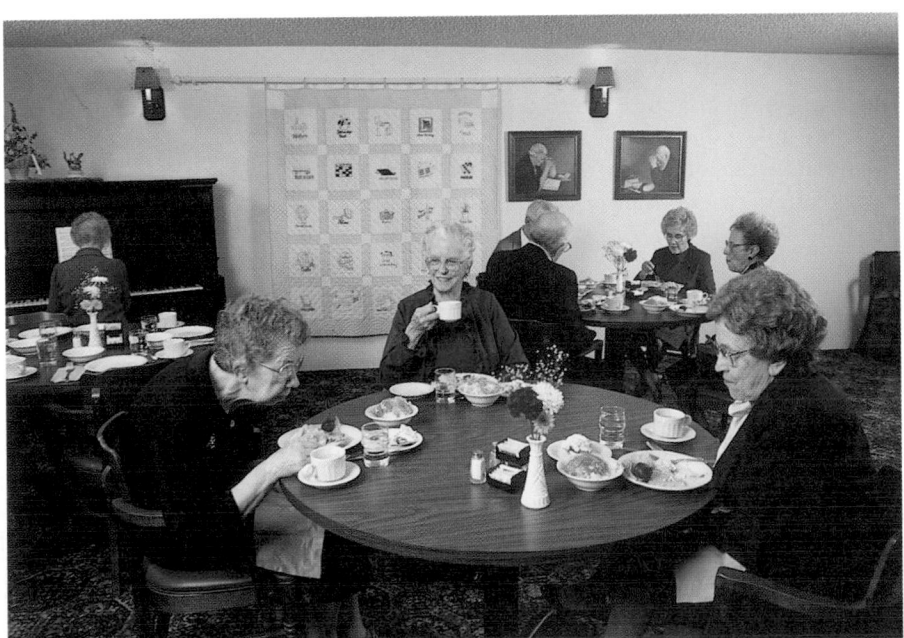

Figure 16.10

Many older people live in assisted living facilities and nursing homes where their meals are prepared for them.
(© Blair Seitz/Photo Researchers)

older adults may be unable to get to markets and food programs, restricting the types of food available to them. While a social support system consisting of family members, friends, and other caregivers can help many people stay at home, others may require assisted-living facilities, where they have their own apartments but can obtain assistance around the clock. For some, however, the degenerative changes of age require a nursing home to provide the appropriate care.

Those in nursing homes are at increased risk for malnutrition because they are more likely to have medical conditions that increase nutrient needs or that interfere with food intake or nutrient absorption, and because they are dependent on others to provide for their care. In addition, 50% of institutionalized elderly suffer from some form of disorientation or confusion, which further increases the likelihood of decreased nutrient intake. Even when adequate meals are provided, nursing-home residents frequently do not consume all of the food served, increasing the likelihood of fluid and energy deficits.[37]

Depression Social, psychological, and physical factors all contribute to depression in the elderly.[38] Retirement and the death or relocation of friends and family can cause social isolation, which contributes to depression. Physical disability causes loss of independence. The inability to engage in normal daily activities, visit with friends and family easily, and provide for personal needs contributes to depression. Depression can make meals less appetizing and decrease the quantity and quality of foods consumed, thereby increasing the risk of malnutrition.

• NUTRITION FOR OLDER ADULTS

Because of the diversity among older adults, defining nutrient needs is challenging. Meeting the nutritional needs of the elderly requires consideration of each person's medical, psychological, social, and economic circumstances (see *Critical Thinking*: Averting Malnutrition).

Can Nutrition Keep Us Young?

Although nutrition is not the key to immortality, a healthy diet can prevent malnutrition and delay the onset of chronic diseases.

The diseases that are the major causes of disability in older adults—cardiovascular disease, hypertension, diabetes, cancer, and osteoporosis—are all nutrition-related. Exercise and a lifetime of healthy eating will not necessarily prevent these diseases, but they may slow the changes that accumulate over time, postponing the onset of disease symptoms. For example, the risk of developing cardiovascular disease can be decreased by exercise and a diet low in *trans* fat and saturated fat and high in whole grains, fruits, and vegetables. The risk of osteoporosis may be reduced by adequate calcium intake and exercise throughout life. And the likelihood of developing certain types of cancer can be reduced by consuming a diet low in fat and high in whole grains, vegetables, and fruits.

Nutrient Needs of Older Adults

General dietary recommendations are difficult to establish for older adults. For instance, the requirements of a wheelchair-bound 70-year-old are different from those of a more active 70-year-old. Dietary recommendations are developed to meet the needs of the majority of healthy individuals in a population, but "healthy" is difficult to define in such a diverse group. The DRIs divide adulthood into four age categories: young adulthood, ages 19 through 30; middle age, 31 through 50 years; adulthood, ages 51 through 70; and older adults, those over 70 years of age. This recognizes the possibly higher nutrient intake needs of younger adults, the decline with age in the need for nutrients involved in energy metabolism, and the variability in the functional capacity of older adults.

Energy and Macronutrient Needs Energy needs are typically reduced in the elderly. With age, there is a decrease in lean body mass that causes a reduction in basal metabolic rate (BMR). This reduction in BMR significantly reduces total energy expenditure. For example, the EER for an 80-year-old man is almost 600 kcalories per day less than that for a 20-year-old man of the same height, weight, and physical activity level. For women, the difference in EER between an 80- and a 20-year-old of the same height, weight, and physical activity level is about 400 kcalories per day.[39] The decrease in EER that occurs with age is even greater if activity level declines, which it typically does. A decrease in activity also contributes to the reduction in lean body mass and BMR. Exercise can reduce the loss of lean body mass, maintain fitness and independence, and allow an increase in food intake without weight gain so micronutrient needs are more easily met. Therefore, maintaining regular physical activity remains important throughout life (Figure 16.11).

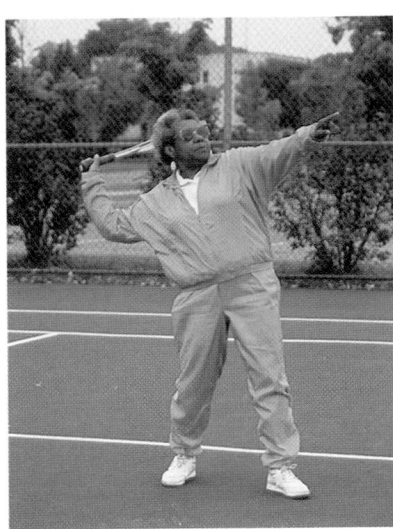

Figure 16.11
Exercise increases energy needs and helps to maintain lean body mass.
(© CLEO/PhotoEdit)

Protein Unlike energy requirements, the need for protein does not decline with age. Therefore, an adequate diet for older adults must be somewhat higher in protein relative to energy intake. Although the RDA for older adults is no different than that for younger adults, actual need depends on the individual. In some, the protein requirement may be less than the RDA because there is less lean body mass to maintain, whereas in others it may be greater than the RDA because protein absorption or utilization is reduced.

Fat The digestion and absorption of fat does not change in older adults; therefore the recommendations regarding dietary fat apply to older as well as younger adults. A diet with 20 to 35% of energy from fat that contains adequate amouts of the essential fatty acids; limits saturated fat, *trans* fat, and cholesterol is recommended. Following these recommendations will allow older adults to meet their nutrient needs without exceeding their energy requirements and may delay the onset of chronic disease. However, there are certain situations, such as being underweight, where greater fat intake may be warranted.

Fiber The recommendations for fiber intake for older adults are slightly lower than for younger adults because the AIs for fiber are based on total energy needs.[39] Fiber, when consumed with adequate fluid, helps prevent constipation, hemorrhoids, and diverticulosis—conditions that are common in older adults. High-fiber diets may also be beneficial in the prevention and management of diabetes, cardiovascular disease, and obesity.

Water The recommended water intake for older adults is the same as that for younger adults; however, changes in the homeostatic mechanisms that regulate water balance may make meeting these needs more challenging. With age there is a reduction in the sense of thirst, which can decrease fluid intake.[37] Changes in mobility may limit access to water even in the presence of thirst. In addition, the kidneys are no longer as efficient at conserving water, so water loss increases. Depression, which decreases water intake, and medications that increase water loss, such as laxatives and diuretics, also increase the risk of dehydration in the elderly. Inadequate fluid intake increases problems with constipation.

Micronutrient Needs The recommended intake for many of the micronutrients is not changed for older adults (Figure 16.12); however, the risk of micronutrient deficiencies increases in this age group due to deficient intakes as well as changes in digestion, absorption, and metabolism.

B Vitamins The only B vitamins for which recommendations differ between older and younger adults are vitamins B_6 and B_{12}. The RDA for vitamin B_6 is greater in individuals age 51 and older than for younger adults, because higher dietary intakes

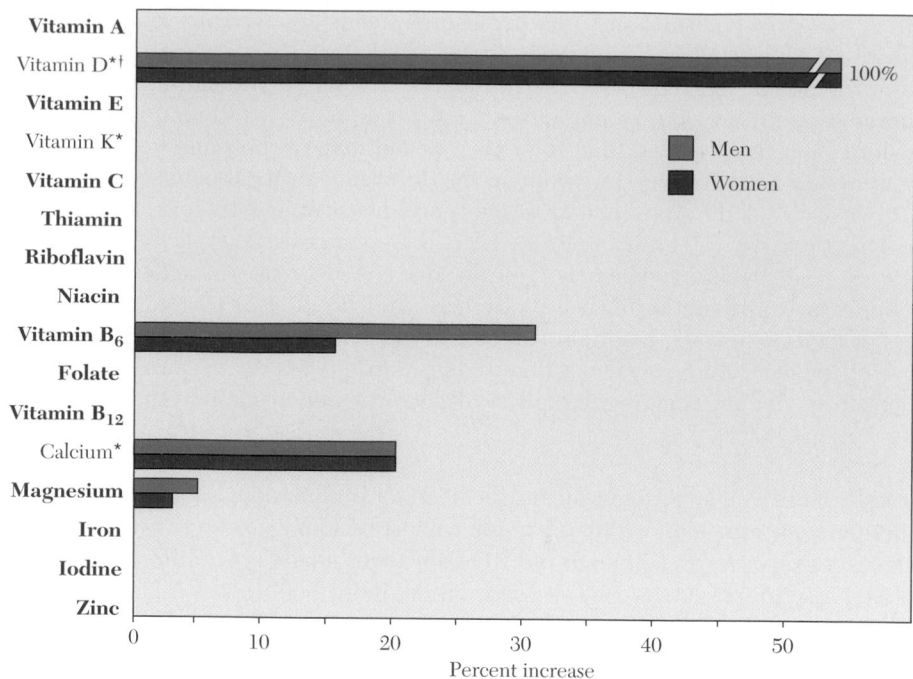

Figure 16.12
The nutrient needs of older adults are not drastically different from those of young adults. This graph illustrates the percentage increase in micronutrient recommendations for adults age 51 and older compared to those of young adults ages 19 through 30. The RDA for vitamin B_{12} is not increased, but it is recommended that vitamin B_{12} be obtained from fortified foods or supplements. Nutrients in bold are RDA values, and those in plain text with an asterisk are AI values. (The RDA for iron for women over 50 years of age is reduced by 50%.)

†This represents the AI for individuals 51 to 70 years old. For those over age 70 the AI is increased by 200%

are needed to maintain the same functional levels in the body. Vitamin B_{12} is a nutrient of concern for older adults because of both reduced absorption of food-bound B_{12} and low dietary intakes, especially among the poor. The RDA for vitamin B_{12} is not increased, but it is recommended that individuals over the age of 50 meet their RDA for vitamin B_{12}, by consuming foods fortified with vitamin B_{12} such as breakfast cereals or soy-based products, or by taking a supplement containing vitamin B_{12}. This recommendation is made because food-bound vitamin B_{12} is not absorbed efficiently in many elderly due to atrophic gastritis, which affects 10 to 30% of individuals over age 50.[12] The vitamin B_{12} in fortified foods and supplements is not bound to proteins, so it is absorbed even when stomach acid is low.

Vitamin D and Calcium Because vitamin D is necessary for calcium absorption, a deficiency may contribute to osteoporosis. Intakes of this vitamin are often low in the elderly population, usually due to limited consumption of dairy products. And, exposure to sunlight, which is necessary for the formation of provitamin D in the skin, is often limited in the elderly because they spend less time outdoors or tend to wear clothing that covers or shades their skin when they go out. Vitamin D deficiency is also a concern because the capacity to synthesize provitamin D in the skin and to form active vitamin D in the kidney decreases with age. Using bone loss as an indicator of adequacy, the AI for men and women aged 51 to 70 has been doubled from that of younger age groups to a value of 10 μg per day. For individuals over age 70, this is further increased to 15 μg per day.

Calcium status is a problem in the elderly because intakes are low and intestinal absorption decreases with age. The current AI for adults over age 51 is 1200 mg, greater than the AI of 1000 mg set for younger adults.[40] Although the decrease in estrogen that occurs at menopause causes bone loss, it cannot be prevented by increasing calcium intake, so the AIs for men and women are not different.

Antioxidant Nutrients: Do They Slow Aging? The hypothesis that aging is caused by oxidative damage has led to the popular conclusion that high dietary intakes of antioxidants will retard the aging process. In reality, antioxidant nutrients will not keep you young, but adequate intakes may reduce the incidence of disease. Antioxidants, including vitamin E, vitamin C, and β-carotene, have been found to improve immune function and may therefore help protect the body from infectious disease.[27] And there is evidence that antioxidant intake is correlated with a reduced incidence of various chronic diseases. High intakes of β-carotene and vitamin E have been associated with a reduced risk of heart disease,[41–43] Diets high in antioxidants are also associated with a reduced incidence of certain types of cancer as well as macular degeneration and cataracts.[44] The evidence that antioxidants in supplement form will have these effects is not as strong as the evidence supporting a diet plentiful in foods high in these nutrients (Figure 16.13). When these nutrients are obtained from foods, they bring with them phytochemicals, some of which offer additional antioxidant protection and some of which protect us from chronic disease in other ways.

Meeting the Nutrient Needs of Older Adults

Despite the fact that the nutrient needs of older adults are not drastically different from those of young adults, it is more challenging to meet these needs. One reason for this is that energy needs are reduced while most micronutrient needs remain the same or increase. A modified Food Guide Pyramid has been developed to emphasize the nutrients and food selections that are of particular concern for older adults. In some cases, nutrient supplements may be necessary to meet needs. Changes in health and social and economic conditions also make meeting nutrient needs difficult.

A Modified Food Guide Pyramid The modified Food Guide Pyramid shown in Figure 16.14 has been designed to help plan diets that will meet the special needs of older adults. This modified pyramid is built on a base of water—eight 8-ounce glasses per day. This helps emphasize that dehydration is a common problem and that older adults need to be more conscious of water consumption. This pyramid also has a narrower base than the traditional USDA Food Guide Pyramid to illustrate that energy needs are typically reduced among the elderly.[45] The recommended numbers of servings are equal to or greater than the minimums recommended by the Food Guide Pyramid, and nutrient-dense choices from each food group are recommended. To highlight the importance of fiber in the diets of older adults, the pyramid for seniors includes a fiber icon in the food groups containing high-fiber foods such as grains, fruits, vegetables, and beans, nuts, and seeds. Another key difference in this pyramid is a flag at the top that indicates the possible need for dietary supplements.

Dietary Supplements Many older adults may benefit from supplementing some nutrients. Vitamin D supplements may be beneficial because production of this vitamin in the skin is decreased and exposure to sunlight may be limited. A calcium supplement may be necessary to meet needs particularly in elderly women because it can be difficult to consume 1200 mg of calcium from food without exceeding energy needs. Supplemental vitamin B_{12} from pills or fortified foods is recommended for older adults because the absorption of vitamin B_{12} decreases with age. However, supplements should not take the place of a balanced, nutrient-dense diet high in grains, fruits, and vegetables. These foods also contain phytochemicals and other substances that may protect against disease. Older adults should be cautious to avoid overdoses, and the resulting toxicities, when selecting supplements.

A multivitamin and mineral supplement containing no more than 100% of the Daily Value for any nutrient is the safest way to supplement the diet. Supplements containing megadoses or nonnutrient substances should be avoided. Most of these provide no proven benefit, many are costly, and others can be toxic. For example, lecithin is claimed to lower cholesterol and to treat Alzheimer's disease, but there is no proof that it does either. RNA is claimed to rejuvenate old cells, improve memory, and prevent wrinkling, but there are no controlled studies to support any of these claims. Superoxide dismutase (SOD), an enzyme that protects against oxidative damage, is said to slow aging and treat Alzheimer's disease. However, SOD is a pro-

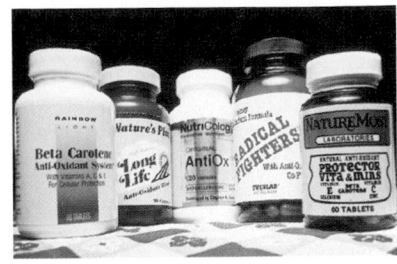

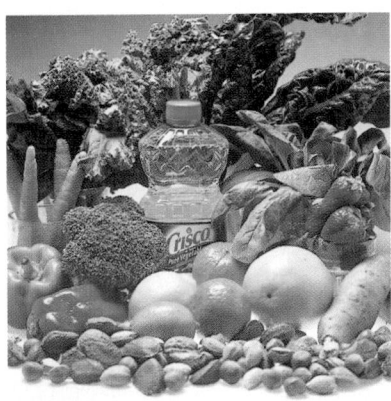

Figure 16.13

(*a*) Supplements are often consumed to increase antioxidant intake. (Charles D. Winters) (*b*) Foods that are good sources of antioxidants such as β-carotene, vitamin C, vitamin E, and selenium also provide fiber, energy, other micronutrients, and phytochemcials. (Charles D. WInters)

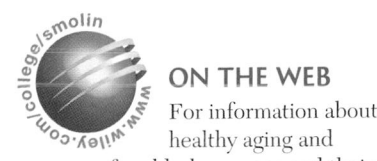

ON THE WEB

For information about healthy aging and resources for elderly persons and their families, go to the Administration on Aging at

www.aoa.dhhs.gov/

and the National Institute on Aging at

www.nih.gov/nia/.

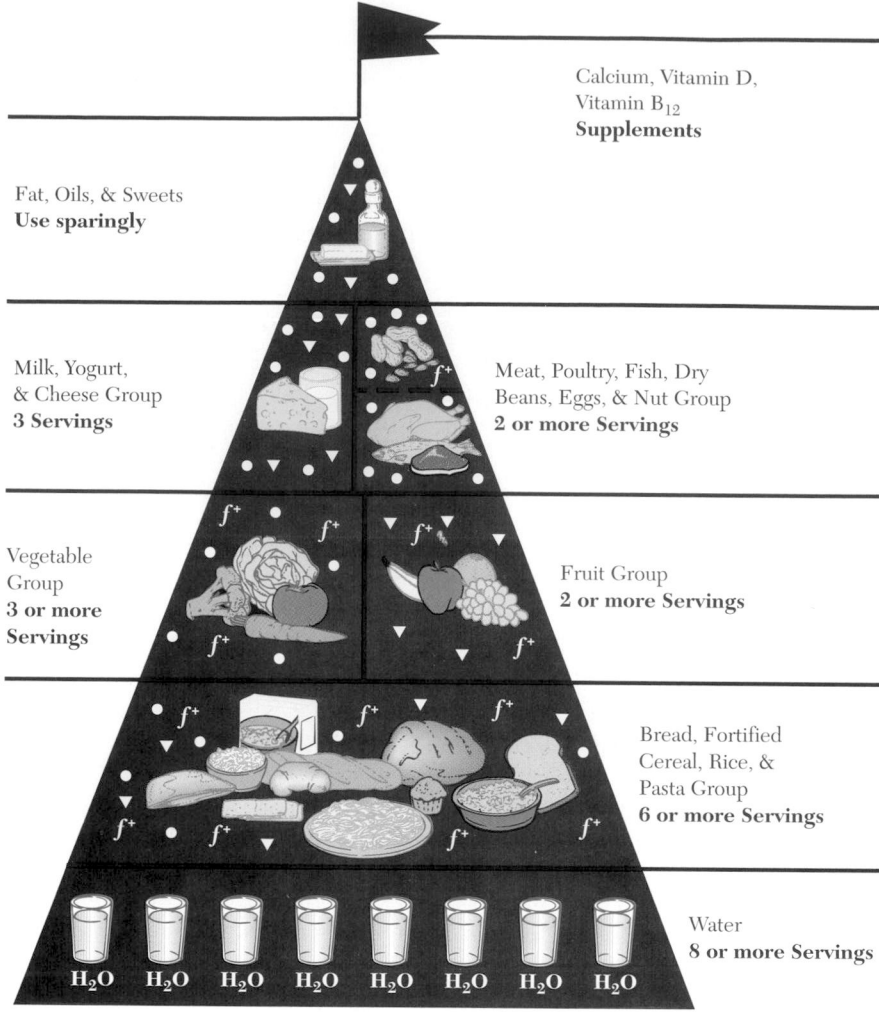

Calcium, Vitamin D, Vitamin B₁₂
Supplements

Fat, Oils, & Sweets
Use sparingly

Milk, Yogurt, & Cheese Group
3 Servings

Meat, Poultry, Fish, Dry Beans, Eggs, & Nut Group
2 or more Servings

Vegetable Group
3 or more Servings

Fruit Group
2 or more Servings

Bread, Fortified Cereal, Rice, & Pasta Group
6 or more Servings

Water
8 or more Servings

H₂O   H₂O   H₂O   H₂O   H₂O   H₂O   H₂O   H₂O

Figure 16.14

This modification of the Food Guide Pyramid targets the needs of healthy mobile seniors (over age 70) and is not designed to meet the needs of those with special dietary needs or significant health problems.

● fat (naturally occurring and added)
▼ sugars (added)
f^+ fiber (should be present)

These symbols show fat, added sugars, and fiber in foods.

tein that is broken down to amino acids in the GI tract, so oral supplements will not increase blood or tissue levels of this enzyme. Coenzyme Q, a synthetic version of a compound in the electron transport chain, is marketed to older adults as a way to slow aging by enhancing the immune system. However, it does not boost immune function and may pose a risk to people with poor circulation.

Preventing Food Insecurity There are many reasons why older individuals may experience food insecurity and therefore not be able to meet their nutrient needs. Ensuring adequate nutrient intake may involve providing nutrient-dense meals or providing education on nutrient needs, economics, and food preparation. Or it may require providing assistance with shopping and food preparation.

Overcoming Economic Limitations Being able to afford a healthy diet is a problem for many older individuals. Reduced-cost food and meals at senior centers, food stamps, food banks, soup kitchens, and commodity foods are available to people on limited incomes. Programs that provide education about low-cost nutritious food choices can also help reduce food costs.

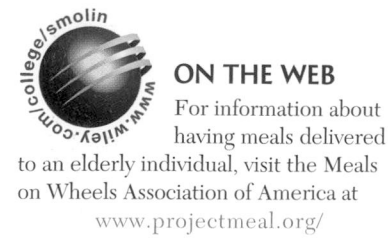

ON THE WEB
For information about having meals delivered to an elderly individual, visit the Meals on Wheels Association of America at
www.projectmeal.org/

Overcoming Social Limitations Another problem that contributes to poor nutrient intake is loneliness. Living, cooking, and eating alone can decrease interest in food. This can be a problem not only for the elderly but for anyone who typically eats alone.

Buying single servings of food is an option, although it can be expensive. To avoid spoilage of perishable items, grocers can be asked to break up packages of meat, eggs, fruits, and vegetables so small amounts can be purchased. Large packages can be purchased and shared among friends. Cooking larger portions and freezing foods in meal-size batches can be helpful not only with cost but also to relieve the boredom of eating the same leftovers several days in a row. Creativity and flexibility in what defines a meal can also help. An easy single meal can be prepared by topping a potato with cooked vegetables and cheese, or with leftover chili or spaghetti sauce (Figure 16.15). Yogurt or a bowl of cereal with fruit and milk is also a nutritious dinner option.

Overcoming Physical Limitations Difficulty in cooking due to limited mobility can also reduce food intake. Precooked foods, frozen dinners, or salad bar items, as well as instant foods such as cereals, rice and noodle dishes, and soups that just require adding water, can provide a meal with almost no preparation. Medical nutritional products such as Ensure or Boost, can also be used to supplement intake. These canned, fortified products have a long shelf life and can meet nutrient needs with a small volume. Frozen meals and canned foods are helpful too. Food can also be ordered by phone if it is affordable. Eating out at senior centers or low-cost restaurants or sharing shopping and cooking chores with a friend can reduce cooking demand and increase social interaction. Home health services can help with cooking and eating, and most senior centers, health departments, or social service agencies offer meals, rides, and in-home care.

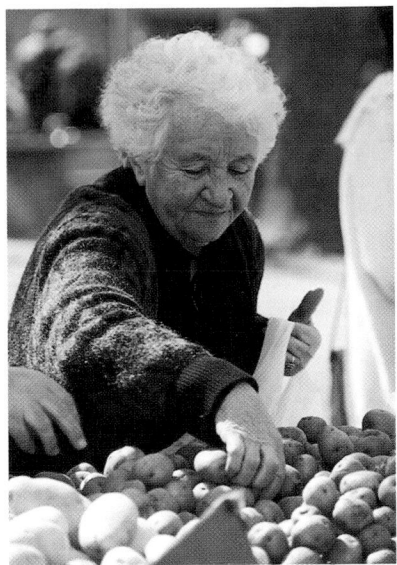

Figure 16.15
Selecting acceptable foods that are nutritious and easy to prepare is important in meeting the needs of the elderly. (© Tony Freeman/PhotoEdit)

Overcoming Medical Limitations Medical conditions and the use of medications often affect food choices. Meals need to be appealing and easy to prepare and consume, as well as compatible with medical conditions. For instance, an individual with dental problems may not be able to chew fresh fruits and vegetables. Therefore, a texture modification is required. Fully cooked, canned, or soft fruit and fruit juices can be substituted for hard-to-chew fruits, and cooked vegetables can replace raw ones. Eggs and stewed meats can provide easy-to-chew protein sources. To overcome changes in the sense of taste and smell, spicy or acidic foods may be limited or emphasized, depending on individual tastes.

Medical conditions often require special diets. These diets may contribute to malnutrition if they restrict favorite foods and if individuals prescribed the diet are not provided with enough information about how to substitute foods that will provide adequate energy, nutrients, and eating pleasure. Education about what foods are appropriate and how to read food labels can help identify products that fit within dietary restrictions.

The use of prescription or over-the-counter medications to treat medical conditions can also affect eating habits. Physicians, pharmacists, and dietitians can provide information about possible effects on food intake. Purchasing all prescription medications from the same pharmacy will ensure that the pharmacist is aware of all medications taken and can advise of possible interactions. Health-care providers also need to be informed about all nonprescription medications and vitamin, mineral, or other dietary supplements used and whether or not medications are taken according to the prescription instructions.

Nutrition Programs for the Elderly The federal Older Americans Act provides nutrition services to older individuals who are in economic need, particularly low-income minorities. Programs that provide nutritious meals in communal settings promote social interaction and can improve nutrient intake. The Congregate and

Table 16.4 *National Programs Promoting Better Nutrition Among Older Americans*

Older Americans Act—Title III Congregate and Home-Delivered Nutrition Programs

Serves at least one meal five days a week to persons 60 years and older. Meals are served at home or in churches, schools, senior centers, or other facilities.

Older Americans Act—Title VI Congregate and Home-Delivered Nutrition Programs

Provides home-delivered and congregate meals to Native American organizations.

Older Americans Act—Title III Health Promotion and Disease Prevention Program

Provides health-promotion and disease-prevention services in areas where there are large numbers of economically needy older adults.

Nutrition Screening Initiative

Promotes nutritional screening and more attention to nutrition in all health-care and social-service settings that provide for older adults.

Food Stamp Program

Provides food stamps to low-income individuals including the elderly. These can be used instead of cash to purchase food.

Nutrition Program for the Elderly

Provides grants, cash, and commodity foods to states and tribes to supplement congregate and home-delivered meal programs.

Commodity Supplemental Food Program—Elderly

Provides food, nutrition education, and health-service referrals to individuals with low incomes, including the elderly.

Child and Adult Care Food Program (Adult Day Care)

Provides cash reimbursements and food commodities to community day-care centers that serve meals and snacks to children and elderly with special needs.

Food Distribution Program on Indian Reservations

Distributes commodity foods to low-income persons including the elderly, living on or near Indian reservations.

Home-Delivered Nutrition Programs established by the Older Americans Act provide congregate meals at locations such as senior centers, community centers, schools, and churches. For those who are unable to attend congregate meals, home-delivered meals are available.

Although such programs are a first step in meeting nutritional needs, currently most provide only one meal a day for five days a week. Each meal served must provide at least a third of the 1989 RDA.[46] In practice, participants in these elder nutrition programs are receiving 40 to 50% of their daily intake from the meal consumed.[47] Studies have shown that individuals who receive these meals have a better-quality diet and fewer hospitalizations than those who do not.[48] These and other programs addressing the nutritional needs of older adults are described in Table 16.4.

CRITICAL THINKING

Averting Malnutrition

Shirley is 82 years old. She lives alone in the city. Recently, her teeth were extracted because of periodontal disease. As a result of her dental problems, she had eaten only cottage cheese and milk for the past few weeks. Even though she is now feeling better, her granddaughter, Anna, begins to worry about Shirley's nutrition. Anna decides to review the DETERMINE checklist with her grandmother to see if she is at risk of malnutrition.

Checklist	Grandma Shirley
Disease	She has high blood pressure, arthritis, periodontal disease, and cataracts.
Eating poorly	She has only eaten cottage cheese and milk for a week; she doesn't like to cook for herself.
Tooth loss or mouth pain	Yes.
Economic hardship	None.
Reduced social support	Anna visits regularly but Shirley has few friends.
Multiple medicines	She takes estrogen, as well as blood pressure and arthritis medications.
Involuntary weight loss/gain	She thinks she has lost about 10 pounds since her dental problems began.
Needs assistance in self-care	She needs help shopping and cleaning.
Elder above age 80	She is 82 years old.

Eight of the items on the DETERMINE checklist apply to Anna's grandmother, confirming her concerns about the risk of malnutrition. Anna takes her to a dietitian who asks her to recall the diet she ate before her teeth were extracted.

Shirley's Original Diet

Food	Amount
Breakfast	
Bran flakes	3/4 cup
Lowfat milk	1 cup
Coffee	1 cup
Lowfat milk	1 Tbsp
Sugar	2 tsp
Lunch	
Gefilte fish	1 oz
Chicken soup	1 cup
Matzoh	1 piece
Apple	1 small
Dinner	
Lowfat milk	1 cup
Instant rice	1 cup
Beef	3 oz
Peas	1 cup
Total energy (kcal)	**1035**

How does Shirley's diet compare to the recommendations of the Food Guide Pyramid for people over 70?

▼

- The bran flakes she has for breakfast are a good source of fiber but are not fortified with vitamin B$_{12}$, a vitamin that is poorly absorbed from food in many older adults.
- She consumes only about 4 cups of fluid and one serving is coffee, which contains caffeine and can therefore contribute to fluid loss.
- Other answers:

Suggest foods Shirley could add to improve her diet without increasing the time she spends cooking.

▼

Answer:

What other factors need to be considered when recommending a diet for Shirley?

▼

Shirley needs a diet that includes foods that are not only easy to prepare and carry home on the bus but that are also easy to chew. Anna can take Shirley shopping once a month for the heavy, bulky items like paper goods, laundry soap, rice, cereal, and canned foods. Shirley will be able to handle the smaller, more perishable items when she takes the bus to the store.

• APPLICATIONS •

1. Use one day of the food record you kept in Chapter 2 and compare it with the EER for a person who is your height, weight, and activity level but is 75 years old. Modify your food choices to meet the recommendations of the Senior Pyramid (shown in Figure 16.14) while not exceeding what your energy needs would be at age 75.

2. Many elderly people have medical conditions and dietary restrictions and modifications. How might you modify your food choices to accommodate:

    a. a low-sodium diet?
    b. restriction of protein to 0.6 gram per kilogram of body weight?
    c. loss of smell and taste?
    d. a dry mouth and poorly fitting dentures?

3. Using the Internet, assess what kind of nutrition information is available to individuals planning for the care of their elderly parents or relatives.

    a. What types of services are available?
    b. What are the costs?

SUMMARY

1. Aging is the accumulation of changes over time that results in an ever-increasing susceptibility to disease and death. A combination of genetic, environmental, and lifestyle factors determines how long we live and how long we remain healthy.

2. As a population, we are living longer but not necessarily healthier lives. Compression of morbidity, that is, increasing the number of healthy years, is an important public health goal. The elderly are the fastest-growing segment of the American population.

3. Life span is a characteristic of a species. The average age to which people in a population live, or life expectancy, is a characteristic of a population. An individual's longevity is affected by genetic background, diet, and lifestyle.

4. The risk of malnutrition increases with age due to the physical, psychological, social, and economic changes that accompany aging. The DETERMINE checklist helps identify older adults who are at risk for malnutrition.

5. As the body ages, reserve capacity decreases, causing organ function to decline. There are changes in vision and the sense of smell, affecting the ability to eat as well as the appeal of food; changes in digestion and absorption, decreasing the intake and absorption of nutrients; changes in metabolism, affecting nutrient utilization; changes in hormonal patterns, affecting body function; and changes in mobility and mental capacity, limiting the ability to acquire, prepare, and consume food.

6. The incidence of disease increases with increasing age. Both infectious and chronic diseases affect nutrient requirements and the ability to consume a nutritious diet. The medications used to treat disease also affect nutrition, especially when the medications are taken over long periods of time and when multiple medications are taken simultaneously.

7. A healthy diet and lifestyle cannot stop aging but can postpone the onset of many of the changes and diseases that are common in older adults.

8. Energy needs are decreased with age, but the need for protein, fluid, and most micronutrients remains the same. Meals for the elderly must be nutrient-dense and consider individual medical, psychological, social, and economic circumstances. In some cases, assistance with shopping and meal preparation may be needed.

9. The federal Older Americans Act includes programs that provide older adults with low-cost or free meals in their homes or in a social setting. Although these programs are helpful, they do not ensure adequate nutrition for all elderly.

REVIEW QUESTIONS

1. How long can each of us expect to live?

2. What is meant by compression of morbidity?

3. What factors determine at what age the consequences of aging become apparent?

4. Why are older adults at risk for malnutrition?

5. List three physiological changes that occur with aging.

6. List three ways in which medication use and nutrition interact.

7. What social and economic factors increase nutritional risk among the elderly?

8. What causes the energy needs of older adults to be reduced?

9. Why is it so important that elderly individuals consume a nutrient-dense diet?

10. How do recommendations such as the Dietary Guidelines for Americans apply to individuals over the age of 65 years?

REFERENCES

1. U.S. Department of Health and Human Services, Administration on Aging. Profile of Older Americans. 1998. Available online at www.aoa.dhhs.gov/aoa/stats/profile/default.htm Accessed August 2, 2002.

2. Kirkwood, T. B. L. Comparative life spans of species: Why do species have the life spans they do? *Am. J. Clin. Nutr.* 55(Suppl.):1191S–1195S, 1992.

3. Shoaf, L. R., and Bishirjina, K. O. Standards of practice for gerontological nutritionists: a mandate for action. *J. Am. Diet. Assoc.* 95:1433–1438, 1995.

4. U.S. Department of Health and Human Services, Administration on Aging. 1997 Census Estimates of the Older Population. Available online at www.aoa.dhhs.gov/aoa/stats/99pop/default.htm Accessed February 17, 2001.

5. Healthy People 2010. *National Health Promotion and Disease Prevention Objectives.* Washington, D.C.: U.S. Department of Health and Human Services, 1998. Available online at web.health.gov/healthypeople/default.htm Accessed August 2, 2002.

6. Blumberg, J. Nutritional needs of seniors. *J. Am. Coll. Nutr.* 16:517–523, 1997.

7. Wellman, N. S., Weddle, D. O., Brain, C. T., and Kranz, S. Elder insecurities: poverty, hunger, and malnutrition. *J. Am. Diet. Assoc.* 97:S120–S122, 1997.

8. American Academy of Family Physicians. Nutrition Screening Initiative. Available online at www.aafp.org/nsi/index.html Accessed August 2, 2002.

9. Duffy, V. B., Backstrand, J. R., and Ferris, A. M. Olfactory dysfunction and related nutritional risk in free-living elderly women. *J. Am. Diet. Assoc.* 95:879–884, 1995.

10. Morley, J. E. Anorexia of aging: physiologic and pathologic. *Am. J. Clin. Nutr.* 66:760–773, 1997.

11. Christen, W. G. Antioxidant vitamins and age-related eye disease. *Proc. Assoc. Am. Physicians* 111:16–21, 1999.

12. Institute of Medicine, Food and Nutrition Board. *Dietary Reference Intakes for Thiamin, Riboflavin, Niacin, Vitamin B6, Folate, Vitamin B12, Pantothenic Acid, Biotin, and Choline.* Washington, D.C.: National Academy Press, 1998.

13. Russell, R. M. New views on the RDAs for older adults. *J. Am. Diet. Assoc.* 97:515–518, 1997.

14. van Asselt, D. Z., van den Broek, W. J., Lamers, C. B., et al. Free and protein-bound cobalamin absorption in healthy middle-aged and older subjects. *J. Am. Geriatr. Soc.* 44:949–953, 1996.

15. Harari, D., Gurwitz, J. H., Avorn, J., et al. Bowel habits in relation to age and gender: findings from the National Health Interview Survey and clinical implications. *Arch. Intern. Med.* 156:315–320, 1996.

16. Brucker, M. C., and Faucher, M. A. Pharmacologic management of common gastrointestinal health problems in women. *J. Nurse-Midwifery* 42:145–162, May/June 1997.

17. Lubran, M. M. Renal function in the elderly. *Ann. Clin. Lab. Sci.* 25:122–133, 1995.

18. Lamberts, S. W. J., van den Beld, A. W., and van der Lely, A-J. The endocrinology of aging. *Science* 278:419–424, 1998.

19. Stevens, J., Cai, J., Pamuk, E. R., et al. The effect of age on the association between body-mass index and mortality. *N. Engl. J. Med.* 338:1–7, 1998.

20. Proctor, D. N., Balagopal, P., and Nair, K. S. Age-related sarcopenia in humans is associated with reduced synthetic rates of specific muscle proteins. *J. Nutr.* 128:351S–355S, 1998.

21. Evans, W. J., and Cyr-Campbell, D. Nutrition, exercise and healthy aging. *J. Am. Diet. Assoc.* 97:632–638, 1997.

22. Wallace, J. I., and Schwartz, R. S. Involuntary weight loss in elderly outpatients: recognition, etiologies and treatment. *Clin. Geriatr. Med.* 13:717–735, 1997.

23. Masoro, E. J. Possible mechanisms underlying the antiaging actions of caloric restriction. *Toxicol. Pathol.* 24:738–741, 1996.

24. Butler, R. N., Fossel, M., Pan, C. X., et al. Efficacy and safety of hormones and antioxidants. *Geriatrics* 55:48–52, 2000.

25. Bastianetto, S., and Quirion, R. Any facts behind the DHEA hype? *Trends Pharmacol. Sci.* 18:447–449, 1997.

26. Rieter, R. J. The pineal gland and melatonin in relation to aging: a summary of the theories and the data. *Exp. Gerontol.* 30:199–212, 1995.

27. Lesourd, B. M., Mazari, L., and Ferry, M. The role of nutrition in immunity in the aged. *Nutr. Rev.* 56 (II):S113–S125, 1998.

28. Bogden, J. D. Studies on micronutrient supplements and immunity in older people. *Nutr. Rev.* 53:S59–S65, 1995.

29. Stabler, S. P., Lindenbaum, J., and Allen, R. H. Vitamin B12 deficiency in the elderly: Current dilemmas. *Am. J. Clin. Nutr.* 66:741–749, 1997.

30. Vogel, G. Tau protein mutations confirmed as neuron killers. *Science* 280:1524–1525, 1998.

31. American Academy of Family Physicians. *The Nutrition Checklist.* Available online at http:www.aafp.org/nsi Accessed August 2, 2002.

32. Hingley, A. T. Preventing childhood poisoning. *FDA Consumer* 30:7–11, March 1996.

33. Hingley, A. T. Preventing childhood poisoning. *FDA Consumer* 30:7–11, March 1996.

34. U.S. Department of Agriculture, U.S. Department of Health and Human Services. *Nutrition and Your Health: Dietary Guidelines for Americans,* 5th ed., 2000. Item Number 147-G. Hyattsville, Md.: U.S. Government Printing Office, 2000.

35. Cleophas, T. J. Wine, beer and spirits and the risk of myocardial infarction: a systematic review. *Biomed. Pharmacother.* 53:417–423, 1999.

36. Ruh, J. C. Wine and polyphenols related to platelet aggregation and atherosclerosis. *Drugs Exp. Clin. Res.* 25:125–131, 1999.

37. Chidester, J. C., and Spangler, A. A. Fluid intake in the institutionalized elderly. *J. Am. Diet. Assoc.* 97:23–28, 1997.

38. Cui, X. J., and Vaillant, G. E. Antecedents and consequences of negative life events in adulthood: A longitudinal study. *Am. J. Psychiatry* 153:21–26, 1996.

39. Institute of Medicine, Food and Nutrition Board. *Dietary Reference Intakes for Energy, Carbohydrate, Fiber, Fat, Protein and Amino Acids.* Washington, D.C.: National Academy Press, 2002.

40. Institute of Medicine, Food and Nutrition Board. *Dietary Reference Intakes: Calcium, Phosphorus, Magnesium, Vitamin D, and Fluoride.* Washington, D.C.: National Academy Press, 1997.

41. Kohlmeier, L., and Hastings, S. B. Epidemiologic evidence of a role of carotenoids in cardiovascular disease prevention. *Am. J. Clin Nutr.* 62(Suppl.):1370S–1376S, 1995.

42. Rimm, E. B., Stampfer, M. J., Ascherio, A., et al. Vitamin E consumption and the risk of heart disease in men. *N. Engl. J. Med.* 328:1450–1456, 1993.

43. Stampfer, M. J., Hennekens, C. H., Manson, J. E., et al. Vitamin E consumption and the risk of heart disease in women. *N. Engl. J. Med.* 328:1487–1489, 1993.

44. Taylor, A., Jacques, P. F., and Epstein, E. M. Relations among aging, antioxidant status and cataract. *Am. J. Clin. Nutr.* 62(Suppl.):1439S–1447S, 1995.

45. Russell, R. M., Rasmussen, H., and Lichtenstein, A. H. Modified food guide pyramid for people over seventy years of age. *J. Nutr.* 129: 751–753, 1999.

46. Fogler-Levitt, E., Lau, D., Csima, A., et al. Utilization of home-delivered meals by recipients 75 years of age or older. *J. Am. Diet. Assoc.* 95:552–557, 1995.

47. U.S. Department of Health and Human Services, Administration on Aging. Elderly Nutrition Program. Available online at www.aoa.gov/nutrition/default.htm Accessed August 2, 2002.

48. Roe, D. A. Development and current status of home-delivered meals programs in the United States: are the right elderly served? *Nutr. Rev.* 52:29–33, 1994.

49. Diplock, A. T. Safety of antioxidant vitamins and beta-carotene. *Am. J. Clin. Nutr.* 62(Suppl.):1510S-1516S, 1995.

How Safe Is Our Food Supply?

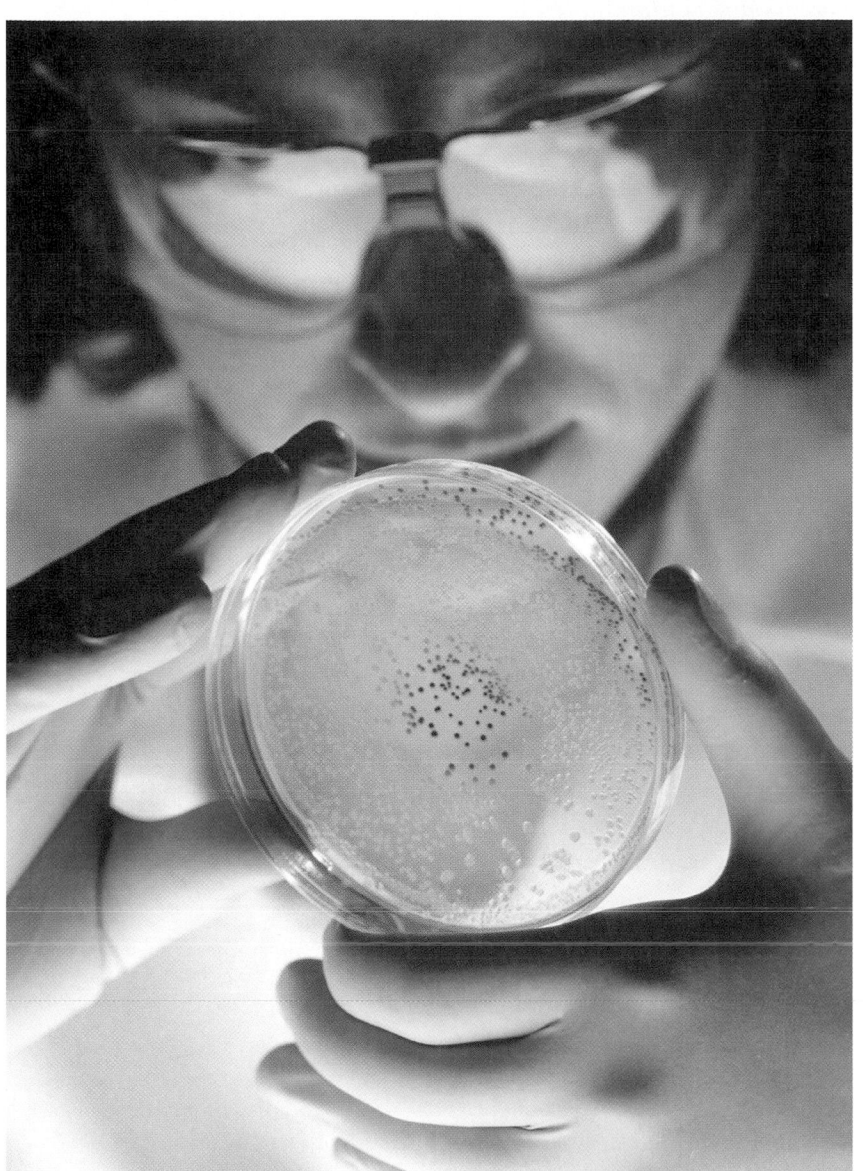

Chapter 17

(© Ted Horowitz/Corbis Stock Market)

Chapter Outline

WEIGHING THE RISKS AND BENEFITS
The Causes of Food-Borne Illness
Safeguarding Our Food Supply

PATHOGENS IN FOOD
Bacteria
Viruses
Molds
Parasites
Reducing the Risks:
  From Store to Table

CHEMICAL CONTAMINANTS IN FOOD
Risks and Benefits of Pesticides
Antibiotics and Hormones in Food
Contamination from Industrial Wastes
Choosing Wisely to Reduce Risk

FOOD TECHNOLOGY
Food Additives
Processing and Packaging
Biotechnology

Chapter Concepts

✔ Public health concern about the safety of the food supply has led to the initiation of programs to prevent or limit the spread of food-borne illness.

✔ Microbial contamination is the number one cause of food-borne illness in the United States.

✔ Bacteria, viruses, molds, and parasites all contaminate food and have the potential to cause food-borne illness.

✔ Care in choosing, preparing, cooking, handling, and storing food can reduce the risk of consuming contaminants.

✔ Chemicals used in agriculture and industry can contaminate the environment and make their way into the food supply.

✔ Food additives are used to protect foods from microbial contamination, enhance food's appeal and nutrient content, increase shelf life, and aid in food processing.

✔ Packaging and processing can improve the safety of the food supply but may also pose risks.

✔ Biotechnology creates new foods and products by manipulating DNA.

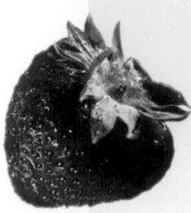

Just a Taste

Is it safe to eat hamburgers cooked medium rare?

Can you tell if your food is contaminated with bacteria?

Do food additives make the food supply safer?

The American food supply is the most carefully monitored in the world; nonetheless, *Salmonella* bacteria contaminate chicken sold in the United States, pesticide residues are found on our fruit, and industrial waste has polluted some of our waterways. Headlines announce *E. coli* in meat and apple juice; *Salmonella* in eggs, on vegetables, and in cereal; *Cyclospora* on fruit; *Cryptosporidium* in drinking water; and hepatitis A in frozen strawberries. In 1997, 25 million pounds of hamburger suspected of harboring a disease-causing strain of *E. coli*—*E. coli* O157:H7—were voluntarily recalled by the food distributor. Although the American food supply may in fact be the safest in the world, it is not risk free or beyond improvement. It is estimated that 76 million people in the United States become ill, 325, 000 are hospitalized and 5,000 die each year from food-related illness.[1,2]

If given a choice, most people would elect to consume food that contains no harmful substances. However, it is nearly impossible to choose a diet that is free of all potential hazards. Food has always carried the risks of bacterial contamination and naturally occurring toxins. In the modern world, changes in agricultural technology, trade patterns, food processing, and dietary habits have increased the risks associated with bacterial contamination and introduced new risks. Regulatory agencies, food manufacturers and retailers, as well as consumers, must work together to maximize the safety of the food supply.

• WEIGHING THE RISKS AND BENEFITS

People need to eat to stay alive. However, an unsafe food supply can cause illness and even death. The risks of consuming a contaminated food must be weighed against the benefits that food provides. Risk-benefit analyses are done by regulatory agencies when they evaluate the safety and sanitation of food processing methods and food service establishments. Consumers must also consider the risks and benefits when they choose which foods to buy, which to eat, and how to handle, store, and cook these foods (Figure 17.1).

The Causes of Food-Borne Illness

Food-borne illness in the broadest sense is any illness that is related to the consumption of food or contaminants or toxins in food. However, most of the food-borne illness in the United States is caused by the contamination of food with **pathogens**, that is, microorganisms or microbes that can cause disease. **Toxins** produced by these microorganisms, as well as those present in the environment and those used in the processing and packaging of food, can also contaminate food and increase risk to the consumer.

Where Does Food Get Contaminated? Many foods are contaminated where they are grown or produced. *Salmonella enteritidis* may enter eggs directly from the hen. Fish and seafood may be contaminated by agricultural runoff, sewage, and other toxins

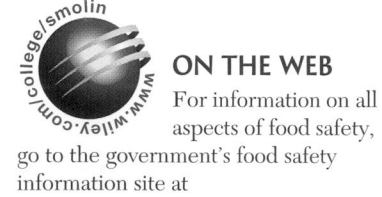

ON THE WEB
For information on all aspects of food safety, go to the government's food safety information site at
www.foodsafety.gov

Food-borne illness An illness caused by consumption of food containing a toxin or disease-causing microorganism.

Pathogen An organism capable of causing disease.

Toxins Substances that can cause harm at some level of exposure.

484

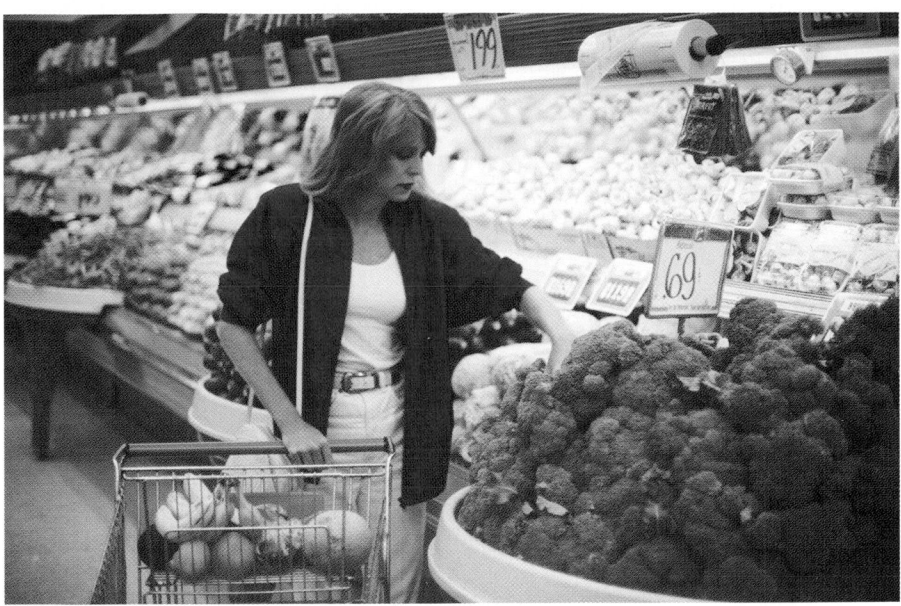

Figure 17.1
Choosing safe, nutritious foods is one way that consumers help control the safety of the foods they eat. (© 1999 PhotoDisc, Inc.)

in our waterways. Molds grow on grains during unusually wet or dry growing seasons. Food can also be contaminated during processing or storage, at retail facilities, and even at home. This often occurs by **cross-contamination** from a contaminated food or utensil to an uninfected one. For example, *E. coli* from a single cow can contaminate thousands of pounds of hamburger during processing. However, careful sanitation and handling can control most of these sources of food-borne illness. Regardless of the original source of contamination, most of the cases of food-borne illness are caused by foods prepared at home and can be prevented by safe food-handling procedures.[3]

Cross-contamination The transfer of contaminants from one food to another.

When Do Contaminants Make Us Sick? Even when a food is contaminated, it does not cause every individual who consumes it to become ill. The potential of a substance to cause harm depends on how potent it is, the amount or dose that is consumed, how frequently it is consumed, and who consumes it. Some contaminants in food cause harm even when minute amounts are consumed, and almost any substance can be toxic if a large enough amount is consumed. Many substances have a **threshold effect**; that is, they are harmless up to a certain dose or threshold, after which negative effects increase with increasing intake. Body size, nutritional status, and how a substance is metabolized by the body can affect toxicity. Small doses are more dangerous in children and small adults because the amount of toxin per unit of body weight is greater. Poor nutritional or health status may decrease the body's natural ability to detoxify harmful substances. Substances that are stored in the body are more likely to be toxic because they accumulate over time. They are deposited in bone, adipose tissue, the liver, or other organs until toxicity symptoms occur. Substances that are easily excreted when consumed in excess are less likely to cause toxicity. The interaction of toxins with one another and with other dietary factors also affects toxicity. For example, mercury, which is extremely toxic, is not absorbed well if the diet is high in selenium, and the absorption of lead is decreased by the presence of iron and calcium in the diet.

Threshold effect A reaction that occurs at a certain level of ingestion and increases as the dose increases. Below that level there is no reaction.

Safeguarding Our Food Supply

Concern about the safety of our food supply is not new. In the early 1900s, a novel by Upton Sinclair, *The Jungle*, caused a public outcry by its description of Chicago's meatpacking industry. Repulsive conditions in the rat-infested processing plants, where spoiled meat was processed alongside fresh, were revealed. This led to the passage of the nation's first food regulations, and since then the government has been involved in safeguarding the food supply.

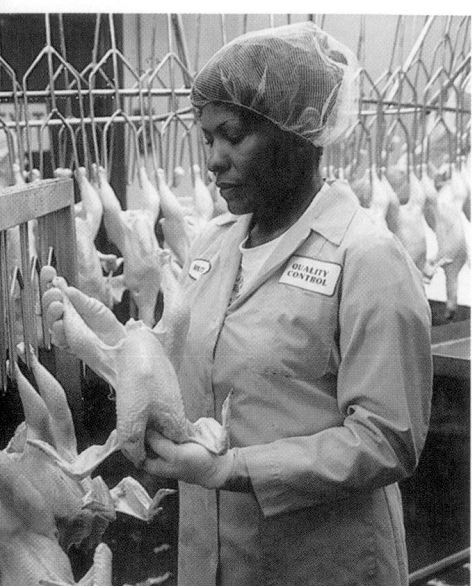

Figure 17.2
Traditional methods of protecting the food supply rely on spot-checks by food safety inspectors. (© Don Smetzer/Stone.)

Hazard Analysis Critical Control Point (HACCP) A food safety system that focuses on identifying and preventing hazards that could cause food-borne illness.

Critical control points Possible points in food production, manufacturing, and transportation at which contamination could occur or be prevented.

Pasteurization The process of heating food products to kill disease-causing organisms.

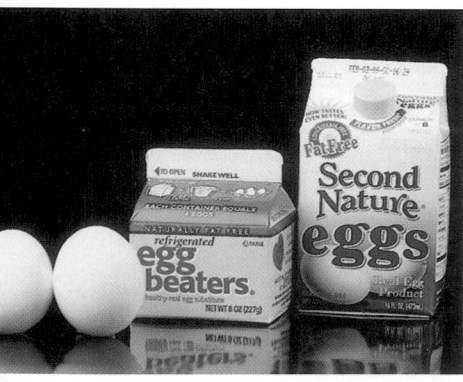

Figure 17.3
Salmonella contamination is a concern in the production of frozen eggs. (George Semple)

Traditional methods for monitoring food safety involve conducting spot-checks of manufacturing conditions and products (Figure 17.2). These spot-checks often rely on visual inspection to detect contamination. Recently, media coverage of large outbreaks of food-borne illnesses has heightened concern about food safety and encouraged regulatory agencies and food manufacturers to establish a better system for safeguarding the food supply. These concerns have been addressed at the federal level in the National Food Safety Initiative, which targets all aspects of food safety from the farm to the table. This program promotes the implementation of a system called **Hazard Analysis Critical Control Point (HACCP)**. HACCP is designed to prevent food contamination rather than catch it after it occurs.

National Food Safety Initiative The National Food Safety Initiative was conceived to reduce the incidence of food-borne illness by improving food safety practices and policies throughout the United States. The focus is on reducing the risk of microbial food-borne illness. However, the initiative also recognizes that chemical contaminants can cause food-borne illness.[4]

The Food Safety Initiative also established a national computer network linking public health laboratories. This enables epidemiologists to quickly respond to serious and widespread food contamination problems.[5] With this system, the distinctive DNA fingerprint of a pathogenic strain of a microorganism can be tracked. For example, if outbreaks of food-borne illness in Ohio and Minnesota are both caused by the same strain of an organism, epidemiologists know that the outbreaks were caused by the same food source. They can focus their search for the source of contamination on foods distributed to both locations. To confirm the source, the DNA fingerprint isolated from the organisms found in victims can be matched to the DNA fingerprint from a contaminated food source.

HACCP The HACCP approach to food safety involves establishing standardized procedures to prevent, control, or eliminate contamination before food reaches the consumers. It is based on identifying points in the handling of food, called **critical control points**, where chemical, physical, or microbial contamination can occur.

The HACCP system allows companies to anticipate where contamination will occur and to prevent the food hazard from reaching the consumer. For example, contamination with *Salmonella* has been identified as a risk in the production of shelled frozen eggs. To produce this product, eggs are removed from their shells; mixed together in large vats; heated, in a process called **pasteurization**, to kill *Salmonella* and other microbial contaminants; packaged; and then frozen (Figure 17.3). The critical control point for preventing contaminated eggs from getting to consumers is the pasteurization process. To monitor the effectiveness of pasteurization in the frozen egg industry, bacterial tests are performed on samples of eggs following pasteurization. All the eggs are held refrigerated or frozen until the results of the bacterial tests have been obtained. If the eggs are *Salmonella*-free, they are released to the market. If they contain *Salmonella*, the entire batch of eggs cannot be sold and pasteurization conditions are adjusted to ensure that *Salmonella* is killed in the next batch. Extensive record keeping enables the manufacturer to trace which eggs were pasteurized when, for how long, and at what temperature, and when and where they were shipped in the event of an outbreak of food-borne illness.

The advantages of the HACCP system over standard inspections by the FDA are that the plan is preventative rather than punitive, oversight is easier, and the responsibility for food safety is placed on the manufacturer, not the regulatory agencies.

Monitoring Foods from Farm to Table The safety of the food supply is monitored by agencies at the international, federal, state, and local levels (Table 17.1). International cooperation on food inspection and regulatory standards helps to ensure the safety of imported foods. Approximately 40 different nations are now partners

Table 17.1 *Agencies Responsible for Food Safety*

Agency	Responsibility
World Health Organization (WHO)	Develops international food safety policies, food inspection programs, and standards for hygienic food preparation; promotes technologies that improve food safety and consumer education about safe food practices.
Food and Drug Administration (FDA) at the Department of Health and Human Services (DHHS)	Ensures the safety and wholesomeness of all foods sold across state lines with the exception of red meat (beef, veal, pork, and lamb), poultry, and egg products; inspects food-processing plants; inspects imported foods with the exception of red meat, poultry, and egg products; sets standards for food composition; oversees use of drugs and feed in food-producing animals; and enforces regulations for food labeling, food and color additives, and food sanitation.
Food Safety and Inspection Service (FSIA) at the U.S. Department of Agriculture) (USDA)	Enforces standards for the wholesomeness and quality of red meat, poultry, and egg products, including that imported from other countries. If a food is suspect, it can be tested for contamination, and entry into the country can be denied.
Environmental Protection Agency (EPA)	Regulates pesticide levels and must approve all pesticides before they can be sold in the United States; establishes water quality standards.
National Marine Fisheries Service at the Department of Commerce	Oversees the management of fisheries and fish harvesting. Operates a voluntary program of inspection and grading of fish products.
Animal and Plant Health Inspection Service (APHIS) at the USDA	Monitors disease in food-producing animals.
Centers for Disease Control and Prevention (CDC) at DHHS	Monitors and investigates the incidence and causes of food-borne diseases.
Bureau of Alcohol, Tobacco, and Firearms (ATF) at the Department of the Treasury	Enforces laws regulating the production, distribution, and labeling of alcoholic beverages.
State and local governments	Inspect food-processing plants, grocery stores, restaurants, and institutions such as schools and hospitals.

with the United States in ensuring food safety through agreements that regulate a variety of food products. In the United States, federal agencies monitor various segments of the food supply. These agencies set standards and establish regulations for the safe and sanitary handling of food and water. They also set standards for safe-handling information on food labels. They regulate the use of agricultural chemicals, additives, and packaging materials; inspect food processing and storage facilities; monitor both domestic and imported foods for contamination; and investigate outbreaks of food-borne illness (see *Off the Shelf*: Mad Cow Disease: Should You Be Concerned?). State agencies have the primary responsibility for milk safety and the inspection of restaurants, retail food stores, dairies, grain mills, and other food-related establishments within their borders (Figure 17.4). As a result, regulations vary from state to state. However, the U.S. Food and Drug Administration (FDA) publishes the **Food Code** which provides recommendations for safeguarding public health when food is offered to the consumer.

Consumers must also be actively involved in preventing food-borne illness. Individuals must decide what foods they will consume and evaluate the risks involved. A food that has been manufactured, packaged, and transported with the greatest care can still cause food-borne illness if it is not carefully handled at home. For example, contaminated foods such as eggs, chicken, or hamburger can cause microbial food-borne illness if they are not thoroughly cooked. Consumers can also protect them-

Food Code A set of recommendations published by the FDA for the handling and service of food sold in restaurants and other establishments that serve food.

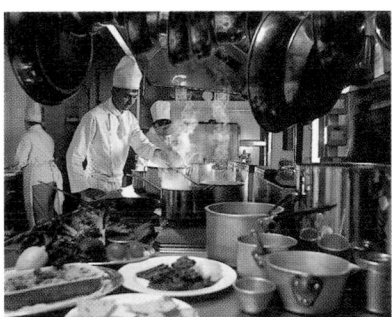

Figure 17.4
State and local governments are responsible for regulating the safety of food sold at restaurants. (John Miller/ Stone)

Off the Shelf
Mad Cow Disease—Should You Be Concerned?

Mad cow disease, or bovine spongiform encephalopathy (BSE), is a degenerative neurological disease that affects cattle. Symptoms begin with weight loss and changes in temperament. Within weeks or months, the animal is dead. It was first diagnosed in England in 1986 and has now spread to other parts of Europe. Within 10 years of its appearance in cattle, a human form of this untreatable, incurable, and always fatal disease was identified. How concerned should U.S. residents be?

Bovine Spongiform Encephalopathy

BSE belongs to a group of diseases called transmissible spongiform encephalopathies (TSEs). These include scrapie in sheep, chronic wasting syndrome in elk and deer, and kuru and Creutzfeldt-Jakob Disease (CJD) in humans. These diseases are characterized by a long incubation period, up to 20 years, during which there is no sign of infection. They cause changes that give the brain a spongelike appearance. Epidemiological research has determined that BSE originated from sheep that carried scrapie, which has been present in British sheep for about 200 years. It is believed to have moved into cattle when the remains of slaughtered diseased sheep began to be included in protein supplements that were fed to cattle. These supplements were banned in the UK in 1988 to prevent further spread of BSE. However, due to the long incubation period, the frequency of new cases did not start to decline until late 1993.

From Cows to Humans

In March 1996, ten cases of the human disease CJD were reported in Britain. CJD is a degenerative disease of the nervous system that may begin with mood swings and numbness and always progresses to dementia and death.[1] There is a genetic form of CJD, but most cases occur sporadically around the world at a rate of about one case per million per year. The ten British cases resembled classical forms of CJD, but there were

differences. This now-termed variant form of CJD (vCJD) affected younger patients (average age of 29 years, as opposed to 65 years), and the course of the disease was slower (a median of 14 months from first symptoms until death as opposed to 4.5 months). In addition, vCJD was linked to exposure to BSE, probably through food. Thus, within 10 years, BSE had crossed the species barrier to humans. As of early December 2000, the CJD surveillance unit for the United Kingdom had reported 81 cases of vCJD.[2]

A New Infectious Agent?

For many years the cause of TSEs was unknown. In 1972, Dr. Stanley Prusiner at the University of California began searching for the infectious agent that causes CJD. He was expecting to find a virus, but 10 years later he had isolated a protein that he called a prion, short for proteinaceous infectious particle. The scientific community did not readily accept his discovery because prions challenge a basic principle of biology—that every entity capable of reproducing itself must contain either DNA or RNA. A prion would have to carry, in a protein alone, information that could be transferred from one protein to another. Prusiner was awarded the 1997 Nobel Prize in Medicine for his work.

The aberrant prions identified in TSEs can be thought of as the "evil twin" of a normal protein that is present in healthy nerve cells. The difference between the normal protein and its evil twin lies in the way the protein is folded. The abnormal prion proteins are not degraded normally, so they accumulate, forming clumps called plaques. These plaques damage nerve tissue. The aberrant prions can be passed on to an uninfected host, most likely from consumption of a food product containing central nervous system tissue from a diseased animal.[3] It has been shown that prions are stable to freezing, drying, irradiation, and heating. Thus far, meat and milk have not been demonstrated to transmit BSE or vCJD, and direct transmission from one human to another is thought to be unlikely.

Should We Be Concerned?

As of this writing, BSE has not been diagnosed in U.S. cattle. The reason for this is a combination of luck and vigilance by government agencies. In the 1950s the United States banned the import of sheep and goats from Britain. This ruling, which was imposed to prevent the spread of scrapie, most likely also prevented BSE from entering the country. In 1989, three years after BSE was identified in Britain, the USDA placed restrictions on the import of all ruminants from countries where BSE was known to exist. And in 1997, the USDA took further steps by restricting the import of ruminants and most ruminant products from all of Europe.[4] In addition to blocking the entry of products potentially carrying this disease, the United States has taken steps to block transmission. To prevent animal-to-animal transmission, mammalian proteins cannot be used in protein supplements for animal feeds. To prevent human-to-human exposure, blood donations are not accepted from individuals who spent substantial time in Europe in the 1980s. In addition, it has been recommended that vaccine manufacturers not use bovine products from countries where BSE has been reported. Because of these precautions, the risk of animals being exposed to BSE and humans contracting vCJD in the United States remains extremely low.

[1]U.S. Department of Agriculture, Animal and Plant Health Inspection Service. Bovine Spongiform Encephalopathy. Available online at www.aphis.usda.gov/oa/bse/ Accessed March 2, 2001.

[2]World Health Organization. Variant Creutzfeldt-Jakob Disease (vCJD) Fact Sheet. Revised December 2000. Available online at www.who.int/inf-fs/en/fact180.html/ Accessed March 4, 2001.

[3]Mad cow and human prion disease. *Neuro News*, May 18, 1998. Available online at neuroscience.about.com/science/neuroscience/library/weekly/aa051898.htm/ Accessed March 5, 2001.

[4]Bren, L. Trying to keep mad cow disease out of U.S. herds. *FDA Consumer*, March/April 2001. Available online at www.fda.gov/fdac/features/2001/201_cow.html/ Accessed March 6, 2001.

Table 17.2   *How to Report an Incident Involving Unsanitary, Unsafe, Deceptive, or Mislabeled Food*

First, get all the facts. Have you used the product as intended and according to the manufacturer's instructions? Check to be sure the item is not being used past its expiration date. Once these steps have been taken, **report the incident to the appropriate agency:**

- **Problems relating to any food except meat and poultry,** including adverse reactions, should be reported to the FDA Food and Seafood Information line (1–800–332–4010). If it is an emergency requiring immediate action, such as a case of food-borne illness, call the FDA's emergency number (1–301–443–1240). For a problem not requiring immediate attention, the FDA district office consumer complaint coordinator for your geographic area can be contacted.[1]

- **Issues relating to meat and poultry** should be reported first to your state's department of agriculture and then to the USDA hotline (1–800–535–4555).

- **Restaurant food and sanitation** problems can be reported directly to local or state health departments.

- **Issues related to alcoholic beverages** should be reported to the Department of the Treasury's Bureau of Alcohol, Tobacco, and Firearms.

- **Accidental poisonings** should be reported to state or local poison control centers or hospitals before calling the Centers for Disease Control and Prevention.

- **Pesticide, air, and water pollution** should be reported first to your state's environmental protection department and then to the EPA.

- **Products purchased at the grocery store** should be returned to the store. Grocery stores are concerned with the safety of the foods they sell, and they will take the responsibility of tracking down and correcting the problem as well as refunding your money or replacing the product with one that is safe.

- **Hazardous household products** are the responsibility of the state department of consumer protection and, federally, the Consumer Product Safety Commission (www.cpsc.gov/).

- **False advertising** should be reported first to your state's department of consumer protection and then to the Federal Trade Commission.

- **Unsolicited products in the mail** should be reported to the U.S. Postal Service.

[1]How to report adverse reactions and other problems with products regulated by FDA. *FDA Backgrounder*, April 29, 1998. Online at www.fda.gov/opacom/backgrounders/problem.html

selves and others by reporting incidents involving unsanitary, unsafe, deceptive, or mislabeled food to the appropriate agencies (Table 17.2).

• PATHOGENS IN FOOD

Food-borne illness can be caused by consuming food contaminated with bacteria, viruses, molds, or parasites, or by consuming foods contaminated with toxins produced by these organisms (Table 17.3). In most cases, the symptoms of a microbial food-borne illness include abdominal pain, nausea, diarrhea, and vomiting. These relatively mild symptoms are often mistaken for the flu. Food-borne illness can also cause more severe symptoms such as spontaneous abortion; hemolytic uremia syndrome, which can lead to kidney failure and death; and long-lasting conditions like arthritis and Guillain-Barré syndrome, which is the most common cause of acute paralysis in adults and children. Young children, pregnant women, elderly persons, and individuals with compromised immune systems, such as AIDS and cancer patients, are most susceptible to severe reactions.[1] Avoiding microbial food-borne illness requires a knowledge of how contamination occurs and how to handle, store, and prepare food safely.

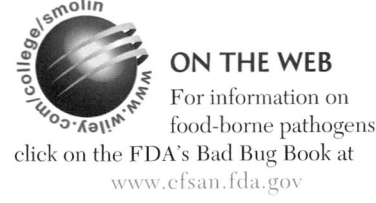

ON THE WEB
For information on food-borne pathogens click on the FDA's Bad Bug Book at
www.cfsan.fda.gov

Bacteria

Bacteria are present in the soil, on our skin, on most surfaces in our homes, and in the food we eat. Most of the bacteria in our environment are harmless, some are

Table 17.3 *Which Bug Has You Down?*

Microbe	Sources	Symptoms	Onset	Duration
Bacteria				
Salmonella	Fecal contamination, raw or undercooked eggs and meat, especially poultry	Nausea, abdominal pain, diarrhea, headache, fever	6–48 hrs	1–2 days
Campylobacter jejuni	Unpasteurized milk, undercooked meat and poultry	Fever, headache, diarrhea, abdominal pain	2–5 days	1–2 wks
Listeria monocytogenes	Raw milk products, raw and undercooked poultry and meats, raw and smoked fish, produce	Fever, headache, stiff neck, chills, nausea, vomiting	Days to weeks	6 wks
Vibrio vulnificus	Raw seafood from contaminated water	Cramps, abdominal pain, weakness, watery diarrhea, fever, chills	15–24 hrs	2–4 days
Staphylococcus aureus	Human contamination from coughs and sneezes, eggs, meat, potato and macaroni salads	Severe nausea, vomiting, diarrhea	2–8 hrs	24–48 hrs
Escherichia coli O157:H7	Fecal contamination, undercooked ground beef	Abdominal pain, bloody diarrhea, kidney failure	5–48 hrs	3 days to 2 wks or longer
Clostridium perfringens	Fecal contamination, deep-dish casseroles	Fever, nausea, diarrhea, abdominal pain	8–22 hrs	6–24 hrs
Clostridium botulinum	Canned foods, deep casseroles, honey	Lassitude, weakness, vertigo, dizziness, respiratory failure, paralysis	18–36 hrs	10 days or longer (must administer antitoxin)
Shigella	Fecal contamination of water or foods, especially salads such as chicken, tuna, shrimp, and potato salad	Diarrhea, abdominal pain, fever, vomiting	12–50 hrs	5–6 days
Yersinia enterocolitica	Pork, dairy products, and produce	Diarrhea, vomiting, fever, abdominal pain; often mistaken for appendicitis	24–48 hrs	Weeks
Viruses				
Norwalk virus	Fecal contamination of seafood	Diarrhea, nausea, vomiting	1–2 days	2–6 days
Hepatitis A virus	Human fecal contamination of food or water, raw shellfish	Jaundice, liver inflammation, fatigue, fever, nausea, anorexia, abdominal discomfort	10–50 days	1–2 wks to several months
Parasites				
Giardia lamblia	Fecal contamination of water and uncooked foods	Diarrhea, abdominal pain, gas, anorexia, nausea, vomiting	5–25 days	1–2 wks but may become chronic
Cryptosporidium parvum	Fecal contamination of food or water	Severe watery diarrhea	Hours	2–4 days but sometimes weeks
Trichinella spiralis	Undercooked pork, game meat	Muscle weakness, flu symptoms	Weeks	Months
Anisakis simplex	Raw fish	Severe abdominal pain	1 hr to 2 wks	3 wks
Toxoplasma gondii	Meat, primarily pork	Toxoplasmosis (can cause central nervous system disorders, flu-like symptoms, and birth defects in women exposed during pregnancy)	10–23 days	May become chronic carrier

Source: U.S. Food and Drug Administration, Center for Food Safety and Nutrition. Foodborne Pathogenic Microorganisms and Natural Toxins Handbook: The "Bad Bug Book." Online at vm.cfsan.fda.gov/~mow/intro.html

beneficial, and some are pathogenic, causing disease either by growing in the gastrointestinal tract or by producing toxins.

Food-borne infection Illness produced by the ingestion of food containing microorganisms that can multiply inside the body and produce injurious effects.

Bacterial Food-Borne Infection **Food-borne infection** is caused when a food containing pathogenic bacteria is ingested and the bacteria grow in the gastrointestinal tract. These bacteria may also grow in other tissues or produce toxins within the body. Usually a large number of bacteria must be consumed to cause illness. Some common causes of bacterial infections include *Salmonella*, *Escherichia coli*, *Campylobacter jejuni*, *Listeria monocytogenes*, and *Vibrio vulnificus*.

It is estimated that 1.4 million people are infected with *Salmonella* each year in the United States. Most of these people just experience diarrhea, but sometimes more serious infections can be fatal. *Salmonella* is found in animal and human feces and infects food through contaminated water or improper handling. *Salmonella* outbreaks have been caused by contaminated meat, meat products, dairy products, seafood, fresh vegetables, and cereal, but poultry and eggs are the most common food sources. Poultry products are often contaminated because poultry farms house large numbers of chickens in close proximity, allowing one infected chicken to infect thousands of others. A new way to reduce infection is to spray chicks with beneficial bacteria (Figure 17.5). The FDA has approved the use of a spray that includes 29 types of living, nontoxic bacteria that are present in the normal gut of adult chickens. The chicks ingest the bacteria when they preen their feathers and the bacteria colonize the digestive tract, leaving no room for pathogens. The spray prevents chicks from being infected with *Salmonella*, *Listeria*, and *E. coli O157:H7*.

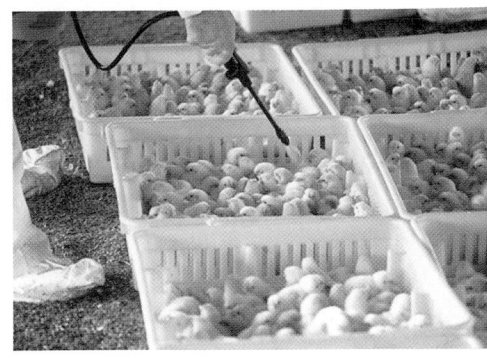

Figure 17.5

A shower of beneficial bacteria prevents chicks from being infected with bacteria that are pathogenic to humans. (Agricultural Research Service/USDA)

Even if food contaminated with *Salmonella* is brought into the kitchen, careful handling and cooking of the food can prevent the organisms from causing illness. Washing hands, cutting boards, and utensils can prevent cross-contamination. If a contaminated food is stored in the refrigerator, the multiplication of the *Salmonella* will be slowed. If a contaminated food is left at room temperature, the *Salmonella* will multiply rapidly, and when the food is ingested, large numbers of bacteria will be ingested with it. *Salmonella* is killed by heat—so foods likely to be contaminated, such as poultry and eggs, should be cooked thoroughly.

Escherichia coli (*E. coli*) is a bacterium that inhabits the gastrointestinal tracts of humans and other animals. It comes in contact with food through fecal contamination of water or unsanitary handling of food. Some strains of *E coli* are harmless, but others can cause serious food-borne illness. One strain of *E. coli*, found in water contaminated by human or animal feces, is the cause of "travelers' diarrhea." Another strain, *E. coli O157:H7*, produces a toxin that causes abdominal pain, bloody diarrhea, and, in severe cases, kidney failure and even death. This strain was responsible for the deaths of several children who consumed undercooked, contaminated hamburgers from a fast-food chain in 1993. In 1996, unpasteurized apple juice contaminated with *E. coli O157:H7* caused illness in 66 people and the death of one child.

Although *E. coli* on food can multiply slowly even at refrigerator temperatures, if a contaminated food is thoroughly cooked to 160°F, both the bacteria and the toxin are destroyed. Ground beef contaminated with *E. coli O157:H7* is a particular risk because, unlike other meats that are likely only to be contaminated on the surface, the grinding mixes the bacteria throughout the meat. The *E. coli* on the outside of the meat are quickly killed during cooking, but those in the interior survive if the meat is not cooked thoroughly. Transmission of *E. coli* is a risk at day-care centers from cross-contamination if caregivers do not carefully wash their hands after diaper changes.

Two species of *Campylobacter*, *Campylobacter jejuni* and *Campylobacter coli*, also cause food-borne infection. *Campylobacter* is the most frequent cause of acute infectious diarrhea in developed countries.[3] Common sources are undercooked chicken, unpasteurized milk, and untreated water. This organism grows slowly in the cold and is killed by heat, so, as with *Salmonella*, thorough cooking and careful storage help prevent infection.

Another cause of bacterial infection is *Listeria monocytogenes*. Although most cases of *Listeria* infection result in flu-like symptoms, in high-risk groups such as pregnant women, children, the elderly, and the ill, it can cause meningitis and serious blood infections and has one of the highest fatality rates of all food-borne illnesses. *Listeria* is a very resistant organism that survives at higher and lower temperatures than most bacteria; it can survive and grow at refrigerator temperatures. *Listeria* frequently contaminates dairy products, but it is destroyed by pasteurization. It is found in processed ready-to-eat foods such as hot dogs and lunchmeats. Because consumers consider ready-to-eat foods safe, they often do not handle them as carefully as raw foods. To prevent infection, ready-to-eat meats should be heated to steaming and unpasteurized dairy products should be avoided.

Vibrio vulnificus infection usually causes gastrointestinal upset but can be deadly in vulnerable populations. The bacteria are most common in mollusks such as oysters, clams, and mussels harvested from the Gulf of Mexico in the summer when the water is most likely to be contaminated with human fecal matter. Foods that pose a risk include raw and undercooked seafood.

Food-borne intoxication Illness caused by consuming a food containing a toxin.

Bacterial Food-Borne Intoxication **Food-borne intoxication** is caused by consuming food containing toxins produced by microbes. The symptoms of food-borne intoxication are caused by the toxin, not the organism itself. Unlike food infections, which are usually caused by ingesting large numbers of bacteria, intoxication can be caused by only a few microorganisms that have produced a toxin. Although the bacteria are fairly easy to kill, some food toxins may be difficult to destroy.

Staphylococcus aureus is a common cause of microbial food-borne intoxication. These bacteria live in human nasal passages and can be transferred through coughing or sneezing when handling food. Foods that are common sources include cooked ham, salads, bakery products, and dairy products.

The bacterium *Clostridium perfringens* may cause illness by both infection and intoxication. It is found in soil and in the intestines of animals and humans. It thrives in conditions with little oxygen (anaerobic conditions) and is difficult to kill because it forms heat-resistant **spores**, which are a stage of bacterial life that remains dormant until environmental conditions favor growth. *Clostridium perfringens* is often called the "cafeteria germ" because foods stored in large containers have anaerobic centers that provide an excellent growth environment. Sources include improperly prepared roast beef, turkey, pork, chicken, and ground beef.

Spore A dormant state of some bacteria that is resistant to heat but can germinate and produce a new organism when environmental conditions are favorable.

Another strain of *Clostridium*, *Clostridium botulinum*, produces the deadliest bacterial food toxin. Although the bacteria themselves are not harmful, the toxin, produced as the spores begin to grow and develop, blocks nerve function, resulting in vomiting, abdominal pain, double vision, dizziness, and paralysis causing respiratory failure. If untreated, botulism poisoning is often fatal, but today modern detection methods and rapid administration of antitoxin have reduced mortality. Low-acid foods, such as potatoes or stew, that are held in anaerobic conditions provide optimal conditions for botulism spores to germinate. Canned foods, particularly improperly home-canned foods, can also be a source of botulism. Canned foods should be discarded if the can is bulging because this indicates the presence of gas produced by bacteria as they grow. Once formed, botulism toxin can be destroyed by boiling, but if the safety of a food is in question, it should be discarded; even a taste of botulism toxin can be deadly.

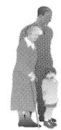

The most common form of botulism is infant botulism.[6] It occurs when ingested botulism spores germinate in the body, producing toxin, some of which is absorbed into the bloodstream causing weakness, paralysis, and respiratory problems. Only infants are affected because in adults competing intestinal microflora prevent spore germinations. Because botulism spores can contaminate honey, it should never be fed to infants under one year of age.

Viruses

Viruses Minute particles not visible under an ordinary microscope that depend on cells for their metabolic and reproductive needs.

Viruses are easily spread. They come in contact with food when it is contaminated with human or animal feces. To reproduce, viruses require living cells. Although the viruses that cause human disease cannot grow and reproduce in foods, they can contaminate foods and then infect the consumer.

Shellfish are notorious carriers of viral infections. Norwalk virus, found in water polluted with human or animal feces, causes most of the gastrointestinal illness that results from eating mollusks and other shellfish.[7] Because Norwalk virus is destroyed by cooking, water and uncooked foods such as raw shellfish and salads are the most common cause of food-borne illness from this virus.

Hepatitis A is a highly contagious viral disorder that can be contracted from food contaminated by unsanitary handling or from eating raw or undercooked shellfish caught in sewage-contaminated waters. Hepatitis A can require a long recovery period and, in some cases, results in permanent liver damage. Individuals who have contracted the hepatitis A virus may remain carriers for years. Hepatitis in drinking water is destroyed by chlorination. Cooking destroys the virus in food, and good sanitation can prevent its spread (Figure 17.6).

Molds

Many types of **molds** grow on foods such as bread, cheese, and fruit. Molds produce toxins that can lead to food intoxication. Aflatoxin is a mold toxin that is among the most potent mutagens and carcinogens known. Another mold toxin that contaminates grain, particularly rye, is ergot. It causes hallucinations and is a natural source of the hallucinogenic drug LSD. Today, modern milling removes the part of the grain that harbors the mold, so the disease ergotism is rare. Cooking and freezing stops mold growth but does not destroy the mold toxins that have already been produced. If a food is moldy, it should be discarded, the area where it was stored should be cleaned, and neighboring foods should be checked to see if they have also become contaminated.

Parasites

Some **parasites** are single-celled animals, while others are worms that can be seen with the naked eye. Parasites are killed by thorough cooking. Most infections occur by exposing fresh food to contaminated water. *Giardia lamblia* is a single-celled parasite that is the most frequent cause of diarrhea not due to bacteria.[8] *Giardia* is sometimes contracted by hikers who drink untreated water from streams contaminated with animal feces, and it is becoming a problem from cross-contamination in day-care centers. *Cryptosporidium parvum* is another parasite that is commonly spread by contaminated water, but cases have also been reported from unpasteurized apple juice and homemade chicken salad.[9,10]

Trichinella spiralis is a parasite found in raw and undercooked pork, pork products, and game meats, particularly bear. Once ingested, these small, wormlike organisms find their way to the muscles, where they grow, causing flu-like symptoms, muscle weakness, fever, and fluid retention. Trichinosis, the disease caused by *Trichinella* infection, can be prevented by thoroughly cooking meat to kill the parasite before it is ingested. The parasites are also destroyed by curing, smoking, canning, or freezing.

Fish are a common source of parasitic infections. Fish can carry the larvae (a wormlike stage of an organism's life cycle) of parasites such as roundworms, flatworms, flukes, and tapeworms. One such infection, Anisakis disease, is caused by the larval form of the small roundworm *Anisakis simplex,* or herring worm, found in raw fish.[8] Once consumed, these parasites invade the stomach and intestinal tract, causing severe abdominal pain. As the popularity of eating raw fish has increased, so has the incidence of parasitic infections from fish. The fresher the fish is when it is eviscerated, the less likely it is to cause this disease because the larvae move from the fish's stomach to its flesh only after the fish dies. Parasitic infections from fish can be avoided by consuming cooked fish or freezing fish for 72 hours before consumption. If raw fish is consumed, it should be very fresh (Figure 17.7).

Reducing the Risks: From Store to Table

Despite the variety of organisms that can cause food-borne illness, most cases can be avoided if food is handled properly. Just as manufacturers are asked to identify critical control points in food handling where contamination can be prevented and monitored, consumers can take a similar approach in selecting, storing, preparing, and serving food and leftovers (Figure 17.8; see Table 17.4).

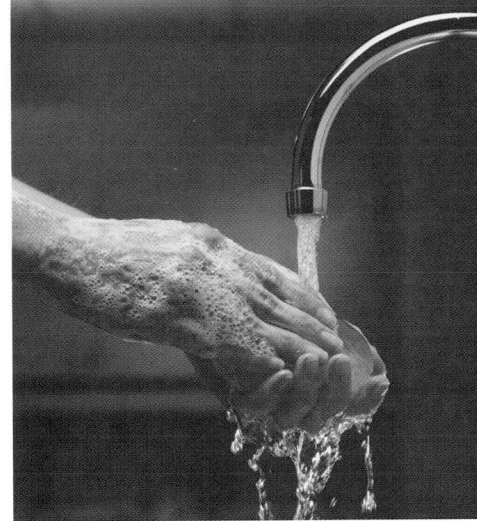

Figure 17.6
Good sanitation when preparing food is important for preventing food-borne illness. (© Dick Clintsman/Corbis)

Molds Multicellular fungi that form a filamentous branching growth.

Parasites Organisms that live at the expense of others without contributing to the survival of the host.

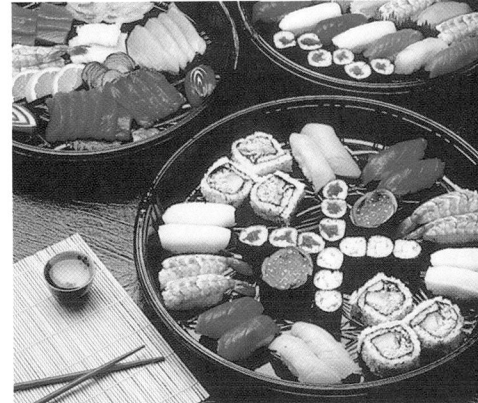

Figure 17.7
The incidence of parasitic infections has increased with the popularity of raw fish, such as this sushi. (R. Pleasant/FPG International)

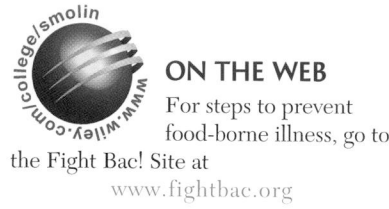

FIGHT BAC!

Keep Food Safe From Bacteria

Separate Don't cross-contaminate.

Clean Wash hands and surfaces often.

Chill Refrigerate promptly.

Cook Cook to proper temperatures.

Figure 17.8

The Fight Bac! Educational campaign recommends that consumers follow four steps—clean, separate, cook, and chill—to prevent food-borne illness.

ON THE WEB

For steps to prevent food-borne illness, go to the Fight Bac! Site at www.fightbac.org

www.wiley.com/college/smolin

Selecting Safe Foods The first critical control point in preventing food-borne illness is making safe selections at the store to reduce the contaminants that are brought into the home. Food should come from reputable vendors and appear fresh. Frozen foods should not contain frost or ice crystals, and food packaging should be secure. Foods that are discolored or smell contaminated and those in damaged packages should not be purchased or consumed. Most packaged products are dated as either "sell by" or "use by." A "sell by" date indicates when the grocery store should take the product off the shelf. A "use by" date indicates the date by which the product should be consumed. Although dates are helpful, they do not ensure food safety.

Table 17.4 *Tips for Handling Food Safely*

Choose wisely

Jars should be closed and seals unbroken. Cans should not be rusted, dented, or bulging. Check product expiration dates. Select frozen foods from below the frost line in the freezer.

Store foods properly

Fresh or frozen foods brought from the store should be refrigerated or frozen immediately. Food that has been in your refrigerator for longer than is safe should be discarded.

Wash

Hands, cooking utensils, and surfaces should be washed with warm soapy water before each food preparation step. This will prevent cross-contamination.

Thaw

Thaw foods in the refrigerator or microwave.

Cook thoroughly

Thorough cooking destroys most bacteria, toxins, viruses, and parasites. Use a meat thermometer.

Refrigerate promptly

Cooked food can be recontaminated, so it should be refrigerated as soon as possible after it is served.

Reheat thoroughly

Thorough reheating to 165°F will destroy microorganisms that have recontaminated cooked foods and toxins that have been produced.

When in doubt, throw it out.

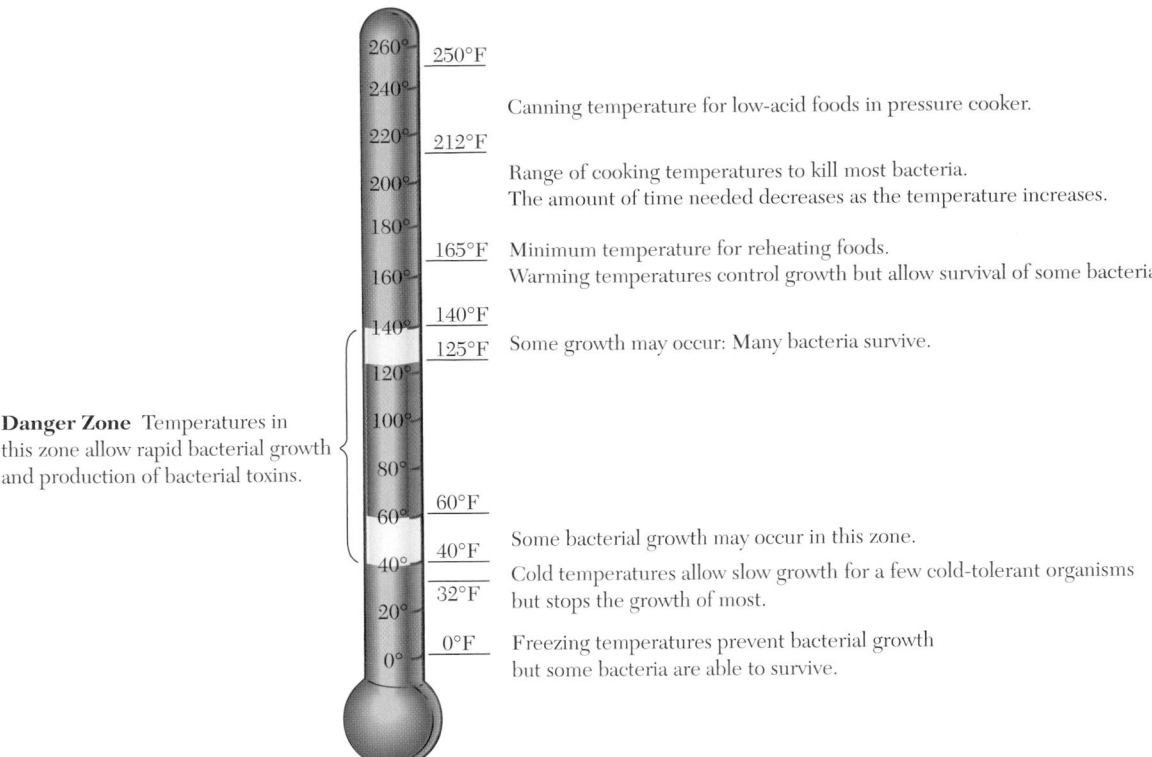

Figure 17.9
The effect of temperature on bacterial growth.

Safe Food Storage Storage is another critical control point in the home. Proper storage both before and after cooking can reduce the risk of food-borne illness. When shopping, cold foods should be purchased last and refrigerated or frozen as quickly as possible. Cold foods should be kept cold, at 40°F or less, and hot foods should be kept hot, greater than 140°F. The goal is to keep foods from setting at temperatures which promote bacterial growth (Figure 17.9). Refrigerator temperature should be set between 38° and 40°F and freezers at 0°F. Produce should be stored in the refrigerator. Fresh meat, poultry, and fish should be frozen immediately if it will not be used within a day or two. Processed meats such as hot dogs and bologna must also be kept refrigerated but can be kept longer than fresh meat.

Preparing and Serving Food Safely The next critical control point is preparation. A clean kitchen is essential for safe food preparation. Hands, countertops, cutting boards, and utensils should be washed with warm soapy water before each food preparation step. Food should be thawed in the refrigerator, in the microwave oven, or under running water—not at room temperature. Foods that are going to be cooked should not be prepared on the same surfaces as foods that are eaten raw. For example, if a chicken contaminated with *Salmonella* is cut up on a cutting board and the unwashed cutting board is then used to chop vegetables for a salad, the vegetables will become contaminated with *Salmonella*. When the chicken is cooked, the bacteria will be killed, but the contaminated vegetables are not cooked, so the bacteria can grow and cause food-borne illness. Cross-contamination can also occur when uncooked foods containing live microbes come in contact with foods that have already been cooked. Therefore, cooked meat should never be returned to the same dish that held the raw meat, and sauces used to marinate uncooked foods should never be used as a sauce on cooked food. Meat packaging is labeled with safe handling guidelines (Figure 17.10).

Cooking food thoroughly is one of the most important control points in the home because heat will destroy most harmful microorganisms. A meat thermometer

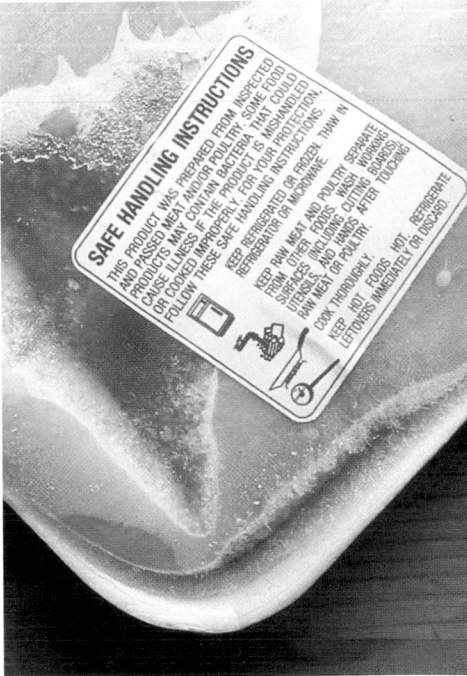

Figure 17.10
Meat carries labels offering safe handling guidelines. (Dennis Drenner)

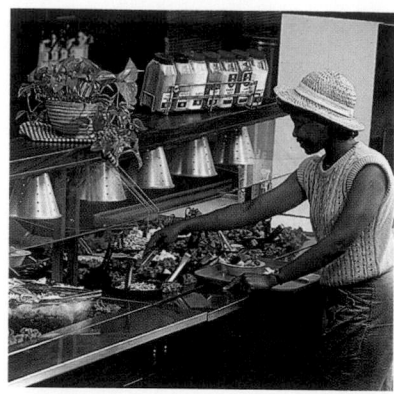

Figure 17.11
Clear plastic shields, or "sneeze guards," above salad bars prevent customers from contaminating food with microorganisms transmitted by coughs and sneezes. (© Charles Gupton/Stone)

should be used because color is not a good indicator of safety. Red meat and fish should be cooked to an internal temperature of 160°F and poultry to 180°F. Shellfish should be cooked to an internal temperature of 145°C for 15 seconds. Eggs should not be eaten raw, since *Salmonella* can contaminate the inside of the shell; they should be boiled for 7 minutes, poached for 5 minutes, or fried for 3 minutes on a side.

Handling of Leftovers Cooked food should be refrigerated as soon as possible after serving. The best temperatures for bacterial growth are the temperatures at which food usually sets between service and storage. Large portions of food should be divided before refrigeration so they will cool quickly. When leftovers are reheated, they should be heated thoroughly to destroy any bacteria that may have grown in them.

Food Safety Away from Home Although most of the food-borne illness in the United States is caused by food prepared in homes, an outbreak in a commercial or institutional establishment usually involves more people at a time and is more likely to be reported. Food in retail establishments has many opportunities to be contaminated because of the large volume of food that is handled and the large number of people involved in food preparation.

Even when a restaurant uses extreme care in food preparation, customers can be a source of contamination. Because customers serve themselves at salad bars, cross-contamination from one customer to another is a risk. Salad and dessert bars in restaurants are usually equipped with "sneeze guards"—clear plastic shields placed above the food to prevent contamination from coughs and sneezes (Figure 17.11). Customers are also asked to use a clean plate if they go back for second helpings.

Picnics and other large events where food is served provide a prime opportunity for microbes to flourish because food is often left at room temperature or in the sun for hours before it is consumed. Foods that last well without refrigeration, such as fresh fruits and vegetables, breads, and crackers, should be selected for these occasions.

Any food that is transported should be kept cold. Lunches should be transported to and from work or school in a cooler or an insulated bag. They should be refrigerated upon arrival or kept cold with ice packs. Most foods that are brought home from work or school uneaten should be thrown out and not saved for another day (see *Critical Thinking*: Are These Choices Safe?).

CRITICAL THINKING

Are These Choices Safe?

Eleanor is in charge of organizing a potluck dinner. Because food at a potluck usually sits at room temperature for several hours and many people serve themselves from the same serving dishes, Eleanor is concerned about the potential for food-borne illness. She collects the following list of food items that her friends intend to bring:

Chicken salad	Cheese and crackers
Tamales	Cheesecake
Fruit salad	Cookies
Raw vegetables	Mushrooms stuffed with crab meat
Chips and onion dip	Lasagna

Do the foods on this list pose a risk of food-borne illness?

▼

The more food is handled, the more likely it is to be contaminated. The chicken salad, tamales, mushrooms, and lasagna pose a risk because they are handled extensively in preparation. The lasagna and stuffed mushrooms are cooked, but when left at room temperature, the inside may stay warm enough to provide a good environment for microbial growth. The raw fruits and vegetables are safe if they are not contaminated during handling. The cookies, chips, and cheese and crackers are safe choices. The onion dip and cheesecake are probably safe during the party as long as they have been refrigerated beforehand.

How might raw vegetables and fruit salad become contaminated?

▼

Answer:

What suggestions might Eleanor make that would decrease the chances of microbial contamination?

▼

Foods such as cheese and crackers that are designed to be served at room temperature are safest, but a potluck without both hot and cold dishes is missing out on variety and taste. To prevent food from becoming contaminated before the potluck, safe kitchen food handling and preparation practices should be followed. Once at the potluck, hot dishes like the lasagna should be kept on a hot plate to ensure that they remain hot. Cold dishes like the fruit salad can be placed in a bowl of ice. Store-bought dips are a good choice because they can remain unopened until the party begins. Acidic dips such as tomato-based salsa are safe. Layer cakes and fruit pies keep better at room temperature than cheesecake.

After the party is over, what foods would you consider safe to keep as leftovers and what would you throw out?

▼

Answer:

• CHEMICAL CONTAMINANTS IN FOOD

Compounds used in agricultural production and industrial wastes contaminate the environment. These are taken up by plants and consumed by small animals. These plants and animals are then eaten by larger animals, which are in turn eaten by still larger animals, thus passing the contaminants up through the food chain to all levels of the food supply. Contaminants are found in the greatest concentration in foods of animal origin because animals are at the top of the food chain (Figure 17.12).

Risks and Benefits of Pesticides

Pesticides are used to prevent plant diseases and insect infestations. They are applied to crops growing in the fields as well as after harvesting to prevent spoilage and extend the shelf life of produce. Crops grown using pesticides generally produce higher yields and look more appealing because insect damage is limited. Some

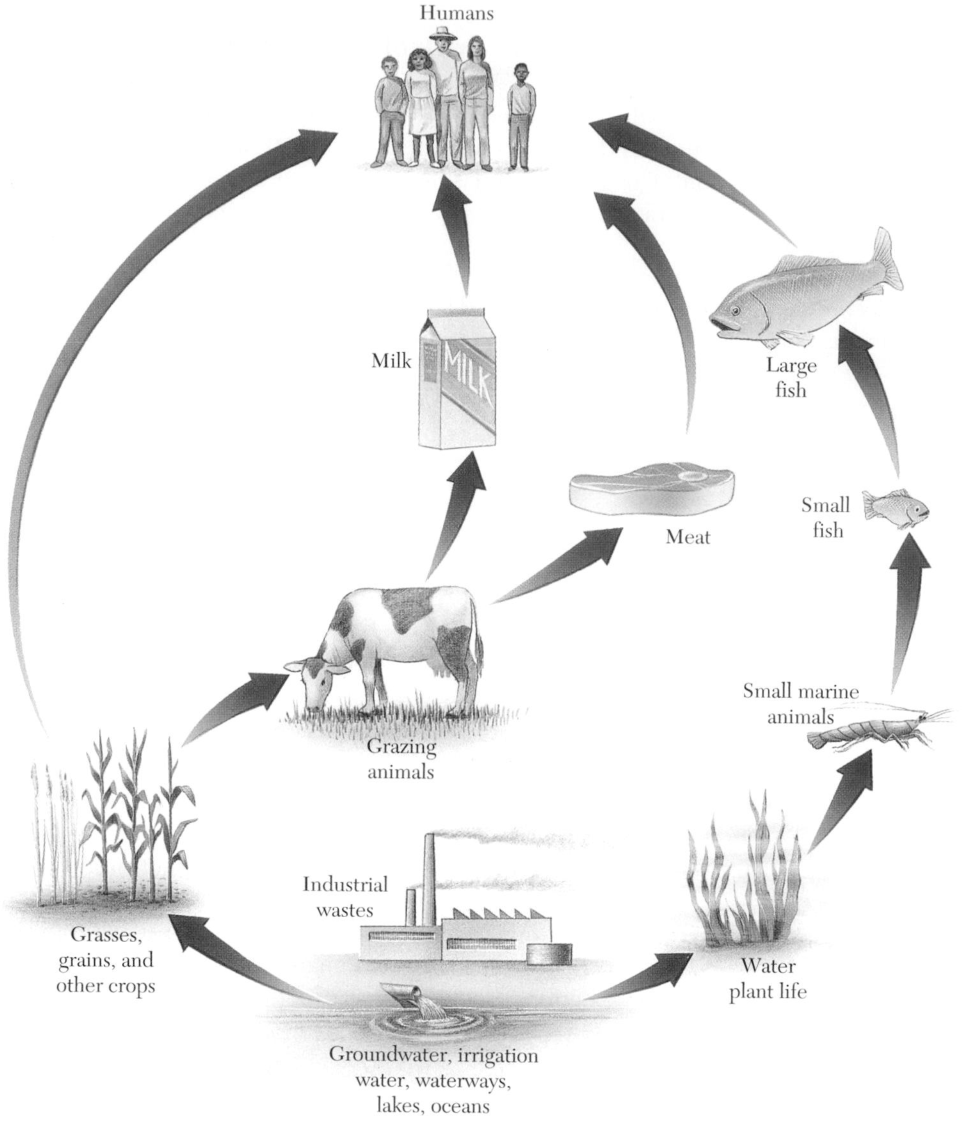

Figure 17.12
Industrial pollutants that contaminate the water supply become more and more concentrated as they are passed up the food chain. Large organisms like cattle and large fish may have high levels of these contaminants in their adipose tissue.

residues of these chemicals remain on the food when it arrives at our tables, and pesticides may travel from the fields where they are applied into water supplies, soil, and other parts of the environment. For instance, pesticides are found not only on treated produce but also in meat, poultry, fish, dairy products, and lard, as well as in groundwater.[11]

The potential risks of pesticides to consumers depend on the type and amount consumed as well as who consumes it. In general, the small amounts of pesticides that remain in the food supply will cause no immediate reaction but could cause health problems if consumed over a long period.

Regulating Pesticide Use The types of pesticides that can be used on food crops and the amounts of residues that can remain when foods reach consumers are regulated. The EPA must approve and register pesticides that are used in food production and establish allowable limits, or **tolerances**. The FDA and USDA then monitor pesticide levels in foods. To establish tolerances for pesticides, the risk of toxicity is weighed against the benefit that the pesticide provides. The risks are

Tolerances The maximum amount of pesticide residues that may legally remain in food, set by the EPA.

based on the known incidence of toxicity and the predicted exposure that consumers will have to the toxin. Tolerance levels are then set at the minimum amount of the pesticide needed to be effective; these levels are often several hundred times lower than the level found to cause reactions in test animals.[12] To protect children, for whom the same amount of pesticide provides a larger dose per unit of body weight, the EPA is required to set tolerances that are safe for children as well as adults.[13]

In general, the amounts of pesticides to which people are exposed through foods are small. According to the FDA's pesticide residue monitoring program, less than 2% of the food samples studied had residues of pesticides that either exceeded tolerance levels or contained pesticides for which there is no legal tolerance.[14] A report by the National Research Council in 1996 concluded that the majority of synthetic chemicals, including pesticides, in the diet are present at levels below which any significant adverse biological effect is likely and that they are unlikely to pose a cancer risk.[14] Although special-interest groups concerned with overuse of pesticides disagree with this conclusion,[15] the fact remains that repeated consumption of large doses of any one pesticide is unlikely because most people consume a variety of foods produced in many different locations.

Reducing Pesticide Risks New, more effective chemical pesticides are being developed, and the use of older, more toxic products is decreasing in the United States. Genetically engineered pesticides use insect-killing proteins that are produced by bacteria. The bacteria containing the pesticides are killed and then sprayed on plants. In addition to developing safer pesticides, production methods are being implemented to make low-pesticide and pesticide-free produce available to the consumer. **Integrated pest management (IPM)** is a method of agricultural pest control that combines chemical and nonchemical methods. It emphasizes the use of natural toxins and more effective pesticide application.

Integrated pest management (IPM) A method of agricultural pest control that integrates nonchemical and chemical techniques.

Exploiting Natural Toxins Many toxins that occur naturally in plants function as natural pesticides that offer protection from bacteria, molds, and insect pests. These naturally pest-resistant crops are advantageous in developing countries because they thrive without the use of expensive added pesticides. Plants high in natural pesticides are being produced through special breeding programs as well as **genetic engineering**. The natural toxins in plants can also be isolated and applied to crops like synthetic pesticides.

As with all chemical toxins, natural toxins move through the food supply. For example, a cow that has foraged on toxic plants can pass the toxin into her milk and poison the consumer of the milk. Abraham Lincoln's mother died from drinking milk from a cow that had eaten poisonous snakeroot plants. The potential for toxicity, however, depends on the dose of toxin and the health of the consumer. Most natural toxins in the food supply are consumed in doses that pose little risk to the consumer.

Genetic engineering A set of techniques used to manipulate DNA for the purpose of changing the characteristics of an organism or creating a new product.

Using Organic Techniques **Organic food** production is based on biological methods that avoid the use of synthetic pesticides, herbicides, or fertilizers. Consumer demand for these products has been increasing due in part to the belief that organic foods are safer or superior in quality, taste, or nutrient content to conventionally grown foods; however, this is not necessarily the case.

The production methods used in organic farming are more ecologically sound than the standard methods used today. They foster the recycling of resources and conserve biodiversity. Organic farming techniques reduce the exposure of farm workers to pesticides and decrease the quantity of pesticides introduced into the food supply and the environment. However, organic foods are not risk-free. Manure is often used for fertilizer. If the manure is not treated properly, it can increase the risks of microbial food-borne illness associated with the food, and runoff can pollute lakes and streams. Irrigation water, rain, and a variety of other sources can introduce

Organic Food Food produced without the use of synthetic fertilizers or pesticides, sewage sludge, irradiation or genetically modified ingredients according to the standards of the USDA's National Organic Program.

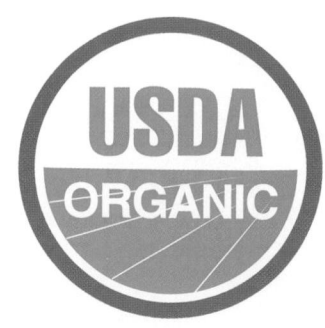

Figure 17.13

The USDA organic seal can appear on the label of agricultural products that meet the definition of "100% organic" or "organic."

traces of synthetic pesticides and other agricultural chemicals not approved for organic use into organically grown foods. The threshold for pesticide residues in organic foods is set at 5% of the EPA's pesticide-residue tolerance.[16] In addition, organic foods are usually more expensive and available in less variety than conventionally grown foods.

Recently, the USDA's National Organic Program developed standards for organic foods.[17] These national standards define both substances approved for and prohibited from use in organic food production. For example, an organic food may not include ingredients that are treated with irradiation, produced by genetic modification, or grown using sewage sludge or industrially synthesized fertilizers and pesticides. Certain natural pesticides and other manufactured agents are permitted. Farming and processing operations that produce and handle foods labeled as organic must be certified by the USDA. Products meeting the definition of "100% organic" or "organic" may display the USDA "Organic" seal shown in Figure 17.13 (See Table 17.5).

Antibiotics and Hormones in Food

Antibiotics are used in animal production to treat and prevent disease and to promote growth. Animals treated with antibiotics can produce greater yields at lower costs, but if used improperly, residues of these drugs can remain in the meat. The FDA regulates which drugs can be used to treat animals used for food production and when they can be administered.[17] The USDA monitors tissue samples for drug residues.

Perhaps a more important concern than drug residues is that antibiotic use in animals may result in the creation of antibiotic-resistant bacteria. When bacteria are exposed to an antibiotic, those that are resistant to that antibiotic survive and produce offspring that are also resistant to the antibiotic. If these resistant bacteria infect humans, the resulting illness cannot be treated with that antibiotic. Since nearly half the antibiotics produced in the United States are used to prevent disease in animals, this use is suspected of being a major contributor to the development of antibiotic-resistant strains of bacteria.[18]

Hormones are used to increase weight gain in sheep and cattle and milk production in dairy cows. Some naturally occurring hormones such as estrogen and testosterone are used in slow-release form, and levels in the animals are no higher than in untreated animals. Before synthetic hormones can be used, it must be demonstrated that residues in meat are within the safe limits. A synthetic hormone that has created public concern is genetically engineered bovine somatotropin (bST) (Figure 17.14*a*). Cows naturally produce somatotropin, a hormone that stimulates milk production. Genetically engineered bST is produced by bacteria and injected into cows to increase their milk production. Consumer groups contend that genetically engineered bST causes health problems for the cows and for humans who consume milk or meat from the cows. An FDA review of the effect of bST concluded that it causes no seri-

Table 17.5 *Labeling of Organic Foods*

Labeling Term	Meaning
100% organic	Contains (by weight or fluid volume, excluding water and salt) 100% organically produced raw or processed ingredients. May display USDA seal.
Organic	Contains (by weight or fluid volume excluding water and salt) not less than 95% organically produced raw or processed agricultural products. May display USDA seal.
Made with organic ingredients (specified ingredients or food groups)	Contains (by weight or fluid volume excluding water and salt) at least 70% organically produced ingredients

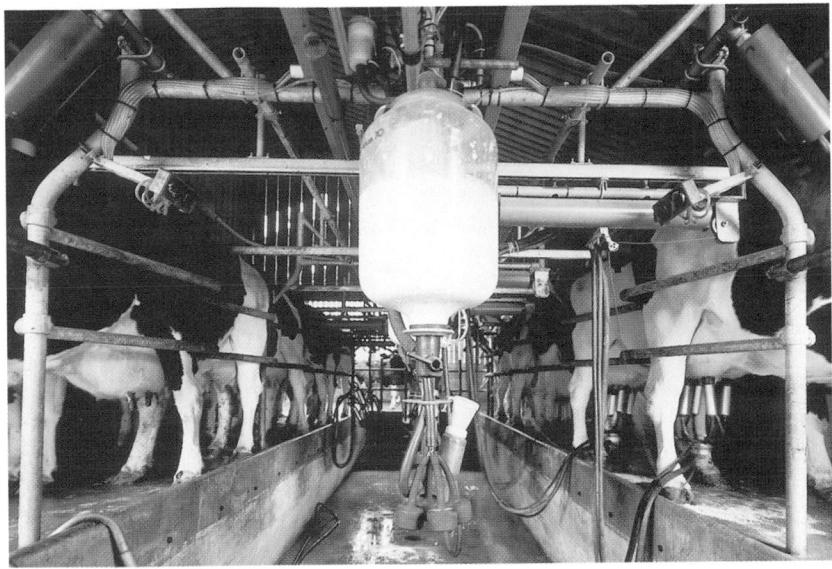 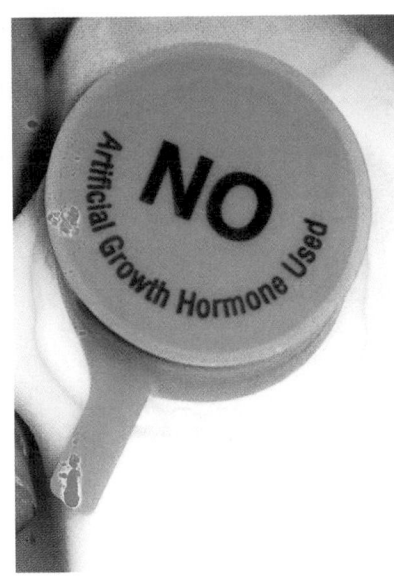

(a)　　　　　　　　　　　　　　　　　　　　　　　(b)

Figure 17.14

(a) When administered to cattle, genetically engineered bovine somatotropin increases milk production. (b) Milk from cows treated with genetically engineered bovine somatotropin is indistinguishable from other milk, but dairies that do not use bovine somatotropin may choose to indicate this on the label. (a, Graeme Norways/Stone; b, Lori Smolin)

ous long-term health effects in cows and that milk and meat from bST-treated cows are not health risks to consumers.[19] The FDA does not require milk from bST-treated cows to be specially labeled, but companies may voluntarily label their products as long as the labeling is truthful and not misleading (Figure 17.14b).

Contamination from Industrial Wastes

Industrial chemicals that contaminate the environment find their way into the food supply. Fish accumulate substances that are in the waters where they live and feed. Pollutants in the water can also contaminate crops and move up the food chain into meat and milk.

One group of carcinogenic chemicals that pollutes the environment is **polychlorinated biphenyls (PCBs)**. These were used in the manufacture of electrical capacitors and transformers, plasticizers, waxes, and paper. In the past, PCBs in runoff from manufacturing plants contaminated water, particularly near the Great Lakes. Although they are no longer produced, these compounds do not degrade and so are still found in the environment. Fish accumulate PCBs in their adipose tissue; humans who consume large quantities of contaminated fish accumulate PCBs in their adipose tissue.

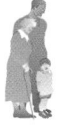

PCBs are a particular problem for mothers and infants. Prenatal exposure can damage the nervous system and cause learning deficits in children.[20,21] Because PCBs are secreted in breast milk, the American Academy of Pediatrics recommends that breast-feeding women in areas where high exposures of PCBs have occurred check with their local health department for recommendations on fish consumption. However, they have concluded that the benefits of breast-feeding outweigh the risks of low levels of PCBs.[22]

Other contaminants from manufacturing, such as chlordane (used to control termites), radioactive substances such as strontium-90, and toxic metals such as cadmium, lead, arsenic, and mercury have also found their way into fish and shellfish. Cadmium and lead can interfere with the absorption of other minerals, as well as have a direct toxic effect: Cadmium can cause kidney damage; lead can impair brain development. Arsenic is believed to contribute to cancer development, and mercury,

Polychlorinated biphenyls (PCBs) Carcinogenic industrial compounds that have found their way into the environment and, subsequently, the food supply. Repeated ingestion causes them to accumulate in biological tissues over time.

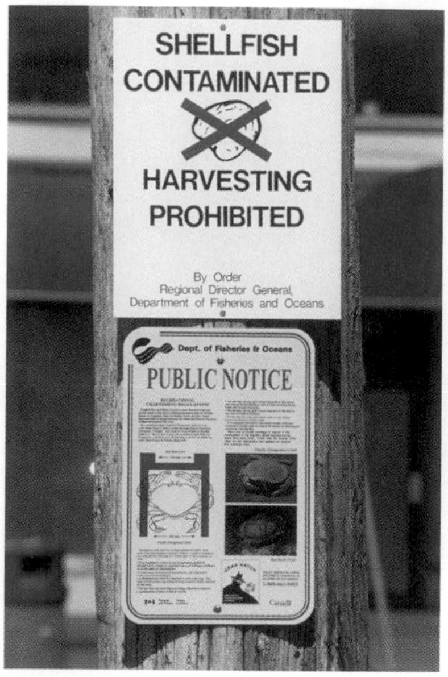

Figure 17.15

It is unsafe to consume shellfish from contaminated waters. (Paul A. Souders/Corbis)

which has been found in large fish, particularly swordfish and shark, damages nerve cells.[23] Large fish at the top of the food chain are more likely to contain high levels of industrial contaminants, but shellfish also accumulate contaminants because they feed by passing large volumes of water through their bodies (Figure 17.15).

Choosing Wisely to Reduce Risk

Even though individual consumers cannot detect chemicals in food, care in selection and preparation can reduce the amounts that are consumed. One of the easiest ways to reduce risk is to choose a wide variety of foods, avoiding excessive consumption of any one food. Although some consumers are concerned about the consumption of pesticide residues, the health risk of eliminating foods from the diet that may contain pesticide residues, such as fresh fruits and vegetables, is probably greater than that of the pesticide exposure. To reduce exposure, consumers can choose locally grown produce which is likely to contain fewer pesticides because it does not contain pesticides used to prevent spoilage and extend the shelf life of produce that is shipped. Foods produced organically or using IPM are also likely to contain fewer pesticide residues.

Pesticides can be removed or reduced on conventionally grown produce by peeling or washing with tap water and scrubbing with a brush if appropriate. For leafy vegetables such as lettuce and cabbage, the outer leaves can be removed and discarded. Some produce, such as cucumbers, apples, eggplant, squash, and tomatoes, are coated with wax to maintain freshness by sealing in moisture, but wax also seals in pesticides. Much of the wax can be removed by rinsing produce in warm water and scrubbing it with a brush, but to eliminate all wax, the produce must be peeled. Although peeling fruits and vegetables eliminates some pesticides, it also eliminates fiber and some micronutrients.

The risk of ingesting chemical pollutants from fish can be minimized by choosing wisely. Small fish are lower on the food chain and therefore will have lower levels of contaminants than larger fish. The safest fish are saltwater varieties caught well offshore, away from polluted waters. Freshwater fish and saltwater fish that live near shore or spend part of their life cycle in freshwater are more likely to contain contaminants. Migratory fish such as striped bass and bluefish are a problem because they may contain contaminants even when they are caught in clean water well offshore. Consuming a variety of fish rather than just one or two kinds can also reduce the risk of ingesting dangerous amounts of contaminants from fish. Most toxins concentrate in adipose tissue, so amounts can be reduced by trimming all fat from fish (and meat) before cooking or eating. Internal organs such as the green-colored "tomale" in lobster and the "mustard" in blue crabs should not be consumed because toxins such as PCBs and cadmium accumulate in these organs.

• FOOD TECHNOLOGY

Advances in food and agricultural technology have improved the safety and availability of foods. This technology includes techniques to preserve food and develop new food products. It can keep food fresh for many seasons; it can add nutrients lacking in the diet, and it can introduce disease-resistant high-yield crops. It has helped ensure that food is available even if the local growing season is not ideal. Without modern techniques, we would be forced to rely on locally grown foods and to eat them soon after harvest or slaughter. While this has some appeal, it would limit the variety of foods in our diet, particularly during the winter months, and place us at risk for malnutrition if food production were interrupted by a natural or man-made disaster. While technology offers many benefits, it also creates risks.

Food Additives

The technology used to improve food availability and safety may intentionally add some substances to foods, while other substances may contaminate food unintentionally. Substances added to preserve or enhance the appeal of food products are called **food additives** (Figure 17.16). By legal definition, a food additive is a substance that can reasonably be expected to become a component of a food during processing. This includes **direct food additives,** which are substances intentionally added during the preparation, packaging, transport, and holding of food. It also includes **indirect food additives**, which are substances known to enter food, although unintentionally, during processing. Food additives are regulated by the FDA. If foods or packaging materials are handled improperly, unexpected substances may accidentally enter food. These **accidental contaminants** are not regulated.

When a manufacturer wants to use a new food additive, a petition must be submitted to the FDA. The petition describes the chemical composition of the additive, how it is manufactured, and how it is detected and measured in food. The manufacturer must prove that the additive will be effective for its intended purpose at the proposed levels, that it is safe for its intended use, and that its use is necessary. Additives may not be used to disguise inferior products or deceive consumers. They cannot be used if they significantly destroy nutrients or where the same effect can be achieved by sound manufacturing processes.

When the 1958 Food Additives Amendment was passed, over 600 chemicals defined as food additives were already in common use. To accommodate these substances, the amendment added a category of materials that were considered **generally recognized as safe (GRAS)**. GRAS substances are exempt from the regulations applied to substances defined as food additives, color additives, or pesticides. If the safety of a substance on the GRAS list is questioned, the FDA must provide evidence that the substance is unsafe before it can be removed from the list.

The 1958 Food Additives Amendment also included the **Delaney Clause**, which was designed to protect the public from additives found to be carcinogenic. The Delaney Clause states that a substance that induces cancer in either an animal species or humans at any dosage, no matter how large, may not be added to food. Currently, support is growing to amend the Delaney Clause to allow the use of substances that are added at a level so low that they would not represent a significant health risk.

Additives to Maintain or Improve Nutritional Quality Many nutrients are added to foods. As discussed in Chapter 8, refined grains are enriched with iron and some of the B vitamins that are lost in processing. In other cases, food is fortified with nutrients typically lacking in the diet. For instance, grains are fortified with folic acid.

Fortification benefits the population by increasing the nutrient content of the diet, but it can also increase the risk of nutrient toxicities. For example, high intakes of foods fortified with folic acid can mask the symptoms of a vitamin B_{12} deficiency.

Additives to Maintain Product Quality Many substances are added to prevent bacteria and molds from causing food spoilage, to extend shelf life, or to protect natural color and flavor. Sugar and salt are two of the oldest **preservatives**. They prevent microbial growth by decreasing the water availability in the product; without adequate water, microbes cannot grow. For example, the high concentration of sugar in jams and jellies draws water away from the microbial cells and prevents them from growing.

Most preservatives have little documented risk. However, for some, the risks have been carefully weighed against the benefits. For example, nitrites and nitrates are used in cured meats such as ham and hot dogs to retard the growth of bacteria, particularly *Clostridium botulinum*, which causes deadly botulism poisoning. However, they also react with amino acids to form **nitrosamines** in the body. Nitrosamines are known to be carcinogenic in animals, but there is little evidence that they pose a serious risk in the amounts consumed in the human diet.[24] To minimize any risk of nitrosamines without increasing the risk of bacterial illness, the FDA has limited the amount of nitrites that can be added to food and has required the addition of antioxidants, which reduce nitrosamine formation, to foods containing

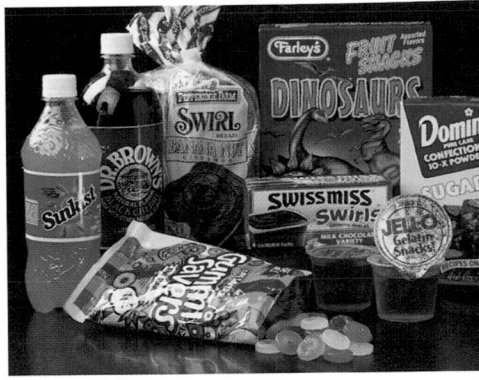

Figure 17.16

The additives in these foods prevent the bread from molding, the fruit snacks from hardening, and the powdered sugar from clumping; they also smooth the texture of the pudding and give color and flavor to soft drinks and candy. (George Semple)

Food additives Substances that can reasonably be expected to become a component of a food during processing. The foods that may contain them and the amounts that may be present are regulated by the FDA.

Direct food additives Substances intentionally added to foods. They are regulated by the FDA.

Indirect food additives Substances that are expected to unintentionally enter foods during manufacturing or from packaging. They are regulated by the FDA.

Accidental contaminants Substances not regulated by the FDA that unexpectedly enter the food supply.

Generally recognized as safe (GRAS) A group of chemical additives that are generally recognized as safe based on their long-standing presence in the food supply without obvious harmful effects.

Delaney Clause A clause added to the 1958 Food Additives Amendment of the Pure Food and Drug Act that prohibits the intentional addition to foods of any compound that has been shown to induce cancer in animals or humans at any dose.

Preservatives Compounds that extend the shelf life of a product by retarding chemical, physical, or microbiological changes.

Nitrosamines Carcinogenic compounds produced by reactions between nitrites and amino acids.

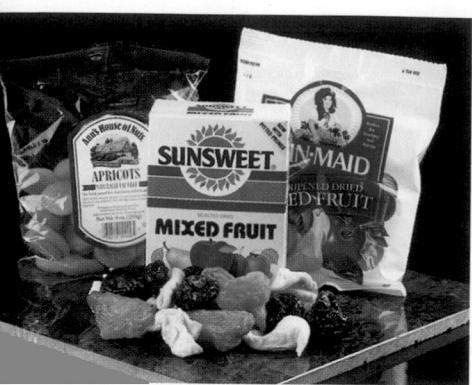

Figure 17.17
Sulfites are used in products such as dried fruit, but they can cause deadly reactions in sulfite-sensitive individuals. (George Semple)

nitrites. Consumers can reduce the risk of nitrites by limiting cured meat consumption to 3 to 4 ounces per week and maintaining adequate intakes of vitamins C and E.

Sulfites are another preservative that can be a health risk to consumers. The use of sulfites is restricted because some individuals are sulfite sensitive—in them, exposure may cause symptoms that range from stomachache and hives to severe asthmatic reactions. Sulfite use is prohibited on foods intended to be eaten raw, but they may be used to prevent discoloration in dried fruits and fresh-cut potatoes, to control black spots in freshly caught shrimp, and to prevent discoloration, bacterial growth, and fermentation in wine (Figure 17.17).

Additives That Aid in Processing or Preparation Many different types of additives are used in product processing and preparation. Emulsifiers improve the homogeneity, stability, and consistency of products such as ice cream. Stabilizers, thickeners, and texturizers, such as pectins and gums, are used to improve consistency or texture in pudding and to stabilize emulsions in foods such as salad dressing. Leavening agents are added to incorporate gas into breads and cakes, causing them to rise. Acids are added as flavor enhancers, preservatives, and antioxidants. Humectants, such as propylene glycol, cause moisture to be retained so products stay fresh. Anticaking agents prevent crystalline products such as powdered sugar from absorbing moisture and caking or lumping.

Additives to Affect Color and Flavor Additives are also used to enhance the flavor and color of foods. Flavor additives may supplement, magnify, or modify the original taste or aroma of a food. For example, both natural and artificial sweeteners are added to enhance the flavor of foods (see Chapter 4).

Colors can be used to make foods appear more appetizing; however, they cannot be used as deception to conceal inferiority. The FDA's list of permitted colors includes two categories: certified food colors and those exempt from certification. Certified food colors are synthetic dyes derived primarily from petroleum and coal sources. Certification means that each batch of the color is tested to ensure safety, quality, consistency, and strength of color. About 10% of the food consumed in the United States contains certified food colors. Colors derived from plant, animal, and certain mineral sources are exempt from certification. Examples include beet juice, caramel, and paprika extract. Colors found to be potential hazards have been removed from the list of permissible additives.[25] However, the certified food color FD&C Yellow No. 5, which may cause itching and hives in hypersensitive individuals, was not considered a great enough risk to be removed from the food supply (see *Off the Label*: Identifying Things Added to Your Food).

Standards of identity Regulations that define the allowable ingredients, composition, and other characteristics of foods.

Regulating What Gets into Food According to the Pure Food and Drug Act of 1906, only additives that were proven to be safe and effective could be used in foods. In 1938, the federal Food, Drug, and Cosmetic Act provided exemptions and safe tolerance levels for additives that were necessary or unavoidable in production. This law established **standards of identity** for foods. These prescribed recipes define exactly the ingredients that can be contained in certain foods such as mayonnaise, jelly, and orange juice. The Food, Drug, and Cosmetic Act also gave the FDA the responsibility of testing food additives for safety. Because the FDA could not possibly test all additives, the 1958 Food Additives Amendment transferred the responsibility for testing from the FDA to the manufacturer.

Processing and Packaging

Fermentation A process in which microorganisms metabolize components of a food and therefore change the composition, taste, and storage properties of the food.

For thousands of years, humans have been treating foods in order to protect them from spoilage by microorganisms. Most of the oldest methods of food preservation—including drying, smoking, **fermentation**, the addition of sugar or salt, and the use of heat or cold—are still used today. In addition, new methods, such as irradiation and specialized packaging are used to enhance the safety of the food supply.

Temperature Cooking food is one of the oldest methods of ensuring food safety. It kills disease-causing organisms and destroys toxins. Cooling food with refrigeration or freezing also protects us by slowing or stopping microbial growth. Other preservation techniques that rely on temperature include canning, pasteurization, sterilization, and aseptic processing. **Aseptic processing** heats foods to temperatures that result in sterilization. Sterilized foods are placed in sterilized packages using sterilized packaging equipment.[26] Aseptic processing is currently used to produce boxes of sterile milk and juices. These can remain free of microbial growth at room temperature for years.

Techniques that rely on temperature benefit us by providing appealing safe food, but they are not risk free, particularly if used incorrectly. If foods are not heated long enough or to a high enough temperature, or if they are not kept cold enough, there is a risk of food-borne illness. In addition, some types of cooking can also generate food hazards such as mutagens and carcinogens. These are considered accidental contaminants, so they are not regulated by the FDA. The most familiar group of chemicals produced during cooking is the **polycyclic aromatic hydrocarbons (PAHs)**. Grilled meats are high in PAHs because they are formed when fat drips onto the flame of a grill. Eating grilled fatty meat every day is not recommended, but occasional grilling, particularly with lowfat meat, presents little risk.

Broiled foods, which are cooked with the heat source at the top, are low in PAHs. However, broiled and pan-fried meats contain another potential hazard—**heterocyclic amines (HAs)**, such as benzopyrene, which are formed from the burning of amino acids and other substances in meats. Well-done meat and meat cooked using hotter temperatures contain greater amounts. The cooking temperatures recommended by the FDA are designed to prevent microbial food-borne illness and minimize the production of heterocyclic amines. The levels of heterocyclic amines can be reduced by precooking meat in the microwave and discarding the juice.

Food Irradiation **Irradiation**, also called cold pasteurization, is a process that exposes food to a high dose of x-rays, gamma radiation, or high-energy electrons. It kills microorganisms and insects and inactivates enzymes that cause germination and ripening of fruits and vegetables. It may, therefore, be used in place of chemicals to reduce insect and microbial contamination and to slow ripening during food storage. It is used in more than 40 countries to treat everything from frog legs to rice. It is one of the technologies singled out in the National Food Safety Initiative because of its potential for improving the safety of food and reducing the incidence of food-borne illness.

Food irradiation is used relatively infrequently in the United States. Part of the reason for its underuse is lack of irradiation facilities, but public fear and suspicion of the technology also limit its use. The word "irradiation" fosters the belief that the food itself becomes radioactive. Opponents to food irradiation claim that it introduces carcinogens, depletes the nutritional value of food, and is used to allow the sale of previously contaminated foods. Irradiated food is not radioactive and scientific studies conducted over the past 50 years have found that the benefits of irradiation outweigh the potential risks.[27] It increases the safety and shelf life of foods and does not compromise nutritional quality or noticeably change food texture, taste, or appearance as long as it is properly applied to a suitable product.[28] Irradiation can benefit the environment by reducing the use of chemicals to kill microbes and insects. Irradiation can decrease the amounts of certain nutrients; as much as 10% of vitamin A, thiamin, vitamin E, and vitamin K in a food can be destroyed. But this is similar to the losses that occur with canning or cold storage.[29]

The FDA has approved irradiation to destroy pathogens in red meat and poultry and contaminants in spices; prevent insect infestation in flour and spices; increase the shelf life of potatoes; eliminate *Trichinella* in pork; control insects in fruits, vegetables, and grains; and slow the ripening and spoilage of some produce. Irradiated foods must be labeled with the radura symbol (Figure 17.18) and the statement "treated with radiation" or "treated by irradiation." Products that contain irradiated

Aseptic processing A method that places sterilized food in a sterilized package using a sterile process.

Polycyclic aromatic hydrocarbons (PAHs) A class of mutagenic substances produced during cooking when there is incomplete combustion of organic materials—such as when fat drips on a grill.

Heterocyclic amines (HAs) A class of mutagenic substances produced when there is incomplete combustion of amino acids during the cooking of meats—such as when meat is charred.

Irradiation A process also called cold pasteurization, that exposes foods to radiation to kill contaminating organisms and retard ripening and spoilage of fruits and vegetables.

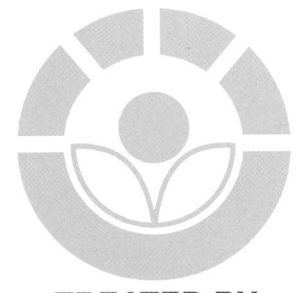

TREATED BY IRRADIATION

Figure 17.18

Foods that have been treated with irradiation can be identified by the radura symbol.

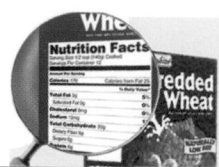

Off the Label
Identifying Things Added to Your Food

For many of us, the ingredients listed on food labels sound like a chemical soup. Calcium propionate is added to bread, disodium EDTA is added to canned kidney beans, and BHA is in potato chips. Are these chemical additives necessary in our food supply?

For most individuals, concerns about food additives are unfounded. Food additives are not approved by the FDA unless they are safe for most consumers. Understanding what these chemicals are used for can help make the ingredient list a source of information rather than a cause for concern. Food additives are used to make food safer; improve color, flavor, or texture; aid in processing; and enhance nutritional value. The table to the right provides some examples of food additives that might appear on food labels, the type of additive each is, and what it does in particular foods.

For individuals who are sensitive or allergic to certain additives, such as preservatives or colors, ingredient lists provide essential information that can be lifesaving. Sulfites are preservatives used in many foods—for example, baked goods, canned

vegetables, condiments, and maraschino cherries. Sulfites allowed in packaged foods include sulfur dioxide, sodium sulfite, sodium and potassium bisulfite, and sodium and potassium metabisulfite.[1] In sensitive individuals, they can cause deadly asthmatic reactions. Individuals sensitive to sulfites should read food labels to identify foods that contain them, and should be aware that foods served in restaurants could contain sulfites. For example, a potato dish served in a restaurant may be prepared using potatoes that were peeled and soaked in a sulfite solution before cooking.

Food colors can also cause reactions in sensitive individuals. For instance, the color additive FD&C Yellow No. 5, which is listed as tartrazine on medicine labels, may cause itching and hives in sensitive people. It is found in beverages, desserts, and processed vegetables. The ingredient list of the food label can be used to identify the presence of color additives. All foods that contain FDA-certified color additives must list them by name in the ingredient list. Colors that are exempt from certification, such as dehydrated beets and

carotenoids, do not have to be specifically identified and may be listed on the label collectively as "artificial color."[2]

Reactions to food ingredients are relatively rare. The FDA estimates that 1 in 100 people are sulfite-sensitive and that sensitivity to FD&C Yellow No. 5 occurs in fewer than 1 in 10,000 people. The FDA monitors problems related to food additives using the Adverse Reaction Monitoring System (ARMS). Adverse reactions can be reported by contacting the FDA district office listed in your phone directory or by writing to:

ARMS
HFS-636
Food and Drug Administration
200 C Street, N.W.
Washington, DC 20204

[1]Papazian, R. Sulfites: safe for most, dangerous for some. *FDA Consumer* 30:11–14, December 1996. Available online at www.fda.gov/fdac/featues/096sulf.html/ Accessed August 2, 2002.

[2]U.S. Food and Drug Administration. Food Color Facts. January 1993. Available online at vm.cfsan.fda.gov/~lrd/colorfac.html/ Accessed August 2, 2002.

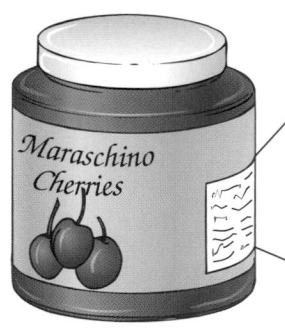

INGREDIENTS: CHERRIES, WATER, CORN SYRUP, SUGAR, CITRIC ACID, NATURAL AND ARTIFICIAL FLAVOR, POTASSIUM SORBATE AND SODIUM BENZOATE ADDED AS PRESERVATIVE, FD&C RED #40 (ARTIFICIAL COLOR), AND SULFUR DIOXIDE (PRESERVATIVE).

spices or other irradiated ingredients do not need to display this symbol, and irradiation labeling requirements do not apply to restaurant food.[28] Because irradiation produces unique compounds in irradiated foods, it is treated as a food additive, and the level of radiation that may be used is regulated by the FDA and USDA. At the allowed levels of radiation, the amounts of these unique compounds produced are almost negligible and have not been found to be a risk to consumers. Irradiated foods may cost more because of the cost of adding an extra processing step, but in

Additive	Function	Example of Use
Acetic acid	Provides acidity	Gives tartness to dressings and sauces.
Ascorbic acid	Preservative, nutrient	Keeps fruit from darkening, inhibits rancidity in fatty foods, enhances nutritional value of beverages.
Baking soda (sodium bicarbonate)	Leavening agent	Generates gas so ensures baked goods rise.
Beet extract	Natural color	Gives deep red color to foods.
BHA (butylated hydroxyanisole)	Preservative	Acts as an antioxidant to prevent rancidity of fats, oils, and dried meats; keeps baked goods fresh.
BHT (butylated hydroxytoluene)	Preservative	Acts as an antioxidant to prevent rancidity in potato flakes, enriched rice, and shortenings.
Calcium silicate	Anticaking agent	Absorbs moisture to keep powdered foods like baking powder free-flowing.
Carrageenan	Stabilizer, texturizer	Improves consistency and texture of chocolate milk, frozen desserts, puddings, and syrup.
Citric acid	Preservative, provides acidity	Provides acidity in beverages and dessert products.
FD&C colors	Color	Adds color to foods, drugs, and cosmetics.
Gelatin	Thickener	Provides texture to desserts, confectionery products, and canned meat products.
Glycerides (monoglycerides and diglycerides)	Emulsifier	Prevents ice cream from separating while melting, keeps oil in peanut butter from separating.
Glycerine (glycerol)	Humectant	Binds water to prevent moisture losses in flaked coconut, marshmallows, and toaster foods.
Guar gum	Thickener	Thickens liquids such as gravies and sauces.
Gum arabic	Stabilizer, emulsifier	Keeps butter mixed in buttered syrups and stabilizes flavors in dry-mix food products.
Lactic acid	Preservative	Controls molds in pickles, sauerkraut, cheese, buttermilk, and yogurt.
Lecithin	Emulsifier	Prevents separation of oil and vinegar in mayonnaise.
Magnesium stearate	Anticaking agent	Prevents clumping in flour.
Pectin	Thickener	Gels jams, jellies, and preserves.
Potassium sorbate	Preservative	Controls surface molds on cheese, syrups, margarine, and mayonnaise.
Propylene glycol	Humectant	Improves texture of foods by holding moisture.
Sodium benzoate	Preservative	Controls molds in syrup, margarine, soft drinks, and fruit products.
Sodium chloride	Preservative, flavor agent	Prevents microbial growth in cured meats, adds flavor to soups.
Sodium nitrite	Preservative	Prevents botulism growth in cured meats, fish, and poultry.
Sorbitol	Sweetener, humectant	Keeps fruit snacks and gummy candies soft.
Sulfites (sulfur dioxide, sodium sulfide, sodium and potassium bisulfite, and sodium and potassium metabisulfite)	Preservative	Acts as an antioxidant to prevent discoloration in fruits and vegetables like dried apples and dehydrated potatoes.
Tartaric acid	Increases acidity	Adds tartness to carbonated fruit-flavored drinks.

the future this may be offset by a longer shelf life (Figure 17.19). Irradiation should be used to complement, not replace, proper food handling by producers, processors, and consumers.

Packaging Consumer demand for fresh foods has led to a new generation of fresh refrigerated foods such as pasta, vegetables, fish, chicken, and beef. To make fresh refrigerated foods—for example, beef teriyaki—the raw ingredients are sealed in

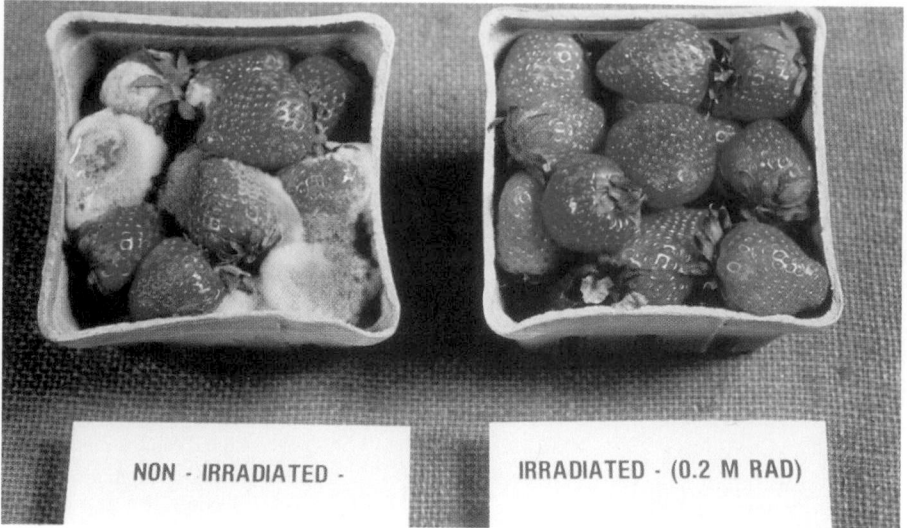

NON - IRRADIATED -   IRRADIATED - (0.2 M RAD)

Figure 17.19
After two weeks in cold storage, the strawberries treated by irradiation remain free of mold (*right*), whereas the untreated strawberries picked at the same time are covered with mold (*left*). (Council for Agricultural Science and Technology)

plastic pouches, the air is vacuumed out, and the pouch and its contents are partially precooked and immediately refrigerated. This type of processing eliminates the need for the extreme cold of freezing or the extreme heat of canning, so flavor and nutrients are better preserved. Unlike canned foods, fresh refrigerated products are not heated to sufficient temperatures to kill all bacteria, and unlike frozen foods, they are not kept at temperatures low enough to prevent all bacteria from growing. In some products, the oxygen in the package is replaced with a gas such as carbon dioxide or nitrogen, in which microbes are unlikely to grow. This is called **modified atmosphere packaging (MAP)**. These foods should be purchased only from reputable vendors, used by the expiration date printed on the package, refrigerated constantly until use, and heated according to the time and temperature on the package directions.

Packaging can protect food from spoilage, but even the best packaging can introduce risk if it becomes a part of the food. A variety of substances leach into foods from plastics, paper, and even dishes. Substances that are known to contaminate foods are indirect food additives and the amounts and types are regulated by EPA tolerance levels and FDA inspections. However, these regulations apply only to the intended use of the product. When used improperly, packaging can migrate into food and become an accidental contaminant. For instance, some plastics migrate into food when heated in a microwave oven. Thus only packages designed for microwave cooking should be used.

Modified atmosphere packaging (MAP) A type of food packaging in which the gases inside the package control or retard chemical, physical, and microbiological changes.

Biotechnology

The term **biotechnology** refers to the use of genetic modification or genetic engineering to alter the DNA of plants, animals, or other life forms to produce selected traits. Traditional plant and animal breeding has been used for centuries to select traits that improve the characteristics of crops and livestock. Planting seeds from the best crops and breeding only the strongest animals allows the most desirable traits to be passed on to the next generation, but it can take many generations to produce the desired results. Biotechnology, which selects specific genes in the laboratory, has significantly sped up this process and removed certain limitations.

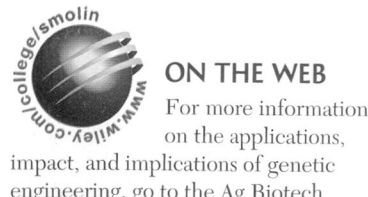

ON THE WEB
For more information on the applications, impact, and implications of genetic engineering, go to the Ag Biotech InfoNet at
www.biotech-info.net/
or to the Council for Biotechnology Information at
www.whybiotech.com

Biotechnology in Food Production Most of the biotechnology used in food production involves the genetic modification of plants. The first step in the production of a genetically modified plant is to identify a stretch of DNA, or gene, for a given desirable trait, such as resistance to a particular disease. This gene could be in a plant, an animal, or a bacterial cell. The gene can be clipped out with specific DNA-cutting enzymes and then transferred into the cells of the plant that is to be modified

Biotechnology A process that involves genetic engineering to alter—and, ideally, to improve—the characteristics of plants, animals, and other life forms.

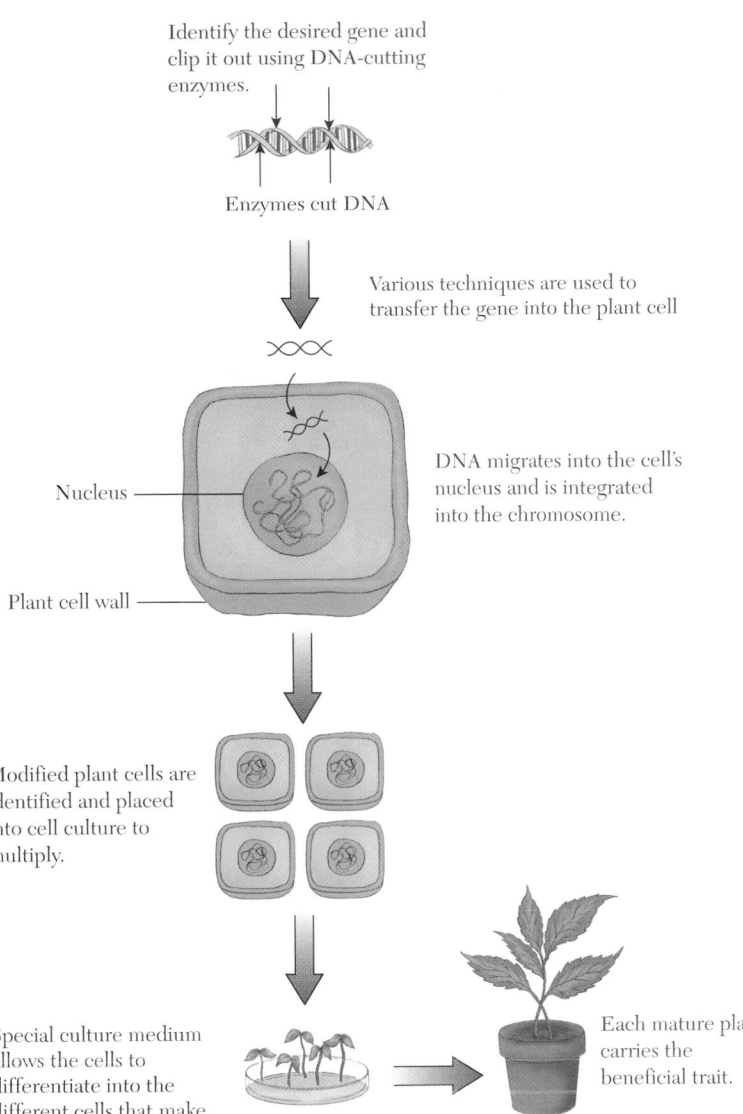

Identify the desired gene and clip it out using DNA-cutting enzymes.

Enzymes cut DNA

Various techniques are used to transfer the gene into the plant cell

DNA migrates into the cell's nucleus and is integrated into the chromosome.

Nucleus

Plant cell wall

Modified plant cells are identified and placed into cell culture to multiply.

Special culture medium allows the cells to differentiate into the different cells that make up a whole plant.

Each mature plant carries the beneficial trait.

Figure 17.20
Genetic engineering involves inserting a gene for a desired trait into the cell of an organism, such as a plant. When this cell divides, the daughter cells also contain the new gene and produce the protein for which it codes.

(Figure 17.20). Once inside the plant cell, the new DNA migrates to the nucleus, where the gene for the new trait is integrated into the plant's DNA. The DNA is then referred to as **recombinant DNA** because the new DNA has been combined with the plant's DNA. The modified plant cells are then allowed to multiply. As they do, the new gene is reproduced with them. The cells are then placed in a special culture medium that allows them to differentiate into the different types of cells that make up a whole plant. Each new plant that grows contains the new gene and therefore the trait, such as disease resistance, coded for by that gene.

Recombinant DNA DNA produced by joining DNA from different sources to create a unique combination of genes.

The Benefits of Biotechnology The techniques of biotechnology can be used in a variety of ways in both food production and processing to alter the quantity, quality, cost, safety, and shelf life of the food supply. Crop yields can be increased either directly, by inserting genes that improve the efficiency with which plants convert sunlight into food, or indirectly, by creating plants that are resistant to herbicides, insects, and plant diseases, thus reducing crop losses. Genes that impart herbicide and insect resistance also help the environment because they allow farmers to achieve weed-free fields and insect-free crops with fewer herbicides and pesticides. One way that insect-resistant plants are produced is to use a gene from the bacterium *Bacillus thuringiensis* (Bt) that produces a protein that is toxic to certain

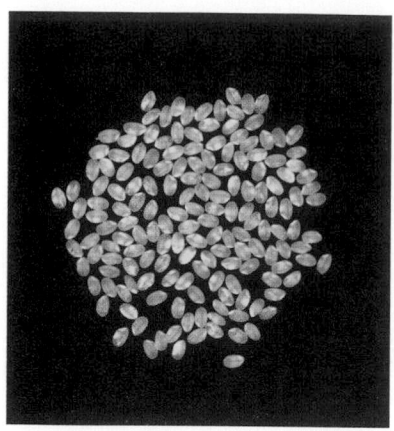

Figure 17.21
This genetically modified rice, called Golden rice, contains beta-carotene and could be used to help prevent vitamin A deficiency in regions where rice is a staple in the diet. (Courtesy of Peter Beyer, University of Freiburg, Germany.)

insects but safe for humans and other animals. When the gene for this protein is inserted into plant cells, the result is plants that manufacture their own insecticide. Corn and cotton are just two crops that have been modified to contain the Bt gene. Genetic modification has also increased crop yields by creating virus-resistant strains of potatoes, squash, cucumbers, watermelons, and papaya.[30]

Biotechnology can also affect plant characteristics that are of benefit after harvest, such as ease-of-transport, longer shelf lives, and slower ripening. It can address nutrient deficiencies in populations by changing the nutrient content of foods. For example, genes that code for enzymes needed to synthesize β-carotene have been inserted into rice.[31] Consuming about 2 cups a day of this genetically modified "Golden rice" provides enough beta-carotene to prevent vitamin A deficiency (Figure 17.21). Biotechnology is also being used to provide foods that may help prevent chronic disease. Vegetable oils that have lower amounts of saturated fat are being developed, as are oils that contain more of the antioxidant vitamin E than the traditional varieties.[32] Biotechnology has even been used to develop potatoes that are denser and have less water so they absorb less oil when fried—lowering the fat content.

Biotechnology is being used to develop environmentally friendly pesticides and safer food additives such as colors, preservatives, and enzymes used in food processing. It is also being used to enhance growth efficiency and fertility in food animals and to improve the prevention, diagnosis, and treatment of animal as well as human diseases. For example, genetically modified bacterial cells are used to produce human medicines such as insulin used to treat diabetes.

Does Biotechnology Carry Risks? Many people are concerned that the rapid advancement of biotechnology has created the potential for health problems and environmental damage. Scientific evaluation of these concerns has concluded that the risks posed by biotechnology are the same as those of products produced by traditional plant breeding.[33] In the two decades since the emergence of agricultural biotechnology, genetically engineered food products have not been shown to cause harm to humans or to the environment.[30] Despite this, many believe that conclusions regarding the environmental and the health impact of these relatively new products are premature and that the impact of this booming technology has not yet become apparent.

Consumer Safety Issues Safety concerns related to bioengineered foods include the possibility that an allergen or toxin may have inadvertently been introduced into a previously safe food, or that the nutrient content of a food has been negatively affected. For example, if DNA from fish or peanuts—foods that commonly cause allergic reactions—is introduced into tomatoes or corn, these foods that were previously safe could cause allergic reactions. Or, if tomatoes, which are a good source of vitamin C, were modified to have no vitamin C, people who rely on tomatoes for the vitamin would develop a deficiency. Because genetically engineered foods appear no different from other foods, it is difficult to tell which foods are produced using these techniques. Special labeling is not required unless the food poses a potential risk. The difficulty of tracking all genetically modified ingredients was brought to the public's attention in 2000 when genetically modified corn that had not been approved for human consumption was used to make taco shells. The product had to be recalled from grocery shelves.[34] The taco shells caused no health problems but this incident served to highlight the fact that it is difficult to identify the presence of genetically modified ingredients and to segregate crops at all phases of food production. Another potential health concern is that the antibiotic resistance genes used in biotechnology may promote the development of antibiotic-resistant strains of bacteria. If bacteria that cause human disease acquire the antibiotic-resistant traits, then the effectiveness of antibiotic treatments will be reduced.

Environmental Concerns One of the arguments against the use of genetically modified crops is that they will harm the environment by reducing diversity, promoting the evolution of pesticide-resistant insects, and creating "superweeds" that will overgrow our agricultural and forest lands. Diversity is a concern because the ability of populations of organisms to adapt to new conditions, diseases, or other hazards depends on the presence of many different species that provide a diversity of genes. If farmers only plant new insect-resistant high-yielding varieties of crops other varieties may eventually become extinct. This is a concern with genetically engineered crops, but no more so than with crops developed by traditional plant breeding.

The evolution of pesticide-resistant insects is also a concern. An illustration of this problem involves insects that are resistant to the Bt toxin. As more and more of the insect's food supply is made up of plants that produce this pesticide, only insects that carry genes making them resistant to Bt can survive and reproduce. This increases the number of Bt-resistant insects and therefore reduces the effectiveness of Bt as a method of pest control. Although an important concern, the risk of this occurring is no greater for genetically modified crops than for pesticides that are sprayed on crops.

Concern about the development of super weeds has arisen because it is hypothesized that traits introduced into domesticated plant species might be passed on to wild relatives, causing them to become fast-growing weeds. Although this is unlikely to occur, as a safeguard plant developers are avoiding introducing traits that could increase plant competitiveness or other undesirable properties of weedy relatives.

Regulation The government sets guidelines to help researchers address safety and environmental issues at all stages of the process, from the early development of genetically engineered plants through field-testing and, eventually, commercialization. Companies that develop new plant varieties must provide data to support the safety and wholesomeness of their products. Crops created by both traditional breeding and biotechnology methods must be field-tested for several seasons to make sure only desirable changes have been made. Plants are examined to ensure that they look right, grow right, and produce food that is safe, not nutritionally altered, and tastes right.[35] The FDA, USDA, and EPA are all involved in overseeing plant biotechnology.

The FDA regulates the safety and labeling of foods derived from genetically modified crops. The FDA policy is that the safety of a food product should be determined based on the characteristics of the food or food product, not the method used to produce it. Foods developed using biotechnology are therefore evaluated to determine their equivalence to foods produced by traditional plant breeding. Emphasis is placed on whether the food creates a new or increased allergenic risk, has an increased level of a naturally occurring toxin, contains a substance not previously present in the food supply, or is nutritionally different from the traditional plant. Currently, premarket approval is required only when the new food contains substances not commonly found in foods or contains a substance that does not have a history of safe use in foods. However, the FDA has proposed a rule regarding plant-derived bioengineered foods that, if approved, would mandate that developers of such foods notify the FDA 120 days prior to the date at which they intend to market the food. The new rule would also require that specific information be submitted to help the FDA determine whether the foods pose any potential safety, labeling, or adulteration issues.[36]

The USDA regulates agricultural products and research concerning the development of new plant varieties. The Animal and Plant Health Inspection Service (APHIS) of the USDA helps to ensure that the cultivation of a new plant variety poses no risk to agricultural production or to the environment. For example, if there is a high probability that a new plant variety will crossbreed with a weed and that the transfer of the new trait could allow the weed plant to survive better, APHIS may not allow further development of this plant. If a plant has been studied and tested and does not pose environmental risks, field-testing is allowed. APHIS continues to oversee the testing until it is determined that the plant is safe.

The EPA regulates any pesticides that may be present in foods and sets tolerance levels for these pesticides. This includes genetically modified plants containing proteins that protect them from insects or disease. The EPA assesses the safety of these proteins for human consumption, for other organisms, and for the environment.

Despite current regulations, a group of scientists who are still concerned about the potential risks of biotechnology have recommended that the government be more careful, and more public, with its review of the environmental impact of genetically altered plants. Genetically engineered foods are one part of the solution to the challenge of producing more food of better quality, but they urge that this technology be used with caution to avoid health or environmental impacts that outweigh the benefits (see *Critical Thinking*: Individual Risk-Benefit Analysis).

CRITICAL THINKING

Individual Risk-Benefit Analysis

After reading a newspaper article about a child who died of food-borne illness contracted by eating an undercooked hamburger, Rex became concerned about the safety of the foods his family was eating. He thought more carefully about other food safety issues, such as eggs and poultry contaminated with Salmonella; pesticide residues on fruits and vegetables; and fish contaminated with industrial pollutants, bacteria, viruses, and parasites. He started to think it was too risky to eat at all but then decided to look at the foods his family eats and see if the benefits they provide are worth the risk.

In general his family eats a healthy diet and is rarely sick, but he knows that a few of the things they like carry risks. He enjoys his meat rare, his son is an athlete who drinks protein shakes containing raw eggs, his young daughter likes to lick the bowl where cookie dough containing raw eggs is mixed, and he and his wife enjoy eating sushi and raw oysters. He made the following list of foods and then recorded the risks and benefits of each:

Food	Risk	Benefit
Hamburger	Can be contaminated with pathogenic *E. coli*.	A good source of protein and iron in the diet.
Chicken	Is often contaminated with *Salmonella*.	An economical source of protein that is low in fat.
Eggs	Can contain *Salmonella* or *Campylobacter*.	An inexpensive source of protein.
Fish	Can be contaminated with environmental pollutants such as PCBs and toxic metals.	A lowfat source of high-quality protein. Consumption has been associated with a reduced risk of cardiovascular disease.
Raw fish and shellfish	May be a source of bacterial, viral, and parasitic infections.	A lowfat source of high-quality protein and omega-3 fatty acids.
Fruits and vegetables	May contain pesticide residues.	An excellent source of fiber and vitamins in the diet. They also contain health-promoting phytochemicals.

After reviewing the risks and benefits of his family's diet, Rex realizes he can minimize the risk of eating hamburger and chicken by thoroughly cooking them because *E. coli* and its toxins and *Salmonella* are destroyed by heat.

What other changes can Rex make to minimize the risks associated with his family's typical diet while including foods that are beneficial?

▼

Answer:

• APPLICATIONS •

1. After 67 people became ill from consuming food at a company picnic, investigators determined that the tossed salad, the egg salad, and the turkey slices were all contaminated with *Salmonella*. Invent a scenario that would explain how all three became contaminated.

2. Use the Internet to go to www.fda.gov/and find the exercise called "Can Your Kitchen Pass the Food Safety Test?" Complete the exercise and answer the following.

a. Based on how you answered these questions, what changes should you make in the way you store and handle foods in your kitchen?

b. Based on how you answered these questions, are there foods that you will eliminate from your diet?

3. A new plant variety that provides readily absorbable iron has been produced by genetic engineering. It is being used as a staple of the diet in a developing country.

a. What are the potential benefits of this product?

b. What are the potential risks?

SUMMARY

1. The safety of the food supply can be affected by biological as well as chemical contamination. The harm caused by contaminants in the food supply depends on the type of toxin, the dose, the length of time over which it is consumed, and the size and health status of the consumer.

2. The food supply is monitored for safety by food manufacturers and regulatory agencies at the international, federal, state, and local levels. In addition, consumers play an important role in limiting the risks of developing food-borne illness.

3. The use of HACCP (Hazard Analysis Critical Control Point) offers a method for preventing food contamination, monitoring food processing methods, and tracking contaminated foods to prevent food-borne illness.

4. The most common cause of food-borne illness is microbial contamination, which often produces acute gastrointestinal symptoms. Some bacteria cause food-borne infection because they are able to grow in the gastrointestinal tract when ingested. Others produce toxins in food and when the toxin is consumed cause food-borne intoxication. Viruses consumed in food can also cause food-borne illness, as can toxins produced by molds that grow on foods, and parasites consumed in contaminated water or food.

5. The risk of food-borne illness can be decreased by proper food selection, preparation, and storage. Consumers should choose the freshest meats and produce, select frozen foods that have been kept at constant temperatures, and avoid packages with broken seals or contents that appear spoiled. Once in the home, foods should be cooked thoroughly and leftovers stored properly. Kitchen surfaces, hands, and cooking utensils should be cleaned between preparation steps.

6. Contaminants such as pesticides applied to crops, drugs given to animals, and industrial wastes that leach into water may find their way into the food supply.

7. To decrease the potential risk of pesticides, safer ones are being developed and American farmers are reducing the amounts applied by using integrated pest management and organic methods.

8. Industrial pollutants such as PCBs, radioactive substances, and toxic metals have contaminated some waterways and the fish that live in them. As these contaminants move up the food chain, their concentrations increase.

9. Consumers can reduce the amounts of pesticides and other environmental contaminants in food by careful selection and handling of produce; selection of lowfat saltwater varieties of fish caught well offshore in unpolluted waters; and trimming fat from meat, poultry, and fish before cooking.

10. Food additives include all substances that can reasonably be expected to find their way into a food during processing. This includes direct food additives, which are used to preserve or enhance the appeal of food, and indirect food additives, which are substances known to find their way into food during cooking, processing, and packaging. Direct and indirect food additives are regulated by the FDA. Accidental contaminants that enter food when it is used or prepared incorrectly are not regulated by the FDA.

11. Processing and packaging techniques are used to prevent food spoilage. Cold temperatures slow or prevent microbial growth. High temperatures used in canning, pasteurization, sterilization, and cooking kill microorganisms. Packaging also preserves foods. Aseptic processing sterilizes the food and the package; modified atmosphere packaging reduces the oxygen available for microbial growth. However, cooking and packaging can also introduce hazards into foods.

12. Irradiation preserves food by exposing it to x-rays, gamma radiation, or high-energy electrons. It kills microorganisms, destroys insects, and slows the germination and ripening of fruits and vegetables.

13. New foods and products can be produced using biotechnology. These techniques alter the DNA of plants or animals to produce new varieties with desired traits, such as disease resistance, increased nutrient content, or delayed spoilage.

14. Genetically engineered products are carefully monitored to ensure the safety of the consumer and the environment. Health concerns include the potential to introduce allergens or toxins into foods or to negatively affect nutrient content. Environmental concerns include reducing biologic diversity, the evolution of pesticide-resistant insects, and the creation of super weeds.

REVIEW QUESTIONS

1. What is the major cause of food-borne illness in the United States today?

2. List three factors that affect the toxicity of a substance.

3. Explain what HACCP is and how it can prevent food contamination.

4. List three ways in which the federal government is involved in providing a safe food supply.

5. List three common bacterial food contaminants. What can be done to avoid the food-borne illnesses caused by them?

6. What temperature range allows the most rapid bacterial growth?

7. What is the difference between a food-borne infection and a food-borne intoxication?

8. How do pesticides applied to crops find their way into animal products?

9. List some ways in which food processing reduces food-borne illnesses.

10. What is the GRAS list?

11. List four reasons for using food additives.

12. What is food irradiation? Is it safe?

13. How does genetic engineering introduce new traits into plants?

14. List three benefits of food biotechnology and three potential risks.

REFERENCES

1. Mead, P. S., Slutsker, L., Dietz, V., et al. Food-related illness and death in the United States. *Emerg. Infect. Dis.* 5:607–625, 1999.

2. National Academy of Sciences. *Ensuring Safe Food from Production to Consumption.* Washington, D.C.: National Academy Press, 1998.

3. Knabel, S. J. Institute of Food Technologists Scientific Status Summary: Foodborne illness: Role of home food handling practices. *Food Technol.* 49:119–131, 1995.

4. U.S. Food and Drug Administration, Department of Agriculture, and Environmental Protection Agency. Food Safety from Farm to Table: A New Strategy for the 21st Century. February 21, 1997. Available online at vm.cfsan.fda.gov/~dms/fs-draft.html Accessed August 3, 2002.

5. U.S. Department of Health and Human Services. National computer network in place to combat foodborne illness (press release). May 22, 1998. Available online at www.cdc.gov/od/oc/media/pressrel/r980522.htm Accessed August 3, 2002.

6. Cerington, M. Clinical spectrum of botulism. *Muscle Nerve* 21:701–710, 1998.

7. Kohn, M. A., Farley, T. A., Ando, T., et al. An outbreak of Norwalk virus gastroenteritis associated with eating raw oysters: implications for maintaining safe oyster beds. *JAMA* 273:466–471, 1995.

8. U.S. Food and Drug Administration, Center for Food Safety and Nutrition. Foodborne Pathogenic Microoganisms and Natual Toxins Handbook: The "Bad Bug Book." Available online at vm.cfsan.fda.gov/~mow/intro.html Accessed August 3, 2002.

9. Outbreaks of *Escherichia coli* O157:H7 infection and cryptosporidosis associated with drinking unpasteurized apple cider—Connecticut and New York, October 1996. *MMWR Morb. Mortal. Wkly. Rep.* 46:4–8, 1997.

10. Foodborne outbreak of diarrheal illness associated with *Cryptosporidium parvum*—Minnesota, 1995. MMWR *Morb. Mortal. Wkly. Rep.* 45:783–784, 1996.

11. Kolpin, D. W., Barbash, J. E., and Gilliom, R. J. Occurrence of pesticides in shallow groundwater of the United States—initial results from the National Water-Quality Assessment Program. *Environ. Sci. Technol.* 32:558–566, 1998.

12. Foulke, J. E. FDA reports on pesticides in foods. *FDA Consumer* 27:29–32, June 1993.

13. Cooney, C. M. New pesticide law drops "zero-tolerance" standard, focuses on exposure to children. *Environ. Sci. Technol.* 30:380A, September 1996.

14. National Research Council, Committee on Comparative Toxicology of Naturally Occurring Carcinogens. Individual chemicals in the diet generally pose no risk to Americans, NRC concludes. *Food Chem. News* 37:32–33, February 19, 1996.

15. Acquavella, J., Burns, C., Flaherty, D., et al. A critique of the World Resource Institute's report "Pesticides and the Immune System: The Public Health Risks." *Environ. Health Perspect.* 106:51–54, 1998.

16. U.S. Department of Agriculture, Agricultural Marketing Service. National Organic Program: Final Rule. Available online at www.ams.usda.gov/nop/nop2000/nop/finalrulepages/finalrulemap.htm/ Accessed March 1, 2001.

17. U.S. Food and Drug Administration, Center for Veterinary Medicine Communications and Education Branch. Monitoring for Residues in Food Animals. Revised March 1994. Available online at www.fda.gov/cvm/index/memos/cvmm19.html/ Accessed March 2, 2001.

18. Kaneene, J. B., and Miller, R. Problems associated with drug residues in beef from feeds and therapy. *Rev. Sci. Tech.* 16:694–708, 1997.

19. Ropp, K. L. New animal drug increases milk production. *FDA Consumer* 28:24–27, May 1994.

20. Clarkson, T. W. Environmental contaminants in the food chain. *Am. J. Clin. Nutr.* 61(suppl):682S–686S, 1995.

21. Jacobson, J. L., and Jacobson, S. W. Intellectual impairment in children exposed to polychlorinated biphenyls in utero. *N. Engl. J. Med.* 335:783–789, 1996.

22. American Academy of Pediatrics, Committee on Environmental Health. PCBs in breast milk. *Pediatrics* 84:122–123, 1994.

23. Foulke, J. E. Mercury in fish: cause for concern? *FDA Consumer* 28:5–8, September 1994.

24. Eichholzer, M., and Gutzwiller, F. Dietary nitrates, nitrites, and N-nitroso compounds and cancer risk: A review of the epidemiologic evidence. *Nutr. Rev.* 56:95–105, 1998.

25. U.S. Food and Drug Administration. Food Color Facts. January 1993. Available online at vm.cfsan.fda.gov/~lrd/colorfac.html Accessed December 15, 2000.

26. Gould, G. W. Methods of preservation and extension of shelf life. *Int. J. Food Microbiol.* 33: 51–64, 1996.

27. U.S. General Accounting Office. Food Irradiation: Available Research Indicates That Benefits Outweigh Risks. Washington D.C., August, 2000. Available online at www.foodsafety.gov/~fsg/irradiat.html/ Accessed March 6, 2001.

28. Henkel, J. Irradiation: a safe measure for safer food. *FDA Consumer* 32:12–17, May/June 1998.

29. Skerrett, P. J. Food irradiation: will it keep the doctor away? *Technol. Rev.* 100:28–36, November/December 1997.

30. Smith, N. Seeds of opportunity: An assessment of the benefits, safety and oversight of plant genomics and agricultural biotechnology. U.S. House of Representatives report, 13 April 2000. Available online at www.house.gov/science/documents.htm/ Accessed October 25, 2000.

31. Ye, X., Al-Babili, S., Kloti, A., et al. Engineering the provitamin A (beta-carotene) biosynthetic pathway into (carotenoid-free) rice endosperm. *Science* 303–305, 2000.

32. Shintani, D., and DellaPenna, D. Elevating the vitamin E content of plants through metabolic engineering. *Science* 282:2098–2100, 1998.

33. National Academy of Sciences, National Research Council. *Genetically Modified Pest-Protected Plants: Science and Regulation.* Washington, D.C.: National Academy Press, 2000.

34. FDA Recalls and Field Corrections of Foods, Class I Enforcement Report. November 1, 2000. Available online at www.fda.gov/bbs/topics/enforce/enf00666.htm#Star/ Accessed 15 December 2000.

35. Thompson, L. Are bioengineered foods safe? *FDA Consumer* 18–23, January/February 2000.

36. Formanek. R., Proposed Rules Issued for Bioengineered Foods *FDA Consumer* March–April, 2001, Available Online at www.fda.gov/fdac/features/2001/201_food.html/ Accessed May 14, 2002.

18 The Global View: Feeding the World

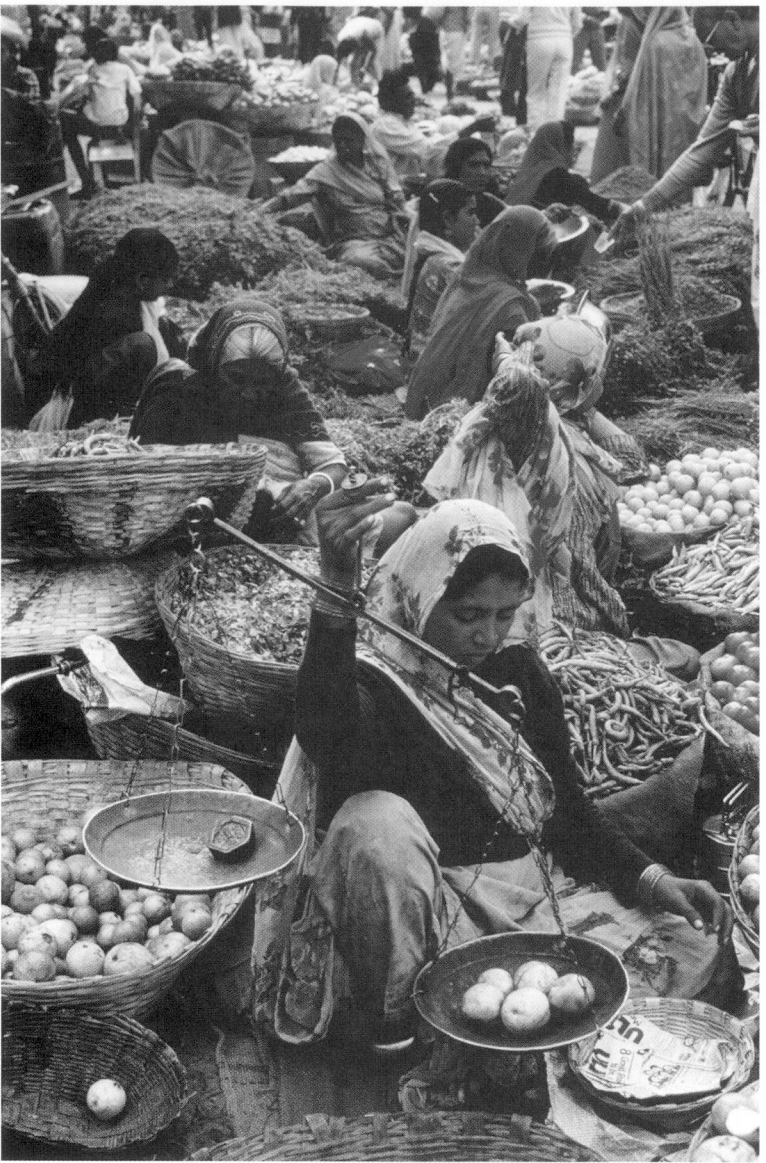

(© Nicholas De Vove/Stone)

Chapter Outline

UNDERNUTRITION:
A WORLD HEALTH PROBLEM
The Cycle of Malnutrition
Food Shortage
Poor Quality Diets
Solutions to World Hunger

FOOD INSECURITY AT HOME
Causes of Food Insecurity
Solutions to Food Insecurity

NUTRITION TRANSITION: THE GROWING
PROBLEM OF OVERNUTRITION

Chapter Concepts

✔ Overnutrition is prevalent in developed countries; undernutrition is a problem in much of the developing world.

✔ When food and nutrients are limited, a cycle of malnutrition produces poorly nourished infants who are at risk for infection, illness, and early death. Those who survive often grow to be unhealthy adults.

✔ Food shortages are caused by natural and man-made disasters and by overpopulation, inequitable distribution of money and other resources, and poor agricultural practices that damage the environment.

✔ Poor-quality diets and increased nutrient needs cause malnutrition even in populations with adequate food supplies.

✔ Solutions to the problem of worldwide undernutrition include short-term programs to feed the hungry and long-term programs that balance population size with resources.

✔ In the United States, the majority of the population is at risk for overnutrition, but some segments suffer from undernutrition.

✔ Solutions to hunger at home involve providing access to affordable food, education, and medical care.

✔ Overnutrition, with the resulting increase in the incidence of chronic disease, is a growing international problem.

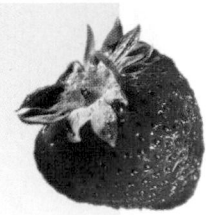

Just a Taste

Is there enough food to feed the world?

Is hunger a problem in the United States?

Can the food choices you make affect the environment?

In developed nations today, the majority of nutritional problems are related to overconsumption. Yet people around the world are starving. Undernutrition is the major form of malnutrition in developing nations, where almost 800 million people are chronically undernourished.[1] In addition, there are pockets of undernutrition in developed countries, including the United States.

Why are there two faces of malnutrition in the world? There are many reasons, but the underlying one is that the food produced in the world is not distributed equitably, so that in some places there is plenty and in others there is not enough. Overpopulation, inefficient land use, and inequitable distribution of land, wealth, and food cause populations and individuals within populations to be malnourished. Solving these problems involves controlling population growth, providing food, and changing agricultural, political, social, and economic systems.

Feeding the world involves every aspect of nutrition. It requires understanding nutrient needs and how to meet these needs. It involves the politics and economics of providing food. It involves technology to increase food production and environmental consciousness to maintain resources for future generations.

• UNDERNUTRITION: A WORLD HEALTH PROBLEM

Hunger is one of the first images that comes to mind when the topic of global nutrition is raised (Figure 18.1). Over time, hunger leads to undernutrition—a lack of energy or one or more nutrients. Undernutrition is the result of either not enough food or the wrong combination of foods to meet nutrient needs. Solutions to the

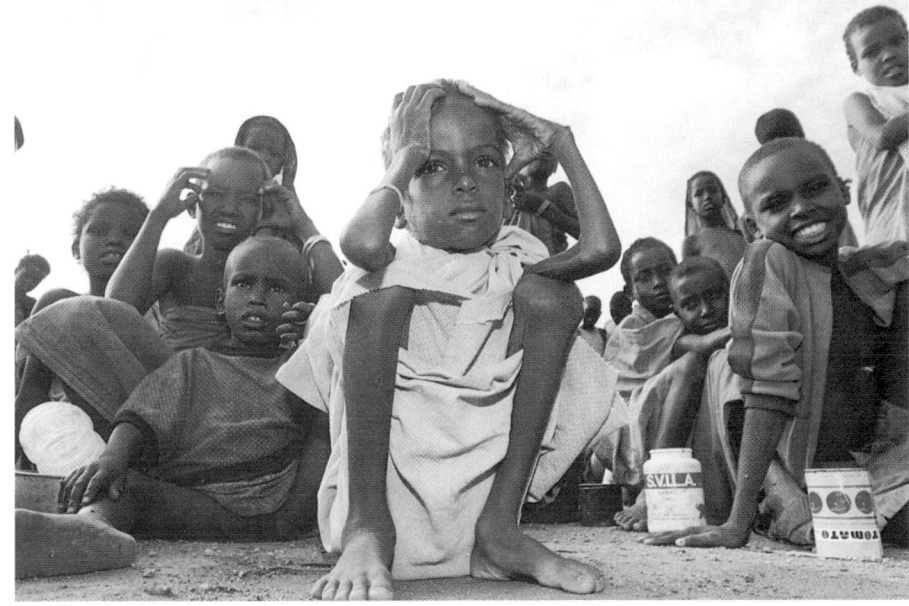

Figure 18.1
Undernutrition is more common in developing nations, especially among children because of their high nutrient needs. (Reuters/Corbis Bettmann)

517

problem of undernutrition must first feed the hungry and then develop strategies to promote a balance between the size of the population, the production of food, and the use of environmental resources.

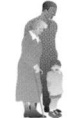

The Cycle of Malnutrition

In populations where undernutrition is a chronic problem, a **cycle of malnutrition** exists (Figure 18.2). The cycle of malnutrition begins when women consume a deficient diet during pregnancy. These women are more likely to give birth to low birth weight infants who are susceptible to illness and early death. The children who do survive may be small and weakened physically and mentally. They grow into undernourished adults unable to contribute optimally to economic and social development. Thus, the women in this next generation also begin their pregnancies poorly nourished and are therefore likely to give birth to low birth weight infants. Interruption of this cycle of malnutrition at any point can benefit the individuals and the society. Healthy children can then grow into healthy adults who produce healthy offspring and can contribute fully to society.

Low Birth Weight and Infant Mortality Low birth weight infants—those weighing less than 2500 grams (about 5.5 pounds) at birth—are at greater risk of complications, illness, and early death. A higher number of low birth weight infants means a higher **infant mortality rate**, the number of deaths per 1000 live births in a population. The infant mortality rate and the number of low birth weight births are indicators of the health and nutritional status of a population. The average infant mortality rate worldwide is about 51 per 1000, but in developing nations the average rate is 89 per 1000, as compared to only 9 per 1000 in more developed countries.[2] Low birth weight infants who do survive require extra nutrients, which are usually not available. Malnutrition in infancy and childhood has a profound effect on growth and development as well as susceptibility to infectious disease.

Stunting Malnourished children grow poorly. The prevalence of decreased linear growth, referred to as **stunting**, is used as an indicator of the well-being of popula-

Cycle of malnutrition A cycle in which malnutrition is perpetuated by an inability to meet nutrient needs at all life stages.

Infant mortality rate The number of deaths during the first year of life per 1000 live births.

Stunting A decrease in linear growth rate, which is an indicator of the nutritional well-being in populations of children.

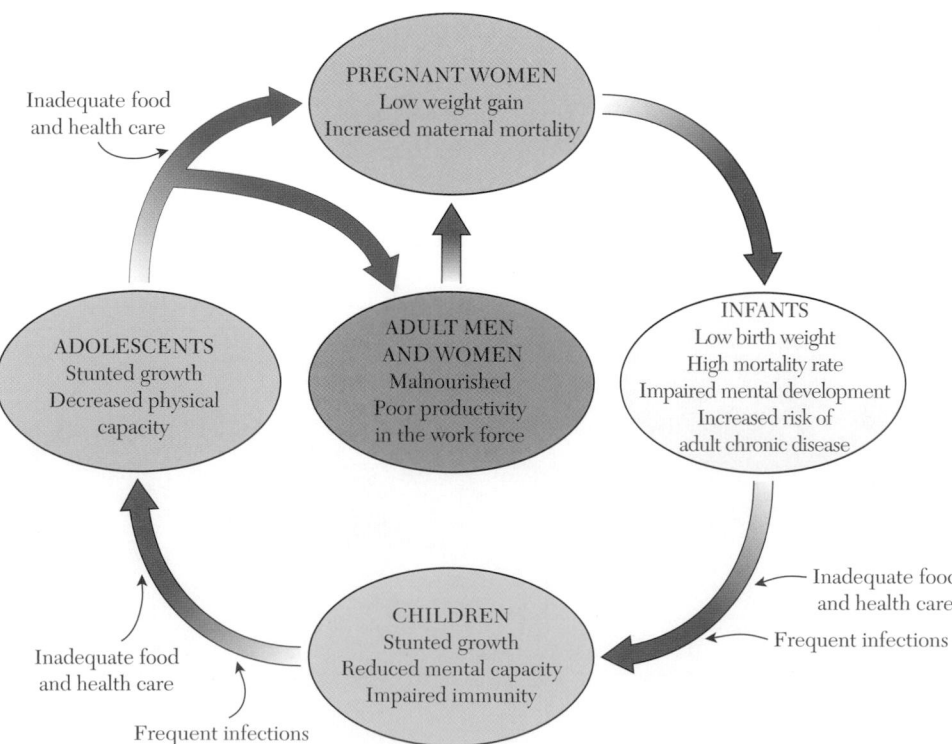

Figure 18.2
Malnutrition affects individuals at every stage of life. It often begins in the womb, continues through infancy and childhood, and extends into adolescent and adult life. This cycle of malnutrition affects both the health and the productivity of a population.

tions of children.[3] It is estimated that 32% of children under 5 years of age in developing countries suffer from stunting.[4] Deficiencies of energy, protein, iron, and zinc, as well as prolonged infections, have been implicated as causes. Stunting in childhood produces smaller adults who have a reduced work capacity. Stunted women are more likely to give birth to low birth weight babies.

Infectious Disease Undernourished children have depressed immune systems, which reduces their ability to resist infection. Of the 50 million deaths that occur worldwide each year, 80% are in developing countries, and half of mortality is due to infectious diseases and parasites.[5] Undernourished children may die of infectious diseases that would not be life-threatening in well-nourished children. Even immunization programs, designed to reduce the incidence of infectious disease, may be ineffective because the immune systems of undernourished individuals cannot respond normally. Mortality is increased even among children with mild to moderate malnutrition.[6]

Food Shortage

While much of the world currently has an abundant supply of food, there are areas where the total amount of food available is insufficient to feed the population. These **food shortages** cause widespread protein-energy malnutrition in local populations. Shortages of food occur for many reasons. The most obvious example of a food shortage is **famine**, which is a widespread failure in the food supply due to a collapse in the food production and marketing systems. Drought, floods, earthquakes, and crop destruction by diseases or pests are natural causes of famines (Figure 18.3). Man-made causes include wars and civil conflicts. Regions that produce barely enough food for survival under normal conditions are vulnerable to the disaster of famine. This situation is analogous to a man standing in water up to his nostrils: If all is calm, he can breathe, but if there is a ripple, he will drown. When a ripple such as a natural or civil disaster occurs, it cuts the margin of survival and creates famine.

Food shortage due to famine is very visible because it causes many deaths in one area during a short period of time. More chronic food shortages occur when the food supply is insufficient to feed the population; when cultural practices limit food choices; when economic inequities result in lack of money, health care, and education for individuals or populations; and when environmental resources are misused, limiting the ability to continue to produce food.

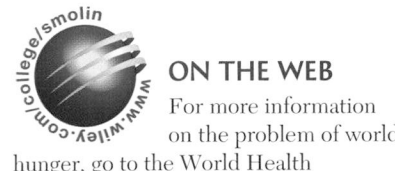

ON THE WEB
For more information
on the problem of world
hunger, go to the World Health
Organization at
　　　www.who.int/
the Food and Agriculture Organization
of the United Nations at
　　　www.fao.org/,
or UNICEF at
　　　www.unicef.org/.

Food shortage Insufficient food to feed a population.

Famine A widespread lack of access to food due to a disaster that causes a collapse in the food production and marketing systems.

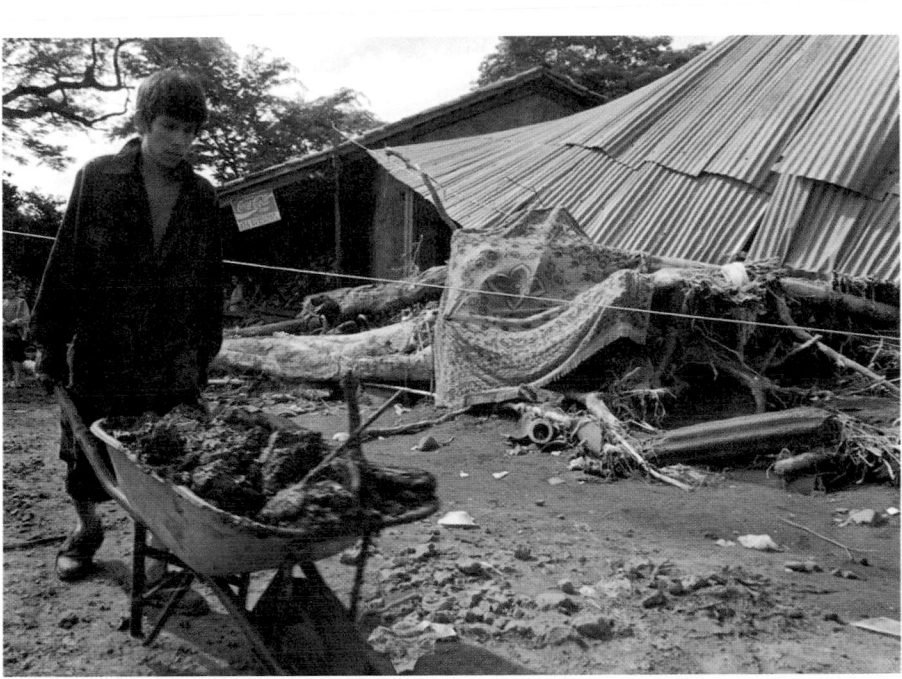

Figure 18.3
Natural disasters, such as hurricanes, destroy homes, farms, and infrastructure and can lead to famine. (© AP Photo/Luis Romero)

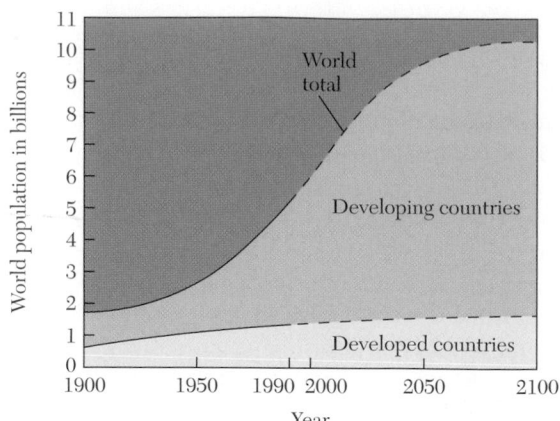

Figure 18.4
Since 1950, most of the increase in world population has occurred in developing countries, and this trend is expected to continue.

Overpopulation   Overpopulation exists when a region has more people than its natural resources can support. A fertile river valley can support more people per acre than can a desert environment. But even in fertile regions of the world, if the number of people increases too much, resources are overwhelmed and food shortages occur.

The human population is currently growing at a rate of more than 80 million persons per year, and most of this growth is occurring in developing countries (Figure 18.4). These countries cannot escape from poverty because their economy cannot keep pace with such fast population growth.[7] Efforts to produce enough food can damage the soil and deplete environmental resources, further reducing the capacity to produce food in the future. The problem of hunger today is due primarily to the unequal distribution of resources, but it is estimated that, worldwide, food production has begun to lag behind population growth.[8] If this trend continues, there will soon be too little food in the world to feed the population.

Culture   In some cultures, access to food may be limited for certain individuals within households. For example, women and girls may receive less food than men and boys because culturally they are viewed as less important. How much food is available to an individual within a household depends on gender, control of income, education, age, birth order, and genetic endowments.[9]

The cultural acceptability or unacceptability of foods also contributes to food shortages and malnutrition. If available foods are culturally unacceptable, a food shortage exists unless the population can be educated to use and accept the new food. For example, insects are eaten in some cultures and provide an excellent source of protein, but they are unacceptable to others.

Economics   About a quarter of the world's population lives in poverty, surviving on less than a dollar a day.[1] Poverty is at the root of the problem of undernutrition. The link between hunger and poverty is so strong that in most parts of the world their incidence is almost identical (Figure 18.5). Poverty can be viewed as the cause as well as the result of inadequate food production, distribution, and storage; of inappropriate utilization of resources; of unsanitary living conditions; and of lack of health care and education. Poverty and food insecurity (the inability to obtain food for any reason) occur in countries, in households, and among individuals when food and resources are not distributed equitably. And food insecurity increases the risk of malnutrition.

Economic Policies   On the national level, lack of money limits the ability to produce, transport, and distribute food. Nations have traditionally grown **subsistence crops**, the crops they need to feed their people. However, colonialism and the development of modern trade practices has shifted the emphasis from producing food for local

Subsistence crops   Crops grown as food for the local population.

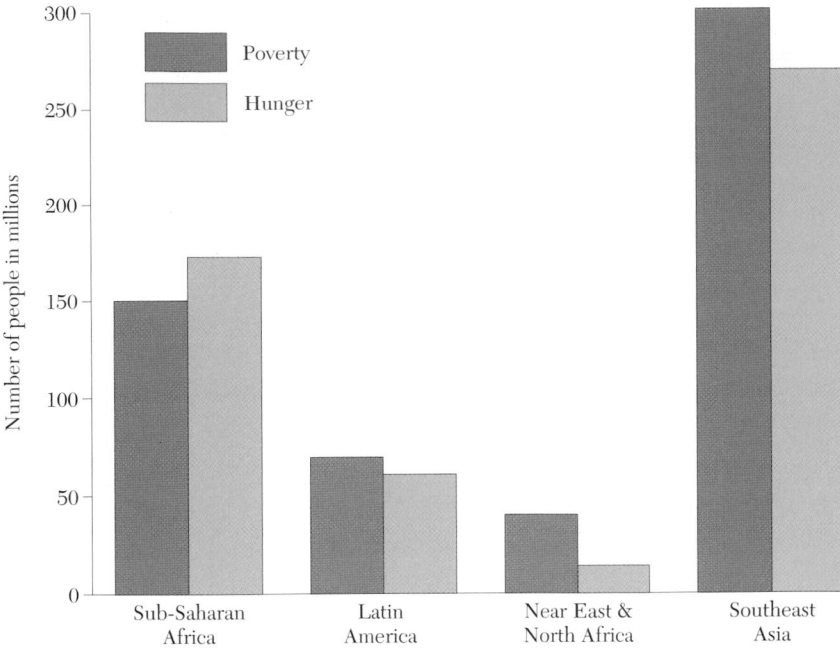

Figure 18.5
The incidences of hunger and poverty are almost identical in most parts of the world. (Adapted from Uvin, P. The state of world hunger. *Nutr. Rev.* 52:151–161, 1994.)

consumption to producing **cash crops**, which can be sold on the national and international market. This improves the cash flow of the country but uses local resources to produce crops for export and leaves the least fertile land to grow food for local consumption.

Household and Individual Poverty At the household and individual level, if money is scarce, food cannot be obtained and malnutrition increases. The poorest poor do not own land to grow food and do not have money to buy enough food or enough of the right kinds of food to meet nutritional needs.

The poor also have less access to health care. Malnutrition increases the incidence of disease and disability, and, in turn, disease further increases malnutrition. Because health care is unavailable, diseases go untreated—which can increase nutrient needs and limit the ability to acquire food. Lack of health care also increases infant mortality and the incidence of low birth weight births. Lack of immunizations and treatment for infections and other illnesses results in an increased incidence and morbidity from infectious disease and a decrease in survival rates from chronic diseases such as cancer.

Lack of education and subsequent illiteracy go hand in hand with poverty, reducing opportunities to escape poverty and increasing the risk of undernutrition and disease (Table 18.1). Inadequate education leads to inadequate care for infants, children, and pregnant women. A lack of education about food preparation and storage can affect food safety and the health of the household—unsanitary food preparation increases the incidence of gastrointestinal diseases, which contribute to malnutrition.

Environment The land and resources available for food production are limited. Some resources, such as minerals and fossil fuels, are present in the earth in limited amounts and are nonrenewable—that is, once used they cannot be replaced in a reasonable amount of time. Technology will need to find substitutes for these resources. Other resources are **renewable** if they are not damaged and are used at a rate at which the earth can restore them. For example, if agricultural land is used wisely—crops rotated, erosion prevented, contamination limited—it can be reused almost endlessly. However, if this land is not used carefully, soil erosion, nutrient depletion, and accumulation of pollutants in soil and water may occur at a rate that exceeds the earth's ability to restore and repair these resources. As agricultural lands are depleted,

Cash crops Crops grown to be sold for monetary return rather than to be used for food locally.

Renewable resources Resources that are restored and replaced by natural processes and that can therefore be used forever.

Table 18.1 *Indicators of Poverty and Malnutrition*

	Infant Mortality (deaths per 1000 live births)	Life Expectancy (years)	Illiteracy (percent of population)	Access to Medical Care (people per physician)
More Developed Countries	20	76	3	680
Less Developed Countries				
Sierra Leone	182	37.2	66.7	———
Central Africa	113	44.9	57.6	25,920
Ghana	67	60	33.6	22,970
Ivory Coast	81	46.7	57.4	11,739
El Salvador	31	69.6	23	848
Cuba	7	76	4.1	176
Haiti	71	54.1	54.2	4,000
India	70	62.6	46.5	2,459
Bangladesh	79	58.1	61	12,884

Global cardiovascular disease information base: cvdinfobase.ic.gc.ca/gcvi/default/htm, and World Bank: www.worldbank.org/data/wdi2000/pdfs/tab2_18.pdf.

forests are cut down to create more agricultural land. This contributes to soil erosion. Deforestation combined with air pollution contributes to global climate changes. Lack of water and pollution of existing water limit agricultural productivity, and overgrazing destroys rangelands. Whether animal products, agricultural crops, or fish or seafood are being produced and distributed, the environmental cost could be high. To maintain adequate agricultural land and water resources, those available must be used in ways that will sustain them for continued use.

Environmental Cost of Meat Production Modern meat production is an example of the inefficient use of natural resources. Modern methods of raising cattle use grain, water, and fossil fuels, and create both air and water pollution. Cattle raised in the United States spend most of their lives eating grass from grazing lands; then, for about their last 100 days, the animals are kept in stockyards and fed grain to increase their body fat (Figure 18.6). A large proportion of the grain produced in the United States is used for this purpose. To produce this feed grain, fertilizers and pesticides are used, soil is eroded, and groundwater is contaminated. Much of the grain is grown on land that must be irrigated, so water supplies are depleted as well (about 87% of the fresh water in the world today is consumed by agriculture[10]). The animals themselves produce methane gas in their gastrointestinal tracts, which enters the air and contributes to the greenhouse effect. And when animal sewage is stored in ponds and heaps, it decomposes anaerobically, producing more methane (see *Off the Shelf*: Do Vegetarian Diets Help the Environment?).

Environmental Cost of Agricultural Crops The environmental cost of producing plant-based foods is lower than that of animal products, but it may still be substantial. For example, growing a head of lettuce in California using pesticides and fertilizer and then trucking it in a refrigerated car to New York requires a great deal of energy. The price of our food may reflect some of these costs, but the cost of the damage to soil, groundwater, and farm workers caused by pesticides and fertilizers is not included.

Overfishing and Water Pollution Throughout human history fish have been an important source of protein. However, increases in population have increased de-

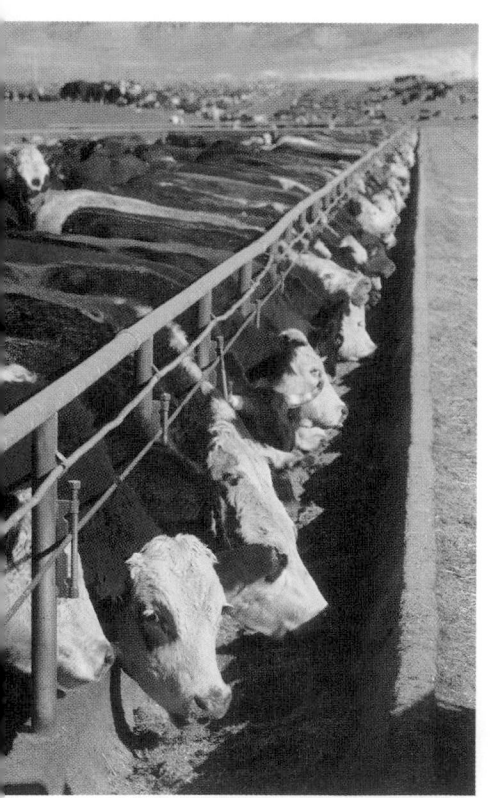

Figure 18.6
Housing large numbers of cattle in stockyards is environmentally costly. They are fed grain, which uses many resources to produce, and they generate wastes that can contaminate the environment. (© Corbis Stock Market)

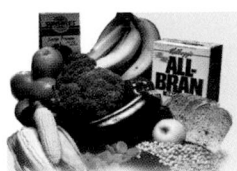

Off the Shelf

Do Vegetarian Diets Help the Environment?

One of the reasons people choose to adopt vegetarian diets is concern about the environment. They argue that producing animal products consumes large amounts of energy, destroys forests and grazing lands, and pollutes the air and water. Although these arguments are valid in some instances, the impact of food animals on the ecosystem depends on how they are integrated into the environment.

For thousands of years, animals were raised on small farms or grazed on open land. The drive to produce animals more efficiently and more profitably has moved them off the family farm and into large agribusinesses. This has had an impact on energy use, land and water use, and air quality.

On a small farm, animals can consume crop wastes, kitchen scraps, and cellulose grasses that people cannot eat, and turn them into meat, milk, and eggs that make important contributions to the human diet. But animals raised in agribusinesses are fed grain rather than grasses and kitchen scraps. This is inefficient because humans who eat the animals get back only a fraction of the energy they could have gotten from eating the grain. For every 100 kcalories of plant material a cow eats, only 10 kcalories are stored in the cow and can be consumed by humans.[1] In the United States, 1 pound of pork provides 1000 to 2000 kcalories in the diet and costs 14,000 kcalories to produce. Worldwide, 38% of the total grain produced is fed to chickens, pigs, and cows. In the United States, as much as 70% of grain grown is fed to animals. Livestock production also uses water—430 gallons to produce 1 pound of pork in the United States. For the world to adopt an American-type diet would require "more grain than the world can grow and more energy, water, and land than the world can supply."[2]

Management of animal waste materials also affects the environment. On small farms, manure is used for fertilizer in local fields, but when thousands of animals are confined to a small area, manure builds up rapidly and the runoff may pollute nearby rivers and lakes. This can cause algae overgrowth that kills other aquatic life and causes nitrate pollution of drinking water. Animal wastes also produce gases that are released into the atmosphere, contributing to acid rain and global warming.

The sheer number of domestic animals is also destructive to the environment. When pastures are overstocked and grazing lands are overgrazed, it reduces the potential to continue to use these lands. Forests such as those in the Amazon are being cut down to create new grazing land for cattle. Forests serve to absorb carbon dioxide; therefore, deforestation allows carbon dioxide to accumulate in the atmosphere and contributes to global warming. Whether domestic animals are confined or free, the natural resources of the Earth are no longer able to sustain their increasing numbers without serious ecological consequences.

Is the elimination of animal foods the answer to feeding the world and saving the planet? Not really. Animal foods make important contributions to the human diet. In parts of the developing world, small amounts of meat and milk in the diet mean the difference between survival and starvation. In the United States, animal foods provide important sources of vitamin B_{12}, calcium, and highly absorbable forms of iron and zinc. Eliminating animal products entirely would reduce both the variety of food and the nutrient content of the human diet.

If we are to both nourish the world and preserve the environment, sustainable agricultural systems must be adopted. The aim of sustainable agriculture is to produce both plant and animal foods while preserving the long-term fertility and productiveness of the planet. Just as the natural ecosystems of the Earth depend on both plants and animals, so must sustainable agricultural systems. For example, in a sustainable system, fertile land would be used to grow crops for human consumption and cattle and sheep would feed only from grazing lands unsuitable for growing crops. This would utilize both productive and unproductive cropland in an ecologically sound manner. However, this system would also produce many fewer animals than the present system. To absorb the decrease in production, demand for animal products would have to decrease in developed nations. Consuming a diet that is higher in grains, vegetables, and fruits and lower in animal products is therefore a goal that is compatible not only with the recommendations of the Dietary Guidelines but also with the ecology of the planet.

Completely eliminating animal products is neither necessary nor beneficial. Both plants and animals are essential for a diversified ecosystem, and both plant and animal foods make valuable contributions to the diet.

[1]Raven, P. H., Berg, L. R., and Johnson, G. B. *Environment*, 3rd ed. Philadelphia: Harcourt College Publishers, 2001.

[2]Durning, A. T. Fat of the land. *World Watch* 4:7–11; 1991.

---

mand for fish to the point that the earth's oceans are being depleted. Because the ocean is open to fishermen from around the world, its use has been difficult to control. Many marine species have been harvested until their numbers are severely depleted. According to the United Nations Food and Agriculture Organization, 70% of the world's fish stocks are either fully exploited, overexploited, or depleted. Pollution also threatens the world's fishing grounds. Oil spills and deliberate dumping can occur offshore, and sewage, pesticides, organic pollutants, and sediments from erosion wash into coastal waters where most fish spend at least part of their lives.

Poor Quality Diets

Undernutrition can be caused by a poor-quality diet. The typical diet in developing countries is based on high-fiber grain products and has little variety. Adults who are able to consume a relatively large amount of this diet may be able to meet their nutrient needs. But those with increased needs or a limited capacity to consume these foods are at risk for nutrient deficiencies. Children, pregnant women, the elderly, and the ill may not be able to eat enough of this bulky grain diet to meet their needs. Deficiencies of protein, iron, iodine, and vitamin A are common because of poor-quality diets.

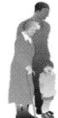 **Protein-Energy Malnutrition** Over 200 million children under the age of five suffer from deficiencies of protein and energy.[11] Protein and energy deficiencies usually occur together. However, in individuals with high protein needs—those who are growing, developing, or healing—protein deficiency can predominate (see Chapter 6). Kwashiorkor (a deficiency of protein but not energy) occurs as a result of the wrong combination of foods rather than of a general lack of food. It is common in children over 18 months of age when the main energy source is a bulky cereal grain low in high-quality protein. Children have small stomachs and are not able to consume enough of this diet to meet their protein needs (Figure 18.7). Other factors such as metabolic changes caused by infection may also play a role in the development of kwashiorkor.

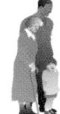 **Iron Deficiency** Iron deficiency anemia is the most common nutritional problem in both developed and developing nations, but the prevalence is almost fourfold higher in the developing world, where it affects 43% of all women and 34% of all men.[3] When the amount of iron available in the diet does not meet individual needs, it causes iron deficiency, which can lead to anemia. It is estimated that a third of the population worldwide, over 2 billion people, suffer from iron deficiency anemia and another 5 billion have low iron stores.[12] Thirty-nine percent of preschool children and 52% of pregnant women are anemic; 90% of these live in developing countries.

Iron deficiency can result from an increased need for iron, chronic loss of iron due to blood loss, or a diet with inadequate amounts of iron-containing foods or one that limits iron bioavailability. Nonheme iron from plant sources is the major dietary source of iron in many parts of the developing world where meat consumption is economically unfeasible. This dietary pattern increases the risk for iron deficiency because nonheme iron is poorly absorbed. Also, intestinal parasites, especially hookworm infections, cause gastrointestinal blood loss, which leads to iron deficiency anemia. The greater rates of both acute and chronic infections, such as malaria, in the developing world aggravate dietary iron deficiency.

Iron deficiency can have a major impact on the health and productivity of a population. Anemia during pregnancy increases the risk of maternal and fetal mortality, premature delivery, and low birth weight. Iron deficiency in infants and children can stunt growth and retard mental development, decrease resistance to infection, and increase morbidity due to disease.[13] In older children and adults it causes fatigue and decreased productivity (see Chapter 11).

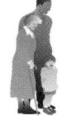 **Iodine Deficiency Diseases** Iodine is a trace element that is an essential constituent of the thyroid hormones. It is estimated that 1.6 billion people live in areas considered to be at risk for iodine deficiency and that about 655 million, or 12% of the global population, have goiter, a sympton of iron deficiency.[14] Iodine deficiency occurs in regions with iodine-deficient soil that rely extensively on locally produced food. Iodine-deficiency disorders affect virtually all members of a community and worldwide are believed to be the greatest single cause of preventable brain damage and mental retardation.[15] During pregnancy iodine deficiency increases the incidence of stillbirths, spontaneous abortions, and developmental abnormalities such as cretinism. Cretinism is characterized by irreversible mental and physical retardation. Iodine-deficient chil-

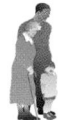

dren have lower IQs and impaired school performance.[16] In children and adults it is associated with apathy and decreased initiative and decision-making capabilities.

Vitamin A Deficiency It is estimated that 3 to 10 million children worldwide suffer from vitamin A deficiency.[17] It causes blindness; depresses immune function, which increases the risk of infections; retards growth; and is often accompanied by anemia.

Vitamin A deficiency can be caused by a low intake of the vitamin in relation to need. Obtaining sufficient vitamin A is a particular problem during periods of rapid growth and development, such as infancy, early childhood, pregnancy, and lactation. Need is increased by frequent infections, such as those causing diarrhea, and illnesses such as measles.[3] Deficiencies of other nutrients, including fat, protein, and zinc, can contribute to vitamin A deficiency because they are needed to absorb and transport the vitamin in the body.

Solutions to World Hunger

Solving the problem of world hunger is a daunting task. It involves controlling population growth, meeting the nutritional needs of a large and diverse population with culturally acceptable foods, increasing food production, and maintaining the global ecosystem. It requires international cooperation, commitment from national and local governments, and the involvement of local populations. The solutions involve economic policies, technical advancement, education, and legislative measures. They require input from politicians, nutrition scientists, economists, and the food industry.

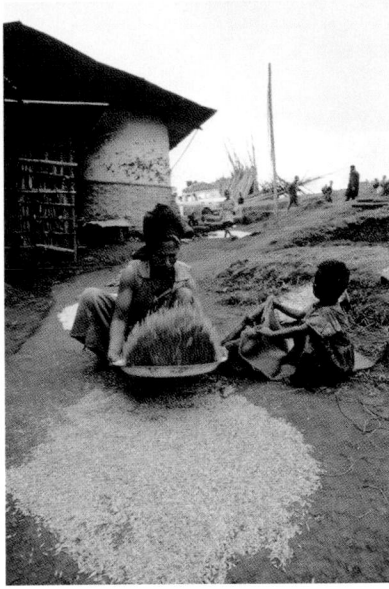

Figure 18.7
Because of their size, children are often unable to eat enough of a bulky grain diet to meet their nutrient needs. (Corbis/Jim Sugar Photography)

The World Food Summit In the 1900s a series of global conferences were held to address the problems of hunger and undernutrition throughout the world. One of these conferences, the 1996 World Food Summit, worked to develop plans that would promote food security, defined as a condition in which "all people, at all times, have physical and economic access to sufficient, safe, and nutritious food to meet their dietary needs and food preferences for an active and healthy life."[18] They pledged to cut in half the number of hungry people in the world by the year 2015. There is agreement on this goal, but opinions differ as to how it should be achieved. Some view food security as a supply problem that could be solved by controlling population growth and increasing agricultural production. Others see food security as a demand problem that could be solved by more equitable food distribution, reducing overconsumption in certain areas, and improving food self-sufficiency by reducing the industrialization of farming. However the problem is viewed, programs and policies must first provide food and then establish **sustainable** programs to allow continued production and distribution.

Sustainable Refers to methods of using resources that prevent overuse of natural systems and allow the environment to be maintained indefinitely without a decline.

Short-Term Solutions: Responding to Emergency Situations The first step in resolving undernutrition is to provide short-term food and medical aid. The standard approach has been to bring food into the stricken area (Figure 18.8). These foods generally consist of agricultural surpluses from other countries and often are not well planned in terms of their nutrient content.[19] Although this type of relief is necessary for a population to survive an immediate crisis such as famine, it does little to prevent future hunger.

There are many international, national, and private organizations working toward the goal of relieving world hunger. The World Health Organization, the United Nations (UN) Food and Agriculture Organization (FAO), and the World Bank provide food and economic relief. The emphasis of the FAO is on the production, intake, and distribution of food. WHO targets community health centers and emphasizes the prevention of nutrition problems, such as micronutrient deficiencies. The World Bank finances projects such as supplementation and fortification to foster economic development. The United Nations Children's Fund (UNICEF), which relies on volunteer support, distributes food to all countries in need with a goal of assisting developing countries that occasionally suffer periods of starvation. The Red Cross, the UN Disaster Relief

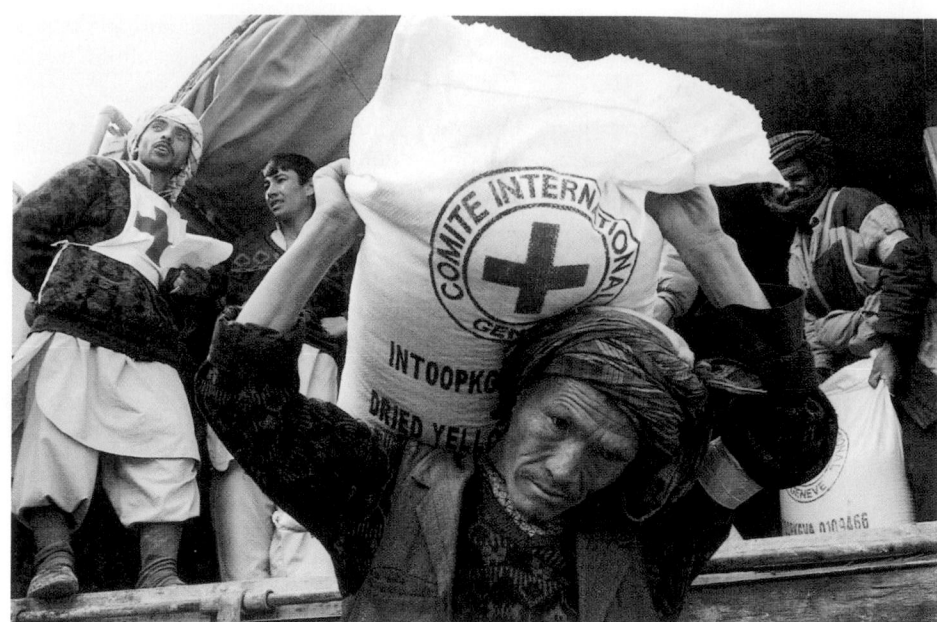

Figure 18.8
There are many international relief organizations that provide food to hungry people throughout the world. (© AP Wide World Photos)

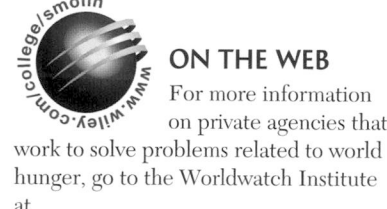

ON THE WEB
For more information on private agencies that work to solve problems related to world hunger, go to the Worldwatch Institute at

www.worldwatch.org/,
or Food First at
www.foodfirst.org/.

Organization, and the UN High Commissioner for Refugees concentrate on famine relief. The Peace Corps focuses more on fostering long-range development. More and more agencies are engaging in both development and relief. A few examples include the U.S. Agency for International Development, Oxfam, the Hunger Project, and Catholic Relief Services.

Long-Term Solutions: Increasing the Ratio of Food to People Long-term solutions to hunger and undernutrition need to be based on the cultural and economic needs of the local population. Local governments need to work to increase the ratio of food to people by controlling population growth and increasing food production.

Controlling Population The problem of world hunger can be solved only by bringing the population into line with the ability to produce food. One solution is to decrease the rate of population growth by controlling birthrates. Although the rate of population growth worldwide has slowed from more than 6 children per woman in 1950 to 3.3 in 1998, the world's population is still growing faster than the food supply.[7]

A direct method of controlling population growth is family planning. To be successful, family-planning efforts must be acceptable to the population and compatible with their cultural and religious needs. A number of approaches, such as provision of contraceptives, education, and economic incentives, have been used to decrease population growth. In Singapore, Thailand, Colombia, and Costa Rica, programs that provide contraceptive information, services, and supplies have been somewhat successful in slowing population growth. In some countries, population-control education is being integrated into the school curriculum, and in Mexico and Egypt popular television shows carry family-planning messages.

Increasing the general level of education has also been shown to reduce population growth.[9] When the social and economic status of women is improved, birthrates decrease.[20] Women with more education tend to marry later and have fewer children. Education also increases the likelihood that women will have control over their fertility, provides knowledge to improve family health, decreases infant and child mortality rates, and offers options other than having numerous children.

Changes in economic policies can help reduce population growth. In many areas, children provide economic security. They are needed to work the farms, support the elders, and otherwise contribute to the economic survival of the family. Thus people are resistant to family-planning messages because of high infant mortal-

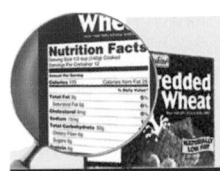

Off the Label
Food Labels: An International Perspective

Importing foods from other countries can enhance the nutrient content and diversity of a nation's food supply. Foods imported to the United States must meet U.S. standards, including those for food labeling. Likewise, foods we export to other countries must meet the labeling guidelines from those nations. Over the last decade, an increase in the international trade of both raw agricultural commodities and processed foods has made food labeling an international issue.[1]

Food labels appear to be simply a source of nutrition information. So why are they an issue? The information on the label is actually of interest at the national, cultural, economic, and consumer levels.[2] Governments want labeling information to be compatible with their national nutrition and food-safety guidelines, such as regulations for food additives, standards for composition of common products, and limits or thresholds of ingredients. Businesses want labels to emphasize features that give the product a competitive advantage. Consumers want labels to tell them how foods fit into their diets. Achieving all of these goals among countries is a difficult task. Despite the high priority of setting international standards for trade, a standard food label is unlikely to be agreed upon.

Without standardized food labels, food for export must be specially labeled. This is expensive even when the labeling guidelines are not too different between countries. For example, if a Canadian food manufacturer wants to export cookies to the United States, it must relabel its product to meet all of the specifications of the U.S. Nutrition Labeling and Education Act. The amount of each nutrient must be adjusted to U.S. serving sizes, and the percent Daily Values must be added. For countries with no labeling guidelines, even getting the information about product composition may be costly.

Currently there are some minimum standards for international labeling of prepackaged foods. They are determined by the Codex Alimentarius Commission (Latin for "code concerned with nourishment") and state simply that "prepackaged foods should not be described or presented on any label or in any labeling material in a manner that is false, misleading, or deceptive or is likely to create an erroneous impression regarding its character in any respect." Guidelines also state that when a nutrition claim or representation is made on the label, the declaration of a standardized list of nutrients becomes mandatory. Canadian and European nutrition labeling systems are similar to Codex guidelines. Labeling regulations in the United States are not contradictory to these but are much more stringent.

Harmonization of food labels and requirements for composition, formulations, and allowable additives would permit manufacturers to produce and label foods for sale in any country. Without some standardization of labeling, the burden of specially labeling foods for export will limit what foods are sold in the United States and therefore limit consumer choices, corporate choices, and government choices.

[1]Potter, N. N., and Hotchkiss, J. H. *Food Science*, 5th ed. New York: Chapman & Hall, 1995.
[2]Food labeling: a Canadian and international perspective. *Nutr. Rev.* 53:103–105, 1995.

---

ity rates—they choose to have many children to ensure that some will survive. Programs that foster economic development and ensure access to food, shelter, and medical care have been shown to cause a decline in birthrates. For example, a reduction in birthrates occurred along with economic success in South Korea.

Stabilizing the Food Supply In order to provide long-term food security, populations must develop manageable systems for producing acceptable, sustainable sources of food. Increasing the level of **food self-sufficiency**, a country's capacity to feed its population, can help to prevent food shortages.

Trade policies often determine what crops will be grown on a nation's arable land. A decision to grow a cash crop instead of food for local consumption may mean that less food is available for the local diet. If, however, the cash from the crop is used to purchase nutritious foods from other countries, this decision may help alleviate undernutrition. Countries that have few natural resources must rely on international trade to distribute world resources more equitably. Trade can provide an economic advantage if food is imported and other products on which a good monetary return is obtained are exported. The newly industrialized countries of Asia such as Japan and Korea are examples of how an increase in food imports can decrease the number of hungry people. In general, the countries of the world are becoming more interdependent on food imports and on exports to pay for this food. Policies and practices in each nation must be developed to ensure that the local population can be fed (see *Off the Label*: Food Labels: An International Perspective).

Food self-sufficiency The ability of an area to produce enough food to feed its population.

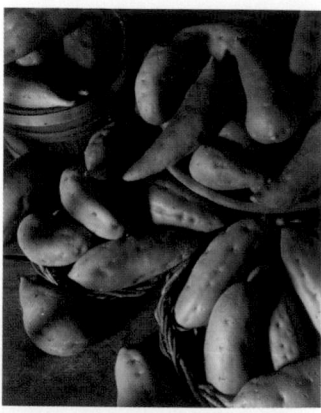

Figure 18.9
The white yam is a poor source of beta-carotene, but the yellow yam supplies the requirement for vitamin A in a single serving. (© Ross Durant/Foodpix)

Alleviating Poverty Although controlling population growth and ensuring adequate food are essential steps in eliminating world hunger, hunger will still exist as long as there is poverty. Even when food is plentiful in a region, the poor do not have access to enough of the right foods to maintain their nutritional health. Economic development that guarantees safe and sanitary housing, access to health care and education, and the resources to acquire enough food are essential to eliminate hunger. Poor, hungry people have little influence on government policies, but these policies can result in higher incomes, lower food prices, or feeding programs for the poor, all of which can improve food security.

Providing Education Educational programs as well as technology may be necessary to make food available and safe. Providing food or technology does little if individuals do not know how to use it. For example, a new crop variety is not beneficial unless local farmers know how to grow it and the population accepts it as a food source and knows how to prepare it for consumption. For instance, white yams are common in some regions but are a poor source of provitamin A. If the yellow yam, which is rich in provitamin A, became an acceptable choice, the provitamin A content of the diet would increase (Figure 18.9). Food safety is also a concern when changing traditional dietary practices. For example, introducing papaya to the diet as a source of vitamin A will not improve nutritional status if it is washed in unsanitary water and causes dysentery among the people it is meant to nourish.

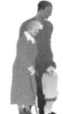

Education to encourage breast feeding can also improve nutritional status and health. Breast feeding reduces the risk of infectious diseases in infants. When infants are not breast fed, education about nutritious breast milk substitutes and safe preparation of formulas is essential.

Solutions for the Life of the Planet: Environmental Awareness The resources needed to support food production depend on the methods used. In developing nations, the resources used by a single person are small, but the number of people is large so it is difficult to produce sufficient food without depleting natural resources. Solutions to the problem of providing enough food must assure that natural resources are conserved to allow continued food production for future generations.

Sustainable Food Production Maintaining the world food supply for the long term requires development of policies that promote sustainable agriculture. Sustainable methods produce food while allowing the environment to restore itself so food can be produced indefinitely. Renewable resources such as fertile agricultural land; grazing land; fish in lakes, rivers, and oceans; fresh water; and clean air can be used forever if they are not exploited. For instance, rotating the crops grown in a field prevents the depletion of specific nutrients in the soil, whereas growing the same crop year after year depletes the soil and increases the need for added fertilizers. Producing these fertilizers uses resources, and applying fertilizers increases water pollution. Pollution of the water reduces the amount available to irrigate the crops and nourish the population. Restoring water once it has become polluted takes long periods of time or expensive resources.

Techniques of sustainable food production rely on ecological principles and normal biological processes such as natural predator-prey relationships and disease-resistant crops. Chemical fertilizers can be avoided or minimized by using integrated pest-management and fertilizing with animal manure. Crop rotation, plowing techniques, and terracing maintain soil fertility and prevent soil erosion (Figure 18.10). Other techniques include agroforestry, in which techniques from forestry and agriculture are used together to restore degraded areas; natural systems agriculture, which attempts to develop agricultural systems that include many types of plants and therefore function like natural ecosystems; and the technique of reducing fertilizer use by matching nutrient resources with the demands of the plant.[20,21]

Water and energy are conserved by relying more on labor-intensive agricultural methods, which produce less food in the short term but will protect water and land

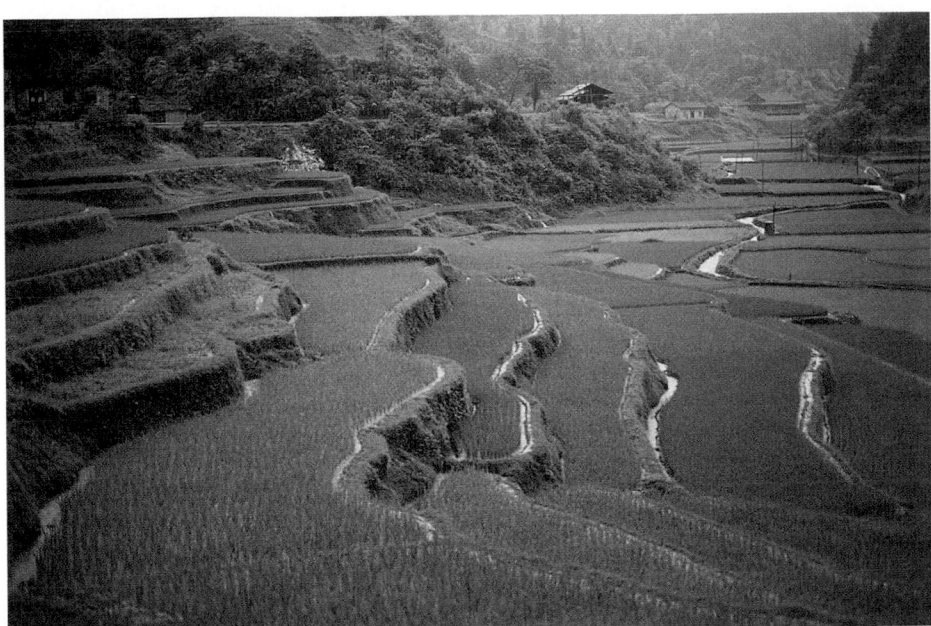

Figure 18.10
Terracing and contour-plowing help sustain the environment by preventing soil erosion. (© Joseph Sohm; ChromoSohm, Inc./Corbis)

resources in the long term. These methods are often more appropriate in developing nations than are high-technology methods because these areas typically have large populations but little access to modern machinery such as tractors and pumps.

Technology to Improve Food Production New technologies are needed to increase food production without damaging the environment. Technological advances such as high-yielding crop varieties, irrigation, and mechanization have dramatically increased our ability to produce food. For example, corn yields in eastern Colorado have increased by 400 to 500% since 1940.[21]

Genetic engineering is one technology that is being implemented to increase food production while minimizing environmental damage. Genetic engineering is in reality just a more sophisticated approach to the traditional plant and animal breeding techniques that have been used for centuries, but it has the advantage of being faster, more precise, and more powerful (see Chapter 17). Biotechnology is being used to help meet the world's nutrient needs by creating safer pesticides, disease-resistant crops, foods with greater nutrient density, and products to increase the intake of deficient nutrients.

In order to increase food production, technology must fit with a nation's cultural and economic structure. For example, providing tractors to help increase food production is ineffective in places where fuel is not available.

Providing the Right Combination of Nutrients In addition to sufficient energy, the right mix of nutrients is necessary to ensure the nutritional health of the population. If the foods and crops that are grown or imported do not meet all nutrient needs, the quality of the diet will be poor and malnutrition will occur. If the right mix of foods is not available, either dietary patterns must be changed or nutrients must be added to the diet by fortifying foods or including dietary supplements.

Nutrification **Nutrification** is the process of adding one or more nutrients to commonly consumed foods with the goal of adding to the nutrient intake of a population. Nutrification will not provide energy to a hungry population, but it can increase the protein quality of the diet and eliminate micronutrient deficiencies.

In order for nutrification to solve a nutritional problem in a population, it must be implemented wisely. Nutrification works if vulnerable groups consume centrally processed foods. The foods selected for nutrification should be among those

Nutrification The process of adding one or more nutrients to commonly consumed foods with the goal of adding to the nutrient intake of a group of people.

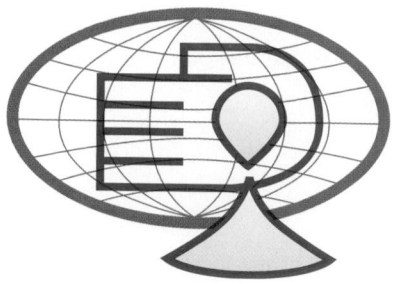

Figure 18.11
This global iodized salt logo can be recognized around the world as an indicator of iodized salt.

consistently consumed by the majority of the population so that extensive promotion and re-education are not needed to encourage their consumption. The nutrient should be added uniformly and in a form that optimizes its utilization. Nutrification has been used successfully in preventing health problems in the United States. The fortification of cow's milk to increase vitamin D intake was a major factor in the elimination of infantile rickets (see Chapter 9), and the enrichment of grains with niacin helped eliminate pellagra. The most recent program is the fortification of grains with folate to reduce neural tube defects in newborns (see Chapters 8 and 14). Nutrification has also been used successfully in developing countries. The use of iodized salt to prevent iodine deficiency has more than tripled over the past decade in developing countries (Figure 18.11).[22] Likewise, the fortification of foods such as margarine and sugar with vitamin A has helped reduce vitamin A deficiencies.

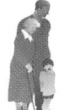

Supplementation Supplementation can also be used to reduce the prevalence of micronutrient malnutrition. Of countries where vitamin A deficiency is a public health problem, 78% have policies supporting regular vitamin A supplementation in children. Many have also adopted the World Health Organization recommendation to provide all breast-feeding women with a high-dose supplement of vitamin A within eight weeks of delivery. This improves maternal vitamin A status and raises the amount of vitamin A that is in breast milk and therefore passed to the infant.[23] Supplementation, along with regular deworming programs, is also used to reduce iron deficiency anemia. Many countries have adopted programs to supplement children older than 6 months with iron and pregnant women with iron and folate.

Education In order for any of these programs to work, consumers must use the foods that have been fortified or change their diets to include natural sources of nutrients that are deficient. Education to modify dietary patterns may promote the use of produce from home gardens. This education must include information about which foods are good nutrient sources so choices made when purchasing foods or growing vegetables at home can meet micronutrient needs.

• FOOD INSECURITY AT HOME

In the United States, most of the nutritional problems are related to overnutrition. It is estimated that approximately 61% of adults in the United States are overweight.[24] Heart disease, hypertension, and cancer—all related to obesity—are the leading causes of death. While much of the population is concerned with consuming a diet to lower the risks for these chronic diseases, hungry families are standing in line at soup kitchens. Problems such as poverty and unemployment lead to food insecurity in a land of plenty (Figure 18.12). Government food and nutrition policy must be concerned with improving economic security as well as providing food to the hungry and maintaining the food supply at an affordable level—at the same time policy must promote healthy diets to reduce diseases related to overconsumption.

Causes of Food Insecurity

In the United States, general food shortage is not the cause of undernutrition, but food insecurity, hunger, and undernutrition are still problems for vulnerable individuals and groups within the population. Thirty-three million people, including 13 million children, live in households that experience food insecurity. This represents about 10% of all U.S. households.[25] About 3.1% of American households experience hunger during the course of the year, and 7.3% are at risk of hunger because they have poor quality diets or they cannot always afford the food they need. Poverty, the main cause of food insecurity, reduces access to food, education, and health care. Despite the relationship between poverty and food insecurity, it cannot be assumed that everyone living in poverty is food-insecure, or that those above the poverty line

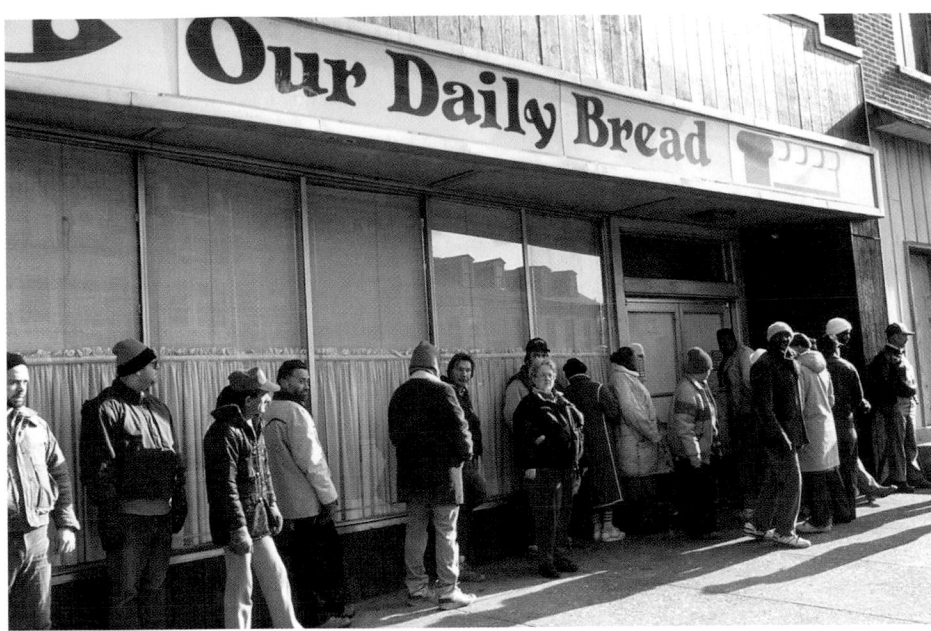

Figure 18.12
Despite the plentiful supply of food in the United States, food insecurity remains a problem. (© Steven Rubin/The Image Works)

have plenty to eat. Illness, disability, a sudden decrease in income, or high living expenses can put anyone at risk for food insecurity.

Economic Insecurity and Limited Access to Food About 13.8% of Americans live at or below the poverty level, and 20.8% of children live in households below the poverty level.[26] The poor have less money to spend on food and often have less access to affordable food. Lower profits have driven supermarkets out of the cities and into the suburbs. Because many low-income families do not own cars, they must shop at small, expensive corner stores or pay cab fares to take advantage of less expensive bulk items that are difficult to transport.

Lack of education, a cause and consequence of poverty, also contributes to food insecurity. For people at or below the poverty level, educational opportunities are fewer and lower in quality. In the short term, lack of knowledge about food selection, food safety, and home economics can contribute to malnutrition. Too little food may cause the diet to be deficient in energy or particular nutrients, but poor food choices also allow food insecurity to coexist with obesity. Lack of education about food safety can also increase the incidence of food-borne illness. In the long term, lack of education prevents people from getting well-paying jobs, which allow them to escape from poverty.

Poverty limits access to health care, leading to poorer health status. Iron deficiency is more than twice as frequent in low-income children, and the incidence of heart disease, cancer, hypertension, and obesity increases with decreasing income.[26] As in developing nations, poverty is reflected in infant mortality rates. Average infant mortality in the United States population is about 7.1 per 1000 live births. However, there are groups within the population that have infant mortality rates as high as those in impoverished nations. Among African Americans, the infant mortality rate is 14.6 per 1000 live births—twice that of the general population.[27] This difference mirrors the the higher poverty rate in this group.

Many find themselves trapped in a cycle of poverty (Figure 18.13). As the U.S. economy has shifted from manufacturing- to service-based, many factories have closed and manufacturing facilities have moved abroad where labor costs are lower. Former employees often lack the experience or education to move on to other types of work. Unable to find well-paying jobs, they must work longer hours at lower-paying jobs. Low incomes reduce access to transportation and child care, which can also limit access to better jobs. Long work hours reduce the amount of time available

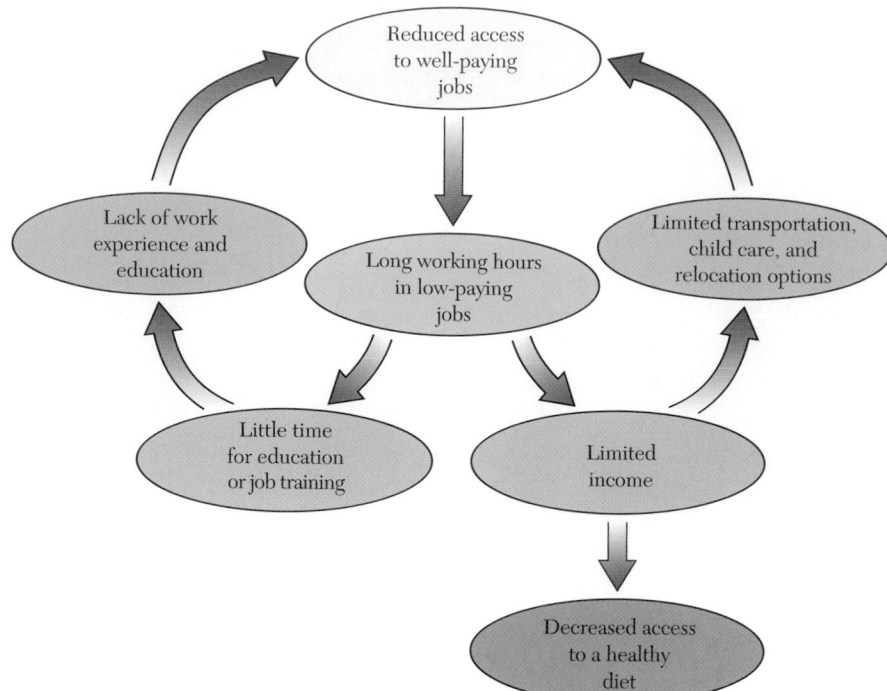

Figure 18.13

Many Americans are trapped in a cycle of poverty because they are unable to acquire the education, training, or resources necessary to obtain better-paying jobs.

to pursue the additional education or training necessary to find better-paying jobs. Limited income and transportation prohibit relocation to areas where better jobs are available.

Vulnerable Populations Certain subgroups within the U.S. population are at increased risk of hunger and undernutrition. These include the homeless; women, infants, and children; the elderly; Native Americans and Alaska Natives; and migrant and seasonal workers. According to a 1997 survey by the hunger-relief organization Second Harvest, 62% of people who rely on emergency food assistance are women, 38% are children under age 18, and 16% are over 65.[28] Considering that children make up only 27% of the U.S. population and the elderly 13%, a disproportionate number of children and elderly are seeking food assistance.

The Homeless The poor must use most of their income to pay for shelter. It is estimated that people who live in poverty spend about 80% of their income on housing, which seriously reduces the chances that their families will be adequately fed.[29] The high cost of housing not only limits food budgets but also has created a growing problem of homelessness in the United States. It is estimated that over half a million Americans are homeless, and one of the major health problems of the homeless population is malnutrition.[30] The homeless are at high risk of food insecurity because they lack not only money but also cooking and food storage facilities. Without cooking facilities, they must rely on ready-to-eat foods. Without storage facilities, they cannot use less expensive staples such as rice and dried beans, which can be purchased in bulk. Homeless individuals often rely on soup kitchens and shelters to obtain adequate food. A study of homeless preschool children found that several times each month the children did not have enough food to eat and that they rarely consumed the recommended amounts of grains, fruits, vegetables, or dairy products.[31]

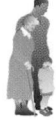

Women and Children Almost a third of households with children headed by single women live below the poverty line.[25] Poverty and food insecurity place these women and children at risk of malnutrition, and their special nutritional needs magnify this risk. Because of their increased need for some nutrients, malnutrition may occur in pregnant women, infants, and children even when the rest of the household is ade-

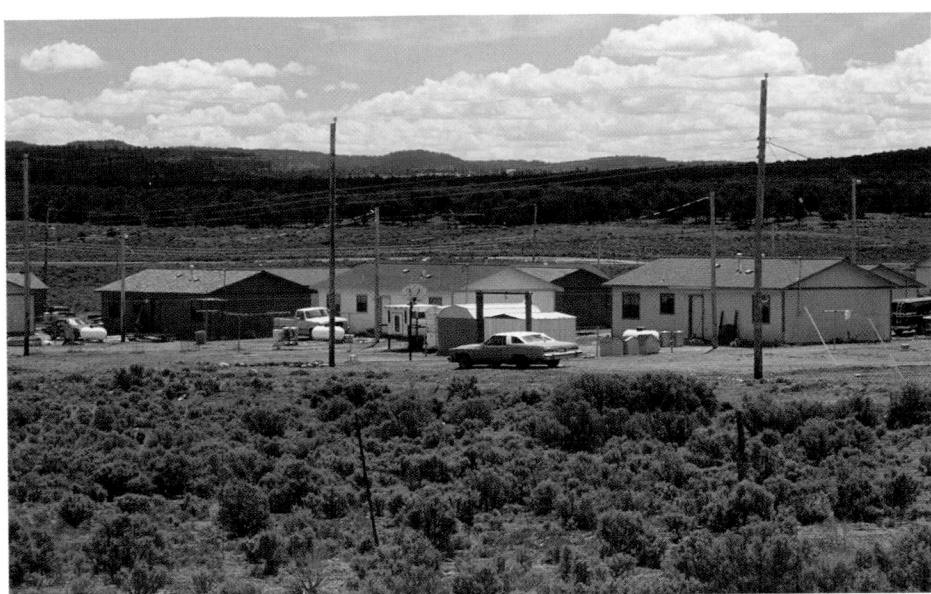

Figure 18.14
Native Americans living on reservations in remote locations have limited access to food, jobs, and education. (© Joe Sohm/The Image Works)

quately fed. For example, the amount of iron in the family diet may be enough to prevent anemia in all but a pregnant teenager.

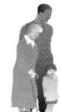

The Elderly Due to diseases and disabilities, the elderly may be limited in their ability to purchase, prepare, and physically ingest food. This puts the elderly, especially the elderly poor, at risk for malnutrition. A recent survey found that 8 to 14% of older adults experience food insecurity at some point in a six-month period.[30] Greater nutritional risk among older adults is associated with more hospital admissions and hence greater health-care costs. The number of individuals over age 85 is expected to quadruple by the year 2050; as the number of elderly increases so will the number at risk of food insecurity. Thus providing food security for older adults both improves their quality of life and reduces health-care costs for the public health system (see Chapter 16).[30]

Native Americans and Alaska Natives Many Native Americans and Alaska Natives live in remote locations, which reduces access to food (Figure 18.14). The unemployment and poverty rates are high among these groups. Unemployment for the United States as a whole was 5.6% in 1995 but was 35% among Native Americans living on or adjacent to reservations; only 29% of those employed earned more than $9048 a year.[26]

Migrant and Seasonal Farm Workers Migrant workers have limited access to food because labor camps are in remote locations and transportation is limited. Low incomes and difficult working and living conditions limit their ability to purchase food and prepare adequate meals.

Solutions to Food Insecurity

Solving the problem of undernutrition in the United States requires alleviating poverty and providing access to an adequate nutritious food supply at a reasonable cost. Historically, many approaches have been attempted to meet this goal. Some have met with success and others have done little to increase access to a nutritious diet for all. Programs that provide access to affordable food and promote healthy eating have been referred to as a nutrition safety net for the American population.

A Historical Perspective Government response to hunger first occurred in the United States during the Great Depression of the 1930s with the distribution of farm surpluses by the Federal Supplies Relief Corporation.[32] Awareness of undernutrition in the United States was again aroused during World War II, when it was determined that 70% of the men rejected from the military draft had poor nutritional histories. At this time, the School Lunch Program (see Chapter 15) was initiated to improve the nutritional status of American youth and create the potential for a strong military.[30]

Between 1952 and 1960 the government showed little interest in the problems of hunger and malnutrition—an attitude that may have stemmed from the assumption that every citizen was well-fed in a land overflowing with food. In the 1960s, the Food Stamp Program and the Commodity Program were developed in response to the hunger witnessed by John F. Kennedy on his travels through the United States during his presidential campaign. At the same time, Martin Luther King Jr.'s Southern Christian Leadership Conference cited areas of hunger in cotton-growing states, where replacement of cotton by corn and soybeans had put many field hands out of work. Reports of hunger also began to appear from other parts of the country, such as Appalachia, northern Maine, Indian reservations in the Southwest, ghettos in large cities, and Native sections of Alaska. In 1967, teams of nutritionists and physicians were sent around the country to assess the problem of hunger. The resulting report indicated widespread malnutrition in every ethnic group in every part of the country, urban and rural. The report was brought to Congress and broadcast on prime-time television in the CBS documentary "Hunger in America." It was a rude awakening for the American public, and the awareness prompted interested organizations to coalesce into the National Council on Hunger and Malnutrition in the United States. The U.S. Senate formed the Senate Select Committee on Nutrition and Human Needs, and a White House Conference on Food, Nutrition, and Health was convened in 1969 to develop workable, implementable recommendations. There were 1800 such recommendations relating to poverty programs, diet, health, and consumer concerns. The Commodity Program was expanded, the Food Stamp Program was made permanent, the Special Supplemental Food Program for Women, Infants, and Children (WIC) was developed, child nutrition programs were expanded, and nutrition programs for the elderly were created.[30]

In 1977, a follow-up survey to assess hunger in America found that although poverty had not changed, the number of hungry people had decreased. There had been a major improvement in the diets of poor people from 1965–66 to 1977. This change was attributed solely to federal food assistance programs. The reduction in hunger was a major social advance, but as times change, so do political agendas. Many of the attempted solutions of the 1960s and 1970s fell by the wayside in the 1980s and 1990s. However, a key group of programs still provide access to food and nutrition education to the poor and other at-risk groups. In addition, nutrition guidelines, such as the Dietary Guidelines and the Food Guide Pyramid, have been developed to promote the consumption of not only an adequate diet but one that will reduce the risk of chronic disease.

As we move further into the 21st century, the structure of the nutrition safety net is being influenced by measures designed to reduce the number of welfare recipients in the United States. The federal Personal Responsibility and Work Opportunity Reconciliation Act of 1996 will not affect WIC or the School Breakfast and Lunch Program, but other components of the nutrition safety net will be changed drastically. For instance, the maximum food-stamp benefits that a family can receive will be reduced, and the length of time able-bodied adults can receive food stamps will be limited to 3 months out of every 36 unless the adult is working or engaged in a work-related program.[33] Only time will reveal the effects of these types of changes in federal assistance programs. If net household income is decreased by these changes, the number of individuals who are at risk for food insecurity at any given time may increase. If, on the other hand, these changes move people out of poverty, the result may be to promote long-term food and financial security.

Programs to Provide Access to Food In the United States the two major programs designed to make sure that all people have access to an adequate diet are the Food Stamp Program and the Emergency Food Assistance Program (Table 18.2). The Food Stamp Program provides monthly benefits in the form of coupons or elec-

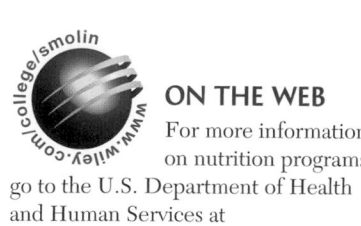

ON THE WEB

For more information on nutrition programs, go to the U.S. Department of Health and Human Services at www.dhhs.gov/, the USDA Food and Nutrition Service at www.fns.usda.gov/fns/, or Bread for the World at www.bread.org/.

Table 18.2 *Programs to Prevent Undernutrition in the United States*

Program	Target Population	Goals and Methods
Food Stamp Program	Low-income individuals	Increases access to food by providing coupons that can be used to purchase food at the grocery store.
Commodity Supplemental Food Program	Low-income pregnant women, breast-feeding, and non-breast-feeding postpartum women, infants and children under six years of age, and the elderly	Provides food by distributing USDA commodity foods.
Special Supplemental Nutrition Program for Women, Infants, and Children (WIC)	Low-income pregnant women, breast-feeding, and non-breast-feeding postpartum women, and infants and children under five years of age	Increases access to the right mix of foods by providing coupons for purchasing foods that are good sources of those nutrients at risk of deficiency in these groups.
WIC Farmers Market Nutrition Program	WIC participants	Increases access to fresh produce by providing coupons to purchase produce at authorized local farmers' markets.
National School Breakfast Program	Low-income children	Provides free or low-cost breakfasts to improve the nutritional status of children.
National School Lunch Program	Low-income children	Provides free or low-cost lunches at school to improve the nutritional status of children.
Special Milk Program	Low-income children	Provides milk for children in schools, camps, and child-care institutions with no federally supported meal program.
Summer Food Service Program	Low-income children	Provides meals for children during the summer months.
Child and Adult Care Food Program	Children up to age 12 and handicapped adults	Provides cash reimbursements and food commodities to child-care programs and community adult day-care centers.
Head Start	Low-income preschool children and their families	Provides education, including nutrition education, to low-income children and their families.
Nutrition Program for the Elderly	Individuals age 60 or over and their spouses	Provides free congregate meals in churches, schools, senior centers, or other facilities, and home-delivers to the homebound.
Homeless Children Nutrition Program	Preschoolers living in shelters	Reimburses providers for meals served to homeless preschool children in shelters.
Emergency Food Assistance Program	Low-income people	Provides commodities to soup kitchens, food banks, and individuals for home use.
Healthy People 2010	U.S. population	Sets national health promotion objectives to improve the health of the U.S. population through health-care system and industry involvement, and individual actions.
Expanded Food and Nutrition Education Program (EFNEP)	Low-income families	Provides education in all aspects of food preparation and nutrition.
Nutrition Education and Training Program (NET)	Children, parents, teachers, and food service personnel	Provides a comprehensive, school-based nutrition education program.
Temporary Assistance for Needy Families (TANF)	Low-income households	Provides money to ensure housing, food, and clothing to low-income families. Exact requirements and provisions are determined by the states.

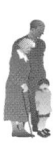

tronic transfers using a plastic card that can be used to purchase food, thereby supplementing the food budgets of low-income individuals and families. The Emergency Food Assistance Program distributes USDA food commodities to individuals for home use as well as to organized programs. Available commodities vary depending on market conditions. Products that are typically available include canned and dried fruits, canned vegetables, canned meats, peanut butter, and pasta products.

Because women, infants, children, the elderly, and the homeless are at highest risk of malnutrition, a number of programs target these particular groups. The WIC program (see Chapter 14) provides coupons to purchase nutrient-dense foods for pregnant women, lactating and non-breast-feeding postpartum women, and infants and children (Figure 18.15).[34] Preschool and school meal programs provide meals to children once they reach preschool age (Figure 18.16; see also Chapter 15). And the Nutrition Program for the Elderly helps prevent malnutrition in the elderly by providing nutritious meals in congregate settings and by home delivery (see Chapter 16).

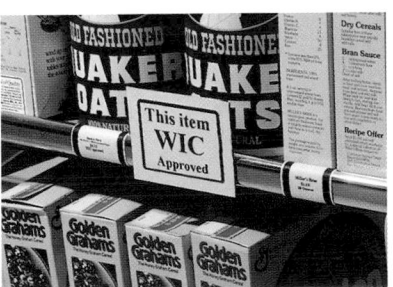

Figure 18.15
WIC supplies vouchers for foods that provide nutrients needed for healthy pregnancy and childhood. (Tony Freeman/PhotoEdit)

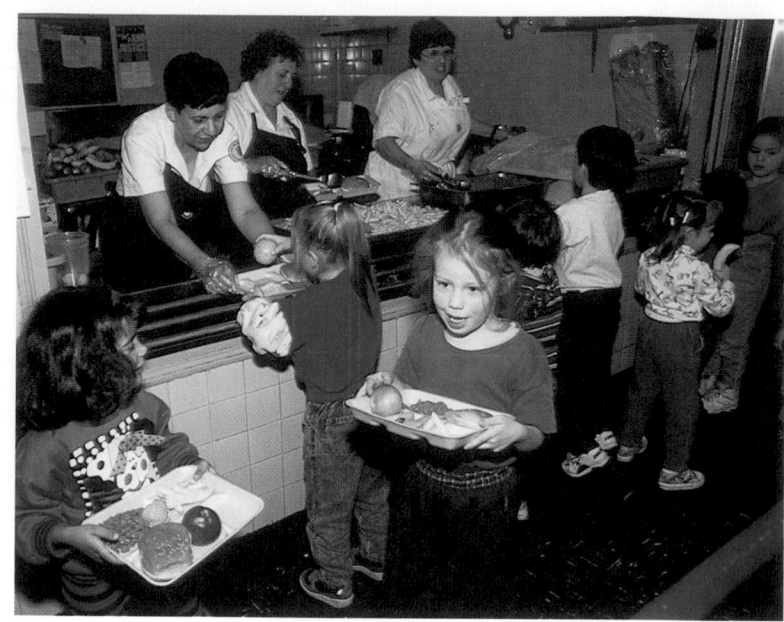

Figure 18.16
The School Lunch Program provides nutritious meals to school-age children.

There are few specific programs that serve the homeless. In 1991 the Healthy Meals for Healthy Americans Act created the Homeless Children Nutrition Program to provide meals for homeless preschool-age children living in shelters. Most of the homeless rely on food banks, feeding centers, and other community resource agencies to provide food; however, this does not guarantee an adequate nutrient intake. Often meals at feeding centers are based more on the types of foods donated than the definition of an adequate diet.

Even with federal assistance programs, many individuals still rely on church, community, and charitable emergency food shelters to provide for their basic nutritional needs. Second Harvest, the nation's largest charitable hunger relief organization, provided food to 23.3 million people in 2000, an increase of over 2 million since 1997.[35]

Nutrition Education The link between nutrition education and diet quality is strong. People with more nutrition information and more awareness of the relationship between diet and health consume healthier diets.[36] Healthy diets not only improve current health by optimizing growth, productivity, and well-being, but are essential for preventing chronic diseases in the future. Increasing nutrition knowledge can reduce medical care costs and improve the quality of life. Education can help individuals with lower incomes stretch limited food dollars by making wise choices at the store and reducing food waste at home. Education can promote community gardens to increase the availability of seasonal vegetables. It can teach people how to prepare foods that become available through commodity distribution and food banks. It can teach safe food handling and food preparation methods. Knowing which foods to choose and how to handle them safely is as important in preventing malnutrition as having the money to buy enough food.

There are a number of government programs designed to provide nutrition education. One of the goals of Healthy People 2010 is to increase the nutrition education provided by schools as well as by work sites. The Expanded Food and Nutrition Education Program (EFNEP) provides education in all aspects of food preparation and nutrition to low-income families. The Family Nutrition Program provides funding to develop and provide nutrition education programs for people on food stamps. In addition, the Dietary Guidelines for Americans, the Food Guide Pyramid, and food labels educate the general public about making wise food choices.

Policies to Control Food Costs The price of food depends on the amount produced and the consumer demand, so controlling the supply of food is important in determining cost. If the supply is large, prices will be low, but if supply forces prices to drop too much, the profit to the farmer and food industry may be too low to justify harvesting the crop. Government policy has tried to prevent this by controlling agricultural production with programs like the Grain Reserve Program and the Price Support Program. The Grain Reserve Program draws surplus grain off the market when excess is produced or prices decline. This practice keeps grain prices more stable and saves food for times when the harvest is not as plentiful. The Price Support Program also protects farmers from the drop in prices that results from overproduction. While these programs protect farmers, moderate food prices, and limit what reaches the marketplace, they may not provide incentive for farmers to limit production when demand is low. Federal programs also have the potential to support sustainable agriculture by regulating the use of natural resources and agricultural chemicals (see *Critical Thinking*: What Can You Do?).

CRITICAL THINKING

What Can You Do?

Keesha is concerned about the problems of hunger, malnutrition, and global ecology. Although she is a college student who cannot afford to make monetary contributions to relief organizations, she would like to contribute in other ways. She enjoys working with children, so she arranges to spend one afternoon a week helping with nutrition education programs for children. She also volunteers to spend one evening a week helping to prepare and serve food in a church soup kitchen near campus.

To be more ecological, Keesha buys a canvas bag to take to the grocery store. This will reduce the amount of waste she generates by eliminating the need for a new paper or plastic bag each time she shops. She asks her grocer to wrap the meat and chicken she buys in recyclable paper, and she begins recycling cans, bottles, and paper goods and tries to avoid purchasing products in nonrecyclable containers. This will reduce the amount of nonrecyclable, nonbiodegradable waste she generates.

What impact will the following changes Keesha makes have on the environment?

▼

Action	Impact
Instead of driving her car the 2 miles from home to campus, she rides her bike, takes the bus, or carpools with a friend.	This reduces the use of fossil fuels and reduces air pollution.
She contacts her local utility company to come and do an energy audit of her home and make energy-saving suggestions.	This will reduce energy usage in her home.
Instead of buying nonrecyclable juice boxes for her lunch, she brings juice in a thermos.	Answer:
She decides to begin composting the leftover vegetable scraps and other plant matter from her kitchen.	Answer:
When she can afford it, she chooses organically grown produce.	Answer:
She selects locally grown foods when possible.	Answer:

Suggest some other changes Keesha could make to decrease her impact on the environment.

▼

Answer:

Policies to Affect the Foods Produced Food policy can have an effect on what foods are produced and consumed by the population. For example, the grading of meat is based on the fat content, which is associated with flavor and tenderness. The greater the fat content, the higher the grade and the greater the cost. Beef labeled "prime" is higher in fat and cost than that labeled "choice" or "select." A change in grading policy could encourage the production of lower-fat meats.

An example of how policy can affect production is pricing in the dairy industry. For years the USDA milk pricing system favored the production of milk high in fat and protein. To respond to the health needs of the consumer, the USDA is now changing its policy—lowering the price it pays farmers for butterfat and increasing the price it pays for skim milk. The goal is to provide less of an incentive for farmers to produce milk with a high butterfat content. Thus changes in technology and policy affect what foods are produced and in turn consumed, which can then affect the nutritional health of the population.

• NUTRITION TRANSITION: THE GROWING PROBLEM OF OVERNUTRITION

Undernutrition is not the only world nutrition problem. Problems of overnutrition coexist with undernutrition in both industrialized and developing nations. Nutrition-related noncommunicable diseases such as cardiovascular disease, cancer, diabetes, and osteoporosis are newly appearing, rapidly rising, or already established in every country around the world. The reason for the growing problem of overnutrition is the change in diet and lifestyle that occur as economic conditions improve. Traditional diets in developing countries are based on a limited number of foods—primarily starchy root vegetables. As incomes increase, the diet becomes more varied to include more meat, milk, fat, and sugar. Along with these dietary transitions come changes in lifestyle that decrease activity. There is a shift toward less physically demanding occupations, an increase in the use of transportation to get to work or school, more labor-saving technology in the home, and more passive leisure time (Figure 18.17).

Nutrition transition The shift in dietary pattern that occurs as incomes increase—from a diet high in complex carbohydrates and fiber to a more varied diet higher in fats, saturated fat, and sugar.

Some of the effects of this economic and **nutrition transition** are positive. Shifts in diet are accompanied both by increases in life expectancy and by decreases in the birthrate and in the incidence of infectious diseases and nutrient deficiencies. However, at the same time, rates of heart disease, cancer, diabetes, obesity, and childhood obesity increase.[37] The increased reliance on animal proteins as well as on refined and processed foods also increases the use of energy and natural resources, which may damage the environment and deplete nonrenewable resources.

A problem facing international development agencies is how to promote economic growth and reduce undernutrition and infectious disease while at the same time preventing the undesirable effects of nutrition transition. To address these growing health concerns, individual countries have developed public health campaigns and policies to prevent overnutrition and promote healthy lifestyles (see Appendix G). International programs also target these issues. One such program is Interhealth, developed by the World Health Organization to work toward the prevention and control of chronic noncommunicable diseases.[38,39] Each country in-

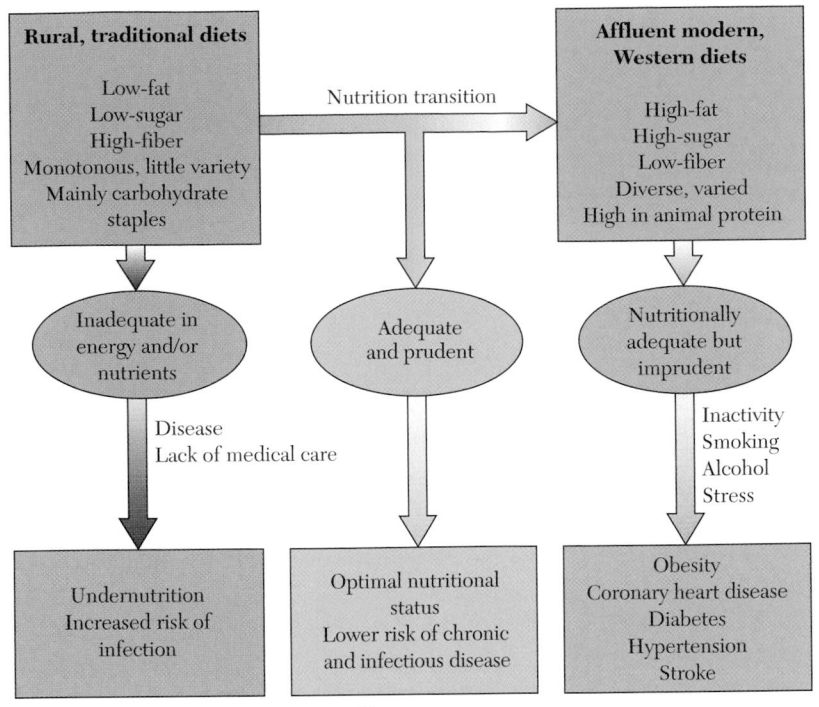

Figure 18.17

This schematic represents the dietary changes that occur with nutrition transition and the health consequences associated with these changes. A diet that falls somewhere between the traditional rural diet that may be inadequate in energy, protein, or micronutrients and the affluent Western diet that meets nutrient needs but is high in fat and sugar and low in fiber is optimal for health. (Adapted from Vorster, H. H., Bourne, L. T., Venter, C. S., and Oosthuizen, W. Contribution of nutrition to the health transition in developing countries: a framework for research and intervention. *Nutr. Rev.* 57: 341–349, 1999.)

volved in Interhealth must assess its nutritional behaviors and intakes, physical activity levels, blood pressure and blood cholesterol levels, as well as other risk factors for chronic diseases such as smoking, alcohol consumption, and obesity. The country must then implement strategies for reducing these risk factors, monitor trends in mortality, and evaluate the success of their programs.

A component of the Interhealth program, called the Interhealth Nutrition Initiative, was developed to collect information about global population and nutrition trends and to evaluate programs related to food and nutrition. Nutrition goals for countries involved must emphasize the availability of a safe and adequate food supply, as well as the promotion of dietary practices to reduce chronic disease risk. For countries where chronic disease rates are low and infectious disease rates and undernutrition are high, programs directed toward feeding the population are emphasized. For countries with high chronic disease risks, nutrition recommendations similar to the Dietary Guidelines for Americans encourage maintenance of appropriate body weight; decreased consumption of *trans* fat, saturated fat, cholesterol, and sodium; increased consumption of fiber-rich foods and complex carbohydrates; and moderate alcohol intake.

• APPLICATIONS •

1. Keep a record of how much money you spend on food in a day and use this to estimate your monthly food costs.
   a. Suggest specific changes in the foods you choose that will reduce your food costs.
   b. How do these changes affect the nutrient content of your diet?
   c. Modify your choices so that your food cost for the day is $3.00.
   d. Would this modified diet meet your nutrient needs? Which nutrients are deficient? Which are excessive?

2. World Food Day is October 16. List some ideas for campus-wide programs to increase awareness of global nutrition issues.

3. Use the Internet to locate Web sites for organizations such as Worldwatch or Bread for the World Institute. Research one area of the world where hunger and undernutrition are a major problem:
   a. What is the cause of undernutrition in this area?
   b. What solutions are in place or proposed to solve these problems?

SUMMARY

1. Both insufficient amounts of food and poor quality diets cause undernutrition—the predominant nutritional problem worldwide.

2. In poorly nourished populations, a cycle of malnutrition exists in which poorly nourished women give birth to low birth weight infants at risk of disease and early death. If these children survive, they grow into adults who are physically unable to fully contribute to society. Indicators of the nutritional status of a population are the infant mortality rate and the incidence of low birth weight and stunting.

3. Hunger and undernutrition occur when there is a shortage of food. Short-term food shortage, such as famine, may result from a natural or man-made disaster. Chronic food shortage occurs when overpopulation and limited natural resources create a situation in which there are more people than food. The inequitable distribution of food and resources caused by poverty creates food insecurity within a population even if there is enough total food.

4. Malnutrition also occurs when the quality of the diet is poor. High-risk groups such as pregnant women, children, the elderly, and the ill may not be able to meet their nutrient needs. Protein, iron, iodine, and vitamin A deficiencies are common worldwide.

5. Short-term solutions to undernutrition provide food through relief at the local, national, and international levels. Long-term solutions include control of population growth, economic and agricultural policies that promote self-sufficiency and alleviate poverty, improvements in the quality of the food supply, and the development of sustainable systems that will provide food without damaging the environment.

6. Technology can help solve the problems of world hunger by providing environmentally safe pesticides, disease-resistant crops, and foods with greater nutrient density.

7. Both undernutrition and overnutrition are problems in the United States. As in developing nations, undernutrition is associated with poverty, but food insecurity can also occur when income is adequate. The homeless, women, children, the elderly, and minority groups are most often food insecure.

8. Nutrition programs in the United States focus on maintaining a nutrition safety net which will provide access to affordable food and promote healthy eating in the United States. Some programs designed to help feed the hungry address the general population, whereas others focus on specific high-risk groups. Most programs provide access to food and some provide nutrition education.

9. Problems of overnutrition coexist with undernutrition in both developed and developing nations. Policies and education must work to feed the population when hunger is prevalent, prevent the population from adopting dietary and lifestyle patterns that result in an increase in chronic disease, and reduce the incidence of chronic diseases where they are a problem.

REVIEW QUESTIONS

1. What is the cycle of malnutrition?

2. How does overpopulation contribute to food shortage?

3. How does poverty contribute to world hunger?

4. How are economic growth and population growth related?

5. What segments of the world population are at greatest risk for undernutrition?

6. List three micronutrient deficiencies that are world health problems.

7. Why are environmental issues important in maintaining the world's food supply?

8. How does sustainable agriculture reduce environmental damage?

9. How can nutrification help eliminate malnutrition?

10. List four groups in the United States population that are at risk for undernutrition.

11. List three federal programs that address malnutrition in the United States.

12. Why is overnutrition a concern in all countries around the world?

REFERENCES

1. Bread for the World Institute. Hunger Basics: International Facts on Hunger and Poverty. Available online at www.bread.org/hungerbasics/international.html/ Accessed May 22, 2002.

2. Infant Mortality Rates of the World and Its Major Regions, 1950–20250. Available online at www.un.org/Depts/eca/divis/fssd/worldmor.htm#95/ Accessed May 22, 2002.

3. United Nations, Administrative Committee on Coordination, Sub-Committee on Nutrition, *Third Report on the World Nutrition Situation*. Geneva: ACC/SCN, December 1997.

4. United Nations Administrative Committee on Coordination, Sub-Committee on Nutrition. *Fourth Symposium of the World Nutrition Situation: Nutrition Throughout the Life Cycle*. Geneva: ACC/SCN, in collaboration with IFPRI, 2000.

5. Bengoa, J. M. A half-century perspective on world nutrition and the international nutrition agencies. *Nutr. Rev.* 55:309–314, 1997.

6. Pelletier, D. L. The potentiating effects of malnutrition on child mortality: Epidemiologic evidence and policy implications. *Nutr. Rev.* 52:409–415, 1994.

7. National Geographic Society. Millennium in maps: Population. Supplement to *National Geographic Magazine*, October 1998.

8. International Food Policy and Research Institute (IFPRI). *A 2020 Vision for Food, Agriculture, and the Environment: The Vision, Challenge, and Recommended Action*. Washington, D.C.: IFPRI, 1995.

9. Beckman, D., Cohen, M. J., and Kennedy, E. Position of the American Dietetic Association: World hunger. *J. Am. Diet. Assoc.* 95: 1160–1162, 1995.

10. Raloff, J. The human numbers crunch. *Sci. News* 149:396–397, June 22, 1996.

11. Table set thinly as Food Summit pledges to halve world hunger in 20 years. *UN Chronicle*, 33:24–28, 1996.

12. World Health Organization. Nutrition for Health and Development, 1999. Available online at www.who.int.nut /Accessed December 12, 2000.

13. Pollitt, E. Functional significance of the covariance between protein energy malnutrition and iron deficiency anemia. *J. Nutr.* 125: 2272S–2277S, 1995.

14. Ramalingaswami, V. New global perspectives on overcoming malnutrition. *Am. J. Clin. Nutr.* 61:259–263, 1995.

15. Delange, F. The disorders induced by iodine deficiency. *Thyroid* 4:107–128, 1994.

16. Hetzel, B. S., and Clugstrum, G. A. Iodine. In *Modern Nutrition in Health and Disease*, 9th ed. Shils, M. E., Olson, J. A., Shike, M., and Ross, A. C., eds. Baltimore: Williams & Wilkins, 1999, 253–264.

17. World Health Organization. Vitamin A—the good news. Donald McLaren highlights recent developments. Available online at www.who.int/chd/pub/newslet/dialog/9/vitamin_a.htm/ Accessed December 12, 2000.

18. United Nations Food and Agriculture Organization. Rome Declaration on World Food Security and World Food Summit Plan of Action, November 13, 1996. Available online at www.fao.org/ Accessed December 12, 2000.

19. Sloham, J. Emergency feeding programmes: Still not delivering the goods. *Br. J. Med.* 305:596–597, 1992.

20. Raven, P. H., Berg, L. R., and Johnson, G. B. *Environment,* 2nd ed. Philadelphia: Saunders College Publishing, 1998, 185.

21. Matson, P. A., Parton, W. J., Power, A. G., and Swift, M. J. Agricultural intensification and ecosystem properties. *Science* 277:504–509, 1997.

22. UNICEF-The State of the World's Children, 2002. Available online at www.unicef.org/media/sowc02presskit/goal-one.htm/ Accessed May 22, 2002.

23. World Health Organization/United Nation's Children's Fund/International Vitamin A Consultative Group. *Vitamin A Supplements: A Guide to Their Use in the Treatment and Prevention of Vitamin A Deficiency and Xerophthalmia,* 2nd ed. Geneva: WHO, 1997.

24. Obesity and Overweight: A Public Health Epidemic, Centers for Disease Control and Prevention. Available online at www.cdc.gov/nccdphp/dnpa/obesity/epidemic.htm/ Accessed March 20, 2002.

25. ERS Food Assistance and Nutrition Research Report No. (FANRR) 21, United States Department of Agriculture, March 2002. Available online at www.ers.usda.gov/publications/fanrr21/ Accessed May 22, 2002.

26. U.S. Department of Agriculture, Foreign Agricultural Service. Discussion paper on domestic food security, February 13, 1998. Available online at www.fas.usda.gov/icd/summit/discussi.html/ Accessed August 5, 2002.

27. National Center for Health Statistics, National Vital Statistics Report No. 49, No. 8, September 21, 2001. Table 27 Infant, Neonatal, and Postneonatal Mortality Rates By Race and Sex: United States, 1940, 1950, 1960, 1970, and 1975–1999. Available online at www.cdc.gov.nchs/fastats/infmort.html/ Accessed May 22, 2002.

28. Second Harvest. Hunger: the faces and facts: a profile of who is hungry. Available online at www.secondharvest.org/websecha/d_ffla.htm/ Accessed December 12, 2000.

29. Mayer, J. Hunger and undernutrition in the United States. *J. Nutr.* 120:919–923, 1990.

30. American Dietetic Association. Position on domestic food and nutrition security. *J. Am. Diet. Assoc.* 98:337–342, 1998.

31. Taylor, M. L., and Oblinsky, S. A. Food consumption and eating behavior of homeless preschool children. *J. Nutr. Ed.* 26:20–25, 1994.

32. Poppendieck, J. Hunger and public policy lessons from the Great Depression. *J. Nutr. Ed.* 24(Suppl.):6S–10S, 1992.

33. Oliveira, V. Cost of food-assistance programs declined slightly in first half of 1996. *Food Review* 26–33, USDA Food and Consumer Service, September/December 1996.

34. Owen, A. L., and Owen, G. M. Twenty years of WIC: A review of some effects of the program. *J. Am. Diet. Assoc.* 97:777–782, 1997.

35. Hunger in America 2001, America's Second Harvest, Available online at secondharvest.org/whoshungry/hunger_study_intro.html/ Accessed May 22, 2002.

36. U.S. Department of Agriculture, Economic Research Service, USDA Center for Nutrition Policy and Promotion. USDA's healthy eating index and nutrition information. Available online at www.usda.gov/cnpp/usda_healthy_eating_index.htm/ Accessed August 5, 2002.

37. Vorster, H. H., Bourne, L. T., Venter, C. S., and Oosthuizen, W. Contribution of nutrition to the health transition in developing countries: a framework for research and intervention. *Nutr. Rev.* 57:341–349, 1999.

38. Posner, B. M., Franz, M., Quatromoni, P., and the Interhealth steering committee. Nutrition and the global risk for chronic diseases: the Interhealth Nutrition Initiative. *Nutr. Rev.* 52:201–207, 1994.

39. Posner, B. M., Quatromoni, P. A., and Franz, M. Nutrition policies and interventions for chronic disease risk reduction in international settings: the Interhealth Nutrition Initiative. *Nutr. Rev.* 52:179–187, 1994.

Appendices

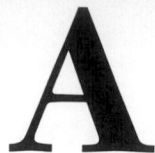

Key: Qty = quantity
Meas = measurement
Wgt = weight
Wtr = water
Cals = kcalories

Prot = protein
Carb = carbohydrate
Fib = fiber
SatF = saturated fat
MonoF = monounsaturated fat

PolyF = polyunsaturated fat
Choles = cholesterol
Calc = calcium
Phos = phosphorus
Sod = sodium

This table of food composition has been prepared for this title and is copyrighted by ESHA Research in Salem, Oregon, developer and publisher of The Food Processor® and Genesis™ nutrition and labeling software systems. The table includes nutrient data for over 3000 foods, including brand-name items, ethnic foods, vegetarian products, nonfat and low-sodium alternatives, baby foods and formulas, and a large selection of common food items. The foods are presented alphabetically with corresponding units of measure. Over 1000 sources of scientific information are researched to provide the most accurate, reliable data available. Government sources of information are the base for all the data: the USDA Handbook series and its cur-

Food Item	Qty	Meas	Wgt (g)	Wtr (g)	Cals	Prot (g)	Carb (g)	Fib (g)	Fat (g)	SatF (g)
Almond butter, plain, unsalted	2	cup	32	0	203	5	7	1.2	19	1.8
Almond chicken	0.5	oz.	121	93	137	10	9	1.9	7	1
Almond, dried, unblanched, whole	0.25	Tbs	36	2	209	7	7	3.9	18	1.8
Almond, dry roasted, unsalted, whole	0.25	cup	34	1	203	6	8	4.7	18	1.7
Almonds, blanched, slices	0.25	cup	26	1	154	5	5	1.8	14	1.3
Almonds, blanched, whole	0.25	cup	36	2	212	7	7	2.4	19	1.8
Almonds, dried, unblanched, chopped	0.25	cup	32	1	191	6	7	3.5	17	1.6
Almonds, dried, unblanched, slivered	0.25	cup	34	1	199	7	7	3.7	18	1.7
Almonds, dry roasted, salted	0.25	cup	34	1	203	6	8	4.7	18	1.7
Almonds, dry roasted, whole	0.25	cup	34	1	206	7	7	3.7	18	1.5
Almonds, natural, whole	0.25	cup	36	2	213	7	7	4.4	18	1.3
Almonds, oil roasted, blanched	0.25	cup	36	1	218	7	6	4	20	1.9
Almonds, oil roasted, salted	0.25	cup	39	1	243	8	6	4.4	23	2.2
Almonds, oil roasted, unsalted	0.25	cup	39	1	243	8	6	4.4	23	2.2
Almonds, oil roasted, whole	0.25	cup	39	1	243	8	6	4.4	23	2.2
Almonds, whole, toasted	1	oz.	28	1	167	6	6	3.2	14	1.4
Amaranth, grain	0.5	cup	98	10	365	14	64	14.8	6	1.6
Apple brown betty	0.75	cup	155	96	264	4	46	3.8	8	4.2
Apple butter	1	Tbs	17	10	30	0	7	0.3	0	0
Apple crisp, recipe	1	cup	282	173	460	5	91	4.8	10	2.1
Apple dumpling	1	each	190	62	670	7	84	2.9	35	8.6
Apple juice, canned/bottled	1	cup	248	218	117	0	29	0.2	0	0
Apple juice, prepared from frozen	1	cup	239	210	112	0	28	0.2	0	0
Apple rings, dried	10	each	64	20	156	1	42	5.6	0	0
Apple slices, canned, sweetened	0.5	cup	102	84	68	0	17	1.7	0	0.1
Apple slices, frozen, heated	0.5	cup	103	90	48	0	12	2	0	0.1
Apple slices, peeled, cooked	0.5	cup	85	72	48	0	12	2.4	0	0.1
Apple strudel	1	each	71	31	195	2	29	1.6	8	1.4
Apple turnover	1	each	82	27	289	3	36	1.2	15	3.7
Apple, baked, unsweetened	1	each	161	133	102	0	26	3.8	1	0.1
Apple, dried, cooked w/o sugar	0.5	cup	128	108	73	0	20	2.6	0	0
Apple, dried, cooked w/sugar	0.5	cup	140	110	116	0	29	2.7	0	0
Apple, no peel	1	each	128	108	73	0	19	2.4	0	0.1
Apple, peeled slices	0.5	cup	55	46	31	0	8	1	0	0
Apple, w/peel	1	each	138	116	81	0	21	3.7	0	0.1

Pot = potassium
Zn = zinc
Magn = magnesium
VitA = vitamin A

VitE = vitamin E
VitC = vitamin C
Thia = thiamin
Ribo = riboflavin

Nia = niacin
B6 = vitamin B6
Fola = folate
B12 = vitamin B12

rent supplemental data, as well as current data from both published and unpublished provisional data. Even with all the government data available, there are still missing values for some nutrients. Dashes in the table appear where there are no data available. Considerable effort has been made to report the most accurate data available and to eliminate missing values. Please be advised that the folate values in this table include the amount added in fortification for all non–brand-name items. Values for brand-name items may or may not include added folic acid. The authors welcome any suggestions or comments for future editions.

MonoF	PolyF	Choles	Calc	Phos	Sod	Pot	Zn	Iron	Magn	VitA	VitE	VitC	Thia	Ribo	Nia	B6	Fola	B12
(g)	(g)	(mg)	(mg)	(mg)	(mg)	(mg)	(mg)	(mg)	(mg)	(µg RE)	(µg α-TE)	(mg)	(mg)	(mg)	(mg)	(mg)	(µg)	(µg)
12.3	4	0	86	167	4	243	1	1.2	97	0	6.5	0	0.04	0.2	0.9	0.02	21	0
2.6	2.9	18	40	119	307	275	0.8	1	30	38	1.32	5	0.04	0.1	4.3	0.21	16	0.12
12	3.9	0	94	185	4	260	1	1.3	105	0	8.52	0	0.08	0.28	1.2	0.04	21	0
11.6	3.7	0	97	189	4	266	1.7	1.3	105	0	1.91	0	0.04	0.21	1	0.03	22	0
9	2.9	0	65	140	3	197	0.8	1	75	0	5.33	0	0.04	0.18	0.8	0.03	10	0
12.4	4	0	90	193	4	272	1.2	1.3	104	0	7.36	0	0.06	0.24	1.2	0.04	14	0
11	3.6	0	86	169	4	238	0.9	1.2	96	0	7.8	0	0.07	0.25	1.1	0.04	19	0
11.4	3.7	0	90	176	4	247	1	1.2	100	0	8.1	0	0.07	0.26	1.1	0.04	20	0
11.6	3.7	0	97	189	269	266	1.7	1.3	105	0	1.91	0	0.04	0.21	1	0.03	22	0
11.5	3.2	0	111	—	1	243	—	—	—	—	7.62	—	0.02	0.49	0.8	—	15	0
11.2	4.1	0	—	—	—	—	—	—	—	—	8.09	—	0.07	0.32	1.1	0.04	16	0
13	4.2	0	69	205	4	246	0.5	1.9	103	0	1.95	0	0.03	0.1	1.4	0.03	22	0
14.7	4.8	0	92	215	306	268	1.9	1.5	119	0	2.18	0	0.05	0.39	1.4	0.03	25	0
14.7	4.8	0	92	215	4	268	1.9	1.5	119	0	2.18	0	0.05	0.39	1.4	0.03	25	0
13.1	5.4	0	120	196	0	232	1.2	1.5	101	—	8.6	—	0.04	0.43	1.4	—	12	0
9.4	3	0	80	156	3	219	1.4	1.4	86	0	4.54	0	0.04	0.17	0.8	0.02	18	0
1.4	2.8	0	149	444	20	357	3.1	7.4	259	0	1	4	0.08	0.2	1.3	0.22	48	0
2.3	0.9	17	70	49	295	147	0.4	1.9	16	61	0.42	0	0.22	0.13	1.9	0.07	7	0.02
0	0	0	2	2	1	16	0	0.1	1	2	0	0	0	0	0	0.01	0	0
4.3	3.3	0	79	70	513	274	0.5	2.1	20	87	—	6	0.24	0.2	2.2	0.12	14	0
15.2	9.2	0	14	75	607	129	0.5	3.1	16	10	3.2	2	0.39	0.3	3.5	0.05	11	0
0	0.1	0	17	17	7	295	0.1	0.9	7	0	0.02	2	0.05	0.04	0.2	0.07	0	0
0	0.1	0	14	17	17	301	0.1	0.6	12	0	0.02	1	0.01	0.04	0.1	0.08	1	0
0	0.1	0	9	24	56	288	0.1	0.9	10	0	0.35	2	0	0.1	0.6	0.08	0	0
0	0.1	0	4	5	3	69	0	0.2	2	5	0.01	0	0.01	0.01	0.1	0.04	0	0
0	0.1	0	5	8	3	78	0.1	0.2	3	2	0.21	0	0.01	0.01	0	0.03	1	0
0	0.1	0	4	7	1	79	0	0.1	3	3	0.01	0	0.01	0.01	0.1	0.04	1	0
2.3	3.8	4	11	23	191	106	0.1	0.3	6	6	2.19	1	0.03	0.02	0.2	0.03	10	0.16
6.6	4	0	6	32	262	56	0.2	1.3	7	4	1.38	1	0.17	0.13	1.5	0.02	5	0
0	0.2	0	12	12	0	179	0.1	0.3	9	7	1.02	8	0.02	0.02	0.1	0.08	3	0
0	0	0	4	12	26	134	0.1	0.4	5	3	0	1	0.01	0.02	0.2	0.06	0	0
0	0	0	4	11	27	137	0.1	0.4	4	3	0.34	1	0.01	0.02	0.2	0.07	0	0
0	0.1	0	5	9	0	145	0.1	0.1	4	5	0.1	5	0.02	0.01	0.1	0.06	1	0
0	0	0	2	4	0	62	0	0	2	2	0.04	2	0.01	0.01	0	0.02	0	0
0	0.1	0	10	10	0	159	0.1	0.2	7	7	0.44	8	0.02	0.02	0.1	0.07	4	0

Food Item	Qty	Meas	Wgt (g)	Wtr (g)	Cals	Prot	Carb (g)	Fib (g)	Fat (g)	SatF (g)
Apple, w/peel, slices	0.5	cup	55	46	32	0	8	1.5	0	0
Applesauce, canned, sweetened	0.5	cup	128	101	97	0	25	1.5	0	0
Applesauce, unsweetened	0.5	cup	122	108	52	0	14	1.5	0	0
Apricot halves w/skin, canned in water	3	each	84	78	23	1	5	1.3	0	0
Apricot halves, dried, cooked	0.5	cup	125	94	106	2	27	4	0	0
Apricot halves, dried, sulfured	10	each	35	11	83	1	22	3.2	0	0
Apricot nectar, canned	1	cup	251	213	141	1	36	1.5	0	0
Apricot, pitted, fresh	3	cup	106	92	51	1	12	2.5	0	0
Apricot, w/skin, canned in heavy syrup	0.5	each	129	100	107	1	28	2.1	0	0
Apricot, w/skin, canned in light syrup	0.5	cup	126	104	80	1	21	2	0	0
Apricot, w/skin, canned w/juice	0.5	cup	124	107	60	1	15	2	0	0
Apricots, frozen, sweetened	0.5	cup	121	89	119	1	30	2.7	0	0
Apricots, halves, fresh	0.5	cup	78	67	37	1	9	1.9	0	0
Apricots, peeled, canned in water	2	cup	90	84	20	1	5	1	0	0
Arby's Bac'n cheddar sandwich, deluxe	1	each	231	136	512	21	39	0.3	32	8.7
Arby's Philly beef'n swiss sandwich	1	each	197	105	467	24	38	—	25	9.6
Arby's Q sandwich	1	each	190	104	389	18	48	—	15	5.4
Arby's chicken sandwich, grilled, deluxe	1	each	230	143	430	24	42	—	20	3.5
Arby's roast beef sandwich, Junior	1	each	89	42	233	12	23	0.5	11	3.8
Arby's roast beef sandwich, regular	1	each	155	72	383	22	35	1.1	18	6.9
Arby's sandwich, light roast beef, deluxe	1	each	182	118	294	18	33	—	10	3.4
Arby's sandwich, light roast chicken, deluxe	1	each	195	129	276	24	33	—	7	1.7
Arby's sauce	0.5	each	14	10	15	0	3	—	0	0
Arby's sub sandwich, Italian	1	oz.	297	174	671	34	47	—	39	12.8
Arby's sub sandwich, roast beef	1	each	305	185	623	38	47	—	32	11.5
Arby's sub sandwich, tuna	1	each	284	118	663	74	50	—	37	8.2
Arby's sub sandwich, turkey	1	each	277	173	486	33	46	—	19	5.3
Arby's, Cheddar fries	5	each	142	64	399	6	46	—	22	9
Arby's, Steak'n cheddar sandwich	1	oz.	194	96	508	25	43	—	26	7.7
Arby's, curly fries	3.5	each	99	31	337	4	43	—	18	7.4
Arby's, roast chicken club sandwich	1	oz.	238	142	503	30	37	—	27	6.9
Artichoke heart, marinated	6	oz.	170	138	168	4	13	7.5	14	2
Artichoke heart, raw	0.5	cup	84	73	37	2	9	5	0	0
Artichoke, Jerusalem, raw, freshly harvested	0.5	cup	75	58	57	2	13	1.2	0	0
Artichoke, frozen, cooked	9	oz.	240	208	108	7	22	11	1	0.3
Artichoke, globe, cooked	1	each	120	101	60	4	13	6.5	0	0
Arugula leaf, raw	5	each	10	9	2	0	0	0.2	0	0
Arugula, chopped, raw	0.5	cup	10	9	2	0	0	0.2	0	0
Asparagus spears, canned, drained	4	each	80	75	15	2	2	1.3	1	0.1
Asparagus spears, canned, not drained, low sodium	4	each	80	75	12	1	2	0.8	0	0
Asparagus spears, cooked, unsalted	4	each	60	55	14	2	3	1	0	0
Asparagus spears, frozen, cooked	4	each	60	55	17	2	3	1	0	0.1
Asparagus, canned w/liquid, low sodium	0.5	cup	122	115	18	2	3	1.2	0	0.1
Asparagus, frozen, uncooked spears	4	each	58	53	14	2	2	1.1	0	0
Aunt Anne's pretzel, original, soft	1	each	138	—	390	12	84	3	1	0
Aunt Anne's pretzel, whole wheat, soft	1	each	140	—	390	13	82	8	2	0
Avocado cubes	0.5	cup	75	56	121	1	6	3.8	12	1.8
Avocado slices	1	piece	10	7	16	0	1	0.5	2	0.2
Avocado, California	1	each	173	126	306	4	12	8.5	30	4.5
Avocado, California, mashed	0.5	cup	115	84	204	2	8	5.6	20	3
Avocado, Florida	1	each	304	242	340	5	27	16.1	27	5.4
Avocado, Florida, mashed	0.5	cup	115	92	129	2	10	6.1	10	2
Avocado, average	1	each	201	149	324	4	15	10.1	31	4.9
Baby Food, bananas, strained, Heinz	1	Tbs	16	12	16	0	4	0.3	0	0
Baby Food, beef dinner supreme, stage 2, Beech-nut	1	each	128	106	147	2	9	1.1	10	—
Baby Food, beef stew, toddler	1	Tbs	14	12	7	1	1	0.2	0	0.1
Baby Food, carrots, stage 1, Beech-nut	1	oz.	28	26	12	0	2	1	0	0
Baby Food, cereal, mixed, w/formula	1	Tbs	18	14	22	1	3	—	1	—
Baby Food, cereal, rice w/fruit, Gerber	1	Tbs	14	12	11	0	3	0.1	0	—
Baby Food, chicken w/broth, stage 1, jar, Beech-nut	1	each	71	59	70	8	0	0	3	—
Baby Food, chicken-rice dinner, stage 2, Beech-nut	4	oz.	113	100	80	1	9	1	3	—
Baby Food, peaches, strained, Heinz	1	Tbs	16	13	12	0	3	0.4	0	0
Baby Food, pudding, cherry vanilla, Gerber	1	Tbs	14	12	10	0	2	0	0	—
Baby Food, spaghetti w/meat sauce, toddler	1	Tbs	14	12	11	1	2	—	0	—
Baby Food, sweet potatoes, stage 3, jar, Beech-nut	1	each	170	148	110	1	25	1	0	0

MonoF	PolyF	Choles	Calc	Phos	Sod	Pot	Zn	Iron	Magn	VitA	VitE	VitC	Thia	Ribo	Nia	B6	Fola	B12
(g)	(g)	(mg)	(mg)	(mg)	(mg)	(mg)	(mg)	(mg)	(mg)	(µg RE)	(µg α-TE)	(mg)	(mg)	(mg)	(mg)	(mg)	(µg)	(µg)
0	0.1	0	4	4	0	63	0	0.1	3	3	0.18	3	0.01	0.01	0	0.03	2	0
0	0.1	0	5	9	4	78	0.1	0.4	4	1	0.01	2	0.02	0.04	0.2	0.03	1	0
0	0	0	4	9	2	92	0	0.1	4	4	0.01	1	0.02	0.03	0.2	0.03	1	0
0.1	0	0	7	11	3	161	0.1	0.3	6	108	0.75	3	0.02	0.02	0.3	0.04	1	0
0.1	0	0	20	51	4	611	0.3	2.1	21	295	0.62	2	0.01	0.04	1.2	0.14	0	0
0.1	0	0	16	41	4	482	0.3	1.6	16	253	0.52	1	0	0.05	1	0.06	4	0
0.1	0	0	18	23	8	286	0.2	1	13	331	0.2	2	0.02	0.04	0.7	0.06	3	0
0.2	0.1	0	15	20	1	314	0.3	0.6	8	277	0.94	11	0.03	0.04	0.6	0.06	9	0
0	0	0	12	16	5	181	0.1	0.4	9	159	1.15	4	0.03	0.03	0.5	0.07	2	0
0	0	0	14	16	5	175	0.1	0.5	10	167	1.13	3	0.02	0.02	0.4	0.07	2	0
0	0	0	15	25	5	205	0.1	0.4	12	210	1.1	6	0.02	0.02	0.4	0.07	2	0
0.1	0	0	12	23	5	277	0.1	1.1	11	203	1.08	11	0.02	0.05	1	0.07	2	0
0.1	0.1	0	11	15	1	229	0.2	0.4	6	202	0.69	8	0.02	0.03	0.5	0.04	7	0
0	0	0	7	14	10	139	0.1	0.5	8	163	0.8	2	0.02	0.02	0.4	0.05	2	0
12.7	10.1	38	110	—	1094	491	3	4.3	—	40	—	11	0.34	0.46	9.6	—	—	—
10.6	5.1	53	290	—	1144	409	3.8	4.1	—	—	—	19	0.28	0.46	8.8	—	—	—
6.3	3.5	29	70	—	1268	456	—	9.2	—	—	—	—	0.27	0.39	9.2	—	—	—
5.1	4.4	44	70	—	901	659	—	2.5	—	80	—	8	0.32	0.29	13.6	—	—	—
4.8	2.3	22	40	60	519	201	1.5	2.7	8	—	—	—	0.18	0.26	6.6	0.1	7	—
7.9	3.4	43	60	120	936	422	3.8	4.9	16	0	—	1	0.28	0.48	11	0.2	14	—
4.6	2	42	130	—	826	392	—	4.5	—	40	—	8	0.27	0.49	8.4	—	—	—
2.9	2.5	33	130	—	326	392	—	2.9	—	40	—	7	0.44	0.75	9.4	—	—	—
0.1	0.1	0	—	—	113	28	—	0.4	—	—	—	—	—	—	—	—	—	—
15.7	8.5	69	410	—	2062	565	—	4.3	—	100	—	11	0.92	0.49	8.2	—	—	—
13	6.8	73	410	—	1847	708	—	7.7	—	100	—	9	0.56	0.71	10.1	—	—	—
11.8	17	43	410	—	1847	708	—	7.7	—	100	—	9	0.56	0.71	14.2	—	—	—
6	7	51	400	—	2033	500	—	4.7	—	20	—	—	13.2	0.54	18.8	—	—	—
10	1.7	9	80	—	443	742	0.9	1.4	—	—	—	—	0.06	0.14	2	—	—	0
12	6.8	52	150	—	1166	321	3	6.1	—	—	—	1	0.42	0.63	9.8	—	—	0
7.6	1.5	0	20	—	167	724	0.6	1.4	—	0	—	—	0.06	0.07	2	—	—	0
9.8	10.4	46	180	—	1143	534	2.2	2.9	—	—	—	8	0.51	0.71	10.6	—	—	—
3	7.7	0	39	102	899	439	0.5	1.6	48	28	1.87	52	0.06	0.17	1.4	0.15	37	0
0	0.1	0	33	50	55	221	0.3	1.1	33	12	0.17	6	0.05	0.04	1	0.07	37	0
0	0	0	10	58	3	322	0.1	2.6	13	2	0.14	3	0.15	0.04	1	0.06	10	0
0	0.5	0	50	146	127	634	0.9	1.3	74	38	0.46	12	0.15	0.38	2.2	0.21	286	0
0	0.1	0	54	103	114	425	0.6	1.6	72	22	0.23	12	0.08	0.08	1.2	0.13	61	0
0	0	0	16	5	3	37	0	0.1	5	24	0.04	2	0	0.01	0	0.01	10	0
0	0	0	16	5	3	37	0	0.1	5	24	0.04	2	0	0.01	0	0.01	10	0
0	0.2	0	13	34	230	138	0.3	1.5	8	42	0.34	15	0.05	0.08	0.8	0.09	76	0
0	0.1	0	12	30	227	138	0.4	0.5	7	42	1.72	13	0.04	0.07	0.7	0.08	68	0
0	0.1	0	12	32	7	96	0.3	0.4	6	32	0.23	6	0.07	0.08	0.6	0.07	88	0
0	0.1	0	14	33	2	131	0.3	0.4	8	49	0.75	15	0.04	0.06	0.6	0.01	81	0
0	0.1	0	18	46	32	210	0.6	0.7	11	65	0.15	20	0.07	0.11	1	0.12	104	0
0	0.1	0	14	37	5	147	0.3	0.4	8	55	1.25	18	0.07	0.08	0.7	0.06	111	0
—	—	0	40	—	1100	—	—	2.7	—	0	—	—	—	—	—	—	—	—
—	—	0	40	—	1290	—	—	2.7	—	0	—	—	—	—	—	—	—	—
7.2	1.5	0	8	31	8	449	0.3	0.8	29	46	1.01	6	0.08	0.09	1.4	0.21	46	0
1	0.2	0	1	4	1	60	0	0.1	4	6	0.13	1	0.01	0.01	0.2	0.03	6	0
19.4	3.5	0	19	73	21	1096	0.7	2	71	106	2.32	14	0.19	0.21	3.3	0.48	113	0
12.9	2.4	0	13	48	14	729	0.5	1.4	47	70	1.54	9	0.12	0.14	2.2	0.32	75	0
14.8	4.5	0	33	119	15	1483	1.3	1.6	103	185	2.37	24	0.33	0.37	5.8	0.85	162	0
5.6	1.7	0	13	45	6	561	0.5	0.6	39	70	0.9	9	0.12	0.14	2.2	0.32	61	0
19.3	3.9	0	22	82	20	1203	0.8	2	78	123	2.69	16	0.22	0.24	3.9	0.56	124	0
—	—	—	1	3	0	52	0	0.1	—	2	—	6	0	0.02	0.1	0.04	—	—
—	—	—	27	—	51	192	—	0.3	—	813	—	0	0.01	0.06	1	—	—	—
0.1	0	2	1	6	49	20	0.1	0.1	2	36	0.03	0	0	0.01	0.2	0.01	1	0.07
0	0	—	6	—	25	40	—	0	—	300	—	0	0	0	0.1	—	—	—
—	—	—	7	—	3	—	—	0.9	—	7	—	1	0.02	0.02	0.3	0.04	—	—
—	—	—	2	3	1	7	0.1	0.4	1	0	—	1	0.02	0.02	0.3	0.02	—	—
—	—	—	12	—	55	120	—	0.6	—	0	—	0	0.02	0.08	1.2	—	—	—
—	—	—	36	—	70	115	—	0.6	—	1260	—	0	0.02	0.03	0.6	—	—	—
—	—	—	1	1	0	34	0	0.1	—	16	—	10	0	0.01	0.2	0	—	—
—	—	—	1	1	1	6	—	0	0	0	—	0	0	0	0	0	—	—
—	—	—	3	6	51	23	0.1	0.1	2	12	—	1	0.01	0.01	0.2	0.01	5	0.03
0	0	—	12	—	15	360	—	0.3	—	855	—	0	0.03	0.04	0.5	—	—	—

Food Item	Qty	Meas	Wgt (g)	Wtr (g)	Cals	Prot	Carb (g)	Fib (g)	Fat (g)	SatF (g)
Baby Food, tropical fruit medley, Gerber	1	Tbs	14	12	9	0	2	0	0	—
Baby Food, turkey sticks, Gerber	1	each	10	8	13	1	0	0	1	0.3
Baby Formulat, similac, liquid, 27cal/oz, Ross Labs	0.46	cup	114	95	100	3	10	—	5	—
Bacon, Canadian style, grilled	2	piece	47	29	87	11	1	0	4	1.3
Bacon, cooked, regular	3	piece	19	2	109	6	0	0	9	3.3
Bagel chips	2	piece	28	1	119	2	21	2.2	3	0.5
Bagel, 100% whole wheat	1	each	55	16	145	6	31	5.4	1	0.1
Bagel, cinnamon raisin	1	each	71	23	195	7	39	1.6	1	0.2
Bagel, egg	1	each	71	23	197	8	38	1.6	1	0.3
Bagel, oat bran	1	each	71	23	181	8	38	2.6	1	0.1
Bagel, plain	1	each	68	22	187	7	36	1.6	1	0.2
Baking chips, butterscotch	0.5	cup	85	1	458	2	57	0	25	20.5
Baking chips, peanut butter	0.5	cup	85	5	422	16	38	7.1	25	11.1
Baking chips, white chocolate	0.5	cup	85	1	458	5	50	0	27	16.5
Baking chocolate, bar, semi-sweet, Nestle	1	oz.	28	0	142	2	18	4	8	5.1
Baking chocolate, bar, unsweetened, Nestle	1	oz.	28	0	162	4	9	6.1	14	4
Baking chocolate, unsweetened, liquid, pkt	1	each	28	0	134	3	10	5.1	14	7.2
Baking chocolate, unsweetened, premelted, ChocoBake	1	oz.	28	1	162	0	10	6.1	16	10.2
Baking mix, reduced fat, Bisquick	1	cup	120	—	450	9	84	1.5	8	1.5
Baking powder, double acting, Calumet	1	tsp	5	0	2	0	1	0	0	0
Baking powder, low sodium	1	tsp	4	0	4	0	2	0.1	0	0
Baking soda/sodium bicarbonate	1	tsp	5	0	0	0	0	0	0	0
Baklava	1	piece	78	20	333	5	29	1.6	23	9.3
Balsam pear, leaftips, cooked	0.5	cup	29	26	10	1	2	0.6	0	0
Balsam pear, pods, cooked	0.5	cup	62	58	12	1	3	1.2	0	0
Bamboo shoot, sliced, canned	0.5	cup	66	62	12	1	2	0.9	0	0.1
Bamboo shoot, sliced, raw	0.5	cup	76	69	20	2	4	1.7	0	0.1
Bamboo shoots, cooked slices	0.5	cup	60	58	7	1	1	0.6	0	0
Banana	1	each	114	85	105	1	27	2.7	1	0.2
Banana chips, fried	0.5	cup	46	2	239	1	27	3.5	16	13.3
Banana nectar	1	cup	250	202	177	1	46	1.4	0	0.2
Banana split w/whipped cream	1	cup	425	221	1076	15	120	1.2	66	37.9
Banana, chocolate-covered, w/nuts	1	each	145	74	336	7	43	4.6	19	7
Banana, dehydrated	0.5	each	50	2	173	2	44	3.8	1	0.3
Banana, ripe, fried	1	cup	91	54	184	1	24	1.6	11	2.2
Barley, pearled, cooked	0.5	each	78	54	97	2	22	3	0	0.1
Barley, pearled, dry	0.5	cup	100	10	352	10	78	15.6	1	0.2
Barley, whole, cooked	0.5	cup	100	65	135	4	30	6.8	1	0.2
Barley, whole, dry	0.5	cup	92	9	326	12	68	15.9	2	0.4
Bay leaf, crumbled	1	cup	1	0	2	0	0	0.2	0	0
Bean cake, Japanese style	1	tsp	32	7	130	2	16	0.9	7	1
Bean paste, sweetened	1	each	28	13	60	2	14	1.5	0	0
Bean sprouts, mung, canned, drained	0.5	oz.	62	60	8	1	1	0.5	0	0
Bean sprouts, mung, raw	0.5	cup	52	47	16	2	3	0.9	0	0
Bean, Italian green, canned, drained, low sodium	0.5	cup	120	112	24	1	5	2.3	0	0
Bean, winged/goabean, dry, cooked	0.5	cup	86	58	126	9	13	2.1	5	0.7
Beans, Adzuki, canned, sweetened	0.5	cup	145	59	344	6	80	4.2	0	0
Beans, Adzuki, cooked	0.5	cup	115	76	147	9	28	1	0	0
Beans, B & M baked, fat free	0.5	cup	130	—	160	8	31	7	1	0
Beans, baked, canned, vegetarian	0.5	cup	127	92	118	6	26	6.4	1	0.1
Beans, baked, canned, w/pork	0.5	cup	126	90	134	7	25	6.9	2	0.8
Beans, baked, home prepared	0.5	cup	126	82	190	7	27	6.9	6	2.5
Beans, black turtle soup, canned w/liquid	0.5	cup	120	91	109	7	20	8.3	0	0.1
Beans, black turtle soup, cooked	0.5	cup	92	60	120	8	22	4.9	0	0.1
Beans, black, dry, cooked, no added salt	0.5	cup	86	56	114	8	20	7.5	0	0.1
Beans, broadbean/fava dry, cooked	0.5	cup	85	61	94	6	17	4.6	0	0.1
Beans, cranberry, cooked	0.5	cup	88	57	120	8	22	8.8	0	0.1
Beans, french, cooked	0.5	cup	86	57	111	6	21	8.1	1	0.1
Beans, Garbanzo/chickpeas, cooked from dry	0.5	cup	82	49	134	7	22	6.2	2	0.2
Beans Garbanzo/Chickpeas, dry	0.25	cup	50	6	182	10	30	8.7	3	0.3
Beans, great northern, dry, cooked	0.5	cup	88	61	104	7	19	6.2	0	0.1
Beans, green, Italian, canned, drained	0.5	cup	68	63	14	1	3	1.3	0	0
Beans, green, Italian, cooked	0.5	cup	62	56	22	1	5	2	0	0
Beans, green, Italian, frozen, cooked, drained	0.5	cup	68	62	19	1	4	2	0	0
Beans, green, Italian, raw	0.5	cup	55	50	17	1	4	1.9	0	0

MonoF	PolyF	Choles	Calc	Phos	Sod	Pot	Zn	Iron	Magn	VitA	VitE	VitC	Thia	Ribo	Nia	B6	Fola	B12
(g)	(g)	(mg)	(mg)	(mg)	(mg)	(mg)	(mg)	(mg)	(mg)	(µg RE)	(µg α-TE)	(mg)	(mg)	(mg)	(mg)	(mg)	(µg)	(µg)
—	—	—	1	0	1	6	—	0	1	2	—	2	0	0	0	0.01	—	—
—	—	9	10	13	43	12	0.2	0.1	1	0	—	0	0	0.02	0.2	0.01	—	—
—	—	—	90	70	34	132	0.8	0.2	7	90	2.01	9	0.1	0.15	1	0.06	15	0.25
1.9	0.4	27	5	139	727	183	0.8	0.4	10	0	0.12	0	0.39	0.09	3.2	0.21	2	0.37
4.5	1.1	16	2	64	303	92	0.6	0.3	5	0	0.1	0	0.13	0.05	1.4	0.05	1	0.33
0.8	1.4	0	4	58	168	67	0.4	0.6	16	0	0.19	0	0.05	0.05	0.6	0.08	23	0
0.1	0.3	0	16	159	270	190	1.3	1.8	59	0	0.49	0	0.17	0.14	2.8	0.18	40	0
0.1	0.5	0	14	71	229	105	0.8	2.7	20	6	0.11	0	0.27	0.2	2.2	0.04	64	0
0.3	0.5	17	9	60	359	48	0.5	2.8	18	23	0.1	0	0.38	0.17	2.4	0.06	62	0.11
0.2	0.3	0	9	78	360	82	0.6	2.2	22	0	0.1	0	0.24	0.24	2.1	0.03	58	0
0.1	0.5	0	50	65	363	69	0.6	2.4	20	0	0.03	0	0.37	0.21	3.1	0.04	60	0
1.9	0.4	0	29	27	76	159	0.1	0.1	4	0	1.91	0	0.07	0	0.1	0.01	1	0.08
8.2	4.5	0	94	264	213	429	1.7	1.4	94	2	2.55	0	0.04	0.17	7	0.19	82	0.05
7.7	0.9	18	169	150	76	243	0.6	0.2	10	3	1.91	0	0.05	0.24	0.6	0.05	14	0.52
—	—	0	0	—	0	109	—	0.7	—	0	—	0	0.02	0	0.2	—	—	—
5.2	0.7	0	0	—	0	239	—	0	—	0	—	0	0.03	0.04	0.4	—	—	—
2.6	3	0	15	96	3	331	1	1.2	75	0	1.71	0	0.01	0.08	0.6	0.02	5	0
—	—	0	0	—	0	—	—	1.5	—	0	—	0	0.04	0.04	0.4	—	—	—
—	—	0	120	—	1380	90	—	4.3	—	—	—	—	0.45	0.31	4.8	—	—	—
0	0	0	270	101	488	1	0	0.5	1	0	0	0	0	0	0	0	0	0
0	0	0	186	295	4	434	0	0.4	1	0	0	0	0	0	0	0	0	0
0	0	0	0	0	1258	0	0	0	0	0	0	0	0	0	0	0	0	0
8.5	3.8	36	34	88	291	139	0.5	1.7	34	124	1.99	1	0.17	0.13	1.3	0.05	9	0.02
0	0	0	12	22	4	175	0.1	0.3	27	50	0.14	16	0.04	0.08	0.3	0.22	25	0
0	0	0	6	22	4	198	0.5	0.2	10	7	0.43	20	0.03	0.03	0.2	0.02	32	0
0	0.1	0	5	16	5	52	0.4	0.2	3	1	0.25	1	0.02	0.02	0.1	0.09	2	0
0	0.1	0	10	44	3	402	0.8	0.4	2	2	0.76	3	0.11	0.05	0.5	0.18	5	0
0	0.1	0	7	12	2	320	0.3	0.1	2	0	0.4	0	0.01	0.03	0.2	0.06	1	0
0	0.1	0	7	23	1	451	0.2	0.4	33	9	0.31	10	0.05	0.11	0.6	0.66	22	0
0.9	0.3	0	8	26	3	247	0.3	0.6	35	4	2.48	3	0.04	0.01	0.3	0.12	6	0
0	0.1	0	8	18	5	347	0.2	0.3	27	7	0.24	8	0.04	0.09	0.5	0.5	17	0
18.8	5	209	468	477	354	779	2.7	1.5	89	545	0.49	2	0.15	0.9	0.5	0.17	19	1.41
7.5	3.2	0	28	153	7	596	1.8	1.4	93	8	1.92	9	0.1	0.19	3.3	0.63	42	0
0.1	0.2	0	11	37	2	746	0.3	0.6	54	16	0	4	0.09	0.12	1.4	0.22	7	0
4.8	3.4	0	10	23	120	366	0.2	0.3	30	142	1.89	6	0.04	0.1	0.5	0.53	10	0.01
0	0.2	0	9	42	2	73	0.6	1	17	1	0.04	0	0.06	0.05	1.6	0.09	13	0
0.1	0.6	0	29	221	9	280	2.1	2.5	79	2	0.13	0	0.19	0.11	4.6	0.26	23	0
0.1	0.6	0	13	115	1	115	0.8	1	22	0	0.6	0	0.08	0.03	1.4	0.09	8	0
0.3	1	0	30	243	11	416	2.6	3.3	122	2	0.55	0	0.59	0.26	4.2	0.29	18	0
0	0	0	5	1	0	3	0	0.3	1	4	0.01	0	0	0	0	0.01	1	0
2.9	2.6	0	3	21	55	58	0.2	0.7	6	0	1.14	0	0.07	0.05	0.5	0.02	9	0
0	0	0	4	23	30	105	0.2	0.5	9	0	0.04	0	0.03	0.01	0.1	0.03	17	0
0	0	0	9	20	88	17	0.2	0.3	6	1	0.01	0	0.02	0.04	0.1	0.02	6	0
0	0	0	7	28	3	78	0.2	0.5	11	1	0	7	0.04	0.06	0.4	0.05	32	0
0	0.1	0	31	23	2	131	0.3	1.1	16	42	0.17	6	0.02	0.07	0.2	0.04	38	0
1.8	1.3	0	122	132	11	241	1.2	3.7	46	0	0.09	0	0.25	0.11	0.7	0.04	9	0
0	0	0	32	107	316	173	2.3	1.6	45	1	0.04	0	0.15	0.08	0.9	0.12	155	0
0	0	0	32	193	9	612	2	2.3	60	1	0.12	0	0.13	0.07	0.8	0.11	139	0
0	0.5	0	60	—	220	—	—	3.6	—	0	—	0	—	—	—	—	—	—
0	0.2	0	64	132	504	376	1.8	2.1	41	22	0.67	4	0.19	0.08	0.5	0.17	30	0
0.8	0.3	9	67	136	522	389	1.8	2.5	43	23	0.49	3	0.07	0.05	0.6	0.08	46	0
2.7	0.9	6	77	137	532	451	0.9	0.4	54	0	0.66	1	0.17	0.06	0.5	0.11	61	0
0	0.2	0	42	130	461	370	0.6	2.3	42	0	0.31	3	0.17	0.14	0.7	0.07	73	0
0	0.1	0	51	140	3	398	0.7	2.6	45	1	0.28	0	0.21	0.05	0.5	0.07	79	0
0	0.2	0	23	120	1	305	1	1.8	60	1	0.07	0	0.21	0.05	0.4	0.06	128	0
0.1	0.1	0	31	106	4	228	0.9	1.3	37	2	0.08	0	0.08	0.08	0.6	0.06	88	0
0	0.2	0	44	119	1	341	1	1.8	44	0	0.09	0	0.18	0.06	0.5	0.07	182	0
0	0.4	0	54	88	5	318	0.6	0.9	48	0	0.1	1	0.11	0.05	0.5	0.09	64	0
0.5	1	0	40	138	6	239	1.2	2.4	39	2	0.29	1	0.1	0.05	0.4	0.11	141	0
0.7	1.4	0	52	183	12	438	1.7	3.1	58	4	0.41	2	0.24	0.11	0.8	0.27	279	0
0	0.2	0	60	146	2	346	0.8	1.9	44	0	0.27	1	0.14	0.05	0.6	0.1	90	0
0	0	0	18	13	177	74	0.2	0.6	9	24	0.1	3	0.01	0.04	0.1	0.02	22	0
0	0.1	0	29	24	2	187	0.2	0.8	16	42	0.09	6	0.05	0.06	0.4	0.04	21	0
0	0.1	0	33	21	6	85	0.3	0.6	16	27	0.1	3	0.02	0.06	0.3	0.04	16	0
0	0	0	20	21	3	115	0.1	0.6	14	37	0.23	9	0.05	0.06	0.4	0.04	20	0

Food Item	Qty	Meas	Wgt (g)	Wtr (g)	Cals	Prot	Carb (g)	Fib (g)	Fat (g)	SatF (g)
Beans, green, canned, drained, low sodium	0.5	cup	68	63	14	1	3	1.3	0	0
Beans, green, canned, not drained, low sodium	0.5	cup	120	114	18	1	4	1.8	0	0
Beans, green, seasoned, canned	0.5	cup	114	108	18	1	4	1.7	0	0.1
Beans, green, snap/string, canned, drained	0.5	cup	68	63	14	1	3	1.3	0	0
Beans, green, snap/string, frozen, cooked, drained	0.5	cup	68	62	19	1	4	2	0	0
Beans, green, string, pickled	0.5	cup	68	61	19	1	4	1.1	0	0
Beans, green/snap/string, raw	0.5	cup	55	50	17	1	4	1.9	0	0
Beans, green/snap/string, raw, cooked	0.5	cup	62	56	22	1	5	2	0	0
Beans, hyacinth, dry, cooked	0.5	cup	97	67	113	8	20	3.5	1	0.1
Beans, Italian green, canned, not drained, low sodium	0.5	cup	120	114	18	1	4	1.8	0	0
Beans, kidney, California red, cooked	0.5	cup	88	59	109	8	20	8.2	0	0
Beans, kidney, red, canned, drained	0.5	cup	128	88	151	9	28	11.4	1	—
Beans, kidney, red, cooked	0.5	cup	88	59	112	8	20	6.5	0	0.1
Beans, lima, baby, dry	0.25	cup	48	6	159	10	30	9.8	0	0.1
Beans, lima, baby, dry, cooked	0.5	cup	91	61	115	7	21	7	0	0.1
Beans, lima, baby, frozen, cooked	0.5	cup	90	65	94	6	18	5.4	0	0.1
Beans, lima, canned, drained	0.5	cup	85	57	82	5	16	3.7	0	0.1
Beans, lima, fordhook, frozen, cooked	0.5	cup	85	62	85	5	16	4.9	0	0.1
Beans, lima, immature, raw, cooked	0.5	cup	85	57	105	6	20	4.5	0	0.1
Beans, lima, large, dry, cooked	0.5	cup	94	66	108	7	20	6.6	0	0.1
Beans, mung, cooked, unsalted	0.5	cup	101	73	106	7	19	7.7	0	0.1
Beans, mungo, cooked	0.5	cup	90	65	94	7	16	5.8	0	0
Beans, Navy, dry, cooked	0.5	cup	91	58	129	8	24	5.8	1	0.1
Beans, pink, cooked	0.5	cup	84	51	125	8	23	4.4	0	0.1
Beans, pinto, dry, cooked	0.5	cup	86	55	117	7	22	7.4	0	0.1
Beans, red kidney, dry	0.25	cup	46	5	155	10	28	7	0	0.1
Beans, red kidney, dry, cooked	0.5	cup	88	59	112	8	20	5.7	0	0.1
Beans, red mexican, dry, cooked	0.5	cup	112	78	126	8	24	9	0	0.1
Beans, refried/frijoles, canned	1	cup	253	192	238	14	39	13.4	3	1.2
Beans, small white, dry, cooked	0.5	cup	90	57	127	8	23	9.3	1	0.1
Beans, white, dry, cooked, unsalted	0.5	cup	90	57	125	9	23	5.7	0	0.1
Beans, winged/goabean, dry, mature	0.5	cup	91	8	372	27	38	6.2	15	2.1
Beans, yardlong, dry, cooked	0.5	cup	86	59	101	7	18	3.2	0	0.1
Beans, yardlong, dry, mature	0.5	cup	84	7	290	20	52	9.2	1	0.3
Beans, yellow snap, canned, low sodium	0.5	cup	68	63	14	1	3	0.9	0	0
Beans, yellow wax, canned, drained	0.5	cup	68	63	14	1	3	0.9	0	0
Beans, yellow wax, cooked, drained	0.5	cup	62	56	22	1	5	2.1	0	0
Beans, yellow wax, frozen, cooked, drained	0.5	cup	68	62	19	1	4	2	0	0
Beans, yellow, dry, cooked	0.5	cup	88	55	127	8	22	9.2	1	0.2
Beans, yokan adzuki, confection, slices	3	piece	43	15	112	1	26	0.9	0	0
Beechnuts, dried	1	oz.	28	2	163	2	10	1	14	1.6
Beef & noodles, w/tomato sauce, Hamburger Helper	0.5	cup	124	93	140	15	10	1.4	4	1.4
Beef (roast) hash	0.5	cup	95	65	158	11	10	1.1	8	2.5
Beef cube steak, fried, lean	4	oz.	113	63	261	38	0	0	11	3.8
Beef jerky	1	each	20	5	81	7	2	0.4	5	2.2
Beef pot pie, Banquet	1	each	198	134	330	9	38	3	15	7
Beef pot pie, Swanson	1	each	198	120	415	11	41	2	23	9
Beef round steak, fried, lean	4	oz.	113	63	261	38	0	0	11	3.8
Beef sirloin steak, fried, lean	4	oz.	113	63	261	38	0	0	11	3.8
Beef stroganoff	0.5	cup	128	91	202	13	8	0.7	13	5.3
Beef, London Broil, broiled, lean	3	oz.	85	52	176	23	0	0	9	3.7
Beef, bacon, Sizzlean	2	piece	22	6	99	7	0	0	8	3.2
Beef, bottom round, pot roast, braised, lean	3	oz.	85	49	178	27	0	0	7	2.4
Beef, bottom round, pot roast, braised, lean	4	oz.	113	65	237	36	0	0	9	3.1
Beef, brisket, corned, cooked, lean	3	oz.	85	51	213	16	0	0	16	5.4
Beef, chuck, arm pot roast, braised, lean	3	oz.	85	49	184	28	0	0	7	2.6
Beef, corned, canned	4	oz.	113	65	284	31	0	0	17	7
Beef, cube steak, bread/flour fried, lean	4	oz.	113	54	313	30	12	0.7	15	4.5
Beef, filet mignon steak, broiled, lean	4	oz.	113	68	239	32	0	0	11	4.2
Beef, ground, baked, well done, extra lean	4	oz.	113	60	311	34	0	0	18	7.1
Beef, ground, broiled, well done, extra lean	4	oz.	113	61	301	32	0	0	18	7
Beef, ground, broiled, well done, lean	4	oz.	113	60	318	32	0	0	20	7.9
Beef, ground, broiled, well done, regular	4	oz.	113	59	331	31	0	0	22	8.7
Beef, ground, fried, well, extra lean	4	oz.	113	61	298	32	0	0	18	7.1
Beef, ground, patty, baked, well done, lean	1	each	88	45	257	26	0	0	16	6.3

MonoF (g)	PolyF (g)	Choles (mg)	Calc (mg)	Phos (mg)	Sod (mg)	Pot (mg)	Zn (mg)	Iron (mg)	Magn (mg)	VitA (µg RE)	VitE (µg α-TE)	VitC (mg)	Thia (mg)	Ribo (mg)	Nia (mg)	B6 (mg)	Fola (µg)	B12 (µg)
0	0	0	18	13	1	74	0.2	0.6	9	24	0.1	3	0.01	0.04	0.1	0.02	22	0
0	0.1	0	29	23	17	110	0.2	1.1	16	38	0.17	4	0.03	0.06	0.2	0.04	22	0
0	0.1	0	25	18	425	106	0.2	0.5	15	60	0.14	4	0.03	0.06	0.3	0.05	20	0
0	0	0	18	13	177	74	0.2	0.6	9	24	0.1	3	0.01	0.04	0.1	0.02	22	0
0	0.1	0	33	21	6	85	0.3	0.6	16	27	0.1	3	0.02	0.06	0.3	0.04	16	0
0	0	0	22	23	148	127	0.1	0.6	16	38	0.24	8	0.04	0.06	0.4	0.04	18	0
0	0	0	20	21	3	115	0.1	0.6	14	37	0.23	9	0.05	0.06	0.4	0.04	20	0
0	0.1	0	29	24	2	187	0.2	0.8	16	42	0.09	6	0.05	0.06	0.4	0.04	21	0
0.1	0.3	0	39	116	7	327	2.8	4.4	80	0	0.1	0	0.26	0.04	0.4	0.04	4	0
0	0.1	0	29	23	17	110	0.2	1.1	16	38	0.17	4	0.03	0.06	0.2	0.04	22	0
0	0	0	58	121	4	369	0.8	2.6	42	0	0.18	1	0.11	0.06	0.5	0.09	65	0
—	—	0	—	166	—	—	1	—	50	0	—	—	0.19	0.16	0.8	0.04	90	0
0	0.2	0	25	125	2	355	0.9	2.6	40	0	0.07	1	0.14	0.05	0.5	0.11	114	0
0	0.2	0	38	176	6	666	1.2	2.9	89	0	0.19	0	0.27	0.1	0.8	0.16	190	0
0	0.2	0	26	116	3	365	0.9	2.2	48	0	0.16	0	0.15	0.05	0.6	0.07	137	0
0	0.1	0	25	101	26	370	0.5	1.8	50	15	0.58	5	0.06	0.05	0.7	0.1	14	0
0	0.2	0	24	60	201	189	0.8	1.5	35	16	0.26	5	0.03	0.04	0.4	0.02	20	0
0	0.1	0	19	54	45	347	0.4	1.2	29	16	0.25	11	0.06	0.05	0.9	0.1	18	0
0	0.1	0	27	111	14	485	0.7	2.1	63	32	0.12	9	0.12	0.08	0.9	0.16	22	0
0	0.2	0	16	104	2	478	0.9	2.2	40	0	0.17	0	0.15	0.05	0.4	0.15	78	0
0.1	0.1	0	27	100	2	269	0.8	1.4	48	2	0.52	1	0.17	0.06	0.6	0.07	161	0
0	0.3	0	48	140	6	208	0.7	1.6	57	3	0.14	1	0.14	0.07	1.4	0.05	85	0
0	0.2	0	64	143	1	335	1	2.3	54	0	0.36	1	0.18	0.06	0.5	0.15	127	0
0	0.2	0	44	139	2	427	0.8	1.9	55	0	0.33	0	0.22	0.05	0.5	0.15	141	0
0.1	0.2	0	41	137	2	400	0.9	2.2	47	0	0.8	2	0.16	0.08	0.3	0.13	147	0
0	0.3	0	38	187	6	625	1.3	3.1	64	0	0.1	2	0.28	0.1	1	0.18	181	0
0	0.2	0	25	126	2	357	0.9	2.6	40	0	0.19	1	0.14	0.05	0.5	0.11	115	0
0.1	0.2	0	42	139	240	369	0.9	1.9	48	0	0.08	2	0.07	0.07	0.4	0.12	94	0
1.4	0.4	20	89	218	756	676	3	4.2	84	0	0	15	0.21	0.04	0.8	0.36	28	0
0	0.2	0	65	151	2	414	1	2.5	61	0	0.36	0	0.13	0.05	0.2	0.11	123	0
0	0.1	0	81	102	5	505	1.2	3.3	57	0	0.2	0	0.11	0.04	0.1	0.08	73	0
5.5	3.9	0	400	410	35	889	4.1	12.2	163	0	0.26	0	0.94	0.41	2.8	0.16	41	0
0	0.2	0	36	155	4	269	0.9	2.3	84	2	0.24	0	0.18	0.06	0.5	0.08	125	0
0.1	0.5	0	115	467	14	966	2.9	7.2	282	4	0.24	1	0.74	0.2	1.8	0.31	549	0
0	0	0	18	13	1	74	0.2	0.6	9	7	0.2	3	0.01	0.04	0.1	0.02	22	0
0	0	0	18	13	169	74	0.2	0.6	9	7	0.2	3	0.01	0.04	0.1	0.02	22	0
0	0.1	0	29	24	2	187	0.2	0.8	16	5	0.18	6	0.05	0.06	0.4	0.04	21	0
0	0.1	0	33	21	6	85	0.3	0.6	16	7	0.1	3	0.02	0.06	0.3	0.04	16	0
0.1	0.4	0	55	161	4	286	0.9	2.2	65	0	0.44	2	0.16	0.09	0.6	0.11	71	0
0	0	0	12	17	36	19	0	0.5	8	0	0.02	0	0	0	0	0	4	0
6.2	5.7	0	0	0	11	288	0.1	0.7	0	0	—	4	0.09	0.1	0.2	0.19	32	0
1.7	0.3	47	13	144	343	390	2.4	2.1	28	50	0.8	6	0.13	0.16	2.9	0.32	10	1.39
2.9	1.7	29	10	103	427	294	2.5	1.2	18	0	0.62	4	0.08	0.1	1.9	0.25	8	0.91
4.6	1	110	9	317	345	555	6.1	3.9	38	0	0.16	0	0.14	0.34	5.6	0.63	13	4
2.2	0.2	10	4	81	438	118	1.6	1.1	10	0	0.1	0	0.03	0.03	0.3	0.04	26	0.2
—	—	25	20	—	1000	—	—	1.1	—	150	—	0	—	—	—	—	—	—
—	—	25	20	—	740	—	—	1.8	—	150	—	0	—	—	—	—	—	—
4.6	1	110	9	317	345	555	6.1	3.9	38	0	0.16	0	0.14	0.34	5.6	0.63	13	4
4.6	1	110	9	317	345	555	6.1	3.9	38	0	0.16	0	0.14	0.34	5.6	0.63	13	4
3.7	3.3	42	46	153	610	276	2.4	1.8	20	49	0.78	1	0.09	0.19	2.2	0.14	10	1.29
3.5	0.3	57	6	201	71	352	4.1	2.2	20	0	0.14	0	0.09	0.16	4.3	0.29	7	2.76
3.7	0.3	26	2	52	496	91	1.4	0.7	6	0	0.05	0	0.02	0.06	1.4	0.07	2	0.76
3	0.3	82	4	231	43	262	4.7	2.9	21	0	0.12	0	0.06	0.22	3.5	0.31	9	2.1
4.1	0.4	109	6	308	58	349	6.2	3.9	28	0	0.16	0	0.08	0.3	4.6	0.41	12	2.8
7.8	0.6	83	7	106	964	123	3.9	1.6	10	0	0.14	0	0.02	0.14	2.6	0.2	5	1.39
3	0.3	86	8	228	56	246	7.4	3.2	20	0	0.12	0	0.07	0.25	3.2	0.28	9	2.89
6.8	0.7	98	14	126	1140	154	4	2.4	16	0	0.17	0	0.02	0.17	2.8	0.15	10	1.84
5.5	3.7	86	36	260	386	438	5.7	4	35	3	0.55	0	0.17	0.34	4.4	0.44	14	3.23
4.3	0.4	95	8	270	71	475	6.3	4.1	34	0	0.16	0	0.15	0.34	4.4	0.5	8	2.91
7.9	0.7	121	10	184	73	330	7.9	3.4	25	0	0.2	0	0.06	0.35	6.1	0.33	12	2.11
7.8	0.7	112	10	215	93	418	7.3	3.1	28	0	0.2	0	0.08	0.36	6.6	0.36	12	2.9
8.8	0.7	115	14	206	101	396	7	2.8	27	0	0.23	0	0.07	0.27	6.8	0.34	12	3.08
9.7	0.8	115	14	217	105	371	6.6	3.1	25	0	0.26	0	0.04	0.24	7.3	0.34	11	3.72
7.9	0.7	105	9	210	92	408	7.1	3.1	27	0	0.2	0	0.08	0.34	6.2	0.35	11	2.63
7.1	0.6	87	11	144	62	252	5.7	2.3	18	0	0.18	0	0.06	0.21	4.8	0.23	11	1.99

Food Item	Qty	Meas	Wgt (g)	Wtr (g)	Cals	Prot	Carb (g)	Fib (g)	Fat (g)	SatF (g)
Beef, heart, simmered	4	oz.	113	73	198	33	0	0	6	1.9
Beef, liver, fried	3	oz.	85	47	184	23	7	0	7	2.3
Beef, lunchmeat, thin sliced	1	oz.	28	16	50	8	2	0	1	0.5
Beef, meat stick, smoked	1	each	20	4	109	4	1	—	10	4.1
Beef, porterhouse steak, choice, broiled, lean	1	each	170	102	366	44	0	0	20	6.9
Beef, rib eye steak, broiled, lean	4	oz.	113	67	255	32	0	0	13	5.4
Beef, rib, whole, roasted, lean	3	oz.	85	49	207	23	0	0	12	4.8
Beef, rib, whole, roasted, lean & fat	3	oz.	85	39	320	19	0	0	26	10.7
Beef, roast, rump, braised, lean	3	oz.	85	50	167	27	0	0	6	2
Beef, roast, rump, braised, lean	4	oz.	113	66	222	36	0	0	8	2.6
Beef, roast, rump, braised, lean & fat	3	oz.	85	45	220	25	0	0	13	4.8
Beef, round steak, fried, lean & fat	4	oz.	113	57	327	35	0	0	20	7.5
Beef, round tip, sirloin roast, roasted, lean	4	oz.	113	74	210	32	0	0	8	2.7
Beef, round, bottom, braised, lean	3	oz.	85	48	187	27	0	0	8	2.7
Beef, round, broiled, lean & fat	4	oz.	113	62	311	29	0	0	21	9.2
Beef, round, pot roasted, lean & fat	3	oz.	85	44	234	24	0	0	14	5.4
Beef, sandwich steak, Steak Ums	1	each	41	24	105	10	0	0	7	2.6
Beef, short ribs, choice, braised, lean	2	each	102	51	301	31	0	0	18	7.9
Beef, shortrib, braised, lean & fat	4	oz.	113	40	534	24	0	0	48	20.2
Beef, sirloin steak, broiled, lean	3	oz.	85	52	172	26	0	0	7	2.6
Beef, sirloin strip steak, broiled, lean	4	oz.	113	68	235	32	0	0	11	4.1
Beef, stew meat, cooked, lean & fat	4	oz.	113	57	345	32	0	0	23	9.2
Beef, stew meat, cooked, lean only	0.5	cup	70	39	164	22	0	0	8	3
Beef, t-bone steak, broiled, lean	3	oz.	85	52	174	23	0	0	9	3.1
Beef, t-bone steak, broiled, lean & fat	3	oz.	85	44	263	20	0	0	20	7.7
Beef, tenderloin steak, broiled, lean	4	oz.	113	68	239	32	0	0	11	4.2
Beef, top round steak, broiled, lean	4	oz.	113	70	204	36	0	0	6	1.9
Beef, tripe, pickled	1	oz.	28	25	18	3	0	0	0	0.1
Beefalo, roasted	4	oz.	113	70	213	35	0	0	7	3
Beer, Lowenbrau Special	1	cup	237	—	105	1	10	—	0	0
Beer, Milwaukee's Best Ice	1	cup	237	—	90	1	5	—	0	0
Beer, Red Dog	1	cup	237	—	98	0	9	—	0	0
Beer, light	1	cup	236	225	66	0	3	0	0	0
Beer, non-alcoholic, Sharp's	1	cup	237	—	39	0	8	—	0	0
Beer, regular, alcoholic	1	cup	237	219	97	1	9	0.5	0	0
Beerwurst/beer salami	1	piece	23	12	76	3	0	0	7	3
Beet greens, cooked, no added salt	0.5	cup	72	64	19	2	4	2.1	0	0
Beets & onions, pickled	0.5	cup	84	72	42	1	10	1.2	0	0
Beets, canned, drained	0.5	cup	85	77	26	1	6	1.4	0	0
Beets, canned, w/liquid, regular	0.5	cup	123	113	34	1	8	1.5	0	0
Beets, cooked, no added salt	0.5	cup	85	74	37	1	8	1.7	0	0
Beets, pickled slices	0.5	cup	114	93	74	1	19	2.3	0	0
Beets, raw slices	0.5	cup	68	60	29	1	6	1.9	0	0
Beets, w/Harvard sauce	0.5	cup	123	91	135	1	25	1.5	4	0.8
Beets, whole, cooked, no added salt	2	each	100	87	44	2	10	2	0	0
Beets, whole, pickled	1	each	50	41	32	0	8	1	0	0
Berry turnover	1	each	78	25	277	3	36	1.4	14	3.4
Biscuit dough, higher fat, chilled, baked	1	each	27	8	93	2	13	0.4	4	1
Biscuit dough, lower fat, chilled, baked	1	each	21	6	63	2	12	0.4	1	0.3
Biscuit mix, dry, prepared	1	each	28	8	95	2	14	0.5	3	0.8
Biscuit, cheese	1	each	30	8	115	3	12	0.4	6	2.2
Biscuit, homemade	1	each	28	8	101	2	13	0.4	5	1.2
Biscuit, plain, fast food	1	each	74	20	276	4	34	1.4	13	8.7
Biscuit, plain/buttermilk, baked	1	each	35	9	127	2	17	0.5	6	0.9
Biscuit, whole wheat	1	each	63	17	201	6	29	4.8	8	2.2
Bison, roasted	4	oz.	113	75	162	32	0	0	3	1
Blackberries, fresh	0.5	cup	72	62	37	1	9	3.8	0	0
Blackberries, frozen, unsweetened	0.5	cup	76	62	48	1	12	3.8	0	0
Blackberry, canned w/heavy syrup	0.5	cup	128	96	118	2	30	4.4	0	0
Blackeyed cowpeas, frozen, cooked	0.5	cup	85	56	112	7	20	5.4	1	0.1
Blackeyed peas, cooked from raw, drained	0.5	cup	82	62	80	3	17	4.1	0	0.1
Blintz, fruit-filled	1	each	70	44	124	4	17	0.4	5	1.4
Blueberries, canned w/heavy syrup	0.5	cup	128	98	113	1	28	1.9	0	0
Blueberries, fresh	0.5	cup	72	61	41	0	10	2	0	0
Blueberries, frozen, sweetened, pkg	0.5	cup	115	89	93	0	25	2.4	0	0

MonoF	PolyF	Choles	Calc	Phos	Sod	Pot	Zn	Iron	Magn	VitA	VitE	VitC	Thia	Ribo	Nia	B6	Fola	B12
(g)	(g)	(mg)	(mg)	(mg)	(mg)	(mg)	(mg)	(mg)	(mg)	(µg RE)	(µg α-TE)	(mg)	(mg)	(mg)	(mg)	(mg)	(µg)	(µg)
1.4	1.6	219	7	284	71	264	3.6	8.5	28	0	0.82	2	0.16	1.75	4.6	0.24	2	16.2
1.4	1.4	410	9	392	90	309	4.6	5.3	20	9119	0.54	20	0.18	3.52	12.2	1.22	187	95.2
0.5	0.1	12	3	48	409	122	1.1	0.8	5	0	0.05	0	0.02	0.05	1.5	0.1	3	0.73
4.1	0.9	26	14	36	293	51	0.5	0.7	4	34	0.06	1	0.03	0.09	0.9	0.04	0	0.2
8.9	0.6	117	12	359	117	624	9	5.3	46	0	0.24	0	0.19	0.42	7.9	0.68	14	3.86
5.6	0.4	91	15	236	78	447	7.9	2.9	31	0	0.18	0	0.11	0.25	5.4	0.45	9	3.76
5	0.4	68	8	182	61	318	5.9	2.4	21	0	0.12	0	0.07	0.18	3.5	0.23	7	2.47
11.4	0.9	72	9	146	54	252	4.4	2	16	0	0.2	0	0.06	0.14	2.9	0.2	6	2.14
2.5	0.2	82	4	231	43	262	4.7	2.9	21	0	0.08	0	0.06	0.22	3.5	0.31	9	2.1
3.4	0.3	109	6	308	58	349	6.2	3.9	28	0	0.1	0	0.08	0.3	4.6	0.41	12	2.8
5.6	0.5	82	5	210	42	241	4.2	2.7	20	0	0.09	0	0.06	0.2	3.2	0.28	8	2.01
8.4	1.2	110	10	287	340	500	5.5	3.6	34	0	0.2	0	0.13	0.31	5.1	0.57	12	3.71
3.1	0.3	92	6	274	74	438	8	3.3	31	0	0.16	0	0.11	0.31	4.2	0.45	9	3.28
3.5	0.3	82	4	231	43	262	4.7	2.9	21	0	0.15	0	0.06	0.22	3.5	0.31	9	2.1
10.5	0.9	95	8	239	68	415	4.7	2.7	27	0	0.29	0	0.03	0.23	4.2	0.5	10	3.12
6.2	0.5	82	5	208	42	240	4.2	2.6	19	0	0.16	0	0.06	0.2	3.2	0.28	8	2
3	0.2	33	3	66	29	128	2.2	1	9	0	0.07	0	0.02	0.11	1.9	0.11	4	0.82
8.1	0.6	95	11	240	59	319	8	3.4	22	0	0.14	0	0.07	0.21	3.3	0.29	7	3.53
21.4	1.7	107	14	184	57	254	5.5	2.6	17	0	0.33	0	0.06	0.17	2.8	0.25	6	2.97
2.9	0.3	76	9	207	56	343	5.5	2.9	27	0	0.12	0	0.11	0.25	3.6	0.38	8	2.42
4.3	0.4	86	9	247	77	449	5.9	2.8	31	0	0.16	0	0.1	0.23	6.1	0.48	9	2.27
10.1	0.8	113	12	248	333	285	8.5	3.5	23	0	0.2	0	0.08	0.27	3.3	0.32	8	2.78
3.4	0.3	71	7	172	208	193	6.1	2.5	16	0	0.1	0	0.06	0.19	2.2	0.21	5	1.83
3.8	0.3	50	5	183	60	321	4.5	2.7	24	0	0.12	0	0.09	0.21	3.9	0.33	7	1.93
8.7	0.7	57	7	156	54	273	3.8	2.3	20	0	0.18	0	0.08	0.18	3.4	0.28	6	1.81
4.3	0.4	95	8	270	71	475	6.3	4.1	34	0	0.16	0	0.15	0.34	4.4	0.5	8	2.91
2.2	0.2	95	7	279	69	501	6.3	3.3	35	0	0.16	0	0.14	0.31	6.8	0.64	14	2.81
0.1	0	19	36	24	13	5	0.5	0.5	2	0	0.03	0	0	0.04	0.5	0	0	0.26
3	0.2	66	27	284	93	521	7.3	3.5	0	0	0.2	10	0.03	0.12	5.6	0.45	20	2.89
0	0	0	—	—	5	—	—	—	—	—	—	—	—	—	—	—	—	0
0	0	0	—	—	3	—	—	—	—	—	—	—	—	—	—	—	—	0
0	0	0	—	—	3	—	—	—	—	—	—	—	—	—	—	—	—	0
0	0	0	12	28	7	42	0.1	0.1	12	0	0	0	0.02	0.07	0.9	0.08	10	0.02
0	0	0	—	—	2	—	—	—	—	—	—	—	—	—	—	—	—	0
0	0	0	12	28	12	59	0	0.1	14	0	0	0	0.01	0.06	1.1	0.12	14	0.05
3.2	0.3	14	2	22	236	40	0.6	0.3	3	0	0.04	0	0.02	0.03	0.8	0.04	1	0.45
0	0	0	82	30	174	654	0.4	1.4	49	367	0.22	18	0.08	0.21	0.4	0.1	10	0
0	0	0	8	21	209	211	0.2	0.5	27	1	0.22	3	0.02	0.01	0.2	0.02	27	0
0	0	0	13	14	165	126	0.2	1.6	14	1	0.26	3	0.01	0.03	0.1	0.05	26	0
0	0	0	16	20	310	162	0.3	0.8	20	4	0.35	3	0.01	0.05	0.2	0.07	36	0
0	0.1	0	14	32	66	259	0.3	0.7	20	3	0.26	3	0.02	0.03	0.3	0.06	68	0
0	0	0	12	19	301	169	0.3	0.5	17	1	0.15	3	0.01	0.06	0.3	0.06	30	0
0	0	0	11	27	53	221	0.2	0.5	16	3	0.2	3	0.02	0.03	0.2	0.05	74	0
1.7	1.2	0	12	30	287	288	0.2	0.7	36	53	0.87	5	0.03	0.02	0.2	0.03	45	0
0	0.1	0	16	38	77	305	0.4	0.8	23	4	0.3	4	0.03	0.04	0.3	0.07	80	0
0	0	0	6	8	132	74	0.1	0.2	8	0	0.06	1	0	0.02	0.1	0.02	13	0
6.1	3.7	0	6	32	230	54	0.2	1.3	8	2	1.51	3	0.18	0.13	1.5	0.02	6	0
2.2	0.5	0	5	104	325	42	0.1	0.7	4	0	0.49	0	0.09	0.06	0.8	0.01	12	0
0.6	0.2	0	4	98	305	39	0.1	0.6	4	0	0.14	0	0.09	0.05	0.7	0.01	14	0
1.2	1.2	1	52	133	271	53	0.2	0.6	7	7	0.11	0	0.1	0.1	0.9	0.02	2	0.06
2.4	1.2	6	80	70	197	42	0.3	0.7	6	17	0.43	0	0.1	0.1	0.8	0.01	3	0.04
2	1.2	1	67	47	165	34	0.2	0.8	5	7	0.37	0	0.1	0.09	0.8	0.01	17	0.02
3.4	0.5	5	90	260	584	87	0.3	1.6	9	24	0.44	0	0.27	0.18	1.6	0.03	6	0.1
2.4	2.2	0	17	151	368	78	0.2	1.2	6	0	1.03	0	0.15	0.1	1.2	0.02	21	0.05
3	1.9	4	120	177	468	200	1.2	1.5	56	9	0.98	0	0.14	0.12	2.2	0.13	13	0.06
1.1	0.3	93	9	237	65	409	4.2	3.9	30	0	0.16	0	0.11	0.31	4.2	0.45	9	3.24
0	0.2	0	23	15	0	141	0.2	0.4	14	12	0.51	15	0.02	0.03	0.3	0.04	24	0
0	0.2	0	22	23	1	106	0.2	0.6	17	8	0.54	2	0.02	0.04	0.9	0.05	26	0
0	0.1	0	27	18	4	127	0.2	0.8	22	28	0.91	4	0.04	0.05	0.4	0.05	34	0
0.1	0.2	0	20	104	4	319	1.2	1.8	42	7	0.33	2	0.22	0.05	0.6	0.08	120	0
0	0.1	0	106	42	3	345	0.8	0.9	43	65	0.18	2	0.08	0.12	1.2	0.05	105	0
1.8	1	50	33	56	151	75	0.3	0.8	6	78	0.69	1	0.05	0.13	0.3	0.04	8	0.2
0.1	0.2	0	6	13	4	51	0.1	0.4	5	8	1.28	1	0.04	0.07	0.1	0.05	2	0
0	0.1	0	4	7	4	64	0.1	0.1	4	7	0.72	9	0.04	0.04	0.3	0.03	5	0
0	0.1	0	7	8	1	69	0.1	0.4	2	5	0.82	1	0.02	0.06	0.3	0.07	8	0

Food Item	Qty	Meas	Wgt (g)	Wtr (g)	Cals	Prot	Carb (g)	Fib (g)	Fat (g)	SatF (g)
Blueberries, frozen, unsweetened	0.5	cup	78	67	40	0	9	2.1	0	0
Bologna, beef	1	piece	23	13	72	3	0	0	7	2.8
Bologna, beef & pork	1	piece	28	15	90	3	1	0	8	3
Bologna, cured pork	1	piece	23	14	57	4	0	0	5	1.6
Bologna, turkey	1	piece	28	18	56	4	0	0	4	1.4
Boysenberries, canned w/heavy syrup	0.5	cup	128	98	113	1	28	3.3	0	0
Boysenberries, fresh	0.5	cup	72	62	37	1	9	3.8	0	0
Boysenberries, frozen, unsweetened	0.5	cup	66	57	33	1	8	2.6	0	0
Bratwurst, cooked link	1	each	85	48	256	12	2	0	22	7.9
Bread crumbs, dry, grated, plain	0.25	cup	25	2	99	3	18	0.6	1	0.3
Bread crumbs, seasoned, dry, grated	0.25	cup	30	2	110	4	21	1.3	1	0.2
Bread crumbs, soft	0.25	cup	11	4	30	1	6	0.2	1	0.2
Bread stick, w/o salt coating, plain	10	each	100	6	412	12	68	3	10	1.4
Bread stick, w/salt coating	1	each	35	2	134	4	26	0.8	1	0.2
Bread stuffing, homemade	1	cup	203	132	341	8	45	4	15	3
Bread stuffing, mix, prepared	1	cup	140	91	249	4	30	4.1	12	2.4
Bread, 7-grain, Pepperidge Farm	1	piece	38	15	100	3	18	2	2	0
Bread, Armenian	1	piece	20	7	55	2	10	0.6	1	0.1
Bread, Boston brown, canned	1	piece	45	21	88	2	20	2.1	1	0.1
Bread, Cuban-Spanish-Portuguese	1	piece	20	6	58	2	11	0.5	1	0.1
Bread, Cuban-Spanish-Portuguese, toasted	1	piece	18	3	61	2	12	0.6	1	0.1
Bread, French	1	piece	35	12	96	3	18	1	1	0.2
Bread, Hollywood, dark	1	piece	18	7	39	2	8	1.4	0	0.1
Bread, Hollywood, light	1	piece	18	7	41	2	8	0.9	0	0
Bread, Indian fry, 5 inch diameter	1	piece	90	24	296	6	48	1.6	9	2.1
Bread, Italian	1	piece	30	11	81	3	15	0.8	1	0.3
Bread, Spanish coffee	1	each	85	21	292	7	49	1.6	7	1.1
Bread, banana, homemade, w/margarine	1	piece	50	15	163	2	27	0.6	5	1.1
Bread, banana, recipe, w/vegetable shortening	1	piece	60	17	203	3	33	0.8	7	1.8
Bread, barley	1	piece	26	10	69	2	13	1.2	1	0.3
Bread, batter	1	piece	33	12	93	3	15	0.6	2	0.7
Bread, buckwheat	1	piece	27	10	71	2	13	1	1	0.3
Bread, cheese	1	piece	26	10	71	2	12	0.6	1	0.5
Bread, cheese, toasted	1	piece	24	7	71	2	12	0.6	1	0.5
Bread, corn & molasses	1	piece	32	12	86	2	15	0.6	2	0.6
Bread, cracked wheat	1	piece	25	9	65	2	12	1.4	1	0.2
Bread, crumpet biscuit	1	piece	45	24	80	2	17	0.8	0	0.1
Bread, dark pumpernickel, Pepperidge Farm	1	each	32	12	80	3	15	1	1	0.5
Bread, date nut	1	piece	56	12	217	3	30	0.8	10	2.2
Bread, egg/challah	1	piece	23	8	66	2	11	0.5	1	0.4
Bread, fruit, w/o nuts	1	piece	41	10	150	2	23	0.5	6	1.5
Bread, hoecake, 1/8 pone	1	piece	61	29	136	3	25	3.6	3	0.7
Bread, milk & honey	1	piece	28	10	74	2	15	0.6	1	0.2
Bread, mixed grain	1	piece	25	9	62	2	12	1.6	1	0.2
Bread, multigrain, low calorie, high fiber	1	piece	23	10	46	2	10	2.8	1	0
Bread, multigrain, low calorie, high fiber, toasted	1	piece	21	8	47	2	10	2.8	1	0
Bread, oat bran	1	piece	30	13	71	3	12	1.4	1	0.2
Bread, oat bran, low calorie	1	piece	28	13	56	2	12	3.4	1	0.1
Bread, oat bran, low calorie, toasted	1	piece	25	9	60	2	12	3.6	1	0.1
Bread, oatmeal	1	piece	25	9	67	2	12	1	1	0.2
Bread, oatmeal, low calorie	1	piece	23	10	48	2	10	—	1	0.1
Bread, onion cheese	1	piece	26	10	71	2	12	0.6	1	0.5
Bread, pita pocket, white	1	each	60	19	165	5	33	1.3	1	0.1
Bread, pita pocket, whole wheat	1	each	45	14	120	4	25	3.3	1	0.2
Bread, potato	1	piece	26	10	69	2	13	0.6	1	0.2
Bread, protein	1	piece	19	8	47	2	8	0.6	0	0.1
Bread, pumpernickel	1	piece	32	12	80	3	15	2.1	1	0.1
Bread, raisin	1	piece	25	8	68	2	13	1.1	1	0.3
Bread, rice	1	piece	25	9	79	2	10	0.6	4	0.4
Bread, rice bran, low calorie	1	piece	27	11	66	2	12	1.3	1	0.2
Bread, rye	1	piece	25	9	65	2	12	1.4	1	0.2
Bread, rye, low calorie	1	piece	23	11	47	2	9	2.8	1	0.1
Bread, sourdough	1	piece	25	9	68	2	13	0.8	1	0.2
Bread, soy	1	piece	26	10	69	3	12	0.7	1	0.4
Bread, sprouted wheat	1	piece	26	10	68	2	12	1.4	1	0.2

MonoF (g)	PolyF (g)	Choles (mg)	Calc (mg)	Phos (mg)	Sod (mg)	Pot (mg)	Zn (mg)	Iron (mg)	Magn (mg)	VitA (µg RE)	VitE (µg α-TE)	VitC (mg)	Thia (mg)	Ribo (mg)	Nia (mg)	B6 (mg)	Fola (µg)	B12 (µg)
0.1	0.2	0	6	9	1	42	0.1	0.1	4	6	0.78	2	0.02	0.03	0.4	0.05	5	0
3.2	0.3	13	3	20	226	36	0.5	0.4	3	0	0.04	0	0.01	0.02	0.6	0.04	1	0.33
3.8	0.7	16	3	26	289	51	0.6	0.4	3	0	0.06	0	0.05	0.04	0.7	0.05	1	0.38
2.2	0.5	14	3	32	272	65	0.5	0.2	3	0	0.06	0	0.12	0.04	0.9	0.06	1	0.21
1.4	1.2	28	24	37	249	56	0.5	0.4	4	0	0.15	0	0.02	0.05	1	0.06	2	0.08
0	0.1	0	23	13	4	115	0.2	0.6	14	5	0.91	8	0.03	0.04	0.3	0.05	44	0
0	0.2	0	23	15	0	141	0.2	0.4	14	12	0.51	15	0.02	0.03	0.3	0.04	24	0
0	0.1	0	18	18	1	92	0.1	0.6	11	5	0.3	2	0.04	0.02	0.5	0.04	42	0
10.4	2.3	51	37	127	473	180	2	1.1	13	0	0.21	1	0.43	0.16	2.7	0.18	2	0.81
0.6	0.3	0	57	37	216	55	0.3	1.5	12	0	0.14	0	0.19	0.11	1.7	0.02	27	0
0.3	0.2	0	30	40	795	81	0.3	1	11	1	0.04	0	0.05	0.05	0.8	0.04	33	0.01
0.2	0.1	0	9	11	57	12	0.1	0.3	2	0	0.02	0	0.04	0.03	0.4	0	4	0
3.6	3.6	0	22	121	657	124	0.9	4.3	32	0	1.48	0	0.59	0.55	5.3	0.07	122	0
0.4	0.3	1	10	35	586	32	0.2	1.5	7	0	0.04	0	0.23	0.18	2.2	0.01	4	0
6.5	4.3	0	130	100	936	266	0.6	3.3	30	140	2.44	3	0.34	0.29	3.2	0.11	34	0
5.3	3.6	0	45	59	760	104	0.4	1.5	17	113	1.96	0	0.19	0.15	2.1	0.06	141	0.01
0.5	0	0	0	—	180	—	—	0.7	—	0	—	0	0.12	0.07	1.2	—	—	—
0.1	0.3	0	16	15	117	15	0.2	0.6	5	0	0.05	0	0.08	0.05	0.7	0.01	5	0
0.1	0.3	0	32	50	284	143	0.2	0.9	28	5	0.25	0	0.01	0.05	0.5	0.04	5	0
0.2	0.2	0	9	17	116	18	0.1	0.6	4	0	0.02	0	0.08	0.05	0.7	0.01	6	0
0.2	0.2	0	9	18	121	19	0.1	0.6	4	0	0.01	0	0.07	0.05	0.7	0.01	6	0
0.4	0.2	0	26	37	213	40	0.3	0.9	9	0	0.1	0	0.18	0.12	1.7	0.02	33	0
0.1	0.2	0	139	29	92	36	0.3	0.6	12	0	0.02	0	0.08	0.07	0.7	0.02	5	0
0.1	0.2	0	130	15	124	34	0.2	0.6	7	0	0.04	0	0.08	0.06	0.7	0.01	4	0
3.6	2.3	0	210	141	626	67	0.4	3.2	14	0	0.7	0	0.39	0.27	3.3	0.02	67	0
0.2	0.4	0	23	31	175	33	0.3	0.9	8	0	0.11	0	0.14	0.09	1.3	0.01	28	0
4.8	0.8	32	12	81	12	82	0.5	2.6	14	15	1.08	0	0.34	0.31	3	0.05	34	0.06
2.2	1.6	22	10	29	151	67	0.2	0.7	7	60	0.9	1	0.09	0.1	0.7	0.08	16	0.05
3	1.8	26	11	34	119	79	0.2	0.8	8	14	0.84	1	0.1	0.12	0.9	0.09	7	0.05
0.3	0.3	1	10	31	96	39	0.3	0.7	8	2	0.06	0	0.09	0.08	1.1	0.02	9	0.01
0.9	0.5	14	20	41	127	50	0.2	0.9	7	9	0.25	0	0.12	0.13	1	0.03	13	0.05
0.4	0.3	1	11	38	100	57	0.3	0.8	18	2	0.12	0	0.1	0.08	1.2	0.04	10	0.01
0.4	0.3	2	38	32	144	30	0.2	0.7	7	4	0.02	0	0.12	0.09	1	0.01	9	0.01
0.4	0.3	1	38	32	145	30	0.2	0.7	6	4	0.02	0	0.1	0.09	1	0.01	7	0.01
0.7	0.4	2	27	35	261	100	0.2	0.9	16	6	0.17	0	0.11	0.11	1	0.05	11	0.03
0.5	0.2	0	11	38	135	44	0.3	0.7	13	0	0.15	0	0.09	0.06	0.9	0.08	15	0
0	0.2	0	50	72	324	37	0.2	0.4	7	0	0.02	0	0.08	0.01	0.4	0.02	4	0
0	0.5	0	20	—	230	—	—	1.1	—	0	—	0	0.12	0.07	1.2	—	—	—
3.8	3.5	28	47	54	140	100	0.3	1	15	14	0.88	1	0.12	0.12	0.9	0.12	9	0.05
0.5	0.3	12	21	24	113	26	0.2	0.7	4	5	0.14	0	0.1	0.1	1.1	0.02	24	0.02
2.5	1.5	22	34	32	109	62	0.2	0.7	7	11	0.61	0	0.08	0.09	0.7	0.08	5	0.04
1.2	1	0	69	94	245	94	0.6	1.1	41	0	0.27	1	0.1	0.06	1.1	0.09	6	0
0.1	0.2	1	10	29	53	35	0.2	0.9	5	2	0.08	0	0.12	0.1	1	0.02	13	0.01
0.4	0.2	0	23	44	122	51	0.3	0.9	13	0	0.16	0	0.1	0.09	1.1	0.08	20	0.02
0	0.1	2	18	57	117	40	0.5	0.6	20	0	0.04	0	0.1	0.07	0.9	0.03	14	0
0	0.1	2	18	58	118	40	0.5	0.6	20	0	0.04	0	0.08	0.07	0.9	0.03	12	0
0.5	0.5	0	20	42	122	44	0.3	0.9	10	0	0.19	0	0.15	0.1	1.4	0.02	24	0
0.2	0.5	0	16	39	98	29	0.3	0.9	15	0	0.13	0	0.1	0.06	1	0.03	18	0
0.2	0.5	0	17	36	105	30	0.3	0.9	14	0	0.13	0	0.08	0.05	1	0.02	14	0
0.4	0.4	0	16	32	150	36	0.3	0.7	9	0	0.15	0	0.1	0.06	0.8	0.02	16	0.01
0.2	0.3	0	26	23	89	28	0.2	0.5	6	0	0.09	0	0.08	0.06	0.7	0.01	13	0.02
0.4	0.3	2	38	32	144	30	0.2	0.7	7	4	0.02	0	0.12	0.09	1	0.01	9	0.01
0.1	0.3	0	52	58	322	72	0.5	1.6	16	0	0.02	0	0.36	0.2	2.8	0.02	57	0
0.2	0.5	0	7	81	239	76	0.7	1.4	31	0	0.41	0	0.15	0.04	1.3	0.12	22	0
0.3	0.3	0	30	27	143	30	0.2	0.8	6	0	0.01	0	0.12	0.09	1	0.01	9	0
0	0.2	0	24	35	104	61	0.3	0.8	12	0	0.07	0	0.07	0.08	0.8	0.01	20	0
0.3	0.4	0	22	57	215	67	0.5	0.9	17	0	0.14	0	0.1	0.1	1	0.04	26	0
0.6	0.2	0	16	27	98	57	0.2	0.7	6	0	0.13	0	0.08	0.1	0.9	0.02	22	0
0.6	2.7	0	3	52	69	93	0.3	0.3	14	0	1.32	0	0.05	0.04	0.9	0.08	19	0
0.4	0.5	0	19	48	119	58	0.4	1	22	0	0.22	0	0.18	0.08	1.8	0.07	18	0
0.3	0.2	0	18	31	165	42	0.3	0.7	10	0	0.09	0	0.11	0.08	1	0.02	22	0
0.2	0.2	0	18	18	93	22	0.2	0.7	5	0	0.06	0	0.08	0.06	0.6	0.02	11	0.01
0.3	0.2	0	19	26	152	28	0.2	0.6	7	0	0.07	0	0.13	0.08	1.2	0.01	24	0
0.4	0.3	1	23	44	74	110	0.2	0.9	14	3	0.07	0	0.1	0.08	0.9	0.03	12	0.02
0.3	0.4	0	23	33	138	35	0.4	0.7	13	0	0.28	0	0.09	0.06	0.8	0.02	7	0

Food Item	Qty	Meas	Wgt (g)	Wtr (g)	Cals	Prot	Carb (g)	Fib (g)	Fat (g)	SatF (g)
Bread, sunflower meal	1	piece	27	10	75	3	12	0.5	1	0.5
Bread, sweet potato	1	piece	25	8	72	2	12	0.6	2	0.3
Bread, triticale	1	piece	25	9	63	2	12	1.6	1	0.2
Bread, vienna	1	piece	25	9	68	2	13	0.8	1	0.2
Bread, wheat	1	piece	28	10	74	3	13	1.2	1	0.3
Bread, wheat berry	1	piece	26	10	68	2	12	1.1	1	0.2
Bread, wheat bran	1	piece	36	14	89	3	17	1.4	1	0.3
Bread, wheat, low calorie, thin sliced	1	piece	23	10	46	2	10	2.8	1	0.1
Bread, wheat, toasted	1	piece	25	8	70	2	13	1.3	1	0.2
Bread, white, composite, firm & soft	1	piece	25	9	67	2	12	0.6	1	0.2
Bread, white, firm	1	piece	33	12	91	3	17	0.7	1	0.4
Bread, white, low calorie, thin sliced	1	piece	20	9	41	2	9	1.9	0	0.1
Bread, white, recipe, w/2% milk	1	piece	42	15	120	2	21	0.8	2	0.5
Bread, white, recipe, w/nonfat dry milk	1	piece	44	15	121	3	24	0.9	1	0.2
Bread, white, soft	0.25	cup	8	3	20	1	4	0.2	0	0.1
Bread, white, soft	1	piece	28	10	76	2	14	0.6	1	0.4
Bread, white, very low sodium	1	piece	26	10	69	2	13	0.6	1	0.2
Bread, whole wheat	1	piece	35	13	86	3	16	2.4	1	0.3
Bread, whole wheat, recipe	1	piece	23	8	64	2	12	1.4	1	0.2
Breadfruit, raw	0.5	cup	110	78	113	1	30	5.4	0	0.1
Breath Savers, spearmint breath mints	1	each	2	—	10	0	0	0	1	0
Broccoflower, raw	0.5	cup	50	45	16	1	3	1.6	1	0
Broccoflower, steamed	0.5	cup	78	70	25	2	5	2.5	1	0
Broccoli floweret, raw	5	each	55	50	15	2	3	1.6	0	0
Broccoli pieces, cooked, no added salt	0.5	cup	78	71	22	2	4	2.3	0	0
Broccoli pieces, frozen, cooked, no added salt	0.5	cup	92	83	26	3	5	2.8	0	0
Broccoli pieces, raw	0.5	cup	44	40	12	1	2	1.3	0	0
Broccoli pieces, steamed	0.5	cup	62	56	17	2	3	1.9	0	0
Broccoli pieces, stir fried	0.5	cup	78	71	22	2	4	2.3	0	0
Broccoli spears, cooked, no added salt	1	each	180	163	50	5	9	5.2	1	0.1
Broccoli spears, frozen, cooked	1	piece	30	27	8	1	2	0.9	0	0
Broccoli spears, raw	1	each	151	137	42	4	8	4.5	1	0.1
Broccoli, Chinese, Gai Lan	4	oz.	113	104	34	3	5	—	0	—
Broccoli, batter-dipped, fried	0.5	cup	42	32	61	2	4	1	4	0.7
Broccoli, cooked w/cheese sauce	0.5	cup	114	92	110	6	6	2	7	3.5
Broccoli, stalk only, raw	0.5	cup	44	40	12	1	2	1.4	0	0
Broth, beef, fat free, Health Valley	4	oz.	113	111	14	2	1	0	0	0
Broth, chicken, dry, cube	1	each	5	0	10	1	1	0	0	0.1
Broth, chicken, dry, prepared	0.5	cup	122	118	11	1	1	0	1	0.1
Brownie, mix, low calorie, low sodium, prepared	1	each	22	3	84	1	16	0.8	2	1.1
Brownie, mix, w/nuts, prepared	1	each	33	4	140	1	20	0.9	7	1.4
Brownie, peanut butter fudge, Weight Watchers	1	each	35	8	110	2	21	3	2	0.5
Brownie, w/nuts	1	each	25	3	101	1	16	0.5	4	1.1
Brownie, w/walnuts, homemade	1	each	20	3	93	1	10	0.4	6	1.5
Brussels sprouts, cooked, drained	4	each	84	73	33	2	7	2.2	0	0.1
Brussels sprouts, cooked, drained, cup measure	0.5	cup	78	68	30	2	7	2	0	0.1
Brussels sprouts, frozen, cooked	0.5	cup	78	67	33	3	6	3.2	0	0.1
Brussels sprouts, raw	4	each	76	65	33	3	7	2.9	0	0
Brussels sprouts, raw, cup measure	0.5	cup	44	38	19	1	4	1.7	0	0
Buckwheat groats, roasted/cooked	0.5	cup	99	75	91	3	20	2.7	1	0.1
Bulgur wheat, cooked	0.5	cup	91	71	76	3	17	4.1	0	0
Bun, hamburger	1	each	45	15	129	4	23	1.2	2	0.5
Bun, hamburger/hot dog, low calorie, extra fiber	1	each	43	20	84	4	18	2.7	1	0.1
Bun, hamburger/hot dog, mixed grain	1	each	43	16	113	4	19	1.6	3	0.4
Bun, hotdog/frankfurter	1	each	40	14	114	3	20	1.1	2	0.5
Burger King, BK broiler, chicken sandwich	1	each	248	146	550	30	41	2	29	6
Burger King, Whopper sandwich	1	each	270	157	640	27	45	3	39	11
Burger King, Whopper sandwich, w/cheese	1	each	294	167	730	33	46	3	46	16
Burger King, cheeseburger, double	1	each	213	104	609	42	28	1	36	17.2
Burger King, chicken sandwich	1	each	229	104	710	26	54	2	43	9
Burger King, fish fillet sandwich, Ocean Catch	1	each	255	130	700	26	56	3	41	6
Burger King, whopper Jr. w/cheese	1	each	180	96	468	23	30	2	28	10.2
Burger King, whopper junior sandwich	1	each	168	90	430	22	30	2	25	8.2
Burrito, apple, small	1	each	155	55	484	5	73	—	20	9.6
Burrito, bean & cheese	2	each	186	100	378	15	55	—	12	6.8

MonoF	PolyF	Choles	Calc	Phos	Sod	Pot	Zn	Iron	Magn	VitA	VitE	VitC	Thia	Ribo	Nia	B6	Fola	B12
(g)	(g)	(mg)	(mg)	(mg)	(mg)	(mg)	(mg)	(mg)	(mg)	(µg RE)	(µg α-TE)	(mg)	(mg)	(mg)	(mg)	(mg)	(µg)	(µg)
0.5	0.4	1	17	40	61	34	0.3	0.8	13	3	0.12	0	0.15	0.09	1.2	0.03	10	0.02
0.6	0.4	14	5	28	228	40	0.2	0.8	5	50	0.3	1	0.09	0.1	0.9	0.03	14	0.03
0.2	0.4	0	22	47	136	52	0.4	0.7	17	0	0.06	0	0.07	0.04	0.7	0.02	12	0
0.3	0.2	0	19	26	152	28	0.2	0.6	7	0	0.07	0	0.13	0.08	1.2	0.01	24	0
0.5	0.3	0	30	43	151	57	0.3	0.9	13	0	0.15	0	0.12	0.08	1.2	0.03	22	0
0.4	0.2	0	27	39	138	52	0.3	0.9	12	0	0.14	0	0.11	0.07	1.1	0.02	20	0
0.6	0.2	0	27	67	175	82	0.5	1.1	29	0	0.17	0	0.14	0.1	1.6	0.06	25	0
0.1	0.2	0	18	24	118	28	0.3	0.7	9	0	0.03	0	0.1	0.07	0.9	0.03	16	0
0.5	0.2	0	28	41	144	54	0.3	0.9	12	0	0.15	0	0.09	0.07	1	0.02	16	0
0.4	0.2	0	27	24	135	30	0.2	0.8	6	0	0.1	0	0.12	0.08	1	0.02	24	0.01
0.5	0.2	1	32	34	163	40	0.2	0.9	7	0	0.25	0	0.13	0.08	1.1	0.01	12	0
0.2	0.1	0	19	24	91	15	0.3	0.6	5	0	0.03	0	0.08	0.06	0.7	0.01	19	0.06
0.5	1.2	1	24	48	151	61	0.3	1.2	8	9	0.36	0	0.17	0.16	1.5	0.02	38	0.03
0.2	0.6	0	14	42	148	49	0.3	1.4	7	5	0.17	0	0.19	0.16	1.6	0.02	37	0.01
0.1	0.1	0	6	7	38	8	0	0.2	2	0	0.01	0	0.03	0.02	0.2	0	3	0
0.5	0.2	1	24	28	143	30	0.2	0.8	6	0	0.05	0	0.11	0.07	0.9	0.01	10	0
0.4	0.2	0	28	24	7	31	0.2	0.8	6	0	0.1	0	0.12	0.09	1	0.02	25	0.01
0.6	0.4	0	25	80	184	88	0.7	1.2	30	0	0.3	0	0.12	0.07	1.3	0.06	18	0
0.3	0.7	0	8	43	80	72	0.3	0.7	19	0	0.31	0	0.07	0.05	0.9	0.05	14	0
0	0.1	0	19	33	2	539	0.1	0.6	28	4	1.23	32	0.12	0.03	1	0.11	15	0
0	0	0	—	—	0	0	—	—	—	—	—	—	—	—	—	—	—	—
0	0.1	0	16	32	12	161	0.2	0	10	4	0.15	37	0.04	0.05	0.4	0.1	28	0
0	0.1	0	25	50	18	251	0.4	0.5	16	5	0.23	49	0.06	0.07	0.6	0.14	38	0
0	0.1	0	26	36	15	179	0.2	0.5	14	165	0.91	51	0.04	0.06	0.4	0.09	39	0
0	0.1	0	36	46	20	228	0.3	0.7	19	108	1.32	58	0.04	0.09	0.4	0.11	39	0
0	0.1	0	47	51	22	166	0.3	0.6	18	174	1.52	37	0.05	0.08	0.4	0.12	52	0
0	0.1	0	21	29	12	143	0.2	0.4	11	68	0.73	41	0.03	0.05	0.3	0.07	31	0
0	0.1	0	30	41	17	201	0.2	0.5	16	91	0.3	49	0.04	0.07	0.4	0.09	37	0
0	0.1	0	37	51	21	253	0.3	0.7	20	108	0.37	62	0.05	0.09	0.5	0.12	44	0
0	0.3	0	83	106	47	526	0.7	1.5	43	250	3.04	134	0.1	0.2	1	0.26	90	0
0	0	0	15	16	7	54	0.1	0.2	6	57	0.31	12	0.02	0.02	0.1	0.04	9	0
0	0.3	0	72	100	41	491	0.6	1.3	38	233	2.51	141	0.1	0.18	1	0.24	107	0
—	—	—	—	—	—	—	—	—	—	186	—	32	—	—	—	—	—	0
1.1	2.4	8	34	35	31	121	0.2	0.5	10	51	1.05	27	0.04	0.07	0.4	0.06	22	0.03
2.4	1	15	148	128	365	269	0.7	0.8	24	176	0.76	57	0.06	0.17	0.5	0.13	41	0.18
0	0.1	0	21	29	12	143	0.2	0.4	11	18	0.73	41	0.03	0.05	0.3	0.07	31	0
0	0	0	0	—	76	93	0	—	0	—	0	2	—	—	0.5	—	—	—
0.1	0.1	1	9	9	1152	18	0	0.1	3	4	0.04	0	0.01	0.02	0.2	0	2	0.01
0.2	0.2	0	7	6	742	12	0	0	2	6	0.01	0	0	0.02	0.1	0	1	0.01
1	0.2	0	3	11	21	69	0	0.3	1	0	0.36	0	0.02	0.03	0.2	0	7	0
2	2.8	9	6	26	83	61	0.2	0.6	11	4	0.66	0	0.04	0.05	0.5	0.01	3	0.02
—	—	0	20	—	140	100	—	1.1	—	0	—	0	—	—	—	—	—	—
2.2	0.6	4	7	25	78	37	0.2	0.6	8	2	0.52	0	0.06	0.05	0.4	0.01	5	0.02
2.2	1.9	15	11	26	69	35	0.2	0.4	11	40	0.58	0	0.03	0.04	0.2	0.02	6	0.03
0	0.2	0	30	47	18	266	0.3	1	17	60	0.71	52	0.09	0.07	0.5	0.15	50	0
0	0.2	0	28	44	16	247	0.3	0.9	16	56	0.66	48	0.08	0.06	0.5	0.14	47	0
0	0.2	0	19	42	18	252	0.3	0.6	19	46	0.45	35	0.08	0.09	0.4	0.22	78	0
0	0.1	0	32	52	19	296	0.3	1.1	18	67	0.67	65	0.11	0.07	0.6	0.17	46	0
0	0.1	0	18	30	11	171	0.2	0.6	10	39	0.39	37	0.06	0.04	0.3	0.1	27	0
0.2	0.2	0	7	69	4	87	0.6	0.8	50	0	0.23	0	0.04	0.04	0.9	0.08	14	0
0	0.1	0	9	36	5	62	0.5	0.9	29	0	0.03	0	0.05	0.02	0.9	0.08	16	0
0.4	1.1	0	63	40	252	64	0.3	1.4	9	0	0.7	0	0.22	0.14	1.8	0.02	43	0.03
0.2	0.3	0	25	36	190	34	0.3	1.3	9	0	0.07	0	0.17	0.08	2.1	0.02	41	0.04
0.8	0.4	0	41	52	197	69	0.5	1.7	19	0	0.24	0	0.2	0.13	1.9	0.04	41	0
0.3	1	0	56	35	224	56	0.2	1.3	8	0	0.62	0	0.19	0.12	1.6	0.02	38	0.02
—	—	80	60	—	480	—	—	5.4	—	60	—	6	—	—	—	—	—	—
—	—	90	80	—	870	—	—	4.5	—	100	—	9	0.33	0.41	7	0.35	—	—
—	—	115	250	—	1350	—	—	4.5	—	150	—	9	0.34	0.48	7	0.33	—	—
—	—	137	203	—	1075	—	—	4.6	—	81	—	0	—	—	—	—	—	—
—	—	60	100	—	1400	—	—	3.6	—	0	—	0	—	—	—	—	—	—
—	—	90	60	—	980	—	—	2.7	—	20	—	1	—	—	—	—	—	—
—	—	76	153	—	783	—	—	3.7	—	81	—	5	—	—	—	—	—	—
—	—	62	62	—	543	—	—	3.7	—	41	—	5	—	—	—	—	—	—
7.2	2.2	8	33	31	443	219	0.8	2.2	16	78	—	2	0.36	0.37	3.9	0.16	51	1.07
2.5	1.8	28	214	180	1166	497	1.6	2.3	80	238	—	2	0.22	0.71	3.6	0.24	74	0.89

Food Item	Qty	Meas	Wgt (g)	Wtr (g)	Cals	Prot	Carb (g)	Fib (g)	Fat (g)	SatF (g)
Burrito, black bean, Life Choice	1	each	374	269	410	12	86	13	2	0
Burrito, sausage, Great Starts	1	each	99	52	240	9	24	1	12	4
Butter replacement, dry (Butter Buds)	1	Tbs	5	0	19	0	4	0	0	0
Butter, lightly salted	1	Tbs	14	2	102	0	0	0	12	7.2
Butter, regular, salted	1	Tbs	14	2	100	0	0	0	11	7.1
Butter, regular, salted, pat	1	each	5	1	36	0	0	0	4	2.5
Butter, unsalted	1	Tbs	14	3	102	0	0	0	12	7.2
Butter, whipped	1	Tbs	9	2	68	0	0	0	8	4.8
Butter/vegetable oil blend, Blue Bonnet spread	1	Tbs	14	2	102	0	0	0	12	4
Butterbur (fuki), canned pieces	0.5	cup	62	61	2	0	0	—	0	—
Butterbur (fuki), raw	0.5	cup	47	44	7	0	2	0.6	0	—
Butterbur (fuki), stalks, cooked	3	each	45	44	4	0	1	0.6	0	—
Buttermilk, skim, cultured	1	cup	245	221	99	8	12	0	2	1.3
Butternuts, dried	1	oz.	28	1	174	7	3	1.3	16	0.4
Butterscotch morsels, Toll House	0.25	cup	42	0	243	0	30	0	12	12.3
Cabbage, Chinese, steamed	0.5	cup	85	81	11	1	2	0.8	0	0
Cabbage, Japanese, pickled	0.5	cup	75	69	16	1	3	2.3	0	0
Cabbage, bok choy, cooked, drained	0.5	cup	85	81	10	1	2	1.4	0	0
Cabbage, bok choy, shredded, raw	0.5	cup	35	33	5	1	1	0.4	0	0
Cabbage, head, cooked, no added salt, drained	1	each	1262	1181	278	13	56	29	5	0.7
Cabbage, head, raw	1	each	908	837	227	13	49	20.9	2	0.3
Cabbage, kim chee style	0.5	cup	75	69	16	1	3	0.9	0	0
Cabbage, mustard, salted	0.5	cup	64	59	13	1	3	2	0	0
Cabbage, pe tsai, chopped, raw	0.5	cup	38	36	6	0	1	1.2	0	0
Cabbage, pe tsai, cooked, drained	0.5	cup	60	57	8	1	1	1.6	0	0
Cabbage, raw, fresh harvest	0.5	cup	35	32	8	0	2	0.8	0	0
Cabbage, red, cooked, drained	0.5	cup	75	70	16	1	3	1.5	0	0
Cabbage, red, pickled	0.5	cup	75	45	110	0	29	0.6	0	0
Cabbage, red, raw	0.5	cup	35	32	9	0	2	0.7	0	0
Cabbage, red, sweet & sour	0.5	cup	75	45	110	0	29	0.6	0	0
Cabbage, savoy, cooked, drained	0.5	cup	72	67	17	1	4	2	0	0
Cabbage, savoy, raw	0.5	cup	35	32	9	1	2	1.1	0	0
Cabbage, shredded, cooked, no added salt, drained	0.5	cup	75	70	16	1	3	1.7	0	0
Cabbage, shredded, raw	0.5	cup	35	32	9	1	2	0.8	0	0
Cactus pad/nopales, cooked	1	each	29	25	12	1	3	1	0	0
Cactus/nopales, raw	0.5	cup	59	52	24	0	6	2.1	0	0.1
Cake, German chocolate, mix, prepared, w/frosting	1	piece	111	30	404	4	55	1.5	21	5.3
Cake, angel food	1	piece	53	18	137	3	31	0.8	0	0.1
Cake, apple spice crumb, fat free, Entenmann's	1	piece	50	—	130	2	30	2	0	0
Cake, applesauce w/nuts & icing	1	piece	108	21	399	3	70	1.5	13	3.2
Cake, applesauce, no icing	1	piece	87	19	313	3	52	1.7	11	2.9
Cake, apricot, no icing	1	piece	87	19	313	3	52	1.7	11	2.9
Cake, banana loaf, fat free, Entenmann's	1	piece	57	—	150	2	34	1	0	0
Cake, banana w/icing	1	piece	108	37	309	3	58	1.1	8	1.6
Cake, banana, no icing	1	piece	87	32	245	3	43	1.1	7	1.6
Cake, blackberry, no icing	1	piece	87	19	313	3	52	1.7	11	2.9
Cake, carrot w/cream cheese frosting, recipe	1	piece	112	23	488	5	53	1.3	30	5.5
Cake, carrot, mix, prepared, no frosting	1	piece	70	22	239	4	33	1.4	11	1.8
Cake, cherry fudge, w/chocolate frosting	1	piece	71	33	187	2	27	0.9	9	3.6
Cake, chocolate crunch, fat free, Entenmann's	1	piece	50	—	130	2	32	2	0	0
Cake, chocolate w/fluffy white icing	1	piece	91	30	262	4	48	1	8	1.8
Cake, chocolate, mix, prepared	1	piece	65	21	198	4	32	1.4	8	1.8
Cake, chocolate, mix, pudding type, prepared	1	piece	77	23	270	4	34	1.5	14	3
Cake, chocolate, recipe, no frosting	1	piece	95	23	340	5	51	1.5	14	5.2
Cake, chocolate, w/chocolate icing-commercial	1	piece	69	16	253	3	38	1.9	11	3.3
Cake, chocolate, w/cream cheese icing	1	piece	103	26	355	4	57	1	14	3.7
Cake, chocolate, w/vanilla icing	1	piece	103	26	358	4	58	1	14	3.6
Cake, coffee, cheese	1	piece	76	24	258	5	34	0.8	12	4.1
Cake, coffee, cheese, Entenmann's	1	piece	54	17	190	4	24	0	8	3.5
Cake, coffee, cinnamon, w/crumb topping	1	piece	63	14	263	4	29	1.3	15	3.6
Cake, coffee, cinnamon, w/crumb topping, recipe	1	piece	60	13	240	4	30	0.9	12	2.2
Cake, coffee, creme filled, w/chocolate frosting	1	piece	90	26	298	4	48	1.8	10	2.6
Cake, coffee, fruit	1	piece	50	16	156	3	26	1.2	5	1.2
Cake, coffee, mix, prepared	1	piece	72	22	229	4	38	0.9	7	1.3
Cake, date pudding	1	piece	42	14	131	2	19	0.9	6	3

MonoF	PolyF	Choles	Calc	Phos	Sod	Pot	Zn	Iron	Magn	VitA	VitE	VitC	Thia	Ribo	Nia	B6	Fola	B12
(g)	(g)	(mg)	(mg)	(mg)	(mg)	(mg)	(mg)	(mg)	(mg)	(μg RE)	(μg α-TE)	(mg)	(mg)	(mg)	(mg)	(mg)	(μg)	(μg)
—	—	0	150	—	570	—	—	3.6	—	20	—	9	—	—	—	—	—	—
—	—	90	60	—	500	—	—	1.4	—	20	—	1	—	—	—	—	—	—
0	0	0	1	0	60	0	0	0.1	0	0	0	0	0	0	0	0	0	0
3.5	0.4	31	3	3	106	4	0	0	0	107	0.22	0	0	0	0	0	0	0.02
3.4	0.4	31	3	3	116	4	0	0	0	106	0.22	0	0	0	0	0	0	0.02
1.2	0.2	11	1	1	41	1	0	0	0	38	0.08	0	0	0	0	0	0	0.01
3.3	0.4	31	3	3	2	4	0	0	0	107	0.22	0	0	0	0	0	0	0.02
2.2	0.3	21	2	2	78	2	0	0	0	71	0.15	0	0	0	0	0	0	0.01
4.7	2.3	12	4	3	127	5	0	0	0	113	1.08	0	0	0	0	0	0	0.01
—	—	0	21	2	2	7	0	0.4	1	0	—	7	0	0	0.1	0.02	2	0
—	—	0	48	6	3	308	0.1	0	7	2	—	15	0.01	0.01	0.1	0.04	5	0
—	—	0	27	3	2	159	0	0	4	1	—	9	0	0	0	0.02	2	0
0.6	0.1	9	284	219	257	370	1	0.1	27	20	0.15	2	0.08	0.38	0.1	0.08	12	0.54
3	12.1	0	15	126	0	119	0.9	1.1	67	3	0.99	1	0.11	0.04	0.3	0.16	19	0
0	0	0	0	—	46	79	—	0	—	0	—	0	0.03	0.04	0	—	—	—
0	0.1	0	89	31	55	213	0.2	0.7	16	8	0.1	3	0.03	0.06	0.4	0.15	47	0
0	0	0	36	32	208	640	0.2	0.4	9	14	0.09	1	0	0.03	0.1	0.08	32	0
0	0.1	0	79	25	29	315	0.1	0.9	9	218	0.1	22	0.03	0.05	0.4	0.14	34	0
0	0	0	37	13	23	88	0.1	0.3	7	105	0.04	16	0.01	0.02	0.2	0.07	23	0
0.4	2.5	0	391	189	101	1224	1.1	2.2	101	164	1.33	254	0.72	0.69	3.6	1.43	252	0
0.2	1.1	0	427	209	163	2233	1.6	5.4	136	118	0.95	292	0.45	0.36	2.7	0.87	390	0
0	0.1	0	73	30	498	188	0.2	0.6	14	213	0.12	40	0.04	0.05	0.4	0.17	44	0
0	0	0	43	17	459	157	0.2	0.4	10	62	0.01	0	0.03	0.06	0.5	0.19	46	0
0	0	0	29	11	3	90	0.1	0.1	5	46	0.05	10	0.02	0.02	0.2	0.09	30	0
0	0	0	19	23	5	134	0.1	0.2	6	58	0.07	9	0.03	0.03	0.3	0.1	32	0
0	0	0	16	8	6	86	0.1	0.2	5	5	0.04	18	0.02	0.01	0.1	0.03	20	0
0	0.1	0	28	22	6	105	0.1	0.3	8	2	0.09	26	0.03	0.02	0.2	0.1	9	0
0	0	0	36	16	14	153	0.1	0.6	13	1	0.03	9	0.01	0.01	0.1	0.06	4	0
0	0	0	18	15	4	72	0.1	0.2	5	1	0.04	20	0.02	0.01	0.1	0.07	7	0
0	0	0	36	16	14	153	0.1	0.6	13	1	0.03	9	0.01	0.01	0.1	0.06	4	0
0	0	0	22	24	17	133	0.2	0.3	17	64	0.08	12	0.04	0.02	0	0.11	34	0
0	0	0	12	15	10	80	0.1	0.1	10	35	0.04	11	0.02	0.01	0.1	0.07	28	0
0	0.1	0	23	11	6	73	0.1	0.1	6	10	0.08	15	0.04	0.04	0.2	0.08	15	0
0	0	0	16	8	6	86	0.1	0.2	5	5	0.04	11	0.02	0.01	0.1	0.03	15	0
0	0.1	0	15	7	68	57	0	0.1	24	1	0	3	0	0.02	0.1	0.02	1	0
0.1	0.1	0	33	14	3	130	0.1	0.2	50	3	0.01	8	0.01	0.04	0.3	0.04	4	0
8.7	5.5	53	53	173	369	151	0.5	1.2	19	23	1.18	0	0.11	0.14	1.1	0.02	4	0.1
0	0.2	0	74	17	397	49	0	0.3	6	0	0.05	0	0.05	0.26	0.5	0.02	19	0.03
0	0	0	0	—	140	65	—	0	—	20	—	0	—	—	—	—	—	—
5.7	3.6	21	20	45	293	137	0.2	1.3	10	49	1.5	1	0.12	0.12	1	0.05	5	0.05
4.9	2.9	22	17	46	285	145	0.2	1.4	11	10	1.15	1	0.14	0.13	1.1	0.06	6	0.04
4.9	2.9	22	17	46	285	145	0.2	1.4	11	10	1.15	1	0.14	0.13	1.1	0.06	6	0.04
0	0	0	20	—	190	140	—	0	—	0	—	0	—	—	—	—	—	—
3.2	2.3	31	28	48	292	198	0.3	1	17	105	1.36	4	0.13	0.18	1.1	0.25	12	0.08
3.1	2.2	29	26	46	257	186	0.3	1	16	100	1.3	3	0.12	0.16	1	0.24	12	0.07
4.9	2.9	22	17	46	285	145	0.2	1.4	11	10	1.15	1	0.14	0.13	1.1	0.06	6	0.04
7.3	15.2	60	28	80	276	125	0.5	1.4	20	430	4.73	1	0.15	0.18	1.1	0.08	13	0.11
3.4	5	51	77	123	249	84	0.2	0.9	5	173	2.94	2	0.09	0.12	0.8	0.06	8	0.81
3.1	1.7	30	34	75	160	118	0.2	0.8	14	72	0.85	10	0.02	0.14	0.5	0.04	7	0.15
0	0	0	0	—	170	200	—	1.1	—	0	—	0	—	—	—	—	—	—
3.1	2.3	35	71	133	411	173	0.5	2.1	22	16	—	0	0.06	0.11	0.8	0.02	8	0.07
3.1	2.3	35	70	132	370	153	0.4	2.1	22	16	1.14	0	0.06	0.1	0.6	0.02	7	0.06
4.7	5.9	53	64	146	402	161	0.5	1.4	19	24	1.37	0	0.08	0.13	0.9	0.03	8	0.32
5.7	2.6	55	57	101	299	133	0.7	1.5	30	38	1.51	0	0.13	0.2	1.1	0.04	26	0.15
6	1.3	29	30	84	230	138	0.5	1.5	24	17	1.17	0	0.02	0.09	0.4	0.03	12	0.1
6.5	3.2	35	71	133	460	167	0.4	2.2	22	60	—	0	0.06	0.1	0.6	0.02	7	0.06
6.4	3.2	35	71	147	404	168	0.4	2.1	22	102	—	0	0.06	0.1	0.6	0.02	7	0.06
5.4	1.2	65	45	77	258	220	0.4	0.5	11	66	1.19	0	0.08	0.1	0.5	0.04	30	0.26
—	—	30	40	—	160	55	—	0	—	20	—	0	—	—	—	—	—	—
8.2	2	20	34	68	221	78	0.5	1.2	14	21	2.15	0	0.13	0.14	1.1	0.02	38	0.11
4.6	4.6	36	67	83	233	143	0.5	1.3	24	99	1.5	0	0.11	0.12	0.7	0.06	9	0.09
5.1	1.3	62	34	68	291	70	0.4	0.5	14	33	1.62	0	0.07	0.07	0.8	0.04	37	0.18
2.8	0.7	4	22	59	193	45	0.3	1.2	8	10	0.43	0	0.02	0.1	1.3	0.02	24	0.01
2.8	2.3	35	98	155	303	81	0.3	1	13	29	1.2	0	0.12	0.13	1.1	0.04	49	0.1
1.9	0.3	16	40	35	56	196	0.2	0.8	23	8	0.26	0	0.04	0.06	0.4	0.08	3	0.05

Food Item	Qty	Meas	Wgt (g)	Wtr (g)	Cals	Prot	Carb (g)	Fib (g)	Fat (g)	SatF (g)
Cake, fruit, recipe	1	piece	43	8	155	2	28	1.6	5	0.6
Cake, funnel, 6 inch diameter	1	each	90	37	285	7	29	0.9	15	3.9
Cake, gingerbread, mix, prepared	1	piece	63	21	195	3	32	0.7	6	1.6
Cake, gingerbread, recipe	1	piece	110	31	392	4	54	0.9	18	4.5
Cake, golden loaf, fat free, Entenmann's	1	piece	48	—	120	2	28	0.5	0	0
Cake, graham cracker	1	piece	45	13	156	3	22	0.4	7	1.7
Cake, ice cream roll, chocolate	1	each	340	134	1015	14	136	3.5	50	22
Cake, lemon, w/icing, 2-layer	1	piece	109	23	388	3	70	0.5	11	2.6
Cake, marble w/chocolate icing	1	piece	111	28	404	3	59	0.9	19	4.4
Cake, marble, mix, pudding type, dry	1	oz.	28	1	118	1	22	0.8	3	0.7
Cake, mix, Angel Food, prepared	1	piece	53	5	192	5	43	0	0	0
Cake, mix, Devil's Food, prep w/oil & egg	1	piece	44	6	210	3	25	0	10	3
Cake, oatmeal w/icing	1	piece	110	21	410	3	70	1.5	14	3.4
Cake, pineapple upside-down cake, recipe	1	piece	115	37	367	4	58	0.9	14	3.4
Cake, plum pudding	1	piece	42	14	131	2	19	0.9	6	3
Cake, poppyseed, no icing	1	piece	90	21	354	7	43	1	18	6.5
Cake, pound, commercial, not w/butter	1	piece	30	7	117	2	16	0.3	5	1.4
Cake, pound, old fashion, w/butter	1	piece	53	11	229	3	25	0.4	13	7.6
Cake, raisin loaf, fat free, Entenmann's	1	piece	53	—	140	2	33	1	0	0
Cake, rhubarb, no icing	1	piece	87	19	313	3	52	1.7	11	2.9
Cake, shortcake, biscuit type, recipe	1	each	65	18	225	4	32	0.8	9	2.5
Cake, snack, chocolate, creme filled, w/icing	1	each	28	6	107	1	17	0.2	4	0.8
Cake, snack, cream filled, Twinkie	1	each	42	8	153	1	27	0.2	5	1.1
Cake, spice, w/icing	1	piece	109	27	374	4	65	1	11	3.8
Cake, sponge, chocolate, no icing	1	piece	66	20	195	5	36	1	4	1.4
Cake, sponge, recipe	1	piece	63	18	187	5	36	0.4	3	0.8
Cake, white, mix, low sodium, prepared	1	piece	38	10	118	1	23	0.2	2	0.4
Cake, white, mix, prepared, pkg	1	each	739	228	2261	30	409	4.9	57	8.6
Cake, white, mix, pudding type, prepared	1	each	826	235	2915	30	427	3.7	122	23.1
Cake, white, no yolk, chocolate icing	1	piece	109	22	397	3	70	1.2	12	5.7
Cake, white, w/coconut frosting, recipe	1	piece	70	14	249	3	44	0.7	7	2.7
Cake, white, w/white frosting	1	piece	71	14	266	2	45	0.7	10	4.3
Cake, yellow, mix, prepared	1	piece	69	21	221	3	38	0.6	6	1.1
Cake, yellow, w/chocolate frosting, commercial	1	piece	69	15	262	3	38	1.2	12	3.2
Cake, yellow, w/vanilla frosting	1	piece	121	27	451	4	71	0.4	18	2.9
Candy, milk chocolate-covered peanuts	0.25	cup	42	1	221	6	21	2	14	6.2
Candy, 3 Musketeers bar	1	each	60	4	251	2	46	1	8	3.9
Candy, 3 Musketeers bar, snack size	1	each	18	1	75	1	14	0.3	2	1.2
Candy, 5th Avenue bar	1	each	56	1	276	5	37	1.2	12	4.4
Candy, Almond Joy bar	1	each	49	5	229	2	29	2.4	13	8.5
Candy, Alpine White bar, w/almonds	1	each	35	0	193	3	18	1.9	13	7
Candy, Baby Ruth bar	1	each	60	3	289	4	39	1.7	13	7.1
Candy, Bar None bar	1	each	42	2	219	3	22	1.4	14	9.2
Candy, Bit-o-Honey chews	6	piece	48	3	186	1	39	—	4	—
Candy, Butterfinger bar	1	each	61	1	293	8	40	1.5	11	6.3
Candy, Butterfinger bar, snack size	1	each	21	0	101	3	14	0.5	4	2.2
Candy, Caramello bar	1	each	45	3	213	3	28	0.7	10	6.3
Candy, Chunky bar, small	1	each	35	1	173	3	20	1.7	10	8.1
Candy, Crisped Rice bar, almond	1	each	28	2	130	2	18	1	6	1.1
Candy, Crisped Rice bar, chocolate chip	1	each	28	2	115	1	21	0.6	4	1.5
Candy, Demet's Turtles	10	piece	170	10	825	11	99	4.4	47	18.4
Candy, English toffee bar, Skor	1	each	39	1	217	2	22	0.6	13	8.5
Candy, Golden Almond Solitaires	1	each	85	2	484	10	40	3.7	32	12.9
Candy, Golden Almond bar	1	each	85	2	488	10	39	4.1	32	13.9
Candy, Golden III bar	1	each	91	3	471	6	51	5.2	30	—
Candy, Kit Kat bar	1	each	42	1	216	3	27	0.8	11	6.8
Candy, Krackel bar	1	each	41	1	218	3	25	0.9	12	7.4
Candy, M&M's, peanut, pieces	10	piece	20	0	103	2	12	0.7	5	2.1
Candy, M&M's, plain, pieces	10	piece	7	0	34	0	5	0.2	1	0.9
Candy, Mars almond bar	1	each	50	2	234	4	31	1	12	3.6
Candy, Milky Way bar	1	each	61	4	258	3	44	1	10	4.8
Candy, Milky Way bar, snack size	1	each	18	1	76	1	13	0.3	3	1.4
Candy, Mounds bar	1	each	53	6	253	2	31	3.1	13	10.8
Candy, Mr. Goodbar bar	1	each	49	0	267	5	25	1.7	17	7.3
Candy, Nestle 100 Grand bar	1	each	42	2	198	2	30	0.6	8	4.8

MonoF (g)	PolyF (g)	Choles (mg)	Calc (mg)	Phos (mg)	Sod (mg)	Pot (mg)	Zn (mg)	Iron (mg)	Magn (mg)	VitA (µg RE)	VitE (µg α-TE)	VitC (mg)	Thia (mg)	Ribo (mg)	Nia (mg)	B6 (mg)	Fola (µg)	B12 (µg)
2	2	12	28	34	62	133	0.3	0.8	15	6	1.08	2	0.07	0.05	0.5	0.04	4	0.02
4.5	5.9	66	115	128	236	153	0.6	1.8	18	46	1	0	0.24	0.32	1.9	0.05	14	0.24
3.6	0.8	22	44	106	289	152	0.3	2.1	10	10	0.86	0	0.12	0.12	1	0.02	6	0.04
7.8	4.6	35	78	59	360	483	0.4	3.2	77	15	2.64	0	0.21	0.18	1.9	0.21	36	0.07
0	0	0	0	—	160	75	—	0	—	20	—	0	—	—	—	—	—	—
3	1.8	34	44	52	176	78	0.3	0.7	8	80	1.12	0	0.04	0.14	0.6	0.02	5	0.09
18.4	7	156	431	380	688	569	2.4	4.7	90	215	2.47	1	0.4	0.71	3	0.14	23	0.79
5.2	2.7	33	70	136	248	55	0.2	0.9	6	79	2.09	1	0.1	0.12	0.8	0.02	6	0.07
7.4	6.2	53	43	172	311	143	0.4	1.4	18	99	—	0	0.07	0.12	0.7	0.03	7	0.1
1.4	1.1	0	22	78	147	35	0.1	0.5	5	0	0.51	0	0.05	0.04	0.4	0.01	10	0
0	0	0	24	—	320	56	—	0	—	0	—	0	0	0	0	—	—	—
3	3.5	25	20	—	270	170	—	1.1	—	0	—	0	0.09	0.1	0.4	—	—	—
6.1	3.8	20	20	56	257	135	0.3	1.8	14	57	1.56	1	0.15	0.11	1.1	0.05	5	0.05
6	3.8	25	138	94	367	129	0.4	1.7	15	75	1.54	1	0.18	0.18	1.4	0.04	30	0.09
1.9	0.3	16	40	35	56	196	0.2	0.8	23	8	0.26	0	0.04	0.06	0.4	0.08	3	0.05
4.6	5.3	79	107	122	251	138	0.7	1.7	20	94	1.03	1	0.25	0.29	1.7	0.05	16	0.18
3	0.7	17	19	40	120	32	0.1	0.5	4	10	0.72	0	0.04	0.08	0.4	0.01	11	0.04
3.9	0.7	92	13	44	153	37	0.3	0.9	5	134	0.4	0	0.1	0.14	0.8	0.02	8	0.13
0	0	0	20	—	150	120	—	0	—	20	—	0	—	—	—	—	—	—
4.9	2.9	22	17	46	285	145	0.2	1.4	11	10	1.15	1	0.14	0.13	1.1	0.06	6	0.04
4	2.4	2	133	93	329	69	0.3	1.6	10	12	1.3	0	0.2	0.18	1.7	0.02	6	0.05
1.6	1.5	5	21	26	121	35	0.1	1	12	1	0.96	0	0.06	0.08	0.7	0.01	8	0.02
1.7	1.4	7	19	78	153	36	0.1	0.5	3	2	0.85	0	0.06	0.06	0.5	0.01	12	0.05
5.1	1.4	48	77	201	271	150	0.4	1.6	15	40	2.2	0	0.13	0.18	1.1	0.04	9	0.11
1.5	0.5	141	22	89	115	98	0.6	1.6	20	63	0.7	1	0.09	0.21	0.7	0.05	14	0.26
1	0.4	107	26	63	144	89	0.4	1	6	48	0.32	0	0.1	0.19	0.8	0.04	25	0.23
1	0.9	0	8	87	83	50	0.1	0.6	3	0	0.39	0	0.07	0.07	0.6	0	2	0.01
23.8	21.4	0	1019	1780	3591	702	2.5	7.3	66	1	9.53	1	0.99	1.19	5.2	0.13	37	0.66
45.4	48.9	0	421	1470	3650	504	1.4	7.2	58	0	14.1	1	1.18	1.25	11.6	0.11	33	0.58
3.9	1.9	20	84	144	336	78	0.2	0.7	6	64	1.06	0	0.08	0.1	0.4	0.01	3	0.07
2.6	1.5	1	63	49	199	69	0.2	0.8	8	8	0.5	0	0.09	0.13	0.7	0.02	15	0.04
3.8	1	6	34	46	166	41	0.1	0.6	4	23	1.28	0	0.07	0.09	0.6	0.01	4	0.04
2.7	2.2	40	70	165	327	50	0.2	0.9	6	17	1.07	0	0.08	0.13	0.8	0.05	6	0.13
6.6	1.5	38	26	111	233	123	0.4	1.4	21	23	1.57	0	0.08	0.11	0.9	0.02	15	0.12
7.4	6.2	67	75	173	416	64	0.3	1.3	7	23	2.3	0	0.12	0.08	0.6	0.03	33	0.18
5.5	1.8	4	44	90	17	213	0.8	0.6	40	0	1.08	0	0.05	0.07	1.8	0.09	3	0.12
2.6	0.3	7	51	55	117	80	0.3	0.4	18	14	0.38	0	0.02	0.08	0.1	0.01	0	0.1
0.8	0.1	2	15	16	35	24	0.1	0.1	5	4	0.11	0	0.01	0.02	0	0	0	0.03
5.6	1.9	3	41	86	92	166	0.7	0.7	36	8	1.29	0	0.08	0.07	1.9	0.05	21	0.07
3.2	0.7	2	30	69	72	121	0.4	0.7	32	2	1.1	0	0.02	0.07	0.2	0.03	—	0.06
5	0.9	4	81	82	26	146	0.4	0.2	13	9	1.33	0	0.03	0.15	0.3	0.03	5	0.3
3.7	1.9	2	25	91	136	238	0.8	0.1	48	0	1.13	0	0.06	0.06	1.7	0.04	19	0.03
3.3	0.9	7	61	84	44	164	0.5	0.5	30	10	0.63	0	0.02	0.11	0.7	0.03	12	0.18
—	—	0	27	32	124	60	0.2	0.1	10	0	—	0	0	0.12	0	0.01	2	0
3.4	1.7	1	16	80	121	232	0.7	0.5	48	0	0.99	0	0.05	0.04	1.5	0.04	16	0.01
1.2	0.6	0	6	28	42	80	0.2	0.2	17	0	0.34	0	0.02	0.02	0.5	0.01	6	0
3.2	0.3	12	83	72	62	153	0.4	0.3	19	35	0.76	0	0.02	0.18	0.5	0.02	—	0.28
0.1	1.5	4	50	73	19	187	0.6	0.4	26	4	0.52	0	0.03	0.14	0.7	0.04	8	0.13
2.1	2.2	0	21	47	66	65	1.5	1.8	20	75	—	3	0.37	0.42	5	0.5	0	0
1.1	1	0	6	38	79	48	0.2	1.8	14	50	0.03	0	0.15	0.17	2	0.2	40	0
18.9	7.9	37	269	335	160	524	2.4	2.3	89	58	—	1	0.26	0.41	0.6	0.09	17	0.68
4.3	0.5	20	51	58	108	93	0.3	0.2	13	27	0.53	0	0.01	0.13	0	0.01	—	0.11
15	3.6	11	160	255	48	428	1.6	2	100	8	1.93	0	0.05	0.42	0.9	0.04	—	0.4
15	3.3	13	190	230	57	400	1.4	1.5	94	32	0.51	0	0.05	0.45	0.9	0.04	—	0.37
—	—	17	275	200	79	413	1	0.5	61	20	1.18	1	0.06	0.26	0.1	0.1	11	0.41
3.1	0.3	3	69	100	32	122	0.5	0.4	16	20	0.34	0	0.07	0.23	1.1	0.05	60	0.07
3.9	0.4	8	72	91	57	140	0.5	0.4	23	5	0.53	0	0.02	0.12	0.2	0.01	—	0.24
2.2	0.8	2	20	46	10	69	0.5	0.2	15	5	0.49	0	0.02	0.03	0.8	0.02	7	0.04
0.5	0	1	7	10	4	19	0.1	0.1	3	4	0.06	0	0	0.02	0	0	0	0.02
5.4	2	8	84	117	85	163	0.6	0.6	36	25	2.33	0	0.02	0.16	0.5	0.03	10	0.18
3.7	0.4	9	79	88	146	147	0.4	0.5	21	20	0.4	1	0.02	0.14	0.2	0.03	6	0.2
1.1	0.1	3	23	26	43	43	0.1	0.1	6	6	0.12	0	0.01	0.04	0.1	0.01	2	0.06
2.3	0.3	1	8	48	79	131	0.5	1.1	30	1	0.36	0	0.02	0.03	0.2	0.05	2	0
5.7	2.4	4	53	122	73	219	0.9	0.6	42	18	1.34	0	0.08	0.12	1.6	0.04	19	0.15
2.5	0.3	8	48	57	88	96	0.4	0.1	16	10	0.31	0	0.12	0.18	1.4	0.14	30	0.11

Food Item	Qty	Meas	Wgt (g)	Wtr (g)	Cals	Prot	Carb (g)	Fib (g)	Fat (g)	SatF (g)
Candy, Nestle Crunch bar	1	each	40	0	209	2	26	1	10	6.1
Candy, Nestle Crunch bar, snack size	1	each	10	0	52	1	7	0.3	3	1.5
Candy, Oh Henry! bar	1	each	57	3	246	6	37	2	10	3.8
Candy, Planter's peanut bar	1.5	oz.	43	1	222	7	20	1.4	14	1.8
Candy, Reese's Pieces	10	piece	8	0	39	1	5	0.2	2	1.4
Candy, Reese's peanut butter cups	2	each	45	1	243	5	25	1.4	14	5
Candy, Rolo chocolate-covered caramels	10	piece	55	11	225	3	29	0.4	11	6.7
Candy, Skittles, bite size	10	piece	11	0	45	0	10	0	0	0.1
Candy, Snickers bar, 2.2 oz	1	each	59	3	281	5	35	1.5	14	5.3
Candy, Special Dark Sweet bar	1	each	41	0	226	2	25	2	13	8.3
Candy, Starburst fruit chews	6	piece	59	4	232	0	50	0	5	0.7
Candy, Symphony bar	1	each	42	0	232	3	24	0.8	14	—
Candy, Twix Cookie bar, caramel	1	each	57	2	283	3	37	0.6	14	5
Candy, Twix Cookie bar, peanut butter	1	each	48	1	257	5	26	1.6	16	5.5
Candy, Whatchamacallit bar	1	each	48	5	214	4	29	1	9	4.5
Candy, Y&S Nibs, cherry	1	oz.	28	0	106	1	26	0	1	—
Candy, York Peppermint Patty	1	each	42	4	165	1	34	0.8	3	1.8
Candy, almonds, chocolate-coated	0.25	cup	41	1	234	5	16	3.5	18	3
Candy, butterscotch	5	piece	30	0	119	0	29	0	1	0.3
Candy, caramel, plain or chocolate	5	piece	40	3	153	2	31	0.5	3	2.6
Candy, carob bar	1	each	87	1	470	7	49	3.3	27	25.2
Candy, cherries, chocolate-covered	2	each	28	2	102	1	22	0.3	3	1.5
Candy, chewing gum	1	piece	4	0	14	0	4	0	0	0
Candy, chewing gum, uncoated, sugarless	1	piece	4	0	11	0	4	0	0	0
Candy, chocolate Kisses	6	piece	28	0	145	2	17	0.8	9	5.2
Candy, chocolate, sweet	1	each	41	0	207	2	24	2.3	14	8.2
Candy, chocolate-covered mint patty	1	each	11	1	40	0	9	0.2	1	0.6
Candy, divinity, no nuts	1	piece	20	2	70	0	18	0	0	0
Candy, fondant/candy corn	1	cup	200	14	716	0	186	0	0	0
Candy, fudge, brown sugar w/nuts, recipe	1	piece	14	1	55	0	11	0.1	1	0.2
Candy, fudge, chocolate marshmallow, recipe	1	piece	20	2	84	0	14	0	3	2
Candy, fudge, chocolate w/nuts, recipe	1	piece	19	1	81	1	14	0.2	3	1.1
Candy, fudge, chocolate, recipe	1	piece	17	2	65	0	14	0.1	1	0.9
Candy, fudge, peanut butter, recipe	1	piece	16	2	59	1	12	0.1	1	0.2
Candy, fudge, vanilla, recipe	1	piece	16	2	59	0	13	0	1	0.5
Candy, gumdrops	10	piece	35	0	135	0	35	0	0	0
Candy, gummy bears	10	each	35	0	135	0	35	0	0	0
Candy, hard, all flavor	1	oz.	28	0	112	0	28	0	0	0
Candy, hard, dietetic	1	piece	3	0	11	0	3	0	0	0
Candy, jellybeans	10	piece	11	1	40	0	10	0	0	0
Candy, licorice	1	oz.	28	1	120	0	24	0	3	3.1
Candy, lollipop	1	each	6	0	24	0	6	0	0	0
Candy, malted milk balls, Whoppers	10	each	29	1	144	2	18	0.8	8	4.6
Candy, milk chocolate bar	1	each	44	1	226	3	26	1.5	14	8.1
Candy, milk chocolate bar w/almonds	1	each	41	1	216	4	22	2.5	14	7
Candy, milk chocolate w/peanuts	1	each	43	1	238	7	17	2.4	18	5.2
Candy, milk chocolate w/rice cereal	1	each	40	1	198	3	25	1.2	11	6.4
Candy, milk chocolate-covered peanuts, Goobers	10	piece	10	0	51	1	5	0.6	3	1.2
Candy, milk chocolate-covered raisins	0.25	cup	48	5	185	2	32	2	7	4.2
Candy, peanut brittle, recipe	0.25	cup	37	1	166	3	26	0.7	7	1.8
Candy, praline, recipe	1	piece	39	4	177	1	24	1	9	0.7
Candy, sesame crunch	20	piece	35	1	181	4	18	2.8	12	1.6
Candy, sugar-coated almonds, Jordan	7	each	28	1	129	2	20	1.3	5	0.4
Candy, taffy, recipe	1	piece	15	1	56	0	14	0	0	0.3
Candy, toffee, Almond Roca	1	piece	11	1	48	1	7	0.3	2	1.1
Candy, toffee, recipe	4	piece	48	1	260	1	31	0	16	9.8
Candy, tootsie roll, bite size	7	each	35	3	126	1	31	0.2	1	0.2
Candy, yogurt-covered peanuts	0.25	cup	42	2	193	4	16	1.8	13	2.5
Candy, yogurt-covered raisins	0.25	cup	48	4	190	2	34	1.5	6	3.6
Candy, truffle, recipe	1	piece	12	2	59	1	5	0.3	4	2.1
Capers	1	tsp	5	4	0	0	0	0.2	0	—
Carambola, raw (starfruit)	1	each	127	115	42	1	10	3.4	0	0
Carissa, raw (natal plum)	1	each	20	17	12	0	3	—	0	—
Carob chips, unsweetened	0.25	cup	42	—	201	6	23	0	9	8.4
Carob flavor mix, prepared w/milk	1	cup	256	215	195	8	22	1	8	5.1

MonoF (g)	PolyF (g)	Choles (mg)	Calc (mg)	Phos (mg)	Sod (mg)	Pot (mg)	Zn (mg)	Iron (mg)	Magn (mg)	VitA (µg RE)	VitE (µg α-TE)	VitC (mg)	Thia (mg)	Ribo (mg)	Nia (mg)	B6 (mg)	Fola (µg)	B12 (µg)
3.4	0.3	5	68	81	53	138	0.6	0.2	23	8	0.44	0	0.14	0.22	1.6	0.16	32	0.15
0.9	0.1	1	17	20	13	34	0.1	0	6	2	0.11	0	0.03	0.06	0.4	0.04	8	0.04
3.8	1.6	5	62	94	135	185	0.7	0.3	35	5	1.08	0	0.01	0.09	1.6	0.04	17	0.12
7.1	4.5	3	33	65	102	173	0.6	0.4	32	22	0.41	0	0.04	0.06	3.4	0.04	26	0.01
0.2	0.1	0	7	11	12	18	0.1	0.1	4	0	0.17	0	0.01	0.01	0.2	0.01	2	0.02
5.9	2.5	2	35	91	143	158	0.8	0.5	40	9	1.83	0	0.11	0.08	2.1	0.07	25	0.07
3.4	0.3	10	84	82	96	136	0.5	0.3	21	20	0.46	0	0.03	0.12	0.1	0.02	3	0.15
0.3	0	0	0	0	2	1	0	0	0	0	0.03	7	0	0	0	0	0	0
6.2	2.9	8	55	130	156	190	1.4	0.4	42	23	0.9	0	0.06	0.09	2.5	0.05	24	0.09
4.6	0.4	0	11	62	3	123	0.6	1	46	2	0.18	0	0.01	0.03	0.2	0.01	1	0
2.1	1.8	0	2	4	33	1	0	0.1	1	0	0.89	31	0	0	0	0	0	0
—	—	9	90	105	39	162	0.5	0.5	23	5	0.52	0	0.04	0.16	0.1	0.02	—	0.16
7.6	0.5	3	51	68	109	115	0.4	0.5	18	14	0.69	0	0.09	0.13	0.7	0.02	14	0.1
7.2	2	2	37	92	132	173	0.7	0.4	36	9	0.54	0	0.05	0.07	2	0.07	12	0.06
2.8	1.5	5	55	87	99	148	0.6	0.3	29	9	0.71	0	0.22	0.29	3.5	0.27	5	0.16
—	—	0	18	88	67	18	0	0.2	2	1	0.17	0	0.01	0.01	0	0	0	0
1	0.1	0	6	40	10	54	0.3	0.4	26	0	0.13	0	0.01	0.04	0.4	0	—	0.01
12	3.2	0	83	141	24	225	1	1.2	91	0	5.21	0	0.05	0.22	0.7	0.03	32	0
0.2	0	3	1	1	110	1	0	0	0	10	0.02	0	0	0	0	0	0	0
0.3	0.1	3	55	46	98	86	0.2	0.1	7	3	0.18	0	0	0.07	0.1	0.01	2	0
0.4	0.3	3	264	110	93	551	3.1	1.1	31	7	1.37	0	0.09	0.16	0.9	0.11	24	0.87
0.9	0.1	0	5	27	7	47	0.1	0.4	18	1	0.1	0	0.01	0.02	0.2	0	0	0
0	0	0	0	0	0	0	0	0	0	0	0	0	0	0	0	0	0	0
0	0	0	1	0	0	0	0	0	0	0	0	0	0	0	0	0	0	0
2.8	0.3	6	54	61	23	109	0.4	0.4	17	14	0.35	0	0.02	0.08	0.1	0.01	2	0.11
4.6	0.4	0	10	60	7	119	0.6	1.1	46	1	0.49	0	0.01	0.1	0.3	0.02	1	0
0.3	0	0	2	10	3	18	0	0.2	7	0	0.04	0	0	0.01	0.1	0	0	0
0	0	0	0	1	9	4	0	0	0	0	—	0	0	0.01	0	0	0	0
0	0	0	4	4	80	32	0.1	0.1	2	1	0	0	0	0.03	0	0	0	0
0.3	0.8	1	16	12	14	52	0.1	0.3	7	2	—	0	0.01	0.01	0	0.02	2	0
1	0.1	5	9	13	21	28	0.1	0.2	7	16	—	0	0	0.02	0	0	0	0.01
0.8	1	3	10	18	11	30	0.1	0.1	9	9	0.08	0	0.01	0.02	0	0.02	2	0.01
0.4	0.1	2	7	10	10	18	0.1	0.1	4	8	0.02	0	0	0.01	0	0	0	0.01
0.5	0.3	1	7	10	12	21	0.1	0	4	2	—	0	0	0.01	0.2	0.01	2	0.01
0.2	0	3	6	5	11	8	0	0	1	8	0.03	0	0	0.01	0	0	0	0.01
0	0	0	1	0	15	2	0	0.1	0	0	0	0	0	0	0	0	0	0
0	0	0	1	0	15	2	0	0.1	0	0	0	0	0	0	0	0	0	0
0	0	0	1	1	11	1	0	0.1	1	0	0	0	0	0	0	0	0	0
0	0	0	0	0	0	0	0	0	0	0	0	0	0	0	0	0	0	0
0	0	0	0	0	3	4	0	0.1	0	0	0	0	0	0	0	0	0	0
—	—	0	0	—	80	54	0.1	0	3	0	—	0	—	—	—	—	—	
0	0	0	0	0	2	0	0	0	0	0	0	0	0	0	0	0	0	0
2.5	0.2	6	50	56	42	100	0.3	0.2	14	3	0.36	0	0.02	0.08	0.1	0.02	3	0.11
4.4	0.5	10	84	95	36	169	0.6	0.6	26	24	0.55	0	0.04	0.13	0.1	0.02	4	0.17
5.5	0.9	8	92	108	30	182	0.5	0.7	37	6	0.78	0	0.02	0.18	0.3	0.02	5	0.14
7.8	3.9	4	50	126	17	230	1	0.8	53	9	1.99	0	0.12	0.08	3.2	0.07	36	0.08
3.5	0.3	8	68	77	58	137	0.4	0.3	20	4	0.44	0	0.02	0.12	0.2	0.02	4	0.14
1.5	0.5	1	13	30	4	50	0.2	0.1	12	0	0.26	0	0.01	0.02	0.5	0.02	1	0.03
2.2	0.2	1	41	68	17	244	0.4	0.8	21	3	0.46	0	0.04	0.08	0.2	0.04	2	0.09
3.1	1.7	5	11	41	166	76	0.4	0.5	18	17	0.6	0	0.07	0.02	1.3	0.04	26	0
5.9	2.4	0	12	42	24	82	0.8	0.5	20	2	0.58	0	0.12	0.02	0.1	0.03	5	0
4.4	5.1	0	229	148	58	113	1.3	1.5	88	0	0.53	0	0.19	0.06	1.3	0.19	23	0
3.6	1.1	0	28	47	6	72	0.5	0.5	46	0	0.52	0	0.01	0.08	0.3	0.02	16	0
0.1	0	1	0	0	13	1	0	0	0	5	0.08	0	0	0	0	0	0	0
0.6	0.2	1	16	19	20	34	0.1	0.1	5	2	0.17	0	0.01	0.02	0.2	0.01	3	0.01
4.6	0.6	50	16	16	90	24	0.1	0	2	153	0.96	0	0	0.03	0	0	1	0.03
0.4	0.3	0	9	14	28	36	0.2	0.1	11	1	0.08	0	0.01	0.03	0	0.01	0	0.02
6.4	3.5	1	17	63	14	107	0.9	0.5	25	10	2.04	1	0.05	0.03	2.4	0.05	48	0.17
1.9	0.2	4	55	65	21	269	0.2	0.6	10	13	0.64	1	0.05	0.08	0.3	0.08	4	0.15
1.8	0.2	6	19	21	9	37	0.1	0.1	6	17	0.14	0	0.01	0.03	0	0	0	0.04
—	—	0	2	—	105	—	—	0.1	—	1	—	0	—	—	—	—	—	0
0	0.2	0	5	20	3	207	0.1	0.3	11	62	0.47	27	0.04	0.03	0.5	0.13	18	0
—	—	0	2	1	1	52	—	0.3	3	1	—	8	0.01	0.01	0	—	—	0
—	—	4	269	—	187	—	—	0.4	—	5	—	2	—	—	—	—	—	—
2.4	0.3	33	292	228	133	369	0.9	0.7	33	77	0.1	2	0.1	0.39	0.3	0.12	12	0.87

Food Item	Qty	Meas	Wgt (g)	Wtr (g)	Cals	Prot	Carb (g)	Fib (g)	Fat (g)	SatF (g)
Carrot chips, dried	0.5	cup	37	1	136	3	27	7.3	1	0.1
Carrot juice, canned	1	cup	246	219	98	2	23	2	0	0.1
Carrot slices, cooked, no added salt, drained	0.5	cup	78	68	35	1	8	2.6	0	0
Carrot slices, steamed	0.5	cup	78	68	34	1	8	2.3	0	0
Carrot slices, stir fried	0.5	cup	78	68	34	1	8	2.3	0	0
Carrot, baby, raw (2.75 inch)	1	each	10	9	4	0	1	0.2	0	0
Carrot, glazed	0.5	cup	80	56	117	1	17	2.1	6	1.1
Carrot, raw, grated	0.5	cup	55	48	24	1	6	1.6	0	0
Carrot, whole, raw	1	each	72	63	31	1	7	2.2	0	0
Carrots, canned, drained	0.5	cup	73	68	18	0	4	1.1	0	0
Carrots, frozen, cooked	0.5	cup	73	66	26	1	6	2.6	0	0
Carrots, julienne	0.5	cup	55	48	24	1	6	1.7	0	0
Carrots, whole, cooked, no added salt, drained	1	each	46	40	21	1	5	1.5	0	0
Cashew butter, salted	1	Tbs	16	0	94	3	4	0.3	8	1.6
Cashew chicken	1	cup	162	91	409	27	11	2	29	4.8
Cashew, dry roasted, salted	0.25	cup	34	1	197	5	11	1	16	3.1
Cashews, dry roasted, unsalted	0.25	cup	34	1	197	5	11	1	16	3.1
Cashews, oil roasted, salted	0.25	cup	32	1	187	5	9	1.2	16	3.1
Cashews, oil roasted, unsalted	0.25	cup	32	1	187	5	9	1.2	16	3.1
Cassava (yuca blanca), pieces, cooked	0.5	cup	68	46	82	2	18	0.1	0	0.1
Cassava, raw	4	oz.	113	68	181	2	43	2	0	0.1
Catsup/ketchup	1	Tbs	15	10	16	0	4	0.2	0	0
Catsup/ketchup, packet	1	each	6	4	6	0	2	0.1	0	0
Cauliflower flowerets, cooked, drained	3	each	54	50	12	1	2	1.5	0	0
Cauliflower, cooked, drained, cup measure	0.5	cup	62	58	14	1	3	1.7	0	0
Cauliflower, flowerets, batter-dipped, fried	5	piece	130	89	250	6	13	2.1	20	4.8
Cauliflower, flowerets, pickled	3	each	81	71	34	1	8	1.5	0	0
Cauliflower, frozen, cooked, drained	0.5	cup	90	85	17	1	3	2.4	0	0
Cauliflower, raw flowerets	3	each	56	52	14	1	3	1.4	0	0
Cauliflower, raw, cup measure	0.5	cup	50	46	12	1	3	1.2	0	0
Cauliflower, w/cheese sauce	0.5	cup	81	67	73	3	5	0.9	5	2.2
Celeriac/celery root, cooked	0.5	cup	78	72	21	1	5	0.9	0	0
Celery pieces, cooked, no added salt	0.5	cup	75	71	14	1	3	1.2	0	0
Celery, chopped, raw	0.5	cup	60	57	10	0	2	1	0	0
Celery, chopped, steamed	0.5	cup	75	71	12	1	3	1.3	0	0
Celery, chopped, stir fried	0.5	cup	75	71	12	1	3	1.3	0	0
Celery, pickled	0.5	cup	75	71	11	0	3	1.1	0	0
Celery, raw, large outer stalk	1	each	40	38	6	0	1	0.7	0	0
Celery, stuffed w/cheese	1	piece	32	25	44	2	1	0.3	4	2.4
Cereal, 100% Bran	0.5	cup	33	1	89	4	24	9.8	2	0.3
Cereal, 100% Natural	0.5	cup	52	1	231	5	36	3.9	9	3.7
Cereal, 100% Natural w/apple cinnamon	0.5	cup	52	1	239	6	35	3.4	10	7.8
Cereal, 100% Natural w/raisins & dates	0.5	cup	55	2	248	6	36	3.6	10	6.8
Cereal, All Bran	0.5	cup	43	1	114	5	33	13.9	1	0.3
Cereal, Alpha Bits	1	cup	28	0	111	2	25	1.2	1	0.1
Cereal, Amaranth flakes	0.5	cup	19	1	67	2	13	1.8	2	0.5
Cereal, Apple Jacks	1	cup	28	1	109	1	25	0.5	0	0.1
Cereal, Bran Buds	0.5	cup	43	1	119	4	34	17.1	1	0.2
Cereal, Bran Chex	1	cup	49	1	156	5	39	7.9	1	0.2
Cereal, Bran Flakes, Kellogg's	1	cup	39	1	128	4	31	6.2	1	0.2
Cereal, Bran Flakes, Post	1	cup	47	1	152	5	37	9.2	1	0.1
Cereal, Bran'ola raisin, Post	1	cup	110	3	400	8	88	10	6	1
Cereal, C.W. Post w/raisins	1	cup	103	4	446	9	74	13.6	15	11
Cereal, C.W. Post, plain	1	cup	97	2	421	9	73	7.2	13	1.7
Cereal, Cap'n Crunch	1	cup	37	1	147	2	32	1.2	2	0.5
Cereal, Cap'n Crunch, peanut butter	1	cup	35	1	146	3	28	1	3	0.7
Cereal, Cap'n Crunchberries	1	cup	35	1	140	2	30	0.8	2	0.5
Cereal, Cheerios	1	cup	23	1	83	2	17	2	1	0.3
Cereal, Clusters	0.5	cup	28	1	111	4	20	2.9	3	0.4
Cereal, Cocoa Krispies	1	cup	36	1	140	2	32	0.5	1	0.7
Cereal, Cocoa Pebbles	1	cup	32	1	131	2	28	0.5	2	1.1
Cereal, Corn Bran	1	cup	36	1	120	2	30	6.4	1	0.3
Cereal, Corn Chex	1	cup	28	1	111	2	25	0.5	0	0
Cereal, Corn Flakes, USDA	1	cup	25	1	91	2	22	0.7	0	0
Cereal, Corn Pops USDA	1	cup	28	1	108	1	26	0.4	0	0.1

MonoF	PolyF	Choles	Calc	Phos	Sod	Pot	Zn	Iron	Magn	VitA	VitE	VitC	Thia	Ribo	Nia	B6	Fola	B12
(g)	(g)	(mg)	(mg)	(mg)	(mg)	(mg)	(mg)	(mg)	(mg)	(µg RE)	(µg α-TE)	(mg)	(mg)	(mg)	(mg)	(mg)	(µg)	(µg)
0	0.3	0	81	125	111	921	0.6	1.5	45	3699	0.14	21	0.26	0.18	2.6	0.44	31	0
0	0.2	0	59	103	71	718	0.4	1.1	34	2693	0.02	21	0.23	0.14	1	0.53	9	0
0	0.1	0	24	23	52	177	0.2	0.5	10	1914	0.33	2	0.03	0.04	0.4	0.19	11	0
0	0.1	0	21	34	27	252	0.2	0.4	12	1977	0.33	5	0.07	0.04	0.7	0.11	10	0
0	0.1	0	21	34	27	252	0.2	0.4	12	1977	0.33	6	0.07	0.04	0.7	0.11	10	0
0	0	0	2	4	4	28	0	0.1	1	150	0.04	1	0	0	0.1	0.01	3	0
2.5	1.8	0	31	24	131	189	0.2	0.6	12	1717	1.16	2	0.02	0.04	0.3	0.17	9	0.01
0	0	0	15	24	19	178	0.1	0.3	8	1547	0.25	5	0.05	0.03	0.5	0.08	8	0
0	0.1	0	19	32	25	233	0.1	0.4	11	2025	0.33	7	0.07	0.04	0.7	0.11	10	0
0	0.1	0	18	18	177	131	0.2	0.5	6	1005	0.31	2	0.01	0.02	0.4	0.08	7	0
0	0	0	20	19	43	115	0.2	0.3	7	1292	0.31	2	0.02	0.03	0.3	0.09	8	0
0	0	0	15	24	19	178	0.1	0.3	8	1554	0.25	5	0.05	0.03	0.5	0.08	8	0
0	0	0	14	14	30	104	0.1	0.3	6	1129	0.19	1	0.02	0.03	0.2	0.11	6	0
4.7	1.3	0	7	73	98	87	0.8	0.8	41	0	0.25	0	0.05	0.03	0.3	0.04	11	0
13	9.1	60	47	249	988	415	1.4	1.9	60	93	3.65	9	0.14	0.14	12.5	0.56	40	0.24
9.4	2.7	0	15	168	219	194	1.9	2.1	89	0	0.2	0	0.07	0.07	0.5	0.09	24	0
9.4	2.7	0	15	168	5	194	1.9	2.1	89	0	0.2	0	0.07	0.07	0.5	0.09	24	0
9.2	2.6	0	13	138	203	172	1.5	1.3	83	0	0.51	0	0.14	0.06	0.6	0.08	22	0
9.2	2.6	0	13	138	6	172	1.5	1.3	83	0	0.51	0	0.14	0.06	0.6	0.08	22	0
0.1	0.1	0	60	43	165	473	0.2	2.4	43	1	0.13	22	0.12	0.06	0.9	0.19	10	0
0.1	0.1	0	18	31	16	307	0.4	0.3	24	2	0.22	23	0.1	0.05	1	0.1	31	0
0	0	0	3	6	182	74	0	0.1	3	16	0.22	2	0.01	0.01	0.2	0.03	2	0
0	0	0	1	2	71	29	0	0	1	6	0.09	1	0	0	0.1	0.01	1	0
0	0.1	0	9	17	8	77	0.1	0.2	5	1	0.02	24	0.02	0.03	0.2	0.09	24	0
0	0.1	0	10	20	9	88	0.1	0.2	6	1	0.02	28	0.03	0.03	0.3	0.11	27	0
5.2	9.1	30	167	173	239	332	0.6	0.9	19	45	3.43	47	0.1	0.16	0.7	0.19	40	0.17
0.1	0.1	0	20	28	129	192	0.1	0.4	10	30	0.08	35	0.04	0.03	0.3	0.12	24	0
0	0.1	0	15	22	16	125	0.1	0.4	8	2	0.04	28	0.03	0.05	0.3	0.08	37	0
0	0.1	0	12	25	17	170	0.2	0.2	8	1	0.02	26	0.03	0.04	0.3	0.12	32	0
0	0	0	11	22	15	152	0.1	0.2	8	1	0.02	23	0.03	0.03	0.3	0.11	28	0
1.7	0.8	10	88	73	258	183	0.4	0.2	10	41	0.29	21	0.04	0.1	0.3	0.1	22	0.17
0	0.1	0	20	51	47	134	0.2	0.3	9	0	0.16	3	0.02	0.03	0.3	0.08	3	0
0	0.1	0	32	19	68	213	0.1	0.3	9	10	0.27	5	0.03	0.04	0.2	0.06	16	0
0	0	0	24	15	52	172	0.1	0.2	7	8	0.22	4	0.03	0.03	0.2	0.05	17	0
0	0.1	0	30	19	65	216	0.1	0.3	8	10	0.27	4	0.1	0.03	0.2	0.06	18	0
0	0.1	0	30	19	65	215	0.1	0.3	8	9	0.27	4	0.1	0.03	0.2	0.06	17	0
0	0	0	26	15	183	177	0.1	0.3	8	8	0.24	3	0.02	0.03	0.2	0.05	12	0
0	0	0	16	10	35	115	0.1	0.2	4	5	0.14	3	0.02	0.02	0.1	0.04	11	0
1.1	0.1	12	45	50	110	75	0.2	0.2	4	46	0.16	2	0.01	0.04	0.1	0.02	7	0.06
0.3	0.9	0	23	401	229	326	2.9	4.1	156	0	0.77	31	0.79	0.89	10.5	1.06	23	3.14
3.7	1.1	1	50	161	14	228	1.2	1.6	55	1	0.59	0	0.18	0.08	0.9	0.09	13	0.06
0.9	0.7	0	78	175	26	257	1	1.4	36	3	0.36	1	0.17	0.29	0.9	0.05	8	0.15
1.9	0.9	0	80	174	24	269	1.1	1.6	62	3	0.38	0	0.15	0.32	1	0.08	23	0.07
0.3	0.8	0	152	422	87	490	5.4	6.4	185	323	0.79	22	0.56	0.6	7.2	0.73	129	2.15
0.2	0.2	0	8	51	180	55	1.5	2.7	17	376	0.02	0	0.37	0.43	5	0.51	100	1.51
0.4	0.9	0	3	63	7	67	0	0.3	5	2	1.61	0	0.01	0.02	0.5	0.01	2	0
0.1	0.2	0	3	28	127	30	3.5	4.2	8	213	0.05	14	0.37	0.4	4.7	0.48	100	0
0.2	0.6	0	29	238	286	386	9.2	6.4	119	323	0.68	22	0.56	0.6	7.2	0.73	129	0
0.3	0.7	0	29	173	345	216	6.5	14	69	11	0.56	26	0.64	0.26	8.6	0.88	173	2.6
0.2	0.5	0	19	202	304	236	5	10.9	81	488	7.22	20	0.51	0.58	6.7	0.66	138	1.95
0.1	0.4	0	21	296	431	251	2.5	13.4	102	622	0.54	0	0.61	0.7	8.3	0.85	166	2.49
—	—	0	0	200	440	440	3	9	80	751	—	0	0.75	0.85	10	1	200	3
1.7	1.4	0	50	232	161	261	1.6	16.4	74	1363	0.72	0	1.34	1.55	18.1	1.85	364	5.46
6	4.7	0	47	224	167	198	1.6	15.4	67	1284	0.68	0	1.26	1.46	17.1	1.75	342	5.14
0.4	0.3	0	7	39	286	47	5.1	6.2	13	5	0.18	0	0.51	0.58	6.8	0.68	137	0
1.1	0.7	0	4	67	264	80	4.9	5.8	24	5	0.19	0	0.49	0.55	6.5	0.65	130	0
0.4	0.3	0	9	40	256	49	5.4	6.1	13	6	0.25	0	0.5	0.57	6.7	0.67	135	0.01
0.5	0.2	0	42	86	215	67	2.8	6.1	25	284	0.16	11	0.28	0.32	3.8	0.38	76	0
1.4	1.4	0	51	106	135	137	0.4	4.5	27	373	0.97	16	0.39	0.48	6	0.52	100	0
0.1	0.1	0	5	34	244	70	1.7	2.1	13	261	0.17	17	0.43	0.5	5.8	0.58	108	0
0.4	0.1	0	5	25	180	53	1.7	2	13	424	0.04	0	0.42	0.48	5.6	0.58	113	1.7
0.3	0.4	0	27	48	338	75	5	10.1	19	5	0.19	0	0.1	0.56	6.7	0.67	134	0
0	0	0	3	11	310	23	0.1	8.1	4	14	0.07	15	0.37	0.07	5	0.51	100	1.5
0	0.1	0	1	10	266	23	0.2	7.8	3	188	0.03	12	0.32	0.35	4.2	0.42	88	0
0.1	0	0	2	6	113	21	1.4	1.7	2	213	0.03	14	0.37	0.4	4.7	0.48	100	0

Food Item	Qty	Meas	Wgt (g)	Wtr (g)	Cals	Prot	Carb (g)	Fib (g)	Fat (g)	SatF (g)
Cereal, Cracklin' Oat Bran	0.5	cup	30	1	123	3	22	3.6	4	1.6
Cereal, Crispy Wheat 'N Raisins	1	cup	43	3	150	3	35	2.7	1	0.1
Cereal, Farina, enriched, cooked	0.5	cup	116	102	58	2	12	1.6	0	0
Cereal, Froot Loops	1	cup	28	1	111	1	25	0.5	1	0.4
Cereal, Frosted Flakes	1	cup	38	1	146	1	34	0.8	0	0.1
Cereal, Fruit & Fibre, date-raisin-nut	0.5	cup	28	3	96	2	22	3.8	1	0.2
Cereal, Fruity Pebbles	1	cup	32	1	130	1	28	0.4	2	1.4
Cereal, Golden Grahams	1	cup	39	1	150	2	33	1.2	1	0.2
Cereal, Granola, Nature Valley	0.5	cup	56	2	255	6	37	3.6	10	1.3
Cereal, Granola, low fat	0.5	cup	47	1	182	5	38	3	3	0
Cereal, Grape Nuts	0.5	cup	54	2	195	7	45	5.4	0	0
Cereal, Grape Nuts Flakes	1	cup	39	1	144	4	32	3.9	1	0.6
Cereal, Heartwise, plain	1	cup	39	1	113	4	31	8.6	1	0.2
Cereal, Honey & Nut Corn Flakes	667	cup	28	1	115	2	24	0.5	1	0.3
Cereal, Honey Bran	1	cup	35	1	119	3	29	3.9	1	0.3
Cereal, Honey Buckwheat Crisp	1	cup	38	2	147	4	31	3.4	1	0.2
Cereal, Honey Bunches of Oats	1	cup	43	1	173	3	36	2.1	2	0.5
Cereal, Honey Comb	1	cup	22	0	86	1	20	0.6	0	0.2
Cereal, Honey Nut Cheerios	1	cup	33	1	126	3	27	1.7	1	0.3
Cereal, Honey Smacks	1	cup	38	1	144	2	33	1.3	1	0.4
Cereal, Just Right	1	cup	43	1	152	5	36	3	1	0.2
Cereal, King Vitaman	1	cup	21	0	81	2	18	0.8	1	0.2
Cereal, Kix	1	cup	19	0	72	1	16	0.5	0	0.1
Cereal, Life, plain/cinnamon	1	cup	44	2	167	4	35	2.8	2	0.3
Cereal, Lucky Charms	1	cup	32	1	124	2	27	1.3	1	0.2
Cereal, Maypo, cooked, no salt added	0.5	cup	120	99	85	3	16	2.9	1	0.2
Cereal, Most	1	cup	52	2	175	7	40	7.3	1	0.1
Cereal, Mueslix Five Grain Muesli	0.5	cup	41	2	139	4	32	3.7	2	0.3
Cereal, Multi-grain, cooked	0.5	cup	123	96	100	3	20	2	1	0.2
Cereal, Oat flakes, fortified	1	cup	48	1	180	8	36	1.4	1	0.2
Cereal, Oatmeal, instant, packet, prepared, plain	1	each	177	151	104	4	18	3	2	0.3
Cereal, Post Toasties	1	cup	24	1	93	2	21	0.8	0	0
Cereal, Product 19	1	cup	33	1	121	3	28	1.1	0	0
Cereal, Quisp	1	cup	30	1	121	2	26	0.8	2	0.5
Cereal, Raisin Bran, Kellogg's	1	cup	56	5	171	5	43	7.5	1	0
Cereal, Raisin Bran, Post	1	cup	56	5	172	5	42	7.9	1	0.2
Cereal, Raisin Nut Bran	1	cup	57	3	221	4	42	5.6	6	1
Cereal, Ralston, cooked	0.5	cup	126	109	67	3	14	3	0	0.1
Cereal, Rice Chex	1	cup	25	1	99	1	22	0.5	0	0
Cereal, Rice Krispies	1	cup	28	1	111	2	25	0.3	0	0
Cereal, Roman meal, cooked	0.5	cup	120	99	73	3	16	4.1	0	0.1
Cereal, Shredded Wheat, large biscuit	1	each	24	1	85	3	19	2.3	0	0.1
Cereal, Shredded Wheat, small	1	cup	43	2	152	5	34	4.2	1	0.1
Cereal, Special K	1	cup	28	1	105	6	20	0.9	0	0
Cereal, Super Golden Crisp	1	cup	33	0	123	2	30	0.5	0	0.1
Cereal, Team Rice	1	cup	42	2	164	3	36	0.5	1	0.1
Cereal, Total, wheat	1	cup	33	1	116	3	26	2.9	1	0.2
Cereal, Trix	1	cup	28	1	114	1	24	0.7	2	0.4
Cereal, Uncle Sam's High Fiber	0.5	cup	55	3	213	8	40	14.5	2	0.2
Cereal, Wheat Chex	1	cup	46	1	169	5	38	4.1	1	0.2
Cereal, Wheatena, cooked, unsalted	0.5	cup	122	104	68	2	14	3.3	1	0.1
Cereal, Wheaties	1	cup	29	1	106	3	23	2	1	0.2
Cereal, cream of rye, cooked	0.5	cup	126	111	54	1	12	2.2	0	0
Cereal, cream of wheat, cooked	0.5	cup	122	106	66	2	14	0.6	0	0
Cereal, cream of wheat, mix'n eat, prep, plain	1	each	142	117	102	3	21	0.4	0	0
Cereal, farina, unenriched, cooked w/o salt	0.5	cup	116	102	58	2	12	1.6	0	0
Cereal, frosted mini wheats, biscuits	4	each	31	2	105	3	26	3.3	0	0.1
Cereal, frosted rice krispies	1	cup	19	0	71	1	17	0.2	0	0
Cereal, honey cluster flake crunch, fat free	1	cup	41	1	173	4	35	5.3	0	0
Cereal, malt-o-meal, plain, cooked	0.5	cup	120	105	61	2	13	0.5	0	0
Cereal, oat bran, cooked, Mother's brand	0.5	cup	121	109	31	2	8	2	1	0.2
Cereal, oatmeal, cooked	0.5	cup	117	100	72	3	13	2	1	0.2
Cereal, oatmeal, instant packet, prepared, apple-ci	1	each	149	117	125	3	26	2.5	1	0.3
Cereal, oatmeal, instant packet, prepared, cinn-spi	1	each	161	118	177	5	35	2.6	2	0.4
Cereal, oatmeal, instant packet, prepared, maple	1	each	155	116	153	4	32	2.6	2	0.4

MonoF (g)	PolyF (g)	Choles (mg)	Calc (mg)	Phos (mg)	Sod (mg)	Pot (mg)	Zn (mg)	Iron (mg)	Magn (mg)	VitA (µg RE)	VitE (µg α-TE)	VitC (mg)	Thia (mg)	Ribo (mg)	Nia (mg)	B6 (mg)	Fola (µg)	B12 (µg)
1.8	0.4	0	14	102	107	139	0.9	1.1	42	138	0.2	9	0.23	0.26	3.1	0.31	83	0
0.1	0.1	0	54	110	223	180	0.8	3.5	33	293	0.45	0	0.29	0.33	3.9	0.39	78	0
0	0	0	2	14	0	15	0.1	0.6	2	0	0.02	0	0.09	0.06	0.6	0.01	27	0
0.2	0.3	0	3	20	133	30	3.5	4	8	200	0.1	13	0.37	0.4	4.7	0.48	85	0
0	0.1	0	1	10	244	25	0.2	5.5	3	274	0.05	18	0.45	0.53	6.1	0.6	113	0
0.6	0.5	0	15	110	134	167	1.5	5.1	40	361	0.66	0	0.38	0.43	5	0.5	100	1.5
0.1	0.1	0	4	19	178	24	1.7	2	9	424	0.03	0	0.42	0.48	5.6	0.58	113	1.7
0.4	0.2	0	19	47	357	69	4.9	5.8	12	293	0.29	20	0.49	0.55	6.5	0.65	130	0
6.7	1.9	0	42	164	92	188	1.1	1.8	54	0	3.98	0	0.18	0.06	0.6	0.08	8	0
—	—	0	—	121	91	144	5.7	2.7	36	227	7.61	—	0.57	0.64	7.6	0.76	152	2.27
0	0.1	0	5	137	379	182	1.2	15.6	36	722	0.14	0	0.71	0.82	9.6	0.98	192	2.89
0.1	0.2	0	16	116	220	136	0.8	11.2	43	516	0.1	0	0.51	0.58	6.9	0.7	138	2.07
0.3	0.4	0	30	154	168	265	2.1	6.2	55	310	0.02	0	0.52	0.58	7	0.69	137	1.95
0.6	0.4	0	3	19	191	31	0.2	2.3	3	116	0.07	8	0.2	0.23	2.6	0.26	57	0
0.1	0.3	0	16	132	202	151	0.9	5.6	46	463	0.81	19	0.46	0.52	6.2	0.63	24	1.86
0.3	0.6	0	53	107	359	141	0.7	10.8	43	908	8.94	36	0.9	1.02	12	1.87	11	3.6
1.4	0.3	0	8	66	272	77	0.7	6	24	838	0.3	0	0.55	0.74	8.3	1.04	196	3.67
0.1	0.1	0	4	22	124	25	1.2	2.1	7	291	0.09	0	0.29	0.33	3.9	0.4	78	1.17
0.5	0.2	0	22	113	285	94	4.1	5	32	248	0.34	16	0.41	0.47	5.5	0.55	110	0
0.1	0.3	0	4	56	71	59	0.5	2.5	22	315	0.19	21	0.53	0.6	7	0.72	140	0
0.2	0.4	0	11	94	288	98	22.8	27.3	29	341	45.6	0	2.27	2.58	30.3	3.03	607	9.1
0.3	0.2	0	3	54	176	58	2.6	5.9	18	212	1.42	8	0.26	0.3	3.5	0.35	71	1.06
0.1	0	0	27	26	166	26	2.4	5.1	6	236	0.05	9	0.24	0.27	3.2	0.32	63	0
0.6	0.8	0	134	187	240	109	5.5	12.3	43	2	0.22	0	0.55	0.62	7.4	0.73	147	0
0.4	0.2	0	35	81	217	58	4	4.8	21	240	0.14	16	0.4	0.45	5.3	0.53	107	0
0.4	0.4	0	62	124	5	106	0.7	4.2	25	352	0.84	14	0.36	0.36	4.7	0.48	5	1.44
0.2	0.3	0	79	361	276	340	2.8	33	103	2753	55	110	2.76	3.13	36.7	3.69	734	11
0.5	0.6	0	19	107	53	185	3.7	4.5	41	374	4.47	0	0.37	0.42	4.9	0.5	98	1.64
0.5	0.3	0	35	92	380	68	0.5	2.7	33	57	1.71	0	0.2	0.23	2.2	0.23	9	0
0.3	0.4	0	68	176	220	228	2.5	13.7	58	636	0.34	0	0.62	0.72	8.4	0.86	169	2.54
0.6	0.7	0	163	133	285	99	0.9	6.3	42	453	0.21	0	0.53	0.28	5.5	0.74	150	0
0	0	0	1	11	252	28	0.1	0.6	4	318	0.06	0	0.31	0.36	4.2	0.43	85	1.27
0.2	0.2	0	3	36	238	45	16.5	19.8	14	248	24.4	66	1.65	1.88	22	2.21	429	6.6
0.4	0.2	0	6	47	216	40	4.3	5.1	15	4	0.16	0	0.42	0.48	5.7	0.56	113	0
0.2	0.7	0	32	197	325	401	3.8	4.6	82	230	0.51	0	0.39	0.45	5.1	0.5	112	1.51
0.1	0.5	0	26	235	365	345	3	8.9	95	741	1.3	0	0.73	0.84	9.9	1.01	198	2.97
1.6	2.9	0	80	201	302	302	1.7	9	64	753	1.32	0	0.75	0.86	10.1	1	201	0
0.1	0.2	0	6	73	3	77	0.7	0.8	29	0	0.13	0	0.1	0.09	1	0.06	9	0.05
0	0	0	4	25	210	29	0.3	7.2	6	2	0.03	13	0.33	0.01	4.4	0.45	89	1.33
0	0	0	5	30	206	27	0.5	0.7	12	371	0.03	15	0.52	0.59	6.9	0.69	138	0.08
0.1	0.2	0	14	107	1	150	0.9	1.1	54	0	0.22	0	0.12	0.06	1.5	0.06	12	0
0.1	0.2	0	10	86	0	77	0.6	0.7	40	0	0.12	0	0.07	0.07	1.1	0.06	12	0
0.1	0.4	0	16	151	4	154	1.4	1.8	56	0	0.23	0	0.11	0.12	2.2	0.11	21	0
0	0.2	0	4	46	229	50	3.4	8	16	206	0.07	14	0.48	0.54	6.4	0.65	85	0
0.1	0.1	0	7	44	51	48	1.8	2.1	20	437	0.12	0	0.43	0.5	5.8	0.59	116	1.75
0.2	0.3	0	6	65	260	71	0.6	12	12	556	0.1	22	0.55	0.63	7.4	0.76	7	2.23
0.1	0.1	0	284	232	218	107	16.5	19.8	35	413	25.8	66	1.65	1.87	22.1	2.2	440	8.45
0.8	0.3	0	30	24	184	16	3.5	4.2	3	210	0.56	14	0.35	0.4	4.7	0.47	93	0
0.5	1.5	0	38	208	125	259	1.5	2	67	0	0.79	0	1.31	1.39	11.6	0.07	43	0
0.1	0.5	0	18	182	308	173	1.2	13.2	58	0	0.17	24	0.6	0.17	8.1	0.83	162	2.44
0.1	0.3	0	5	73	2	94	0.8	0.7	24	0	0.45	0	0.01	0.02	0.7	0.02	9	0
0.2	0.1	0	53	92	215	101	0.7	7.8	31	218	0.36	14	0.36	0.41	4.8	0.48	97	0
0	0.1	0	6	27	175	33	0.3	0.3	11	0	0.08	0	0.04	0.01	0.1	0.03	2	0
0	0.1	0	26	51	71	23	0.2	5.2	6	0	0.02	0	0.12	0	0.7	0.02	55	0
0	0.2	0	20	20	241	38	0.2	8.1	7	376	0.02	0	0.43	0.28	5	0.57	101	0
0	0	0	2	14	0	15	0.1	0	2	0	0.02	0	0.01	0.01	0.1	0.01	2	0
0.1	0.3	0	11	90	1	103	0.9	8.7	31	0	0.28	0	0.22	0.25	3	0.28	62	0.9
0	0.1	0	1	15	138	15	0.2	1.3	5	164	0.02	11	0.26	0.3	3.6	0.36	76	0
0	0	0	0	—	27	—	—	0.5	—	40	—	2	—	—	—	—	—	—
0	0	0	2	12	1	16	0.1	4.8	2	0	0.02	0	0.24	0.12	2.9	0.01	2	0
0.3	0.4	0	10	89	127	69	0.4	0.7	31	0	0.22	0	0.12	0.02	0.1	0.02	5	0
0.4	0.4	0	9	89	1	66	0.6	0.8	28	2	0.12	0	0.13	0.02	0.2	0.02	5	0
0.5	0.6	0	104	113	121	106	0.7	3.9	30	305	0.12	0	0.3	0.35	4.1	0.41	94	0
0.6	0.7	0	172	145	280	105	1	6.6	52	473	0.35	0	0.56	0.34	5.6	0.77	153	0
0.6	0.7	0	105	132	234	112	0.9	3.9	39	302	0.16	0	0.3	0.34	4	0.4	81	0

Food Item	Qty	Meas	Wgt (g)	Wtr (g)	Cals	Prot	Carb (g)	Fib (g)	Fat (g)	SatF (g)
Cereal, oatmeal, instant, prepared, raisin-spice	1	each	158	119	161	4	32	2.2	2	0.3
Cereal, puffed rice, fortified	1	cup	14	1	54	1	12	0.2	0	0
Cereal, puffed wheat, fortified	1	cup	12	0	44	2	9	1.1	0	0
Cereal, rolled wheat, cooked	0.5	cup	120	100	74	2	16	1.9	0	0.1
Cerealm, Tasteeos	1	cup	24	1	94	3	19	2.5	1	0.2
Chayote fruit, raw	1	each	203	191	39	2	9	3.4	0	0.1
Chayote, cooked pieces	0.5	cup	80	75	19	0	4	2.2	0	0.1
Cheese food, American cold pack	1	oz.	28	12	94	6	2	0	7	4.4
Cheese food, swiss processed, slice	1	piece	21	9	68	5	1	0	5	3.3
Cheese product, nonfat (Kraft Free Singles)	1	piece	19	12	30	4	3	0	0	0
Cheese puffs (Cheetos)	1	cup	20	0	111	2	11	0.2	7	1.3
Cheese spread, American	1	Tbs	15	7	44	2	1	0	3	2
Cheese spread, Velveeta	1	oz.	28	13	80	5	3	0	6	4
Cheese spread, lowfat, low sodium (Velveeta)	1	Tbs	15	9	27	4	1	0	1	0.7
Cheese, American food slice	1	piece	21	9	69	4	2	0	5	3.2
Cheese, American processed	1	piece	21	8	79	5	0	0	7	4.1
Cheese, American processed, lowfat	1	oz.	28	17	51	7	1	0	2	1.2
Cheese, Mexican, nonfat, Lifetime	1	oz.	28	18	40	8	1	0	0	0
Cheese, asiago, shredded	0.25	cup	27	10	102	8	1	0	7	4.8
Cheese, beer	1	oz.	28	12	105	7	1	0	8	5.3
Cheese, blue	1	oz.	28	12	100	6	1	0	8	5.3
Cheese, brick w/salami	1	oz.	28	12	102	6	1	0	8	5
Cheese, brick, shredded	0.25	cup	28	12	105	7	1	0	8	5.3
Cheese, brick, shredded	1	oz.	28	12	105	7	1	0	8	5.3
Cheese, brie, sliced	1	oz.	28	14	95	6	0	0	8	4.9
Cheese, camembert	0.25	cup	28	15	85	6	0	0	7	4.3
Cheese, camembert	1	oz.	28	15	85	6	0	0	7	4.3
Cheese, caraway	1	piece	28	11	107	7	1	0	8	5.3
Cheese, cheddar, low fat, Alpine Lace	1	oz.	28	14	81	9	1	0	5	3
Cheese, cheddar, low sodium	1	oz.	28	11	113	7	1	0	9	5.9
Cheese, cheddar, lowfat, low sodium	0.25	cup	28	18	49	7	1	0	2	1.2
Cheese, cheddar, nonfat, Lifetime	1	oz.	28	18	40	8	1	0	0	0
Cheese, cheddar, shredded	0.25	cup	28	10	114	7	0	0	9	6
Cheese, cheshire	1	oz.	28	11	110	7	1	0	9	5.5
Cheese, colby, cubed	0.25	cup	33	13	130	8	1	0	11	6.7
Cheese, colby, cubed	1	oz.	28	11	112	7	1	0	9	5.7
Cheese, colby, low sodium	1	oz.	28	11	113	7	1	0	9	5.9
Cheese, colby, lowfat, low sodium	1	oz.	28	18	49	7	1	0	2	1.3
Cheese, colby, shredded	0.25	cup	28	11	111	7	1	0	9	5.7
Cheese, cottage, 1% lowfat	0.5	cup	113	93	82	14	3	0	1	0.7
Cheese, cottage, 2% lowfat	0.5	cup	101	89	101	15	4	0	2	1.4
Cheese, cottage, creamed w/fruit	0.5	cup	113	82	140	11	15	0	4	2.4
Cheese, cottage, creamed, large curd	0.5	cup	113	89	116	14	3	0	5	3.2
Cheese, cottage, lowfat, low sodium	0.5	cup	112	94	81	14	3	0	1	0.7
Cheese, cottage, nonfat (Knudsen)	0.5	cup	122	103	80	15	4	0	0	0
Cheese, cottage, small curd	0.5	cup	105	83	108	13	3	0	5	3
Cheese, cream	2	Tbs	29	16	101	2	1	0	10	6.4
Cheese, cream, lowfat	2	Tbs	30	19	69	3	2	0	5	3.3
Cheese, cream, nonfat (Philadelphia Free)	2	Tbs	33	26	30	5	2	0	0	0
Cheese, cream, soft (Philadelphia)	2	Tbs	30	17	100	2	1	0	10	7
Cheese, edam	1	oz.	28	12	101	7	0	0	8	5
Cheese, feta, shredded	0.25	cup	62	34	162	9	3	0	13	9.2
Cheese, fontina	1	oz.	28	11	110	7	0	0	9	5.4
Cheese, goat, hard	1	oz.	28	8	128	9	1	0	10	7
Cheese, goat, soft	0.5	cup	62	37	165	11	1	0	13	9
Cheese, goat, soft	1	oz.	28	17	76	5	0	0	6	4.1
Cheese, gouda	1	oz.	28	12	101	7	1	0	8	5
Cheese, gruyere	1	oz.	28	9	117	8	0	0	9	5.4
Cheese, havarti	1	oz.	28	12	105	7	1	0	8	5.3
Cheese, imitation mozzarella, shredded	0.25	cup	28	17	51	4	3	0	2	1.3
Cheese, light neufchatel (Kraft Philadelphia)	1	oz.	28	18	71	3	1	1	6	4
Cheese, limburger	1	oz.	33	14	93	6	0	0	8	4.7
Cheese, monterey jack, cubed	0.25	cup	28	14	123	8	0	0	10	6.3
Cheese, monterey jack, nonfat, Lifetime	1	oz.	35	18	40	8	1	0	0	0
Cheese, mozzarella nuggets, Banquet	8	piece	28	15	110	5	8	0	6	2.5

MonoF	PolyF	Choles	Calc	Phos	Sod	Pot	Zn	Iron	Magn	VitA	VitE	VitC	Thia	Ribo	Nia	B6	Fola	B12
(g)	(g)	(mg)	(mg)	(mg)	(mg)	(mg)	(mg)	(mg)	(mg)	(µg RE)	(µg α-TE)	(mg)	(mg)	(mg)	(mg)	(mg)	(µg)	(µg)
0.6	0.6	0	166	133	226	150	0.7	6.6	36	441	0.16	0	0.51	0.36	5.5	0.75	150	0
0	0	0	1	16	1	16	0.2	0.4	4	0	0.01	0	0.06	0.01	0.9	0	1	0
0	0.1	0	3	40	1	44	0.4	0.6	16	0	0.08	0	0.05	0.03	1.4	0.02	4	0.05
0.1	0.2	0	8	83	0	85	0.6	0.7	26	0	0.24	0	0.08	0.06	1.1	0.09	13	0
0.2	0.2	0	11	96	183	71	0.7	6.9	26	318	0.17	13	0.31	0.36	4.2	0.43	85	1.27
0	0.1	0	34	36	4	254	1.5	0.7	24	12	0.24	16	0.05	0.06	1	0.15	189	0
0	0.2	0	10	23	1	138	0.2	0.2	10	4	0.1	6	0.02	0.03	0.3	0.09	14	0
2	0.2	18	141	113	274	103	0.9	0.2	8	57	0.19	0	0.01	0.13	0	0.04	2	0.36
1.4	0.1	17	152	110	326	60	0.7	0.1	6	51	0.14	0	0	0.08	0	0.01	1	0.48
0	0	2	150	714	290	55	—	0	—	86	0	0	—	0.07	—	—	—	—
4.1	1	1	12	22	210	33	0.1	0.5	4	7	1.02	0	0.05	0.07	0.6	0.03	24	0.03
0.9	0.1	8	84	107	202	36	0.4	0	4	28	0.11	0	0.01	0.06	0	0.02	1	0.06
—	—	20	150	250	420	80	0.6	0	8	86	—	0	—	0.14	—	—	—	0.24
0.3	0	5	103	124	1	27	0.5	0.1	4	10	0.08	0	0	0.06	0	0.01	1	0.12
1.5	0.2	13	121	96	250	59	0.6	0.2	6	46	0.15	0	0.01	0.09	0	0.03	2	0.24
1.9	0.2	20	129	156	300	34	0.6	0.1	5	61	0.1	0	0.01	0.07	0	0.02	2	0.15
0.6	0.1	10	194	234	405	51	0.9	0.1	7	18	0.14	0	0.01	0.11	0	0.02	3	0.22
0	0	5	405	—	223	—	—	—	—	87	—	0	—	—	—	—	—	—
2	0.3	25	259	163	70	30	1	0	10	68	0.14	0	0.01	0.1	0	0.02	2	0.45
2.4	0.2	27	191	128	159	39	0.7	0.1	7	86	0.14	0	0	0.1	0	0.02	6	0.36
2.2	0.2	21	150	110	395	73	0.8	0.1	6	65	0.18	0	0.01	0.1	0.1	0.02	5	0.42
2.4	0.3	26	172	118	173	40	0.7	0.2	7	77	0.13	0	0.01	0.1	0.1	0.02	5	0.42
2.4	0.2	27	190	127	158	38	0.7	0.1	7	85	0.14	0	0	0.1	0	0.02	6	0.36
2.4	0.2	27	190	127	158	38	0.7	0.1	7	85	0.14	0	0	0.1	0	0.02	6	0.36
2.3	0.2	28	52	53	178	43	0.7	0.1	6	52	0.19	0	0.02	0.15	0.1	0.07	18	0.47
2	0.2	20	110	98	238	53	0.7	0.1	6	71	0.18	0	0.01	0.14	0.2	0.06	18	0.37
2	0.2	20	110	98	239	53	0.7	0.1	6	71	0.19	0	0.01	0.14	0.2	0.06	18	0.37
2.4	0.2	26	191	139	196	26	0.8	0.2	6	82	0.14	0	0.01	0.13	0.1	0.02	5	0.08
—	—	15	253	—	96	—	—	0.4	—	87	—	1	—	—	—	—	—	—
2.6	0.3	28	199	137	6	32	0.9	0.2	8	82	0.1	0	0.01	0.11	0	0.02	5	0.24
0.6	0.1	6	199	137	6	32	0.9	0.2	8	18	0.05	0	0.01	0.01	0	0.02	5	0.23
0	0	5	405	—	223	—	—	—	—	87	—	—	—	—	—	—	—	—
2.6	0.3	30	204	145	175	28	0.9	0.2	8	78	0.1	0	0.01	0.11	0	0.02	5	0.23
2.5	0.2	29	183	132	199	27	0.8	0.1	6	70	0.18	0	0.01	0.08	0	0.02	5	0.24
3.1	0.3	31	226	151	199	42	1	0.3	9	91	0.12	0	0	0.12	0	0.03	6	0.27
2.6	0.3	27	194	130	171	36	0.9	0.2	7	78	0.1	0	0	0.11	0	0.02	5	0.23
2.6	0.3	28	199	137	6	32	0.9	0.2	8	82	0.1	0	0.01	0.11	0	0.02	5	0.24
0.6	0.1	6	199	137	6	32	0.9	0.2	8	18	0.05	0	0.01	0.01	0	0.02	5	0.24
2.6	0.3	27	194	129	171	36	0.9	0.2	7	78	0.1	0	0	0.11	0	0.02	5	0.23
0.3	0	5	69	151	459	97	0.4	0.2	6	12	0.12	0	0.02	0.19	0.1	0.08	14	0.72
0.6	.07	9.5	77	171	459	109	0.5	0.2	7	23	0.3	0	0.03	0.21	0.06	0.09	15	0.8
1.1	0.1	13	54	119	458	76	0.3	0.1	5	41	0.1	0	0.02	0.15	0.1	0.06	11	0.56
1.5	0.2	17	68	149	458	95	0.4	0.2	6	54	0.14	0	0.02	0.18	0.1	0.08	14	0.7
0.3	0	4	69	151	15	97	0.4	0.2	6	12	0.12	0	0.02	0.18	0.1	0.08	14	0.71
0	0	10	60	150	370	75	—	0	—	57	—	0	0	0.17	—	0.03	—	0.6
1.4	0.1	16	63	139	425	88	0.4	0.1	6	50	0.13	0	0.02	0.17	0.1	0.07	13	0.65
2.8	0.4	32	23	30	86	34	0.2	0.3	2	111	0.27	0	0	0.06	0	0.01	4	0.12
1.7	0.2	17	34	44	89	50	0.2	0.5	2	66	0.14	0	0.01	0.08	0	0.02	5	0.18
0	0	2	100	150	160	65	0.3	0	0	143	—	0	—	0.34	—	—	—	0.12
—	—	30	20	20	100	40	0	0	0	86	—	0	—	0.03	—	—	—	0
2.3	0.2	25	207	152	274	53	1.1	0.1	8	72	0.21	0	0.01	0.11	0	0.02	5	0.44
2.8	0.4	55	303	207	686	38	1.8	0.4	12	79	0.02	0	0.1	0.52	0.6	0.26	20	1.04
2.5	0.2	33	156	98	227	18	1	0.1	4	82	0.1	0	0.01	0.06	0	0.02	2	0.48
2.3	0.5	30	254	207	98	14	0.5	0.5	15	135	0.22	0	0.04	0.34	0.7	0.02	1	0.03
3	0.3	28	86	157	226	16	0.6	1.2	10	174	0.28	0	0.04	0.23	0.3	0.15	7	0.12
1.4	0.1	13	40	73	104	7	0.3	0.5	5	80	0.13	0	0.02	0.11	0.1	0.07	3	0.05
2.2	0.2	32	198	155	232	34	1.1	0.1	8	49	0.1	0	0.01	0.1	0	0.02	6	0.44
2.8	0.5	31	287	172	95	23	1.1	0	10	85	0.1	0	0.02	0.08	0	0.02	3	0.45
2.4	0.2	27	191	128	159	39	0.7	0.1	7	86	0.14	0	0	0.1	0	0.02	6	0.36
0.6	0.1	5	161	206	324	65	0.7	0	8	23	0.05	0	0.01	0.11	0.1	0.04	1	0.13
—	—	20	20	40	122	30	0	0	0	58	—	0	—	0.03	—	—	—	0
2.4	0.1	26	141	111	227	36	0.6	0	6	90	0.18	0	0.02	0.14	0	0.02	16	0.3
2.9	0.3	29	246	147	177	27	1	0.2	9	84	0.11	0	0	0.13	0	0.03	6	0.27
0	0	5	405	—	223	—	—	—	—	87	—	—	—	—	—	—	—	—
—	—	10	100	290	200	60	—	0.4	—	0	—	0	0.06	0.1	0.2	—	—	—

Food Item	Qty	Meas	Wgt (g)	Wtr (g)	Cals	Prot	Carb (g)	Fib (g)	Fat (g)	SatF (g)
Cheese, mozzarella sting/stick	1	each	28	15	72	7	1	0	5	2.9
Cheese, mozzarella, low sodium	1	oz.	28	14	79	8	1	0	5	3.1
Cheese, mozzarella, low sodium string/stick	1	each	28	14	79	8	1	0	5	3.1
Cheese, mozzarella, lowfat, shredded	0.25	cup	28	14	79	8	1	0	5	3.1
Cheese, mozzarella, nonfat, Lifetime	1	oz.	28	18	40	8	1	0	0	0
Cheese, mozzarella, part skim, shredded	0.25	cup	28	15	72	7	1	0	4	2.8
Cheese, mozzarella, whole milk, low moisture	0.25	cup	28	14	90	6	1	0	7	4.4
Cheese, mozzarella, whole milk, shredded	0.25	cup	28	15	79	5	1	0	6	3.7
Cheese, muenster	0.25	cup	28	12	104	7	0	0	8	5.4
Cheese, neufchatel	1	oz.	28	18	74	3	1	0	7	4.2
Cheese, parmesan, grated	1	Tbs	6	1	28	3	0	0	2	1.2
Cheese, parmesan, low sodium, grated	0.25	cup	25	6	114	10	1	0	8	4.9
Cheese, parmesan, shredded	2	oz.	57	14	235	22	2	0	16	9.9
Cheese, pimento processed	1	oz.	28	11	106	6	0	0	9	5.6
Cheese, port du salut	1	oz.	28	13	100	7	0	0	8	4.7
Cheese, provolone	0.25	cup	33	14	116	8	1	0	9	5.6
Cheese, ricotta, part skim	1	oz.	28	21	39	3	1	0	2	1.4
Cheese, ricotta, whole milk	0.33	cup	82	59	143	9	2	0	11	6.8
Cheese, romano, grated	0.33	cup	33	10	128	10	1	0	9	5.6
Cheese, roquefort, crumbled	0.25	cup	34	13	125	7	1	0	10	6.5
Cheese, roquefort, cubed	1	oz.	28	11	105	6	1	0	9	5.5
Cheese, sharp cheddar, nonfat, Lifetime	1	oz.	28	18	40	8	1	0	0	0
Cheese, swiss	1	oz.	28	10	107	8	1	0	8	5
Cheese, swiss, low fat, Alpine Lace	1	oz.	28	12	91	8	1	0	6	4
Cheese, swiss, low sodium	1	oz.	28	11	107	8	1	0	8	5
Cheese, swiss, nonfat, Lifetime	1	oz.	28	18	40	8	1	0	0	0
Cheese, swiss, shredded	0.25	cup	27	10	102	8	1	0	7	4.8
Cheese, tilsit, whole milk	1	oz.	28	12	96	7	1	0	7	4.8
Cheese, white, fat free, Apine Lace	1	oz.	28	18	25	5	1	0	0	0
Cheese, yogurt	1	oz.	28	21	22	2	3	0	0	0
Cherimoya, raw	1	each	547	402	514	7	131	13.1	2	—
Cherries, maraschino	0.5	cup	80	56	93	0	24	—	0	0
Cherries, sour, canned in extra heavy syrup	0.5	cup	130	91	149	1	38	1	0	0
Cherries, sour, canned in water	0.5	cup	122	110	44	1	11	1.3	0	0
Cherries, sour, frozen, unsweetened	0.5	cup	78	68	36	1	9	1.2	0	0.1
Cherries, sour, red, fresh, pitted	0.5	cup	78	67	39	1	9	1.2	0	0.1
Cherries, sweet, canned in heavy syrup	0.5	cup	128	100	107	1	27	1.9	0	0
Cherries, sweet, canned in juice	0.5	cup	125	106	68	1	17	1.9	0	0
Cherries, sweet, fresh	10	each	68	55	49	1	11	1.6	1	0.1
Cherries, sweet, frozen, sweetened	0.5	cup	130	98	115	1	29	2.7	0	0
Cherry crisp	1	cup	246	97	710	5	112	2.3	28	6.2
Cherry crisp, piece, 3x3 in	1	piece	138	106	146	2	24	1.3	5	0.9
Cherry turnover	1	each	78	32	238	3	31	0.9	12	2.9
Chervil, dried	0.25	tsp	0	0	0	0	0	0	0	0
Chestnuts, Chinese, cooked	1	oz.	28	18	43	1	10	0.3	0	0
Chestnuts, Chinese, raw	1	oz.	28	12	64	1	14	0.4	0	0
Chestnuts, Chinese, roasted	1	oz.	28	11	68	1	15	0.4	0	0
Chestnuts, European, cooked	1	oz.	28	19	37	1	8	1.4	0	0.1
Chestnuts, European, raw, peeled	1	oz.	28	15	56	0	12	2.2	0	0.1
Chestnuts, European, roasted, cup measure	0.25	cup	36	14	88	1	19	1.8	1	0.1
Chestnuts, European, roasted, whole	17	each	143	58	350	5	76	7.3	3	0.6
Chex party mix	1	oz.	28	1	120	3	18	1.6	5	1.5
Chia seeds, dried	1	oz.	28	2	134	5	14	7.2	7	3
Chicken & dumplings, Chicken Helper	0.5	cup	122	87	187	13	10	0.3	10	2.9
Chicken & noodles, recipe	1	cup	240	171	367	22	26	1.8	18	5.9
Chicken hearts, simmered	1	each	3	2	6	1	0	0	0	0.1
Chicken nuggets, fast food serving	1	each	102	52	276	17	15	0	16	3.5
Chicken parmigiana	1	piece	182	120	317	28	15	1.4	16	5.4
Chicken patty, breaded, cooked	1	each	75	37	213	12	11	0.3	13	4.1
Chicken pot pie, Banquet	1	each	198	133	350	10	36	3	18	7
Chicken salad, w/celery	0.5	cup	78	41	268	11	1	0.2	25	3.1
Chicken teriyaki, breast	1	each	128	85	176	26	7	0.2	4	0.9
Chicken teriyaki, drumstick	1	each	68	45	93	14	4	0.1	2	0.5
Chicken, back, skinless, fried	0.5	each	58	28	167	17	3	0	9	2.4
Chicken, back, skinless, roasted	0.5	each	40	24	96	11	0	0	5	1.4

MonoF	PolyF	Choles	Calc	Phos	Sod	Pot	Zn	Iron	Magn	VitA	VitE	VitC	Thia	Ribo	Nia	B6	Fola	B12
(g)	(g)	(mg)	(mg)	(mg)	(mg)	(mg)	(mg)	(mg)	(mg)	(µg RE)	(µg α-TE)	(mg)	(mg)	(mg)	(mg)	(mg)	(µg)	(µg)
1.3	0.1	16	183	131	132	24	0.8	0.1	7	50	0.12	0	0	0.09	0	0.02	2	0.23
1.4	0.1	15	207	149	5	27	0.9	0.1	7	54	0.13	0	0.01	0.1	0	0.02	3	0.26
1.4	0.1	15	207	149	5	27	0.9	0.1	7	54	0.13	0	0.01	0.1	0	0.02	3	0.26
1.4	0.1	15	207	148	149	27	0.9	0.1	7	54	0.13	0	0.01	0.1	0	0.02	3	0.26
0	0	5	405	—	223	—	—	—	—	87	—	—	—	—	—	—	—	—
1.3	0.1	16	182	131	132	24	0.8	0.1	7	50	0.12	0	0	0.09	0	0.02	2	0.23
2	0.2	25	162	116	117	21	0.7	0.1	6	77	0.19	0	0	0.08	0	0.02	2	0.2
1.9	0.2	22	146	105	105	19	0.6	0.1	5	68	0.1	0	0	0.07	0	0.02	2	0.18
2.5	0.2	27	203	132	177	38	0.8	0.1	8	89	0.13	0	0	0.09	0	0.02	3	0.42
1.9	0.2	22	21	39	113	32	0.1	0.1	2	85	0.27	0	0	0.06	0	0.01	3	0.08
0.5	0	5	86	50	116	7	0.2	0.1	3	11	0.05	0	0	0.02	0	0.01	0	0.09
2.2	0.2	20	344	202	16	27	0.8	0.2	13	43	0.2	0	0.01	0.1	0.1	0.02	2	0.35
5	0.4	41	710	417	962	55	1.8	0.5	29	98	0.48	0	0.02	0.2	0.2	0.06	5	0.79
2.5	0.3	27	174	211	405	46	0.8	0.1	6	91	0.13	0	0.01	0.1	0	0.02	5	0.2
2.6	0.2	35	184	102	151	39	0.7	0.1	7	105	0.14	0	0	0.07	0	0.02	5	0.42
2.4	0.3	23	249	164	289	46	1.1	0.2	9	87	0.12	1	0.01	0.11	0.1	0.02	3	0.48
0.7	0.1	9	77	52	35	35	0.4	0.1	4	32	0.06	0	0.01	0.05	0	0.01	4	0.08
3	0.3	42	170	130	69	86	1	0.3	9	110	0.29	0	0.01	0.16	0.1	0.04	10	0.28
2.6	0.2	34	351	251	396	28	0.9	0.3	14	46	0.24	0	0.01	0.12	0	0.03	2	0.37
2.9	0.4	30	223	132	611	31	0.7	0.2	10	101	0.26	0	0.01	0.2	0.2	0.04	16	0.22
2.4	0.4	26	188	111	513	26	0.6	0.2	8	85	0.22	0	0.01	0.17	0.2	0.04	14	0.18
0	0	5	405	—	223	—	—	—	—	87	—	—	—	—	—	—	—	—
2.1	0.3	26	272	172	74	32	1.1	0	10	72	0.14	0	0.01	0.1	0	0.02	2	0.48
—	—	20	253	—	35	—	—	0.4	—	87	—	1	—	—	—	—	—	—
2.1	0.3	26	272	172	4	32	1.1	0	10	72	0.14	0	0.01	0.1	0	0.02	2	0.48
0	0	5	405	—	223	—	—	—	—	87	—	—	—	—	—	—	—	—
2	0.3	25	259	163	70	30	1	0	10	68	0.14	0	0.01	0.1	0	0.02	2	0.45
2	0.2	29	198	142	213	18	1	0.1	4	82	0.2	0	0.02	0.1	0.1	0.02	6	0.6
0	0	5	150	—	420	—	—	0.4	—	57	—	1	—	—	—	—	—	—
0	0	1	56	44	22	72	0.3	0	5	1	0	0	0.01	0.06	0	0.01	3	0.17
—	—	0	126	219	16	—	—	2.7	—	5	—	49	0.55	0.6	7.1	—	—	0
0	0	0	12	10	1	101	—	0.2	—	0	0.1	0	0	0	0	—	—	0
0	0	0	13	12	9	119	0.1	1.6	7	91	0.16	2	0.02	0.05	0.2	0.06	10	0
0	0	0	13	12	9	120	0.1	1.7	7	92	0.16	3	0.02	0.05	0.2	0.05	10	0
0.1	0.1	0	10	12	1	96	0.1	0.4	7	67	0.1	1	0.03	0.03	0.1	0.05	3	0
0.1	0.1	0	12	12	2	134	0.1	0.2	7	99	0.1	8	0.02	0.03	0.3	0.03	6	0
0.1	0.1	0	12	23	4	186	0.1	0.4	12	19	0.08	5	0.03	0.05	0.5	0.04	5	0
0	0	0	18	28	4	164	0.1	0.7	15	16	0.12	3	0.02	0.03	0.5	0.04	5	0
0.2	0.2	0	10	13	0	152	0	0.3	7	14	0.09	5	0.03	0.04	0.3	0.05	3	0
0	0.1	0	16	21	1	258	0.1	0.5	13	25	0.17	1	0.04	0.06	0.2	0.05	5	0.02
13.2	7.3	0	157	284	592	223	0.3	3.7	20	305	5.26	3	0.27	0.27	2.2	0.09	16	0.01
2.5	1.8	0	26	23	74	154	0.2	2.1	11	150	0.93	3	0.06	0.08	0.6	0.06	11	0
5.1	3.1	0	8	28	212	58	0.2	1.6	7	27	1.09	1	0.14	0.11	1.2	0.02	6	0
0	0	0	2	1	0	8	0	0.1	0	1	0	0	0	0	0	0	0	0
0.1	0.1	0	3	19	1	87	0.2	0.3	16	4	0.11	7	0.03	0.08	0.2	0.08	13	0
0.2	0.1	0	5	27	1	127	0.2	0.4	24	6	0.17	10	0.04	0.05	0.2	0.12	19	0
0.2	0.1	0	5	29	1	135	0.3	0.4	26	0	0.17	11	0.04	0.03	0.4	0.12	20	0
0.1	0.2	0	13	28	8	203	0.1	0.5	15	1	0.2	8	0.04	0.03	0.2	0.07	11	0
0.1	0.1	0	5	11	1	137	0.1	0.3	9	1	0.2	11	0.04	0	0.3	0.1	16	0
0.3	0.3	0	10	38	1	212	0.2	0.3	12	1	0.43	9	0.09	0.06	0.5	0.18	25	0
1.1	1.2	0	42	153	3	847	0.8	1.3	47	3	1.72	37	0.35	0.25	1.9	0.71	100	0
2.6	0.7	0	10	53	288	76	0.6	7	18	4	0.07	14	0.44	0.14	4.8	0.44	0	3.52
2.1	2.1	0	150	171	11	292	1.5	2.8	22	1	—	4	0.25	0.05	1.6	0.2	32	0
4	2.2	47	55	125	503	151	1	1.1	17	24	0.37	1	0.11	0.15	4.8	0.15	5	0.16
7.1	3.5	96	26	247	600	149	1.5	2.2	26	10	—	0	0.05	0.17	4.3	0.19	10	0.25
0.1	0.1	8	1	7	2	4	0.2	0.3	1	0	0.05	0	0	0.02	0.1	0.01	3	0.24
7.1	3.4	59	13	278	494	294	1	0.9	24	0	1.35	0	0.11	0.15	7.2	0.3	30	0.3
4.4	4.3	138	189	317	767	463	2.3	2.1	44	146	1.84	9	0.15	0.33	8.2	0.36	18	0.43
6.4	1.6	45	12	150	399	185	0.8	0.9	15	22	1.46	0	0.07	0.1	5	0.23	8	0.22
—	—	40	20	—	950	—	—	1.1	—	200	—	0	—	—	3.3	0.34	8	0.19
4.5	15.8	48	16	80	201	138	0.8	0.6	11	31	6.27	1	0.03	0.07	8.7	0.46	13	0.28
1	0.9	80	27	199	1866	309	1.9	1.8	36	16	0.35	3	0.08	0.2	4.6	0.24	7	0.15
0.6	0.5	43	14	105	991	164	1	0.9	19	8	0.18	2	0.04	0.1	4.4	0.2	5	0.18
3.3	2.1	54	15	102	57	146	1.6	1	14	17	0.34	0	0.06	0.15	2.8	0.14	3	0.12
1.9	1.2	36	10	66	38	95	1.1	0.6	9	11	0.11	0	0.03	0.09				

Food Item	Qty	Meas	Wgt (g)	Wtr (g)	Cals	Prot	Carb (g)	Fib (g)	Fat (g)	SatF (g)
Chicken, back, w/skin, flour fried	1	each	72	32	238	20	5	0.1	15	4
Chicken, back, w/skin, roasted	1	each	53	28	159	14	0	0	11	3.1
Chicken, breast meat, skinless, stewed	1	each	95	65	143	28	0	0	3	0.8
Chicken, breast w/skin, roasted	1	each	98	61	193	29	0	0	8	2.2
Chicken, breast, skinless, fried	1	each	86	52	161	29	0	0	4	1.1
Chicken, breast, skinless, roasted	1	each	86	56	142	27	0	0	3	0.9
Chicken, breast, w/skin, flour fried	1	each	98	56	218	31	2	0.1	9	2.4
Chicken, breast, w/skin, stewed	1	each	110	73	202	30	0	0	8	2.3
Chicken, canned in water, Swanson	0.5	cup	124	94	131	24	2	0	2	1.1
Chicken, canned, diced, dark meat	0.5	cup	102	70	169	22	0	0	8	2.3
Chicken, canned, diced, light & dark meat	0.5	cup	102	70	169	22	0	0	8	2.3
Chicken, canned, diced, light meat	0.5	cup	102	70	169	22	0	0	8	2.3
Chicken, dark meat, skinless, fried	4	oz.	113	63	271	33	3	0	13	3.5
Chicken, dark meat, skinless, roasted	4	oz.	113	72	232	31	0	0	11	3
Chicken, drumstick, batter fried	1	each	72	38	193	16	6	0.2	11	3
Chicken, drumstick, flour fried	1	each	49	28	120	13	1	0	7	1.8
Chicken, drumstick, roasted	1	each	52	33	112	14	0	0	6	1.6
Chicken, drumstick, skinless, fried	1	each	42	26	82	12	0	0	3	0.9
Chicken, drumstick, skinless, roasted	1	each	44	29	76	12	0	0	2	0.7
Chicken, fried, dark meat, 2 piece serving	1	each	148	72	431	30	16	0.9	27	7
Chicken, fried, white meat, 2 piece serving	1	each	163	74	494	36	20	1.1	30	7.8
Chicken, gizzard, simmered	1	each	22	15	34	6	0	0	1	0.2
Chicken, light meat, skinless, fried	4	oz.	113	68	218	37	0	0	6	1.7
Chicken, light meat, skinless, roasted	4	oz.	113	74	196	35	0	0	5	1.4
Chicken, liver pate, canned	0.5	cup	104	68	209	14	7	0.2	14	4.2
Chicken, liver, simmered	7	each	140	96	220	34	1	0	8	2.6
Chicken, meat, all types, skinless, fried	4	oz.	113	65	248	35	2	0.1	10	2.8
Chicken, meat, all types, skinless, roasted	4	oz.	113	72	215	33	0	0	8	2.3
Chicken, meat, all types, skinless, stewed	0.5	cup	70	47	124	19	0	0	5	1.3
Chicken, roaster, skinless, roasted	4	oz.	113	76	189	28	0	0	8	2
Chicken, skinless, stewed	0.5	cup	70	40	166	21	0	0	8	2.2
Chicken, stewer w/giblets, cooked	1	each	593	322	1636	157	0	0	107	29.1
Chicken, thigh, skinless, fried	1	each	52	31	113	15	1	0	5	1.4
Chicken, thigh, skinless, roasted	1	each	52	33	109	14	0	0	6	1.6
Chicken, thigh, w/skin, flour fried	1	each	62	34	162	17	2	0.1	9	2.5
Chicken, thigh, w/skin, roasted	1	each	62	37	153	16	0	0	10	2.7
Chicken, whole, roasted	1	each	598	356	1429	163	0	0	81	22.7
Chicken, whole, stewed	1	each	668	427	1462	165	0	0	84	23.4
Chicken, wing, flour fried	1	each	32	16	103	8	1	0	7	1.9
Chicken, wing, skinless, fried	1	each	20	12	42	6	0	0	2	0.5
Chicken, wing, skinless, roasted	1	each	21	13	43	6	0	0	2	0.5
Chicken, wing, w/skin, roasted	3	each	102	56	296	27	0	0	20	5.6
Chicken, wings, buffalo type/spicy	1	piece	16	8	49	4	0	0	3	0.9
Chile, banana, cooked	4	oz.	113	101	17	1	4	1.8	0	—
Chile, banana, raw	0.5	cup	75	68	10	1	3	1	0	—
Chiles rellenos	1	each	143	75	425	23	7	1	35	17
Chili & beans, canned	1	cups	255	193	286	15	30	11.2	14	6
Chili pepper, dried, Foran Spice	0.5	gram	0	0	2	0	0	0.1	0	—
Chilies, green, canned, Santiago	1	each	62	58	13	0	3	0.7	0	0
Chilies, green, whole, Old El Paso	1	each	35	33	10	0	2	1	0	0
Chimichanga, beef	1	each	174	88	425	20	43	2	20	8.5
Chimichanga, beef & bean	1	each	118	68	249	11	26	3.1	12	3.4
Chocolate chips, milk chocolate	0.25	cup	42	1	218	3	25	1.4	13	7.9
Chocolate chips, semi-sweet	0.25	cup	42	0	204	2	27	2.5	13	7.6
Chocolate, baking, unsweetened, square	1	each	28	0	148	3	8	4.4	16	9.2
Chocolate, bittersweet, square	1	each	28	1	135	2	13	0.9	11	6.3
Chow mein entree, chicken, Chun King	1	each	369	292	370	16	45	4	14	5
Chow mein, chicken, canned	1	cup	250	222	95	6	18	2	1	0
Chow mein, pork, no noodles	0.5	cup	110	83	144	11	6	1.2	8	2.2
Chowder, Manhattan clam, chunky, RTS	0.5	cup	120	103	67	4	9	1.4	2	1.1
Chowder, Manhattan clam, w/water	0.5	cup	122	112	39	1	6	0.7	1	0.2
Chowder, New England clam, w/milk	0.5	cup	124	106	82	5	8	0.7	3	1.5
Chowder, New England clam, w/water	0.5	cup	122	110	48	2	6	0.7	1	0.2
Chowder, fish/seafood	0.5	cup	122	100	98	12	6	0.3	3	1.5
Chutney	1	Tbs	17	10	26	0	7	0.4	0	0

MonoF (g)	PolyF (g)	Choles (mg)	Calc (mg)	Phos (mg)	Sod (mg)	Pot (mg)	Zn (mg)	Iron (mg)	Magn (mg)	VitA (μg RE)	VitE (μg α-TE)	VitC (mg)	Thia (mg)	Ribo (mg)	Nia (mg)	B6 (mg)	Fola (μg)	B12 (μg)
5.9	3.5	64	17	120	65	163	1.8	1.2	17	27	0.6	0	0.08	0.17	5.3	0.22	11	0.2
4.4	2.4	47	11	82	46	111	1.2	0.8	11	52	0.14	0	0.03	0.1	3.6	0.14	3	0.14
1	0.6	73	12	157	60	178	0.9	0.8	23	6	0.25	0	0.04	0.11	8	0.31	3	0.22
3	1.6	82	14	210	70	240	1	1	26	26	0.26	0	0.06	0.12	12.4	0.55	4	0.31
1.5	0.9	78	14	212	68	237	0.9	1	27	6	0.36	0	0.07	0.11	12.7	0.55	3	0.32
1.1	0.7	73	13	196	64	220	0.9	0.9	25	5	0.23	0	0.06	0.1	11.8	0.52	3	0.29
3.4	1.9	87	16	228	74	254	1.1	1.2	29	15	0.56	0	0.08	0.13	13.4	0.57	6	0.33
3.2	1.7	82	14	172	68	196	1.1	1	24	26	0.29	0	0.04	0.13	8.6	0.32	3	0.23
—	—	54	0	—	500	—	—	0	—	0	—	0	—	—	—	—	—	—
3.2	1.8	64	14	114	516	141	1.4	1.6	12	35	0.22	2	0.02	0.13	6.5	0.36	4	0.3
3.2	1.8	64	14	114	516	141	1.4	1.6	12	35	0.22	2	0.02	0.13	6.5	0.36	4	0.3
3.2	1.8	64	14	114	516	141	1.4	1.6	12	35	0.22	2	0.02	0.13	6.5	0.36	4	0.3
4.9	3.1	109	20	212	110	287	3.3	1.7	28	27	0.66	0	0.1	0.28	8	0.42	10	0.37
4	2.6	105	17	203	105	272	3.2	1.5	26	25	0.3	0	0.08	0.26	7.4	0.41	9	0.36
4.6	2.7	62	12	106	194	134	1.7	1	14	19	0.88	0	0.08	0.16	3.7	0.19	13	0.2
2.7	1.6	44	6	86	44	112	1.4	0.7	11	12	0.41	0	0.04	0.11	3	0.17	5	0.16
2.2	1.3	47	6	91	47	119	1.5	0.7	12	16	0.14	0	0.04	0.11	3.1	0.18	4	0.17
1.2	0.8	40	5	78	40	105	1.4	0.6	10	8	0.21	0	0.03	0.1	2.6	0.16	4	0.15
0.8	0.6	41	5	81	42	108	1.4	0.6	11	8	0.12	0	0.03	0.1	2.7	0.17	4	0.15
10.9	6.3	166	36	240	755	445	3.2	1.6	37	67	1.33	0	0.13	0.43	7.2	0.33	25	0.83
12.2	6.8	148	60	306	975	566	1.6	1.5	38	59	1.52	0	0.15	0.29	12	0.57	29	0.67
0.2	0.2	43	2	34	15	39	1	0.9	4	12	0.26	0	0.01	0.05	0.9	0.03	12	0.43
2.2	1.4	102	18	262	92	298	1.4	1.3	33	10	0.34	0	0.08	0.14	15.2	0.71	5	0.41
1.8	1.1	96	17	245	87	280	1.4	1.2	31	10	0.3	0	0.07	0.13	14.1	0.68	5	0.39
5.5	2.6	407	10	182	401	99	2.2	9.6	14	226	1.02	10	0.05	1.46	7.8	0.27	334	8.4
1.9	1.3	883	20	437	71	196	6.1	11.9	29	6878	2.02	22	0.21	2.45	6.2	0.81	1078	27.2
3.8	2.4	107	19	232	103	291	2.5	1.5	31	20	0.52	0	0.1	0.22	11	0.54	8	0.39
3	1.9	101	17	221	98	276	2.4	1.4	28	18	0.3	0	0.08	0.2	10.4	0.53	7	0.37
1.7	1.1	58	10	105	49	126	1.4	0.8	15	10	0.19	0	0.03	0.11	4.3	0.18	4	0.15
2.8	1.7	85	14	218	85	260	1.7	1.4	24	14	0.47	0	0.07	0.17	8.9	0.46	6	0.33
2.8	2	58	9	143	55	141	1.4	1	15	23	0.21	0	0.08	0.19	4.5	0.22	4	0.18
40.5	23.8	605	77	1079	421	1049	12	10.9	119	1630	2.09	3	0.55	1.8	33.4	1.54	213	5.93
2	1.3	53	7	103	49	135	1.4	0.8	14	11	0.3	0	0.05	0.13	3.7	0.2	5	0.17
2.2	1.3	49	6	95	46	124	1.3	0.7	12	10	0.14	0	0.04	0.12	3.4	0.18	4	0.16
3.6	2.1	60	9	116	55	147	1.6	0.9	16	18	0.52	0	0.06	0.15	4.3	0.2	7	0.19
3.8	2.1	58	7	108	52	138	1.5	0.8	14	30	0.16	0	0.04	0.13	4	0.19	4	0.18
31.9	17.8	526	90	1088	490	1333	11.6	7.5	138	281	1.58	0	0.38	1	50.8	2.39	30	1.79
32.9	18.3	521	87	929	448	1108	11.8	7.8	127	281	1.77	0	0.31	0.99	37.3	1.47	33	1.34
2.8	1.6	26	5	48	25	57	0.6	0.4	6	12	0.18	0	0.02	0.04	2.1	0.13	2	0.09
0.6	0.4	17	3	33	18	42	0.4	0.2	4	4	0.06	0	0.01	0.03	1.4	0.12	1	0.07
0.5	0.4	18	3	35	19	44	0.4	0.2	4	4	0.06	0	0.01	0.03	1.5	0.12	1	0.07
7.8	4.2	86	15	154	84	188	1.9	1.3	19	48	0.27	0	0.04	0.13	6.8	0.43	3	0.3
1.4	0.8	13	2	24	30	29	0.3	0.2	3	9	0.12	0	0.01	0.02	1	0.07	0	0.04
—	—	0	23	—	5	255	0.5	0.5	19	10	—	136	0.06	0.04	0.7	—	—	0
—	—	0	16	—	3	188	0.3	0.3	14	8	—	113	0.04	0.03	0.5	—	—	0
10.2	5.4	165	595	409	620	337	2.8	1.6	39	641	1.84	88	0.07	0.46	0.8	0.22	29	0.54
5.9	0.9	43	120	393	1331	931	5.1	8.8	115	87	1.87	4	0.12	0.27	0.9	0.34	58	0
—	—	0	0	2	0	10	—	0	—	26	—	0	0	0.01	0.1	—	—	0
0	0.1	0	39	9	122	77	—	0.8	—	35	—	23	0.01	0.01	0.3	0.3	—	0
0	0	0	0	—	230	—	—	—	—	20	—	9	—	—	—	—	—	0
8.1	1.1	9	63	124	910	586	5	4.5	63	16	—	5	0.49	0.64	5.8	0.28	84	1.51
4.9	2.3	24	46	132	242	386	1.8	2.6	34	40	1.73	9	0.2	0.17	2.8	0.18	55	0.69
4.2	0.5	9	81	92	35	164	0.6	0.6	26	23	0.53	0	0.03	0.13	0.1	0.02	3	0.17
4.2	0.4	0	14	56	5	155	0.7	1.3	49	1	0.51	0	0.02	0.04	0.2	0.02	1	0
5.2	0.5	0	21	118	4	236	1.1	1.8	88	3	0.35	0	0.02	0.05	0.3	0.03	2	0
4.2	0.2	0	16	80	1	174	1.1	1.4	28	3	0.35	0	0.01	0.05	0.3	0.01	3	0
—	—	45	40	200	2010	260	—	1.4	—	100	—	9	1.5	0.17	3	—	—	—
0.1	0.8	8	45	85	725	418	1.3	1.2	14	28	0.05	12	0.05	0.1	1	0.09	12	0.05
3.7	1.9	28	24	113	385	264	1.2	0.9	20	77	1.07	12	0.32	0.17	2.4	0.22	20	0.24
0.5	0.1	7	34	42	500	192	0.8	1.3	10	164	0.05	6	0.03	0.03	0.9	0.13	5	3.96
0.2	0.6	1	13	21	289	94	0.5	0.8	6	49	0.37	2	0.02	0.02	0.4	0.05	5	2.03
1.1	0.5	11	93	78	496	150	0.4	0.7	11	20	0.07	2	0.03	0.12	0.5	0.06	5	5.12
0.6	0.5	2	22	27	458	73	0.4	0.7	4	0	0.04	1	0.01	0.02	0.5	0.04	2	4
1	0.3	30	73	146	251	351	0.5	0.3	24	22	0.19	4	0.08	0.13	1.4	0.18	8	0.61
0	0	0	5	7	38	65	0	0.2	4	8	0.1	3	0.01	0.01	0.1	0.02	2	0

Food Item	Qty	Meas	Wgt (g)	Wtr (g)	Cals	Prot	Carb (g)	Fib (g)	Fat (g)	SatF (g)
Citron, candied, chopped	2	Tbs	28	5	89	0	23	0.4	0	0
Citrus juice drink, Citrus Hill	1	cup	240	210	112	1	28	0.1	0	0
Clam nectar, canned	1	cup	240	234	5	1	0	0	0	0
Clam patty	1	each	120	33	429	24	40	1.2	18	4.4
Clam, baked/broiled, small	15	each	150	108	209	22	5	0	10	1.9
Cobbler, apple, piece, 3 x 3	1	piece	104	59	199	2	35	2.1	6	1.2
Cobbler, berry	1	cup	217	103	506	6	92	3.8	14	3.7
Cobbler, cherry	1	cup	217	120	430	5	78	2	12	3.1
Cobbler, cherry, piece, 3 x 3	1	piece	129	85	198	2	34	1.2	6	1.2
Cobbler, peach, piece, 3x3 in	1	piece	130	84	204	2	36	1.7	6	1.2
Cobbler, plum	1	cup	217	115	446	5	84	3	11	2.9
Cobbler, rhubarb	1	cup	217	93	548	5	102	2.9	15	3.6
Cocoa mix, prep w/water, sugar free	1	cup	250	231	62	5	11	0.5	0	0.3
Cocoa mix, w/water (fortified)	1	cup	279	237	159	3	32	1.1	4	2.4
Cocoa powder w/lowfat milk added	1	cup	250	205	186	8	30	1.2	5	3.1
Cocoa powder w/skim milk added	1	cup	250	208	152	8	30	1.2	1	0.6
Cocoa powder, dutch processed, unsweetened	1	Tbs	5	0	12	1	3	1.6	1	0.4
Cocoa powder, unsweetened	1	Tbs	5	0	12	1	3	1.8	1	0.4
Cocoa, baking type	1	oz.	28	1	85	6	16	11.3	3	0
Cocoa, dry, low fat	1	oz.	28	1	53	6	16	—	2	1.1
Cocoa, sugar free w/lowfat milk (Swiss Miss)	1	cup	250	218	136	9	14	1.5	6	3.3
Coconut cream, canned	0.5	cup	148	105	284	4	12	3.3	26	23.2
Coconut milk, raw	1	cup	240	162	552	6	13	5.3	57	50.6
Coconut water, raw	1	cup	240	228	46	2	9	2.6	0	0.4
Coconut, dried, sweetened, shredded	0.25	cup	23	3	116	1	11	1	8	7.3
Coconut, dried, toasted	1	oz.	28	0	168	2	13	1.8	13	11.8
Coconut, dried, unsweetened	0.25	cup	20	1	129	1	5	3.2	13	11.2
Coconut, fresh, grated	0.25	cup	20	9	71	1	3	1.8	7	5.9
Coffee substitute, dry, prepared, Postum	1	cup	240	237	12	0	2	0	0	0
Coffee, brewed	1	cup	240	238	5	0	1	0	0	0
Coffee, brewed. decaffeinated	1	cup	240	238	5	0	1	0	0	0
Coffee, cappuccino, mix, prepared	1	cup	256	237	82	1	14	0	3	2.4
Coffee, chicory, instant, dry	1	Tbs	3	0	9	0	2	0	0	0
Coffee, chicory, instant, prepared	1	cup	239	236	10	0	2	0	0	0
Coffee, decaffeinated, instant, prepared	1	cup	239	236	5	0	1	0	0	0
Coffee, demi tasse	1	cup	240	238	5	0	1	0	0	0
Coffee, espresso	1	cup	240	238	5	0	1	0	0	0
Coffee, espresso, decaffeinated	1	cup	240	238	5	0	1	0	0	0
Coffee, french, mix, prepared	1	cup	252	237	76	1	9	0	5	3.9
Coffee, mocha, instant, dry	1	Tbs	9	0	38	0	6	0.1	1	1.2
Coffee, mocha, mix, prepared	1	cup	251	236	68	1	11	0.3	3	2.2
Coffee, prepared from instant	1	cup	240	238	5	0	1	0	0	0
Coffee, swiss mocha, mix, prepared	1	cup	251	235	67	1	11	0.2	2	2.2
Coffee, vending machine, creamer	1	each	180	174	27	0	3	0	2	1.5
Coffee, vending machine, sugared	1	each	180	172	28	0	7	0	0	0
Coffee, vending machine, sugared, creamed	1	each	180	168	51	0	9	0	2	1.4
Coleslaw salad	0.5	cup	60	44	89	1	8	1	7	1
Collard greens, cooked, no added salt	0.5	cup	64	59	17	1	3	1.8	0	0
Collard greens, frozen, cooked, no added salt	0.5	cup	85	75	31	3	6	2.4	0	0.1
Consomme, beef, w/gelatin, prep w/water	0.5	cup	120	116	14	3	1	0	0	0
Cookie crust, chocolate, recipe, baked	1	each	219	12	1130	11	122	3.4	69	15
Cookie dough, chocolate chip, refrigerated	4	each	48	6	213	2	30	0.7	10	3.2
Cookie mix, oatmeal, dry	8	oz.	227	12	1047	15	153	6.4	44	10.8
Cookie mix, oatmeal, dry, prepared	2	each	32	2	148	2	21	1.2	6	1.6
Cookie, Fig bar	4	each	56	9	195	2	40	2.6	4	0.6
Cookie, Ladyfinger	2	each	22	4	80	2	13	0.2	2	0.7
Cookie, Nilla wafers	7	each	28	—	124	1	21	0.4	4	0.9
Cookie, almond	2	each	20	1	104	2	10	0.5	6	1
Cookie, animal, small box	1	each	67	3	299	4	50	—	9	3.5
Cookie, apple filled oatmeal, Archway	1	each	28	4	111	1	18	0.6	4	0.8
Cookie, applesauce, large	2	each	36	6	133	2	23	1.1	4	0.9
Cookie, apricot filled, Archway	1	each	28	4	112	1	18	0.4	4	1.5
Cookie, blueberry filled, Archway	1	each	28	—	110	1	19	0.5	4	1.5
Cookie, butter, commercially prepared	5	each	25	1	117	2	17	0.2	5	2.8
Cookie, butterscotch brownie	1	each	34	4	149	2	22	0.3	7	1.2

MonoF (g)	PolyF (g)	Choles (mg)	Calc (mg)	Phos (mg)	Sod (mg)	Pot (mg)	Zn (mg)	Iron (mg)	Magn (mg)	VitA (µg RE)	VitE (µg α-TE)	VitC (mg)	Thia (mg)	Ribo (mg)	Nia (mg)	B6 (mg)	Fola (µg)	B12 (µg)
0	0	0	24	7	82	34	—	0.2	—	0	—	0	0	0	0	0	—	0
0	0	0	316	20	4	196	0.1	0.2	17	1	0.07	80	0.06	0.03	0.3	0.06	5	0
0	0	7	31	274	516	358	0.2	0.7	26	22	2.4	2	0.02	0.05	0.4	0.02	5	12
7.5	4.8	117	191	336	567	496	2.4	21.2	24	168	2.57	12	0.37	0.56	4.6	0.11	29	56.7
4.1	3.3	60	84	299	622	556	2.4	24.5	16	253	3.16	22	0.13	0.3	2.9	0.1	27	82.4
2.8	2	1	22	30	288	106	0.2	0.8	6	76	1.11	0	0.1	0.09	0.7	0.04	3	0.04
5.8	3.6	4	141	105	347	189	0.5	2	19	18	2.35	12	0.29	0.28	2.4	0.06	12	0.06
5	3	3	118	86	354	195	0.4	3.4	18	106	1.29	2	0.21	0.23	1.8	0.08	12	0.05
2.8	2	1	28	34	294	133	0.2	1.8	9	135	1.01	2	0.1	0.11	0.8	0.05	9	0.04
2.8	1.9	1	24	40	291	159	0.2	0.9	10	105	1.16	3	0.09	0.09	1.2	0.03	6	0.04
4.9	2.7	3	107	85	258	291	0.4	1.5	20	42	1.74	10	0.24	0.3	2.2	0.12	8	0.05
6.2	4	3	184	89	408	356	0.4	1.9	24	83	1.84	6	0.24	0.23	2.1	0.04	11	0.05
0.2	0	2	118	175	225	528	0.7	1	42	0	0.08	0	0.05	0.27	0.2	0.06	3	0.38
1.3	0.1	0	139	148	276	541	0.4	2.4	31	201	0.11	8	0.2	0.23	2.7	0.05	0	0.56
1.5	0.2	17	287	245	158	476	1.2	0.8	52	131	0.24	2	0.1	0.41	0.3	0.1	13	0.84
0.3	0	4	291	258	162	502	1.2	0.7	46	140	0.18	2	0.09	0.35	0.3	0.1	13	0.87
0.2	0	0	6	39	1	135	0.3	0.8	26	0	0.02	0	0.01	0.02	0.1	0.01	2	0
0.2	0	0	7	40	1	82	0.4	0.7	27	0	0.02	0	0	0.01	0.1	0.01	2	0
0.9	0.1	0	0	—	0	493	—	2	—	0	—	0	0.05	0.07	0.7	—	—	—
0.9	0.2	0	43	213	2	431	—	3	—	0	—	0	0.03	0.13	0.7	—	—	—
1.6	0.3	18	303	268	160	495	1.3	0.8	56	140	0.22	2	0.1	0.44	0.3	0.12	14	0.9
1.1	0.3	0	1	33	74	149	0.9	0.8	25	0	1.08	3	0.03	0.06	0.1	0.04	21	0
2.4	0.6	0	38	240	36	631	1.6	3.9	89	0	1.75	7	0.06	0	1.8	0.08	39	0
0	0	0	58	48	252	600	0.2	0.7	60	0	0	6	0.07	0.14	0.2	0.08	6	0
0.4	0.1	0	3	25	61	78	0.4	0.4	12	0	0.31	0	0.01	0	0.1	0.06	2	0
0.6	0.1	0	8	60	10	157	0.6	1	26	0	0.28	0	0.02	0.03	0.2	0.09	3	0
0.5	0.1	0	5	40	7	106	0.4	0.6	18	0	0.26	0	0.01	0.02	0.1	0.06	2	0
0.3	0.1	0	3	23	4	71	0.2	0.5	6	0	0.15	1	0.01	0	0.1	0.01	5	0
0	0	0	7	17	10	58	0.1	0.1	10	0	0	0	0.02	0	0.5	0.03	1	0
0	0	0	5	2	5	130	0	0.1	12	0	0	0	0	0	0.5	0	0	0
0	0	0	5	2	5	130	0	0.1	12	0	0	0	0	0	0.5	0	0	0
0.2	0.1	0	10	36	138	159	0.1	0.2	13	0	0.1	0	0.02	0.01	0.4	0	0	0
0	0	0	3	7	7	92	0	0.1	6	0	0	0	0	0.01	0.6	0	0	0
0	0	0	7	7	14	81	0.1	0.1	7	0	0	0	0	0.01	0.5	0	0	0
0	0	0	7	7	7	84	0.1	0.1	10	0	0	0	0	0.03	0.7	0	0	0
0	0	0	5	2	5	130	0	0.1	12	0	0	0	0	0	0.5	0	0	0
0	0	0	5	2	5	130	0	0.1	12	0	0	0	0	0	0.5	0	0	0
0	0	0	5	2	5	130	0	0.1	12	0	0	0	0	0	0.5	0	0	0
0.3	0.1	0	10	55	40	181	0	0	3	0	0	0	0	0	0.9	0	0	0
0.1	0	0	3	22	23	89	0.1	0.2	6	0	0	0	0	0	0.2	0	0	0
0.1	0	0	10	38	48	158	0.2	0.3	12	0	0.02	0	0	0	0.3	0	0	0
0	0	0	7	7	7	86	0.1	0.1	10	0	0	0	0	0	0.7	0	0	0
0.1	0	0	10	38	48	158	0.2	0.3	13	0	0	0	0	0	0.3	0	0	0
0	0	0	6	22	14	72	0.1	0.1	5	1	0.01	0	0	0.01	0.3	0	0	0
0	0	0	5	3	6	35	0.1	0.1	5	0	0	0	0	0	0.3	0	0	0
0	0	0	6	21	13	70	0.1	0.1	5	1	0.01	0	0	0.01	0.3	0	0	0
1.5	3.9	3	20	22	162	107	0.1	0.4	5	30	2.4	5	0.02	0.02	0	0.07	23	0.11
0	0.1	0	76	17	6	166	0.3	0.3	11	200	0.56	12	0.03	0.07	0.4	0.08	60	0
0	0.2	0	179	23	42	213	0.2	1	26	508	0.42	22	0.04	0.1	0.5	0.1	65	0
0	0	0	5	16	318	77	0.2	0.3	0	0	0.01	0	0.01	0.01	0.4	0.01	1	0
32.9	17.2	4	68	234	1502	374	1.8	6.7	90	488	—	0	0.34	0.46	4.8	0	0	0.04
5	1	12	12	33	100	86	0.2	1.1	12	8	1.11	0	0.09	0.09	1	0.02	27	0.04
24	6.3	0	57	370	1072	415	1.8	5	109	5	5.9	0	0.32	0.32	3	0.1	113	0
3.4	0.9	13	9	56	150	60	0.3	0.7	15	7	0.9	0	0.09	0.05	0.4	0.02	4	0.03
1.7	1.6	0	36	35	196	116	0.2	1.6	15	2	0.7	0	0.09	0.12	1	0.04	15	0.05
0.9	0.3	80	10	38	32	25	0.3	0.8	3	37	0.28	1	0.06	0.09	0.5	0.03	17	0.16
1.3	0	2	18	—	89	27	—	1	—	—	—	—	—	—	—	—	—	—
3.2	1.8	9	15	34	49	42	0.2	0.5	14	57	1.7	0	0.05	0.07	0.5	0.01	4	0.02
3.8	1	11	11	64	273	56	0.3	1.5	11	8	0.32	1	0.25	0.24	2.5	0.02	81	0.05
1.4	0.3	2	8	—	116	51	—	0.9	—	1	—	0	0.07	0.04	0.5	—	15	—
1.9	1.4	9	22	44	109	76	0.2	0.7	11	55	0.74	0	0.07	0.05	0.4	0.03	3	0.02
1.2	0.2	8	6	—	9	35	—	0.6	—	3	—	0	0.07	0.06	0.5	—	—	—
—	—	5	0	—	115	—	—	0.7	—	0	—	0	—	—	—	—	—	—
1.4	0.2	29	7	26	88	28	0.1	0.6	3	42	0.13	0	0.09	0.08	0.8	0.01	10	0.09
2.6	2.3	18	24	26	96	80	0.2	0.7	10	76	0.96	0	0.05	0.06	0.4	0.02	4	0.04

Food Item	Qty	Meas	Wgt (g)	Wtr (g)	Cals	Prot	Carb (g)	Fib (g)	Fat (g)	SatF (g)
Cookie, carob	2	each	26	1	103	2	17	1.6	4	0.8
Cookie, chocolate brownie, fat-free, Entenmann's	1	each	12	1	40	0	10	0.5	0	0
Cookie, chocolate chip, Archway	3	each	27	—	130	1	17	0	7	2
Cookie, chocolate chip, commercial	1	each	10	0	45	1	7	0.4	2	0.4
Cookie, chocolate chip, homemade, w/butter	2	each	32	2	156	2	19	0.8	9	4.5
Cookie, chocolate chip, homemade, w/margarine	2	each	20	1	98	1	12	0.6	6	1.6
Cookie, chocolate chip, mix, prepared	2	each	32	1	159	2	20	0.4	8	2.7
Cookie, chocolate chip, no sodium, w/fructose	4	each	28	1	126	1	21	0.4	5	1.2
Cookie, chocolate chip, refrigerated dough, baked	2	each	24	1	118	1	16	0.4	5	1.9
Cookie, chocolate chip, soft	2	each	21	2	96	1	12	0.7	5	1.6
Cookie, chocolate sandwich, Snackwell's	1	oz.	28	1	116	1	22	0.7	3	0.7
Cookie, chocolate sandwich, creme-filled	2	each	20	0	94	1	14	0.6	4	0.7
Cookie, chocolate sandwich, low sodium, w/fructose	3	each	30	1	138	1	20	1.2	7	1.2
Cookie, chocolate sandwich, w/chocolate icing	2	each	34	1	164	1	22	1.8	9	2.5
Cookie, chocolate sandwich, w/extra creme	2	each	26	0	130	1	18	0.5	7	1
Cookie, chocolate wafer	4	each	24	1	104	2	17	0.8	3	1
Cookie, cinnamon honey, fat free, Archway	3	each	30	3	106	1	25	0.4	0	0.1
Cookie, coconut macaroon, Archway	1	each	23	2	111	1	13	0.5	6	5.7
Cookie, coconut macaroon, recipe	1	each	24	3	97	1	17	0.4	3	2.7
Cookie, date filled oatmeal, Archway	1	each	28	4	111	1	19	0.8	3	0.8
Cookie, devil's food, Snackwell's	1	oz.	28	5	97	1	22	0.4	0	0
Cookie, double fudge, fat free, Snackwell's	1	oz.	28	4	94	1	21	0.5	0	0.2
Cookie, fortune	4	each	32	3	121	1	27	0.5	1	0.2
Cookie, fruit bar, no fat, Archway	1	each	28	—	90	2	21	0	0	0
Cookie, fudge cake type	1	each	21	2	73	1	16	0.6	1	0.2
Cookie, fudge, fat free, Snackwell's	2	each	32	5	106	2	24	0.6	0	0.2
Cookie, gingerbread, iced, Archway	3	each	32	1	149	1	23	0.4	6	1.8
Cookie, gingersnap	4	each	28	1	116	2	22	0.6	3	0.7
Cookie, graham cracker, chocolate-coated	2	each	28	1	136	2	19	0.9	6	3.8
Cookie, granola	2	each	26	1	119	2	17	1.1	4	3.7
Cookie, lemon bar	2	each	32	4	139	2	20	0.3	6	1.2
Cookie, marshmallow, chocolate-coated	2	each	26	3	109	1	18	0.5	4	1.2
Cookie, molasses	2	each	30	2	129	2	22	0.3	4	1
Cookie, molasses, old fashioned, Archway	1	each	28	3	113	1	20	0.3	3	0.8
Cookie, oatmeal	2	each	36	2	162	2	25	1	7	1.6
Cookie, oatmeal chocolate chip, fat free, Entenmann	1	each	12	—	40	0	10	0.5	0	0
Cookie, oatmeal raisin, Archway	1	each	28	—	110	2	19	0.5	4	1
Cookie, oatmeal raisin, fat free, Entenmann's	1	each	24	4	80	1	18	0.5	0	0
Cookie, oatmeal raisin, no fat, Archway	1	each	28	4	96	1	22	0.9	0	0.1
Cookie, oatmeal raisin, recipe	2	each	26	2	113	2	18	0.8	4	0.8
Cookie, oatmeal raisin, w/fructose, no sodium	4	each	28	2	126	1	20	0.8	5	0.8
Cookie, oatmeal w/raisins, dietetic	3	each	33	3	144	2	21	0.8	6	1.5
Cookie, oatmeal, Archway	1	each	27	3	115	2	18	0.8	4	0.9
Cookie, oatmeal, chilled dough, baked	2	each	24	1	113	1	16	0.7	5	1.3
Cookie, oatmeal, recipe	2	each	30	2	134	2	20	0.9	5	1.1
Cookie, oatmeal, soft	2	each	30	3	123	2	20	0.8	4	1.1
Cookie, oreo sandwich	2	each	28	—	138	2	20	0.9	6	1.3
Cookie, peanut butter sandwich	2	each	28	1	134	2	18	0.5	6	1.4
Cookie, peanut butter sandwich, low sodium, w/fructose	3	each	30	1	161	3	15	0.5	10	1.5
Cookie, peanut butter, Archway	1	each	28	2	134	3	16	0.8	7	1.5
Cookie, peanut butter, chilled dough, baked	2	each	24	1	121	2	14	0.3	7	1.5
Cookie, peanut butter, homemade	2	each	24	1	114	2	14	0.5	6	1.1
Cookie, peanut butter, soft type	2	each	30	3	137	2	17	0.5	7	1.8
Cookie, pecan sandies	2	each	30	1	149	2	20	0.5	7	1.8
Cookie, pecan shortbread	2	each	28	1	152	1	16	0.5	9	2.3
Cookie, raisin oatmeal, Archway	3	each	28	—	130	2	19	1	6	1.5
Cookie, raisin, soft type	2	each	30	4	120	1	20	0.4	4	1
Cookie, raspberry filled, Archway	1	each	28	4	113	1	18	0.4	4	1.5
Cookie, raspberry oatmeal, no fat, Archway	1	each	28	3	98	1	22	0.9	0	0.1
Cookie, sandwich-type, dietetic	3	each	33	4	151	2	18	0.3	8	2
Cookie, shortbread, commercial, plain	4	each	32	1	161	2	21	0.6	8	2
Cookie, shortbread, homemade, w/butter	2	each	28	1	155	2	16	0.4	9	5.8
Cookie, shortbread, homemade, w/margarine	3	each	33	1	180	2	19	0.5	11	2.1
Cookie, snickerdoodle	1	each	20	4	81	1	12	0.4	3	2.1
Cookie, sugar	2	each	30	1	143	2	20	0.2	6	1.6

MonoF	PolyF	Choles	Calc	Phos	Sod	Pot	Zn	Iron	Magn	VitA	VitE	VitC	Thia	Ribo	Nia	B6	Fola	B12
(g)	(g)	(mg)	(mg)	(mg)	(mg)	(mg)	(mg)	(mg)	(mg)	(µg RE)	(µg α-TE)	(mg)	(mg)	(mg)	(mg)	(mg)	(µg)	(µg)
2	1.4	16	70	59	80	140	0.4	0.6	17	7	0.7	0	0.04	0.09	0.5	0.05	6	0.08
0	0	0	0	—	45	62	—	0.4	—	0	—	0	—	—	—	—	—	—
—	—	10	0	—	70	—	—	0.7	—	0	—	0	—	—	—	—	—	—
0.6	0.5	0	2	8	38	12	0.1	0.3	3	0	0.18	0	0.03	0.03	0.3	0.03	7	0
2.6	1.4	22	12	32	109	71	0.3	0.8	18	47	0.29	0	0.06	0.06	0.4	0.03	11	0.03
2.1	1.7	6	8	20	72	45	0.2	0.5	11	33	0.57	0	0.04	0.04	0.3	0.02	7	0.02
4.2	0.9	13	15	30	94	68	0.2	0.7	12	6	0.83	0	0.05	0.07	0.6	0.01	3	0.03
1.9	1.4	0	13	30	3	56	0.1	1	6	0	0.69	0	0.1	0.05	0.8	0	13	0
2.7	0.6	6	7	18	56	48	0.1	0.6	6	4	0.49	0	0.04	0.05	0.5	0	2	0.02
2.7	0.7	0	3	10	68	20	0.1	0.5	7	0	0.61	0	0.02	0.04	0.3	0.03	8	0
0.8	0.2	0	16	58	217	45	0.2	0.8	13	0	—	0	0.04	0.05	0.6	0.01	—	0
1.7	1.4	0	5	20	121	35	0.2	0.8	9	0	0.69	0	0.02	0.04	0.4	0	9	0.01
2.8	2.4	0	29	60	73	88	0.2	1.4	8	0	1.13	0	0.16	0.09	1.2	0.01	19	0.01
5	1	0	12	31	111	82	0.2	1.1	13	0	1.13	0	0.03	0.07	0.5	0.02	6	0.02
2.8	2.4	0	6	24	128	32	0.2	0.7	9	0	1.17	0	0.02	0.04	0.4	0.01	11	0
1.2	1	0	7	32	139	50	0.3	1	13	1	0.38	0	0.05	0.06	0.7	0.01	12	0.02
0.1	0.1	0	6	—	123	20	—	0.8	—	0	—	0	0.1	0.06	0.8	—	24	—
0.4	0.1	0	4	—	40	6	—	0.4	—	0	—	0	0.01	0.01	0.1	—	1	—
0.1	0	0	2	10	59	37	0.2	0.2	5	0	0.07	0	0	0.03	0	0.02	1	0.01
1.3	0.3	4	10	—	110	59	—	0.6	—	1	—	0	0.07	0.05	0.5	—	—	—
0.2	0	0	9	22	48	30	0.1	0.4	6	0	—	0	0.03	0.04	0.4	0.01	—	0.02
0.1	0.1	0	5	20	125	47	0.1	0.5	9	0	0	0	0.03	0.03	0.5	0.01	—	0
0.4	0.1	1	4	11	88	13	0.1	0.5	2	0	0.11	0	0.06	0.04	0.6	0	18	0
0	0	0	0	—	95	—	—	0.4	—	0	0.01	0	—	—	—	—	—	—
0.4	0.1	0	7	17	40	29	0.1	0.5	7	0	0.12	0	0.05	0.04	0.3	0.01	9	0.02
0.1	0.1	0	6	22	141	53	0.2	0.6	10	0	0	0	0.03	0.04	0.5	0.01	—	0
1.9	0.7	0	7	—	114	22	—	0.1	—	0	—	0	0.06	0.09	0.8	—	22	—
1.5	0.4	0	22	23	183	97	0.2	1.8	14	0	0.36	0	0.06	0.08	0.9	0.03	20	0
2.2	0.3	0	16	38	82	58	0.3	1	16	0	0.32	0	0.04	0.06	0.6	0.02	5	0
0.3	0.1	0	18	93	86	94	0.4	0.8	26	0	0.03	0	0.16	0.06	0.5	0.09	21	0
2.6	1.8	25	12	22	78	22	0.1	0.5	3	83	1	1	0.06	0.07	0.4	0.01	4	0.05
2.4	0.5	0	12	25	44	47	0.2	0.7	9	0	0.56	0	0.02	0.05	0.2	0.02	5	0.04
2.1	0.5	0	22	28	138	104	0.1	1.9	16	0	0.51	0	0.11	0.08	0.9	0.03	22	0
1.2	0.2	9	10	—	148	32	—	1.3	—	3	—	0	0.08	0.07	0.7	—	—	—
3.6	0.9	0	13	50	138	51	0.3	0.9	12	1	0.91	0	0.1	0.08	0.8	0.02	16	0
0	0	0	0	—	55	40	—	0.2	—	0	—	0	—	—	—	—	—	—
—	—	2	0	—	115	—	—	1.1	—	0	—	0	—	—	—	—	—	—
0	0	0	0	—	120	60	—	0	—	0	—	0	—	—	—	—	—	—
0.1	0.2	0	10	—	149	79	—	0.9	—	0	—	0	0.07	0.04	0.5	—	13	—
1.8	1.3	9	26	42	140	62	0.2	0.7	11	43	0.65	0	0.06	0.04	0.3	0.02	8	0.02
2.1	1.9	0	15	34	3	49	0.1	1.1	5	0	0.9	0	0.13	0.06	0.9	0.01	15	0
2.6	1.6	1	7	46	1	55	0.3	0.7	9	0	0.82	0	0.08	0.03	0.3	0.01	4	0.04
1.5	0.4	3	8	—	94	50	—	0.6	—	1	—	0	0.08	0.05	0.5	—	—	—
2.8	0.7	6	8	28	78	39	0.2	0.6	8	3	0.72	0	0.05	0.04	0.4	0.01	2	0.01
2.3	1.7	11	32	50	179	55	0.3	0.8	13	55	0.81	0	0.08	0.05	0.4	0.02	10	0.03
2.4	0.7	2	27	63	105	40	0.1	0.8	9	2	0.6	0	0.06	0.07	0.5	0.03	10	0
2.6	0.4	0	—	—	189	52	—	0.6	—	—	—	—	—	—	—	—	—	—
3.1	1.1	0	15	53	103	54	0.3	0.7	14	0	0.91	0	0.09	0.07	1	0.04	12	0.06
4.6	3.6	0	13	46	124	88	0.3	0.8	15	0	1.72	0	0.1	0.04	1.6	0.02	16	0
2.9	1.2	10	10	—	113	59	—	0.8	—	3	—	0	0.07	0.06	1.2	—	—	—
3.5	1.2	7	27	63	105	81	0.2	0.4	10	3	0.96	0	0.04	0.04	1	0.02	2	0.01
2.6	1.7	7	9	28	124	55	0.2	0.5	9	37	0.91	0	0.05	0.05	0.8	0.02	13	0.02
4.1	1	0	4	26	101	32	0.2	0.3	10	0	1.17	0	0.07	0.05	0.6	0.01	20	0
3.9	0.9	10	21	47	18	20	0.1	0.9	5	7	0.89	0	0.14	0.08	0.9	0.01	3	0.02
5.2	1.2	9	8	24	79	20	0.2	0.7	5	0	1.06	0	0.08	0.06	0.7	0.01	18	0
—	—	10	0	—	55	—	—	0.7	—	0	—	0	—	—	—	—	—	—
2.3	0.5	1	14	25	101	42	0.1	0.7	6	0	0.58	0	0.06	0.06	0.6	0.02	13	0.01
1.2	0.2	8	7	—	94	35	—	0.6	—	2	—	0	0.09	0.06	0.5	—	—	—
0.2	0.2	0	11	—	150	80	—	0.9	—	0	—	0	0.08	0.04	0.5	—	13	—
3.6	2.2	0	12	21	4	32	0.2	0.4	10	0	1.32	0	0.05	0.05	0.4	0.01	2	0
4.3	1	6	11	35	146	32	0.2	0.9	5	4	1.03	0	0.11	0.1	1.1	0.03	19	0.03
2.7	0.4	25	5	20	132	20	0.1	0.7	4	87	0.23	0	0.1	0.07	0.8	0.01	3	0.01
4.8	3.5	0	7	23	169	25	0.1	0.9	4	114	1.65	0	0.12	0.08	1	0.01	4	0.01
1	0.2	9	8	10	74	24	0.1	0.5	2	32	0.1	0	0.05	0.04	0.4	0.01	2	0.02
3.5	0.8	15	6	24	107	19	0.1	0.6	4	8	0.85	0	0.07	0.06	0.8	0.02	14	0.06

Food Item	Qty	Meas	Wgt (g)	Wtr (g)	Cals	Prot	Carb (g)	Fib (g)	Fat (g)	SatF (g)
Cookie, sugar wafer, cream-filled w/fructose, no sodium	7	each	28	1	141	1	18	0.5	7	1.1
Cookie, sugar wafer, creme-filled	8	each	28	0	143	1	20	0.2	7	1
Cookie, sugar, Archway	1	each	28	—	120	2	20	0	4	1
Cookie, sugar, homemade, w/butter	2	each	28	2	132	2	17	0.4	7	4
Cookie, sugar, homemade, w/margarine	2	each	28	2	132	2	17	0.3	7	1.3
Cookie, sugar, no sodium, w/fructose	4	each	28	2	121	1	22	0.2	4	0.5
Cookie, sugar, refrigerated dough, baked	2	each	24	1	116	1	16	0.2	6	1.4
Cookie, sugar, soft, Archway	1	each	28	3	115	1	19	0.3	4	0.9
Cookie, sugar/plain, dietetic	5	each	30	3	139	1	18	0.1	7	1.4
Cookie, vanilla sandwich	3	each	30	1	145	1	22	0.4	6	0.9
Cookie, vanilla sandwich, Snackwell's	1	oz.	28	1	119	1	23	0.6	3	0.6
Cookie, vanilla wafer, Archway	5	each	30	—	130	2	22	0	4	1
Cookie, vanilla wafer, made w/egg	7	each	28	1	123	1	21	0.5	4	1.1
Cookie, vanilla wafer, no egg	4	each	24	1	114	1	17	0.5	5	1.2
Cookie, whole wheat fruit & nut	2	each	28	4	121	2	16	1.3	6	1
Cooking wine, red, Fleischmann's	1	Tbs	15	13	10	0	0	0	0	0
Cooking wine, white, Fleischmann's	1	Tbs	15	13	10	0	0	0	0	0
Coriander/cilantro, fresh	0.25	cup	4	4	1	0	0	0.1	0	0
Corn chips, BBQ flavor	10	piece	18	0	94	1	10	0.9	6	0.8
Corn chips/Fritos	1	cup	26	0	140	2	15	1.3	9	1.2
Corn cones, nacho flavor, Bugles	1	oz.	28	1	152	2	16	0.3	9	7.6
Corn cones, plain, Bugles	1	oz.	28	1	145	2	18	0.3	8	6.5
Corn grits, white, enriched, cooked	0.5	cup	121	103	73	2	16	0.2	0	0
Corn grits, white, packet, prepared	1	each	137	113	89	2	21	1.2	0	0
Corn grits, white, unenriched, cooked	0.5	cup	121	103	73	2	16	0.2	0	0
Corn grits, yellow, enriched, cooked	0.5	cup	121	103	73	2	16	0.2	0	0
Corn grits, yellow, enriched, dry	0.5	cup	78	8	289	7	62	1.2	1	0.1
Corn on cob, small, frozen, cooked	1	each	77	56	72	2	17	2.2	1	0.1
Corn w/sweet peppers, canned, w/liquid	0.5	cup	114	88	85	3	21	2.3	1	0.1
Corn, canned, not drained	0.5	cup	128	104	82	2	20	2.2	1	0.1
Corn, creamed, canned	0.5	cup	128	101	92	2	23	1.5	1	0.1
Corn, sweet, yellow, canned, drained	0.5	cup	82	63	66	2	15	1.6	1	0.1
Corn, white, canned, drained, salted	0.5	cup	82	63	66	2	15	1.6	1	0.1
Corn, white, cream style, canned, drained, salted	0.5	cup	128	101	92	2	23	1.5	1	0.1
Corn, white, cream style, canned, w/salt	0.5	cup	128	101	92	2	23	1.5	1	0.1
Corn, white, fresh, cooked	0.5	cup	82	57	89	3	21	2.2	1	0.2
Corn, white, kernel, frozen, cooked	0.5	cup	82	63	66	2	16	2	0	0.1
Corn, yellow, creamed, low sodium	0.5	cup	128	101	92	2	23	1.5	1	0.1
Corn, yellow, fresh, cooked	0.5	cup	82	57	89	3	21	2.3	1	0.2
Corn, yellow, frozen, cooked, no added salt	0.5	cup	82	63	66	2	16	2	0	0.1
Corn, yellow, on cob, cooked ear	1	each	77	54	83	3	19	2.2	1	0.2
Cornbread mix, dry, prepared	1	piece	60	19	188	4	29	1.4	6	1.6
Cornbread, dry, recipe, w/2% milk, 1/6th	1	piece	60	24	160	4	26	1.7	4	0.9
Cornbread, dry, recipe, w/whole milk, 1/9th	1	piece	65	25	176	4	28	2.3	5	1.2
Corndog (hotdog w/coating)	1	each	175	82	460	17	56	—	19	5.2
Corndog, chicken	1	each	113	59	272	13	26	—	13	—
Corned beef hash, canned	0.5	cup	110	74	199	10	12	0.6	12	6
Cornish game hen, whole, roasted (20 oz hen)	1	each	306	181	727	83	0	0	41	11.5
Cornmeal mush, fried slice	1	piece	51	32	84	2	15	0.8	2	0.4
Cornmeal mush, made w/milk	0.5	cup	120	80	180	7	25	1.2	6	3.3
Cornmeal, yellow, degermed, enriched	0.5	cup	69	8	253	6	54	5.1	1	0.2
Cornmeal, yellow, self rising, degermed	1	cup	138	14	490	12	103	9.8	2	0.3
Cornmeal, yellow, whole grain	0.5	cup	61	6	221	5	47	4.4	2	0.3
Cornnuts, BBQ flavor	10	piece	18	0	78	2	13	1.5	3	0.5
Cornnuts, plain	10	piece	18	0	79	2	13	1.2	3	0.5
Couscous, cooked	0.5	cup	90	65	100	3	21	1.2	0	0
Cowpea, catjang, dry, cooked	0.5	cup	86	60	101	7	18	3.1	1	0.2
Crab cake, blue crab	1	each	60	43	93	12	0	0	5	0.9
Crab imperial	0.5	cup	130	94	196	20	4	0.2	10	2.5
Crab salad	0.5	cup	104	76	142	14	6	0.3	7	1
Crab thermidor	0.5	cup	122	75	306	15	5	0.1	25	14.8
Crab, deviled	0.5	cup	88	54	171	11	12	0.7	9	1.8
Crabapple, raw, slices	0.5	cup	55	43	42	0	11	0.6	0	0
Cracker bread, Armenian/Ak Mak	4	piece	24	1	94	3	20	0.7	0	0
Cracker, Better Cheddar, low sodium	4	each	5	0	25	1	3	0	1	0.4

MonoF	PolyF	Choles	Calc	Phos	Sod	Pot	Zn	Iron	Magn	VitA	VitE	VitC	Thia	Ribo	Nia	B6	Fola	B12
(g)	(g)	(mg)	(mg)	(mg)	(mg)	(mg)	(mg)	(mg)	(mg)	(µg RE)	(µg α-TE)	(mg)	(mg)	(mg)	(mg)	(mg)	(µg)	(µg)
3	2.7	0	15	10	3	17	0.1	0.4	2	0	1.13	0	0.05	0.03	0.4	0	12	0
2.9	2.6	0	5	16	41	16	0.1	0.5	3	0	1.23	0	0.03	0.06	0.7	0	12	0
—	—	2	0	—	190	—	—	0.7	—	0	—	0	—	—	—	—	—	—
1.9	0.3	24	20	25	129	20	0.1	0.7	3	62	0.2	0	0.08	0.07	0.7	0.01	3	0.02
2.9	2	7	20	25	137	22	0.1	0.7	3	70	1.02	0	0.08	0.07	0.7	0.01	15	0.02
1.5	1.3	0	7	20	1	29	0.1	1.1	3	0	0.62	0	0.14	0.06	1	0	16	0
3.1	0.7	8	22	45	112	39	0.1	0.4	2	3	0.77	0	0.04	0.03	0.6	0.01	13	0.02
1.3	0.2	6	9	—	189	23	—	0.6	—	2	—	0	0.09	0.06	0.7	—	—	—
3.1	2.2	18	2	11	0	12	0.1	0.4	4	0	0.96	0	0.06	0.03	0.4	0.01	3	0.03
2.5	2.3	0	8	22	105	27	0.1	0.7	4	0	1.08	0	0.08	0.07	0.8	0	18	0
0.8	0.2	0	19	40	104	31	0.2	0.7	5	0	—	0	0.05	0.07	0.7	0.01	—	0.02
—	—	5	0	—	130	—	—	1.1	—	0	—	0	—	—	—	—	—	—
1.8	1.1	14	13	29	87	27	0.1	0.7	4	2	0.36	0	0.08	0.09	0.9	0.02	14	0.04
2.7	0.6	0	6	15	73	26	0.1	0.5	3	0	0.34	0	0.09	0.05	0.7	0.01	10	0.01
2.2	2.7	15	18	49	59	111	0.4	0.7	20	50	0.81	0	0.05	0.04	0.5	0.06	6	0.03
0	0	—	1	2	90	12	—	0.1	—	0	—	0	0.08	0.08	0.1	—	—	0
0	0	0	1	2	90	13	—	0.1	—	0	—	0	0.08	0.08	0.1	—	—	0
0	0	0	4	1	1	22	0	0.1	1	11	0.1	0	0	0	0	0	0	0
1.7	2.9	0	24	37	137	42	0.2	0.3	14	11	0.24	0	0.01	0.04	0.3	0.04	7	0
2.5	4.3	0	33	48	164	37	0.3	0.3	20	2	0.35	0	0.01	0.04	0.3	0.06	5	0
0.6	0.2	1	10	22	270	35	0.1	0.4	7	11	0.6	0	0.06	0.03	0.4	0.03	1	0
0.5	0.2	0	1	12	290	23	0.1	0.7	3	9	0.54	0	0.09	0.07	0.4	0.01	1	0
0.1	0.1	0	0	14	0	27	0.1	0.8	5	0	0.06	0	0.12	0.07	1	0.03	38	0
0	0.1	0	8	29	289	38	0.2	8.2	11	0	0.03	0	0.15	0.08	1.4	0.06	47	0
0.1	0.1	0	0	14	0	27	0.1	0.2	5	0	0.06	0	0.02	0.01	0.2	0.03	1	0
0.1	0.1	0	0	14	0	27	0.1	0.8	5	7	0.06	0	0.12	0.07	1	0.03	38	0
0.2	0.4	0	2	57	1	107	0.3	3	21	34	0.2	0	0.5	0.3	3.9	0.12	146	0
0.2	0.3	0	2	58	3	193	0.5	0.5	22	16	0.07	4	0.13	0.05	1.2	0.17	24	0
0.2	0.3	0	6	70	394	174	0.4	0.9	28	26	1.25	10	0.02	0.09	1.1	0.11	38	0
0.2	0.3	0	5	65	273	210	0.5	0.5	20	19	0.15	7	0.03	0.08	1.2	0.05	49	0
0.2	0.3	0	4	65	365	172	0.7	0.5	22	13	0.12	6	0.03	0.07	1.2	0.08	57	0
0.2	0.4	0	4	53	175	160	0.3	0.7	16	13	0.12	7	0.03	0.06	1	0.04	40	0
0.2	0.4	0	4	53	265	160	0.3	0.7	16	0	0.07	7	0.03	0.06	1	0.04	40	0
0.2	0.3	0	4	65	4	172	0.7	0.5	22	0	0.12	6	0.03	0.07	1.2	0.08	57	0
0.2	0.3	0	4	65	365	172	0.7	0.5	22	0	0.12	6	0.03	0.07	1.2	0.08	57	0
0.3	0.5	0	2	84	14	204	0.4	0.5	26	0	0.07	5	0.18	0.06	1.3	0.05	38	0
0.1	0.2	0	3	47	4	121	0.3	0.3	16	0	0.07	3	0.07	0.06	1.1	0.11	25	0
0.2	0.3	0	4	65	4	172	0.7	0.5	22	13	0.12	6	0.03	0.07	1.2	0.08	57	0
0.3	0.5	0	2	84	14	204	0.4	0.5	26	18	0.07	5	0.18	0.06	1.3	0.05	38	0
0.1	0.2	0	3	47	4	121	0.3	0.3	16	18	0.07	3	0.07	0.06	1.1	0.11	25	0
0.3	0.5	0	2	79	13	192	0.4	0.5	25	17	0.07	5	0.17	0.06	1.2	0.05	36	0
3.1	0.7	37	44	226	467	77	0.4	1.1	12	26	0.72	0	0.15	0.16	1.2	0.06	7	0.1
1.1	1.9	24	149	101	395	88	0.4	1.5	15	32	0.54	0	0.18	0.18	1.4	0.07	38	0.09
1.3	2.1	28	161	109	428	95	0.4	1.6	16	28	0.65	0	0.19	0.19	1.5	0.07	12	0.1
9.1	3.5	79	102	166	973	263	1.3	6.2	18	37	0.7	0	0.28	0.7	4.2	0.09	103	0.44
—	—	65	—	—	670	—	—	—	—	—	—	0	—	—	—	—	—	—
5.5	0.4	36	14	74	594	220	1.6	2.2	18	0	0.24	0	0.01	0.1	2.3	0.22	10	0.67
16.2	9	268	46	554	957	678	5.9	3.8	70	143	0.8	0	0.19	0.51	25.8	1.22	15	0.91
0.8	0.5	0	2	20	265	23	0.3	0.8	11	7	0.31	0	0.06	0.05	0.6	0.04	3	0
1.6	0.4	21	187	165	262	273	0.8	1	30	57	0.23	1	0.18	0.34	1.2	0.11	14	0.44
0.3	0.5	0	3	58	2	112	0.5	2.8	28	28	0.23	0	0.49	0.28	3.5	0.18	129	0
0.6	1	0	483	860	1860	235	1.4	6.5	68	57	0.28	0	0.94	0.53	6.3	0.54	258	0
0.6	1	0	4	147	21	175	1.1	2.1	78	29	0.41	0	0.24	0.12	2.2	0.18	16	0
1.3	0.6	0	3	51	176	52	0.3	0.3	20	6	0.18	0	0.06	0.03	0.3	0.03	0	0
1.3	0.6	0	2	50	99	50	0.3	0.3	20	0	0.18	0	0.01	0.02	0.3	0.04	0	0
0	0.1	0	7	20	4	52	0.2	0.3	7	0	0.01	0	0.06	0.02	0.9	0.05	13	0
0.1	0.3	0	22	122	16	323	1.6	2.6	83	1	0.32	0	0.14	0.04	0.6	0.08	122	0
1.7	1.4	90	63	128	198	194	2.4	0.6	20	49	0.9	2	0.05	0.05	1.7	0.1	32	3.56
4	2.8	162	125	229	336	345	3.8	1.2	34	125	2.23	7	0.13	0.19	2.8	0.19	49	6.27
1.8	3.6	72	79	147	513	266	2.9	0.7	24	18	1.43	3	0.08	0.05	2.3	0.14	40	4.93
7.3	1.3	212	124	193	446	266	2	1.2	27	263	1.49	1	0.07	0.2	1.5	0.11	22	2.48
3.5	2.6	81	70	126	576	255	2	1.1	23	121	1.91	6	0.11	0.12	2	0.12	31	3.17
0	0	0	10	8	1	107	—	0.2	4	2	0.32	4	0.02	0.01	0.1	—	—	0
0	0.1	0	4	28	120	27	0.2	1.2	6	0	0.1	0	0.16	0.11	1.4	0.01	5	0
0.5	0.1	2	18	16	24	6	0	0.2	1	2	0.03	0	0.02	0.02	0.2	0.01	1	0.02

Food Item	Qty	Meas	Wgt (g)	Wtr (g)	Cals	Prot	Carb (g)	Fib (g)	Fat (g)	SatF (g)
Cracker, Cuban	4	each	20	1	80	2	15	0.4	1	0.3
Cracker, Finn Ry Krisp, thin	3	each	6	0	21	1	5	0.5	0	0
Cracker, Matzoh, egg	1	each	28	2	111	3	22	0.8	1	0.2
Cracker, Matzoh, plain	1	each	28	1	112	3	24	0.9	0	0.1
Cracker, Matzoh, whole wheat	1	each	28	1	100	4	22	3.4	0	0.1
Cracker, Melba Toast, unsalted	4	piece	20	1	78	2	15	1.3	1	0.1
Cracker, Melba Toast, wheat	2	piece	10	1	37	1	8	0.7	0	0
Cracker, Melba toast, plain	1	piece	5	0	20	1	4	0.3	0	0
Cracker, Norwegian flatbread	4	each	23	1	85	2	19	3.8	0	0
Cracker, Premium, unsalted tops	4	each	12	—	50	2	8	0	1	0
Cracker, Saltine, unsalted top	4	each	20	1	87	2	14	0.6	2	0.6
Cracker, Saltine, whole wheat	4	each	12	0	52	1	8	0.8	2	0.4
Cracker, Wasa rye crispbread	2	piece	17	1	58	2	13	1.5	0	0
Cracker, Wheatsworth	6	each	18	1	86	1	12	1	4	1.6
Cracker, buttery, Ritz	10	each	30	1	151	2	18	0.5	8	1.1
Cracker, cheese w/peanut butter filling	4	each	30	1	145	4	17	0.8	7	1.6
Cracker, crispbread, Wasa extra crisp	4	each	24	1	95	3	18	1.7	2	0.4
Cracker, crispbread, wheat	4	each	24	1	94	3	20	0.7	0	0
Cracker, crispbread, white/rye, fat added	4	each	24	1	95	3	18	1.7	2	0.4
Cracker, graham, crumbs	0.25	cup	30	1	127	2	23	0.8	3	0.5
Cracker, graham, crust, baked	1	piece	54	2	268	2	35	0.8	14	2.8
Cracker, graham, plain/honey	2	each	14	1	59	1	11	0.4	1	0.2
Cracker, milk, New England Biscuit	2	each	22	1	100	2	15	0.4	3	0.7
Cracker, oat bran-oat thins	3	each	6	0	26	1	4	0.3	1	0.1
Cracker, rusk toast	2	each	20	1	81	3	14	0.4	1	0.3
Cracker, rye crispbread	3	each	30	2	110	2	25	5	0	0
Cracker, rye, Melba Toast	2	each	10	0	39	1	8	0.8	0	0
Cracker, rye, cheese filled	4	each	28	1	135	3	17	1	6	1.7
Cracker, rye, seasoned, triple	1	each	22	1	84	2	16	4.6	2	0.3
Cracker, sesame seed	8	each	24	1	120	2	15	0.4	6	0.9
Cracker, snack type, cheese-filled	4	each	28	1	134	3	17	0.5	6	1.7
Cracker, snack type, peanut butter-filled	4	each	28	1	137	3	16	0.8	7	1.6
Cracker, wheat	15	each	30	1	142	3	20	1.4	6	1.6
Cracker, wheat thin type, low sodium	10	each	20	1	92	2	14	0.4	4	1.1
Cracker, wheat'n bran, Triscuits	4	each	16	1	64	1	11	1.7	2	0.4
Cracker, wheat, 100% stoned wheat	4	each	16	1	64	1	11	1.7	2	0.4
Cracker, wheat, cheese-filled	4	each	28	1	139	3	16	0.9	7	1.2
Cracker, wheat, peanut butter-filled	4	each	28	1	139	4	15	1.2	7	1.3
Cracker, wheat, thin type	10	each	20	1	95	1	13	1.1	4	1.8
Cracker, whole wheat, Triscuit	2	each	9	0	40	1	6	0.9	2	0.3
Crackers, Cracked Pepper, Snackwell's	1	oz.	28	0	113	3	24	0.9	1	0.2
Crackers, Fire, chilis and cheese, fat free, Health Valley	6	each	15	1	50	2	11	2	0	0
Crackers, Pizza, zesty cheese, fat free, Health Valley	6	each	15	1	50	2	11	2	0	0
Crackers, buttery snack type (Club/Waverly)	7	each	28	1	141	2	17	0.4	7	1.1
Crackers, cheese, Cheez-its	10	each	10	0	50	1	6	0.2	3	0.9
Crackers, cheese, reduced fat, Snackwell's	1	oz.	28	1	119	3	22	0.9	2	0.6
Crackers, classic golden, reduced fat, Snackwell's	1	oz.	28	0	117	2	23	0.7	2	0.4
Crackers, cracked pepper, Snackwell's	1	each	15	0	60	2	12	0.5	0	0.1
Crackers, oyster	1	each	1	0	4	0	1	0	0	0
Crackers, saltine	4	each	12	0	52	1	9	0.4	1	0.4
Crackers, wheat, fat free, Snackwell's	1	oz.	28	0	113	3	23	1.2	1	0.2
Crackers, whole grain rye, Ry Krisp	2	each	14	1	47	1	11	3.2	0	0
Cranberries, fresh	0.5	cup	48	41	23	0	6	2	0	0
Cranberries, fresh, cooked, sauce	0.5	cup	138	84	209	0	54	1.4	0	0
Cranberry juice cocktail	1	cup	253	216	144	0	36	0.3	0	0
Cranberry-apple drink, w/vitamin C, bottled	1	cup	237	209	170	0	43	0.3	0	0
Cranberry-apple juice drink, low calorie	1	cup	253	228	46	0	11	0.2	0	0
Cranberry-blackberry juice drink, low calorie	1	cup	240	228	46	0	11	0.2	0	0
Cream of tartar	0.25	tsp	1	0	2	0	1	0	0	0
Cream puff shell, recipe	1	each	66	27	239	6	15	0.5	17	3.7
Cream puff, custard-filled	1	each	110	59	284	7	25	0.4	17	4
Cream, coffee/table	1	Tbs	15	11	29	0	1	0	3	1.8
Cream, half & half	2	Tbs	30	24	39	1	1	0	3	2.2
Cream, sour, cultured	2	Tbs	29	20	62	1	1	0	6	3.7
Cream, sour, imitation, IMO	2	Tbs	29	20	60	1	2	0	6	5.1

MonoF	PolyF	Choles	Calc	Phos	Sod	Pot	Zn	Iron	Magn	VitA	VitE	VitC	Thia	Ribo	Nia	B6	Fola	B12
(g)	(g)	(mg)	(mg)	(mg)	(mg)	(mg)	(mg)	(mg)	(mg)	(µg RE)	(µg α-TE)	(mg)	(mg)	(mg)	(mg)	(mg)	(µg)	(µg)
0.7	0.2	0	15	18	52	52	0.1	0.3	9	0	0.22	0	0.02	0.01	0.2	0.02	3	0
0	0	0	3	23	53	36	0.2	0.2	7	0	0.11	0	0.02	0.02	0.1	0.02	3	0
0.2	0.1	24	11	42	6	42	0.2	0.8	7	4	0.28	0	0.22	0.18	1.4	0.02	33	0.05
0	0.2	0	4	25	1	32	0.2	0.9	7	0	0.02	0	0.11	0.08	1.1	0.03	33	0
0.1	0.2	0	7	86	1	90	0.7	1.3	38	0	0.38	0	0.1	0.08	1.5	0.04	14	0
0.2	0.3	0	19	39	4	40	0.4	0.7	12	0	0.01	0	0.08	0.06	0.8	0.02	25	0
0.1	0.1	0	4	16	84	15	0.2	0.4	6	0	0.04	0	0.04	0.03	0.5	0.01	13	0
0	0.1	0	5	10	42	10	0.1	0.2	3	0	0	0	0.02	0.01	0.2	0	6	0
0	0.1	0	7	62	61	74	0.6	0.6	18	0	0.31	0	0.06	0.03	0.2	0.05	11	0
0	0	0	—	—	100	10	—	0.7	—	—	0.2	—	—	—	—	—	—	—
1.3	0.3	0	24	21	127	145	0.2	1.1	5	0	0.31	0	0.11	0.09	1	0.01	25	0
0.9	0.2	0	3	23	124	26	0.2	0.5	8	0	0.28	0	0.06	0.04	0.6	0.02	3	0
0	0.1	0	9	66	150	102	0.5	0.7	20	0	0.32	0	0.05	0.04	0.2	0.05	8	0
1.8	0.4	4	6	32	157	36	0.3	0.6	11	1	0.05	0	0.09	0.06	0.8	0.02	3	0.08
3.2	2.9	0	36	68	254	40	0.2	1.1	8	0	1.36	0	0.12	0.1	1.2	0.02	23	0
3.5	1.4	2	24	97	298	74	0.3	0.9	17	10	1.12	0	0.12	0.1	2	0.45	26	0
0.8	0.3	0	20	45	153	68	0.3	0.8	11	0	0.34	0	0.1	0.08	0.8	0.03	4	0.03
0	0.1	0	4	28	120	27	0.2	1.2	6	0	0.1	0	0.16	0.11	1.4	0.01	5	0
0.8	0.3	0	20	45	153	68	0.3	0.8	11	0	0.34	0	0.1	0.08	0.8	0.03	4	0.03
1.2	1.2	0	7	31	182	40	0.2	1.1	9	0	0.61	0	0.07	0.09	1.2	0.02	18	0
6.2	3.8	0	11	35	309	48	0.3	1.2	10	109	2.21	0	0.06	0.1	1.2	0.02	13	0.01
0.6	0.5	0	3	15	85	19	0.1	0.5	4	0	0.29	0	0.03	0.04	0.6	0.01	8	0
1.9	0.5	2	38	67	130	25	0.1	0.8	5	2	0.6	0	0.12	0.09	1	0.01	18	0.02
0.3	0.3	0	5	17	36	12	0.1	0.2	4	0	0.14	0	0.03	0.02	0.2	0	1	0
0.6	0.5	16	5	31	51	49	0.2	0.5	7	2	0.1	0	0.08	0.08	0.9	0.01	17	0.04
0	0.2	0	9	81	79	96	0.7	0.7	23	0	0.4	0	0.07	0.04	0.3	0.06	14	0
0.1	0.1	0	8	18	90	19	0.1	0.4	4	0	0.06	0	0.05	0.03	0.5	0.01	8	0
3.4	0.8	3	62	95	292	96	0.2	0.7	10	11	0.56	0	0.17	0.14	1	0.02	23	0.03
0.7	0.8	0	10	68	195	100	0.6	0.7	23	0	0.44	0	0.07	0.05	0.5	0.04	3	0
2.5	2.3	0	29	55	203	32	0.2	0.9	6	0	1.08	0	0.1	0.08	1	0.01	18	0
3.2	0.7	1	72	114	392	120	0.2	0.7	10	5	0.14	0	0.12	0.19	1.1	0.01	24	0.03
3.5	1.2	0	27	68	264	62	0.3	0.9	15	0	1.04	0	0.12	0.09	1.6	0.03	24	0
3.4	0.8	0	15	66	239	55	0.5	1.3	19	0	0.97	0	0.15	0.1	1.5	0.04	13	0
1.3	0.9	0	6	38	50	43	0.2	0.8	10	3	0.12	0	0.1	0.07	0.9	0.03	5	0
1.2	0.3	0	4	32	86	22	0.2	0.5	11	0	0.59	0	0.08	0.05	0.7	0.02	4	0.15
1.2	0.3	0	4	30	88	19	0.2	0.5	10	0	0.59	0	0.08	0.05	0.7	0.02	4	0.16
2.9	2.6	2	57	107	256	86	0.2	0.7	15	3	0.17	0	0.1	0.12	0.9	0.07	18	0.03
3.3	2.5	0	48	97	226	83	0.2	0.7	11	0	0.17	0	0.11	0.08	1.6	0.04	20	0
2	0.5	4	6	36	174	40	0.3	0.7	13	1	0.05	0	0.1	0.07	0.8	0.03	4	0.08
0.5	0.6	0	4	27	59	27	0.2	0.3	9	0	0.1	0	0.02	0.01	0.4	0.02	4	0
0.1	0.3	0	49	96	280	36	0.3	1.4	7	0	—	0	0.1	0.12	1.5	0.02	—	—
0	0	0	0	—	80	—	—	0	—	20	—	1	—	—	—	—	—	—
0	0	0	0	—	140	—	—	0	—	20	—	1	—	—	—	—	—	—
3	2.7	0	34	64	237	37	0.2	1	8	0	1.27	0	0.11	0.1	1.1	0.02	22	0
1.2	0.2	1	15	22	100	14	0.1	0.5	4	3	0.26	0	0.06	0.04	0.5	0.06	8	0.05
0.6	0.2	2	18	45	320	43	0.3	1.4	8	12	—	0	0.11	0.16	1.8	0.03	—	0.01
0.6	0.2	0	56	104	292	31	0.2	1.2	6	0	—	0	0.18	0.12	1.4	0.02	—	0.01
0	0.1	0	26	51	148	19	0.1	0.7	4	0	—	0	0.05	0.06	0.8	0.01	—	—
0.1	0	0	1	1	13	1	0	0.1	0	0	0.02	0	0.01	0	0.1	0	1	0
0.8	0.2	0	14	13	156	15	0.1	0.6	3	0	0.19	0	0.07	0.06	0.6	0	15	0
0.2	0.3	0	52	116	320	81	0.4	1.1	13	0	—	0	0.08	0.14	1.4	0.03	—	0.04
0	0.1	0	6	47	111	69	0.4	0.8	17	0	0.2	0	0.06	0.04	0.2	0.04	2	0
0	0	0	3	4	0	34	0.1	0.1	2	2	0.05	6	0.01	0.01	0	0.03	1	0
0	0.1	0	6	8	40	36	0.1	0.3	4	3	0.14	3	0.02	0.03	0.1	0.02	1	0
0	0.1	0	8	5	5	46	0.2	0.4	5	1	0	90	0.02	0.02	0.1	0.05	1	0
0	0	0	18	8	5	68	0.1	0.2	5	1	0	81	0.01	0.05	0.2	0.05	1	0
0	0	0	17	7	5	65	0.1	0.1	5	1	0	77	0	0.05	0.1	0.05	1	0
0	0	0	17	7	5	65	0.1	0.1	5	1	0	77	0	0.05	0.1	0.05	0	0
0	0	0	0	0	0	137	0	0	0	0	0	0	0	0	0	0	0	0
7.3	4.9	129	24	78	368	64	0.5	1.3	8	203	2.54	0	0.14	0.24	1	0.05	32	0.26
7.2	4.6	147	73	120	375	127	0.7	1.3	13	219	2.43	0	0.13	0.31	0.9	0.07	31	0.4
0.8	0.1	10	14	12	6	18	0	0	1	27	0.02	0	0	0.02	0	0	0	0.03
1	0.1	11	32	29	12	39	0.2	0	3	32	0.03	0	0.01	0.04	0	0.01	1	0.1
1.7	0.2	13	33	24	15	41	0.1	0	3	56	0.16	0	0.01	0.04	0	0	3	0.09
0.2	0	0	1	13	29	46	0.3	0.1	2	0	0.04	0	0	0	0	0	0	0

Food Item	Qty	Meas	Wgt (g)	Wtr (g)	Cals	Prot	Carb (g)	Fib (g)	Fat (g)	SatF (g)
Cream, whipped, pressurized	2	Tbs	8	5	19	0	1	0	2	1
Cream, whipping, heavy	2	Tbs	30	17	103	1	1	0	11	6.8
Cream, whipping, light	1	Tbs	30	19	87	1	1	0	9	5.8
Creamer, non-dairy, Cremora	1	tsp	2	—	10	0	1	—	0	0.5
Creamer, non-dairy, Mocha Mix	1	Tbs	14	11	19	0	1	0	2	0.3
Creamer, non-dairy, powdered coffee whitener	1	tsp	2	0	11	0	1	0	1	0.6
Crepe suzette w/sauce	1	each	66	36	161	4	16	0.3	9	4.2
Crepe, chocolate-filled	1	each	78	53	119	4	15	0.6	5	2
Crepe, fruit-filled	1	each	78	49	131	4	21	0.9	4	1.2
Cress, garden, cooked, drained	0.5	cup	68	62	16	1	3	0.5	0	0
Cress, garden, raw	0.5	cup	25	22	8	1	1	0.3	0	0
Croissant, apple	1	each	57	26	145	4	21	1.4	5	2.8
Croissant, butter	1	each	57	13	231	5	26	1.5	12	6.7
Croissant, cheese	1	each	57	12	236	5	27	1.5	12	6
Croissant, chocolate	1	each	56	12	233	5	23	1.6	14	8.2
Croissant, egg & cheese	1	each	127	58	368	13	24	—	25	14.1
Croutons, dry	0.25	cup	8	0	30	1	6	0.4	0	0.1
Croutons, seasoned	3	Tbs	7	0	33	1	4	0.4	1	0.4
Cucumber salad, cucumber & vinegar	0.5	cup	80	72	24	0	6	0.6	0	0
Cucumber, kim chee	0.5	cup	75	68	16	1	4	1.1	0	0
Cucumber, w/peel, raw slices	0.5	cup	52	50	7	0	1	0.4	0	0
Cucumber, w/peel, raw, whole	1	each	301	289	39	2	8	2.4	0	0.1
Cumin seed	0.25	tsp	0	0	2	0	0	0.1	0	0
Cupcake, chocolate w/chocolate icing-commercial	1	each	42	10	154	2	23	1.2	7	2
Currants, black, fresh	0.5	cup	56	46	35	1	9	4.1	0	0
Currants, dried (Zante)	0.5	cup	72	14	204	3	53	4.9	0	0
Currants, red/white, fresh	0.5	cup	56	47	31	1	8	2.4	0	0
Custard apple, raw	4	oz.	113	81	115	2	29	4.2	1	0.1
Custard, egg, baked, recipe	0.5	cup	141	111	148	7	15	0	7	3.3
Custard, egg, mix, w/2% milk	0.5	cup	133	99	149	6	24	0	4	1.9
Custard, egg, prepared mix w/whole milk	0.5	cup	133	97	162	5	23	0	5	3
Dairy Queen blizzard, heath, regular size	1	each	404	236	820	14	119	1	33	20
Dairy Queen breeze, heath, frozen yogurt	1	each	379	229	666	14	115	0.9	17	10.3
Dairy Queen shake, chocolate	1	each	397	273	567	12	96	0	15	9.6
Dairy Queen, Buster bar	1	each	149	67	450	10	41	2	28	12
Dairy Queen, Dilly Bar	1	each	85	47	210	3	21	0	13	7
Dairy Queen, Mr. Misty, regular size	1	each	330	267	250	0	63	0	0	0
Dairy Queen, banana split	1	each	369	249	510	8	96	3	12	8
Dairy Queen, blizzard, strawberry	1	each	383	259	570	12	95	1	16	11
Dairy Queen, breeze, strawberry frozen yogurt	1	each	354	246	425	12	92	0.9	1	0.9
Dairy Queen, cheeseburger, single	1	each	156	86	349	20	30	2	17	8.2
Dairy Queen, choc dipped vanilla cone, regular	1	each	156	92	340	6	42	0.7	17	8.7
Dairy Queen, chocolate cone, regular	1	each	142	90	240	6	37	0	7	5.3
Dairy Queen, hamburger, single	1	each	142	80	298	18	30	2.1	12	5.1
Dairy Queen, hot fudge brownie delight	1	each	305	160	710	11	102	0.6	29	14
Dairy Queen, hotdog	1	each	99	57	240	9	19	1	14	5
Dairy Queen, hotdog, w/cheese	1	each	113	62	290	12	20	1	18	8
Dairy Queen, malt, vanilla, regular size	1	each	418	285	610	13	106	0.3	14	8
Dairy Queen, peanut buster parfait	1	each	305	156	730	16	99	2	31	17
Dairy Queen, quarter pound super hotdog	1	each	198	98	590	20	41	—	38	16
Dairy Queen, sundae, chocolate, regular	1	each	177	110	301	6	54	0	7	4.4
Dairy Queen, sundae, nutty double fudge	1	each	276	—	570	10	85	—	22	10
Dairy Queen, ultimate burger, double bacon-cheese	1	each	276	159	687	41	30	2	44	19.5
Dandelion greens, cooked, drained	0.5	cup	52	47	17	1	3	1.5	0	0.1
Danish pastry, cheese	1	each	91	31	353	6	29	—	25	5.1
Danish pastry, cinnamon	1	each	88	18	349	5	47	0.3	17	3.5
Danish pastry, fruit filled	1	each	94	27	335	5	45	—	16	3.3
Dates, chopped	0.5	cup	89	20	245	2	65	6.7	0	0.2
Dates, whole	10	each	83	19	228	2	61	6.2	0	0.2
Deer/venison steak, fried	1	each	85	52	146	28	0	0	3	1.2
Deer/venison, roasted	4	oz.	113	74	179	34	0	0	4	1.4
Dessert topping, low cal, mix, prepared	1	Tbs	5	4	3	0	1	0	0	0.3
Dessert topping, mix w/whole milk (Dream Whip)	1	Tbs	5	3	9	0	1	0	1	0.5
Dessert topping, non-dairy, frozen (Cool Whip)	1	Tbs	5	2	15	0	1	0	1	1
Dessert topping, non-dairy, pressurized	1	Tbs	4	3	12	0	1	0	1	0.8

MonoF	PolyF	Choles	Calc	Phos	Sod	Pot	Zn	Iron	Magn	VitA	VitE	VitC	Thia	Ribo	Nia	B6	Fola	B12
(g)	(g)	(mg)	(mg)	(mg)	(mg)	(mg)	(mg)	(mg)	(mg)	(µg RE)	(µg α-TE)	(mg)	(mg)	(mg)	(mg)	(mg)	(µg)	(µg)
0.5	0.1	6	8	7	10	11	0	0	1	16	0.04	0	0	0	0	0	0	0.02
3.2	0.4	41	19	19	11	22	0.1	0	2	125	0.19	0	0.01	0.03	0	0.01	1	0.05
2.7	0.3	33	21	18	10	29	0.1	0	2	88	0.18	0	0.01	0.04	0	0.01	1	0.06
—	—	—	—	—	5	15	—	—	—	—	—	—	—	—	—	—	—	—
0	0.7	0	1	8	7	20	—	—	0	0	0	0	0	0	0	0	0	0
0	0	0	0	8	4	16	0	0	0	0	0	0	0	0	0	0	0	0
3.2	1.2	84	45	68	163	84	0.4	0.8	8	76	0.72	3	0.08	0.17	0.6	0.04	11	0.22
1.7	0.7	58	81	89	148	126	0.5	0.7	12	58	0.52	0	0.07	0.2	0.4	0.04	8	0.27
1.5	0.8	63	38	59	124	90	0.3	0.7	8	59	0.92	4	0.08	0.16	0.6	0.04	9	0.19
0.1	0.1	0	41	32	5	238	0.1	0.5	18	520	0.47	16	0.04	0.11	0.5	0.11	25	0
0.1	0.1	0	20	19	4	152	0.1	0.3	10	233	0.18	17	0.02	0.06	0.2	0.06	20	0
1.4	0.4	18	17	33	156	51	0.6	0.6	7	56	0.11	0	0.13	0.09	0.9	0.02	32	0.11
3.2	0.6	38	21	60	424	67	0.4	1.2	9	106	0.25	0	0.22	0.14	1.2	0.03	35	0.09
3.7	1.4	32	30	74	316	75	0.5	1.2	14	112	0.59	0	0.3	0.18	1.2	0.04	42	0.18
4.2	0.7	56	31	82	257	113	0.6	1.7	28	105	0.42	0	0.19	0.21	2	0.05	19	0.1
7.5	1.4	216	244	348	551	174	1.8	2.2	22	255	—	0	0.19	0.38	1.5	0.1	47	0.78
0.2	0.1	0	6	9	52	9	0.1	0.3	2	0	0.02	0	0.05	0.02	0.4	0	10	0
0.4	0.2	0	7	10	87	13	0.1	0.2	3	1	0.15	0	0.04	0.03	0.3	0.01	6	0.01
0	0	0	10	13	175	105	0.1	0.3	10	2	0.05	3	0.02	0.01	0.2	0.04	8	0
0	0	0	7	10	766	88	0.4	3.6	6	25	0.12	3	0.02	0.02	0.3	0.08	17	0
0	0	0	7	10	1	75	0.1	0.1	6	11	0.04	3	0.01	0.01	0.1	0.02	7	0
0	0.2	0	42	60	6	433	0.6	0.8	33	63	0.24	16	0.07	0.07	0.7	0.13	39	0
0.1	0	0	5	2	1	9	0	0.3	2	1	0	0	0	0	0	0	0	0
3.7	0.8	18	18	51	140	84	0.3	0.9	14	10	0.71	0	0.01	0.06	0.2	0.02	7	0.06
0	0.1	0	31	33	1	180	0.2	0.9	13	13	0.06	101	0.03	0.03	0.2	0.04	2	0
0	0.1	0	62	90	6	642	0.5	2.4	30	5	0.07	3	0.12	0.1	1.2	0.21	7	0
0	0	0	18	25	1	154	0.1	0.6	7	7	0.06	23	0.02	0.03	0.1	0.04	4	0
0.2	0.1	0	34	24	5	433	0.5	0.8	20	3	—	22	0.09	0.11	0.6	0.25	—	0
2.1	0.5	123	158	159	109	216	0.7	0.4	20	85	0.34	1	0.05	0.32	0.1	0.07	14	0.44
1.2	0.3	74	197	176	200	287	0.7	0.3	27	74	0.27	1	0.07	0.29	0.2	0.08	11	0.61
1.7	0.3	81	194	174	198	283	0.7	0.3	25	44	0.13	1	0.07	0.29	0.2	0.08	11	0.6
—	—	60	450	450	580	730	—	1.8	—	300	—	1	0.15	0.76	—	—	—	—
—	—	19	422	449	544	539	—	2.5	—	19	—	2	0.12	0.76	—	—	—	—
—	—	52	442	400	309	600	—	2	—	295	—	2	0.12	0.59	0.8	—	—	—
—	—	15	150	250	280	400	—	1.1	—	80	—	0	0.09	0.17	3	0.08	—	—
3	3	10	100	80	75	170	—	0.4	—	60	—	0	0.03	0.14	—	0.06	—	—
0	0	0	0	—	10	—	—	0	—	0	—	2	0	0	—	0	—	—
—	—	30	250	40	180	860	—	1.8	—	200	—	15	0.15	0.26	0.4	0.2	—	—
—	—	50	450	350	260	700	—	1.8	—	300	—	9	0.15	0.68	—	—	—	—
0	0	9	416	349	250	490	—	2.5	—	0	—	8	0.12	0.68	—	—	—	—
—	—	56	154	249	872	270	—	3.7	—	62	—	4	0.3	0.34	4	—	—	—
—	—	20	200	150	133	290	—	1.2	—	100	—	2	0.06	0.26	0.1	0.09	—	—
—	—	20	167	200	120	350	—	1.2	—	133	—	1	0.06	0.26	—	—	—	—
6.2	1	46	62	149	648	259	—	2.8	—	41	—	4	0.3	0.25	4	—	—	—
12	2	35	300	600	340	510	—	5.4	—	80	—	1	0.15	0.68	0.3	0.18	—	—
—	—	25	60	60	730	170	—	1.8	—	20	—	4	0.22	0.14	2	—	—	—
8	2	40	150	150	950	180	—	1.8	—	60	—	4	0.22	0.17	2	—	—	—
2	2	45	400	350	230	570	—	1.4	—	80	—	0	0.12	0.6	0.8	0.19	—	—
—	—	35	300	450	400	660	—	1.8	—	150	—	1	0.15	0.51	3	0.22	—	—
16	4	60	100	150	1360	340	—	2.7	—	—	—	—	0.45	0.34	5	—	—	—
—	—	22	184	150	154	289	—	1.1	—	110	—	0	0.06	0.26	0.3	0.14	—	—
9	3	35	300	300	170	450	—	3.6	—	60	—	0	0.12	0.6	—	—	—	—
—	—	139	616	399	1241	479	—	2.8	—	41	—	4	0.44	0.5	7.9	—	—	—
0	0.1	0	74	22	23	122	0.1	0.9	13	614	1.31	9	0.07	0.09	0.3	0.08	7	0
15.6	2.4	20	70	80	319	116	0.6	1.8	16	43	—	3	0.26	0.21	2.6	0.06	55	0.23
10.6	1.6	27	37	74	326	96	0.5	1.8	14	5	0.79	3	0.26	0.19	2.2	0.05	55	0.22
10.1	1.6	19	22	69	333	110	0.5	1.4	14	24	0.85	2	0.29	0.21	1.8	0.06	31	0.24
0.1	0	0	28	36	3	580	0.3	1	31	4	0.09	0	0.08	0.09	2	0.17	11	0
0.1	0	0	27	33	2	541	0.2	1	29	4	0.08	0	0.08	0.08	1.8	0.16	10	0
0.9	0.6	102	6	206	331	305	2.5	4.1	24	0	0.24	0	0.14	0.55	5.7	0.22	5	5.3
1	0.7	127	8	256	61	380	3.1	5.1	27	0	0.28	0	0.2	0.68	7.6	0.43	5	3.61
0	0	0	0	2	5	1	0	0	0	0	0	0	0	0	0	0	0	0
0	0	0	5	4	3	8	0	0	0	2	0.01	0	0	0.01	0	0	0	0.01
0.1	0	0	0	0	1	1	0	0	0	4	0.01	0	0	0	0	0	0	0
0.1	0	0	0	1	3	1	0	0	0	2	0.01	0	0	0	0	0	0	0

Food Item	Qty	Meas	Wgt (g)	Wtr (g)	Cals	Prot	Carb (g)	Fib (g)	Fat (g)	SatF (g)
Dip, Jalapeno pepper bean	1	Tbs	33	22	46	2	6	2.2	2	0.2
Dip, caramel, Marie's	2	cup	35	5	150	0	24	1	5	4
Dip, sour cream, buttermilk/onion	2	Tbs	30	20	67	1	2	0.2	6	3.7
Dip, sour cream, low calorie	2	Tbs	30	22	44	1	2	0.2	3	2.1
Distilled spirits, 80 proof, all	1	oz.	28	19	66	0	0	0	0	0
Distilled spirits, 86 proof, all	1	oz.	28	18	71	0	0	0	0	0
Distilled spirits, 94 proof	1	oz.	28	17	78	0	0	0	0	0
Dock/sorrel greens, cooked	0.5	cup	50	47	10	1	1	1.3	0	—
Domino's pizza, pepperoni, deep dish	2	piece	218	94	622	26	63	3.3	29	11.3
Domino's pizza, pepperoni, hand tossed	2	piece	159	72	406	18	50	2.6	15	6.5
Domino's pizza, pepperoni, thin crust	1	piece	59	26	169	7	15	0.8	9	3.5
Domino's pizza, sausage mushroom, deep dish	2	piece	236	111	618	26	66	3.8	28	10.8
Domino's pizza, vegetarian, hand tossed	2	piece	176	95	360	15	52	3	10	4.6
Domino's pizza, veggie, deep dish	2	piece	236	117	576	24	65	3.8	25	9.2
Domino's pizza, veggie, thin crust	1	piece	68	37	146	6	16	1	6	2.4
Doo Dads, original flavor	0.5	cup	28	1	129	3	18	1.9	5	1
Doughnut, Eclair, chocolate, custard-filled	1	each	94	49	246	6	23	0.6	15	3.9
Doughnut, French cruller, glazed	1	each	41	7	169	1	24	0.5	8	1.9
Doughnut, Mexican crueller	1	each	26	6	116	1	12	0.2	7	1.4
Doughnut, cake, chocolate-iced	1	each	43	6	204	2	21	0.9	13	3.5
Doughnut, cake, plain	1	each	50	10	211	2	25	0.8	12	1.8
Doughnut, cake, sugared/glazed	1	each	45	9	192	2	23	0.7	10	2.7
Doughnut, custard filled, Bismarck	1	each	70	20	261	3	34	1	13	5.9
Doughnut, eggless, carob-coated, raised	1	each	78	21	285	5	32	5.4	18	2.6
Doughnut, fritter, apple	1	each	24	9	87	1	8	0.3	6	1.6
Doughnut, oriental, Okinawan	1	each	18	3	75	1	10	0.2	4	0.9
Doughnut, wheat, sugared/glazed	1	each	45	13	162	3	19	1	9	1.4
Doughnut, yeast, chocolate, w/choc icing	1	each	71	20	273	4	30	2.5	16	7.5
Doughnut, yeast, creme-filled	1	each	85	32	307	5	26	0.7	21	4.6
Doughnut, yeast, glazed	1	each	60	15	242	4	27	0.7	14	3.5
Doughnut, yeast, jelly-filled	1	each	65	23	221	4	25	0.6	12	3.2
Drink mix, citrus, Crystal Light	1	cup	238	237	5	0	0	0	0	0
Duck meat, skinless, roasted	4	oz.	113	73	228	27	0	0	13	4.7
Duck, domestic, w/skin, roasted	4	oz.	113	59	382	22	0	0	32	11
Dumpling, apple	1	each	151	78	357	2	53	2.5	16	3.6
Dumpling, plain, medium	1	each	32	22	42	1	7	0.2	1	0.4
Egg Beaters, Fleischmann's	0.5	cup	122	—	60	12	2	0	0	0
Egg Delight, frozen, prepared	0.5	cup	70	51	92	9	5	0	4	0.7
Egg foo yung patty	1	each	86	67	113	6	3	0.6	8	1.9
Egg omelet, ham & cheese, 1 egg	1	each	78	55	142	10	1	0	11	3.9
Egg omelet, mushroom, 1 egg	1	each	69	54	91	6	1	0.1	7	2.6
Egg omelet, onion, peppper, tomato, mushroom, 3 egg	1	each	145	122	125	5	7	1.6	9	2
Egg omelet, plain, 1 large egg	1	each	59	45	90	6	1	0	7	1.9
Egg omelet, sausage & mushroom, 1 egg	1	each	95	68	172	11	1	0.2	13	4.9
Egg omelet, spanish, 1 egg	1	each	145	122	125	5	7	1.6	9	2
Egg omelet, spinach, 1 egg	1	each	84	68	95	7	2	0.7	7	2.2
Egg roll, chicken, Chun King	6	piece	106	62	210	6	30	3	7	1.5
Egg roll, shrimp, Chun King	6	piece	106	65	190	5	29	3	6	1
Egg salad	0.5	cup	92	52	293	8	1	0	28	5.3
Egg substitute, frozen	0.25	cup	60	44	96	7	2	0	7	1.2
Egg substitute, liquid	0.25	cup	63	52	53	8	0	0	2	0.4
Egg substitute, liquid, prepared	0.5	cup	105	84	100	14	1	0	4	0.8
Egg white, cooked	1	each	33	29	17	4	0	0	0	0
Egg white, fresh or frozen, raw, large	1	each	33	29	17	4	0	0	0	0
Egg yolk, cooked	1	each	17	8	59	3	0	0	5	1.6
Egg yolk, fresh, raw, large	1	each	17	8	59	3	0	0	5	1.6
Egg yolk, frozen, raw, salted	0.5	cup	122	62	333	17	2	0	28	8.5
Egg, Second Nature, prepared	0.5	cup	105	84	100	14	1	0	4	0.8
Egg, creamed	1	each	145	107	230	11	8	0.2	17	5.2
Egg, deviled	2	each	62	43	125	7	1	0	10	2.5
Egg, hard cooked, extra large	1	each	58	43	90	7	1	0	6	1.9
Egg, hard cooked/boiled, large	1	each	50	37	78	6	1	0	5	1.6
Egg, hard cooked/boiled, medium	1	each	44	33	68	6	0	0	5	1.4
Egg, poached, large	1	each	50	38	74	6	1	0	5	1.6
Egg, poached, medium size	1	each	44	33	66	5	1	0	4	1.4

MonoF	PolyF	Choles	Calc	Phos	Sod	Pot	Zn	Iron	Magn	VitA	VitE	VitC	Thia	Ribo	Nia	B6	Fola	B12
(g)	(g)	(mg)	(mg)	(mg)	(mg)	(mg)	(mg)	(mg)	(mg)	(µg RE)	(µg α-TE)	(mg)	(mg)	(mg)	(mg)	(mg)	(µg)	(µg)
0.4	1	0	11	34	382	96	0.2	0.5	12	18	0.38	4	0.03	0.02	0.1	0.03	23	0
—	—	5	20	—	75	—	—	0	—	0	—	0	—	—	—	—	—	—
1.8	0.2	13	36	32	228	56	0.1	0.1	5	55	0.18	0	0.02	0.06	0.1	0.01	3	0.08
1	0.1	11	32	34	212	51	0.2	0.1	4	31	0.11	0	0.02	0.06	0.1	0.01	3	0.08
0	0	0	0	1	0	1	0	0	0	0	0	0	0	0	0	0	0	0
0	0	0	0	1	0	1	0	0	0	0	0	0	0	0	0	0	0	0
0	0	0	0	1	0	1	0	0	0	0	0	0	0	0	0	0	0	0
—	—	0	19	26	2	161	0.1	1	44	174	0.5	13	0.02	0.04	0.2	0.05	4	0
—	—	44	456	—	1382	—	—	5	—	155	—	3	—	—	—	—	—	—
—	—	32	282	—	1179	—	—	4.3	—	94	—	3	—	—	—	—	—	—
—	—	16	162	—	484	—	—	0.7	—	44	—	1	—	—	—	—	—	—
—	—	43	460	—	1355	—	—	5.2	—	158	—	4	—	—	—	—	—	—
—	—	19	286	—	1028	—	—	4.4	—	99	—	13	—	—	—	—	—	—
—	—	32	460	—	1232	—	—	5.2	—	160	—	13	—	—	—	—	—	—
—	—	10	164	—	408	—	—	0.7	—	47	—	6	—	—	—	—	—	—
3.2	0.9	0	21	84	360	78	0.6	0.7	17	12	0.04	0	0.1	0.07	1.5	0.06	11	0
6.1	3.7	119	59	101	317	110	0.6	1.1	14	180	1.97	0	0.11	0.25	0.8	0.06	26	0.32
4.3	0.9	5	11	50	141	32	0.1	1	5	1	1.02	0	0.07	0.09	0.9	0.01	14	0.02
3	2.6	2	2	8	37	8	0.1	0.3	2	6	1.11	0	0.04	0.03	0.4	0	1	0
7.5	1.6	26	15	87	184	84	0.3	1.1	17	5	1.79	0	0.06	0.04	0.6	0.02	12	0.1
4.6	3.9	18	22	135	273	64	0.3	1	10	8	1.92	0	0.11	0.12	0.9	0.03	24	0.14
5.7	1.3	14	27	53	181	46	0.2	0.5	8	1	0.45	0	0.1	0.09	0.7	0.01	21	0.11
5.3	0.9	20	27	43	125	50	0.6	1	13	4	1.91	0	0.11	0.12	0.9	0.04	13	0.17
6.4	7.4	0	77	146	74	218	1.1	1.6	56	0	2.74	0	0.14	0.13	2.3	0.16	30	0
2.4	1.4	21	13	22	10	34	0.1	0.3	3	12	0.55	0	0.04	0.06	0.3	0.02	3	0.06
1.5	0.9	13	19	19	49	15	0.1	0.4	2	7	0.34	0	0.04	0.05	0.4	0.01	2	0.03
3.6	3.2	9	22	47	160	67	0.3	0.5	10	7	1.62	0	0.1	0.11	0.8	0.04	9	0.08
6.5	1.2	22	31	74	129	110	0.9	1.6	35	10	2.17	0	0.12	0.14	1	0.04	15	0.18
10.3	2.6	20	21	65	263	68	0.7	1.6	17	16	2.35	0	0.29	0.13	1.9	0.06	54	0.12
7.7	1.7	4	26	56	205	65	0.5	1.2	13	2	1.84	0	0.22	0.13	1.7	0.03	26	0.05
6.6	1.6	17	16	55	190	51	0.5	1.1	13	10	1.6	0	0.2	0.09	1.4	0.06	40	0.14
0	0	0	0	—	0	45	—	0	—	0	—	6	—	—	—	—	—	0
4.2	1.6	101	14	230	74	286	3	3.1	23	26	0.79	0	0.3	0.53	5.8	0.28	11	0.45
14.6	4.1	95	12	177	67	231	2.1	3.1	18	71	0.79	0	0.2	0.3	5.5	0.2	7	0.34
8.2	3.4	0	50	38	302	212	0.2	1.3	16	94	3.24	5	0.1	0.07	0.8	0.07	6	0.01
0.4	0.2	1	33	22	105	21	0.1	0.4	3	2	0.1	0	0.06	0.05	0.5	0.01	2	0.02
0	0	0	80	—	200	170	—	2.2	—	80	0.59	—	—	—	—	—	—	—
1.6	1.2	46	12	21	113	103	0.1	0.2	7	172	0.59	0	0.01	0.21	0.1	0.01	12	0.12
3.4	2.1	184	31	93	310	118	0.7	1	12	86	1.57	5	0.04	0.26	0.4	0.09	30	0.37
4.1	1.6	231	70	163	368	98	1	0.8	9	138	1.69	0	0.08	0.29	0.4	0.1	19	0.54
2.6	1.3	204	25	97	158	99	0.6	0.8	6	109	1.53	0	0.04	0.28	0.5	0.07	19	0.41
3.6	2.3	126	28	118	251	325	0.7	1.2	15	147	1.88	14	0.09	0.34	1.9	0.15	28	0.26
2.7	1.3	207	25	87	159	60	0.5	0.7	5	110	0.76	0	0.03	0.24	0	0.06	17	0.41
5.6	2.2	254	35	140	454	145	1.1	1.1	10	128	1.82	0	0.17	0.32	1	0.14	21	0.79
3.6	2.3	126	28	118	251	325	0.7	1.2	15	147	1.88	14	0.09	0.34	1.9	0.15	28	0.26
3	1.4	201	44	101	201	152	0.7	1.2	16	198	1.69	16	0.04	0.27	0.2	0.11	38	0.4
—	—	10	20	90	260	120	—	0.4	—	3	—	1	0.1	0.06	0.7	—	—	—
—	—	10	20	50	360	80	—	0.4	—	20	—	4	0.09	0.03	0.4	—	—	—
8.7	12.1	287	37	117	333	90	0.7	0.9	7	130	4.44	0	0.04	0.33	0	0.23	31	0.79
1.5	3.7	1	44	43	119	128	0.6	1.2	9	81	1.27	0	0.07	0.23	0.1	0.08	10	0.2
0.6	1	1	33	76	111	207	0.8	1.3	5	136	0.3	0	0.07	0.19	0.1	0	9	0.19
1.1	1.9	1	63	144	211	394	1.6	2.5	10	258	0.58	0	0.11	0.34	0.1	0	13	0.3
0	0	0	2	4	106	48	0	0	4	0	0	0	0	0.14	0	0	1	0.06
0	0	0	2	4	55	48	0	0	4	0	0	0	0	0.15	0	0	1	0.07
1.9	0.7	212	23	81	33	16	0.5	0.6	1	97	0.49	0	0.02	0.1	0	0.06	18	0.44
1.9	0.7	213	23	81	7	16	0.5	0.6	1	97	0.52	0	0.03	0.11	0	0.06	24	0.52
10.8	3.8	1160	139	524	4592	142	3.4	4.6	12	434	2.74	0	0.16	0.52	0	0.32	130	3.06
1.1	1.9	1	63	144	211	394	1.6	2.5	10	258	0.58	0	0.11	0.34	0.1	0	13	0.3
6.7	3.4	281	125	185	484	193	1	0.9	16	216	2.33	1	0.08	0.46	0.3	0.11	33	0.98
3.5	3	242	29	98	187	73	0.6	0.7	6	99	1.72	0	0.04	0.29	0	0.1	26	0.65
2.4	0.8	246	29	100	72	73	0.6	0.7	6	97	0.61	0	0.04	0.3	0	0.07	26	0.64
2	0.7	212	25	86	62	63	0.5	0.6	5	84	0.52	0	0.03	0.26	0	0.06	22	0.56
1.8	0.6	187	22	76	55	55	0.5	0.5	4	74	0.46	0	0.03	0.23	0	0.05	19	0.49
1.9	0.7	212	24	88	140	60	0.6	0.7	5	95	0.52	0	0.02	0.22	0	0.06	18	0.4
1.7	0.6	186	22	78	123	53	0.5	0.6	4	84	0.46	0	0.02	0.19	0	0.05	15	0.35

Food Item	Qty	Meas	Wgt (g)	Wtr (g)	Cals	Prot	Carb (g)	Fib (g)	Fat (g)	SatF (g)
Egg, scrambled, dry, prepared	0.5	cup	107	73	238	10	1	0	21	5.1
Egg, scrambled, w/cheese, no chol, frozen, prepared	0.5	cup	76	62	64	10	2	0	2	1
Egg, scrambled, w/milk & margarine, large	1	each	61	45	101	7	1	0	7	2.2
Egg, substitute, frozen, prepared	0.5	cup	76	53	139	10	3	0	10	1.7
Egg, whole, fresh or frozen, raw	1	each	50	38	74	6	1	0	5	1.6
Egg, whole, fresh or frozen, raw, jumbo	1	each	65	49	97	8	1	0	6	2
Egg, whole, fresh or frozen, raw, medium	1	each	44	33	66	6	1	0	4	1.4
Egg, whole, fresh or frozen, raw, small	1	each	37	28	55	5	0	0	4	1.2
Egg, whole, fresh or frozen, raw, extra large	1	each	58	44	86	7	1	0	6	1.8
Egg, whole, fried in margarine, large	1	each	46	32	92	6	1	0	7	1.9
Eggnog, made w/2% lowfat milk	1	cup	254	215	189	12	17	0	8	3.8
Eggnog, w/whole milk, commercial	1	cup	254	189	343	10	34	0	19	11.3
Eggplant slices, batter-dipped, fried	1	piece	50	37	75	1	6	1.2	5	1.3
Eggplant slices, cooked, drained, no added salt	1	piece	54	50	15	0	4	1.4	0	0
Eggplant, pieces, steamed	0.5	cup	48	44	12	0	3	1.2	0	0
Eggplant, whole, cooked, drained, no added salt	1	each	538	494	151	4	36	13.5	1	0.2
Eggs, scrambled, plain	2	each	100	75	155	13	1	0	11	3.3
Elderberries, cooked or canned	0.5	cup	128	87	152	1	39	6.6	0	0
Elderberries, raw	0.5	cup	72	58	53	0	13	5.1	0	0
Elk, roasted	4	oz.	113	75	166	34	0	0	2	0.8
Emu, thigh, raw	4	oz.	113	—	105	23	—	—	2	—
Enchilada suiza, chicken, Stouffer's Lean Cuisine	1	each	255	187	290	12	48	5	5	2
Enchilada suiza, chicken, Weight Watchers	1	each	255	203	250	15	28	4	8	3
Enchilada, cheese	1	each	163	103	319	10	28	—	19	10.6
Enchilada, chicken	1	each	120	81	192	13	16	1.9	9	3.5
Enchirito, beef-bean-cheese	1	each	193	121	344	18	34	5.5	16	8
English muffin, cheese	1	each	63	28	148	6	25	1.5	2	1
English muffin, mixed grain	1	each	61	24	143	6	28	1.7	1	0.1
English muffin, plain	1	each	57	24	134	4	26	1.5	1	0.1
English muffin, raisin cinnamon	1	each	57	22	139	4	28	1.6	2	0.2
English muffin, sourdough	1	each	56	24	132	4	26	1.5	1	0.1
English muffin, toasted	1	each	50	19	128	4	25	1.4	1	0.1
English muffin, w/butter, fast food	1	each	63	20	189	4	30	1.9	6	2.4
English muffin, wheat	1	each	57	24	127	5	26	2.6	1	0.2
English muffin, whole wheat	1	each	50	23	102	4	20	3.4	1	0.6
Escarole/curly endive, raw, chopped	0.5	cup	25	24	4	0	1	0.8	0	0
Escargot, snail, steamed	2	each	10	6	18	3	0	0	0	0.1
Fajita, w/beef	1	each	223	140	409	17	46	3.8	18	5.1
Falafel, fava bean patty	1	piece	17	6	57	2	5	0.9	3	0.4
Fat, beef/tallow, drippings	1	Tbs	13	0	116	0	0	0	13	6.4
Fat, chicken	1	Tbs	13	0	115	0	0	0	13	3.8
Feijoa fruit, raw	1	each	50	43	24	1	5	2.1	0	0.1
Fig, canned in heavy syrup	3	each	85	65	75	0	20	1.9	0	0
Figs, canned in water	3	each	80	68	42	0	11	1.8	0	0
Figs, dried	10	each	187	53	477	6	122	22.8	2	0.4
Figs, dried, cooked, unsweetened	0.5	cup	130	90	140	2	36	6.6	1	0.1
Figs, fresh	1	each	50	40	37	0	10	1.6	0	0
Filbert/hazelnut, dried, unblanched, chopped	0.25	cup	29	2	182	4	4	1.8	18	1.3
Filbert/hazelnut, dried, unblanched, whole	0.25	cup	34	2	213	4	5	2.1	21	1.6
Filberts/hazelnuts, dry roasted, unsalted	1	oz.	28	1	188	3	5	2	19	1.4
Filberts/hazelnuts, dry roasted, w/salt	1	oz.	28	1	188	3	5	2.2	19	1.4
Filberts/hazelnuts, oil roasted, salted	1	oz.	28	0	187	4	5	1.8	18	1.3
Filberts/hazelnuts, oil roasted, unsalted	1	oz.	28	0	187	4	5	1.8	18	1.3
Fish ball, cod	1	each	63	39	125	9	8	0.7	7	1.7
Fish cake, cod	1	each	120	74	239	16	15	1.4	13	3.3
Fish cake, fried	1	each	69	41	150	14	5	0.3	8	2
Fish cake, fried, frozen, heated	1	each	85	45	230	8	15	0.8	15	6
Fish dinner, lemon pepper, Healthy Choice	1	each	303	236	320	14	50	5	7	2
Fish patty, heated from frozen	1	each	57	26	155	9	14	0	7	1.8
Fish stick/portion, heated, from frozen	2	each	57	26	155	9	14	0	7	1.8
Fish, Abalone, canned	4	oz.	113	91	91	18	3	0	6	0.3
Fish, Anchovies, canned in oil, drained	10	each	40	20	84	12	0	0	4	0.9
Fish, Gefiltefish, sweet, commercial	1	piece	42	34	35	4	3	0	1	0.2
Fish, Kamaboko (Japanese fish cake)	1	piece	16	11	18	2	2	0	0	0
Fish, King Crab leg, baked/broiled	1	each	119	87	164	23	0	0	8	1.4

MonoF (g)	PolyF (g)	Choles (mg)	Calc (mg)	Phos (mg)	Sod (mg)	Pot (mg)	Zn (mg)	Iron (mg)	Magn (mg)	VitA (μg RE)	VitE (μg α-TE)	VitC (mg)	Thia (mg)	Ribo (mg)	Nia (mg)	B6 (mg)	Fola (μg)	B12 (μg)
9.3	5.1	411	52	149	468	111	1.2	1.7	11	291	3.13	0	0.06	0.24	0.1	0.08	30	1.83
0.4	0	4	66	87	271	135	0.3	0.1	12	14	0.04	0	0.01	0.37	0.1	0.01	2	0.15
2.9	1.3	215	43	104	171	84	0.6	0.7	7	119	0.8	0	0.03	0.27	0	0.07	18	0.47
2.1	5.4	2	63	62	173	185	0.9	1.7	13	117	1.84	0	0.09	0.32	0.1	0.11	11	0.25
1.9	0.7	213	24	89	63	60	0.6	0.7	5	96	0.52	0	0.03	0.25	0	0.07	24	0.5
2.5	0.9	276	32	116	82	79	0.7	0.9	6	124	0.68	0	0.04	0.33	0	0.09	31	0.65
1.7	0.6	187	22	78	55	53	0.5	0.6	4	84	0.46	0	0.03	0.22	0	0.06	21	0.44
1.4	0.5	157	18	66	47	45	0.4	0.5	4	71	0.39	0	0.02	0.19	0	0.05	17	0.37
2.2	0.8	247	28	103	73	70	0.6	0.8	6	111	0.61	0	0.04	0.3	0	0.08	27	0.58
2.8	1.3	211	25	89	162	61	0.5	0.7	5	114	0.75	0	0.03	0.24	0	0.07	18	0.42
2.7	0.7	194	269	269	155	367	1.3	0.7	32	197	1.01	2	0.11	0.55	0.2	0.15	30	1.17
5.7	0.9	149	330	277	138	419	1.2	0.5	47	203	0.58	4	0.09	0.48	0.3	0.13	2	1.14
2.3	1.5	9	27	26	31	107	0.1	0.5	6	5	0.45	1	0.06	0.04	0.5	0.04	7	0.06
0	0	0	3	12	2	134	0.1	0.2	7	3	0.02	1	0.04	0.01	0.3	0.05	8	0
0	0	0	3	11	1	104	0.1	0.1	5	3	0.01	1	0.04	0.01	0.3	0.04	9	0
0.1	0.5	0	32	118	16	1334	0.8	1.9	70	32	0.16	7	0.41	0.11	3.2	0.46	78	0
4.1	1.4	424	50	172	124	126	1	1.2	10	168	1.05	0	0.07	0.51	0.1	0.12	44	1.11
0.1	0.2	0	34	37	6	236	0.1	1.5	5	42	0.94	24	0.05	0.06	0.4	0.19	3	0
0.1	0.2	0	28	28	4	203	0.1	1.2	4	44	0.72	26	0.05	0.04	0.4	0.17	4	0
0.5	0.5	83	6	204	69	372	3.6	4.1	27	0	0.03	0	0.25	0.91	6.6	0.28	5	7.37
—	—	56	—	—	—	—	—	5.7	—	—	—	—	—	—	—	—	—	—
1.5	1.5	25	150	—	530	360	—	0.7	—	60	—	4	—	—	—	—	—	—
—	—	25	300	—	570	470	—	1.4	—	40	—	1	0.15	0.26	4	—	—	—
6.3	0.8	44	324	134	784	240	2.5	1.3	50	186	1.47	1	0.08	0.42	1.9	0.39	65	0.75
2.5	2	36	159	212	307	199	1.3	1	34	108	0.73	16	0.08	0.13	3.1	0.25	15	0.2
6.5	0.3	50	218	224	1250	560	2.8	2.4	71	133	1.54	5	0.17	0.7	3	0.21	60	1.62
0.7	0.5	3	118	78	184	80	0.6	1.8	14	10	0.1	0	0.26	0.27	3	0.1	55	0.02
0.5	0.3	0	120	49	254	95	0.8	1.8	25	0	0.17	0	0.26	0.19	2.2	0.02	49	0
0.2	0.5	0	99	76	264	75	0.4	1.4	12	0	0.1	0	0.25	0.16	2.2	0.02	46	0.02
0.3	0.8	0	84	39	255	119	0.6	1.4	9	0	0.23	0	0.22	0.17	2	0.04	46	0
0.2	0.5	0	97	74	260	73	0.4	1.4	12	0	0.1	0	0.25	0.16	2.2	0.02	45	0.02
0.2	0.5	0	94	72	252	72	0.4	1.4	11	0	0.09	0	0.19	0.14	1.9	0.02	37	0.02
1.5	1.4	13	103	85	386	69	0.4	1.6	13	33	0.13	1	0.25	0.32	2.6	0.04	57	0.02
0.2	0.5	0	101	61	218	106	0.6	1.6	21	0	0.28	0	0.25	0.17	1.9	0.05	31	0
0.4	0	0	133	141	319	105	0.8	1.2	36	0	0.35	0	0.15	0.07	1.7	0.08	21	0
0	0	0	13	7	6	78	0.2	0.2	4	51	0.11	2	0.02	0.02	0.1	0	36	0
0.1	0.1	10	2	38	12	54	0.2	0.6	42	5	1	0	0	0.02	0.2	0.02	1	0.06
7.6	3.9	26	76	200	850	427	2.4	3.7	38	52	2.08	29	0.46	0.3	4.7	0.32	25	1.18
1.7	0.7	0	9	33	50	100	0.3	0.6	14	0	0.19	0	0.02	0.03	0.2	0.02	16	0
5.4	0.5	14	0	0	0	0	0	0	0	0	0.35	0	0	0	0	0	0	0
5.7	2.7	11	0	0	0	0	0	0	0	0	0.35	0	0	0	0	0	0	0
0	0.2	0	8	10	2	78	0	0	4	0	—	10	0	0.02	0.1	0.02	19	0
0	0	0	23	8	1	84	0.1	0.2	8	3	0.76	1	0.02	0.03	0.4	0.06	2	0
0	0	0	22	8	1	82	0.1	0.2	8	3	0.71	1	0.02	0.03	0.4	0.06	2	0
0.5	1	0	269	127	21	1331	1	4.2	110	24	0	2	0.13	0.16	1.3	0.42	14	0
0.1	0.3	0	79	38	6	390	0.3	1.2	32	21	0	6	0.01	0.14	0.8	0.17	1	0
0	0.1	0	18	7	0	116	0.1	0.2	8	7	0.44	1	0.03	0.02	0.2	0.06	3	0
14.1	1.7	0	54	90	1	128	0.7	0.9	82	2	6.87	0	0.14	0.03	0.3	0.18	21	0
16.6	2	0	64	105	1	150	0.8	1.1	96	2	8.07	0	0.17	0.04	0.4	0.21	24	0
14.7	1.8	0	55	92	1	131	0.7	1	84	2	6.78	0	0.06	0.06	0.8	0.18	21	0
14.7	1.8	0	55	92	221	131	0.7	1	84	0	7.09	0	0.06	0.06	0.8	0.18	21	0
14.1	1.7	0	56	92	223	132	0.7	1	84	2	7.09	0	0.06	0.06	0.8	0.18	21	0
14.1	1.7	0	56	92	1	132	0.7	1	84	2	6.78	0	0.06	0.06	0.8	0.18	21	0
2.8	1.7	35	18	108	175	274	0.3	0.4	20	13	0.64	2	0.07	0.07	1.3	0.16	7	0.33
5.3	3.2	66	34	206	333	522	0.7	0.8	38	25	1.21	5	0.13	0.13	2.5	0.31	13	0.63
3.2	2	47	24	139	267	255	0.4	0.6	24	13	1.89	1	0.07	0.09	2.2	0.13	8	0.94
3.4	3.4	22	9	142	150	296	0.3	0.3	15	17	0.51	0	0.03	0.06	1.4	0.04	10	0.85
—	—	30	20	—	480	—	—	1.1	—	100	—	30	—	—	—	—	—	—
2.9	1.8	64	11	103	332	149	0.4	0.4	14	18	0.78	0	0.07	0.1	1.2	0.03	10	1.03
2.9	1.8	64	11	103	332	149	0.4	0.4	14	18	0.78	0	0.07	0.1	1.2	0.03	10	1.03
2.6	3.6	91	16	145	794	318	1	2.6	57	2	5.67	1	0.14	0.08	2	0.17	2	0.79
1.5	1	34	93	101	1467	218	1	1.8	28	8	2	0	0.03	0.14	8	0.08	5	0.35
0.3	0.1	13	10	31	220	38	0.3	1	4	11	0.06	0	0.03	0.02	0.4	0.03	1	0.35
0	0.1	8	7	24	135	39	0.1	0.1	7	1	0.02	0	0	0.02	0.4	0.03	0	0.33
2.8	2.5	111	118	231	642	364	4.7	1	37	78	2.01	4	0.11	0.06	3.7	0.2	57	8.13

Food Item	Qty	Meas	Wgt (g)	Wtr (g)	Cals	Prot	Carb (g)	Fib (g)	Fat (g)	SatF (g)
Fish, Lingcod, baked/broiled fillet	0.5	each	151	114	165	34	0	0	2	0.4
Fish, Queen crab, baked/broiled	0.5	cup	59	44	68	14	0	0	1	0.1
Fish, Snow Crab leg, baked/broiled	1	each	10	7	14	2	0	0	1	0.1
Fish, Spiny lobster, steamed	1	each	229	153	327	60	7	0	4	0.7
Fish, abalone, floured, fried	4	oz.	113	68	214	22	13	0	8	1.9
Fish, abalone, fried	4	oz.	113	68	214	22	13	0	8	1.9
Fish, abalone, mixed species, raw	4	oz.	113	85	119	19	7	0	1	0.2
Fish, abalone, steamed/poached	4	oz.	113	56	238	39	14	0	2	0.3
Fish, butterfish, baked/broiled fillet	3	oz.	85	57	159	19	0	0	9	2.6
Fish, calamari, dried	1	oz.	28	6	95	16	3	0	1	0.4
Fish, carp, baked/broiled fillet	3	oz.	85	59	138	20	0	0	6	1.2
Fish, catfish, breaded fried fillet	3	oz.	85	50	195	15	7	0.6	11	2.8
Fish, catfish, steamed/poached	4	oz.	113	78	191	22	0	0	11	2.5
Fish, caviar, black/red, granular	2	Tbs	32	15	81	8	1	0	6	1.3
Fish, clam, breaded, fried	0.5	cup	75	46	152	11	8	0.1	8	2
Fish, clam, smoked, canned in oil	10	each	100	69	175	14	3	0	12	2.7
Fish, clams, canned, drained	4	oz.	113	72	168	29	6	0	2	0.2
Fish, clams, steamed, large	8	each	150	95	222	38	8	0	3	0.3
Fish, clams, steamed, small	20	each	90	57	133	23	5	0	2	0.2
Fish, cod, Pacific, baked/broiled fillet	1	each	90	68	94	21	0	0	1	0.1
Fish, cod, Pacific, baked/broiled fillet	3	oz.	85	65	89	20	0	0	1	0.1
Fish, cod, batter fried pieces	3	piece	48	32	83	8	3	0.1	4	0.9
Fish, cod, steamed/poached	4	oz.	113	87	116	25	0	0	1	0.2
Fish, crab leg, Alaskan King, steamed	1	each	134	104	130	26	0	0	2	0.2
Fish, crab, baked/broiled	0.5	cup	59	43	81	11	0	0	4	0.7
Fish, crab, blue, canned meat	4	oz.	113	86	112	23	0	0	1	0.3
Fish, crab, blue, steamed, whole	1	each	48	37	49	10	0	0	1	0.1
Fish, crab, dungeness, steamed	4	oz.	113	83	125	25	1	0	1	0.2
Fish, crab, imitation	4	oz.	113	84	116	14	12	0	1	0.3
Fish, crab, soft shell, floured/breaded, fried	1	each	65	26	217	13	11	0.5	13	3.2
Fish, crayfish/Crawdads, steamed	4	oz.	113	90	93	19	0	0	1	0.2
Fish, crayfish/crawdads wild, raw	8	each	27	22	21	4	0	0	0	0
Fish, cuttlefish, steamed	4	oz.	113	69	179	37	2	0	2	0.3
Fish, eel, steamed/poached	4	oz.	113	68	261	26	0	0	16	3.3
Fish, grouper, baked/broiled fillet	3	oz.	85	62	100	21	0	0	1	0.3
Fish, haddock patty	1	each	120	74	239	16	15	1.4	13	3.3
Fish, haddock, baked/broiled fillet	3	oz.	85	63	95	21	0	0	1	0.1
Fish, haddock, breaded, fried fillet	3	oz.	85	47	199	16	11	0.6	10	2.4
Fish, haddock, steamed/poached	3	oz.	85	64	92	20	0	0	1	0.1
Fish, halibut, Pacific, steamed	4	oz.	113	81	159	30	0	0	3	0.5
Fish, herring, Atlantic, baked/broiled fillet	3	oz.	85	55	173	20	0	0	10	2.2
Fish, herring, Atlantic, pickled	6	piece	90	50	236	13	9	0	16	2.1
Fish, jellyfish, pickled	0.5	cup	29	20	10	2	0	0	0	0.1
Fish, lobster pieces, baked/broiled	0.5	cup	72	54	84	14	1	0	2	1.2
Fish, lobster tail, baked/broiled	1	each	125	92	145	25	2	0	4	2
Fish, lobster, battered, fried	3	oz.	85	51	180	16	7	0.2	9	2.3
Fish, lobster, northern, raw	3	oz.	85	65	76	16	0	0	1	0.2
Fish, lobster, northern, steamed	4	oz.	113	86	111	23	1	0	1	0.1
Fish, lobster, w/butter sauce	0.5	cup	94	59	224	15	1	0	18	10.9
Fish, mackerel, Atlantic, baked/broiled fillet	3	oz.	85	45	223	20	0	0	15	3.6
Fish, mackerel, Jack, canned, drained	1	cup	190	131	296	44	0	0	12	3.5
Fish, moochim, Korean (dried fish & soy sauce)	0.5	cup	40	9	133	15	4	0.2	6	0.9
Fish, mullet, baked/broiled fillet	3	oz.	85	60	128	21	0	0	4	1.2
Fish, mussels, blue, raw	4	oz.	113	91	98	14	4	0	3	0.5
Fish, mussels, blue, steamed	4	oz.	113	69	195	27	8	0	5	1
Fish, mussels, smoked, canned, in oil, drained	0.5	cup	75	46	146	16	3	0	8	—
Fish, mussels, w/tomato-based sauce	0.5	cup	120	87	134	15	12	1.8	3	0.6
Fish, octopus, cooked	4	oz.	113	69	186	34	5	0	2	0.5
Fish, octopus, dried	0.5	cup	26	5	90	15	3	0	1	0.3
Fish, octopus, dried, cooked	0.5	cup	53	30	97	16	3	0	1	0.4
Fish, octopus, raw	4	oz.	113	91	93	17	2	0	1	0.3
Fish, octopus, smoked	4	oz.	113	75	158	29	4	0	2	0.4
Fish, orange roughy baked/broiled	0.5	cup	66	46	59	12	0	0	1	0
Fish, oyster, Eastern, breaded, fried, cup measure	1	cup	131	85	258	12	15	0.2	16	4.2
Fish, oyster, Pacific, raw	1	each	50	41	40	5	2	0	1	0.3

MonoF (g)	PolyF (g)	Choles (mg)	Calc (mg)	Phos (mg)	Sod (mg)	Pot (mg)	Zn (mg)	Iron (mg)	Magn (mg)	VitA (µg RE)	VitE (µg α-TE)	VitC (mg)	Thia (mg)	Ribo (mg)	Nia (mg)	B6 (mg)	Fola (µg)	B12 (µg)
0.7	0.6	101	27	390	115	846	0.9	0.6	50	26	0.44	0	0.05	0.21	3.5	0.52	15	6.27
0.2	0.3	42	20	76	408	118	2.1	1.7	37	31	0.67	4	0.06	0.14	1.7	0.1	25	6.14
0.2	0.2	9	10	19	54	31	0.4	0.1	3	7	0.17	0	0.01	0	0.3	0.02	5	0.68
0.8	1.7	206	144	524	520	476	16.6	3.2	117	14	4.58	5	0.02	0.13	11.2	0.4	2	9.25
3.1	1.9	107	42	246	670	322	1.1	4.3	64	2	6.8	2	0.25	0.15	2.2	0.17	16	0.78
3.1	1.9	107	42	246	670	322	1.1	4.3	64	2	6.8	2	0.25	0.15	2.2	0.17	16	0.78
0.1	0.1	96	35	215	341	284	0.9	3.6	54	2	4.54	2	0.22	0.11	1.7	0.17	6	0.83
0.2	0.2	193	67	302	580	397	1.9	6.5	92	4	9.07	3	0.39	0.17	2.6	0.29	9	0.99
3.1	2.7	71	24	262	97	409	0.8	0.5	27	28	0.52	0	0.12	0.16	4.9	0.29	14	1.56
0.1	0.5	240	33	228	165	253	1.6	0.7	34	9	1.24	4	0.02	0.42	2.2	0.06	5	1.27
2.5	1.6	71	44	451	54	363	1.6	1.4	32	8	0.91	1	0.12	0.06	1.8	0.19	15	1.25
4.8	2.8	69	37	184	238	289	0.7	1.2	23	7	1.09	0	0.06	0.11	1.9	0.16	26	1.62
5.1	2.2	67	13	258	68	360	1	0.7	29	17	1.7	1	0.41	0.1	2.8	0.21	11	2.98
1.5	2.4	188	88	114	480	58	0.3	3.8	96	179	2.24	0	0.06	0.2	0	0.1	16	6.4
3.4	2.2	46	47	141	273	245	1.1	10.4	10	68	1.88	8	0.08	0.18	1.6	0.04	27	30.2
4.8	3.1	38	52	188	321	349	1.5	15.6	10	100	1.97	14	0.08	0.24	2	0.07	18	55
0.2	0.6	76	104	383	127	712	3.1	31.8	20	194	1.13	25	0.17	0.48	3.8	0.12	33	112
0.3	0.8	101	138	507	168	942	4.1	42	27	257	2.94	33	0.22	0.64	5	0.16	43	148
0.2	0.5	60	83	304	101	565	2.5	25.2	16	154	1.76	20	0.14	0.38	3	0.1	26	89
0.1	0.3	42	8	201	82	465	0.5	0.3	28	9	0.31	3	0.02	0.05	2.2	0.42	7	0.94
0.1	0.3	40	8	190	77	439	0.4	0.3	26	8	0.29	3	0.02	0.04	2.1	0.39	7	0.88
1.5	1.1	27	18	98	52	188	0.3	0.4	15	7	0.39	0	0.05	0.06	1.1	0.1	4	0.41
0.1	0.3	61	23	259	69	498	0.6	0.5	41	14	0.32	1	0.09	0.08	2.5	0.28	8	1.09
0.2	0.7	71	79	375	1436	351	10.2	1	84	12	1.21	10	0.07	0.07	1.8	0.24	68	15.4
1.4	1.2	55	59	115	319	180	2.3	0.5	18	38	0.99	2	0.06	0.03	1.8	0.1	28	4.03
0.2	0.5	101	115	295	378	424	4.6	1	44	2	1.13	3	0.09	0.1	1.6	0.17	48	0.52
0.1	0.3	48	50	99	134	156	2	0.4	16	1	0.48	2	0.05	0.02	1.6	0.09	24	3.5
0.2	0.5	86	67	198	429	463	6.2	0.5	66	35	1.28	4	0.06	0.23	4.1	0.2	48	11.8
0.2	0.8	23	15	320	954	102	0.4	0.4	49	23	0.11	0	0.04	0.03	0.2	0.03	2	1.81
5.4	3.4	80	71	141	336	203	2.4	1.2	23	14	1.63	1	0.13	0.12	2.4	0.1	28	3.34
0.3	0.4	151	68	306	107	336	2	0.9	37	17	1.7	1	0.06	0.1	2.6	0.09	50	2.44
0	0.1	31	7	69	16	82	0.4	0.2	7	4	0.77	0	0.02	0.01	0.6	0.03	10	0.54
0.2	0.3	254	204	658	844	722	3.9	12.2	68	230	5.1	10	0.02	1.96	2.5	0.31	27	6.12
10.2	1.3	179	28	276	65	328	2.3	0.7	26	1256	5.67	2	0.17	0.05	4.2	0.08	17	3.61
0.2	0.3	40	18	122	45	404	0.4	1	32	42	0.53	0	0.07	0	0.3	0.3	9	0.59
5.3	3.2	66	34	206	333	522	0.7	0.8	38	25	1.21	5	0.13	0.13	2.5	0.31	13	0.63
0.1	0.3	63	36	205	74	339	0.4	1.2	42	16	0.42	0	0.03	0.04	3.9	0.29	11	1.18
4	2.5	72	48	171	393	259	0.4	1.4	35	25	1.17	0	0.06	0.11	3.4	0.21	15	0.85
0.1	0.3	61	35	180	65	281	0.4	1.1	37	14	0.41	0	0.03	0.04	3.4	0.26	10	1.09
1.1	1.1	46	68	323	78	653	0.6	1.2	121	61	1.24	0	0.08	0.1	8.1	0.45	16	1.55
4.1	2.3	66	63	258	98	356	1.1	1.2	35	26	1.14	1	0.1	0.25	3.5	0.3	10	11.1
10.7	1.5	12	69	80	783	62	0.5	1.1	7	232	0.9	0	0.03	0.12	3	0.15	2	3.84
0.1	0.2	1	1	6	2809	1	0.1	0.7	1	1	0.01	0	0	0	0.1	0	0	0.01
0.6	0.1	55	43	130	451	247	2	0.3	24	35	0.73	0	0	0.05	0.7	0.05	8	2.18
1.1	0.2	95	75	224	777	425	3.5	0.5	42	60	1.27	0	0.01	0.08	1.3	0.09	14	3.75
4	2.6	68	64	155	326	278	2.2	0.7	28	23	1.46	0	0.05	0.1	1.1	0.06	8	2.02
0.2	0.1	81	41	122	252	234	2.6	0.3	23	18	1.25	0	0	0.04	1.2	0.05	8	0.79
0.2	0.1	82	69	210	431	399	3.3	0.4	40	30	1.13	0	0.01	0.08	1.2	0.09	13	3.53
5.1	0.7	99	49	139	453	261	2.1	0.3	26	180	1.06	0	0.01	0.06	0.8	0.06	9	2.29
6	3.7	64	13	236	71	341	0.8	1.3	82	46	1.57	0	0.14	0.35	5.8	0.39	1	16.2
4.2	3.1	150	458	572	720	369	1.9	3.9	70	247	2.66	2	0.08	0.4	11.7	0.4	10	13.2
2.3	2.5	34	54	230	2015	349	0.5	1	38	9	0.37	1	0.08	0.07	2	0.22	8	2.22
1.2	0.8	54	26	207	60	389	0.7	1.2	28	36	1.04	1	0.08	0.08	5.4	0.42	8	0.21
0.6	0.7	32	30	223	324	363	1.8	4.5	39	54	0.84	9	0.18	0.24	1.8	0.06	48	13.6
1.2	1.4	64	37	323	418	304	3	7.6	42	103	1.64	15	0.34	0.48	3.4	0.11	86	27.2
—	—	69	51	—	341	104	2.8	7	74	90	—	0	—	0.36	1.7	—	—	—
0.6	0.7	34	37	193	745	457	2	4.5	44	72	1.91	12	0.21	0.26	2.2	0.1	52	13
0.4	0.5	109	120	316	522	714	3.8	10.8	68	92	1.36	9	0.06	0.09	4.3	0.74	27	40.8
0.1	0.5	227	31	215	156	240	1.5	0.7	32	9	1.17	4	0.02	0.4	2.1	0.05	5	1.2
0.1	0.6	246	34	233	169	259	1.6	0.7	35	9	1.26	4	0.02	0.43	2.3	0.06	5	1.3
0.2	0.3	54	60	211	261	397	1.9	6	34	51	1.36	6	0.03	0.04	2.4	0.41	18	22.7
0.3	0.5	93	102	359	444	676	3.2	10.2	58	78	2.32	8	0.06	0.08	4.1	0.66	29	36.7
0.4	0	17	25	169	54	254	0.6	0.2	25	16	0.42	0	0.08	0.12	2.4	0.23	5	1.52
6.2	4.3	106	81	208	546	320	114	9.1	76	118	2.99	5	0.2	0.26	2.2	0.08	41	20.4
0.2	0.4	25	4	80	53	83	8.2	2.5	11	40	0.42	4	0.03	0.12	1	0.02	5	7.94

Food Item	Qty	Meas	Wgt (g)	Wtr (g)	Cals	Prot	Carb (g)	Fib (g)	Fat (g)	SatF (g)
Fish, oyster, baked/broiled	4	oz.	113	94	82	9	5	0	2	0.6
Fish, oyster, eastern, canned, w/liquid	0.5	cup	124	106	86	9	5	0	3	0.8
Fish, oyster, eastern, raw	4	oz.	113	97	77	8	4	0	3	0.9
Fish, oyster, eastern, steamed	6	each	42	30	58	6	3	0	2	0.6
Fish, oysters, Pacific, steamed/boiled	4	oz.	113	73	185	21	11	0	5	1.2
Fish, perch, mixed, baked/broiled fillet	1	each	46	34	54	12	0	0	1	0.1
Fish, perch, mixed, baked/broiled fillet	3	oz.	85	62	100	21	0	0	1	0.2
Fish, pollock, walleye, baked/broiled	1	each	60	44	68	14	0	0	1	0.1
Fish, pollock, walleye, baked/broiled	3	oz.	85	63	96	20	0	0	1	0.2
Fish, salmon cake/patty	1	each	120	71	261	16	14	1.3	16	4.1
Fish, salmon croquette	1	each	63	37	137	9	7	0.7	8	2.2
Fish, salmon loaf	3	oz.	85	51	170	13	7	0.3	9	2.5
Fish, salmon, Atlantic, baked/broiled fillet	3	oz.	85	51	155	22	0	0	7	1.1
Fish, salmon, chinook, baked/broiled	4	oz.	113	74	262	29	0	0	15	3.6
Fish, salmon, chinook, smoked/lox	4	oz.	113	82	133	21	0	0	5	1
Fish, salmon, chum, baked/broiled	4	oz.	113	78	175	29	0	0	5	1.2
Fish, salmon, chum, canned, drained	0.5	cup	75	53	106	16	0	0	4	1.1
Fish, salmon, coho, steamed/poached fillet	3	oz.	85	56	156	23	0	0	6	1.4
Fish, salmon, pink, baked/broiled	4	oz.	113	79	169	29	0	0	5	0.8
Fish, salmon, sockeye, canned, drained	0.5	cup	75	52	115	15	0	0	5	1.2
Fish, sardine, Atlantic, canned in oil, drained	4	each	48	29	100	12	0	0	6	0.7
Fish, sardines, Pacific, canned in tomato sauce	2	each	76	52	135	12	0	0	9	2.4
Fish, sardines, canned, w/mustard	4	oz.	113	73	222	21	2	0	14	4.4
Fish, sardines, skinless, water pack	4	each	84	50	182	21	0	0	10	2.3
Fish, scallop, battered, fried	10	each	80	44	184	14	11	0.4	9	2.2
Fish, scallops, baked/broiled	4	each	100	70	133	21	3	0	4	0.7
Fish, scallops, breaded, fried, large	2	each	31	18	67	6	3	0	3	0.8
Fish, scallops, imitation, from surimi	4	oz.	113	84	112	14	12	0	0	0.1
Fish, scallops, steamed	4	oz.	113	86	121	18	3	0	4	0.6
Fish, sea bass, baked/broiled fillet	3	oz.	85	61	105	20	0	0	2	0.6
Fish, shark, baked/broiled w/marg, lemon juice, salt	4	oz.	113	74	203	28	0	0	9	1.9
Fish, shark, batter fried	4	oz.	113	68	259	21	7	0	16	3.6
Fish, shrimp cocktail	0.5	cup	115	89	98	13	10	2.1	1	0.3
Fish, shrimp w/butter sauce	0.5	cup	68	47	110	15	1	0	5	2.6
Fish, shrimp, baked/broiled, medium size	2	each	10	7	16	2	0	0	1	0.1
Fish, shrimp, batter fried	12	each	90	48	218	19	10	0.3	11	1.9
Fish, shrimp, canned, drained	10	each	32	23	38	7	0	0	1	0.1
Fish, shrimp, dried	1	cup	38	12	115	22	1	0	2	0.4
Fish, shrimp, dried, whole	60	each	30	9	91	18	1	0	1	0.3
Fish, shrimp, imitation, made from surimi	4	oz.	113	85	115	14	10	0	2	0.3
Fish, shrimp, large/prawns, breaded, fried	5	each	85	45	206	18	10	0.3	10	1.8
Fish, shrimp, large/prawns, steamed	10	each	55	42	54	12	0	0	1	0.2
Fish, shrimp, popcorn, baked/broiled	15	each	15	10	23	4	0	0	1	0.1
Fish, shrimp, small, breaded, fried	12	each	72	38	174	15	8	0.3	9	1.5
Fish, shrimp, small, steamed	10	each	40	31	40	8	0	0	0	0.1
Fish, shrimp, sweet & sour	0.5	cup	88	42	240	9	21	0.4	14	2.1
Fish, smelt, rainbow, baked/broiled	4	oz.	113	83	141	26	0	0	4	0.7
Fish, snapper, baked/broiled fillet	4	oz.	113	80	145	30	0	0	2	0.4
Fish, sole/flounder, baked/broiled fillet	3	oz.	85	62	100	21	0	0	1	0.3
Fish, sole/flounder, breaded, fried fillet	3	oz.	85	50	185	17	7	0.4	10	2.4
Fish, sole/flounder, steamed/poached	4	oz.	113	84	129	27	0	0	2	0.4
Fish, squid, canned	0.5	cup	94	70	99	17	3	0	1	0.4
Fish, squid, flour fried	0.5	cup	75	48	131	13	6	0	6	1.4
Fish, squid, pickled	4	oz.	113	85	104	17	5	0	2	0.4
Fish, squid/calamari, baked/broiled	4	oz.	113	80	156	21	4	0	5	1.2
Fish, steelhead, baked/broiled fillet	3	oz.	85	61	113	18	0	0	4	1.1
Fish, sturgeon, baked/broiled	4	oz.	113	79	153	24	0	0	6	1.3
Fish, sturgeon, smoked	4	oz.	113	71	196	35	0	0	5	1.2
Fish, surimi (processed pollock)	4	oz.	113	86	112	17	8	0	1	0.2
Fish, swordfish, broiled/baked	3	oz.	85	58	132	22	0	0	4	1.2
Fish, swordfish, steamed/poached	4	oz.	113	78	174	28	0	0	6	1.6
Fish, trout, mixed, baked/broiled	4	oz.	113	72	215	30	0	0	10	1.7
Fish, trout, rainbow, baked/broiled fillet	3	oz.	85	60	128	20	0	0	5	1.4
Fish, tuna, bluefin, baked/broiled	4	oz.	113	67	209	34	0	0	7	1.8
Fish, tuna, light, canned in oil, drained	1	cup	146	87	289	42	0	0	12	2.2

MonoF	PolyF	Choles	Calc	Phos	Sod	Pot	Zn	Iron	Magn	VitA	VitE	VitC	Thia	Ribo	Nia	B6	Fola	B12
(g)	(g)	(mg)	(mg)	(mg)	(mg)	(mg)	(mg)	(mg)	(mg)	(µg RE)	(µg α-TE)	(mg)	(mg)	(mg)	(mg)	(mg)	(µg)	(µg)
0.3	0.9	56	51	154	277	191	83.5	4.9	52	0	0.96	5	0.1	0.09	1.9	0.11	20	31.5
0.3	0.9	68	56	172	139	284	113	8.3	67	112	1.05	6	0.19	0.21	1.5	0.12	11	23.7
0.4	1.1	60	51	153	239	177	103	7.6	53	34	0.96	4	0.11	0.11	1.6	0.07	11	22.1
0.3	0.8	44	38	85	177	118	76.4	5	40	23	0.67	3	0.08	0.08	1	0.05	6	14.7
0.8	2	113	18	276	240	342	37.6	10.4	50	166	2.01	14	0.14	0.5	4.1	0.1	17	32.7
0.1	0.2	53	47	118	36	158	0.7	0.5	18	5	0.7	1	0.04	0.06	0.9	0.06	3	1.01
0.2	0.4	98	87	218	67	292	1.2	1	32	8	1.28	1	0.07	0.1	1.6	0.12	5	1.87
0.1	0.3	58	4	289	70	232	0.4	0.2	44	14	0.12	0	0.04	0.05	1	0.04	2	2.52
0.1	0.4	82	5	410	99	329	0.5	0.2	62	20	0.17	0	0.06	0.06	1.4	0.06	3	3.57
6.4	4	56	180	275	657	385	0.9	0.9	32	27	2.11	4	0.09	0.18	5.4	0.37	20	2.19
3.4	2.1	30	95	144	345	202	0.5	0.5	17	14	1.11	2	0.05	0.1	2.9	0.2	10	1.15
3.5	2.6	99	153	223	640	234	0.8	1	25	97	1.63	2	0.07	0.24	3.7	0.18	18	1.9
2.3	2.8	60	13	218	48	534	0.7	0.9	32	11	1.07	0	0.23	0.41	8.6	0.8	25	2.59
6.5	3	96	32	421	68	573	0.6	1	138	169	1.94	5	0.05	0.18	11.3	0.52	40	3.25
2.3	1.1	26	12	186	2268	198	0.4	1	20	30	1.53	0	0.03	0.12	5.4	0.32	2	3.7
2.2	1.3	108	16	412	73	624	0.7	0.8	32	39	1.94	0	0.1	0.25	9.7	0.52	6	3.92
1.4	1.1	29	187	266	365	225	0.8	0.5	22	14	1.2	0	0.02	0.12	5.2	0.28	15	3.3
2.3	2.1	48	39	253	45	387	0.4	0.6	30	27	0.69	1	0.1	0.14	6.6	0.47	8	3.81
1.4	2	76	19	335	98	469	0.8	1.1	37	46	1.43	0	0.22	0.08	9.7	0.26	6	3.92
2.4	1.4	33	179	245	404	283	0.8	0.8	22	40	1.2	0	0.01	0.14	4.1	0.22	7	0.22
1.9	2.5	68	183	235	242	191	0.6	1.4	19	32	0.14	0	0.04	0.11	2.5	0.08	6	4.29
4.2	1.8	46	182	278	315	259	1.1	1.8	26	53	2.81	1	0.03	0.18	3.2	0.09	18	6.84
4.8	3.2	125	344	401	862	295	0.6	5.9	11	10	1.13	1	0.03	0.23	6.1	0.14	18	7.94
4.3	2.4	69	71	273	771	375	1.1	1.3	39	33	0.84	1	0.11	0.27	3.7	0.35	12	15.7
3.7	2.3	65	29	182	374	248	0.8	0.9	43	29	1.55	2	0.07	0.14	1.3	0.11	15	0.98
1.4	1.3	40	30	265	511	390	1.2	0.4	68	56	1.69	3	0.01	0.06	1.3	0.17	18	1.75
1.4	0.9	19	13	73	144	103	0.3	0.3	18	7	0.59	1	0.01	0.03	0.5	0.04	12	0.41
0.1	0.2	25	9	320	902	117	0.4	0.4	49	23	0.12	0	0.01	0.02	0.4	0.03	2	1.81
1.3	1.2	36	28	180	465	318	1	0.3	61	52	1.53	3	0.01	0.07	1.1	0.16	13	1.51
0.5	0.8	45	11	211	74	279	0.4	0.3	45	54	0.54	0	0.11	0.13	1.6	0.39	5	0.26
3.5	3	68	47	279	455	219	0.6	1.1	65	124	1.86	2	0.05	0.08	3.9	0.48	4	1.48
6.7	4.2	67	57	220	138	176	0.5	1.3	49	61	1.19	0	0.08	0.11	3.2	0.34	17	1.37
0.2	0.4	87	43	138	496	277	0.7	1.7	27	36	2.32	12	0.05	0.05	1.9	0.12	27	0.56
1.3	0.6	120	38	149	146	134	0.8	1.7	26	47	1.66	1	0.02	0.02	1.8	0.07	1	0.72
0.2	0.2	18	6	25	50	22	0.1	0.3	4	10	0.39	0	0	0	0.3	0.01	0	0.13
3.4	4.6	159	60	196	310	203	1.2	1.1	36	50	1.35	1	0.12	0.12	2.8	0.09	7	1.68
0.1	0.2	55	19	75	54	67	0.4	0.9	13	6	0.3	1	0.01	0.01	0.9	0.04	1	0.36
0.3	0.7	166	57	224	163	202	1.2	2.6	39	17	2.41	2	0.03	0.04	2.6	0.11	2	1.08
0.2	0.6	131	45	177	128	159	1	2.1	31	14	1.9	2	0.02	0.03	2.1	0.08	1	0.85
0.2	0.9	41	22	320	799	101	0.4	0.7	49	23	0.12	0	0.03	0.04	0.2	0.03	2	1.81
3.2	4.3	150	57	185	292	191	1.2	1.1	34	48	1.28	1	0.11	0.12	2.6	0.08	7	1.59
0.1	0.2	107	22	75	123	100	0.9	1.7	19	36	0.28	1	0.02	0.02	1.4	0.07	2	0.82
0.2	0.3	28	10	37	75	34	0.2	0.4	7	14	0.59	0	0	0	0.4	0.02	1	0.2
2.7	3.7	127	48	157	248	162	1	0.9	29	40	1.08	1	0.09	0.1	2.2	0.07	6	1.35
0.1	0.2	78	16	55	90	73	0.6	1.2	14	26	0.2	1	0.01	0.01	1	0.05	1	0.6
3.3	8.2	60	29	98	409	183	0.6	1.5	23	25	2.07	5	0.03	0.04	1.4	0.1	3	0.39
0.9	1.3	102	87	335	87	422	2.4	1.3	43	19	0.71	0	0.01	0.17	2	0.19	5	4.5
0.4	0.7	53	45	228	65	592	0.5	0.3	42	40	0.71	2	0.06	0	0.4	0.52	7	3.97
0.2	0.5	58	15	246	89	292	0.5	0.3	49	9	1.61	0	0.07	0.1	1.8	0.2	8	2.13
4	2.5	58	30	171	329	315	0.5	0.7	29	16	2.33	1	0.09	0.11	2.8	0.16	10	1.16
0.3	0.5	68	26	235	103	435	0.6	0.5	40	11	2.68	2	0.1	0.1	3.5	0.24	9	1.83
0.1	0.6	250	35	190	292	211	1.6	0.7	32	9	1.29	4	0.02	0.35	1.9	0.04	4	1.05
2.1	1.6	195	29	188	230	209	1.3	0.8	28	8	1.39	3	0.04	0.34	2	0.04	10	0.92
0.1	0.6	254	37	229	1585	273	1.7	0.7	36	10	1.31	4	0.02	0.45	2.2	0.05	5	1.35
1.7	1.8	318	45	303	420	338	2.1	0.9	45	58	2.19	6	0.02	0.45	2.8	0.07	6	1.69
1	0.8	90	19	273	63	371	0.5	0.3	34	30	0.21	0	0.06	0.18	2.5	0.39	5	2.94
2.8	1	87	19	307	78	413	0.6	1	51	274	0.85	0	0.09	0.1	11.5	0.26	20	2.84
2.7	0.5	91	19	319	838	430	0.6	1	53	318	0.57	0	0.1	0.1	12.6	0.31	23	3.29
0.2	0.5	34	10	320	162	127	0.4	0.3	49	23	0.28	0	0.02	0.02	0.2	0.03	2	1.81
1.7	1	42	5	286	98	314	1.2	0.9	29	35	0.54	1	0.04	0.1	10	0.32	2	1.72
2.2	1.3	56	6	340	116	351	1.6	1.2	35	44	0.72	1	0.04	0.12	11.8	0.38	2	2.14
4.7	2.2	84	62	356	76	525	1	2.2	32	22	0.3	1	0.48	0.48	6.5	0.26	17	8.49
1.5	1.6	59	73	229	48	381	0.4	0.3	26	13	0.43	2	0.13	0.08	4.9	0.29	16	5.36
2.3	2.1	56	11	370	57	366	0.9	1.5	73	857	1.43	0	0.32	0.35	11.9	0.6	2	12.4
4.3	4.2	26	19	454	517	302	1.3	2	45	34	1.75	0	0.06	0.18	18.1	0.16	8	3.21

Food Item	Qty	Meas	Wgt (g)	Wtr (g)	Cals	Prot	Carb (g)	Fib (g)	Fat (g)	SatF (g)
Fish, tuna, skipjack, baked/broiled	4	oz.	113	71	150	32	0	0	1	0.5
Fish, tuna, yellowfin, baked/broiled	4	oz.	113	71	158	34	0	0	1	0.3
Fish, whelk, steamed	4	oz.	113	36	312	54	18	0	1	0.1
Fish, whiting, baked/broiled	4	oz.	113	85	132	27	0	0	2	0.5
Flan caramel custard mix w/2% milk	0.5	cup	133	100	136	4	26	0.1	2	1.5
Flan caramel custard mix w/whole milk	0.5	cup	133	99	150	4	25	0.1	4	2.5
Flauta, beef	1	each	113	55	360	16	13	1.7	27	4.9
Flauta, chicken	1	each	113	59	343	14	13	1.7	27	4.3
Flour, bread, white, Pillsbury	1	cup	113	16	396	14	81	2.7	1	0.3
Flour, brown rice	1	cup	158	19	574	11	121	7.3	4	0.9
Flour, buckwheat, whole groat	1	cup	98	11	328	12	69	9.8	3	0.7
Flour, carob	1	cup	103	4	229	5	92	41	1	0.1
Flour, chickpea	1	cup	85	8	313	17	51	3.1	6	—
Flour, corn, yellow	1	cup	114	10	416	11	87	15.3	4	0.6
Flour, corn/masa harina, enriched	1	cup	114	10	416	11	87	10.9	4	0.6
Flour, gluten	1	cup	140	12	529	58	66	1.2	3	0
Flour, potato	1	cup	179	12	639	12	149	10.6	1	0.2
Flour, rye, dark	1	cup	128	14	415	18	88	28.9	3	0.4
Flour, rye, light	1	cup	102	9	374	9	82	14.9	1	0.1
Flour, rye, medium	1	cup	102	10	361	10	79	14.9	2	0.2
Flour, sesame, partially defatted	1	oz.	28	2	108	11	10	1.7	2	0.5
Flour, shake and blend, Pillsbury	1	cup	216	30	756	23	158	5.8	3	1.1
Flour, sunflower seed, partially defatted	1	cup	80	6	261	38	29	4.2	3	0.1
Flour, triticale, whole grain	1	cup	130	13	439	17	95	19	1	0.4
Flour, white, all purpose, enriched	1	cup	125	15	455	13	95	3.4	2	0.2
Flour, white, all purpose, enriched, unbleached	1	cup	125	15	455	13	95	3.4	1	0.2
Flour, white, all purpose, sifted	1	cup	115	14	419	12	88	3.1	1	0.2
Flour, white, cake, enriched, sifted	1	cup	96	12	348	8	75	1.6	1	0.1
Flour, white, self-rising, enriched	1	cup	125	13	443	12	93	3.4	1	0.2
Flour, whole wheat	1	cup	120	12	407	16	87	14.6	2	0.4
Forza energy bar	1	each	70	12	231	10	45	4	1	—
French toast, homemade, w/2% milk	1	piece	65	36	149	5	16	0.6	7	1.8
French toast, recipe, w/whole milk	1	piece	65	35	151	5	16	0.5	7	2
Fritter, banana	1	each	34	13	116	2	11	0.4	7	2
Fritter, berry	1	each	34	15	111	2	10	0.6	7	1.9
Fritter, wheat, no syrup	1	each	22	8	99	2	4	0.1	9	2
Frog legs, steamed	2	each	100	74	106	24	0	0	0	0.1
Frosting, chocolate cream, recipe, w/margarine	2	Tbs	34	3	138	0	27	0.6	4	0.9
Frosting, chocolate, creamy, ready to eat, can	1	each	462	78	1834	5	292	2.8	81	25.5
Frosting, chocolate, creamy, w/butter	2	Tbs	34	5	131	0	25	0.6	4	1.9
Frosting, chocolate, creamy, w/margarine	2	Tbs	34	5	132	0	25	0.6	4	0.6
Frosting, coconut nut, ready to eat, can	1	each	462	97	1903	7	244	6.5	111	32.5
Frosting, cream cheese flavor, ready to eat	1	each	462	70	1908	0	308	0	80	23.3
Frosting, creamy chocolate butter, recipe	2	Tbs	34	3	138	0	27	0.6	4	2.4
Frosting, french vanilla supreme, Pillsbury	2	Tbs	38	6	158	0	26	0	6	1.7
Frosting, lite, milk chocolate, Pillsbury	2	Tbs	58	11	209	1	41	1.6	5	1.4
Frosting, lite, vanilla, Pillsbury	2	Tbs	32	5	121	0	24	0.1	3	0.7
Frosting, seven minute, recipe	0.25	cup	80	14	254	1	64	0	0	0
Frosting, sour cream flavor, ready to eat, can	1	each	462	66	1903	0	312	0.5	80	23.1
Frosting, vanilla cream, recipe, w/butter	2	Tbs	40	7	137	0	31	0	2	1
Frosting, vanilla cream, recipe, w/margarine	2	Tbs	40	4	162	0	32	0	4	0.9
Frosting/Icing, chocolate, ready to spread	1	oz.	28	5	120	0	18	0	5	2
Frosting/glaze, recipe	0.25	cup	80	14	287	0	59	0	6	1.4
Frosting/icing, creamy vanilla, canned	2	Tbs	31	4	131	0	22	0	5	1.5
Frosting/icing, creamy, mix, prepared	2	Tbs	40	5	169	0	28	0	7	1.3
Frozen dessert bar, Treat, Weight Watchers	1	each	81	58	88	2	19	0	1	0.2
Frozen dessert, Weight Watchers	0.5	cup	66	47	73	3	14	0	1	0.3
Frozen yogurt cone, chocolate	1	each	78	44	157	4	22	1.1	7	3.9
Frozen yogurt cone, not chocolate	1	each	78	47	143	3	22	0.5	5	2.6
Frozen yogurt, chocolate	0.5	cup	96	67	110	5	21	1.5	2	1.2
Frozen yogurt, chocolate-coated	1	each	41	21	109	1	12	0.1	7	5.4
Frozen yogurt, nonfat, chocolate	0.5	cup	96	67	104	5	21	1.5	1	0.5
Frozen yogurt, nonfat, fruit	0.5	cup	96	72	95	5	19	0	0	0.1
Frozen yogurt, soft serve, chocolate	0.5	cup	72	46	115	3	18	1.6	4	2.6
Frozen yogurt, soft serve, vanilla	0.5	cup	72	47	114	3	17	0	4	2.5

MonoF	PolyF	Choles	Calc	Phos	Sod	Pot	Zn	Iron	Magn	VitA	VitE	VitC	Thia	Ribo	Nia	B6	Fola	B12
(g)	(g)	(mg)	(mg)	(mg)	(mg)	(mg)	(mg)	(mg)	(mg)	(µg RE)	(µg α-TE)	(mg)	(mg)	(mg)	(mg)	(mg)	(µg)	(µg)
3.3	0.5	68	42	323	53	592	1.2	1.8	50	20	1.43	1	0.04	0.14	21.3	1.11	11	2.48
0.2	0.4	66	24	278	53	645	0.8	1.1	73	23	0.71	1	0.57	0.06	13.5	1.18	2	0.68
0.1	0.1	147	128	320	467	787	3.7	11.5	195	56	0.3	8	0.06	0.24	2.3	0.74	13	20.5
0.5	0.7	95	70	323	150	492	0.6	0.5	31	39	0.34	0	0.08	0.07	1.9	0.2	17	2.95
0.7	0.1	9	153	116	66	194	0.5	0.1	17	62	0.07	1	0.04	0.2	0.1	0.05	5	0.36
1.2	0.2	16	150	114	65	192	0.5	0.1	16	35	0.13	1	0.04	0.2	0.1	0.05	5	0.35
11.6	9.1	45	50	199	187	292	4.2	2.2	29	15	4	14	0.07	0.15	2.1	0.25	10	1.45
11.1	9.6	37	52	146	189	243	1.2	1	28	22	4.06	14	0.05	0.1	3.2	0.22	8	0.09
—	—	0	23	—	1	—	—	5	—	0	—	0	0.68	0.45	6	—	175	—
1.6	1.6	0	17	532	13	457	3.9	3.1	177	0	1.14	0	0.7	0.13	10	1.16	25	0
0.9	0.9	0	40	330	11	565	3.1	4	246	0	1.01	0	0.41	0.19	6	0.57	53	0
0.2	0.2	0	358	81	36	852	0.9	3	56	1	0.65	0	0.06	0.48	2	0.38	30	0
—	—	—	85	296	—	—	—	6	92	—	—	—	0.1	0.28	0.6	—	—	0
1.1	2	0	161	254	6	340	2	8.2	125	54	0.95	0	1.63	0.09	11.2	0.42	213	0
1.1	2	0	161	254	6	340	2	8.2	125	0	0.28	0	1.63	0.86	11.2	0.42	213	0
0	0	0	56	196	3	84	—	0.6	—	0	—	0	0.04	0.04	0.7	—	30	0
0	0.3	0	116	301	98	1791	1	2.5	116	0	0.45	7	0.41	0.09	6.3	1.38	45	0
0.4	1.5	0	72	809	1	934	7.2	8.3	317	0	3.3	0	0.4	0.32	5.5	0.57	77	0
0.2	0.6	0	21	198	2	238	1.8	1.8	71	0	0.57	0	0.34	0.09	0.8	0.24	22	0
0.2	0.8	0	24	211	3	347	2	2.2	76	0	1.36	0	0.29	0.12	1.8	0.27	19	0
1.2	1.4	0	42	230	12	120	3	4	103	2	0.16	0	0.72	0.08	3.6	0.04	8	0
—	—	0	43	—	2	—	—	9.5	—	0	—	0	1.3	0.86	11.4	—	—	—
0.2	0.7	0	91	551	2	54	4	5.3	277	4	1.3	1	2.55	0.21	5.8	0.6	178	0
0.2	1	0	46	417	3	606	3.5	3.4	199	0	2.48	0	0.49	0.17	3.7	0.52	96	0
0.1	0.5	0	19	135	2	134	0.9	5.8	28	0	0.08	0	0.98	0.62	7.4	0.06	193	0
0.1	0.5	0	19	135	2	134	0.9	5.8	28	0	0.46	0	0.98	0.62	7.4	0.06	193	0
0.1	0.5	0	17	124	2	123	0.8	5.3	25	0	0.07	0	0.9	0.57	6.8	0.05	177	0
0.1	0.4	0	13	82	2	101	0.6	7	15	0	0.06	0	0.86	0.41	6.5	0.03	148	0
0.1	0.5	0	423	744	1587	155	3.5	4.7	166	0	1.48	0	0.54	0.26	7.6	0.41	53	0
0.3	0.9	0	41	415	6	486	3.5	4.7	166	0	1.48	0	0.54	0.26	7.6	0.41	53	0
—	**—**	**0**	**300**	**350**	**65**	**220**	**5.2**	**6.3**	**160**	**—**	**20**	**60**	**1.5**	**1.7**	**20**	**2**	**400**	**6**
2.9	1.7	75	65	76	311	87	0.4	1.1	11	86	0.72	0	0.13	0.21	1.1	0.05	28	0.2
3	1.7	76	64	76	311	86	0.4	1.1	11	81	0.31	0	0.13	0.21	1.1	0.05	15	0.2
3.1	1.8	25	16	29	19	86	0.2	0.4	8	23	0.75	1	0.05	0.09	0.4	0.1	5	0.07
3.1	1.8	25	16	27	20	41	0.2	0.4	4	23	0.87	2	0.05	0.08	0.4	0.02	4	0.08
3.8	2.4	36	6	21	56	17	0.1	0.3	2	67	1.11	0	0.03	0.06	0.3	0.01	4	0.08
0.1	0.2	72	26	160	84	372	1.4	2	29	20	1.45	0	0.19	0.34	1.6	0.16	16	0.52
1.7	1.1	0	6	16	70	32	0.1	0.3	9	38	0.69	0	0	0.01	0	0	1	0.01
41.7	9.8	0	37	365	845	906	1.3	6.6	97	915	10.9	0	0.06	0.08	0.6	0.02	0	0
0.9	0.1	8	4	17	52	49	0.2	0.3	10	21	0.69	0	0	0.01	0	0.02	0	0
1.4	1	0	4	17	56	50	0.2	0.3	10	23	0.69	0	0	0.01	0	0.02	0	0
56.4	15.8	0	60	291	901	859	1.9	2.5	88	0	5.27	1	0.16	0.09	1	0.25	28	0
41.7	10.9	0	14	14	1094	162	0	0.7	9	536	9.33	0	0	0.03	0.1	0	0	0
1.1	0.1	10	6	16	65	31	0.1	0.3	9	34	0.69	0	0	0.01	0	0	1	0.01
—	—	0	1	—	76	—	—	0	—	0	—	0	—	—	—	—	—	—
—	—	0	5	—	144	—	—	0.9	—	0	—	0	—	—	—	—	—	—
—	—	0	1	—	58	—	—	0	—	0	—	0	—	—	—	—	—	—
0	0	0	2	2	136	51	0	0.1	2	0	0	0	0	0.07	0	0	0	0.02
41.5	10.8	0	9	18	942	896	0	0.3	9	564	9.33	0	0.05	0.09	3.1	0.02	5	0.05
0.5	0.1	5	9	7	26	12	0	0	1	15	0.81	0	0	0.01	0	0	0	0.03
1.9	1.3	0	5	4	82	7	0	0	1	45	0.81	0	0	0.01	0	0	0	0.02
2	0	0	0	—	40	40	—	0	—	0	—	0	0	0	0	—	—	0
2.7	1.8	2	18	14	75	24	0.1	0	2	65	0.61	0	0.01	0.02	0	0.01	1	0.06
2.7	0.7	0	1	12	28	12	0	0	0	70	1.47	0	0	0	0	0	0	0
2.7	2.3	0	4	11	88	9	0	0.1	1	43	0.81	0	0.01	0.01	0.1	0	0	0
0.1	0.4	1	82	66	47	111	0.3	0.1	10	38	0.07	1	0.03	0.11	0.1	0.03	3	0.24
0.2	0	3	111	88	61	156	0.3	0.1	10	5	0.01	0	0.03	0.13	0.1	0.03	1	0.44
2.5	0.5	1	115	119	70	193	0.5	0.6	29	42	0.34	1	0.05	0.17	0.3	0.08	6	0.2
1.8	0.4	1	118	107	74	167	0.4	0.4	17	44	0.3	1	0.04	0.17	0.3	0.08	6	0.21
0.6	0.1	5	150	150	56	311	1	0.8	38	13	0.05	1	0.04	0.19	0.2	0.04	10	0.44
0.8	0.2	1	46	43	28	74	0.2	0.1	6	18	0.05	0	0.01	0.07	0.1	0.03	2	0.09
0.3	0	1	163	160	62	327	1.1	0.9	39	2	0.02	1	0.04	0.21	0.2	0.05	11	0.48
0	0	2	167	132	64	214	0.8	0.1	16	2	0	1	0.04	0.2	0.1	0.04	10	0.51
1.3	0.2	4	106	100	71	188	0.4	0.9	19	31	0.1	0	0.03	0.15	0.2	0.05	8	0.21
1.1	0.2	1	103	93	63	152	0.3	0.2	10	41	0.04	1	0.03	0.16	0.2	0.06	4	0.21

Food Item	Qty	Meas	Wgt (g)	Wtr (g)	Cals	Prot	Carb (g)	Fib (g)	Fat (g)	SatF (g)
Frozen yogurt, vanilla	0.5	cup	96	71	102	4	18	0	1	0.8
Frozen yogurt, vanilla/fruit	0.5	cup	96	71	102	4	18	0	1	0.8
Fruit cocktail in light syrup	0.5	cup	126	106	72	1	19	1.3	0	0
Fruit cocktail, canned in heavy syrup	0.5	cup	128	103	93	0	24	1.3	0	0
Fruit cocktail, juice pack	0.5	cup	124	108	57	1	15	1.2	0	0
Fruit cocktail, water pack	0.5	cup	122	111	39	1	10	1.2	0	0
Fruit drink, Crystal Light, prepared	1	cup	240	239	3	0	0	0	0	0
Fruit drink, low calorie, powder, prepared	1	cup	240	228	43	0	11	0	0	0
Fruit drink, powder, prepared (Koolade)	1	cup	240	217	89	0	23	0	0	0
Fruit drink, punch flavor (Hi-C)	1	cup	240	228	43	0	11	0	0	0
Fruit juice bar, frozen	1	each	77	60	63	1	16	0	0	0
Fruit juice bar, w/cream, frozen	1	each	65	43	86	1	19	0.1	1	0.8
Fruit leather/roll ups, small	1	each	14	2	49	0	12	0.5	0	0.1
Fruit punch drink, canned	1	cup	253	223	119	0	30	0.3	0	0
Fruit punch drink, frozen concentrate, prepared	1	cup	247	218	114	0	29	0.2	0	0
Fruit punch juice drink, frozen, prepared	1	cup	248	217	124	0	30	0.2	0	0.1
Fruit punch, powder	1	Tbs	6	0	24	0	6	0	0	0
Fruit salad, canned in light syrup	0.5	cup	126	106	73	0	19	1.3	0	0
Fruit salad, includes citrus	0.5	cup	88	74	50	0	13	1.2	0	0.1
Fruit salad, no citrus	0.5	cup	88	73	51	1	13	1.5	0	0.1
Fruit salad, tropical, canned in heavy syrup	0.5	cup	128	99	111	1	29	1.7	0	0
Fruit spread, strawberry, low calorie, Kraft	1	Tbs	20	—	20	0	5	0	0	0
Garlic clove, fresh	1	each	3	2	4	0	1	0.1	0	0
Gatorade	1	cup	241	93	60	0	15	0	0	0
Gelatin dessert/Jello, prepared	0.5	cup	135	114	80	2	19	0	0	0
Gelatin dessert/Jello, sugar-free	0.5	cup	117	115	8	1	1	0	0	0
Gelatin/Jello dessert w/fruit (Jello)	0.5	cup	106	86	73	1	18	0.6	0	0.1
Gelatin/Jello frozen fruit bar	1	each	44	36	31	1	7	0	0	—
Gherkin in sweetened brine	1	each	19	14	19	0	5	0.4	0	0
Gnocchi, cheese	0.5	cup	35	24	62	3	3	0.1	4	1.6
Gnocchi, potato	0.5	cup	94	68	136	2	17	0.9	7	4.2
Goat meat, cooked	4	oz.	113	66	237	37	0	0	9	3.7
Goose, liver pate, smoked, canned	0.5	cup	104	38	480	12	5	0	46	15.1
Goose, roasted	4	oz.	113	59	346	29	0	0	25	7.8
Goose, skinless, roasted	4	oz.	113	65	270	33	0	0	14	5.2
Gooseberries canned in light syrup	0.5	cup	126	101	92	1	24	3	0	0
Gooseberries, cooked	0.5	cup	126	101	92	1	24	3	0	0
Gooseberries, fresh	0.5	cup	75	66	33	1	8	3.2	0	0
Graham cracker crust, chilled, not baked	1	oz.	28	2	137	1	18	0.4	7	1.4
Granola bar, hard, almond	1	each	24	1	117	2	15	1.1	6	3
Granola bar, hard, chocolate chip	1	each	24	1	103	2	17	1	4	2.7
Granola bar, hard, peanut butter	1	each	24	1	114	2	15	0.7	6	0.8
Granola bar, hard, plain	1	each	28	1	134	3	18	1.5	6	0.7
Granola bar, high fiber, yogurt coating, Fi-Bar	1	each	28	3	96	3	19	2.2	3	1
Granola bar, soft, choc chip w/granola & marshmallow	1	each	28	2	121	2	20	1.1	4	2.6
Granola bar, soft, chocolate chocolate chip	1	each	35	1	165	2	23	1.2	9	5
Granola bar, soft, chocolate peanut butter	1	each	37	1	187	4	20	1	11	6.2
Granola bar, soft, chocolate raisin	1	each	42	3	190	3	28	1.8	8	4.1
Granola bar, soft, nut & raisin	1	each	28	2	129	2	18	1.6	6	2.7
Granola bar, soft, peanut butter	1	each	24	2	101	2	15	1	4	0.9
Granola bar, soft, peanut butter chocolate chip	1	each	28	2	122	3	18	1.2	6	1.6
Granola bar, soft, uncoated, chocolate	1	each	42	2	179	3	29	2	7	4.3
Granola bar, soft, uncoated, plain	1	each	28	2	126	2	19	1.3	5	2
Granola clusters, Nature Valley	1	each	34	1	140	2	24	1.4	5	1.9
Grape drink, canned	1	cup	251	222	113	0	29	0	0	0
Grape drink, low calorie	1	cup	240	228	43	0	11	0	0	0
Grape juice, bottle/canned, unsweetened	1	cup	253	213	154	1	38	0.3	0	0.1
Grape juice, frozen conc w/vit C, prepared	1	cup	250	217	128	0	32	0.2	0	0.1
Grape leaves, raw	1	oz.	28	22	19	1	4	—	0	—
Grape, American type/slip skin, no seeds	0.5	cup	46	37	31	0	8	0.5	0	0.1
Grape, Tokay/Red Flame, seedless, cup measure	0.5	cup	80	64	57	1	14	0.8	0	0.2
Grapefruit juice, canned, unsweetened	1	cup	247	223	94	1	22	0.2	0	0
Grapefruit juice, fresh	1	cup	247	222	96	1	23	0.2	0	0
Grapefruit juice, frozen concentrate, prepared	1	cup	247	221	101	1	24	0.2	0	0
Grapefruit sections canned in juice	0.5	cup	124	112	46	1	12	0.5	0	0

MonoF	PolyF	Choles	Calc	Phos	Sod	Pot	Zn	Iron	Magn	VitA	VitE	VitC	Thia	Ribo	Nia	B6	Fola	B12
(g)	(g)	(mg)	(mg)	(mg)	(mg)	(mg)	(mg)	(mg)	(mg)	(µg RE)	(µg α-TE)	(mg)	(mg)	(mg)	(mg)	(mg)	(µg)	(µg)
0.4	0	5	153	121	59	197	0.8	0.1	15	13	0.04	1	0.04	0.18	0.1	0.04	9	0.47
0.4	0	5	153	121	59	197	0.8	0.1	15	13	0.04	1	0.04	0.18	0.1	0.04	9	0.47
0	0	0	8	14	8	112	0.1	0.4	6	26	0.36	2	0.02	0.02	0.5	0.06	3	0
0	0	0	8	14	8	112	0.1	0.4	6	26	0.37	2	0.02	0.02	0.5	0.06	3	0
0	0	0	10	17	5	118	0.1	0.3	9	38	0.25	3	0.02	0.02	0.5	0.06	3	0
0	0	0	6	14	5	115	0.1	0.3	9	31	0.36	3	0.02	0.01	0.4	0.06	3	0
0	0	0	38	15	7	45	0.1	0	2	0	0	6	0	0	0	0	0	0
0	0	0	17	5	50	50	0.3	0.6	5	2	0	78	0.02	0.05	0	0	5	0
0	0	0	38	48	34	2	0.1	0.1	2	0	0	28	0	0	0	0	0	0
0	0	0	17	5	50	50	0.3	0.6	5	2	0	78	0.02	0.05	0	0	5	0
0	0	0	4	5	3	41	0	0.1	3	2	0	7	0.01	0.01	0.1	0.02	5	0
0.4	0	5	29	5	20	64	0	0.1	2	8	0.03	8	0.01	0.06	0.1	0.03	3	0.05
0.2	0.1	0	4	4	9	41	0	0.1	3	2	0.04	1	0.01	0	0	0.04	1	0
0	0	0	20	3	56	63	0.3	0.5	5	4	0	75	0.06	0.06	0.1	0	3	0
0	0	0	10	2	10	32	0.1	0.2	5	2	0	108	0.02	0.03	0.1	0.02	2	0
0.1	0.1	0	17	0	12	191	0.5	0.6	10	2	0	14	0	0.16	0.1	0.03	3	0
0	0	0	9	13	8	0	0	0	0	0	0	8	0	0	0	0	0	0
0	0	0	9	11	8	103	0.1	0.4	6	54	0.82	3	0.02	0.02	0.5	0.04	3	0
0	0.1	0	8	9	0	154	0.1	0.2	9	7	0.39	14	0.03	0.03	0.2	0.12	7	0
0	0.1	0	7	10	0	164	0.1	0.2	10	17	0.39	7	0.04	0.04	0.4	0.1	7	0
0	0	0	17	9	3	168	0.1	0.7	17	17	0.64	22	0.07	0.06	0.7	0.15	12	0
0	0	0	0	—	20	25	—	0	—	0	—	0	—	—	—	—	—	—
0	0	0	5	5	1	12	0	0.1	1	0	0	1	0.01	0	0	0.04	0	0
0	0	0	0	22	96	26	.05	.12	2	0	0	.01	0	0	0	0	0	0
0	0	0	3	30	57	1	0	0	1	0	0	0	0	0	0	0	0	0
0	0	0	2	32	56	0	0	0	1	0	0	0	0	0	0	0	0	0
0	0.1	0	5	22	30	110	0.1	0.1	7	3	0.11	4	0.03	0.03	0.2	0.13	4	0
—	—	0	1	0	20	1	0	0	0	0	—	0	0	0	0	0	0	0
0	0	0	4	—	99	2	—	0.1	—	1	—	0	0	0	—	0.01	3	0
1.6	0.8	24	68	52	92	25	0.3	0.3	4	52	0.47	0	0.02	0.06	0.2	0.01	4	0.1
1.9	0.3	18	22	39	71	121	0.2	0.7	10	65	0.2	2	0.11	0.09	1.1	0.08	5	0.05
3.3	0.5	192	42	271	368	320	4.9	1.5	30	0	0.44	0	0.07	0.41	11.3	0.29	18	1.83
26.6	0.9	156	73	208	725	144	1	5.7	14	1040	1.79	2	0.09	0.31	2.6	0.06	62	9.78
11.7	2.9	103	15	306	79	373	3	3.2	25	24	1.97	0	0.09	0.37	4.7	0.42	2	0.46
4.9	1.8	109	16	350	86	440	3.6	3.2	28	14	1.76	0	0.1	0.44	4.6	0.53	14	0.56
0	0.1	0	20	9	3	97	0.1	0.4	8	18	0.47	13	0.02	0.07	0.2	0.02	4	0
0	0.1	0	20	9	3	97	0.1	0.4	8	18	0.47	13	0.02	0.07	0.2	0.02	4	0
0	0.2	0	19	20	1	149	0.1	0.2	8	22	0.28	21	0.03	0.02	0.2	0.06	4	0
3.2	1.9	0	6	18	159	24	0.1	0.6	5	56	1.15	0	0.03	0.05	0.6	0.01	10	0.01
1.8	0.9	0	8	54	60	64	0.4	0.6	19	1	0.42	0	0.07	0.02	0.1	0.01	3	0
0.6	0.3	0	18	48	81	59	0.5	0.7	17	1	0.21	0	0.04	0.02	0.1	0.01	3	0
1.6	2.9	0	10	33	67	69	0.3	0.6	13	0	0.31	0	0.05	0.02	0.5	0.02	4	0
1.2	3.4	2	17	79	84	95	0.6	0.8	28	4	0.38	0	0.08	0.03	0.4	0.02	7	0
1	0.7	4	15	107	6	107	0.6	0.7	36	0	0.56	0	0.12	0.05	0.8	0.04	8	0.01
0.8	0.7	0	25	57	90	78	0.4	0.7	20	1	0.26	0	0.04	0.04	0.3	0.01	6	0
2.8	0.6	0	36	70	71	111	0.5	0.8	23	2	0.35	0	0.03	0.09	0.3	0.04	9	0.2
2.4	0.7	0	40	83	71	124	0.5	0.5	25	13	0.48	0	0.04	0.08	1.2	0.04	9	0.08
1.2	1.4	0	43	94	120	154	0.6	1	31	0	0.47	0	0.1	0.07	0.5	0.04	9	0.07
1.2	1.6	0	24	68	72	111	0.5	0.6	26	1	0.31	0	0.05	0.05	0.7	0.03	9	0.05
1.6	1	0	22	59	96	69	0.4	0.5	20	1	0.29	0	0.05	0.04	0.7	0.02	8	0.05
2.4	1.3	0	23	74	93	107	0.5	0.6	25	1	0.37	0	0.03	0.03	0.9	0.03	9	0.13
1.5	0.8	0	40	98	116	145	0.6	1.1	33	2	0.42	0	0.1	0.06	0.4	0.04	9	0.07
1.1	1.5	0	30	65	79	92	0.4	0.7	21	0	0.35	0	0.08	0.05	0.1	0.03	7	0.11
1.1	1.6	0	15	55	48	77	0.5	0.6	16	2	0.58	0	0.08	0.05	0.3	0.05	10	0.01
0	0	0	8	3	15	12	0.3	0.4	5	0	0	86	0.01	0.01	0.1	0.02	1	0
0	0	0	17	5	50	50	0.3	0.6	5	2	0	78	0.02	0.05	0	0	5	0
0	0.1	0	23	28	8	334	0.1	0.6	25	3	0	0	0.07	0.09	0.7	0.16	7	0
0	0.1	0	10	10	5	52	0.1	0.2	10	2	0.12	60	0.04	0.06	0.3	0.1	3	0
—	—	0	203	11	6	72	—	2	—	765	—	3	0.06	0.02	0.3	—	—	0
0	0	0	6	5	1	88	0	0.1	2	5	0.16	2	0.04	0.03	0.1	0.05	2	0
0	0.1	0	9	10	2	148	0	0.2	5	6	0.56	9	0.07	0.05	0.2	0.09	3	0
0	0.1	0	17	27	2	378	0.2	0.5	25	2	0.12	72	0.1	0.05	0.6	0.05	26	0
0	0.1	0	22	37	2	400	0.1	0.5	30	2	0.12	94	0.1	0.05	0.5	0.11	25	0
0	0.1	0	20	35	2	336	0.1	0.3	27	2	0.12	83	0.1	0.05	0.5	0.11	9	0
0	0	0	19	15	9	210	0.1	0.3	14	0	0.31	42	0.04	0.02	0.3	0.02	11	0

Food Item	Qty	Meas	Wgt (g)	Wtr (g)	Cals	Prot	Carb (g)	Fib (g)	Fat (g)	SatF (g)
Grapefruit sections, canned in light syrup	0.5	cup	127	106	76	1	20	0.5	0	0
Grapefruit sections, fresh	1	piece	15	14	5	0	1	0.2	0	0
Grapefruit, pink/red	0.5	each	123	110	46	1	12	1.6	0	0
Grapefruit, white	0.5	each	118	107	39	1	10	1.3	0	0
Grapes, Concord	0.5	cup	46	37	31	0	8	0.5	0	0.1
Grapes, Thompson seedless, canned in heavy syrup	0.5	cup	128	102	93	1	25	0.5	0	0
Gravy, au jus, canned	0.25	cup	60	56	10	1	1	0	0	0.1
Gravy, au jus, dry w/water	0.25	cup	62	59	8	0	1	0	0	0.2
Gravy, beef, canned	0.25	cup	58	51	31	2	3	0.2	1	0.7
Gravy, beef, recipe	0.25	cup	34	29	22	1	2	0.1	1	0.4
Gravy, brown, from dry, w/water	0.25	cup	64	59	19	1	3	0.1	0	0.2
Gravy, chicken giblet, recipe	0.25	cup	32	28	24	2	2	0.1	1	0.3
Gravy, chicken, canned	0.25	cup	60	51	47	1	3	0.2	3	0.8
Gravy, chicken, dry mix w/water	0.25	cup	65	59	21	1	4	0.1	0	0.1
Gravy, mushroom, canned	0.25	cup	60	53	30	1	3	0.2	2	0.2
Gravy, mushroom, dry mix w/water	0.25	cup	64	59	17	1	3	0.3	0	0.1
Gravy, swiss steak	0.25	cup	58	51	31	2	3	0.2	1	0.7
Gravy, turkey, canned	0.25	cup	60	53	30	2	3	0.2	1	0.4
Gravy, turkey, dry, w/water	0.25	cup	65	59	22	1	4	0.3	0	0.1
Green pepper, stuffed	1	each	172	128	229	11	20	1.8	12	5
Guava juice drink, vitamin C added	1	cup	253	218	132	0	34	2	0	0.1
Guava nectar	1	cup	250	211	149	0	38	2	0	0.1
Guava, raw	1	each	90	78	46	1	11	4.9	1	0.2
Ham hocks, diced meat, cooked	0.5	cup	70	33	229	20	0	0	16	5.9
Ham salad spread	0.5	cup	120	75	259	10	13	0	19	6.1
Ham, canned, unheated, extra lean (7% fat)	0.5	cup	70	50	101	13	0	0	5	1.7
Ham, smoked, sliced, 95% fat free	1	oz.	28	—	31	5	0	—	1	0.3
Ham, whole, roasted, lean	4	oz.	28	19	44	7	0	0	2	0.5
Ham, whole, roasted, lean & fat	4	oz.	113	66	276	24	0	0	19	6.8
Hardee's Big Country Breakfast, bacon	1	each	217	66	740	25	81	—	43	13
Hardee's Biscuit 'n gravy	1	each	221	126	510	10	55	—	28	9
Hardee's ham'n cheese sandwich, hot	1	each	201	101	530	18	49	—	30	9
Hardee's mushroom & swiss hamburger	1	each	203	107	520	30	37	—	27	13
Hardee's roast beef sandwich, regular	1	each	124	68	270	15	28	—	11	5
Hardee's sundae, Cool Twist, hot fudge	1	each	156	91	290	7	51	—	6	3
Hardee's, Frisco hamburger	1	each	242	—	760	36	43	—	50	18
Hardee's, ice cream cone, Cool Twist, vanilla/choc	1	each	118	77	180	4	34	—	2	0.7
Hardee's, shake, peach	1	each	345	—	390	10	77	—	4	3
Healthy Choice Meal, Beef Broccoli Bejing	1	each	340	261	300	21	45	5	4	1.5
Healthy Choice Meal, Beef Burrito Ranchero, mild	1	each	306	240	300	13	45	7	7	2.5
Healthy Choice Meal, Beef Macaroni Casserole	1	each	241	191	210	14	34	5	2	0.5
Healthy Choice Meal, Beef Tips Francais	1	each	262	196	280	20	40	4	5	1.5
Healthy Choice Meal, Beef/Peppers Cantonese	1	each	326	264	270	22	32	5	6	2.5
Healthy Choice Meal, Cacciatore Chicken	1	each	354	292	270	22	36	5	4	1
Healthy Choice Meal, Cheddar Broccoli Potatoes	1	each	298	226	330	13	53	6	7	3
Healthy Choice Meal, Cheese Ravioli Parmigiana	1	each	255	195	260	11	44	6	5	2.5
Healthy Choice Meal, Chicken & Vegetable Marsala	1	each	326	270	240	20	32	3	4	2
Healthy Choice Meal, Chicken Broccoli Alfredo	1	each	326	259	300	25	34	2	7	3
Healthy Choice Meal, Chicken Cantonese	1	each	305	242	280	22	34	2	6	3
Healthy Choice Meal, Chicken Con Queso Burrito	1	each	299	218	350	14	60	6	6	2.5
Healthy Choice Meal, Chicken Enchilada Suprema	1	each	320	253	300	13	46	4	7	3
Healthy Choice Meal, Chicken Enchiladas Suiza	1	tsp	284	217	280	14	43	5	6	3
Healthy Choice Meal, Chicken Fettuccini Alfredo	1	each	241	183	260	22	35	3	4	2
Healthy Choice Meal, Chicken Francesca Classic	1	each	354	270	330	23	46	4	6	2.5
Healthy Choice Meal, Country Herb Chicken	1	each	344	293	310	18	44	3	6	2.5
Healthy Choice Meal, Country Inn Roast Turkey	1	each	284	224	250	20	28	4	6	2
Healthy Choice Meal, Country Roast Turkey with Mush	1	each	241	189	230	19	26	2	5	1.5
Healthy Choice Meal, Fiesta Chicken Fajitas	1	each	198	136	260	21	36	5	4	1
Healthy Choice Meal, Garden Potato Casserole	1	each	262	216	210	11	30	6	5	1.5
Healthy Choice Meal, Ginger Chicken Hunan	1	each	357	271	380	24	59	5	5	1
Healthy Choice Meal, Honey Mustard Chicken	1	each	269	205	270	21	38	2	4	1.5
Healthy Choice Meal, Imperial Chicken	1	each	255	201	240	17	31	3	5	1.5
Healthy Choice Meal, Macaroni and Cheese	1	each	255	189	320	15	50	4	7	2.5
Healthy Choice Meal, Mandarin Chicken	1	each	284	216	280	20	44	4	2	0
Healthy Choice Meal, Mesquite Beef Barbeque	1	each	312	239	320	21	38	5	9	3

MonoF	PolyF	Choles	Calc	Phos	Sod	Pot	Zn	Iron	Magn	VitA	VitE	VitC	Thia	Ribo	Nia	B6	Fola	B12
(g)	(g)	(mg)	(mg)	(mg)	(mg)	(mg)	(mg)	(mg)	(mg)	(µg RE)	(µg α-TE)	(mg)	(mg)	(mg)	(mg)	(mg)	(µg)	(µg)
0	0	0	18	13	3	164	0.1	0.5	13	0	0.32	27	0.05	0.02	0.3	0.02	11	0
0	0	0	2	1	0	21	0	0	1	2	0.04	5	0	0	0	0.01	2	0
0	0	0	14	15	1	181	0.1	0.1	11	32	0.31	47	0.04	0.02	0.2	0.05	15	0
0	0	0	14	9	0	175	0.1	0.1	11	1	0.3	39	0.04	0.02	0.3	0.05	12	0
0	0	0	6	5	1	88	0	0.1	2	5	0.16	2	0.04	0.03	0.1	0.05	2	0
0	0	0	13	22	6	132	0.1	1.2	8	8	0.9	1	0.04	0.03	0.2	0.08	3	0
0	0	0	2	18	30	48	0.6	0.4	1	0	0	1	0.01	0.04	0.5	0.01	1	0.06
0.1	0	1	6	0	241	0	0	0	2	0	0	0	0	0	0	0	0	0
0.6	0	2	4	18	326	47	0.6	0.4	1	0	0.04	0	0.02	0.02	0.4	0.01	1	0.06
0.6	0.2	1	4	10	192	32	0.3	0.2	1	19	0.04	0	0.01	0.01	0.2	0	1	0.03
0.2	0	1	17	11	269	14	0.1	0.1	3	0	0.01	0	0.01	0.02	0.2	0	0	0
0.5	0.3	14	4	16	171	38	0.4	0.4	1	82	0.08	0	0.01	0.05	0.4	0.01	12	0.58
1.5	0.9	1	12	17	343	65	0.5	0.3	1	66	0.09	0	0.01	0.03	0.3	0.01	1	0.06
0.2	0.1	1	10	12	283	16	0.1	0.1	3	0	0.01	1	0.01	0.04	0.2	0.01	1	0.04
0.7	0.6	0	4	9	339	63	0.4	0.4	1	0	0.05	0	0.02	0.04	0.4	0.01	7	0
0.1	0	0	12	11	350	14	0.1	0.1	2	0	0.01	0	0.01	0.02	0.2	0.01	1	0.04
0.6	0	2	4	18	326	47	0.6	0.4	1	0	0.04	0	0.02	0.02	0.4	0.01	1	0.06
0.5	0.3	1	2	17	343	65	0.5	0.4	1	0	0.04	0	0.01	0.05	0.8	0.01	1	0.06
0.2	0.1	1	12	12	374	16	0.1	0.1	3	0	0.01	0	0.01	0.03	0.3	0.01	1	0.06
4.9	0.5	34	16	85	201	233	2.3	1.8	20	44	0.75	55	0.15	0.1	2.7	0.3	17	0.67
0	0.1	0	11	10	7	105	0.1	0.1	6	29	0.41	85	0.02	0.02	0.4	0.05	5	0
0	0.1	0	11	10	7	93	0.1	0.2	5	22	0.4	46	0.02	0.02	0.4	0.05	3	0
0	0.2	0	18	22	3	256	0.2	0.3	9	71	1.01	166	0.04	0.04	1.1	0.13	13	0
7.2	1.6	76	13	147	223	257	2.9	1.1	13	2	0.18	0	0.38	0.21	3.6	0.24	3	0.45
8.6	3.2	44	10	144	1094	180	1.3	0.7	12	0	2.09	0	0.52	0.14	2.5	0.18	1	0.91
2.5	0.5	27	4	145	893	234	1.3	0.6	11	0	0.18	0	0.62	0.16	3.2	0.32	4	0.56
0.6	0.3	14	—	—	357	—	—	—	—	0	0.07	0	0.19	0.07	1.4	0.13	1	0.2
0.7	0.2	16	2	64	376	90	0.7	0.3	6	0	0.07	0	0.19	0.07	1.4	0.13	1	0.2
8.9	2	70	8	243	1346	324	2.6	1	22	0	0.3	0	0.68	0.25	5.1	0.43	3	0.73
22	8	305	166	—	1800	530	—	5	—	—	—	—	—	—	—	—	—	—
14	5	15	150	—	1500	210	—	2	—	—	—	—	—	—	—	—	—	—
—	—	65	288	—	—	300	—	3	—	—	—	—	—	—	—	—	—	—
12	2	45	294	—	890	370	—	5	—	—	—	—	—	—	—	—	—	—
4	2	25	105	—	780	260	—	4	—	—	—	—	—	—	—	—	—	—
1.6	0.2	20	152	—	310	173	—	0.4	—	—	—	—	—	—	—	—	—	—
—	—	70	—	—	1280	—	—	—	—	—	—	—	—	—	—	—	—	—
1.3	0	10	123	—	120	180	—	2	—	—	—	—	—	—	—	—	—	—
—	—	25	—	—	290	—	—	—	—	—	—	—	—	—	—	—	—	—
—	—	25	40	—	420	—	—	2.7	—	200	—	12	—	—	—	—	—	—
—	—	15	20	—	480	—	—	1.1	—	40	—	5	—	—	—	—	—	—
—	—	15	40	—	450	—	—	2.7	—	100	—	54	—	—	—	—	—	—
—	—	30	20	—	520	—	—	1.8	—	0	—	0	—	—	—	—	—	—
—	—	55	40	—	480	—	—	1.8	—	100	—	21	—	—	—	—	—	—
—	—	35	40	—	550	—	—	1.8	—	40	—	6	—	—	—	—	—	—
—	—	25	200	—	550	—	—	1.1	—	60	—	27	—	—	—	—	—	—
—	—	30	150	—	290	—	—	1.8	—	60	—	0	—	—	—	—	—	—
—	—	30	40	—	440	—	—	0.7	—	100	—	4	—	—	—	—	—	—
—	—	50	100	—	530	—	—	1.8	—	20	—	2	—	—	—	—	—	—
—	—	50	40	—	480	—	—	1.8	—	600	—	6	—	—	—	—	—	—
—	—	35	40	—	590	—	—	1.8	—	300	—	15	—	—	—	—	—	—
—	—	40	100	—	560	—	—	0.7	—	150	—	18	—	—	—	—	—	—
—	—	40	150	—	440	—	—	1.1	—	60	—	6	—	—	—	—	—	—
—	—	40	100	—	410	—	—	1.4	—	0	—	0	—	—	—	—	—	—
—	—	30	100	—	600	—	—	1.8	—	20	—	15	—	—	—	—	—	—
—	—	45	40	—	540	—	—	0.7	—	250	—	0	—	—	—	—	—	—
—	—	40	40	—	530	—	—	1.8	—	100	—	0	—	—	—	—	—	—
—	—	45	0	—	440	—	—	0.7	—	150	—	0	—	—	—	—	—	—
—	—	30	20	—	410	—	—	1.8	—	150	—	36	—	—	—	—	—	—
—	—	10	100	—	520	—	—	0.7	—	250	—	21	—	—	—	—	—	—
—	—	30	60	—	430	—	—	2.7	—	100	—	0	—	—	—	—	—	—
—	—	40	20	—	520	—	—	0.4	—	200	—	0	—	—	—	—	—	—
—	—	50	20	—	470	—	—	1.4	—	150	—	6	—	—	—	—	—	—
—	—	25	250	—	580	—	—	1.4	—	0	—	0	—	—	—	—	—	—
—	—	35	20	—	520	—	—	0.7	—	150	—	15	—	—	—	—	—	—
—	—	55	40	—	490	—	—	1.1	—	250	—	0	—	—	—	—	—	—

Food Item	Qty	Meas	Wgt (g)	Wtr (g)	Cals	Prot	Carb (g)	Fib (g)	Fat (g)	SatF (g)
Healthy Choice Meal, Mesquite Chicken Barbeque	1	each	298	221	310	18	48	6	5	2
Healthy Choice Meal, Pasta Shells Marinara	1	each	340	252	380	25	55	5	6	3.5
Healthy Choice Meal, Salisbury Steak Classics	1	each	312	255	310	16	40	4	9	3
Healthy Choice Meal, Sesame Chicken Shanghai	1	each	340	268	300	24	40	6	5	1
Healthy Choice Meal, Shrimp & Vegetable Maria	1	each	354	290	290	15	46	5	5	2
Healthy Choice Meal, Shrimp Marinara	1	each	298	243	250	10	44	5	4	2
Healthy Choice Meal, Smokey Chicken Barbeque	1	each	361	273	290	25	57	7	5	3
Healthy Choice Meal, Three Cheese Manicotti	1	each	312	245	300	15	40	5	9	3
Healthy Choice Meal, Traditional Beef Tips	1	each	319	261	280	20	32	4	8	3
Healthy Choice Meal, Vegetable Pasta Italiano	1	each	284	230	250	9	48	6	3	1.5
Healthy Choice Meal, Yankee Pot Roast	1	each	312	249	290	19	38	4	7	3
Healthy Choice Meal, Zucchini Lasagna	1	each	383	318	280	13	47	5	4	2.5
Hi-C, punch	1	cup	240	207	125	0	33	0	0	0
Hickory nuts, dried	1	oz.	28	1	186	4	5	1.8	18	2
Hominy, cooked	0.5	cup	82	62	73	2	17	4.7	1	0.1
Honey	1	Tbs	21	4	64	0	18	0	0	0
Horseradish, prepared	1	tsp	5	4	2	0	1	0.2	0	0
Hot cocoa, homemade, w/whole milk	1	cup	250	203	193	10	30	2	6	3.6
Hot dog, beef, fat free, Oscar Mayer	1	piece	50	39	39	7	3	0	0	0.1
Hot dog, turkey	1	oz.	28	18	64	4	0	0	5	1.7
Hotdog, w/chili	1	each	114	54	296	14	31	—	14	4.9
Hotdog/frankfurter, beef & pork, 8 per pkg	1	each	57	31	182	6	1	0	17	6.2
Hotdog/frankfurter, beef, 8 per pkg	1	each	57	31	180	7	1	0	16	6.9
Hotdog/frankfurter, turkey	1	each	45	28	102	6	1	0	8	2.6
Hummus/hummous	0.5	cup	123	80	210	6	25	6.3	10	1.6
Hungry Man dinner, Mexican	1	each	567	420	690	26	87	13	27	9
Hush puppies, recipe	1	each	22	6	74	2	10	0.6	3	0.5
Ice Cream sundae, hot fudge	1	each	158	94	284	6	48	0	9	5
Ice Cream sundae, strawberry	1	each	153	93	268	6	45	0	8	3.7
Ice cream bar, Creamsicle	1	each	66	44	92	2	18	0	2	1.2
Ice cream bar, Drumstick	1	each	60	29	157	3	18	0.7	9	4.3
Ice cream bar, Fudgesicle	1	each	73	49	90	4	19	0.1	0	0.1
Ice cream bar, Heath	1	each	68	33	206	2	17	0.2	15	11.6
Ice cream bar, Nutty Buddy	1	each	78	37	215	4	23	1.3	13	5.5
Ice cream bar, chocolate coated w/nuts	1	each	54	23	171	2	17	0.3	11	6.4
Ice cream cone, cake/wafer type	1	each	4	0	17	0	3	0.1	0	0
Ice cream cone, chocolate	1	each	78	42	171	3	25	0.6	7	4.4
Ice cream cone, sugar/rolled type	1	each	10	0	40	1	8	0.2	0	0.1
Ice cream cone, vanilla	1	each	78	44	167	3	22	0.1	8	4.9
Ice cream cone, vanilla, choc dipped	1	each	78	41	185	3	24	0.4	9	5.6
Ice cream cookie sandwich, Chipwich	1	each	59	28	144	3	22	0.6	6	3.2
Ice cream sandwich	1	each	59	28	144	3	22	0.6	6	3.2
Ice cream sandwich, mini Oreo	1	each	29	14	71	1	11	0.3	3	1.6
Ice cream, Choc Chip Cookie Dough, Ben & Jerry's	0.5	cup	106	—	270	4	30	0	17	9
Ice cream, Chunky Monkey, Ben & Jerry's	0.5	cup	106	—	280	4	29	1	19	10
Ice cream, brandied cherry, HaagenDaz	0.5	cup	106	—	250	4	24	—	15	0.5
Ice cream, chocolate Dove bar	1	each	101	38	339	3	36	2.1	23	13.8
Ice cream, chocolate chip, low fat, Healthy Choice	0.5	cup	71	44	120	3	21	0.5	2	1
Ice cream, chocolate, regular	0.5	cup	66	37	143	3	19	0.8	7	4.5
Ice cream, cookie & cream, Healthy Choice	0.5	cup	71	44	120	3	21	0.5	2	1.5
Ice cream, deep choc pnut butter, HaagenDaz	0.5	cup	106	—	330	7	25	—	19	—
Ice cream, imitation, chocolate, Mellorine	0.5	cup	66	40	134	3	16	0.5	7	6
Ice cream, imitation, strawberry, Mellorine	0.5	cup	66	41	132	2	16	0	7	5.9
Ice cream, orange sorbet & vanilla, HaagenDaz	0.5	cup	106	62	199	3	30	—	8	4
Ice cream, praline & cream, Healthy Choice	0.5	cup	71	40	130	3	25	0.5	2	0.5
Ice cream, rocky road, low fat, Healthy Choice	0.5	cup	71	37	140	3	28	2	2	1
Ice cream, soft serve, chocolate	0.5	cup	173	100	355	6	48	1.4	17	10.4
Ice cream, soft serve, french vanilla	0.5	cup	86	51	185	4	19	0	11	6.4
Ice cream, strawberry	0.5	cup	66	40	127	2	18	0.2	6	3.4
Ice cream, triple choc chunk, Healthy Choice	0.5	cup	71	44	110	3	21	1	2	1
Ice cream, vanilla	0.5	cup	66	40	133	2	16	0	7	4.5
Ice cream, vanilla, Healthy Choice	0.5	cup	71	47	100	3	18	1	2	0.5
Ice cream, vanilla, rich, 16% fat	0.5	cup	74	42	178	3	17	0	12	7.4
Ice milk, chocolate	0.5	cup	66	43	94	3	17	0.3	2	1.3
Ice milk, vanilla, hard	0.5	cup	66	45	92	3	15	0	3	1.7

MonoF	PolyF	Choles	Calc	Phos	Sod	Pot	Zn	Iron	Magn	VitA	VitE	VitC	Thia	Ribo	Nia	B6	Fola	B12
(g)	(g)	(mg)	(mg)	(mg)	(mg)	(mg)	(mg)	(mg)	(mg)	(µg RE)	(µg α-TE)	(mg)	(mg)	(mg)	(mg)	(mg)	(µg)	(µg)
—	—	55	40	—	480	—	—	1.4	—	350	—	9	—	—	—	—	—	—
—	—	25	400	—	390	—	—	1.8	—	100	—	0	—	—	—	—	—	—
—	—	45	20	—	550	—	—	1.8	—	200	—	0	—	—	—	—	—	—
—	—	40	40	—	550	—	—	1.8	—	150	—	5	—	—	—	—	—	—
—	—	40	40	—	540	—	—	2.7	—	20	—	12	—	—	—	—	—	—
—	—	55	60	—	260	—	—	1.8	—	60	—	1	—	—	—	—	—	—
—	—	50	40	—	450	—	—	1.8	—	450	—	6	—	—	—	—	—	—
—	—	35	250	—	550	—	—	0.2	—	150	—	0	—	—	—	—	—	—
—	—	50	20	—	480	—	—	1.8	—	600	—	42	—	—	—	—	—	—
—	—	10	60	—	480	—	—	2.7	—	100	—	2	—	—	—	—	—	—
—	—	55	40	—	460	—	—	1.8	—	450	—	6	—	—	—	—	—	—
—	—	10	200	—	310	—	—	1.8	—	250	—	0	—	—	—	—	—	—
0	0	—	—	—	29	—	—	—	—	0	—	96	—	—	—	—	—	0
9.2	6.2	0	17	95	0	124	1.2	0.6	49	4	1.48	1	0.25	0.04	0.3	0.05	11	0
0.2	0.5	0	8	35	146	8	0.9	0.8	14	0	0.04	0	0	0	0	0.01	1	0
0	0	0	1	1	1	11	0	0.1	0	0	0	0	0	0.01	0	0	0	0
0	0	0	3	2	16	12	0	0	1	0	0	1	0	0	0	0	3	0
1.7	0.2	20	315	293	128	500	1.5	1.2	70	138	0.26	2	0.1	0.44	0.4	0.12	15	0.92
0.1	0.1	15	10	64	484	234	1.2	1	10	0	—	0	—	—	—	—	—	—
1.6	1.4	30	30	38	404	51	0.9	0.5	4	0	0.18	0	0.01	0.05	1.2	0.06	2	0.08
6.6	1.2	51	19	192	480	166	0.8	3.3	10	6	—	3	0.22	0.4	3.7	0.05	73	0.3
7.8	1.6	28	6	49	638	95	1	0.7	6	0	0.14	0	0.11	0.07	1.5	0.07	2	0.74
7.8	0.8	35	11	50	585	95	1.2	0.8	2	0	0.11	0	0.03	0.06	1.4	0.07	2	0.88
2.5	2.2	48	48	60	642	81	1.4	0.8	6	0	0.28	0	0.02	0.08	1.9	0.1	4	0.13
4.4	3.9	0	62	138	300	214	1.4	1.9	36	2	1.23	10	0.11	0.06	0.5	0.49	73	0
—	—	35	300	—	2170	—	—	3.6	—	300	—	36	—	—	—	—	—	—
0.7	1.6	10	61	42	147	32	0.1	0.7	5	9	0.52	0	0.08	0.07	0.6	0.02	16	0.04
2.3	0.8	20	207	228	182	395	0.9	0.6	33	57	0.66	2	0.06	0.3	1.1	0.13	9	0.65
2.7	1	21	161	155	92	271	0.7	0.3	24	58	0.78	2	0.06	0.28	0.9	0.08	18	0.64
0.6	0.1	7	62	48	42	102	0.4	0.1	7	22	0	1	0.02	0.1	0.1	0.02	4	0.24
3	1	21	72	86	48	151	0.7	0.4	21	55	0.4	0	0.04	0.14	0.9	0.04	7	0.18
0.1	0	1	129	99	55	173	0.3	0.1	14	2	0.01	0	0.03	0.18	0.1	0.05	1	0.62
2.3	0.4	24	70	62	43	126	0.4	0.2	11	63	0.07	0	0.02	0.13	0.1	0.03	3	0.21
5.4	1.3	26	104	123	60	206	0.9	0.6	40	69	0.53	0	0.05	0.25	0.6	0.04	9	0.23
2.6	0.8	1	136	62	50	129	0.3	0.4	16	25	0.36	0	0.02	0.1	0.5	0.12	6	0.2
0.1	0.1	0	1	4	6	4	0	0.1	1	0	0.07	0	0.01	0.01	0.2	0	4	0
2	0.3	18	96	89	51	176	0.4	0.4	17	62	0.22	0	0.04	0.14	0.3	0.03	4	0.27
0.1	0.1	0	4	10	32	14	0.1	0.4	3	0	0.05	0	0.05	0.04	0.5	0	8	0
2.3	0.4	32	102	88	72	158	0.5	0.2	11	84	0.03	0	0.04	0.2	0.3	0.04	4	0.28
2.8	0.4	29	95	89	66	169	0.6	0.4	18	77	0.1	0	0.04	0.19	0.3	0.04	4	0.26
1.7	0.4	20	60	64	36	122	0.4	0.3	13	53	0.09	0	0.03	0.12	0.2	0.03	5	0.18
1.7	0.4	20	60	64	36	122	0.4	0.3	13	53	0.09	0	0.03	0.12	0.2	0.03	5	0.18
0.8	0.2	10	30	31	18	60	0.2	0.1	6	26	0.05	0	0.02	0.06	0.1	0.01	2	0.09
—	—	80	100	—	95	—	—	1.1	—	150	—	1	—	—	—	—	—	—
—	—	70	100	—	50	—	—	1.1	—	100	—	1	—	—	—	—	—	—
7.5	7	100	107	107	80	170	—	—	—	160	—	—	0.16	0.18	—	—	—	—
7.1	0.7	38	74	139	56	260	1.1	1.1	63	95	0.72	0	0.03	0.21	0.3	0.04	2	0.23
1	0	2	100	141	50	240	—	0	—	40	—	0	—	—	—	—	—	—
2.1	0.3	22	72	71	50	164	0.4	0.6	19	78	0.22	0	0.03	0.13	0.1	0.04	11	0.19
0.5	0	2	100	141	90	254	—	—	—	60	—	2	0.03	0.15	—	—	—	—
—	—	—	107	213	90	300	—	1.2	—	21	—	—	0.1	0.14	2.1	—	—	—
0.5	0.1	0	90	81	48	179	0.8	0.3	17	0	0.06	0	0.03	0.15	0.1	0.04	2	0.38
0.4	0.1	0	90	71	48	144	0.7	0.1	10	0	0.05	0	0.03	0.15	0.1	0.04	1	0.39
—	—	60	64	64	30	114	—	0	—	85	—	6	0.03	0.11	0.8	—	—	—
0.1	1.4	2	100	141	70	226	—	0	—	40	—	0	0.03	0.15	—	—	—	—
0.5	0	2	100	9	60	168	—	0	—	40	—	0	0.03	0.15	—	—	—	—
4.9	0.6	43	206	184	89	384	1	0.7	37	147	0.46	1	0.07	0.27	0.2	0.06	9	0.64
3	0.4	78	113	100	52	152	0.4	0.2	10	132	0.32	1	0.04	0.16	0.1	0.04	8	0.43
1.6	0.2	19	79	66	40	124	0.2	0.1	9	52	0.13	5	0.03	0.17	0.1	0.03	8	0.2
—	—	2	100	—	60	—	—	0.4	—	8	—	0	—	—	—	—	—	—
2.1	0.3	29	84	69	53	131	0.5	0.1	9	77	0	0	0.03	0.16	0.1	0.03	3	0.26
1.5	0	5	100	141	50	254	—	—	—	60	—	2	0.05	0.22	—	—	—	—
3.4	0.4	45	87	70	41	118	0.3	0	8	136	0	1	0.03	0.12	0.1	0.03	4	0.27
0.6	0.1	6	94	78	41	155	0.4	0.2	13	18	0.06	0	0.03	0.12	0.1	0.03	4	0.3
0.8	0.1	9	92	72	56	139	0.3	0.1	10	31	0	1	0.04	0.18	0.1	0.04	4	0.44

Food Item	Qty	Meas	Wgt (g)	Wtr (g)	Cals	Prot	Carb (g)	Fib (g)	Fat (g)	SatF (g)
Ice slushy	1	cup	193	129	151	1	63	0	0	0
Ices, fruit flavor, sugar-free	1	each	51	48	12	0	3	0	0	0
Ices, lime	1	cup	192	128	246	1	63	0	0	0
Injera (Ethiopian bread), 12 inch loaf	1	piece	21	13	29	1	6	0.2	0	0.1
Instant breakfast, w/1% milk	1	cup	281	222	233	15	36	0.2	3	2
Instant breakfast, w/2% milk	1	cup	281	220	252	16	36	0.2	5	3.3
Instant breakfast, w/nonfat milk	1	cup	282	225	216	16	36	0.2	1	0.7
Instant breakfast, w/whole milk	1	cup	281	217	280	15	36	0.2	9	5.4
Jack in the Box, BreakfastJack sandwich	1	each	121	59	300	18	30	0	12	4.8
Jack in the Box, Jumbo Jack	1	each	229	126	560	26	41	0	32	10
Jack in the Box, Jumbo Jack w/cheese	1	each	242	133	610	29	41	0	36	12
Jack in the Box, bacon cheeseburger	1	each	242	119	710	35	41	4	45	15
Jack in the Box, chicken caesar pita sandwich	1	each	237	139	520	27	44	0	26	6
Jack in the Box, chicken sandwich	1	each	160	83	400	20	38	0	18	4
Jack in the Box, cinnamon churritos, serving	1	each	75	16	330	3	34	3	21	5
Jack in the Box, fajita, chicken pita	1	each	189	127	290	24	29	3	8	3
Jack in the Box, fried steak sandwich	1	each	153	70	450	14	42	0	25	7
Jack in the Box, hamburger, sourdough, grilled	1	each	223	107	670	32	39	0	43	16
Jack in the Box, monterey roast beef sandwich	1	each	238	135	540	30	40	3	30	9
Jack in the Box, sourdough breakfast sandwich	1	each	147	73	380	21	31	0	20	7
Jack in the Box, ultimate breakfast sandwich	1	each	242	128	620	36	39	—	35	11
Jackfruit, raw	4	oz.	113	83	107	2	27	1.8	0	0.1
Jam/marmalade, artificially sweetened	1	Tbs	20	9	2	0	11	0.5	0	0
Jam/preserves, 1 pkt	1	Tbs	20	7	48	0	13	0.2	0	0
Jam/preserves/marmalade, reduced sugar	1	Tbs	20	10	36	0	9	0.6	0	0
Java plum/jambolan, fresh	3	each	9	7	5	0	1	0.1	0	—
Jelly	1	Tbs	18	5	49	0	13	0.2	0	0
Jelly, reduced sugar, all flavors	1	Tbs	19	10	34	0	9	0.2	0	0
Jicama, raw	0.5	cup	60	54	23	1	5	2.9	0	0
Jicama/Yambean tuber, sliced, cooked	0.5	cup	50	45	19	0	4	2.4	0	0
Juice drink, cranberry apricot, w/vitamin C	1	cup	253	209	170	0	43	0.3	0	0
Juice drink, cranberry blueberry, w/vitamin C	1	cup	253	209	170	0	43	0.3	0	0
Juice drink, cranberry grape, w/vitamin C	1	cup	253	209	170	0	43	0.3	0	0
Juice drink, cranberry raspberry, w/vitamin C	1	cup	253	209	170	0	43	0.3	0	0
Juice drink, orange, CapriSun Natural	1	cup	176	—	83	0	22	0	0	0
Juice, apple, frozen w/vit C, prepared	1	cup	239	210	112	0	28	0.2	0	0
Juice, apple, w/vit C, canned/bottled	1	cup	248	218	117	0	29	0.2	0	0
Juice, apple-cherry	1	cup	250	219	117	1	29	0.8	0	0.1
Juice, apple-grape	1	cup	244	211	128	1	32	0.2	0	0.1
Juice, apple-raspberry	1	cup	239	212	108	0	26	0.2	0	0
Juice, clam and tomato	1	cup	241	210	115	1	26	0.5	0	0.1
Juice, grapefruit, canned, sweetened	0.5	cup	125	109	58	1	14	0.1	0	0
Juice, orange, chilled	1	cup	249	220	110	2	25	0.5	1	0.1
Juice, orange, fresh	1	cup	248	219	112	2	26	0.5	0	0.1
Juice, orange, frozen concentrate, prepared	1	cup	249	219	112	2	27	0.5	0	0
Juice, orange, unsweetened, canned	1	cup	249	222	105	1	24	0.5	0	0
Juice, passion fruit, purple, fresh	0.5	cup	124	106	63	0	17	0.2	0	0
Juice, passion fruit, yellow	0.5	cup	124	104	74	1	18	0.2	0	0
Juice, pineapple, canned, unsweetened	1	cup	250	214	140	1	34	0.5	0	0
Juice, pineapple, frozen concentrate, prepared	1	cup	250	216	130	1	32	0.5	0	0
Juice, pineapple, sweetened	1	cup	252	211	158	1	39	0.2	0	0
Juice, prune, bottled	1	cup	256	208	182	2	45	2.6	0	0
Juice, strawberry	1	cup	237	217	71	1	17	0.2	1	0
Juice, tangerine, canned, sweetened	0.5	cup	124	108	62	1	15	0.2	0	0
Juice, tangerine, fresh, unsweetened	1	cup	247	220	106	1	25	0.5	0	0.1
Juice, tangerine, frozen, sweetened, prepared	1	cup	241	212	111	1	27	0.5	0	0
Juice, tangerine, frozen, unswt, prepared	1	cup	247	220	106	1	25	0.5	0	0.1
Juice, watermelon, fresh	1	cup	238	218	76	1	17	1.2	1	0.1
Jujube fruit, raw	4	oz.	113	88	90	1	23	1.4	0	—
Jute/potherb, cooked	0.5	cup	43	38	16	2	3	0.9	0	0
KFC chicken leg, original	1	each	57	30	152	14	3	0.2	8	2.2
KFC, Chicken Little sandwich	1	each	47	16	169	6	14	0.4	10	2
KFC, Chicken breast, side, original	1	each	90	42	266	20	10	0.2	16	4.5
KFC, Chicken sandwich, Colonel's	1	each	166	76	482	21	39	—	27	6
KFC, Red beans & rice	1	each	111	84	113	4	18	3	3	1

MonoF	PolyF	Choles	Calc	Phos	Sod	Pot	Zn	Iron	Magn	VitA	VitE	VitC	Thia	Ribo	Nia	B6	Fola	B12
(g)	(g)	(mg)	(mg)	(mg)	(mg)	(mg)	(mg)	(mg)	(mg)	(µg RE)	(µg α-TE)	(mg)	(mg)	(mg)	(mg)	(mg)	(µg)	(µg)
0	0	0	4	2	42	6	0	0.3	2	0	0	2	0	0	0	0	0	0
—	—	0	1	0	3	13	0	0.1	1	0	0	0	0	0	0.1	0	0	0
0	0	0	4	2	42	6	0	0.3	2	0	0	2	0.02	0.02	0.3	0.01	6	0
0	0.1	0	12	24	42	12	0.1	6.2	2	698	5.36	31	0.41	0.48	5.5	0.53	118	1.53
0.9	0.1	14	406	393	266	731	4.1	4.9	118	693	5.41	31	0.41	0.48	5.5	0.53	118	1.52
1.5	0.2	23	401	390	264	726	4.1	4.9	112	703	5.3	31	0.4	0.42	5.5	0.52	118	1.56
0.3	0	9	407	406	268	755	4.1	4.8	117	630	5.51	31	0.41	0.47	5.5	0.52	118	1.5
2.5	0.3	185	200	—	890	220	—	2.7	—	80	—	9	0.47	0.41	3	—	—	—
4.8	2.4	65	100	—	700	450	—	4.5	—	40	—	6	0.36	0.29	1.8	—	—	—
13	8	80	200	—	780	460	—	5.4	—	60	—	6	0.36	0.44	1.6	—	—	—
15	9	110	250	—	1240	540	—	5.4	—	80	—	9	0.24	0.48	8.8	0.39	—	—
15.7	8.7	55	250	—	1050	490	—	2.7	—	80	—	2	—	—	—	—	—	—
—	—	45	150	—	1290	180	—	1.8	—	40	—	0	—	—	—	—	—	—
—	—	20	20	—	200	170	—	5.4	—	0	—	0	—	—	—	—	—	—
3.6	1.4	35	250	—	700	430	—	2.7	—	100	—	6	0.75	0.17	6	—	—	—
—	—	35	60	—	890	270	—	2.7	—	20	—	5	—	—	—	—	—	—
17.8	7.9	110	200	—	1140	510	—	4.5	—	150	—	6	0.65	0.48	8	0.33	—	—
—	—	75	300	—	1270	500	—	3.6	—	80	—	5	—	—	—	—	—	—
—	—	235	250	—	1120	260	—	3.6	—	150	—	9	—	—	—	—	—	—
—	—	455	250	—	1800	450	—	4.5	—	150	—	9	—	—	—	—	—	—
0	0.1	0	39	41	3	344	0.5	0.7	42	34	0.17	8	0.03	0.12	0.5	0.12	16	0
0	0	0	2	2	0	14	0	0.1	1	0	0.01	0	0	0	0	0	2	0
0	0	0	4	2	8	15	0	0.1	1	0	0	2	0	0	0	0	7	0
0	0.1	0	1	1	5	12	0	0.2	1	0	0.03	8	0	0.02	0.1	0.03	2	0
—	—	0	2	2	1	7	0	0	1	0	—	1	0	0	0	0	—	0
0	0	0	1	1	6	12	0	0	1	0	0	0	0	0	0	0.01	0	0
0	0	0	1	1	0	13	0	0	1	0	0	0	0	0	0	0	0	0
0	0	0	7	11	2	90	0.1	0.4	7	1	2.74	12	0.01	0.02	0.1	0.02	7	0
0	0	0	6	8	2	68	0.1	0.3	6	1	0.23	7	0.01	0.01	0.1	0.02	4	0
0	0	0	18	8	5	68	0.1	0.2	5	1	0	81	0.01	0.05	0.2	0.05	1	0
0	0	0	18	8	5	68	0.1	0.2	5	1	0	81	0.01	0.05	0.2	0.05	1	0
0	0	0	18	8	5	68	0.1	0.2	5	1	0	81	0.01	0.05	0.2	0.05	1	0
0	0	0	18	8	5	68	0.1	0.2	5	1	0	81	0.01	0.05	0.2	0.05	1	0
0	0	0	0	—	21	92	—	0	—	0	—	0	—	—	—	—	—	0
0	0.1	0	14	17	17	301	0.1	0.6	12	0	0.02	60	0.01	0.04	0.1	0.08	1	0
0	0.1	0	17	17	7	295	0.1	0.9	7	0	0.02	103	0.05	0.04	0.2	0.07	0	0
0.1	0.2	0	21	24	6	308	0.1	0.9	12	13	0.12	3	0.05	0.06	0.5	0.08	4	0
0	0.1	0	19	21	7	303	0.1	0.8	14	1	0.02	1	0.06	0.06	0.4	0.11	3	0
0	0.2	0	19	19	6	309	0.1	1.1	16	7	0.09	6	0.05	0.05	0.3	0.08	5	0
0	0	0	29	188	871	217	2.6	1.4	53	53	1.2	10	0.1	0.07	0.5	0.2	38	73.6
0	0	0	10	14	2	203	0.1	0.4	12	0	0.06	34	0.05	0.03	0.4	0.02	13	0
0.1	0.2	0	25	27	2	473	0.1	0.4	27	20	0.47	82	0.28	0.05	0.7	0.13	45	0
0.1	0.1	0	27	42	2	496	0.1	0.5	27	50	0.22	124	0.22	0.07	1	0.1	75	0
0	0	0	22	40	2	473	0.1	0.2	25	20	0.47	97	0.2	0.04	0.5	0.11	109	0
0.1	0.1	0	20	35	5	436	0.2	1.1	27	45	0.22	86	0.15	0.07	0.8	0.22	45	0
0	0	0	5	16	7	343	0.1	0.3	21	89	0.06	37	0	0.16	1.8	0.06	9	0
0	0.1	0	5	31	7	343	0.1	0.4	21	298	0.06	22	0	0.12	2.8	0.07	10	0
0	0.1	0	42	20	2	335	0.3	0.6	32	1	0.05	27	0.14	0.06	0.6	0.24	58	0
0	0	0	28	20	2	340	0.3	0.8	22	2	0.02	30	0.18	0.05	0.5	0.18	26	0
0	0.1	0	42	20	3	331	0.3	0.6	32	1	0.05	26	0.14	0.06	0.6	0.24	57	0
0.1	0	0	31	64	10	707	0.5	3	36	1	0.03	10	0.04	0.18	2	0.56	1	0
0.1	0.4	0	33	45	2	393	0.3	0.9	24	5	0.33	67	0.05	0.14	0.5	0.12	21	0
0	0	0	22	17	1	222	0	0.2	10	52	0.11	27	0.08	0.02	0.1	0.04	6	0
0.1	0.1	0	44	35	2	440	0.1	0.5	20	104	0.22	77	0.15	0.05	0.2	0.1	11	0
0	0	0	19	19	2	272	0.1	0.2	19	137	0.1	58	0.12	0.05	0.2	0.1	11	0
0.1	0.1	0	44	35	2	440	0.1	0.5	20	104	0.22	77	0.15	0.05	0.2	0.1	11	0
0.3	0.3	0	19	21	5	276	0.2	0.4	26	88	0.36	23	0.19	0.05	0.5	0.34	5	0
—	—	0	24	26	3	284	0.1	0.5	11	5	—	78	0.02	0.04	1	0.09	—	0
0	0	0	91	31	5	237	0.3	1.4	27	223	0.3	14	0.04	0.08	0.4	0.24	45	0
4.1	1.3	75	21	—	269	—	—	1.1	—	15	—	—	0.05	0.12	3.2	—	—	—
4.7	3.4	18	23	—	331	—	—	1.7	—	5	—	—	0.16	0.12	2.2	—	—	—
9.4	2.4	85	74	—	655	—	—	1.3	—	16	—	—	0.06	0.14	7.5	—	—	—
—	—	47	50	—	1060	—	—	1.3	—	15	—	6	—	—	—	—	—	—
—	—	4	10	—	312	—	—	0.7	—	—	—	—	—	—	—	—	—	—

Food Item	Qty	Meas	Wgt (g)	Wtr (g)	Cals	Prot	Carb (g)	Fib (g)	Fat (g)	SatF (g)
KFC, chicken breast, center, original	1	each	115	60	290	28	10	0.1	16	4.2
KFC, chicken breast, crispy	1	each	135	65	378	30	16	0.1	22	5.5
KFC, chicken leg, crispy	1	each	69	34	202	14	6	0.1	13	3.4
KFC, chicken, dark quarter, no skin, rotisserie gold	1	each	117	77	217	27	0	0	12	3.5
KFC, chicken, hot wings pieces (6)	1	each	119	45	415	24	16	—	29	—
KFC, chicken, white quarter, no skin, rotisserie gold	1	each	117	73	199	37	0	0	6	1.7
KFC, chicken, wing, whole, Hot and Spicy	1	each	61	23	220	14	5	—	16	4
Kale, fresh, chopped	0.5	cup	34	28	17	1	3	0.7	0	0
Kale, fresh, cooked, drained, no added salt	0.5	cup	65	59	18	1	4	1.3	0	0
Kale, frozen, cooked, drained, no added salt	0.5	cup	65	59	20	2	3	1.3	0	0
Kiwi fruit, raw slices	10	piece	70	58	43	1	10	2.4	0	0
Kohlrabi slices, raw	0.5	each	70	64	19	1	4	2.5	0	0
Kohlrabi, cooked, drained, no added salt	0.5	cup	82	74	24	1	6	0.9	0	0
Kool-aid, mix, unsweetened, grape, prepared	1	cup	246	221	100	0	25	0	0	0
Kudos nutty fudge snack bar	1	each	37	1	200	3	20	—	12	—
Kumquat, raw	1	each	19	16	12	0	3	1.2	0	0
LJS, chicken plank, 2 piece	1	each	112	62	240	16	22	—	12	3.2
LJS, clam dinner	1	each	361	168	990	24	114	—	52	10.9
LJS, fish & fryes, batter fried, 2 piece	1	each	261	142	610	27	52	—	37	7.9
LJS, fish & more, 2 piece w/fries & slaw	1	each	407	233	890	31	92	—	48	10.1
LJS, fish sandwich, batter dipped	1	each	159	86	340	18	40	—	13	3.1
LJS, fish shrimp chicken dinner	1	each	513	—	1160	45	113	—	65	14.2
LJS, fish w/lemon dinner, 3 piece	1	each	493	352	610	39	86	—	13	2.2
LJS, fish, batter fried, svg	1	each	88	52	180	12	12	—	11	2.7
LJS, fish, light portion dinner	1	each	334	257	330	24	46	—	5	0.9
LJS, fish-shrimp-clams dinner	1	each	512	—	1240	44	123	—	70	15.2
LJS, herb chicken a la carte	1	each	100	74	120	22	—	—	4	1.2
LJS, malt vinegar, serving	1	each	8	—	1	0	0	0	—	—
LJS, seafood gumbo w/cod	1	each	198	175	120	9	4	—	8	2.1
Lamb curry	0.5	cup	118	93	141	14	1	0.3	9	2.2
Lamb kabob meat, broiled, lean	4	oz.	113	72	211	32	0	0	8	3
Lamb stew meat, braised, lean	4	oz.	113	64	253	38	0	0	10	3.6
Lamb, arm chop, broiled, lean	3	oz.	85	53	170	24	0	0	8	2.9
Lamb, chop, loin, broiled, lean	3	oz.	85	52	184	26	0	0	8	3
Lamb, chop, loin, broiled, lean & fat	3	oz.	85	44	269	21	0	0	20	8.4
Lamb, ground, broiled	4	oz.	113	62	321	28	0	0	22	9.2
Lamb, leg, roasted, lean	3	oz.	85	54	162	24	0	0	7	2.4
Lamb, leg, sirloin, roasted, lean & fat	4	oz.	113	61	331	28	0	0	24	9.9
Lamb, rib, roast, cooked, lean	4	oz.	113	68	263	30	0	0	15	5.4
Lamb, rib, roast, cooked, lean & fat	4	oz.	113	54	407	24	0	0	34	14.5
Lamb, shoulder, roasted, lean	4	oz.	113	72	231	28	0	0	12	4.6
Lamb, shoulder, roasted, lean & fat	4	oz.	113	64	313	26	0	0	23	9.6
Lard, pork fat	1	Tbs	13	0	116	0	0	0	13	5.1
Lasagna, w/meat, recipe	1	piece	245	165	382	22	39	3.3	15	7.8
Lasagna, zucchini, Healthy Choice	1	each	397	330	290	14	49	5.2	4	2.6
Leek, whole, drained	1	each	124	113	38	1	9	1.2	0	0
Leeks, chopped, cooked, drained	0.5	cup	52	47	16	0	4	0.5	0	0
Leeks, chopped, raw	0.5	cup	52	43	32	1	7	0.9	0	0
Lemon juice, bottled	1	cup	244	226	51	1	16	1	1	0.1
Lemon juice, fresh	1	cup	244	221	61	1	21	1	0	0
Lemon juice, frozen, unsweetened	1	cup	244	225	54	1	16	1	1	0.1
Lemon peel, candied	1.5	oz.	43	7	134	0	34	—	0	0
Lemon peel, fresh	1	Tbs	6	5	3	0	1	0.6	0	0
Lemon turnover	1	each	78	33	238	3	29	0.6	12	3.1
Lemon, fresh, peeled	1	each	58	52	17	1	5	1.6	0	0
Lemonade flavor drink, dry, prepared	1	cup	266	237	112	0	29	0	0	0
Lemonade, low calorie	1	cup	240	228	43	0	11	0.2	0	0
Lemonade, pink, frozen, prepared	1	cup	248	221	99	0	26	0	0	0
Lemonade, white, frozen, prepared	1	cup	248	221	99	0	26	0.2	0	0
Lentil loaf	1	piece	47	30	82	4	9	3.1	3	0.4
Lentil sprouts, raw	0.5	cup	38	26	41	3	9	1.6	0	0
Lentil, sprouted, stir fried	4	oz.	113	78	115	10	24	4.4	1	0.1
Lentils, dry, cooked	0.5	cup	99	69	115	9	20	7.8	0	0.1
Lettuce, butterhead, chopped	0.5	cup	28	27	4	0	1	0.3	0	0
Lettuce, iceberg/crisphead leaves	1	piece	20	19	2	0	0	0.3	0	0

| MonoF | PolyF | Choles | Calc | Phos | Sod | Pot | Zn | Iron | Magn | VitA | VitE | VitC | Thia | Ribo | Nia | B6 | Fola | B12 |
(g)	(g)	(mg)	(mg)	(mg)	(mg)	(mg)	(mg)	(mg)	(mg)	(µg RE)	(µg α-TE)	(mg)	(mg)	(mg)	(mg)	(mg)	(µg)	(µg)
8.7	2.2	103	34	—	680	—	—	0.8	—	17	—	—	0.1	0.19	12.8	—	—	—
12.4	2.4	86	38	—	847	—	—	0.9	—	17	—	—	0.13	0.15	15	—	—	—
7.7	1.7	69	21	—	329	—	—	0.4	—	32	—	—	0.06	0.13	3.9	—	—	—
—	—	128	10	—	772	—	—	0.2	—	15	—	1	—	—	—	—	—	—
—	—	132	35	—	1084	—	—	2.9	—	13	—	5	—	—	—	—	—	—
—	—	97	10	—	667	—	—	0.2	—	15	—	1	—	—	—	—	—	—
—	—	65	20	—	440	—	—	0.7	—	30	—	—	—	—	—	—	—	—
0	0.1	0	45	19	14	150	0.1	0.6	11	298	0.27	40	0.04	0.04	0.3	0.09	10	0
0	0.1	0	47	18	15	148	0.2	0.6	12	481	0.55	27	0.03	0.05	0.3	0.09	9	0
0	0.2	0	90	18	10	209	0.1	0.6	12	413	0.12	16	0.03	0.07	0.4	0.06	9	0
0	0.2	0	18	28	4	232	0.1	0.3	21	13	0.78	52	0.01	0.04	0.4	0.04	7	0
0	0	0	17	32	14	245	0	0.3	13	3	0.34	43	0.04	0.01	0.3	0.1	11	0
0	0	0	21	37	17	281	0.3	0.3	16	3	1.38	45	0.03	0.02	0.3	0.13	10	0
0	0	0	0	—	15	0	—	0	—	0	—	6	—	—	—	—	—	0
—	—	—	40	—	55	—	—	0.4	—	—	—	—	—	0.1	—	—	—	—
0	0	0	8	4	1	37	0	0.1	2	6	0.05	7	0.02	0.02	0.1	0.01	3	0
8.4	0.2	30	—	—	790	320	0.6	1.1	—	—	—	—	0.15	0.26	7	—	—	—
31.3	9.9	75	200	—	1830	910	3	4.5	—	40	—	12	0.75	0.42	12	—	—	—
23.5	5.3	60	40	—	1480	900	1.2	1.8	—	—	—	9	0.38	0.34	8	—	—	—
28.5	9.5	75	200	—	1790	1230	2.2	3.6	—	40	—	9	0.52	0.51	12	—	—	—
8.9	1	30	80	—	890	370	1.5	3.6	—	—	—	1	0.38	0.34	6	—	—	—
40.3	9.6	135	200	—	2590	1450	3.8	4.5	—	40	—	9	0.75	0.68	16	—	—	—
3.9	5.3	125	200	—	1420	990	2.2	5.4	—	700	—	6	0.75	0.6	24	—	—	—
8.1	0.2	30	—	—	490	260	0.3	0.4	—	—	—	—	0.15	0.17	3	—	—	—
1.6	1.2	75	80	—	640	440	0.9	1.8	—	1000	—	18	0.3	0.26	14	—	—	—
44.2	9.9	140	200	—	2630	1390	3.8	5.4	—	40	—	9	0.9	0.68	16	—	—	—
1.7	1.1	60	—	—	570	270	0.6	0.7	—	—	—	—	0.09	0.26	—	—	—	—
—	—	—	—	—	15	10	—	—	—	—	—	—	—	—	—	—	—	—
3.2	2.6	25	100	—	740	310	1.5	1.8	—	200	—	—	0.15	0.17	3	—	—	—
2.9	2.8	44	15	137	237	235	3.2	1.3	18	0	1	1	0.04	0.14	3.9	0.09	13	1.41
3.4	0.8	102	15	254	86	380	6.5	2.6	35	0	0.23	0	0.12	0.34	7.5	0.16	26	3.44
4	0.9	122	17	232	79	295	7.5	3.2	32	0	0.23	0	0.08	0.27	6.8	0.14	24	3.1
3.1	0.7	78	14	186	70	289	4.9	2	26	0	0.17	0	0.08	0.25	5.8	0.12	20	2.55
3.6	0.5	81	16	192	71	320	3.5	1.7	24	0	0.14	0	0.09	0.24	5.8	0.14	20	2.14
8.2	1.4	85	17	167	66	278	3	1.5	20	0	0.11	0	0.08	0.21	6	0.11	15	2.1
9.4	1.6	110	25	228	92	384	5.3	2	27	0	0.28	0	0.11	0.28	7.6	0.16	22	2.96
2.9	0.4	76	7	175	58	287	4.2	1.8	22	0	0.15	0	0.09	0.25	7.1	0.14	20	2.24
9.9	1.7	110	12	208	77	341	4.7	2.3	25	0	0.15	0	0.12	0.32	7.5	0.16	19	2.87
6.6	1	100	24	221	92	357	5.1	2	26	0	0.17	0	0.1	0.26	7	0.17	25	2.45
14.2	2.5	110	25	188	83	307	4	1.8	23	0	0.11	0	0.1	0.24	7.6	0.12	17	2.53
4.9	1.1	99	22	227	77	301	6.8	2.4	28	0	0.2	0	0.1	0.3	6.5	0.17	28	3.06
9.3	1.8	104	23	209	75	285	5.9	2.2	26	0	0.16	0	0.1	0.27	7	0.15	24	2.99
5.4	1.8	12	0	0	0	0	0	0	0	0	0.15	0	0	0	0	0	0	0
5	0.9	56	258	289	745	461	3.2	3.2	50	158	1.15	16	0.23	0.33	4	0.21	19	0.78
—	—	10	207	—	321	—	—	1.9	—	259	—	0	—	—	—	—	—	—
0	0.1	0	37	21	12	108	0.1	1.4	17	6	0.76	5	0.03	0.02	0.2	0.14	30	0
0	0.1	0	16	9	5	45	0	0.6	7	3	0.32	2	0.01	0.01	0.1	0.06	13	0
0	0.1	0	31	18	10	94	0.1	1.1	15	5	0.48	6	0.03	0.02	0.2	0.12	33	0
0	0.2	0	27	22	51	249	0.1	0.3	20	5	0.22	60	0.1	0.02	0.5	0.1	25	0
0	0	0	17	15	2	303	0.1	0.1	15	5	0.22	112	0.07	0.02	0.2	0.12	32	0
0	0.2	0	20	20	2	217	0.1	0.3	20	2	0.22	77	0.14	0.03	0.3	0.15	23	0
—	—	0	0	0	0	0	—	0	—	0	—	0	0	0	0	—	0	0
0	0	0	8	1	0	10	0	0	1	0	0.01	8	0	0	0	0.01	1	0
5.4	3.2	47	10	41	228	31	0.3	1.1	5	32	1.16	1	0.13	0.12	1.1	0.02	8	0.09
0	0.1	0	15	9	1	80	0	0.3	5	2	0.14	31	0.02	0.01	0.1	0.05	6	0
0	0	0	29	3	19	3	0.1	0.1	3	0	0	34	0	0	0	0	0	0
0	0	0	7	2	7	38	0.1	0.4	5	2	0	16	0.02	0.02	0	0	7	0
0	0	0	7	5	7	37	0.1	0.4	5	0	0	10	0.02	0.05	0	0.02	5	0
0	0	0	7	5	7	37	0.1	0.4	5	5	0	10	0.02	0.05	0	0.02	5	0
0.7	2.1	0	15	88	40	155	0.6	1.4	26	0	2.01	1	0.13	0.04	0.6	0.09	62	0
0	0.1	0	10	67	4	124	0.6	1.2	14	2	0.04	6	0.09	0.05	0.4	0.07	38	0
0.1	0.2	0	16	174	11	322	1.8	3.5	40	5	0.1	14	0.25	0.1	1.4	0.19	76	0
0.1	0.2	0	19	178	2	365	1.3	3.3	36	1	0.11	1	0.17	0.07	1	0.18	179	0
0	0	0	9	6	1	72	0	0.1	4	27	0.12	2	0.02	0.02	0.1	0.01	20	0
0	0	0	4	4	2	32	0	0.1	2	7	0.06	1	0.01	0.01	0	0.01	11	0

Food Item	Qty	Meas	Wgt (g)	Wtr (g)	Cals	Prot	Carb (g)	Fib (g)	Fat (g)	SatF (g)
Lettuce, iceberg/crisphead, chopped	0.5	cup	28	27	3	0	1	0.4	0	0
Lettuce, looseleaf, chopped	0.5	cup	28	26	5	0	1	0.5	0	0
Lettuce, looseleaf, leaves	1	piece	10	9	2	0	0	0.2	0	0
Lettuce, romaine, chopped	0.5	cup	28	27	4	0	1	0.5	0	0
Lettuce, romaine, inner leaf	1	piece	10	9	1	0	0	0.2	0	0
Lime juice, bottled	1	cup	246	228	52	1	16	1	1	0.1
Lime juice, fresh	1	cup	246	222	66	1	22	1	0	0
Lime, fresh, peeled	0.5	each	67	59	20	0	7	1.9	0	0
Limeade, concentrate, frozen	0.5	cup	145	73	272	0	72	0.6	0	0
Limeade, from frozen	1	cup	247	220	101	0	27	0.2	0	0
Liqueur, coffee, 53 proof	1	oz.	28	9	95	0	13	0	1	0
Liqueur, coffee, 63 proof	1	oz.	28	12	87	0	9	0	0	0
Liqueur, de menthe, 72 proof	1	oz.	28	8	105	0	12	0	0	0
Liver, chopped, w/egg & onion	0.5	cup	104	66	230	13	3	0.4	18	5.5
Liverwurst	1	oz.	28	15	92	4	1	0	8	3
Lobster newburg	0.5	cup	122	75	306	15	6	0.1	25	14.8
Loganberries, canned w/heavy syrup	0.5	cup	128	98	113	1	28	3.3	0	0
Loganberries, fresh	0.5	cup	75	64	39	1	10	4	0	0
Loganberries, frozen	0.5	cup	74	62	40	1	10	3.6	0	0
Longan, raw	1	each	3	3	2	0	0	0	0	—
Loquat, raw	1	each	10	9	5	0	1	0.2	0	0
Lotus root, cooked	10	each	89	72	59	1	14	2.8	0	0
Lotus root, slices, raw	10	each	81	64	60	2	14	4	0	0
Lunchmeat, Spam, canned	1	piece	28	14	95	4	1	0.1	9	—
Lunchmeat, chicken/turkey sandwich spread	1	Tbs	13	9	26	2	1	0	2	0.4
Lunchmeat, chopped ham, slices	2	piece	42	27	96	7	0	0	7	2.4
Lunchmeat, pickle & pimento loaf	2	piece	57	32	149	7	3	0	12	4.5
Lychee, raw	1	each	10	8	6	0	2	0.1	0	0
Lychees, canned, sweetened	3.5	oz.	100	76	91	1	23	0.3	0	0.1
Macadamia nut, dried	0.25	cup	34	1	235	3	5	3.1	25	3.7
Macadamia nuts, oil roasted, salted	0.25	cup	34	1	241	2	4	3.1	26	3.8
Macadamia nuts, oil roasted, unsalted	11	each	28	0	204	2	4	2.6	22	3.3
Macaroni & cheese, canned	0.5	cup	120	96	114	5	13	0.7	5	2.1
Macaroni & cheese, recipe, w/margarine	0.5	cup	100	58	215	8	20	0.6	11	4.4
Mamey apple, raw	1	each	846	729	431	4	106	25.4	4	1.2
Mango nectar	1	cup	250	210	147	1	38	2	0	0.1
Mango, fresh slices	0.5	cup	82	67	54	0	14	1.5	0	0.1
Margarine, Blue Bonnet, stick	1	Tbs	14	2	102	0	0	0	11	2.4
Margarine, Fleischmann's corn oil, tub type	1	Tbs	14	2	102	0	0	0	11	2
Margarine, Parkay Squeeze	1	Tbs	14	2	102	0	0	0	11	1.9
Margarine, Parkay, soft, tub	1	Tbs	14	2	102	0	0	0	11	1.9
Margarine, Saffola, stick	1	Tbs	14	2	102	0	0	0	11	1.9
Margarine, Saffola, tub	1	Tbs	14	2	102	0	0	0	11	1.5
Margarine, hard, stick	1	Tbs	14	2	102	0	0	0	11	1.9
Margarine, hard, unsalted	1	Tbs	14	3	101	0	0	0	11	2.1
Margarine, liquid	1	Tbs	14	2	102	0	0	0	11	1.9
Margarine, soft, tub	1	Tbs	14	2	102	0	0	0	11	1.9
Margarine, spread, Blue Bonnet, tub	1	Tbs	14	8	49	0	0	0	6	0.9
Margarine, spread, Fleischmann's light, tub	1	Tbs	14	8	49	0	0	0	6	0.9
Margarine, spread, Shedd's Spread, tub	1	Tbs	14	8	60	0	0	0	6	0.8
Margarine, spread, Touch of Butter, stick	1	Tbs	14	4	90	0	0	0	10	2
Margarine, spread, Weight Watcher's XLight, tub	1	Tbs	14	8	49	0	0	0	6	1.1
Margarine, unsalted, Saffola	1	Tbs	14	3	101	0	0	0	11	2
Marmalade, orange	1	Tbs	20	7	49	0	13	0	0	0
Marshmallow	4	each	28	5	90	1	23	0	0	0
Marshmallow creme, Kraft	1	oz.	28	5	93	0	23	0	0	0
Marshmallow, miniature, not packed	0.5	cup	23	4	73	0	19	0	0	0
Mayonnaise, fat free (Kraft Free)	1	Tbs	16	14	10	0	2	0	0	0
Mayonnaise, imitation	1	Tbs	15	9	35	0	2	0	3	0.5
Mayonnaise, low calorie	1	Tbs	16	10	36	0	2	0	3	0.5
Mayonnaise, soybean, w/salt	1	Tbs	14	2	99	0	0	0	11	1.6
McDonald's Egg McMuffin	1	each	137	78	289	17	27	1.5	13	0.7
McDonald's Fillet-O-Fish sandwich	1	each	145	71	364	14	41	1.5	16	3.7
McDonald's McDonaldland cookies	1	each	56	2	258	4	41	1	9	1.7
McDonald's McLean Deluxe, w/cheese	1	each	228	143	397	26	38	2.2	16	6.8

MonoF (g)	PolyF (g)	Choles (mg)	Calc (mg)	Phos (mg)	Sod (mg)	Pot (mg)	Zn (mg)	Iron (mg)	Magn (mg)	VitA (µg RE)	VitE (µg α-TE)	VitC (mg)	Thia (mg)	Ribo (mg)	Nia (mg)	B6 (mg)	Fola (µg)	B12 (µg)
0	0	0	5	6	3	44	0.1	0.1	3	9	0.08	1	0.01	0.01	0.1	0.01	16	0
0	0	0	19	7	3	74	0.1	0.4	3	53	0.12	5	0.01	0.02	0.1	0.02	14	0
0	0	0	7	2	1	26	0	0.1	1	19	0.04	2	0	0.01	0	0.01	5	0
0	0	0	10	13	2	81	0.1	0.3	2	73	0.12	7	0.03	0.03	0.1	0.01	38	0
0	0	0	4	4	1	29	0	0.1	1	26	0.04	2	0.01	0.01	0	0	14	0
0.1	0.2	0	30	25	39	185	0.1	0.6	17	5	0.17	16	0.08	0.01	0.4	0.07	19	0
0	0.1	0	22	17	2	268	0.1	0.1	15	2	0.22	72	0.05	0.02	0.2	0.11	20	0
0	0	0	22	12	1	68	0.1	0.4	4	1	0.16	20	0.02	0.01	0.1	0.03	5	0
0	0	0	7	9	0	86	0.1	0.1	6	0	0	17	0.02	0.02	0.1	0	6	0
0	0	0	7	2	5	32	0	0.1	2	0	0	7	0	0	0.1	0	2	0
0	0	0	0	2	2	9	0	0	1	0	0	0	0	0	0	0	0	0
0	0	0	0	2	2	9	0	0	1	0	0	0	0	0	0	0	0	0
0	0	0	0	0	1	0	0	0	0	0	0	0	0	0	0	0	0	0
7.4	3.5	367	21	178	1078	125	2.2	4.1	14	2230	1.38	9	0.09	0.88	2	0.31	358	8.89
3.8	0.7	45	7	65	244	48	0.7	1.8	3	2353	0.08	0	0.08	0.29	1.2	0.05	9	3.83
7.3	1.1	184	120	199	323	304	2	0.6	28	261	1	0	0.05	0.21	0.8	0.08	16	2.01
0	0.1	0	23	13	4	115	0.2	0.6	14	5	0.91	8	0.03	0.04	0.3	0.05	44	0
0	0.2	0	24	16	0	146	0.2	0.4	15	12	0.53	16	0.02	0.03	0.3	0.04	25	0
0	0.1	0	19	19	1	107	0.2	0.5	15	3	1.62	11	0.04	0.02	0.6	0.05	19	0
—	—	0	0	1	0	9	0	0	0	0	—	3	0	0	0	—	—	0
0	0	0	2	3	0	26	0	0	1	15	0.09	0	0	0	0	0.01	1	0
0	0	0	23	69	40	323	0.3	0.8	20	0	0.01	24	0.11	0.01	0.3	0.19	7	0
0	0	0	36	81	32	450	0.3	0.9	19	0	0.01	36	0.13	0.18	0.3	0.21	10	0
—	—	16	2	—	445	54	0.7	0.4	3	5	—	—	0.03	0.05	0.9	—	—	0.05
0.4	0.8	4	1	4	49	24	0.1	0.1	1	5	0.29	0	0	0.01	0.2	0.01	1	0.39
3.4	0.9	21	3	65	576	134	0.8	0.3	7	0	0.11	0	0.26	0.09	1.6	0.15	0	0.39
5.5	1.5	21	54	80	792	194	0.8	0.6	10	4	0.14	0	0.17	0.14	1.2	0.11	3	0.67
0	0	0	0	3	0	16	0	0	1	0	0.07	7	0	0.01	0.1	0.01	1	0
0	0.1	0	4	20	1	100	0.1	0.2	7	0	0.45	32	0.01	0.04	0.4	0.06	5	0
19.5	0.4	0	24	46	2	123	0.6	0.8	39	0	0.14	0	0.12	0.04	0.7	0.07	5	0
20.2	0.4	0	15	67	87	110	0.4	0.6	39	0	0.14	0	0.07	0.04	0.7	0.07	5	0
17.1	0.4	0	13	57	2	93	0.3	0.5	33	0	0.12	0	0.06	0.03	0.6	0.06	5	0
1.5	0.7	12	100	91	365	70	0.6	0.5	16	37	0.07	0	0.06	0.12	0.5	0.01	4	0.1
4.4	1.8	21	181	161	543	120	0.6	0.9	18	117	0.06	0	0.1	0.2	0.9	0.02	5	0.15
1.7	0.7	0	93	93	127	398	0.8	5.9	135	195	4.99	118	0.17	0.34	3.4	0.85	118	0
0.1	0.1	0	12	11	6	141	0.1	0.2	10	292	1.12	19	0.05	0.06	0.5	0.12	7	0
0.1	0	0	8	9	2	129	0	0.1	7	321	0.92	23	0.05	0.05	0.5	0.11	12	0
5.6	3	0	4	3	134	6	0	0	0	113	1.48	0	0	0	0	0	0	0.01
4.5	4.4	0	4	3	153	5	0	0	0	113	2.13	0	0	0	0	0	0	0.01
4	5.1	0	9	7	111	13	0	0	1	113	0.74	0	0	0.01	0	0	0	0.03
5.2	3.8	0	4	3	153	5	0	0	0	113	1.85	0	0	0	0	0	0	0.01
3.3	5.8	0	4	3	134	6	0	0	0	113	2.7	0	0	0	0	0	0	0.01
4.4	5	0	4	3	153	5	0	0	0	113	2.41	0	0	0	0	0	0	0.01
5.3	3.7	0	4	3	134	6	—	0	0	113	1.82	0	0	0	0	0	0	0.01
5.2	3.6	0	2	2	0	4	0	0	0	113	1.82	0	0	0	0	0	0	0.01
4	5.1	0	9	7	111	13	0	0	1	113	0.74	0	0	0.01	0	0	0	0.03
5.2	3.8	0	4	3	153	5	0	0	0	113	1.85	0	0	0	0	0	0	0.01
2.4	2	0	3	2	136	4	0	0	0	113	1.21	0	0	0	0	0	0	0.01
2.1	2.3	0	3	2	136	4	0	0	0	113	1.56	0	0	0	0	0	0	0.01
2.4	2.4	0	3	2	110	4	0	0	0	144	0.48	0	0	0	0	0	0	0.01
—	—	0	0	—	110	0	0	0	—	122	—	0	—	—	—	—	0	0.01
2.2	2	0	3	2	136	4	0	0	0	154	0.33	0	0	0	0	0	0	0.01
3	4.6	—	0	—	0	—	—	0	—	52	—	0	—	0	0	0	7	0
0	0	0	8	1	11	7	0	0	0	1	0	1	0	0	0	0	7	0
0	0	0	1	2	13	1	0	0.1	1	0	0	0	0	0	0	0	0	0
0	0	0	0	—	23	0	—	0	—	0	0	0	—	—	—	—	—	0
0	0	0	1	2	11	1	0	0.1	0	0	0	0	0	0	0	0	0	0
0	0	0	0	—	105	5	—	0	—	0	—	0	—	—	—	—	—	0
0.7	1.6	4	0	0	75	2	0	0	0	0	0.96	0	0	0	0	0	0	0
0.7	1.6	4	0	0	78	2	0	0	0	0	1	0	0	0	0	0	0	0
3.1	5.7	8	2	4	78	5	0	0.1	0	12	1.63	0	0	0	0	0.08	1	0.04
4.5	1.6	234	151	270	730	199	1.6	2.4	24	100	0.85	2	0.49	0.45	3.3	0.15	33	0.67
3.8	5.6	37	124	183	708	266	0.7	1.8	32	21	1.52	0	0.32	0.23	2.6	0.07	30	0.58
6.3	0.8	0	10	70	267	62	0.4	1.7	11	0	0.99	0	0.24	0.16	2	0.03	—	—
4.6	1.3	72	139	291	1045	558	5.3	4.3	43	115	0.85	8	0.42	0.39	7.2	0.3	47	2.05

Food Item	Qty	Meas	Wgt (g)	Wtr (g)	Cals	Prot	Carb (g)	Fib (g)	Fat (g)	SatF (g)
McDonald's McLean deluxe	1	each	214	137	345	24	37	2.2	12	4.4
McDonald's Sausage McMuffin	1	each	112	48	361	13	26	1.5	23	8.3
McDonald's cheeseburger	1	each	122	56	319	15	36	1.9	13	5.6
McDonald's frozen yogurt cone, vanilla	1	each	90	61	118	4	24	0.4	1	0.5
McDonald's frozen yogurt shake, small, choc	1	each	295	—	348	13	62	0.9	6	3.5
McDonald's frozen yogurt shake, small, strawberry	1	each	294	—	343	12	63	0.3	5	3.4
McDonald's frozen yogurt shake, small, vanilla	1	each	293	—	308	12	54	0.3	5	3.3
McDonald's hashed browns	1	each	53	29	130	1	14	1.4	8	1.4
McDonald's turnover, apple	1	each	85	40	225	2	32	1.2	11	2.6
McDonald's, Big Mac sandwich	1	each	216	115	510	25	46	3.3	26	9.3
McDonald's, Chicken McNuggets	4	piece	73	37	198	12	10	0	12	2.5
McDonald's, Fajita, chicken	1	each	82	42	190	11	20	1	8	2
McDonald's, McChicken sandwich	1	each	189	98	492	17	42	1.7	29	5.5
McDonald's, Quarter-Pounder	1	each	171	89	415	23	36	1.7	20	7.8
McDonald's, Quarter-Pounder, w/cheese	1	each	199	100	520	28	37	1.7	29	12.6
McDonald's, biscuit w/spread	1	each	76	24	260	4	32	1.1	13	3.8
McDonald's, burrito, breakfast	1	each	105	52	290	12	21	1	17	5
McDonald's, chicken salad, chunky	1	each	296	259	164	23	8	3.2	5	1.3
McDonald's, chicken sandwich, McGrilled	1	each	188	126	254	24	33	2	3	0.7
McDonald's, chicken, drumstick, hot & spicy	1	each	63	29	180	14	6	—	12	3
McDonald's, danish pastry, apple	1	each	105	—	360	5	51	1.5	17	5.2
McDonald's, danish pastry, cinnamon raisin	1	each	105	20	435	5	56	1.4	22	7.4
McDonald's, danish pastry, raspberry	1	each	105	24	396	5	58	1.4	16	5.2
McDonald's, french fries, regular order	1	each	97	37	320	4	36	1.7	17	3.5
McDonald's, hamburger	1	each	108	54	266	12	36	1.9	9	3.2
McDonald's, scrambled eggs, serving	1	each	102	75	170	13	1	0	12	3.6
Meatless hot dog, Tofu Pups, Lightlife	1	each	42	3	60	8	28	0	2	1
Meatless patty, Garden Burger	2.5	oz.	71	41	130	8	18	5	3	1
Meatless patty, Garden Burger, Veggie Medley	2.5	oz.	71	41	130	8	18	5	3	1
Meatless patty, Garden Burger, vegan	2.5	oz.	71	36	140	11	23	4	0	0
Melon balls, mixed, frozen	0.5	cup	86	78	28	1	7	0.6	0	0.1
Melon, cantaloupe, cubes	0.5	cup	80	72	28	1	7	0.6	0	0.1
Melon, casaba/crenshaw cubes	0.5	cup	85	78	22	1	5	0.7	0	0
Melon, honeydew, cubes	0.5	cup	85	76	30	0	8	0.5	0	0
Milk drink, malted, chocolate (Ovaltine)	1	cup	265	215	225	9	29	0.3	9	5.5
Milk drink, malted, chocolate, unfortified	1	cup	265	215	228	9	30	0.3	9	5.5
Milk drink, malted, natural (Ovaltine)	1	cup	265	215	231	10	28	0	9	5.4
Milk, 1% fat, low lactose	1	cup	246	222	103	9	12	0	3	1.6
Milk, 1% lowfat	1	cup	244	220	102	8	12	0	3	1.6
Milk, 1% lowfat, protein fortified	1	cup	246	218	119	10	14	0	3	1.8
Milk, 2% lowfat	1	cup	244	218	121	8	12	0	5	2.9
Milk, 2% lowfat, protein+vitamin A fortified	1	cup	246	216	137	10	14	0	5	3
Milk, Goat	1	cup	244	212	168	9	11	0	10	6.5
Milk, chocolate, 1% lowfat	1	cup	250	211	158	8	26	1.2	2	1.5
Milk, chocolate, 2% lowfat	1	cup	250	209	179	8	26	1.2	5	3.1
Milk, chocolate, nonfat	1	cup	250	211	144	9	27	1.5	1	0.7
Milk, chocolate, whole fat	1	cup	250	206	209	8	26	2	8	5.2
Milk, condensed, sweetened, canned	3	Tbs	57	16	184	5	31	0	5	3.2
Milk, dry, nonfat, instant, w/vitamin A added	1	Tbs	4	0	15	1	2	0	0	0
Milk, evaporated, 2% fat	2	Tbs	32	25	29	2	4	0	1	0.4
Milk, evaporated, skim, canned	0.5	cup	128	101	99	10	14	0	0	0.2
Milk, human breast, mature	1	cup	246	215	171	3	17	0	11	4.9
Milk, imitation, (Vitamite)	1	cup	244	220	112	4	13	0	5	1
Milk, imitation, fluid, soy based	1	cup	244	215	150	4	15	0	8	1.9
Milk, malted, natural, powder, unfortified	1	cup	265	5	1097	30	201	1.6	21	11.1
Milk, nonfat skim	1	cup	245	222	86	8	12	0	0	0.3
Milk, nonfat, dry, reconstituted,	1	cup	245	223	82	8	12	0	0	0.1
Milk, nonfat, low lactose	1	cup	245	222	86	9	12	0	0	0.3
Milk, rice, Arroz con leche	1	cup	245	219	100	0	25	0.2	0	0
Milk, skim, protein fortified	1	cup	245	219	100	10	14	0	1	0.4
Milk, strawberry mix w/milk (Nestle's Quik)	1	cup	250	202	220	8	31	0	8	4.8
Milk, whole, 3.3% fat	1	cup	244	215	150	8	11	0	8	5.1
Milk, whole, extra rich, 3.7% fat	1	cup	244	214	157	8	11	0	9	5.6
Milk, whole, fluid, low sodium	1	cup	244	215	149	8	11	0	8	5.2
Milkshake, chocolate	1	cup	226	162	288	8	46	1.8	8	5.2

MonoF (g)	PolyF (g)	Choles (mg)	Calc (mg)	Phos (mg)	Sod (mg)	Pot (mg)	Zn (mg)	Iron (mg)	Magn (mg)	VitA (µg RE)	VitE (µg α-TE)	VitC (mg)	Thia (mg)	Ribo (mg)	Nia (mg)	B6 (mg)	Fola (µg)	B12 (µg)
3.6	1.2	59	131	226	809	537	4.9	4.3	40	74	0.63	8	0.42	0.34	7.2	0.29	44	1.9
8.2	2.8	46	132	157	751	191	1.5	2.1	22	48	0.66	0	0.56	0.27	3.8	0.14	16	0.5
3.8	1.1	42	134	178	768	282	2.6	2.7	27	64	0.46	2	0.33	0.31	3.8	0.15	24	1.2
0.2	0	3	132	101	84	175	—	0.2	—	4	—	1	0	0.02	0.2	—	—	—
0.1	0.7	24	371	354	241	542	—	1	—	46	—	3	0.12	0.51	0.4	0.1	—	—
0.1	0.6	24	366	329	170	542	—	0.3	—	46	—	3	0.12	0.51	0.4	0.11	—	—
0.1	0.6	24	360	327	194	534	—	0.3	—	45	—	3	0.12	0.51	0.3	—	—	—
2.3	1.9	0	7	51	332	213	0.2	0.3	11	0	0.58	3	0.08	0.02	0.9	0.08	8	0
4.6	2.8	0	6	24	179	67	0.2	1	6	10	1.62	1	0.13	0.09	1	0.03	20	0
7.5	4.1	76	202	267	931	455	4.8	4.3	46	66	1.01	3	0.49	0.44	6.1	0.25	49	2.25
3.7	2.4	42	9	199	353	210	0.7	0.6	17	0	0.96	0	0.08	0.11	5.2	0.21	—	0.21
—	—	35	80	—	310	—	—	0.7	—	20	—	6	—	—	—	—	—	—
8.5	10.2	52	129	223	799	320	1.1	2.5	33	29	6.17	1	0.91	0.24	7.8	0.39	37	0.05
6.7	1.3	70	127	207	692	405	4.7	4.3	34	33	0.36	3	0.39	0.32	6.8	0.24	27	2.58
8.7	1.6	97	143	—	1160	—	—	4.5	—	115	0.81	3	0.39	0.43	6.8	0.26	33	2.89
3.7	0.8	0	68	353	836	105	0.3	1.8	9	2	0.81	0	0.29	0.23	2.2	0.03	5	—
—	—	135	100	—	580	—	—	1.4	—	100	—	6	—	—	—	—	—	—
1.6	1	76	54	277	318	673	1.5	1.6	44	1973	1.28	30	0.51	0.21	8.5	0.52	83	0.28
0.5	1.1	47	117	327	506	433	0.9	2.4	42	46	0.3	5	0.43	0.28	12.1	0.55	38	0.16
—	—	55	—	—	320	—	—	—	—	15	—	6	—	—	—	—	—	—
—	—	42	78	0	291	113	—	1	—	100	—	1	0.3	0.17	2	—	—	—
—	—	51	92	0	280	112	—	1.6	—	100	—	1	0.3	0.26	3	—	—	—
—	—	44	86	0	296	94	—	1	—	101	—	1	0.3	0.17	2	—	—	0
12	1.5	0	14	—	150	—	—	0.7	—	0	—	12	0.23	0	3	—	—	—
2.8	0.9	28	126	113	533	261	2.3	2.7	24	23	0.23	2	0.33	0.26	3.8	0.14	21	1.05
5.3	1.7	424	50	172	143	126	1.1	1.2	10	168	0.92	0	0.07	0.51	0.1	0.12	44	1.11
—	—	0	20	—	140	—	—	1.8	—	0	—	2	—	—	—	—	—	—
1.5	0.5	11	84	132	290	193	0.9	0	30	10	0.2	0	0.11	0.15	1.1	0.08	10	0.11
1.5	0.5	11	84	132	290	193	0.9	0	30	10	0.2	1	0.11	0.15	1.1	0.08	10	0.11
0	0	0	20	—	250	—	—	1.1	—	0	—	0	—	—	—	—	—	—
0	0.1	0	9	10	27	242	0.1	0.3	12	153	0.13	5	0.14	0.02	0.6	0.09	22	0
0	0.1	0	9	14	7	247	0.1	0.2	9	258	0.12	34	0.03	0.02	0.5	0.09	14	0
0	0	0	4	6	10	179	0.1	0.3	7	3	0.13	14	0.05	0.02	0.3	0.1	14	0
0	0	0	5	8	8	230	0.1	0.1	6	3	0.13	21	0.06	0.02	0.5	0.05	5	0
2.6	0.4	34	384	313	244	620	1.2	3.8	53	901	0.32	34	0.73	1.26	10.9	1.02	32	0.88
2.6	0.4	34	305	265	172	498	1.1	0.6	48	80	0.26	3	0.13	0.44	0.6	0.14	16	0.93
2.5	0.4	34	371	307	204	572	1.1	3.6	48	742	0.32	29	0.71	1.14	10.4	0.87	22	1.03
0.8	0.1	10	303	237	124	384	1	0.1	34	145	0.1	2	0.1	0.41	0.2	0.11	12	0.9
0.7	0.1	10	300	235	123	381	1	0.1	34	144	0.1	2	0.1	0.41	0.2	0.1	12	0.9
0.8	0.1	10	349	273	143	443	1.1	0.1	39	145	0.1	3	0.11	0.47	0.2	0.12	14	1.05
1.4	0.2	18	298	232	122	376	1	0.1	33	139	0.17	2	0.1	0.4	0.2	0.1	12	0.89
1.4	0.2	19	352	276	145	448	1.1	0.1	40	140	0.17	3	0.11	0.48	0.2	0.12	15	1.05
2.7	0.4	28	327	271	122	498	0.7	0.1	34	137	0.22	3	0.12	0.34	0.7	0.11	1	0.16
0.8	0.1	7	288	258	152	425	1	0.6	33	148	0.06	2	0.1	0.42	0.3	0.1	12	0.86
1.5	0.2	17	285	255	151	423	1	0.6	33	143	0.13	2	0.09	0.41	0.3	0.1	12	0.85
0.4	0	4	292	265	121	486	1.2	0.7	46	142	0.11	2	0.09	0.34	0.3	0.1	14	0.88
2.5	0.3	30	280	253	149	418	1	0.6	32	72	0.23	2	0.09	0.4	0.3	0.1	12	0.84
1.4	0.2	20	163	145	73	213	0.5	0.1	15	46	0.12	1	0.05	0.24	0.1	0.03	6	0.26
0	0	1	52	42	23	72	0.2	0	5	30	0	0	0.02	0.07	0	0.02	2	0.17
0.2	0	3	90	60	36	103	0.3	0.1	8	41	0.02	0	0.01	0.1	0.1	0.02	3	0.07
0.1	0	5	370	249	147	423	1.2	0.4	34	149	0.01	2	0.06	0.39	0.2	0.07	11	0.3
4.1	1.2	34	79	34	42	126	0.4	0.1	8	157	2.21	12	0.03	0.09	0.4	0.03	13	0.11
2.7	0.9	0	200	244	134	366	0.2	0.2	2	149	0	0	0.03	0.22	0	0	0	0
4.9	1.2	0	79	181	191	278	2.9	1	16	0	2.56	0	0.03	0.22	0	0	0	0
5.4	3.2	53	790	949	1306	2008	2.6	1.9	246	233	1.06	8	1.34	2.44	13.9	1.09	122	2.07
0.1	0	4	301	247	126	407	1	0.1	28	149	0.1	2	0.09	0.34	0.2	0.1	13	0.93
0.1	0	4	284	224	131	388	1.1	0.1	29	162	0	1	0.09	0.4	0.2	0.08	11	0.91
0.1	0	4	302	247	126	406	1	0.1	28	149	0.1	2	0.09	0.34	0.2	0.1	13	0.93
0	0	0	12	5	7	6	0.1	0.3	4	0	0	0	0.02	0.01	0.1	0.01	0	0
0.2	0	5	350	274	144	446	1.1	0.1	39	149	0.1	3	0.11	0.48	0.2	0.12	15	1.05
2.2	0.3	30	275	215	120	348	0.9	0.2	30	70	0.25	2	0.09	0.4	0.2	0.1	12	0.82
2.4	0.3	33	290	228	120	371	0.9	0.1	33	76	0.24	2	0.09	0.4	0.2	0.1	12	0.87
2.6	0.3	35	290	227	119	368	0.9	0.1	33	83	0.24	4	0.09	0.39	0.2	0.1	12	0.87
2.4	0.3	33	246	209	6	617	0.9	0.1	12	78	0.24	2	0.05	0.26	0.1	0.08	12	0.88
2.4	0.3	29	256	231	220	453	0.9	0.7	38	52	0.15	1	0.13	0.56	0.4	0.11	8	0.77

Food Item	Qty	Meas	Wgt (g)	Wtr (g)	Cals	Prot	Carb (g)	Fib (g)	Fat (g)	SatF (g)
Milkshake, strawberry	1	cup	226	168	256	8	43	0.9	6	3.9
Milkshake, vanilla	1	cup	226	169	251	8	40	0.9	7	4.2
Millet, cooked	0.5	cup	120	86	143	4	28	1.6	1	0.2
Miso (soybean)	1	Tbs	17	7	36	2	5	0.9	1	0.2
Miso sauce	0.25	cup	62	36	96	3	18	1.5	2	0.2
Mixed fruit canned in heavy syrup	0.5	cup	128	103	92	0	24	1.3	0	0
Mixed fruit, dried	0.5	cup	68	21	165	2	44	5.3	0	0
Mixed fruit, frozen-sweetened-thawed	0.5	cup	125	92	123	2	30	2.4	0	0
Mixed nuts, no peanuts, oil roasted, salted	0.25	cup	36	1	221	6	8	2	20	3.3
Mixed nuts, no peanuts, oil roasted, unsalted	0.25	cup	36	1	221	6	8	2	20	3.3
Mixed nuts, w/peanuts, dry roasted, salted	0.25	cup	34	1	203	6	9	3.1	18	2.4
Mixed nuts, w/peanuts, dry roasted, unsalted	0.25	cup	34	1	203	6	9	3.1	18	2.4
Mixed nuts, w/peanuts, oil roasted, salted	0.25	cup	36	1	219	6	8	3.2	20	3.1
Mixed nuts, w/peanuts, oil roasted, unsalted	0.5	cup	71	1	438	12	15	7	40	6.2
Mixed vegetables, Chinese, LaChoy	4	oz.	113	108	14	1	3	1.7	0	0
Mixed vegetables, canned, drained	0.5	cup	82	71	38	2	8	2.4	0	0
Mixed vegetables, canned, low sodium	0.5	cup	91	82	33	1	6	2.8	0	0
Mixed vegetables, dried-Salad Crunchies	1	Tbs	6	0	22	1	3	0.8	1	0.1
Mixed vegetables, frozen, cooked	0.5	cup	91	76	54	3	12	4	0	0
Mocha mix, vanilla	1	Tbs	8	5	17	0	2	—	1	0.2
Mock chicken leg, cooked	4	oz.	113	66	262	23	6	0.2	16	4.9
Molasses, blackstrap cane	1	Tbs	20	6	48	0	12	0	0	0
Molasses, light cane	1	Tbs	20	5	54	0	14	0	0	0
Moo goo gai pan	0.5	cup	108	84	140	8	6	1.4	10	2.4
Mothbean, cooked, no salt	0.5	cup	88	61	103	7	18	3.3	0	0.1
Moussaka, lamb & eggplant	1	cup	250	205	237	16	13	3.6	13	4.6
Mousse, chocolate, recipe	0.5	cup	202	125	446	9	33	1.2	33	18.5
Muffin, blueberry, commercial	1	each	57	22	158	3	27	1.5	4	0.8
Muffin, blueberry, mix, prepared	1	each	45	16	135	2	22	0.5	4	0.7
Muffin, blueberry, recipe, w/2% milk	1	each	57	22	162	4	23	1.1	6	1.2
Muffin, blueberry, recipe, w/whole milk	1	each	45	18	131	3	18	0.8	5	1.1
Muffin, buckwheat	1	each	47	16	144	4	20	1.4	6	1.7
Muffin, carrot w/raisins & nuts	1	each	58	20	177	4	26	1	7	1.1
Muffin, cheese	1	each	58	21	184	5	23	0.7	8	3
Muffin, chocolate chip	1	each	58	18	190	4	27	1	8	2.8
Muffin, cornmeal, commercial	1	each	57	19	174	3	29	1.9	5	0.8
Muffin, cornmeal, mix, prepared	1	each	45	14	144	3	22	1.1	5	1.3
Muffin, cornmeal, recipe w/2% milk	1	each	57	19	180	4	25	1.9	7	1.3
Muffin, cornmeal, recipe, w/whole milk	1	each	45	15	144	3	20	1.5	6	1.2
Muffin, cranberry nut	1	each	58	22	164	4	25	0.8	5	1.5
Muffin, egg-bacon-cheese, Great Starts	1	each	116	59	290	14	25	2	15	6
Muffin, oat bran	1	each	57	20	154	4	28	2.6	4	0.6
Muffin, oatmeal	1	each	47	22	112	3	17	0.7	3	1
Muffin, plain, recipe, w/2% milk	1	each	57	22	169	4	24	1.5	6	1.2
Muffin, plain, recipe, w/whole milk	1	each	45	17	135	3	19	1.2	5	1.2
Muffin, pumpkin, w/raisins	1	each	58	16	181	3	34	1.1	4	0.8
Muffin, toaster type, blueberry	1	each	33	10	103	2	18	0.6	3	0.5
Muffin, toaster type, blueberry, toasted	1	each	31	8	103	2	18	0.6	3	0.5
Muffin, toaster type, corn	1	each	33	8	114	2	19	0.5	4	0.6
Muffin, toaster type, cornmeal, toasted	1	each	31	6	114	2	19	0.5	4	0.6
Muffin, toaster type, wheat bran-raisin	1	each	36	11	106	2	19	2.8	3	0.5
Muffin, toaster type, wheat bran-raisin, toasted	1	each	34	9	106	2	19	2.8	3	0.5
Muffin, wheat bran, mix, prepared	1	each	45	16	124	3	21	1.9	4	1.1
Muffin, wheat bran, recipe, w/2% milk	1	each	57	20	161	4	24	2.2	7	1.3
Muffin, wheat bran, recipe, w/whole milk	1	each	45	16	130	3	19	3.2	6	1.2
Muffin, whole wheat	1	each	47	16	142	4	20	2.5	6	1.7
Muffin, zucchini	1	each	58	17	210	3	26	0.8	10	1.7
Mulberries, raw	0.5	cup	70	61	30	1	7	1.2	0	0
Mushroom pieces, cooked, drained	0.5	cup	78	71	21	2	4	1.7	0	0
Mushroom pieces, raw	0.5	cup	35	32	9	1	2	0.4	0	0
Mushroom pieces, steamed	0.5	cup	78	72	20	2	4	0.9	0	0
Mushroom pieces, stir fried, no oil	0.5	cup	78	72	20	2	4	0.9	0	0
Mushroom, batter-dipped, fried	5	each	70	46	148	2	8	0.7	12	2.1
Mushroom, chanterelle, dried	0.5	cup	72	9	246	13	38	14.2	5	0.5
Mushroom, enoki, raw	1	each	3	3	1	0	0	0.1	0	0

MonoF (g)	PolyF (g)	Choles (mg)	Calc (mg)	Phos (mg)	Sod (mg)	Pot (mg)	Zn (mg)	Iron (mg)	Magn (mg)	VitA (µg RE)	VitE (µg α-TE)	VitC (mg)	Thia (mg)	Ribo (mg)	Nia (mg)	B6 (mg)	Fola (µg)	B12 (µg)
1.8	0.3	25	256	226	188	412	0.8	0.2	29	66	0.29	2	0.1	0.44	0.4	0.1	7	0.7
2	0.3	25	276	231	186	394	0.8	0.2	27	72	0.13	2	0.1	0.41	0.4	0.12	7	0.82
0.2	0.6	0	4	120	2	74	1.1	0.8	53	0	0.22	0	0.13	0.1	1.6	0.13	23	0
0.2	0.6	0	11	26	629	28	0.6	0.5	7	2	0	0	0.02	0.04	0.1	0.04	6	0
0.4	0.9	0	19	43	1003	52	0.9	0.8	13	2	0	0	0.03	0.07	0.2	0.06	9	0
0	0.1	0	1	13	5	107	0.1	0.5	6	24	0.51	88	0.02	0.05	0.8	0.05	4	0
0.2	0.1	0	26	52	12	541	0.3	1.8	26	166	0.43	3	0.03	0.11	1.3	0.11	3	0
0	0.1	0	9	15	4	164	0.1	0.4	8	40	0.75	94	0.02	0.04	0.5	0.03	10	0
11.9	4.1	0	38	162	252	196	1.7	0.9	90	1	2.16	0	0.18	0.18	0.7	0.06	20	0
11.9	4.1	0	38	162	4	196	1.7	0.9	90	1	2.16	0	0.18	0.18	0.7	0.06	20	0
10.8	3.7	0	24	149	229	204	1.3	1.3	77	0	2.06	0	0.07	0.07	1.6	0.1	17	0
10.8	3.7	0	24	149	4	204	1.3	1.3	77	0	2.06	0	0.07	0.07	1.6	0.1	17	0
11.3	4.7	0	38	165	231	206	1.8	1.1	83	1	2.13	0	0.18	0.08	1.8	0.08	30	0
22.5	9.4	0	77	329	8	413	3.6	2.3	167	1	4.26	0	0.35	0.16	3.6	0.17	59	0
—	—	0	14	—	59	—	—	0.2	—	1	—	8	—	—	—	—	—	0
0	0.1	0	22	34	121	237	0.3	0.9	13	949	0.49	4	0.04	0.04	0.5	0.06	19	0
0	0.1	0	19	34	24	126	0.5	0.6	14	462	0.19	3	0.03	0.04	0.4	0.07	16	0
0.1	0.4	0	17	23	28	106	0.2	0.8	10	194	0.47	13	0.05	0.03	0.4	0.06	13	0.01
0	0.1	0	23	46	32	154	0.4	0.7	20	389	0.33	3	0.06	0.11	0.8	0.07	17	0
0.3	0.4	0	3	5	10	12	—	0.1	0	0	—	0	0	0	0	—	—	—
6.5	2.6	98	24	211	648	320	3.8	1.3	24	4	0.78	0	0.31	0.34	5.6	0.31	11	1.25
0	0	0	176	8	11	511	0.2	3.6	44	0	0	0	0.01	0.01	0.2	0.14	0	0
0	0	0	42	6	8	300	0.1	1	50	0	0	0	0.01	0	0.2	0.14	0	0
3.2	3.7	19	65	98	163	238	0.8	0.8	16	101	1.03	17	0.07	0.16	2.2	0.16	22	0.18
0	0.2	0	3	132	9	268	0.5	2.8	92	1	0.09	1	0.11	0.02	0.6	0.08	126	0
5.4	1.9	97	68	179	432	557	2.6	1.8	40	105	0.81	6	0.15	0.31	4.1	0.23	45	1.41
10.3	1.7	299	202	259	87	297	1.4	1.3	44	323	0.98	1	0.08	0.41	0.3	0.13	32	0.93
1.1	1.4	17	32	112	255	70	0.3	0.9	9	5	0.6	1	0.08	0.07	0.6	0.01	26	0.33
1.6	1.4	21	11	85	197	35	0.2	0.5	5	10	0.63	1	0.07	0.14	1	0.03	5	0.04
1.5	3.1	21	108	83	251	70	0.3	1.3	9	22	0.97	1	0.16	0.16	1.3	0.02	27	0.08
1.2	2.4	18	85	65	198	55	0.2	1	7	13	0.81	1	0.12	0.13	1	0.02	5	0.06
2.4	1.3	21	88	85	284	106	0.5	1	31	14	0.6	0	0.1	0.12	1.1	0.07	8	0.07
1.6	3.6	18	82	69	251	112	0.3	1.2	10	263	0.61	1	0.15	0.15	1.2	0.04	7	0.08
3	1.4	30	111	115	274	80	0.5	1.3	11	35	0.6	0	0.16	0.2	1.3	0.03	8	0.11
3	1.4	24	74	75	186	92	0.4	1.4	16	17	0.65	0	0.17	0.18	1.4	0.03	7	0.09
1.2	1.8	15	42	162	297	39	0.3	1.6	18	20	1.05	0	0.16	0.19	1.2	0.05	35	0.05
2.4	0.6	28	34	173	358	59	0.3	0.9	9	20	0.68	0	0.11	0.12	0.9	0.05	5	0.07
1.7	3.5	24	148	101	333	83	0.3	1.5	13	29	1.03	0	0.17	0.18	1.4	0.05	35	0.09
1.4	2.8	20	116	79	263	65	0.3	1.2	10	18	0.86	0	0.14	0.14	1.1	0.04	8	0.07
2	1.1	39	81	72	326	71	0.3	1.2	9	23	0.61	0	0.16	0.18	1.3	0.03	8	0.11
—	—	95	150	—	750	—	—	1.8	—	0	—	0	—	—	—	—	—	—
1	2.4	0	36	214	224	289	1	2.4	90	0	0.75	0	0.15	0.05	0.2	0.09	30	0.01
1.2	0.7	18	69	62	161	58	0.3	0.9	10	13	0.32	0	0.13	0.13	0.9	0.02	6	0.07
1.6	3.3	22	114	87	266	69	0.3	1.4	10	23	1.03	0	0.16	0.17	1.3	0.02	29	0.09
1.3	2.6	19	90	68	210	54	0.3	1.1	7	13	0.81	0	0.13	0.14	1	0.02	5	0.07
1	2.1	26	31	40	154	87	0.2	1.1	9	331	0.59	1	0.1	0.11	0.8	0.03	6	0.05
0.7	1.8	2	4	20	158	27	0.1	0.2	4	22	0.57	0	0.08	0.1	0.7	0.01	18	0.01
0.7	1.7	2	4	60	158	27	0.1	0.2	5	20	0.24	0	0.06	0.09	0.6	0.01	15	0
0.9	2.1	4	6	50	142	30	0.1	0.5	5	7	0.53	0	0.1	0.12	0.8	0.02	19	0.01
0.9	1.9	2	6	80	142	30	0.1	0.5	4	6	0.5	0	0.08	0.11	0.7	0.01	3	0.01
0.7	1.7	6	13	71	178	60	0.2	1	11	18	0.62	0	0.09	0.11	0.9	0.04	12	0.01
0.8	1.7	3	13	97	179	60	0.2	1	7	16	0.42	0	0.07	0.1	0.8	0.02	7	0.01
2.1	0.6	31	14	150	210	66	0.5	1.1	26	14	0.68	0	0.09	0.11	1.3	0.08	7	0.06
1.7	3.6	19	107	162	335	181	1.6	2.4	44	143	1.31	4	0.19	0.25	2.3	0.18	30	0.08
1.4	2.8	16	84	128	265	143	1.2	1.9	35	108	1.04	4	0.15	0.2	1.8	0.14	23	0.06
2.3	1.4	21	89	110	283	119	0.7	0.9	31	14	0.7	0	0.08	0.09	1.2	0.07	9	0.07
2.6	5.7	37	41	44	169	69	0.3	1.2	8	22	0.84	1	0.12	0.12	0.9	0.03	9	0.07
0	0.1	0	27	27	7	136	0.1	1.3	13	2	0.32	26	0.02	0.07	0.4	0.04	4	0
0	0.1	0	5	68	2	278	0.7	1.4	9	0	0.09	3	0.06	0.23	3.5	0.07	14	0
0	0.1	0	2	36	1	130	0.3	0.4	4	0	0.04	1	0.04	0.16	1.4	0.03	7	0
0	0.1	0	4	81	3	289	0.6	1	8	0	0.09	2	0.07	0.34	3.1	0.07	14	0
0	0.1	0	4	81	3	289	0.6	1	8	0	0.09	2	0.07	0.33	3.1	0.07	13	0
3	6.4	14	54	103	121	180	0.4	0.8	8	10	0.92	1	0.07	0.22	1.6	0.05	8	0.06
2.3	2	1	34	—	23	—	—	8.2	—	2	—	1	—	—	—	—	—	0
0	0	0	0	3	0	11	0	0	0	0	0	0	0	0	0.1	0	1	0

Food Item	Qty	Meas	Wgt (g)	Wtr (g)	Cals	Prot	Carb (g)	Fib (g)	Fat (g)	SatF (g)
Mushroom, oyster, dried	0.5	cup	72	5	262	20	39	7.5	3	0.4
Mushroom, raw, sliced	0.5	cup	34	31	8	1	2	0.4	0	0
Mushroom, shiitake, cooked pieces	0.5	cup	72	60	40	1	10	1.5	0	0
Mushroom, shiitake, dried	0.5	cup	72	9	241	19	37	9.1	2	0.3
Mushroom, whole, pickled	1	each	12	11	3	0	1	0.1	0	0
Mushrooms, canned, drained	0.5	cup	78	71	19	1	4	1.9	0	0
Mushrooms, whole, cooked, drained	10	each	120	109	32	3	6	2.6	1	0.1
Mushrooms, whole, raw	5	each	90	83	22	2	4	1.1	0	0
Mustard greens, cooked, drained, no added salt	0.5	cup	70	66	10	2	1	1.4	0	0
Mustard greens, frozen, cooked, drained	0.5	cup	75	70	14	2	2	2.1	0	0
Mustard, Chinese Gai Choy	1	tsp	5	5	1	0	0	—	0	—
Mustard, brown, prepared	1	tsp	5	4	5	0	0	0.1	0	0
Mustard, yellow, prepared	1	tsp	5	4	4	0	0	0.1	0	0
Nacho chips, w/cinnamon & sugar	7	piece	109	1	592	7	63	3.3	36	18.2
Nachos, w/cheese	7	piece	113	46	346	9	36	—	19	7.8
Nectarine, fresh	1	each	136	117	67	1	16	2.2	1	0.1
Noodle roni, prepared	0.5	cup	82	55	123	4	20	1.8	3	0.6
Noodles, Japanese soba, buckwheat, cooked	0.5	cup	57	42	56	3	12	0.6	0	0
Noodles, Japanese somen, wheat, cooked	0.5	cup	88	60	115	4	24	1.4	0	0
Noodles, Ramen, cooked	5	cup	114	93	78	3	15	1.4	1	0.2
Noodles, buckwheat, dry, cooked	0.5	cup	70	50	81	2	17	0.1	0	—
Noodles, chow mein, dry	0.25	cup	11	0	59	1	6	0.4	3	0.5
Noodles, egg, enriched, cooked	0.5	cup	80	55	106	4	20	0.9	1	0.2
Noodles, mug-o-lunch, prepared	1	each	198	132	295	9	48	4.2	7	1.5
Noodles, rice, cooked	0.5	cup	80	65	62	0	15	0.1	0	0
Noodles, rice, freshly made	0.5	cup	70	36	142	2	32	0.4	0	—
Oat bran, cooked	1	Tbs	14	12	5	0	2	0.4	0	0
Oat bran, dry	2	Tbs	12	1	29	2	8	1.8	1	0.2
Oats, rolled, baked value	1	cup	80	7	307	13	54	8.5	5	0.9
Oats, rolled, dry	0.25	cup	20	2	78	3	14	2.2	1	0.2
Oats, whole grain	0.5	cup	78	6	303	13	52	8.3	5	1
Oil, almond	1	Tbs	14	0	120	0	0	0	14	1.1
Oil, butter	1	Tbs	13	0	112	0	0	0	13	7.9
Oil, canola	1	Tbs	14	0	120	0	0	0	14	1
Oil, cocoa butter	1	Tbs	14	0	120	0	0	0	14	8.1
Oil, coconut	1	Tbs	14	0	117	0	0	0	14	11.8
Oil, cod liver	1	Tbs	14	0	123	0	0	0	14	3.1
Oil, corn	1	Tbs	14	0	120	0	0	0	14	1.7
Oil, cottonseed	1	Tbs	14	0	120	0	0	0	14	3.5
Oil, grapeseed	1	Tbs	14	0	120	0	0	0	14	1.3
Oil, herring	1	Tbs	14	0	123	0	0	0	14	2.9
Oil, olive	1	Tbs	14	0	119	0	0	0	14	1.8
Oil, palm	1	Tbs	14	0	120	0	0	0	14	6.7
Oil, palm kernel	1	Tbs	14	0	117	0	0	0	14	11.1
Oil, peanut	1	Tbs	14	0	119	0	0	0	14	2.3
Oil, safflower	1	Tbs	14	0	120	0	0	0	14	1.2
Oil, salmon	1	Tbs	14	0	123	0	0	0	14	2.7
Oil, sardine	1	Tbs	14	0	123	0	0	0	14	4.1
Oil, sesame	1	Tbs	14	0	120	0	0	0	14	1.9
Oil, soybean & cottonseed	1	Tbs	14	0	120	0	0	0	14	2.4
Oil, soybean (Crisco/Wesson)	1	Tbs	14	0	120	0	0	0	14	2
Oil, sunflower (Wesson Sunlite)	1	Tbs	14	0	120	0	0	0	14	1.4
Oil, walnut	1	Tbs	14	0	120	0	0	0	14	1.2
Oil, wheat germ	1	Tbs	14	0	120	0	0	0	14	2.6
Okra pods, frozen, cooked, drained	0.5	cup	92	84	26	2	5	2.6	0	0.1
Okra, batter-dipped, fried	0.5	cup	46	32	88	1	6	1	7	1.1
Okra, fresh slices, cooked, drained	0.5	cup	80	72	26	2	6	2	0	0
Olive, green, no pits	10	each	39	30	45	1	1	0.4	5	0.5
Olive, green, stuffed	5	each	20	16	21	0	0	0.2	2	0.2
Olive, ripe, jumbo/super colossal	1	each	15	13	12	0	1	0.4	1	0.1
Olive, ripe, large, no pits	10	each	45	36	52	0	3	1.4	5	0.6
Olives, Calamata	1	oz.	28	16	80	0	3	0.2	7	0.9
Onion rings, breaded, fried, serving	8.5	piece	83	31	276	4	31	—	16	7
Onion rings, heated from frozen	2	each	20	6	81	1	8	0.3	5	1.7
Onion slices, cooked	2	piece	24	21	11	0	2	0.3	0	0

MonoF	PolyF	Choles	Calc	Phos	Sod	Pot	Zn	Iron	Magn	VitA	VitE	VitC	Thia	Ribo	Nia	B6	Fola	B12
(g)	(g)	(mg)	(mg)	(mg)	(mg)	(mg)	(mg)	(mg)	(mg)	(µg RE)	(µg α-TE)	(mg)	(mg)	(mg)	(mg)	(mg)	(µg)	(µg)
0.7	1.9	1	7	—	70	—	—	6.8	—	1	—	5	—	—	—	—	—	0
0	0.1	0	2	35	1	126	0.2	0.4	3	0	0.04	1	0.04	0.15	1.4	0.03	7	0
0	0	0	2	21	3	85	1	0.3	10	0	0.09	0	0.03	0.12	1.1	0.12	15	0
0.1	1.5	1	28	—	61	—	—	11.5	—	1	—	1	—	—	—	—	—	0
0	0	0	1	10	24	36	0.1	0.1	1	0	0.01	0	0.01	0.04	0.4	0.01	1	0
0	0.1	0	9	52	332	101	0.6	0.6	12	0	0.09	0	0.07	0.02	1.2	0.05	10	0
0	0.2	0	7	104	2	427	1	2.1	14	0	0.14	5	0.09	0.36	5.4	0.11	22	0
0	0.2	0	4	94	4	333	0.7	1.1	9	0	0.11	3	0.09	0.4	3.7	0.09	19	0
0.1	0	0	52	29	11	141	0.1	0.5	10	212	1.41	18	0.03	0.04	0.3	0.07	51	0
0.1	0	0	76	18	19	104	0.2	0.8	10	335	1.31	10	0.03	0.04	0.2	0.08	52	0
—	—	—	—	—	—	—	—	—	—	—	—	—	—	—	—	—	—	0
0	0.2	0	6	7	65	6	—	0.1	—	0	—	0	0	0	0	—	—	—
0.2	0	0	4	4	65	7	0	0.1	2	0	0.09	0	0	0	0	0	0	0
11.9	4.1	39	85	33	439	78	0.6	2.9	20	11	—	8	0.18	0.45	3.9	0.17	8	1.72
8	2.2	18	272	276	816	172	1.8	1.3	55	92	—	1	0.19	0.37	1.5	0.2	10	0.82
0.2	0.3	0	7	22	0	288	0.1	0.2	11	101	1.21	7	0.02	0.06	1.4	0.03	5	0
1.2	0.9	26	10	56	163	23	0.5	1.3	15	30	0.34	0	0.15	0.07	1.2	0.03	6	0.07
0	0	0	2	14	34	20	0.1	0.3	5	0	—	0	0.05	0.02	0.3	0.02	4	0
0	0.1	0	7	24	142	26	0.2	0.5	2	0	0.01	0	0.02	0.03	0.1	0.01	2	0
0.2	0.2	19	10	41	675	25	0.4	0.9	12	102	0.04	0	0.11	0.05	0.9	0.03	5	0.05
—	—	—	7	56	—	—	—	0.7	—	—	—	0	0.04	0.02	0.3	—	—	—
0.9	2	0	2	18	49	14	0.2	0.5	6	1	0.02	0	0.06	0.05	0.7	0.01	10	0
0.3	0.3	26	10	55	6	22	0.5	1.3	15	5	0.04	0	0.15	0.07	1.2	0.03	51	0.07
2.8	2.2	63	25	133	391	56	1.2	3	37	72	0.82	0	0.36	0.16	2.8	0.07	14	0.18
0	0	0	5	5	3	1	0.1	0.3	1	0	0.02	0	0.02	0	0	0.01	0	0
—	—	—	7	26	—	—	—	1.7	—	—	—	0	0.03	0.01	0.9	—	—	—
0	0	0	1	16	0	13	0.1	0.1	5	0	0.2	0	0.14	0.03	0.1	0.02	6	0
0.3	0.3	0	7	86	0	66	0.4	3.4	118	8	0.91	0	0.47	0.1	0.6	0.09	18	0
1.6	1.8	0	42	379	3	280	2.5	0.9	30	2	0.14	0	0.15	0.03	0.2	0.02	6	0
0.4	0.5	0	10	96	1	71	0.6	3.7	138	0	0.55	0	0.6	0.11	0.8	0.09	44	0
1.7	2	0	42	408	2	335	3.1	3.7	138	0	0.55	0	0.6	0.11	0.8	0.09	44	0
9.5	2.4	0	0	0	0	0	0	0	0	0	5.36	0	0	0	0	0	0	0
3.7	0.5	33	0	0	0	1	0	0	0	118	0.36	0	0	0	0	0	0	0
8	4	0	0	0	0	0	0	0	0	0	2.86	0	0	0	0	0	0	0
4.5	0.4	0	0	0	0	0	0	0	0	0	0.24	0	0	0	0	0	0	0
0.8	0.2	0	0	0	0	0	0	0	0	0	0.04	0	0	0	0	0	0	0
6.4	3.1	78	0	0	0	0	0	0	0	4080	2.99	0	0	0	0	0	0	0
3.3	8	0	0	0	0	0	0	0	0	0	2.88	0	0	0	0	0	0	0
2.4	7.1	0	0	0	0	0	0	0	0	0	5.22	0	0	0	0	0	0	0
2.2	9.5	0	0	0	0	0	0	0	0	0	4.36	0	0	0	0	0	0	0
7.7	2.1	104	0	0	0	0	0	0	0	0	1.25	0	0	0	0	0	0	0
10	1.1	0	0	0	0	0	0	0.1	0	0	1.67	0	0	0	0	0	0	0
5	1.3	0	0	0	0	0	0	0	0	0	2.97	0	0	0	0	0	0	0
1.6	0.2	0	0	0	0	0	0	0	0	0	0.52	0	0	0	0	0	0	0
6.2	4.3	0	0	0	0	0	0	0	0	0	1.74	0	0	0	0	0	0	0
1.6	10.2	0	0	0	0	0	0	0	0	0	5.87	0	0	0	0	0	0	0
3.9	5.5	66	0	0	0	0	0	0	0	0	2.6	0	0	0	0	0	0	0
4.6	4.3	97	0	0	0	0	0	0	0	0	1.63	0	0	0	0	0	0	0
5.4	5.7	0	0	0	0	0	0	0	0	0	0.56	0	0	0	0	0	0	0
4	6.6	0	0	0	0	0	0	0	0	0	3.84	0	0	0	0	0	0	0
3.2	7.9	0	0	0	0	0	0	0	0	0	2.48	0	0	0	0	0	0	0
2.7	9	0	0	0	0	0	0	0	0	0	6.9	0	0	0	0	0	0	0
3.1	8.6	0	0	0	0	0	0	0	0	0	0.44	0	0	0	0	0	0	0
2	8.4	0	0	0	0	0	0	0	0	0	26.1	0	0	0	0	0	0	0
0	0.1	0	88	42	3	215	0.6	0.6	47	47	0.64	11	0.09	0.11	0.7	0.04	134	0
0	3.6	8	52	53	68	107	0.2	0.4	18	21	1.54	5	0.07	0.05	0.4	0.06	19	0.04
1.7	0	0	50	45	4	258	0.4	0.4	46	46	0.55	13	0.11	0.04	0.7	0.15	37	0
3.8	0.3	0	24	7	936	22	0	0.6	9	12	1.17	0	0	0	0	0.01	0	0
1.6	0.2	0	11	3	413	16	0	0.3	4	12	0.54	3	0	0	0	0.01	1	0
0.8	0.1	0	14	0	136	1	0	0.5	1	5	0.46	0	0	0	0	0	0	0
3.6	0.4	0	40	1	392	4	0.1	1.5	2	18	1.35	0	0	0	0	0	0	0
5.7	0.9	0	10	—	462	—	—	0.2	—	2	—	0	—	—	—	—	—	—
6.6	0.7	14	73	86	430	129	0.3	0.8	16	1	0.33	1	0.08	0.1	0.9	0.06	55	0.12
2.2	1	0	6	16	75	26	0.1	0.3	4	5	0.14	0	0.06	0.03	0.7	0.02	13	0
0	0	0	5	8	1	40	0	0.1	3	0	0.03	1	0.01	0.01	0	0.03	4	0

Food Item	Qty	Meas	Wgt (g)	Wtr (g)	Cals	Prot	Carb (g)	Fib (g)	Fat (g)	SatF (g)
Onion slices, raw	1	piece	14	13	5	0	1	0.3	0	0
Onion, canned w/liquid	1	each	63	59	12	1	3	0.8	0	0
Onion, chopped, frozen, cooked	0.5	cup	105	97	29	1	7	1.9	0	0
Onion, chopped, steamed	0.5	cup	105	94	40	1	9	1.9	0	0
Onion, chopped, stir fried	0.5	cup	105	94	40	1	9	1.9	0	0
Onion, creamed	0.5	cup	114	94	100	3	11	1.3	5	1.7
Onion, pearl, cooked, whole	3	each	45	39	20	1	5	0.7	0	0
Onion, raw, chopped	0.5	cup	80	72	30	1	7	1.4	0	0
Onion, spring/green, chopped	0.5	cup	50	45	16	1	4	1.3	0	0
Onion, spring/green, top only	0.5	cup	50	46	17	1	3	1.2	0	0.1
Onion, whole, frozen, cooked	1	each	63	58	18	0	4	0.9	0	0
Onions, cooked, drained	0.5	cup	105	92	46	1	11	1.5	0	0
Orange & apricot juice drink, canned	1	cup	250	217	128	1	32	0.2	0	0
Orange Julius	1	cup	215	183	133	0	33	0.2	0	0.1
Orange breakfast drink, frozen, prepared	1	cup	248	216	122	0	30	0.2	0	0.1
Orange breakfast drink, prepared w/water	1	cup	248	218	114	0	29	0	0	0
Orange drink, Sunny Delight	1	cup	249	216	127	0	32	0.2	0	0
Orange drink, carbonated	1	cup	248	217	119	0	30	0	0	0
Orange drink, frozen, prepared	1	cup	248	218	112	0	28	0	0	0
Orange peel, candied	1.5	oz.	43	7	134	0	34	—	0	0
Orange peel, fresh, grated	1	Tbs	6	4	6	0	2	0.6	0	0
Orange sections, fresh, cup measure	0.5	cup	90	78	42	1	11	2.2	0	0
Orange, fresh	1	each	131	114	62	1	16	3.1	0	0
Orange, mandarin, canned	0.5	cup	126	113	47	1	12	0.9	0	0
Orange-grapefruit juice, canned	0.5	cup	124	109	53	1	13	0.1	0	0
Oriental snack mix	1	oz.	28	1	56	5	15	3.7	7	1.1
Oysters Rockefeller	0.5	cup	112	84	131	8	11	1.8	6	2.4
Palm heart, cooked slices	0.5	cup	73	51	75	2	19	1.1	0	0.1
Pancake mix, buckwheat, prepared	1	each	27	14	56	2	8	0.6	2	0.5
Pancake, Chinese	1	each	28	14	58	1	13	0.2	0	0
Pancake, French/crepe	1	each	102	57	239	9	22	0.6	12	4
Pancake, Indian	1	each	29	16	52	2	10	0.7	0	0.2
Pancake, blueberry, recipe	2	each	76	40	169	5	22	0.9	7	1.5
Pancake, buttermilk, recipe	2	each	76	40	173	5	22	0.6	7	1.4
Pancake, cornmeal	1	each	21	12	43	1	7	0.3	1	0.3
Pancake, frozen, ready to eat, 6 inch	2	each	146	66	334	8	64	2.6	5	1.1
Pancake, plain, mix, prepared	1	each	27	14	52	1	10	0.4	1	0.1
Pancake, plain, recipe	1	each	27	14	61	2	8	0.4	3	0.6
Pancakes w/butter & syrup, Fast Food	3	each	232	101	582	9	105	2	14	2.5
Pannetone-Italian sweetbread	1	piece	27	8	86	2	15	0.7	2	1.2
Papaya nectar, canned	1	cup	250	213	143	0	36	1.5	0	0.1
Papaya, fresh slices	0.5	cup	70	62	27	0	7	1.3	0	0
Papaya, whole, fresh	1	each	304	270	119	2	30	5.5	0	0.1
Parsnip, cooked from raw, drained	0.5	cup	78	61	63	1	15	3.1	0	0
Passion fruit, purple, fresh	1	each	18	13	18	0	4	1.9	0	0
Pasta, spaghetti, whole wheat, cooked	0.5	cup	70	47	87	4	19	3.2	0	0
Pasta/Noodle, spaghetti, spinach, cooked	0.5	cup	70	48	91	3	18	2.4	0	0.1
Pasta/Noodles, cellophane, cooked	0.5	cup	95	75	80	0	20	0.1	0	0.1
Pasta/Noodles, egg, fried	0.5	cup	84	63	129	2	10	0.4	10	1.7
Pasta/Noodles, egg, spinach, cooked	0.5	cup	80	55	106	4	19	1.8	1	0.3
Pasta/Noodles, fresh, cooked	2	oz.	57	39	74	3	14	1	1	0.1
Pasta/Noodles, homemade w/egg, cooked	0.5	cup	80	55	104	4	19	3.1	1	0.3
Pasta/Noodles, homemade, no egg, cooked	2	oz.	57	39	70	2	14	0.9	1	0.1
Pasta/Noodles, jumbo shells, enriched, cooked	2.5	oz.	70	46	99	3	20	0.9	0	0.1
Pasta/Noodles, lasagna cuts, cooked	0.5	cup	70	46	99	3	20	0.9	0	0.1
Pasta/Noodles, linguini, cooked	0.5	cup	70	46	99	3	20	1.2	0	0.1
Pasta/Noodles, macaroni, enriched, cooked	1	cup	140	92	197	7	40	1.8	1	0.1
Pasta/Noodles, macaroni, vegetable, cooked	0.5	cup	67	46	86	3	18	2.9	0	0
Pasta/Noodles, rotini, enriched, cooked	0.5	cup	70	46	99	3	20	0.9	0	0.1
Pasta/Noodles, small shells, enriched, cooked	0.5	cup	58	38	81	3	16	0.7	0	0.1
Pasta/Noodles, spaghetti, cooked	0.5	cup	70	46	99	3	20	1.2	0	0.1
Pasta/Noodles, spaghetti, cooked w/salt	0.5	cup	70	46	99	3	20	1.2	0	0.1
Pasta/Noodles, spinach, fresh, cooked	2	oz.	57	39	74	3	14	1.3	1	0.1
Pasta/Noodles, spirals, enriched, cooked	0.5	cup	67	44	94	3	19	0.9	0	0.1
Pasta/Noodles, vermicelli, cooked	0.5	cup	70	46	99	3	20	1.2	0	0.1

MonoF (g)	PolyF (g)	Choles (mg)	Calc (mg)	Phos (mg)	Sod (mg)	Pot (mg)	Zn (mg)	Iron (mg)	Magn (mg)	VitA (µg RE)	VitE (µg α-TE)	VitC (mg)	Thia (mg)	Ribo (mg)	Nia (mg)	B6 (mg)	Fola (µg)	B12 (µg)
0	0	0	3	5	0	22	0	0	1	0	0.02	1	0.01	0	0	0.02	3	0
0	0	0	28	18	234	70	0.2	0.1	4	0	0.05	3	0.02	0	0	0.09	6	0
0	0	0	17	20	13	113	0.1	0.3	6	3	0.2	3	0.02	0.03	0.1	0.07	14	0
0	0.1	0	21	35	3	165	0.2	0.2	10	0	0.33	5	0.04	0.02	0.1	0.12	16	0
0	0.1	0	21	35	3	165	0.2	0.2	10	0	0.33	5	0.04	0.02	0.1	0.12	16	0
2.2	1.3	5	65	64	334	177	0.3	0.3	13	58	0.66	4	0.05	0.09	0.2	0.11	13	0.14
0	0	0	10	16	105	74	0.1	0.1	5	0	0.06	2	0.02	0.01	0.1	0.06	7	0
0	0	0	16	26	2	126	0.2	0.2	8	0	0.1	5	0.03	0.02	0.1	0.09	15	0
0	0	0	36	18	8	138	0.2	0.7	10	20	0.06	9	0.03	0.04	0.3	0.03	32	0
0	0.1	0	28	20	4	130	0.1	1.1	10	20	0.15	26	0.04	0.05	0.3	0	40	0
0	0	0	17	1	5	64	0.1	0.2	5	1	0.08	3	0.01	0.01	0.1	0.04	8	0
0	0.1	0	23	37	3	174	0.2	0.3	12	0	0.14	5	0.04	0.02	0.2	0.14	16	0
0.1	0.1	0	12	20	5	200	0.1	0.2	10	145	0	50	0.05	0.02	0.5	0.07	14	0
0	0	0	32	—	8	145	—	0.1	—	0	—	29	0.07	0.07	—	0.04	—	0
0.2	0.1	0	82	55	22	308	0.1	0.2	2	0	0.74	172	0.3	0.09	0	0	56	0
0	0	0	62	37	12	50	0.1	0.2	2	551	0	121	0	0.04	0	0	143	0
0	0	0	15	2	40	45	0.2	0.7	5	5	0	85	0.02	0.01	0.1	0.02	5	0
0	0	0	12	2	30	5	0.2	0.1	2	0	0	0	0	0	0	0	0	0
0	0	0	290	82	25	335	0.1	0.2	27	2	0.01	137	0.26	2.58	0.6	0.18	80	0
—	—	0	0	0	0	0	—	0	—	0	—	0	0	0	0	—	—	—
0	0	0	10	1	0	13	0	0	1	3	0.01	8	0.01	0	0.1	0.01	2	0
0	0	0	36	13	0	163	0.1	0.1	9	19	0.22	48	0.08	0.04	0.3	0.05	27	0
0	0	0	52	18	0	237	0.1	0.1	13	28	0.31	70	0.11	0.05	0.4	0.08	40	0
0	0	0	14	13	6	168	0.6	0.3	14	107	0.63	43	0.1	0.04	0.6	0.05	6	0
0	0	0	10	17	4	195	0.1	0.6	12	15	0.09	36	0.07	0.04	0.4	0.03	18	0
2.8	3	0	15	74	117	93	0.8	0.7	34	0	2.39	0	0.09	0.04	0.9	0.02	11	0
2.1	1	39	89	130	445	331	50.2	5.1	62	423	1.05	16	0.19	0.21	1.8	0.12	64	10.6
0	0	0	13	102	10	1318	2.7	1.2	7	5	0.36	5	0.03	0.12	0.6	0.53	15	0
0.5	0.8	18	69	110	144	63	0.3	0.5	15	18	0.56	0	0.05	0.07	0.4	0.04	5	0.09
0	0	0	5	18	1	18	0.2	0.1	4	0	0.02	0	0.01	0.01	0.3	0.03	1	0
4.9	2.4	163	93	145	274	159	0.8	1.6	17	88	1.43	0	0.17	0.37	1.3	0.08	19	0.48
0.1	0.1	1	29	40	59	84	0.3	0.2	10	2	0.06	0	0.04	0.04	0.3	0.04	9	0.08
1.8	3.2	43	157	115	313	105	0.4	1.3	12	39	0.76	2	0.15	0.21	1.2	0.04	27	0.15
1.8	3.4	44	119	106	397	110	0.5	1.3	11	23	1.06	0	0.16	0.22	1.2	0.03	29	0.14
0.5	0.4	9	25	19	42	21	0.1	0.4	4	19	0.21	0	0.05	0.05	0.4	0.02	3	0.03
1.8	1.4	13	90	543	743	107	1	5.1	20	42	0.58	0	0.55	0.68	5.8	0.12	73	0.26
0.2	0.2	3	34	90	170	47	0.1	0.4	5	2	0.23	0	0.06	0.06	0.5	0.02	2	0.05
0.7	1.2	16	59	43	119	36	0.2	0.5	4	15	0.26	0	0.05	0.08	0.4	0.01	10	0.06
4.9	6.1	11	113	525	780	298	0.6	2.1	28	125	1.25	0	0.25	0.27	2	0.09	0	0.28
0.6	0.2	19	16	39	96	53	0.2	0.8	6	22	0.13	0	0.1	0.12	1	0.05	24	0.05
0.1	0.1	0	25	0	12	78	0.4	0.8	8	28	0.05	8	0.02	0.01	0.4	0.02	5	0
0	0	0	17	4	2	180	0	0.1	7	20	0.78	43	0.02	0.02	0.2	0.01	27	0
0.1	0.1	0	73	15	9	781	0.2	0.3	30	85	3.4	188	0.08	0.1	1	0.06	116	0
0.1	0	0	29	54	8	286	0.2	0.5	23	0	0.78	10	0.06	0.04	0.6	0.07	45	0
0	0.1	0	2	12	5	63	0	0.3	5	13	0.2	5	0	0.02	0.3	0.02	3	0
0.1	0.1	0	10	62	2	31	0.6	0.7	21	0	0.04	0	0.08	0.03	0.5	0.06	4	0
0	0.2	0	21	76	10	41	0.8	0.7	43	10	0.01	0	0.07	0.07	1.1	0.07	8	0
0	0	0	7	7	4	2	0.1	0.5	1	0	0.03	0	0.03	0	0	0.01	0	0
2	2.8	4	5	—	71	24	0.3	0.3	—	2	—	0	0.01	0.01	—	0.01	1	0
0.4	0.3	26	15	46	10	30	0.5	0.9	19	11	0.04	0	0.2	0.1	1.2	0.09	51	0.11
0.1	0.2	19	3	36	3	14	0.3	0.6	10	3	0.08	0	0.12	0.08	0.6	0.02	36	0.08
0.4	0.4	33	8	42	66	17	0.4	0.9	11	14	0.17	0	0.14	0.14	1	0.03	34	0.08
0.1	0.3	0	3	23	42	11	0.2	0.6	8	0	0.08	0	0.1	0.08	0.8	0.02	24	0
0.1	0.2	0	5	38	1	22	0.4	1	13	0	0.02	0	0.14	0.07	1.2	0.02	49	0
0.1	0.2	0	5	38	1	22	0.4	1	13	0	0.02	0	0.14	0.07	1.2	0.02	49	0
0.1	0.2	0	5	38	1	22	0.4	1	13	0	0.04	0	0.14	0.07	1.2	0.02	49	0
0.1	0.4	0	10	76	1	43	0.7	2	25	0	0.04	0	0.29	0.14	2.3	0.05	98	0
0	0	0	7	34	4	21	0.3	0.3	13	3	0.03	0	0.08	0.04	0.7	0.02	44	0
0.1	0.2	0	5	38	1	22	0.4	1	13	0	0.02	0	0.14	0.07	1.2	0.02	49	0
0	0.2	0	4	31	1	18	0.3	0.8	10	0	0.02	0	0.12	0.06	1	0.02	40	0
0.1	0.2	0	5	38	1	22	0.4	1	13	0	0.04	0	0.14	0.07	1.2	0.02	49	0
0.1	0.2	0	5	38	70	22	0.4	1	13	0	0.19	0	0.14	0.07	1.2	0.02	49	0
0.2	0.1	19	10	32	3	21	0.4	0.6	14	8	0.12	0	0.1	0.08	0.6	0.06	36	0.08
0.1	0.2	0	5	36	1	21	0.4	0.9	12	0	0.02	0	0.14	0.07	1.1	0.02	47	0
0.1	0.2	0	5	38	1	22	0.4	1	13	0	0.04	0	0.14	0.07	1.2	0.02	49	0

Food Item	Qty	Meas	Wgt (g)	Wtr (g)	Cals	Prot	Carb (g)	Fib (g)	Fat (g)	SatF (g)
Pasta/Noodles, wagon wheels, enriched, cooked	0.5	cup	70	46	99	3	20	0.9	0	0.1
Pasta/Noodles, whole wheat, lasagna cuts, cooked	0.5	cup	70	47	87	4	19	2	0	0.1
Pasta/Noodles, whole wheat, macaroni, cooked	0.5	cup	70	47	87	4	19	2	0	0.1
Pasta/Noodles, whole wheat, rotini, cooked	0.5	cup	70	47	87	4	19	2	0	0.1
Pasta/Noodles, whole wheat, shells, cooked	0.5	cup	70	47	87	4	19	2	0	0.1
Pasta/Noodles, whole wheat, spirals, cooked	0.5	cup	70	47	87	4	19	2	0	0.1
Pasta/Noodles, whole wheat, wagon wheels, cooked	0.5	cup	70	47	87	4	19	2	0	0.1
Pastrami, turkey	2	piece	57	40	80	10	1	0	4	1
Pastry, Chinese	1	oz.	28	13	67	1	13	0.1	1	0.2
Patty tart shell, frozen, baked	1	each	71	5	396	5	32	1.1	27	3.9
Pea pod (snow pea), stir fried	0.5	cup	82	73	35	2	6	2.2	0	0
Pea sprouts, cooked	4	oz.	113	84	134	8	25	4.9	1	0.1
Pea sprouts, raw	0.5	cup	60	37	77	5	17	2.4	0	0.1
Peach crisp, piece, 3x3 in	1	piece	139	104	155	2	27	2	5	0.9
Peach halves, cooked from dry	0.5	cup	129	101	99	2	25	3.5	0	0
Peach halves, dried	10	each	130	41	311	5	80	10.7	1	0.1
Peach nectar, canned	1	cup	249	213	134	1	35	1.5	0	0
Peach nectar, canned, sweetened	1	cup	249	213	134	1	35	1.5	0	0
Peach slices, frozen, sweetened	1	each	284	212	267	2	68	5.1	0	0
Peach turnover	1	each	78	28	261	3	33	1.3	13	3.3
Peach, fresh, whole (2.5in)	1	each	87	76	37	1	10	1.7	0	0
Peach, peeled slices, fresh	0.5	cup	85	74	37	1	9	1.7	0	0
Peaches, canned in heavy syrup	0.5	cup	128	102	95	1	26	1.7	0	0
Peaches, canned in juice	0.5	cup	124	109	55	1	14	1.6	0	0
Peaches, canned in light syrup	0.5	cup	126	106	68	1	18	1.6	0	0
Peanut butter, chunky, salted	2	Tbs	32	0	188	8	7	2.1	16	3.1
Peanut butter, chunky, unsalted	2	Tbs	32	0	188	8	7	2.1	16	3.1
Peanut butter, natural, salted	2	Tbs	32	0	187	8	7	2.1	16	2.2
Peanut butter, natural, unsalted	2	Tbs	32	0	187	8	7	2.1	16	2.2
Peanut butter, smooth, salted	2	Tbs	32	0	190	8	6	1.9	16	3.3
Peanut butter, smooth, unsalted	2	Tbs	32	0	190	8	6	1.9	16	3.3
Peanut, Spanish, raw	0.5	cup	36	2	208	10	6	3.5	18	2.8
Peanuts, Spanish, oil roasted, unsalted	0.25	cup	37	1	213	10	6	3.3	18	2.8
Peanuts, Valencia, oil roasted, unsalted	0.25	cup	36	1	212	10	6	3.2	18	2.8
Peanuts, Virginia, oil roasted, unsalted	0.25	cup	36	1	207	9	7	3.2	17	2.3
Peanuts, dry roasted, unsalted	0.25	cup	36	1	214	9	8	2.9	18	2.5
Peanuts, oil roasted, unsalted	0.25	cup	36	1	209	10	7	2.5	18	2.5
Pear halves canned in water	1	each	77	71	22	0	6	1.2	0	0
Pear halves, dried	10	each	175	47	459	3	122	13.1	1	0.1
Pear nectar, canned	1	cup	250	210	150	0	40	1.5	0	0
Pear, Asian, raw	1	each	122	108	51	1	13	4.4	0	0
Pear, candied	1.5	oz.	43	9	129	1	32	—	0	0
Pear, canned in heavy syrup	0.5	cup	128	103	94	0	24	2	0	0
Pear, fresh slices	0.5	cup	82	69	49	0	12	2	0	0
Pear, fresh, Bartlett	1	each	166	139	98	1	25	4	1	0
Pears, canned in juice	0.5	cup	124	107	62	0	16	2	0	0
Pears, canned in light syrup	0.5	cup	126	106	72	0	19	2	0	0
Peas & carrots, frozen, cooked	0.5	cup	80	69	38	2	8	2.5	0	0.1
Peas & carrots, frozen, unheated	0.5	cup	70	59	37	2	8	2.4	0	0.1
Peas, edible pod/snow pea, cooked	0.5	cup	80	71	34	3	6	2.2	0	0
Peas, blackeyed/cowpea, dry	0.5	cup	84	10	281	20	50	8.8	1	0.3
Peas, blackeyed/cowpea, dry, cooked	0.5	cup	86	60	99	7	18	5.6	0	0.1
Peas, edible pod/snow pea, frozen, cooked	0.5	cup	80	69	42	3	7	2.5	0	0.1
Peas, edible pod/snow pea, raw	0.5	cup	72	64	30	2	5	1.9	0	0
Peas, edible pods/snow peas, steamed	0.5	cup	82	73	35	2	6	2.2	0	0
Peas, green, canned, drained	0.5	cup	85	69	59	4	11	3.5	0	0.1
Peas, green, canned, low sodium	0.5	cup	85	69	59	4	11	3.5	0	0.1
Peas, green, frozen, cooked	0.5	cup	80	64	62	4	11	4.4	0	0
Peas, green, frozen, unheated	0.5	cup	72	58	55	4	10	3.4	0	0
Peas, green, raw	0.5	cup	72	57	59	4	10	3.7	0	0.1
Peas, green, raw, cooked	0.5	cup	80	62	67	4	12	4.4	0	0
Peas, pigeon/red gram, cooked	0.5	cup	84	58	102	6	20	5.6	0	0.1
Peas, split, dry	0.5	cup	98	11	336	24	60	25.1	1	0.2
Peas, split, dry, cooked	0.5	cup	98	68	116	8	21	8.1	0	0.1
Pecan halves, oil roasted, unsalted	15	each	28	1	194	2	5	1.9	20	1.6

MonoF	PolyF	Choles	Calc	Phos	Sod	Pot	Zn	Iron	Magn	VitA	VitE	VitC	Thia	Ribo	Nia	B6	Fola	B12
(g)	(g)	(mg)	(mg)	(mg)	(mg)	(mg)	(mg)	(mg)	(mg)	(µg RE)	(µg α-TE)	(mg)	(mg)	(mg)	(mg)	(mg)	(µg)	(µg)
0.1	0.2	0	5	38	1	22	0.4	1	13	0	0.02	0	0.14	0.07	1.2	0.02	49	0
0.1	0.1	0	10	62	2	31	0.6	0.7	21	0	0.07	0	0.08	0.03	0.5	0.06	4	0
0.1	0.1	0	10	62	2	31	0.6	0.7	21	0	0.07	0	0.08	0.03	0.5	0.06	4	0
0.1	0.1	0	10	62	2	31	0.6	0.7	21	0	0.07	0	0.08	0.03	0.5	0.06	4	0
0.1	0.1	0	10	62	2	31	0.6	0.7	21	0	0.07	0	0.08	0.03	0.5	0.06	4	0
0.1	0.1	0	10	62	2	31	0.6	0.7	21	0	0.07	0	0.08	0.03	0.5	0.06	4	0
0.1	0.1	0	10	62	2	31	0.6	0.7	21	0	0.07	0	0.08	0.03	0.5	0.06	4	0
1.2	0.9	31	5	114	596	148	1.2	0.9	8	0	0.12	0	0.03	0.14	2	0.15	3	0.14
0.4	0.8	0	8	16	3	28	0.2	0.5	6	0	0.25	0	0.05	0	0.4	0.02	1	0
6.3	15.8	0	7	43	180	44	0.4	1.8	11	0	1.69	0	0.23	0.18	2.7	0.01	33	0
0	0.1	0	36	44	3	165	0.2	1.7	20	11	0.32	42	0.11	0.06	0.5	0.12	28	0
0.1	0.3	0	30	27	3	304	0.9	1.9	46	12	0.01	7	0.24	0.32	1.2	0.14	41	0
0	0.2	0	22	99	12	229	0.6	1.4	34	10	0.01	6	0.14	0.09	1.8	0.16	86	0
2.5	1.8	0	20	31	70	189	0.2	0.9	12	108	1.13	5	0.06	0.05	1.1	0.03	6	0.01
0.1	0.2	0	12	49	3	413	0.2	1.7	17	26	0	5	0.01	0.03	2	0.05	0	0
0.4	0.5	0	36	155	9	1294	0.7	5.3	55	281	0	6	0	0.28	5.7	0.09	0	0
0	0	0	12	15	17	100	0.2	0.5	10	65	0.02	13	0.01	0.04	0.7	0.02	3	0
0	0	0	12	15	17	100	0.2	0.5	10	65	0.02	13	0.01	0.04	0.7	0.02	3	0
0.1	0.2	0	9	31	17	369	0.1	1	14	80	2.53	268	0.04	0.1	1.8	0.05	9	0
5.9	3.5	0	6	32	218	89	0.2	1.2	8	14	1.4	2	0.16	0.13	1.7	0.02	5	0
0	0	0	4	10	0	171	0.1	0.1	6	47	0.61	6	0.02	0.04	0.9	0.02	3	0
0	0	0	4	10	0	167	0.1	0.1	6	46	0.6	6	0.01	0.04	0.8	0.02	3	0
0	0.1	0	4	14	8	118	0.1	0.3	6	42	1.14	4	0.01	0.03	0.8	0.02	4	0
0	0	0	7	21	5	159	0.1	0.3	9	47	1.86	4	0.01	0.02	0.7	0.02	4	0
0	0	0	4	14	6	122	0.1	0.5	6	44	1.12	3	0.01	0.03	0.7	0.02	4	0
7.6	4.5	0	13	101	156	239	0.9	0.6	51	0	2.4	0	0.04	0.04	4.4	0.14	29	0
7.6	4.5	0	13	101	5	239	0.9	0.6	51	0	3.2	0	0.04	0.04	4.4	0.14	29	0
7.9	5	0	17	114	80	210	1.1	0.7	56	0	2.59	0	0.04	0.03	4.3	0.13	46	0
7.9	5	0	17	115	2	211	1.1	0.7	56	0	2.4	0	0.14	0.03	4.3	0.13	46	0
7.8	4.4	0	12	118	149	214	0.9	0.6	51	0	3.2	0	0.03	0.03	4.3	0.14	24	0
7.8	4.4	0	12	118	5	214	0.9	0.6	51	0	3.2	0	0.03	0.03	4.3	0.14	24	0
8.1	6.3	0	39	142	8	272	0.8	1.4	69	0	2.7	0	0.25	0.05	5.8	0.13	88	0
8.1	6.2	0	37	142	2	285	0.7	0.8	62	0	2.72	0	0.12	0.03	5.5	0.09	46	0
8.3	6.4	0	19	115	2	220	1.1	0.6	58	0	2.77	0	0.03	0.06	5.2	0.09	45	0
9	5.3	0	31	181	2	233	2.4	0.6	67	0	2.61	0	0.1	0.04	5.3	0.09	45	0
9	5.7	0	20	131	297	240	1.2	0.8	64	0	2.7	0	0.16	0.04	4.9	0.09	53	0
8.8	5.6	0	32	186	2	246	2.4	0.7	67	0	2.67	0	0.09	0.04	5.2	0.09	45	0
0	0	0	3	5	2	41	0.1	0.2	3	0	0.38	1	0.01	0.01	0	0.01	1	0
0.2	0.3	0	60	103	10	933	0.7	3.7	58	1	0	12	0.01	0.25	2.4	0.13	0	0
0	0	0	12	8	10	32	0.2	0.6	8	0	0.25	3	0	0.03	0.3	0.04	3	0
0.1	0.1	0	5	13	0	148	0	0	10	0	0.61	5	0.01	0.01	0.3	0.03	10	0
—	—	0	15	20	3	244	—	0.6	—	3	—	3	0	0.08	0.3	—	—	—
0	0	0	6	9	6	83	0.1	0.3	5	0	0.64	1	0.01	0.03	0.3	0.02	2	0
0.1	0.1	0	9	9	0	103	0.1	0.2	5	2	0.41	3	0.02	0.03	0.1	0.02	6	0
0.1	0.2	0	18	18	0	208	0.2	0.4	10	3	0.83	7	0.03	0.07	0.2	0.03	12	0
0	0	0	11	15	5	119	0.1	0.4	9	1	0.62	2	0.01	0.01	0.2	0.02	1	0
0	0	0	6	9	6	83	0.1	0.4	5	0	0.63	1	0.01	0.02	0.2	0.02	2	0
0	0.2	0	18	39	54	126	0.4	0.8	13	621	0.26	6	0.18	0.05	0.9	0.07	21	0
0	0.2	0	19	42	55	136	0.4	0.8	13	665	0.22	8	0.13	0.06	1	0.07	25	0
0	0.1	0	34	44	3	192	0.3	1.6	21	10	0.31	38	0.1	0.06	0.4	0.12	23	0
0.1	0.5	0	92	354	13	929	2.8	6.9	154	4	0.33	1	0.71	0.19	1.7	0.3	529	0
0	0.2	0	20	133	3	238	1.1	2.2	45	2	0.24	0	0.17	0.05	0.4	0.09	178	0
0	0.1	0	47	46	4	174	0.4	1.9	22	14	0.17	18	0.05	0.1	0.4	0.14	28	0
0	0.1	0	31	38	3	145	0.2	1.5	17	10	0.28	44	0.11	0.06	0.4	0.12	30	0
0	0.1	0	36	44	3	165	0.2	1.7	20	11	0.32	42	0.11	0.06	0.5	0.12	29	0
0	0.1	0	17	57	214	147	0.6	0.8	14	66	0.32	8	0.1	0.07	0.6	0.05	38	0
0	0.1	0	17	57	2	147	0.6	0.8	14	66	0.32	8	0.1	0.07	0.6	0.05	38	0
0	0.1	0	19	72	70	134	0.8	1.3	23	54	0.14	8	0.23	0.08	1.2	0.09	47	0
0	0.1	0	16	58	81	107	0.6	1.1	18	53	0.12	13	0.19	0.07	1.2	0.09	38	0
0	0.1	0	18	78	4	177	0.9	1.1	24	46	0.28	29	0.19	0.1	1.5	0.12	47	0
0	0.1	0	22	94	2	217	1	1.2	31	48	0.31	11	0.21	0.12	1.6	0.17	51	0
0	0.2	0	36	100	4	323	0.8	0.9	39	0	0.08	0	0.12	0.05	0.7	0.04	93	0
0.2	0.5	0	54	361	15	966	3	4.4	113	15	0.3	2	0.72	0.21	2.8	0.17	270	0
0.1	0.2	0	14	97	2	355	1	1.3	35	1	0.38	0	0.19	0.06	0.9	0.05	64	0
12.6	5	0	10	83	0	102	1.6	0.6	37	4	0.94	1	0.09	0.03	0.3	0.05	11	0

Food Item	Qty	Meas	Wgt (g)	Wtr (g)	Cals	Prot	Carb (g)	Fib (g)	Fat (g)	SatF (g)
Pecan, dry roasted, salted	0.25	cup	28	0	187	2	6	2.6	18	1.5
Pecans, dried halves	0.25	cup	27	1	180	2	5	2	18	1.5
Pecans, dried, chopped	0.25	cup	30	1	198	2	5	2.3	20	1.6
Pecans, dried, ground	0.25	cup	24	1	158	2	4	1.8	16	1.3
Pecans, oil roasted, salted	0.25	cup	28	1	188	2	4	1.8	20	1.6
Pecans, oil roasted, unsalted	0.25	cup	28	1	188	2	4	1.8	20	1.6
Pepper, hot green chili, raw, whole	1	each	45	40	18	1	4	0.7	0	0
Pepper, hot jalapeno, pickled	2	each	16	13	8	0	2	0.2	0	0
Pepper, hot red chili, raw pod	1	each	45	40	18	1	4	0.7	0	0
Pepper, hot red chili, raw, chopped	1	Tbs	9	8	4	0	1	0.1	0	0
Pepper, jalapeno, chopped, canned	1	Tbs	8	8	2	0	0	0.2	0	0
Pepper, jalapeno, raw	1	each	45	40	11	0	2	—	0	—
Pepper, pickled	1	each	20	18	8	0	2	0.3	0	0
Pepper, serrano, raw	1	each	45	40	20	—	—	—	—	—
Pepper, sweet green bell, frozen, cooked	0.5	cup	68	64	12	1	3	0.6	0	0
Pepper, sweet green, chopped, cooked	0.5	cup	68	62	19	1	5	0.8	0	0
Pepper, sweet green, chopped, steamed	0.5	cup	68	63	18	1	4	1.2	0	0
Pepper, sweet green, chopped, stir fried	0.5	cup	68	63	18	1	4	1.2	0	0
Pepper, sweet green, raw, chopped	0.5	cup	50	46	14	0	3	0.9	0	0
Pepper, sweet green, raw, whole	1	each	74	68	20	1	5	1.3	0	0
Pepper, sweet green, whole, cooked	1	each	73	67	20	1	5	0.9	0	0
Pepper, sweet red bell, chopped, cooked	0.5	cup	68	62	19	1	5	0.8	0	0
Pepper, sweet red bell, freeze dried	0.5	cup	3	0	10	1	2	0.7	0	0
Pepper, sweet red bell, frozen, cooked	0.5	cup	68	64	12	1	3	1.1	0	0
Pepper, sweet red bell, steamed	0.5	cup	68	63	18	1	4	1.2	0	0
Pepper, sweet red bell, stir fried, no oil	0.5	cup	68	63	18	1	4	1.2	0	0
Pepper, sweet red, raw, chopped	0.5	cup	50	46	14	0	3	1	0	0
Pepper, sweet yellow, raw, large	1	each	186	171	50	2	12	1.7	0	0.1
Pepperoncini, Italian	1	oz.	28	26	6	0	1	0.2	0	0
Peppers, hot green chili, raw, chopped	1	Tbs	9	8	4	0	1	0.1	0	0
Peppers, sweet cherry	1	oz.	28	24	16	1	2	0.5	0	0.1
Persimmon, Japanese, large, raw	1	each	168	135	118	1	31	6	0	0
Persimmon, native, fresh	1	each	25	16	32	0	8	0.4	0	—
Pickle, chow chow	1	Tbs	15	10	18	0	4	0.2	0	0
Pickle, cucumber, dill, low sodium, slices	4	each	30	28	3	0	1	0.4	0	0
Pickle, cucumber, dill, low sodium, whole	1	each	65	61	7	0	1	0.8	0	0
Pickle, cucumber, fresh slices	4	piece	30	24	22	0	5	0.4	0	0
Pickle, dill	1	each	65	60	12	0	3	0.8	0	0
Pickle, dill, slices	10	piece	60	55	11	0	2	0.7	0	0
Pickle, mustard	0.25	cup	61	42	71	1	16	0.9	1	0
Pickle, sour	1	each	35	33	4	0	1	0.4	0	0
Pickle, sour cucumber, slices	10	piece	70	66	8	0	2	0.8	0	0
Pickle, sour, low sodium	1	each	35	33	4	0	1	0.4	0	0
Pickle, sour, low sodium, slices	10	piece	70	66	8	0	2	0.8	0	0
Pickle, sweet butter chips, low sodium	5	each	30	20	35	0	10	0.4	0	0
Pickle, sweet cucumber, low sodium, slices	5	each	30	20	35	0	10	0.4	0	0
Pickle, sweet relish	1	Tbs	15	10	21	0	5	0.3	0	0
Pickle, sweet, medium size	1	each	35	23	41	0	11	0.4	0	0
Pickles, Japanese, tsukemono	0.5	cup	68	62	14	1	3	1.8	0	0
Pie crust, double, recipe, baked	1	each	320	31	1686	20	152	5.4	111	27.6
Pie crust, frozen, baked	1	piece	21	2	108	1	10	0.2	7	2.2
Pie crust, mix, prepared, baked	1	each	180	19	902	12	91	3.2	55	13.9
Pie crust, single, recipe, baked	1	each	180	18	949	12	86	3	62	15.5
Pie filling, apple	1	cup	255	187	258	0	67	2.6	0	0.1
Pie filling, blueberry	1	cup	262	190	272	2	68	3.7	1	0.1
Pie filling, cherry	1	cup	264	184	304	1	77	1.6	1	0.1
Pie filling, cherry, low calorie	1	cup	264	208	211	2	51	1.6	2	0.4
Pie filling, lemon	1	cup	266	49	927	13	185	1.2	18	4.4
Pie filling, pumpkin, canned	0.5	cup	135	96	140	1	36	11.2	0	0.1
Pie, Boston cream, thaw'n serve, Mrs. Smith	1	piece	106	51	240	3	48	0.8	4	1.5
Pie, banana cream, mix, no bake, prepared	1	piece	737	375	1849	25	233	4.6	95	50.9
Pie, blackberry, 1/5th pie, Banquet	1	each	113	47	300	3	45	3	12	5
Pie, cheesecake	1	piece	92	42	295	5	24	0.4	21	9.1
Pie, cheesecake, chocolate	1	piece	128	37	501	8	48	1.9	32	15.5
Pie, cheesecake, no bake mix, prepared	1	piece	103	46	282	6	37	2	13	6.9

MonoF	PolyF	Choles	Calc	Phos	Sod	Pot	Zn	Iron	Magn	VitA	VitE	VitC	Thia	Ribo	Nia	B6	Fola	B12
(g)	(g)	(mg)	(mg)	(mg)	(mg)	(mg)	(mg)	(mg)	(mg)	(µg RE)	(µg α-TE)	(mg)	(mg)	(mg)	(mg)	(mg)	(µg)	(µg)
11.4	4.5	0	10	86	222	105	1.6	0.6	38	4	0.85	1	0.09	0.03	0.3	0.06	12	0
11.4	4.5	0	10	79	0	106	1.5	0.6	35	4	0.84	1	0.23	0.04	0.2	0.05	11	0
12.6	5	0	11	87	0	117	1.6	0.6	38	4	0.92	1	0.25	0.04	0.3	0.06	12	0
10	4	0	9	69	0	93	1.3	0.5	30	3	0.74	0	0.2	0.03	0.2	0.04	9	0
12.2	4.8	0	9	81	208	99	1.5	0.6	36	4	0.91	1	0.08	0.03	0.2	0.05	11	0
12.2	4.8	0	9	81	0	99	1.5	0.6	36	4	0.91	1	0.08	0.03	0.2	0.05	11	0
0	0	0	8	21	3	153	0.1	0.5	11	35	0.31	109	0.04	0.04	0.4	0.12	10	0
0	0	0	3	6	121	43	0	0.1	3	124	0.08	28	0.01	0.01	0.1	0.03	3	0
0	0	0	8	21	3	153	0.1	0.5	11	484	0.31	109	0.04	0.04	0.4	0.12	10	0
0	0	0	2	4	1	32	0	0.1	2	101	0.06	23	0.01	0.01	0.1	0.03	2	0
0	0	0	2	2	142	16	0	0.2	1	14	0.06	1	0	0	0	0.02	1	0
—	—	—	—	—	2	2	—	—	—	30	0.37	53	—	—	—	—	—	0
0	0	0	2	4	26	31	0	0.1	2	46	0.1	21	0.01	0	0.1	0.04	4	0
—	—	—	—	—	2	2	—	—	—	63	—	37	—	—	—	—	—	0
0	0.1	0	5	9	3	49	0	0.4	5	20	0.42	28	0.04	0.02	0.7	0.07	7	0
0	0.1	0	6	12	1	113	0.1	0.3	7	40	0.47	51	0.04	0.02	0.3	0.16	11	0
0	0.1	0	6	13	1	120	0.1	0.3	7	41	0.47	52	0.04	0.02	0.3	0.15	13	0
0	0.1	0	6	13	1	120	0.1	0.3	7	39	0.47	52	0.04	0.02	0.3	0.15	12	0
0	0.1	0	4	10	1	88	0.1	0.2	5	32	0.34	45	0.03	0.02	0.3	0.12	11	0
0	0.1	0	7	14	1	131	0.1	0.3	7	47	0.51	66	0.05	0.02	0.4	0.18	16	0
0	0.1	0	7	13	1	121	0.1	0.3	7	43	0.5	54	0.04	0.02	0.3	0.17	12	0
0	0.1	0	6	12	1	113	0.1	0.3	7	256	0.47	116	0.04	0.02	0.3	0.16	11	0
0	0.1	0	4	10	6	101	0.1	0.3	6	247	0.14	61	0.04	0.04	0.2	0.07	7	0
0	0.1	0	5	9	3	49	0	0.4	5	227	0.42	28	0.04	0.02	0.7	0.07	7	0
0	0.1	0	6	13	1	120	0.1	0.3	7	368	0.47	110	0.04	0.02	0.3	0.15	13	0
0	0.1	0	6	13	1	120	0.1	0.3	7	349	0.47	110	0.04	0.02	0.3	0.15	12	0
0	0.1	0	4	10	1	88	0.1	0.2	5	285	0.34	95	0.03	0.02	0.3	0.12	11	0
0	0.2	0	20	45	4	394	0.3	0.9	22	45	1.28	342	0.05	0.05	1.7	0.31	48	0
0	0.1	0	14	—	598	—	—	0.4	—	12	—	0	—	—	—	—	—	—
0	0	0	2	4	1	32	0	0.1	2	7	0.06	23	0.01	0.01	0.1	0.03	2	0
0	0.3	0	4	—	323	—	—	0.5	—	52	—	12	—	—	—	—	—	—
0.1	0.1	0	13	29	2	270	0.2	0.3	15	365	0.99	13	0.05	0.03	0.2	0.17	13	0
—	—	0	7	6	0	78	—	0.6	—	0	0.25	16	—	—	—	—	2	0
0.1	0	0	4	3	81	31	0	0.2	3	1	0.02	1	0	0	0	0	1	0
0	0	0	0	4	5	7	0	0.1	1	4	0.02	0	0	0	0	0	0	0
0	0.1	0	0	9	12	15	0	0.3	3	10	0.03	1	0	0.01	0	0.01	0	0
0	0	0	10	8	202	60	0	0.5	2	4	0.05	3	0	0.01	0	0	0	0
0	0	0	6	14	833	75	0.1	0.3	7	22	0.1	1	0.01	0.02	0	0.01	1	0
0	0	0	5	13	769	70	0.1	0.3	7	20	0.1	1	0.01	0.02	0	0.01	1	0
0.3	0.1	0	14	14	323	123	0.1	0.9	13	6	0.1	4	0	0.01	0	0.01	3	0
0	0	0	0	5	423	8	0	0.1	1	5	0.06	0	0	0	0	0	0	0
0	0.1	0	0	10	846	16	0	0.3	3	10	0.11	1	0	0.01	0	0.01	0	0
0	0	0	0	5	6	8	0	0.1	1	5	0.02	0	0	0	0	0	0	0
0	0.1	0	0	10	13	16	0	0.3	3	10	0.04	1	0	0.01	0	0.01	0	0
0	0	0	1	4	5	10	0	0.2	1	4	0.05	0	0	0.01	0.1	0	0	0
0	0	0	1	4	5	10	0	0.2	1	4	0.05	0	0	0.01	0	0	0	0
0	0	0	3	2	109	31	0	0.1	1	2	0.02	1	0	0	0	0	0	0
0	0	0	1	4	329	11	0	0.2	1	5	0.06	0	0	0.01	0.1	0	0	0
0	0.1	0	26	25	360	400	0.1	0.2	7	6	0.04	0	0.01	0.02	0.2	0.07	17	0
48.6	29.2	0	32	214	1734	214	1.4	9.2	45	0	17.7	0	1.25	0.89	10.6	0.08	214	0
3.3	0.8	0	4	12	136	23	0.1	0.5	4	0	1.07	0	0.06	0.08	0.5	0.02	8	0
31.1	6.9	0	108	151	1312	112	0.7	3.9	27	0	9.94	0	0.55	0.34	4.3	0.1	22	0
27.4	16.4	0	18	121	976	121	0.8	5.2	25	0	9.94	0	0.7	0.5	6	0.04	121	0
0	0.1	0	10	18	112	115	0.1	0.7	5	3	0	3	0.03	0.03	0.1	0.04	0	0
0.1	0.3	0	13	26	68	97	0.2	1	10	16	2.45	3	0.08	0.13	0.3	0.08	5	0
0.2	0.2	0	29	40	24	277	0.1	0.6	18	55	0.58	10	0.07	0.04	0.4	0.1	11	0
1	0.7	0	24	21	24	201	0.2	0.6	13	53	0.58	4	0.03	0.08	0.4	0.08	11	0
7.3	4.2	349	58	177	216	198	1.1	2.2	16	284	3.31	28	0.18	0.53	1.2	0.15	38	0.67
0	0	0	50	61	281	186	0.4	1.4	22	1120	1.08	5	0.02	0.16	0.5	0.22	47	0
1.7	0.8	4	43	—	240	105	—	0.5	—	7	—	1	0.02	0.12	0.3	0.05	—	—
33.6	5.6	214	538	1230	2137	833	2.4	3.4	88	737	11.8	4	0.75	1.08	5.2	0.26	155	1.55
—	—	5	80	—	430	—	—	1.1	—	0	—	4	0.02	0.03	0.3	—	—	—
7.9	1.5	51	47	86	190	83	0.5	0.6	10	134	1.45	0	0.03	0.18	0.2	0.05	17	0.16
11	3.9	118	72	144	403	188	0.9	2.2	37	347	2.31	0	0.16	0.29	1.3	0.05	14	0.23
4.7	0.8	30	177	241	391	217	0.5	0.5	20	102	1.13	1	0.12	0.27	0.5	0.05	31	0.32

Food Item	Qty	Meas	Wgt (g)	Wtr (g)	Cals	Prot	Carb	Fib (g)	Fat (g)	SatF (g)
Pie, cheesecake, triple chocolate, svg, Weight Watc	1	piece	89	46	200	7	32	1	5	2.5
Pie, cheesecake, w/cherry topping, recipe	1	piece	142	70	408	7	38	0.6	26	14.5
Pie, cherry, fried, turnover	1	each	85	32	269	3	36	2.2	14	2.1
Pie, chocolate cream, individual	1	each	117	47	357	6	44	1.7	19	6.7
Pie, chocolate mousse, mix, no bake, prepared	1	each	760	378	1976	27	225	—	117	62.3
Pie, coconut cream, mix, no bake, prepared	1	each	754	375	2081	21	215	3.8	133	67.3
Pie, fried, apple, turnover	1	each	85	34	266	2	33	1.5	14	6.5
Pie, pecan, individual, Bama pie	1	each	85	14	366	4	45	1.4	20	3.4
Pimento/pimiento, canned	1	Tbs	12	11	3	0	1	0.2	0	0
Pine nut, pignola, dried	1	oz.	28	2	160	7	4	1.3	14	0
Pine nut, pinon, dried	1	oz.	28	2	178	3	5	3	17	2.2
Pineapple chunks, fresh	0.5	cup	78	67	38	0	10	0.9	0	2.7
Pineapple chunks, frozen, sweetened	0.5	cup	122	94	104	0	27	1.4	0	0
Pineapple grapefruit juice drink, canned	1	cup	250	220	118	0	29	0.2	0	0
Pineapple juice, canned, vit C, unsweetened	1	cup	250	214	140	1	34	0.5	0	0
Pineapple orange drink, canned	1	cup	250	217	125	3	30	0.2	0	0
Pineapple pieces in heavy syrup	0.5	cup	128	101	100	0	26	1	0	0
Pineapple rings in heavy syrup	1	each	58	46	45	0	12	0.5	0	0
Pineapple slices, fresh	1	piece	84	73	41	0	10	1	0	0
Pineapple, canned in juice	0.5	cup	125	104	75	1	20	1	0	0
Pineapple, canned in light syrup	0.5	cup	126	108	66	0	17	1	0	0
Pistachio nut, dried, meat	0.25	cup	32	1	185	7	8	3.5	16	2
Pistachio nuts, dry roasted, unsalted	0.25	cup	32	1	194	5	9	3.5	17	2.1
Pitanga, raw	1	each	7	6	2	0	1	0.1	0	—
Pizza Hut, pizza, cheese, pan	2	piece	205	106	495	23	53	3.8	21	9.5
Pizza Hut, pizza, pepperoni, pan	2	piece	211	103	539	22	57	4.1	24	8.1
Pizza Hut, pizza, supreme, pan	2	piece	255	143	581	28	52	5.6	28	11.2
Pizza Hut, pizza, pepperoni, hand-tossed	2	piece	197	100	452	23	55	3.8	15	7.6
Pizza Hut, pizza, pepperoni, personal pan	1	each	256	128	639	27	69	5	28	10
Pizza Hut, pizza, supreme, personal pan	1	each	264	152	582	27	56	4.8	27	9.7
Pizza Hut, pizza, supreme, thin/crispy	2	piece	200	114	443	24	36	3.4	22	8.6
Pizza, deluxe, Tombstone	2	piece	250	131	597	28	54	3.7	30	13.1
Pizza, supreme, light, Tombstone	2	piece	276	—	540	50	60	4	18	7
Plantain chips	32	piece	35	1	180	1	20	2.7	12	10
Plantain slices, cooked	0.5	cup	77	52	89	1	24	1.8	0	0.1
Plantain slices, raw	0.5	cup	74	48	90	1	24	1.7	0	0.1
Plantain, ripe, fried	0.5	cup	84	40	216	1	30	2.2	12	1.8
Plum slices, fresh	0.5	cup	82	70	45	1	11	1.2	1	0
Plum, fresh	1	each	66	56	36	1	9	1	0	0
Plum, purple, canned in light syrup	0.5	cup	126	105	79	0	20	1.3	0	0
Plums, canned in heavy syrup	0.5	cup	129	98	115	0	30	1.3	0	0
Plums, purple, canned in juice	0.5	cup	126	106	73	1	19	1.3	0	0
Pochito, frank w/chili in tortilla	1	each	122	72	268	9	22	3.3	16	5.9
Pokeberry shoots/poke greens, cooked	0.5	cup	78	72	16	2	2	1.2	0	0.1
Pokeberry shoots/poke greens, cooked, drained	0.5	cup	82	77	16	2	3	1.2	0	0.1
Pomegranate, raw (3.5-in. diameter)	1	each	154	125	105	1	26	0.9	0	0.1
Pop Tarts, raspberry frosted	1	each	52	6	210	2	37	1	6	1
Popcorn cake	1	each	10	0	38	1	8	0.3	0	0
Popcorn, air popped, plain	1	cup	8	0	31	1	6	1.2	0	0
Popcorn, caramel corn	1	cup	35	1	152	1	28	1.8	5	1.3
Popcorn, caramel-coated, w/peanuts, Cracker Jacks	1	oz.	28	1	113	2	23	1.1	2	0.3
Popcorn, cheese-flavored	1	cup	11	0	58	1	6	1.1	4	0.7
Popcorn, cooked in oil, salted	1	cup	11	0	55	1	6	1.1	3	0.5
Popcorn, microwave, lowfat, low sodium	1	cup	6	0	24	1	4	0.8	1	0.1
Popcorn, microwave, pop & serve bag	1	each	87	2	435	8	50	8.7	24	4.2
Popcorn, white, air-popped	1	cup	8	0	31	1	6	1.2	0	0
Popover mix, prepared, 2 x 2	1	each	33	18	67	3	10	0.3	1	0.4
Popover, homemade, w/2% milk	1	each	40	22	88	3	11	0.4	3	0.8
Popover, homemade, w/whole milk	1	each	54	29	122	5	15	0.4	5	1.4
Popsicle/ice pop, double stick	1	each	128	102	92	0	24	0	0	0
Pork & beans, w/sweet sauce, canned	0.5	cup	126	89	140	7	27	6.6	2	0.7
Pork & beans, w/tomato sauce, canned	0.5	cup	126	92	124	7	24	6.1	1	0.5
Pork loin, top roast, prime, roasted, lean	1	piece	42	26	82	13	0	0	3	1.1
Pork skins/rinds, BBQ flavor	1	cup	32	1	172	18	1	—	10	3.7
Pork, blade chop, fried, lean & fat	1	each	89	44	304	19	0	0	25	9.1

MonoF (g)	PolyF (g)	Choles (mg)	Calc (mg)	Phos (mg)	Sod (mg)	Pot (mg)	Zn (mg)	Iron (mg)	Magn (mg)	VitA (µg RE)	VitE (µg α-TE)	VitC (mg)	Thia (mg)	Ribo (mg)	Nia (mg)	B6 (mg)	Fola (µg)	B12 (µg)
—	—	10	80	—	200	170	—	1.1	—	0		0	—	—	—	—	—	—
8.3	2.2	121	61	101	288	132	0.6	1.8	10	342	2.27	1	0.04	0.23	0.5	0.06	14	0.24
6.3	4.6	0	19	37	318	55	0.2	1	8	14	0.37	1	0.12	0.09	1.2	0.03	15	0.07
7.5	3.6	58	81	126	277	169	0.8	1.8	34	41	1.31	0	0.18	0.24	1.5	0.05	12	0.21
38.6	6.2	266	585	1755	3496	2166	4.6	8.2	243	768	11.4	4	0.39	1.12	4.5	0.22	198	1.6
49.4	9.2	173	543	1274	2480	1063	2.9	3	128	754	11.3	5	0.21	0.78	1	0.34	113	1.58
5.8	1.2	13	13	37	325	51	0.2	0.9	8	33	0.37	1	0.1	0.08	1	0.03	4	0.08
10.7	5.1	38	19	83	210	104	1	1.4	27	19	1.47	0	0.23	0.15	1.1	0.05	11	0.07
0	0	0	1	2	2	19	0	0.2	1	32	0.08	10	0	0.01	0.1	0.03	1	0
5.4	6	0	7	144	1	170	1.2	2.6	66	1	0.99	1	0.23	0.05	1	0.03	16	0
6.5	7.3	0	2	10	20	178	1.2	0.9	66	1	0.99	1	0.35	0.06	1.2	0.03	16	0
0	0.1	0	5	5	1	88	0.1	0.3	11	2	0.08	12	0.07	0.03	0.3	0.07	8	0
0	0	0	11	5	2	123	0.1	0.5	12	4	0.12	10	0.12	0.04	0.4	0.09	13	0
0	0.1	0	18	15	35	153	0.2	0.8	15	10	0	115	0.08	0.04	0.7	0.1	26	0
0	0.1	0	42	20	2	335	0.3	0.6	32	1	0.05	60	0.14	0.06	0.6	0.24	58	0
0	0	0	12	10	8	115	0.2	0.7	15	133	0	56	0.08	0.05	0.5	0.12	27	0
0	0.1	0	18	9	1	133	0.2	0.5	20	1	0.13	9	0.12	0.03	0.4	0.09	6	0
0	0	0	8	4	1	60	0.1	0.2	9	1	0.06	4	0.05	0.02	0.2	0.04	3	0
0	0.1	0	6	6	1	95	0.1	0.3	12	2	0.08	13	0.08	0.03	0.4	0.07	9	0
0	0	0	18	8	1	153	0.1	0.4	18	5	0.12	12	0.12	0.02	0.4	0.09	6	0
0	0	0	18	9	1	132	0.2	0.5	20	1	0.13	9	0.12	0.03	0.4	0.09	6	0
10.5	2.3	0	43	161	2	350	0.4	2.2	51	7	1.67	2	0.26	0.06	0.3	0.08	19	0
11.4	2.6	0	22	152	2	310	0.4	1	42	8	1.67	2	0.14	0.08	0.5	0.08	19	0
—	—	0	1	1	0	7	—	0	1	10	—	2	0	0	0	—	—	0
6.4	3.2	48	273	—	951	320	4.1	2.8	60	200	—	7	0.57	0.61	5.2	0.17	—	—
10.1	3.8	49	209	—	1156	405	4.2	3.2	56	193	—	8	0.63	0.49	5.4	0.16	0	—
11.2	3.9	56	219	—	1428	580	5.6	4.3	76	182	—	10	0.8	0.78	6	0.31	—	—
—	—	46	192	—	1307	578	5.7	3	80	177	—	12	0.68	0.53	7.2	—	—	—
11.8	4.5	55	251	—	1344	408	3.8	4	60	234	—	10	0.56	0.66	8.2	0.2	—	—
11.9	4.5	53	223	—	1419	487	3.8	4.2	60	194	—	11	0.59	0.66	8	0.32	—	—
—	—	54	205	—	1371	544	4.7	3.1	68	170	—	10	0.6	0.49	5.4	—	—	—
—	—	56	466	—	1194	—	—	2.7	—	187	—	17	—	—	—	—	—	—
—	—	40	800	—	1420	—	—	3.6	—	400	—	12	—	—	—	—	—	—
0.7	0.2	0	6	19	2	185	0.3	0.4	26	3	1.87	2	0.03	0.01	0.2	0.09	5	0
0	0	0	2	22	4	358	0.1	0.4	25	70	0.11	8	0.04	0.04	0.6	0.18	20	0
0	0.1	0	2	25	3	369	0.1	0.4	27	84	0.2	14	0.04	0.04	0.5	0.22	16	0
2.7	6.6	0	3	32	4	427	0.1	0.6	35	81	0.96	12	0.04	0.05	0.6	0.26	10	0
0.3	0.1	0	3	8	0	142	0.1	0.1	6	26	0.5	8	0.04	0.08	0.4	0.07	2	0
0.3	0.1	0	3	7	0	114	0.1	0.1	5	21	0.4	6	0.03	0.06	0.3	0.05	1	0
0.1	0	0	11	16	25	117	0.1	1.1	6	33	0.88	1	0.02	0.05	0.4	0.03	3	0
0.1	0	0	12	17	24	117	0.1	1.1	6	34	0.9	1	0.02	0.05	0.4	0.04	3	0
0	0	0	13	19	1	194	0.1	0.4	10	127	0.88	4	0.03	0.07	0.6	0.03	3	0
7.3	1.8	30	86	211	728	279	2	2.4	46	20	0.54	10	0.13	0.12	1.7	0.18	16	0.5
0	0.1	0	41	26	14	143	0.1	0.9	11	674	0.66	64	0.05	0.19	0.9	0.09	7	0
0	0.1	0	44	27	15	152	0.2	1	12	718	0.7	68	0.06	0.21	0.9	0.09	7	0
0.1	0.1	0	5	12	5	399	0.2	0.5	5	0	0.85	9	0.05	0.05	0.5	0.16	3	0
—	—	0	0	40	210	—	0.6	1.8	8	150	—	0	0.15	0.17	2	0.2	40	—
0.1	0.1	0	1	28	29	33	0.4	0.2	16	1	0.01	0	0.01	0.02	0.6	0.02	2	0
0.1	0.2	0	1	24	0	24	0.3	0.2	10	2	0.01	0	0.02	0.02	0.2	0.02	2	0
1	1.6	2	15	29	72	38	0.2	0.6	12	4	0.42	0	0.02	0.02	0.8	0.01	1	0
0.8	0.9	0	19	36	84	101	0.4	1.1	23	2	0.42	0	0.01	0.04	0.6	0.05	5	0
1.1	1.7	1	12	40	98	29	0.2	0.2	10	5	0.01	0	0.01	0.03	0.2	0.03	1	0.06
0.9	1.5	0	1	28	97	25	0.3	0.3	12	2	0.01	0	0.02	0.02	0.2	0.02	2	0
0.2	0.3	0	1	15	28	14	0.2	0.1	9	1	0.06	0	0.02	0.01	0.1	0.01	1	0
7.1	11.7	0	9	218	769	196	2.3	2.4	94	13	0.1	0	0.12	0.12	1.4	0.18	15	0
0.1	0.2	0	1	24	0	24	0.3	0.2	10	0	0.01	0	0.02	0.02	0.2	0.02	2	0
0.6	0.2	37	9	30	143	25	0.2	0.6	5	16	0.36	0	0.05	0.06	0.4	0.02	6	0.08
0.9	1	46	38	56	82	65	0.3	0.8	7	34	0.43	0	0.09	0.15	0.7	0.03	7	0.13
1.3	1.4	64	50	75	110	87	0.4	1	10	37	0.2	0	0.12	0.2	1	0.04	10	0.18
0	0	0	0	0	15	5	0	0	1	0	0	0	0	0	0	0	0	0
0.8	0.2	9	77	133	425	336	1.9	2.1	43	14	0.68	4	0.06	0.08	0.4	0.11	47	0
0.6	0.2	9	71	148	557	380	7.4	4.2	44	15	0.68	4	0.07	0.06	0.6	0.09	28	0
1.4	0.2	33	2	93	19	149	1	0.4	10	1	0.15	0	0.27	0.13	2.2	0.17	4	0.23
4.8	1.1	37	14	70	853	58	0.2	0.3	0	58	—	0	0.03	0.14	1.1	0.05	10	0.04
10.4	2.8	76	27	183	60	295	2.8	0.8	19	3	0.23	1	0.55	0.26	3.5	0.3	4	0.75

Food Item	Qty	Meas	Wgt (g)	Wtr (g)	Cals	Prot	Carb (g)	Fib (g)	Fat (g)	SatF (g)
Pork, chop, blade, fried, lean	1	each	62	37	149	15	0	0	9	3.2
Pork, chop, breaded, baked/broiled, lean	1	each	80	44	184	21	5	0.2	8	2.9
Pork, chop, center loin, fried, lean	1	each	67	38	155	22	0	0	7	2.4
Pork, chop, center loin, fried, lean & fat	1	each	89	47	247	27	0	0	15	5.4
Pork, chop, loin, broiled, lean	1	each	66	40	139	19	0	0	6	2.4
Pork, chop, loin, roasted, lean & fat	1	piece	42	24	104	11	0	0	6	2.3
Pork, chop, smoked/cured, cooked, lean	1	each	67	43	114	17	0	0	5	1.6
Pork, loin, slice, roasted, lean	1	piece	42	26	88	12	0	0	4	1.5
Pork, loin, sparerib, braised, lean	4	oz.	113	67	265	30	0	0	15	5.6
Pork, rib, country style, roasted, lean	4	oz.	113	66	280	30	0	0	17	6
Pork, sausage link, cooked	1	each	13	6	48	3	0	0	4	1.4
Pork, sausage patty, cooked	1	each	27	12	100	5	0	0	8	2.9
Pork, shoulder, braised, lean	4	oz.	113	62	281	37	0	0	14	4.7
Pork, sirloin steak, broiled, lean	4	oz.	113	69	242	32	0	0	12	4.1
Pork, sparerib, braised, lean & fat	4	oz.	113	46	450	33	0	0	34	12.6
Pork, steak/cutlet, breaded, fried	4	oz.	113	56	325	26	10	0.6	20	6.2
Pork, tenderloin, roasted, lean & fat	4	oz.	113	74	196	32	0	0	7	2.4
Pork, tenderloin, tipless, roasted, lean	4	oz.	113	75	186	32	0	0	5	1.9
Potato chips	10	piece	20	0	107	1	11	0.9	7	2.2
Potato chips, BBQ flavor	20	piece	26	0	128	2	14	1.1	8	2.1
Potato chips, cheese flavor	1	cup	20	0	99	2	12	1	5	1.7
Potato chips, light	20	piece	40	0	188	3	27	2.3	8	1.7
Potato chips, light, Pringle, can	1	oz.	28	0	142	2	18	1	7	1.4
Potato chips, no salt added	10	each	20	1	105	1	10	1	7	1.8
Potato chips, rippled	10	piece	30	1	161	2	16	1.4	10	3.3
Potato chips, sour cream & onion	1	oz.	28	1	151	2	15	1.5	10	2.5
Potato pancake, large	1	each	76	36	207	5	22	1.5	12	2.3
Potato pieces, canned, drained	0.5	cup	90	76	54	1	12	2.1	0	0
Potato salad w/mayonnaise & eggs	0.5	cup	125	95	179	3	14	1.6	10	1.8
Potato salad, German	0.5	cup	88	68	79	2	15	1.4	2	0.6
Potato skin, cooked	1	each	34	26	26	1	6	1.1	0	0
Potato skins, chips, Tato Skins	10	piece	20	0	112	1	10	0.7	7	1.9
Potato, Tater Tots, frozen, oven heated	10	each	70	37	155	2	21	2.2	7	3.6
Potato, au gratin, prep from dry mix	0.5	cup	122	97	114	3	16	1.1	5	3.2
Potato, au gratin, recipe, w/margarine	0.5	cup	122	91	162	6	14	2.2	9	4.3
Potato, baked, flesh only, medium size	1	each	122	92	113	2	26	1.8	0	0
Potato, boiled in skin, peeled after, diced	0.5	cup	78	60	68	1	16	1.4	0	0
Potato, boiled, peeled after	1	each	136	105	118	3	27	2.4	0	0
Potato, canned, 1 in diam, drained	2	each	70	59	42	1	10	1.6	0	0
Potato, cottage fries, frozen, oven heated	10	each	50	26	109	2	17	1.6	4	2
Potato, flesh, raw, diced	0.5	cup	75	59	59	2	14	1.2	0	0
Potato, french fries, frozen, oven heated	10	piece	50	18	167	2	20	1.6	9	3
Potato, french fries, frozen, restaurant fried	10	each	50	19	158	2	20	1.6	8	1.9
Potato, french fries, fried in animal & veg oil	10	each	50	19	158	2	20	1.6	8	1.9
Potato, hash browns-fast food serving	1	each	65	39	137	2	15	—	8	3.9
Potato, hashed brown patty, frozen, fried	1	each	66	37	144	2	18	1.3	8	3
Potato, hashed brown w/butter sauce, frozen, cooked	0.5	cup	72	46	129	2	18	2.8	6	2.4
Potato, hashed browns, frozen, cooked	0.5	cup	78	44	170	2	22	1.6	9	3.5
Potato, mashed w/milk & margarine	0.5	cup	105	80	111	2	18	2.1	4	1.1
Potato, mashed w/whole milk	0.5	cup	105	82	81	2	18	2.1	1	0.4
Potato, mashed w/whole milk & butter	0.5	cup	105	80	111	2	18	2.1	4	2.9
Potato, mashed, flakes prep w/whole milk & margarine	0.5	cup	110	84	124	2	16	2.5	6	1.6
Potato, mashed, granules w/whole milk & butter	0.5	cup	105	81	113	2	15	2.3	5	3.2
Potato, microwaved w/skin, flesh only, medium size	1	each	92	68	92	2	21	1.5	0	0
Potato, o'brien, frozen, cooked	0.5	cup	97	60	198	2	21	1.6	13	3.2
Potato, o'brien, recipe	0.5	cup	97	77	79	2	15	1	1	0.8
Potato, peeled, boiled, diced	0.5	cup	78	60	67	1	16	1.4	0	0
Potato, peeled, boiled, whole	1	each	135	105	116	2	27	2.4	0	0
Potato, prepared mix, Twice Baked	0.5	cup	118	54	324	8	33	2.7	18	9
Potato, scalloped, prep from dry mix	0.5	cup	122	97	114	3	16	1.4	5	3.2
Potato, scalloped, recipe w/margarine	0.5	cup	122	99	105	4	13	2.3	5	1.7
Potato, small, whole, frozen, cooked	1	each	70	58	46	1	10	1	0	0
Potato, w/skin, medium size, baked	1	each	122	87	133	3	31	2.9	0	0
Potato, w/skin, medium size, microwaved	1	each	93	67	98	2	22	2.1	0	0
Potato, white, roasted	1	each	93	58	132	3	30	2.7	0	0

MonoF (g)	PolyF (g)	Choles (mg)	Calc (mg)	Phos (mg)	Sod (mg)	Pot (mg)	Zn (mg)	Iron (mg)	Magn (mg)	VitA (µg RE)	VitE (µg α-TE)	VitC (mg)	Thia (mg)	Ribo (mg)	Nia (mg)	B6 (mg)	Fola (µg)	B12 (µg)
3.9	1.2	51	14	137	48	226	2.4	0.7	16	1	0.16	0	0.45	0.22	2.8	0.25	2	0.6
3.7	0.9	57	17	197	333	331	1.8	0.8	22	1	0.36	1	0.68	0.25	4	0.36	5	0.52
3	0.9	62	15	182	58	301	1.6	0.7	21	1	0.17	1	0.83	0.22	4	0.34	4	0.51
6.3	1.7	82	24	231	71	378	2.1	0.8	26	2	0.23	1	1.01	0.27	5	0.42	5	0.65
2.9	0.5	52	11	167	42	289	1.6	0.6	19	1	0.17	0	0.61	0.22	3.5	0.32	4	0.48
2.7	0.5	34	8	102	25	171	1	0.4	11	1	0.11	0	0.42	0.13	2.3	0.22	3	0.3
2.2	0.5	32	7	163	825	196	2	0.7	11	0	0.17	0	0.49	0.15	3.2	0.25	3	0.74
1.8	0.3	34	8	105	24	179	1.1	0.5	12	1	0.11	0	0.43	0.14	2.5	0.23	3	0.31
6.7	1.2	98	28	191	71	391	4.5	1.6	20	2	0.5	1	0.62	0.32	4.6	0.41	3	0.84
7.3	1.2	105	33	251	33	396	4.3	1.5	27	2	0.55	0	0.65	0.39	5.3	0.5	6	0.91
2	0.4	11	4	24	168	47	0.3	0.2	2	0	0.03	0	0.1	0.03	0.6	0.04	0	0.23
4.2	0.8	22	9	50	349	98	0.7	0.3	5	0	0.07	0	0.2	0.07	1.2	0.09	1	0.47
6.6	1.3	129	9	256	116	459	5.6	2.2	25	2	0.3	0	0.68	0.41	6.7	0.46	6	0.8
5	1	96	15	291	82	455	3.1	1.2	35	2	0.3	1	1.17	0.42	5.4	0.68	6	0.9
15.3	3.1	137	53	296	105	363	5.2	2.1	27	3	0.3	0	0.46	0.43	6.2	0.4	5	1.22
7.7	3.7	109	44	233	458	343	3.3	1.7	28	15	0.71	1	0.77	0.4	4.4	0.38	11	0.86
2.8	0.6	90	7	291	62	491	3	1.6	31	2	0.3	0	1.05	0.44	5.3	0.47	7	0.62
2.2	0.5	90	7	294	64	496	3	1.7	32	2	0.3	0	1.07	0.44	5.3	0.48	7	0.62
2	2.4	0	5	33	119	255	0.2	0.3	13	0	0.98	6	0.03	0.04	0.8	0.13	9	0
1.7	4.3	0	13	48	195	328	0.2	0.5	20	6	1.3	9	0.06	0.06	1.2	0.16	22	0
1.5	1.9	1	14	60	159	306	0.2	0.4	15	2	0.98	11	0.03	0.03	1	0.07	0	0
1.9	4.4	0	8	77	197	698	0	0.5	36	0	1.16	10	0.08	0.11	2.8	0.27	11	0
1.7	3.8	0	10	44	121	285	0.2	0.4	18	0	1.42	3	0.05	0.02	1.2	0.22	7	0
1.2	3.6	0	5	31	2	260	0.2	0.2	12	0	0.86	8	0.03	0	0.8	0.1	9	0
3	3.7	0	7	50	178	383	0.3	0.5	20	0	1.46	9	0.05	0.06	1.2	0.2	14	0
1.7	4.9	2	20	50	177	377	0.3	0.5	21	6	1.38	11	0.05	0.06	1.1	0.19	18	0.28
3.5	5	73	18	84	386	597	0.6	1.2	25	11	1.52	17	0.1	0.13	1.6	0.29	12	0.14
0	0.1	0	4	25	197	206	0.3	1.1	13	0	0.04	5	0.06	0.01	0.8	0.17	6	0
3.1	4.7	85	24	65	661	318	0.4	0.8	19	41	2.33	12	0.1	0.08	1.1	0.18	8	0
0.7	0.2	3	7	42	201	277	0.3	0.3	18	1	0.07	10	0.09	0.02	1.1	0.21	9	0.05
0	0	0	15	18	5	138	0.2	2.1	10	0	0.01	2	0.01	0.01	0.4	0.08	3	0
1.2	3.9	0	5	31	131	202	0.1	0.3	12	0	0.98	2	0.04	0.02	0.6	0.03	1	0
3	0.6	0	21	34	522	266	0.2	1.1	13	1	0.04	5	0.14	0.05	1.5	0.16	12	0
1.4	0.2	18	102	116	538	268	0.3	0.4	18	38	1.47	4	0.02	0.1	1.2	0.05	8	0
3.2	1.3	18	146	138	530	485	0.8	0.8	24	47	0.65	12	0.08	0.14	1.2	0.21	14	0
0	0.1	0	6	61	6	477	0.4	0.4	30	0	0.05	16	0.13	0.03	1.7	0.37	11	0
0	0	0	4	34	3	296	0.2	0.2	17	0	0.04	10	0.08	0.02	1.1	0.23	8	0
0	0.1	0	7	60	5	515	0.4	0.4	30	0	0.07	18	0.14	0.03	2	0.41	14	0
0	0.1	0	4	20	153	160	0.2	0.9	10	0	0.04	4	0.05	0.01	0.6	0.13	4	0
1.7	0.3	0	5	32	22	240	0.2	0.7	11	0	0.1	5	0.06	0.02	1.2	0.12	8	0
0	0	0	5	34	4	407	0.4	0.6	16	0	0.04	15	0.07	0.03	1.1	0.2	10	0
5.6	0.7	0	6	48	307	270	0.2	0.8	12	0	0.25	3	0.04	0.02	1.3	0.11	11	0
4.7	0.7	0	10	46	108	366	0.2	0.4	17	0	0.25	5	0.09	0.01	1.6	0.12	14	0
4.7	0.7	6	10	46	108	366	0.2	0.4	17	0	0.25	5	0.09	0.01	1.6	0.12	14	0
3.5	0.4	8	.6	62	262	241	0.2	0.4	14	3	0.11	5	0.07	0.01	1	0.15	7	0.01
3.4	0.9	0	10	48	22	288	0.2	1	11	0	0.12	4	0.07	0.01	1.6	0.08	4	0
2.3	1.3	17	24	28	73	237	0.2	0.7	11	12	0.1	3	0.04	0.02	1	0.19	10	0
4	1	0	12	56	26	340	0.2	1.2	13	0	0.15	5	0.09	0.02	1.9	0.1	5	0
1.9	1.3	2	27	48	310	303	0.3	0.3	19	21	0.32	6	0.09	0.04	1.1	0.24	8	0
0.2	0.1	2	27	50	318	314	0.3	0.3	19	6	0.05	7	0.09	0.04	1.2	0.24	9	0
1.2	0.2	13	27	48	310	303	0.3	0.3	19	21	0.32	6	0.09	0.04	1.1	0.24	8	0
2.5	1.7	4	54	62	365	256	0.2	0.2	20	23	0.77	11	0.12	0.06	0.7	0.01	8	0
1.5	0.2	15	37	63	270	151	0.3	0.2	20	20	0.03	6	0.08	0.08	0.8	0.01	8	0
0	0	0	5	100	6	378	0.3	0.4	23	0	0.04	14	0.12	0.02	1.5	0.29	11	0
5.6	3.4	0	19	90	42	459	0.5	0.9	33	18	0.18	10	0.05	0.13	1.4	0.37	12	0
0.3	0.1	4	35	48	210	258	0.3	0.5	18	55	0.12	16	0.07	0.05	1	0.21	8	0
0	0	0	6	31	4	256	0.2	0.2	16	0	0.04	6	0.08	0.02	1	0.21	7	0
0	0.1	0	11	54	7	443	0.4	0.4	27	0	0.07	10	0.13	0.03	1.8	0.36	12	0
6.5	1.3	155	83	153	936	515	0.7	0.8	34	155	1.38	25	0.34	0.26	2.2	0.32	23	0.36
1.5	0.2	14	44	69	418	249	0.3	0.5	17	26	0.18	4	0.02	0.07	1.3	0.05	12	0
1.6	0.9	7	70	77	410	463	0.5	0.7	23	23	0.4	13	0.08	0.11	1.3	0.22	14	0
0	0	0	5	18	14	201	0.2	0.6	8	0	0.04	7	0.07	0.02	0.9	0.14	6	0
0	0.1	0	12	70	10	510	0.4	1.7	33	0	0.06	16	0.13	0.04	2	0.42	13	0
0	0	0	10	98	7	416	0.3	1.2	25	0	0.05	14	0.11	0.03	1.6	0.32	11	0
0	0.1	0	12	77	10	905	0.6	1.3	35	0	0.1	26	0.12	0.06	2.4	0.41	19	0

Food Item	Qty	Meas	Wgt (g)	Wtr (g)	Cals	Prot	Carb (g)	Fib (g)	Fat (g)	SatF (g)
Potato, whole, raw, flesh only	1	each	112	88	88	2	20	1.8	0	0
Power bar	1	each	65	—	230	10	45	3	2	—
Power bar, mocha	1	each	65	7	230	10	45	3	2	1
Power bar, apple cinnamon	1	each	65	7	230	10	45	3	2	0.5
Pretzel, hard twist, unenriched, unsalted	10	each	60	2	229	5	48	1.7	2	0.4
Pretzel, hard, twist	10	each	60	2	229	5	48	1.9	2	0.4
Pretzel, hard, whole wheat	1	oz.	28	1	103	3	23	2.2	1	0.2
Pretzel, soft	1	each	55	8	190	5	38	0.9	2	0.7
Pretzel, sticks	10	each	5	0	19	0	4	0.2	0	0
Pretzel, thick Dutch twist	1	each	16	1	61	1	13	0.5	1	0.1
Pretzel, yogurt-covered	6	each	25	1	115	2	17	0.2	5	3.6
Pretzels, cheddar, Combos snack	10	piece	30	1	139	3	20	—	5	—
Prickly pear fruit, raw	1	each	103	90	42	1	10	3.7	1	0.1
Prunes, canned in heavy syrup	0.5	cup	117	83	123	1	32	4.4	0	0
Prunes, dried	10	each	84	27	201	2	53	6	0	0
Prunes, dry, stewed, no sugar added	0.5	cup	106	74	113	1	30	7	0	0
Pudding pop, chocolate	1	each	47	30	72	2	12	0.2	2	2.1
Pudding pop, vanilla	1	each	47	30	75	2	13	0	2	2.1
Pudding, banana, instant w/2% milk	0.5	cup	147	110	153	4	29	0	2	1.5
Pudding, banana, instant w/whole milk	0.5	cup	147	108	166	4	29	0	4	2.6
Pudding, banana, mix w/whole milk	0.5	cup	140	104	157	4	25	0	4	2.6
Pudding, banana, regular w/2% milk	0.5	cup	140	106	143	4	26	0	2	1.5
Pudding, bread, w/raisins	0.5	cup	126	79	212	7	31	1.3	7	2.9
Pudding, chocolate, instant w/2% milk	0.5	cup	147	110	150	5	28	0.6	3	1.6
Pudding, chocolate, instant w/whole milk	0.5	cup	147	108	163	5	28	1.5	5	2.7
Pudding, chocolate, recipe w/2% milk	0.5	cup	157	106	206	5	40	1.4	4	2
Pudding, chocolate, reg mix w/whole milk	0.5	cup	142	106	158	5	26	1.4	5	3
Pudding, chocolate, regular w/2% milk	0.5	cup	142	105	151	5	28	0.4	3	1.8
Pudding, chocolate, w/whole milk, recipe	0.5	cup	157	105	221	5	40	1.3	6	3.1
Pudding, coconut cream, instant w/2% milk	0.5	cup	147	109	157	4	28	0.1	3	2
Pudding, coconut cream, reg w/2% milk	0.5	cup	140	106	146	4	25	0.3	4	2.5
Pudding, coconut, instant w/whole milk	0.5	cup	147	108	172	4	28	0.1	5	3.1
Pudding, lemon, instant w/2% milk	0.5	cup	147	109	154	4	30	0	2	1.5
Pudding, lemon, instant w/whole milk	0.5	cup	147	108	169	4	30	0	4	2.6
Pudding, lemon, mix+sugar+egg yolk+water	0.5	cup	146	106	164	1	36	0	2	0.6
Pudding, low cal mix w/milk, D-Zerta	0.5	cup	130	110	88	4	12	0	2	1.5
Pudding, low calorie mix w/milk, D-Zerta	0.5	cup	125	108	60	5	11	1	0	0
Pudding, rice w/raisins, recipe	0.5	cup	152	101	217	5	40	0.8	4	2.6
Pudding, rice, mix w/2% milk	0.5	cup	144	105	161	5	30	0.1	2	1.4
Pudding, rice, mix w/whole milk, cooked	0.5	cup	144	104	176	5	30	0.1	4	2.5
Pudding, tapioca, mix w/2% milk	0.5	cup	141	105	147	4	28	0	2	1.5
Pudding, tapioca, reg mix w/whole milk	0.5	cup	141	104	161	4	28	0	4	2.5
Pudding, tapioca, w/whole milk, recipe	0.5	cup	82	60	103	4	14	0	4	1.8
Pudding, vanilla, fat free, snack size, Jell-o	1	each	113	87	100	2	23	0	0	0
Pudding, vanilla, instant w/2% milk	0.5	cup	142	106	148	4	28	0	2	1.4
Pudding, vanilla, instant w/whole milk	0.5	cup	142	104	162	4	28	0	4	2.5
Pudding, vanilla, reg mix w/2% milk	0.5	cup	140	106	141	4	26	0	2	1.5
Pudding, vanilla, reg mix w/whole milk	0.5	cup	140	104	155	4	26	0	4	2.6
Pudding, vanilla, w/whole milk, recipe	0.5	cup	123	94	130	4	20	0	4	2.5
Puff pastry, frozen, baked	1	each	40	3	223	3	18	0.6	15	2.2
Pummelo, raw sections	0.5	cup	95	85	36	1	9	1	0	—
Pumpkin seed kernel, dry roasted, unsalted	0.25	cup	34	2	187	8	6	1.4	16	3
Pumpkin seed kernels, roasted, salted	0.25	cup	57	4	296	19	8	2.2	24	4.5
Pumpkin seed kernels, roasted, unsalted	0.25	cup	57	4	296	19	8	2.2	24	4.5
Pumpkin turnover	1	each	78	41	198	4	20	1.3	11	3.5
Pumpkin, canned, low sodium	0.5	cup	123	111	42	1	10	3.6	0	0.2
Pumpkin, fresh, cooked	0.5	cup	122	115	24	1	6	1.4	0	0
Quesadilla	1	each	54	16	199	6	21	1.2	10	3.6
Quiche Lorraine, 1/8th pie	1	piece	176	95	508	20	20	0.6	39	17.6
Rabbit, domestic, roasted	4	oz.	113	69	223	33	0	0	9	2.7
Radicchio leaf, raw	10	each	80	74	18	1	4	0.7	0	0
Radicchio, raw, shredded	0.5	cup	20	19	5	0	1	0.2	0	0
Radish, Daikon/Chinese, cooked slices	0.5	cup	74	70	12	0	3	1.2	0	0.1
Radish, red	10	each	45	43	9	0	2	0.7	0	0
Radish, white icicle, raw, whole	3	each	51	49	7	1	1	0.7	0	0

MonoF	PolyF	Choles	Calc	Phos	Sod	Pot	Zn	Iron	Magn	VitA	VitE	VitC	Thia	Ribo	Nia	B6	Fola	B12
(g)	(g)	(mg)	(mg)	(mg)	(mg)	(mg)	(mg)	(mg)	(mg)	(µg RE)	(µg α-TE)	(mg)	(mg)	(mg)	(mg)	(mg)	(µg)	(µg)
0	0	0	8	52	7	608	0.4	0.9	24	0	0.07	22	0.1	0.04	1.7	0.29	14	0
—	—	0	300	350	110	150	5.2	5.4	140	—	—	60	1.5	1.7	20	2	400	6
1	0.5	0	300	350	90	145	5.2	6.3	140	0	20	60	1.5	1.7	20	2	400	6
1.5	0.5	0	300	350	90	110	5.2	6.3	140	0	20	60	1.5	1.7	20	2	400	6
0.8	0.7	0	22	68	173	88	0.5	1	21	0	0.13	0	0.11	0.06	1.2	0.07	50	0
0.8	0.7	0	22	68	1029	88	0.5	2.6	21	0	0.13	0	0.28	0.37	3.2	0.07	103	0
0.3	0.2	0	8	35	58	122	0.2	0.8	9	0	0.07	0	0.12	0.08	1.8	0.08	15	0
0.8	0.2	2	13	44	772	48	0.5	2.2	12	0	0.02	0	0.23	0.16	2.4	0.01	8	0
0.1	0.1	0	2	6	86	7	0	0.2	2	0	0.01	0	0.02	0.03	0.3	0.01	9	0
0.2	0.2	0	6	18	274	23	0.1	0.7	6	0	0.03	0	0.07	0.1	0.8	0.02	27	0
0.5	0.1	1	37	36	16	60	0.2	0.4	5	19	0.17	0	0.08	0.09	0.7	0.01	4	0.12
—	—	2	59	43	335	39	0.2	0.3	7	2	0.06	0	0.09	0.17	1	0.01	2	0.04
0.1	0.2	0	58	25	5	227	0.1	0.3	88	5	0.01	14	0.01	0.06	0.5	0.06	6	0
0.2	0	0	20	30	4	264	0.2	0.5	18	94	0.29	3	0.04	0.14	1	0.24	0	0
0.3	0.1	0	43	66	3	626	0.4	2.1	38	167	1.22	3	0.07	0.14	1.6	0.22	3	0
0.2	0.1	0	24	37	2	354	0.3	1.2	21	33	0	3	0.02	0.11	0.8	0.23	0	0
0	0	1	66	53	78	105	0.2	0.2	10	16	0.01	0	0.02	0.08	0.1	0.02	1	0.25
0	0	1	61	48	50	65	0.2	0	5	24	0.01	0	0.02	0.09	0	0.02	2	0.17
0.7	0.2	9	150	318	435	193	0.5	0.1	18	66	0.07	1	0.05	0.2	0.1	0.05	6	0.44
1.2	0.2	16	147	315	434	188	0.5	0.1	18	37	0.07	1	0.05	0.2	0.1	0.05	6	0.44
1.2	0.2	17	151	116	231	189	0.5	0.1	18	38	0.07	1	0.04	0.2	0.1	0.05	6	0.35
0.7	0.1	10	154	118	232	193	0.5	0.1	18	70	0.07	1	0.04	0.2	0.1	0.05	6	0.36
2.7	1.2	83	144	137	291	282	0.7	1.4	24	82	0.63	1	0.12	0.28	0.8	0.09	16	0.33
0.9	0.2	9	153	353	417	247	0.6	0.4	26	56	0.15	1	0.05	0.21	0.1	0.06	6	0.46
1.4	0.3	16	150	351	417	244	0.6	0.4	26	31	0.09	1	0.05	0.21	0.1	0.06	6	0.44
1.3	0.4	9	155	149	138	256	0.8	0.7	39	78	0.11	1	0.05	0.22	0.2	0.05	6	0.36
1.4	0.2	17	158	132	146	231	0.6	0.5	21	37	0.08	1	0.04	0.25	0.1	0.05	6	0.36
0.8	0.1	10	160	138	149	240	0.7	0.5	30	68	0.08	1	0.04	0.21	0.2	0.05	6	0.36
1.8	0.5	17	152	148	137	253	0.8	0.7	38	49	0.14	1	0.05	0.22	0.2	0.05	6	0.34
0.9	0.3	9	150	295	362	194	0.5	0.2	21	69	0.06	1	0.05	0.2	0.1	0.06	6	0.44
0.7	0.1	10	158	125	228	223	0.5	0.3	22	70	0.1	1	0.04	0.2	0.1	0.2	6	0.36
1.4	0.4	16	147	294	362	190	0.5	0.2	21	37	0.09	1	0.05	0.2	0.1	0.05	6	0.44
0.7	0.1	9	148	304	394	190	0.5	0.1	16	69	0.07	1	0.05	0.2	0.1	0.05	6	0.44
1.2	0.2	16	146	301	392	187	0.5	0.1	16	38	0.07	1	0.05	0.2	0.1	0.05	6	0.44
0.7	0.2	77	12	31	93	7	0.2	0.3	3	35	0.07	0	0.01	0.05	0	0.02	9	0.19
0.7	0.1	9	151	211	303	191	0.5	0.1	18	70	0.09	1	0.05	0.2	0.1	0.05	6	0.45
0	0	0	150	210	65	290	0.5	0.4	27	40	0.09	1	0.05	0.2	0.1	0.05	6	0.42
1.2	0.2	17	155	143	85	269	0.7	1	24	38	0.08	1	0.12	0.21	0.8	0.08	6	0.24
0.6	0.1	9	151	127	158	190	0.6	0.5	19	52	0.06	1	0.11	0.2	0.6	0.05	6	0.36
1.2	0.2	16	148	124	157	186	0.5	0.5	19	29	0.09	1	0.11	0.2	0.6	0.05	6	0.35
0.7	0.1	8	149	117	172	189	0.5	0.1	17	69	0.07	1	0.04	0.2	0.1	0.06	6	0.35
1.2	0.2	17	147	116	171	186	0.5	0.1	17	38	0.11	1	0.04	0.2	0.1	0.05	6	0.35
1.2	0.3	68	86	87	157	117	0.4	0.3	11	47	0.07	0	0.03	0.18	0.1	0.04	7	0.3
0	0	0	80	—	240	125	—	0	—	20	—	0	—	—	—	—	—	—
0.7	0.1	9	146	283	406	185	0.5	0.1	17	64	0.07	1	0.05	0.2	0.1	0.05	6	0.43
1.2	0.2	16	143	280	406	182	0.5	0.1	17	36	0.08	1	0.05	0.19	0.1	0.05	6	0.43
0.7	0.1	10	153	118	224	193	0.5	0.1	18	70	0.07	1	0.04	0.2	0.1	0.05	6	0.36
1.2	0.2	17	150	115	224	190	0.5	0.1	18	38	0.08	1	0.04	0.2	0.1	0.05	6	0.35
1.2	0.2	16	145	114	113	185	0.5	0.1	16	37	0.1	1	0.03	0.2	0.1	0.04	5	0.23
3.5	8.9	0	4	24	101	25	0.2	1	6	0	0.95	0	0.13	0.1	1.5	0.01	19	0
—	—	0	4	16	1	205	0.1	0.1	6	0	0.09	58	0.03	0.03	0.2	0.03	25	0
4.9	7.2	0	15	405	6	278	2.6	5.2	185	13	0.34	1	0.07	0.11	0.6	0.08	20	0
7.4	10.9	0	24	665	326	457	4.2	8.5	303	22	0.57	1	0.12	0.18	1	0.05	33	0
7.4	10.9	0	24	665	10	457	4.2	8.5	303	22	0.57	1	0.12	0.18	1	0.05	33	0
4.7	2.5	34	72	84	103	153	0.4	1.3	16	635	1.26	1	0.12	0.19	1	0.04	10	0.07
0	0	0	32	43	6	253	0.2	1.7	28	2713	1.3	5	0.03	0.07	0.5	0.07	15	0
0	0	0	18	37	1	282	0.3	0.7	11	132	1.3	6	0.04	0.1	0.5	0.05	10	0
3.6	2.3	14	123	112	255	66	0.7	1.3	13	55	1.16	3	0.15	0.14	1.2	0.03	5	0.06
13.8	4.9	205	201	271	549	271	1.7	1.9	27	243	1.91	3	0.23	0.44	4.7	0.2	17	0.99
2.5	1.8	93	22	298	53	434	2.6	2.6	24	0	0.96	0	0.1	0.24	9.6	0.53	12	9.41
0	0.1	0	15	32	18	242	0.5	0.5	10	2	1.81	6	0.01	0.02	0.2	0.05	48	0
0	0	0	4	8	4	60	0.1	0.1	3	1	0.45	2	0	0.01	0.1	0.01	12	0
0	0.1	0	12	18	10	209	0.1	0.1	7	0	0	11	0	0.02	0.1	0.03	13	0
0	0	0	9	8	11	104	0.1	0.1	4	0	0	10	0	0.02	0.1	0.03	12	0
0	0	0	14	14	8	143	0.1	0.4	5	0	0	15	0.02	0.01	0.2	0.04	7	0

Food Item	Qty	Meas	Wgt (g)	Wtr (g)	Cals	Prot	Carb (g)	Fib (g)	Fat (g)	SatF (g)
Radishes, Daikon/Chinese, whole, raw	1	each	338	320	61	2	14	5.4	0	0.1
Raisin, seedless, packed	0.5	cup	82	13	248	3	65	3.3	0	0.1
Raisin, seedless, unpacked	0.5	cup	72	11	218	2	57	2.9	0	0.1
Raisins, golden seedless, packed	0.5	cup	82	12	249	3	66	3.3	0	0.1
Raspberries, canned in heavy syrup	0.5	cup	128	96	116	1	30	4.2	0	0
Raspberries, fresh	0.5	cup	62	53	30	1	7	4.2	0	0
Raspberries, frozen, sweetened	10	oz.	284	207	293	2	74	12.5	0	0
Ravioli, cheese-filled, w/tomato sauce, serving	1	each	250	178	336	14	38	2.2	14	6.3
Ravioli, meat filled	0.5	cup	125	85	194	10	18	1.3	9	3
Refried beans/frijoles, w/cheese	8	oz.	167	115	225	11	29	—	8	4.1
Relish, corn	1	Tbs	15	11	13	0	3	0.4	0	0
Relish, cranberry orange	0.5	cup	138	73	245	0	64	0	0	0
Relish, hotdog	1	Tbs	15	10	18	0	4	0.2	0	0
Relish, pickle, sweet	1	Tbs	15	10	21	0	5	0.3	0	0
Relish, vegetable	1	Tbs	9	8	4	0	1	0.1	0	0
Relish/preserves, tomato	1	Tbs	20	10	30	0	8	0.4	0	0
Rennin dessert mix w/2% milk, chocolate	0.5	cup	136	109	110	4	18	0.7	3	1.7
Rennin dessert mix w/2% milk, vanilla	0.5	cup	133	109	101	4	16	0	2	1.5
Rennin dessert mix w/whole milk, chocolate	0.5	cup	136	108	125	4	18	0.7	4	2.8
Rennin dessert mix w/whole milk, vanilla	0.5	cup	133	108	116	4	16	0	4	2.5
Rhubarb crisp	1	cup	246	130	513	3	96	4.2	16	3.1
Rhubarb, frozen, cooked w/sugar	0.5	cup	120	81	139	0	37	2.4	0	0
Rhubarb, raw, diced	0.5	cup	61	57	13	1	3	1.1	0	0
Rice bran, crude	0.25	cup	21	1	66	3	10	4.4	4	0.9
Rice cake, brown, buckwheat	2	each	18	1	68	2	14	0.7	1	0.1
Rice cake, brown, corn	2	each	18	1	69	2	15	0.5	1	0.1
Rice cake, brown, multi-grain	2	each	18	1	70	2	14	0.5	1	0.1
Rice cake, brown, plain	1	each	9	1	35	1	7	0.4	0	0.1
Rice cake, brown, rye	2	each	18	1	70	1	14	0.7	1	0.1
Rice cake, brown, sesame seed	2	each	18	1	71	1	15	1	1	0.1
Rice Krispie bar	1	each	28	3	109	1	21	0.1	3	0.5
Rice paste (mochi)	1	Tbs	17	7	40	1	9	0.3	0	0
Rice pilaf	0.5	cup	103	73	134	2	23	0.6	3	0.7
Rice w/cheddar/broccoli sauce, Lipton	0.5	cup	63	5	250	6	48	1	3	1
Rice, Spanish	0.5	cup	122	95	108	2	21	1.9	2	0.3
Rice, basmati, white, premium, dry	0.25	cup	51	6	183	4	41	0.3	1	0.2
Rice, brown, glutinous	0.5	cup	92	11	333	7	71	0.7	2	—
Rice, brown, long grain, cooked	0.5	cup	98	71	108	3	22	1.8	1	0.2
Rice, brown, med grain, cooked	0.5	cup	98	72	110	2	23	1.8	1	0.2
Rice, fried, meatless	0.5	cup	83	57	132	3	17	0.7	6	0.9
Rice, white, enriched, long grain, cooked, hot	0.5	cup	102	70	133	3	29	0.4	0	0.1
Rice, white, enriched, long grain, dry	0.25	cup	46	5	169	3	37	0.6	0	0.1
Rice, white, glutinous/sticky, cooked	0.5	cup	120	92	117	2	25	1.2	0	0
Rice, white, instant, long grain, cooked, hot	0.5	cup	82	63	81	2	18	0.5	0	0
Rice, white, instant, long grain, dry	0.25	cup	24	2	90	2	20	0.4	0	0
Rice, white, long grain, cooked, cold	0.5	cup	72	50	94	2	20	0.3	0	0.1
Rice, white, long grain, parboiled, dry	0.25	cup	46	5	172	3	38	0.8	0	0.1
Rice, white, med grain, unenriched, cooked	0.5	cup	102	70	133	2	29	0.3	0	0.1
Rice, white, short grain, cooked	1	cup	205	140	267	5	59	2.1	0	0.1
Rice, wild, cooked	0.5	cup	82	61	83	3	18	1.5	0	0
Rockfish, Pacific, baked/broiled	1	each	149	109	180	36	0	0	3	0.7
Roll dough, cinnamon, frosted, refrigerated, baked	1	each	30	7	109	2	17	0.6	4	1
Roll, French	1	each	38	13	105	3	19	1.2	2	0.4
Roll, Mexican bolillo	1	each	117	46	295	10	58	2.2	2	0.4
Roll, Mexican sweet (pan dulce), crumb topping	1	each	79	17	291	5	48	1.1	9	2
Roll, butterhorn	1	each	55	17	174	5	27	0.7	5	1.3
Roll, cheese bread	1	each	41	13	124	4	21	0.7	3	1
Roll, cinnamon w/raisins & nuts, homemade	1	each	57	15	196	4	30	1.1	7	1.4
Roll, dinner	1	each	28	9	85	2	14	0.9	2	0.5
Roll, dinner, bran	1	each	28	10	76	3	14	1.2	2	0.2
Roll, dinner, egg	1	each	35	11	107	3	18	1.3	2	0.6
Roll, dinner, homemade, w/2% milk	1	each	35	10	111	3	19	0.7	3	0.6
Roll, dinner, recipe, w/whole milk	1	each	35	10	112	3	19	1	3	0.8
Roll, dinner, wheat	1	each	28	10	77	2	13	1.1	2	0.4
Roll, dinner, whole wheat	1	each	35	12	93	3	18	2.6	2	0.3

MonoF	PolyF	Choles	Calc	Phos	Sod	Pot	Zn	Iron	Magn	VitA	VitE	VitC	Thia	Ribo	Nia	B6	Fola	B12
(g)	(g)	(mg)	(mg)	(mg)	(mg)	(mg)	(mg)	(mg)	(mg)	(μg RE)	(μg α-TE)	(mg)	(mg)	(mg)	(mg)	(mg)	(μg)	(μg)
0.1	0.2	0	91	78	71	767	0.5	1.4	54	0	0	74	0.07	0.07	0.7	0.16	95	0
0	0.1	0	40	80	10	620	0.2	1.7	27	1	0.58	3	0.13	0.07	0.7	0.2	3	0
0	0.1	0	36	70	9	544	0.2	1.5	24	1	0.51	2	0.11	0.06	0.6	0.18	2	0
0	0.1	0	44	95	10	615	0.3	1.5	29	3	0.58	3	0.01	0.16	0.9	0.27	3	0
0	0.1	0	14	12	4	120	0.2	0.5	15	4	0.58	11	0.03	0.04	0.6	0.05	13	0
0	0.2	0	14	7	0	94	0.3	0.4	11	8	0.28	15	0.02	0.06	0.6	0.04	16	0
0	0.3	0	43	48	3	324	0.5	1.8	37	17	1.28	47	0.05	0.13	0.7	0.1	74	0
4.8	2	160	166	214	1541	400	1.4	3.1	32	245	2.36	9	0.31	0.42	2.9	0.19	30	0.38
3.6	1	84	32	109	619	259	1.7	2	20	94	1.52	11	0.15	0.22	3	0.14	14	0.81
2.6	0.7	37	189	175	882	605	1.7	2.2	85	70	—	2	0.13	0.33	1.5	0.2	112	0.68
0	0	0	2	7	55	28	0	0.1	3	9	0.03	4	0.01	0.01	0.1	0.02	4	0
0	0.1	0	15	11	44	52	0.1	0.3	6	10	0.07	25	0.04	0.03	0.1	0.03	4	0
0.1	0	0	4	3	81	31	0	0.2	3	1	0.02	1	0	0	0	0	1	0
0	0	0	3	2	109	31	0	0.1	1	2	0.02	1	0	0	0	0	0	0
0	0	0	2	2	41	16	0	0	1	2	0.02	1	0	0	0	0	1	0
0	0	0	9	9	452	79	0	0.3	6	25	0.1	10	0.01	0.01	0.1	0.03	2	0
0.8	0.1	10	171	133	71	248	0.7	0.4	27	60	0.07	1	0.05	0.21	0.1	0.06	7	0.45
0.7	0.1	9	161	126	61	189	0.5	0.1	17	69	0.07	1	0.05	0.2	0.1	0.05	7	0.44
1.3	0.2	16	169	132	69	243	0.7	0.4	27	33	0.11	1	0.05	0.21	0.1	0.06	7	0.44
1.2	0.2	17	158	124	61	186	0.5	0.1	16	33	0.11	1	0.05	0.2	0.1	0.05	7	0.44
6.9	5	0	294	46	193	289	0.3	1.8	34	221	2.9	6	0.15	0.14	1.4	0.05	14	0.02
0	0	0	174	10	1	115	0.1	0.3	14	8	0.24	4	0.02	0.03	0.2	0.02	6	0
0	0.1	0	52	9	2	176	0.1	0.1	7	6	0.12	5	0.01	0.02	0.2	0.02	4	0
1.6	1.6	0	12	348	1	308	1.2	3.8	162	0	1.26	0	0.57	0.06	7.1	0.84	13	0
0.2	0.2	0	2	68	21	54	0.4	0.2	27	0	0.02	0	0.01	0.02	1.5	0.02	4	0
0.2	0.2	0	2	58	52	50	0.4	0.2	20	0	0	0	0.01	0.02	1.2	0.02	4	0
0.2	0.3	0	4	67	45	53	0.5	0.4	25	0	0	0	0.01	0.03	1.2	0.02	4	0
0.1	0.1	0	1	32	29	26	0.3	0.1	12	0	0.06	0	0	0.02	0.7	0.01	2	0
0.2	0.3	0	4	68	20	56	0.5	0.3	26	0	0	0	0.02	0.02	1.3	0.03	1	0
0.2	0.2	0	2	68	41	52	0.5	0.3	24	0	0.02	1	0.01	0.02	1.3	0.03	3	0
1.2	0.8	0	3	12	141	11	0.2	0.6	3	103	0.42	5	0.11	0.13	1.5	0.16	30	0
0	0	0	6	16	1	37	0.2	0.6	7	0	0.02	0	0.01	0	0.5	0.02	1	0
1.5	1.1	0	13	39	377	54	0.4	1.2	10	43	0.56	0	0.14	0.02	1.3	0.06	4	0
—	—	2	40	—	940	—	—	1.8	—	0	—	2	—	—	—	—	—	—
0.7	0.7	0	35	47	162	271	0.4	1.2	20	58	0.65	20	0.12	0.04	1.5	0.16	10	0
0.2	0.2	0	4	—	—	—	—	0.2	—	0	—	0	—	—	—	—	—	—
—	—	—	19	225	10	266	—	3.2	—	0	0.48	—	0.28	0.11	4.6	—	—	—
0.3	0.3	0	10	81	5	42	0.6	0.4	42	0	0.7	0	0.09	0.02	1.5	0.14	4	0
0.3	0.3	0	10	76	1	77	0.6	0.5	43	0	0.32	0	0.1	0.01	1.3	0.15	4	0
1.5	3.2	21	15	47	143	67	0.4	0.9	12	10	1.23	2	0.1	0.05	1.1	0.08	11	0.06
0.1	0.1	0	10	44	1	36	0.5	1.2	12	0	0.05	0	0.17	0.01	1.5	0.1	60	0
0.1	0.1	0	13	53	2	53	0.5	2	12	0	0.06	0	0.27	0.02	1.9	0.08	107	0
0.1	0.1	0	2	10	6	12	0.5	0.2	6	0	0.04	0	0.02	0.02	0.3	0.03	1	0
0	0	0	7	12	2	3	0.2	0.5	4	0	0.04	0	0.06	0.04	0.7	0.01	34	0
0	0	0	4	16	1	4	0.2	1	3	0	0.03	0	0.15	0.01	1.3	0.01	55	0
0.1	0.1	0	7	31	1	25	0.4	0.9	9	0	0.04	0	0.12	0.01	1.1	0.07	42	0
0.1	0.1	0	28	63	2	56	0.4	1.6	14	0	0.06	0	0.28	0.03	1.7	0.16	107	0
0.1	0.1	0	3	38	0	30	0.4	1.5	13	0	0.05	0	0.17	0.02	1.9	0.05	60	0
0.1	0.1	0	2	68	0	53	0.8	3	16	0	0.09	0	0.34	0.03	3	0.12	121	0
0	0.2	0	2	67	2	83	1.1	0.5	26	0	0.19	0	0.04	0.07	1.1	0.11	21	0
0.7	0.9	66	18	340	115	775	0.8	0.8	51	98	1.86	0	0.07	0.12	5.8	0.4	16	1.79
2.2	0.5	0	10	104	250	19	0.1	0.8	4	0	0.48	0	0.12	0.07	1.1	0.01	2	0.02
0.7	0.3	0	35	32	231	43	0.3	1	8	0	0.17	0	0.2	0.11	1.6	0.02	36	0
0.2	0.6	1	14	88	347	96	0.8	3.7	22	4	0.05	0	0.67	0.45	6.3	0.06	47	0
3.9	2.7	26	13	56	140	57	0.4	1.8	10	88	1.35	0	0.23	0.21	2	0.04	22	0.06
2.6	0.7	18	58	59	214	68	0.3	1.2	10	12	0.66	0	0.2	0.18	1.2	0.06	17	0
1.3	0.4	2	54	44	210	39	0.3	1.1	9	6	0.04	0	0.16	0.1	1.3	0.02	15	0.01
2.7	2.8	13	36	63	185	123	0.4	1.5	16	60	0.91	0	0.16	0.16	1.3	0.05	18	0.06
1	0.3	0	34	33	148	38	0.2	0.9	7	0	0.25	0	0.14	0.09	1.1	0.02	27	0.02
0.6	0.6	0	6	54	126	53	0.3	0.9	15	0	0.22	0	0.13	0.1	1.1	0.04	22	0
1	0.4	18	21	35	191	36	0.4	1.2	9	3	0.25	0	0.18	0.18	1.2	0.02	37	0.08
1	0.7	12	21	44	145	53	0.2	1	7	32	0.34	0	0.14	0.14	1.2	0.02	32	0.05
1.1	0.7	13	21	44	145	53	0.2	1	7	28	0.35	0	0.14	0.14	1.2	0.02	15	0.05
0.9	0.3	0	50	30	96	33	0.3	1	10	0	0.27	0	0.12	0.08	1.2	0.02	14	0
0.4	0.8	0	37	78	167	95	0.7	0.8	30	0	0.48	0	0.09	0.05	1.3	0.07	11	0

Food Item	Qty	Meas	Wgt (g)	Wtr (g)	Cals	Prot	Carb (g)	Fib (g)	Fat (g)	SatF (g)
Roll, garlic	1	each	35	11	104	3	18	0.7	2	0.5
Roll, hard, white, enriched	1	each	50	16	147	5	26	1.2	2	0.3
Roll, jelly filled	1	each	55	17	173	4	28	0.9	5	1.2
Roll, oatmeal, toasted	1	each	33	14	78	3	13	1.4	2	0.2
Roll, rye, light	1	each	28	9	81	3	15	1.4	1	0.2
Roll, sourdough	1	each	45	14	131	4	25	1.2	1	0.3
Roll, submarine/hoagie	1	each	135	41	392	12	75	3.6	4	0.9
Roll, sweet, cheese	1	each	66	19	238	5	29	0.8	12	4
Roll, sweet, cinnamon raisin, commercial	1	each	39	10	145	2	20	0.9	6	1.2
Rose apple, raw	4	oz.	113	105	28	1	6	1.5	0	—
Rutabaga, cooked cubes	0.5	cup	85	76	33	1	7	1.5	0	0
Rutabaga, cooked, mashed	0.5	cup	120	107	47	2	10	2.2	0	0
Salad dressing, Blue Cheese, low calorie	2	Tbs	31	24	30	2	1	0	2	0.3
Salad dressing, Catalina, fat free, Kraft	2	Tbs	35	4	124	5	24	1.6	1	0.5
Salad dressing, Dijon Vinaigrette Lite	2	Tbs	30	25	32	0	1	0	3	0.4
Salad dressing, Italian, fat free, Kraft	2	Tbs	35	32	11	0	2	0	0	0
Salad dressing, Italian, fat free, Lipton	2	Tbs	30	28	15	0	2	0	0	0
Salad dressing, Seven Seas Viva	2	Tbs	30	12	140	0	3	0	14	2.1
Salad dressing, bacon & tomato, low calorie	2	Tbs	32	24	65	1	1	0.1	7	1.1
Salad dressing, blue cheese	2	Tbs	31	10	154	1	2	0	16	3
Salad dressing, buttermilk, light	2	Tbs	29	21	58	1	2	—	5	—
Salad dressing, caesar's	2	Tbs	23	8	107	3	1	0.1	10	1.9
Salad dressing, caesar, low calorie	2	Tbs	30	22	33	0	6	0	1	0.2
Salad dressing, cooked	2	Tbs	32	22	50	1	5	0	3	0.9
Salad dressing, creamy Italian	2	Tbs	29	11	143	0	2	0	16	2.3
Salad dressing, creamy bacon	2	Tbs	29	11	143	0	2	0	16	2.3
Salad dressing, creamy cucumber	2	Tbs	29	11	143	0	2	0	16	2.3
Salad dressing, creamy cucumber, low calorie	2	Tbs	30	22	48	0	2	0	4	0.6
Salad dressing, creamy, oil free, low calorie	2	Tbs	30	22	48	0	2	0	4	0.6
Salad dressing, french	2	Tbs	31	12	134	0	5	0	13	3
Salad dressing, french, fat free, Kraft	2	Tbs	35	23	40	0	12	0.5	0	0
Salad dressing, french, homemade	2	Tbs	28	7	177	0	1	0	20	3.5
Salad dressing, french, low calorie	2	Tbs	32	23	44	0	7	0	2	0.3
Salad dressing, honey dijon, fat free, Kraft	2	Tbs	35	23	50	0	11	1	0	0
Salad dressing, honey mustard	2	Tbs	31	11	101	0	14	0.2	6	0.8
Salad dressing, Italian	2	Tbs	29	11	137	0	3	0	14	2.1
Salad dressing, Italian, low calorie	2	Tbs	30	25	32	0	1	0	3	0.4
Salad dressing, light, cholesterol free	1	Tbs	15	9	48	0	2	0	4	1.1
Salad dressing, low calorie, Miracle Whip Light	1	Tbs	14	8	36	0	3	0	3	0.4
Salad dressing, mayonnaise type	1	Tbs	15	6	57	0	4	0	5	0.7
Salad dressing, oil free, low calorie	2	Tbs	30	26	7	0	2	0	0	0
Salad dressing, ranch	2	Tbs	30	16	109	1	1	0	11	1.7
Salad dressing, ranch, fat free, Kraft	2	Tbs	35	23	50	0	11	0.5	0	0
Salad dressing, roquefort, low calorie	2	Tbs	31	24	30	2	1	0	2	0.3
Salad dressing, russian	2	Tbs	31	11	151	0	3	0	16	2.2
Salad dressing, russian, low calorie	2	Tbs	33	21	46	0	9	0.1	1	0.2
Salad dressing, sesame seed	2	Tbs	31	12	136	1	3	0.3	14	1.9
Salad dressing, thousand island	2	Tbs	31	14	118	0	5	0	11	1.9
Salad dressing, thousand island, low calorie	2	Tbs	31	21	49	0	5	0.4	3	0.5
Salad dressing, vinaigrette	2	Tbs	29	11	137	0	3	0	14	2.1
Salad dressing, vinegar & oil	2	Tbs	32	15	144	0	1	0	16	2.9
Salad dressing, vinegar & sugar & water	2	Tbs	32	27	16	0	4	0	0	0
Salad dressing, yogurt	2	Tbs	31	26	22	1	2	0	1	0.6
Salad dressing/marinade, Korean	2	Tbs	30	27	10	0	2	0.2	0	0
Salad topping, Bac-O-Bits	2	Tbs	12	1	50	5	3	—	2	—
Salad, carrot raisin	0.5	cup	88	50	202	1	21	2	14	2
Salad, chef style w/turkey+ham+cheese	1.5	cup	326	269	267	26	5	—	16	8.2
Salad, crab, w/imitation crab	0.5	cup	104	72	150	9	14	0.4	6	0.9
Salad, fruit, canned, juice pack	0.5	cup	124	107	62	1	16	1.2	0	0
Salad, mixed greens/lettuce	0.5	cup	28	26	5	0	1	0.5	0	0
Salad, spinach, no dressing	0.5	cup	37	27	44	2	5	0.8	2	0.5
Salad, taco	1.5	cup	198	143	279	13	24	—	15	6.8
Salad, three bean	0.5	cup	75	61	70	2	7	1.5	4	0.6
Salad, tossed green	0.5	cup	69	66	12	1	2	0.8	0	0
Salad, Waldorf	0.5	cup	68	40	204	2	6	1.2	20	2.1

MonoF	PolyF	Choles	Calc	Phos	Sod	Pot	Zn	Iron	Magn	VitA	VitE	VitC	Thia	Ribo	Nia	B6	Fola	B12
(g)	(g)	(mg)	(mg)	(mg)	(mg)	(mg)	(mg)	(mg)	(mg)	(µg RE)	(µg α-TE)	(mg)	(mg)	(mg)	(mg)	(mg)	(µg)	(µg)
1	0.3	0	35	30	176	34	0.3	1	7	0	0.03	0	0.14	0.08	1.2	0.02	13	0
0.6	0.9	0	48	50	272	54	0.5	1.6	14	0	0.16	0	0.24	0.17	2.1	0.02	48	0
2.4	0.7	17	56	58	199	92	0.3	1.2	10	11	0.64	0	0.2	0.17	1.2	0.07	16	0
0.5	0.5	0	28	38	136	40	0.3	1.4	11	0	0.23	0	0.15	0.1	1.6	0.02	31	0
0.4	0.2	0	9	45	253	51	0.3	0.8	15	0	0.1	0	0.11	0.08	1.1	0.02	24	0
0.4	0.5	0	40	38	261	40	0.3	1.3	9	0	0.03	0	0.18	0.11	1.5	0.02	14	0
1.3	1.4	0	122	115	783	122	0.9	3.8	27	0	0.1	0	0.54	0.33	4.5	0.05	40	0.2
6	1.3	50	78	65	236	90	0.4	0.5	12	51	1.25	0	0.1	0.09	0.5	0.05	28	0.06
1.9	2.9	26	28	30	149	43	0.2	0.6	7	25	1.68	1	0.13	0.1	0.9	0.04	20	0
—	—	0	33	9	0	139	0.1	0.1	6	39	—	25	0.02	0.03	0.9	—	—	0
0	0.1	0	41	48	17	277	0.3	0.5	20	48	0.13	16	0.07	0.04	0.6	0.09	13	0
0	0.1	0	58	67	24	391	0.4	0.6	28	67	0.18	23	0.1	0.05	0.9	0.12	18	0
0.9	0.8	0	27	25	367	2	0.1	0.2	2	1	0.28	0	0.01	0.03	0	0.01	1	0.07
0.5	0.3	0	162	188	48	78	2.8	3.4	75	0	10.8	32	0.81	0.92	10.8	1.08	215	3.23
0.6	1.8	2	1	2	236	4	0	0.1	0	0	0.45	0	0	0	0	0	0	0
0	0	0	0	—	327	45	—	0	—	0	—	0	—	—	—	—	—	—
0	0	0	0	—	280	—	—	0	—	0	—	0	—	—	—	—	—	—
3.4	8.4	0	3	2	236	4	0	0.1	0	7	3.12	0	0	0.01	0	0	1	0.05
1.8	3.6	1	1	8	351	35	0.1	0.1	2	9	1.3	3	0.01	0.01	0.2	0.03	0	0.03
3.8	8.5	5	25	23	335	11	0.1	0.1	0	20	2.85	1	0	0.03	0	0.01	2	0.08
—	—	—	—	—	167	35	—	—	—	—	—	—	0.01	0.05	1	0.02	3	0.11
7.2	1	24	43	37	396	40	0.2	0.4	5	13	1.38	1	0.01	0.05	1	0.02	3	0.11
0.6	0.5	1	7	6	323	9	0	0.1	1	1	0.12	0	0	0	0	0	1	0.01
1.2	0.7	18	27	28	235	39	0.1	0.2	3	39	0.61	0	0.02	0.05	0.1	0.01	3	0.11
3.8	8.7	1	4	3	347	8	0	0	1	6	3.15	0	0	0	0	0	0	0.01
3.8	8.7	1	4	3	347	8	0	0	1	6	3.15	0	0	0	0	0	0	0.01
3.8	8.7	1	4	3	347	8	0	0	1	6	3.15	0	0	0	0	0	0	0.01
1.8	1.6	0	2	2	307	11	0	0	1	2	0.57	0	0	0	0	0.01	4	0.02
1.8	1.6	0	2	2	307	11	0	0	1	2	0.57	0	0	0	0	0.01	4	0.02
2.5	6.8	0	3	4	428	25	0	0.1	0	41	2.63	0	0	0	0	0	1	0.04
0	0	0	0	—	300	40	—	0	—	150	—	0	—	—	—	—	—	—
5.8	9.4	0	2	1	184	7	0	0.1	0	43	3.36	0	0	0.01	0	0	0	0
0.5	1.1	0	4	5	256	26	0.1	0.1	0	42	0.39	0	0	0	0	0	0	0
0	0	0	0	—	330	50	—	0.4	—	0	—	0	—	—	—	—	—	—
1.4	3.2	0	6	5	181	20	0.1	0.2	3	0	0.44	0	0	0.01	0.1	0.01	1	0
3.3	8.2	0	3	1	231	4	0	0.1	0	7	3.06	0	0	0.01	0	0	1	0.05
0.6	1.8	2	1	2	236	4	0	0.1	0	0	0.45	0	0	0	0	0	0	0
1.1	2.1	0	0	0	102	0	0	0	0	2	0.64	0	0	0	0	0	0	0
0.7	1.4	4	2	4	99	1	0	0	0	9	0.6	0	0	0	0	0	1	0.03
1.3	2.6	4	2	4	104	1	0	0	0	12	0.59	0	0	0	0	0	1	0.03
0	0	0	2	2	512	15	0	0.1	3	0	0	0	0	0	0	0	0	0
4.8	4.2	12	30	25	131	40	0.1	0.1	3	22	1.19	0	0.01	0.04	0	0.01	2	0.08
0	0	0	0	—	310	50	—	0	—	0	—	0	—	—	—	—	—	—
0.9	0.8	0	27	25	367	2	0.1	0.2	2	1	0.28	0	0.01	0.03	0	0.01	1	0.07
3.6	9	6	6	11	266	48	0.1	0.2	0	63	3.12	2	0.02	0.02	0.2	0.01	3	0.09
0.3	0.8	2	6	12	283	51	0	0.2	0	5	0.25	2	0	0	0	0	1	0.04
3.6	7.7	0	6	11	306	48	0	0.2	0	63	1.53	0	0	0	0	0	2	0.06
2.6	6.2	8	3	5	219	35	0	0.2	1	30	0.36	0	0	0.01	0	0	2	0.06
0.7	1.9	5	3	5	306	35	0	0.2	0	29	0.36	0	0	0.01	0	0	2	0.06
3.3	8.2	0	3	1	231	4	0	0.1	0	7	3.06	0	0	0.01	0	0	1	0.05
4.7	7.7	0	0	0	0	2	0	0	0	0	2.82	0	0	0	0	0	0	0
0	0	0	1	1	331	9	0	0.1	2	0	0	0	0	0	0	0	0	0
0.3	0.2	3	31	24	118	45	0.1	0.1	4	7	0.04	1	0.01	0.04	0	0.01	2	0.09
0	0	0	8	8	77	31	0	0.2	4	41	0.03	9	0.01	0.01	0.2	0.03	3	0
—	—	0	26	—	205	328	—	0.8	—	—	—	—	1.03	0.04	0.2	—	—	—
3.9	7.2	10	26	46	117	315	0.2	0.7	14	1444	5	5	0.08	0.05	0.6	0.22	9	0.05
5.2	1.4	140	235	401	743	401	3.1	2	49	137	—	16	0.39	0.39	6	0.42	101	0.85
1.6	3.4	37	37	110	892	211	0.3	0.4	33	22	0.86	1	0.03	0.1	1.5	0.14	7	1.41
0	0	0	14	17	6	144	0.2	0.3	10	74	0.74	4	0.01	0.02	0.4	0.03	3	0
0	0	0	15	9	7	87	0.1	0.4	7	75	0.18	4	0.02	0.03	0.1	0.02	32	0
0.7	0.4	30	26	37	78	138	0.3	0.8	17	120	0.5	5	0.06	0.13	0.7	0.05	38	0.08
5.2	1.8	44	192	143	762	416	2.7	2.3	52	77	—	4	0.1	0.36	2.5	0.22	83	0.63
1	2.4	0	18	32	257	112	0.3	0.7	13	11	0.98	2	0.04	0.05	0.2	0.02	26	0.01
0	0.1	0	10	16	7	134	0.1	0.3	7	139	0.26	7	0.04	0.03	0.3	0.04	24	0
3.7	13.5	10	21	42	118	135	0.3	0.4	20	20	4.34	3	0.05	0.02	0.2	0.18	14	0.04

Food Item	Qty	Meas	Wgt (g)	Wtr (g)	Cals	Prot	Carb (g)	Fib (g)	Fat (g)	SatF (g)
Salami, beef, cooked	1	piece	23	13	60	3	1	0	5	2.1
Salami, dry, beef & pork	2	piece	20	7	84	5	1	0	7	2.4
Salami, turkey, cooked	2	piece	57	38	112	9	0	0	8	2.3
Salisbury steak, 4-compartment, Swanson	1	each	298	231	325	15	33	5.7	14	5.7
Salsa cruda (uncooked salsa)	2	Tbs	30	28	6	0	1	0.3	0	0
Salsify, cooked, drained	0.5	cup	68	55	46	2	10	2.1	0	0
Salt	0.25	tsp	1	0	0	0	0	0	0	0
Sandwich, BLT, on firm white	1	each	145	75	366	12	35	2	19	4.9
Sandwich, avocado & cheese, on wheat	1	each	196	116	433	14	34	6.5	28	8.4
Sandwich, bologna	1	each	83	34	257	7	26	1.2	14	4.2
Sandwich, chicken frank on bun	1	each	85	38	235	9	24	0.8	11	3
Sandwich, chicken salad, on firm white	1	each	114	45	381	11	34	1.6	22	3.5
Sandwich, corned beef & swiss, on rye	1	each	147	73	396	26	20	0.1	24	8.9
Sandwich, egg salad, on firm white	1	each	121	50	394	10	34	1.5	24	4.2
Sandwich, fish w/tartar sauce & cheese	1	each	183	83	523	21	48	0.4	28	8.1
Sandwich, french dip au jus	1	each	193	118	359	26	34	1.7	12	4.8
Sandwich, grilled cheese, on firm white	1	each	127	46	426	19	34	1.5	24	13.1
Sandwich, grilled chicken, Weight Watchers	1	each	113	65	210	18	24	2	5	2
Sandwich, gyro	1	each	105	67	169	12	20	1.1	4	1.5
Sandwich, ham & swiss, on rye	1	each	145	79	328	22	21	0.1	18	6.3
Sandwich, ham salad, on wheat	1	each	126	60	343	10	34	3.3	19	4.4
Sandwich, ham, on wheat	1	each	123	68	259	17	22	2.7	11	2.2
Sandwich, hotdog, plain	1	each	98	53	242	10	18	—	14	5.1
Sandwich, pastrami	1	each	134	71	334	14	27	1.7	18	6.3
Sandwich, patty melt, on rye	1	each	177	81	546	36	21	2.9	36	12.9
Sandwich, peanut butter & jam, on soft white	1	each	101	26	351	12	47	3	15	3.1
Sandwich, reuben	1	each	181	91	496	23	31	4.1	31	10.6
Sandwich, roast beef, on wheat	1	each	123	57	314	23	25	2.6	13	2.5
Sandwich, submarine w/coldcuts	1	each	228	132	456	22	51	1.7	19	6.8
Sandwich, tuna salad, on firm white	1	each	126	57	342	14	38	1.8	14	2.3
Sandwich, turkey ham & cheese, on wheat	1	each	152	76	385	22	27	3.3	21	8
Sandwich, turkey ham, on rye	1	each	116	70	217	16	16	0.1	10	1.9
Sandwich, turkey, on whole wheat	1	each	136	72	294	21	26	3.5	12	1.8
Sapodilla, raw	1	each	170	133	141	1	34	9	2	0.3
Sapotes, raw	1	each	170	106	228	4	58	4.4	1	0.2
Sauce, Alfredo, Di Girono	0.5	cup	124	—	460	8	4	0	44	20
Sauce, Alfredo, low fat, Di Girono	0.5	cup	138	—	340	10	32	0	20	12
Sauce, Tabasco brand pepper	1	tsp	5	5	1	0	0	0	0	0
Sauce, alfredo, Progresso	0.5	cup	124	81	310	10	5	0	27	15
Sauce, armanino pesto	0.25	cup	58	30	195	4	4	0.9	18	3
Sauce, barbecue	2	Tbs	31	25	23	1	4	0.4	1	0.1
Sauce, bechamel	0.25	cup	72	61	71	1	3	0.2	6	3.7
Sauce, black bean	1	tsp	6	5	5	0	1	0.1	0	0
Sauce, bordelaise	0.25	cup	116	100	104	1	5	0.3	6	3.9
Sauce, cheese	0.25	cup	50	32	110	5	4	0.1	8	4.6
Sauce, cheese, dry mix w/milk	0.25	cup	70	54	77	4	6	0.2	4	2.3
Sauce, cheese, low fat	1	cup	243	177	338	23	16	0.3	20	8.2
Sauce, chili, hot green	1	tsp	5	5	1	0	0	—	0	0
Sauce, chili, tomato base	1	tsp	6	4	6	0	1	0.1	0	0
Sauce, chili, unsalted, bottled	0.25	cup	68	46	71	2	17	—	0	0
Sauce, curry	0.25	cup	58	51	37	1	2	0.1	3	0.5
Sauce, enchilada, green	0.5	cup	62	54	44	1	4	0.7	3	1.8
Sauce, enchilada, red	0.25	cup	62	50	83	1	3	0.6	8	4.1
Sauce, fish/bagoong	0.25	cup	68	44	71	14	0	0	1	0.2
Sauce, hoisin	2	Tbs	34	16	70	1	14	0	2	0
Sauce, hollandaise, dry mix w/water	2	Tbs	32	27	30	1	2	0.1	2	1.4
Sauce, horseradish	1	tsp	5	3	10	0	0	0	1	0.6
Sauce, hot chili/red pepper	1	tsp	5	5	1	0	0	0	0	0
Sauce, lobster	0.25	cup	58	41	95	6	4	0.3	6	1.3
Sauce, marinara tomato	0.5	cup	125	103	85	2	13	—	4	0.6
Sauce, mole poblano	0.25	cup	66	47	109	2	9	2.8	7	2.2
Sauce, mole verde	0.25	cup	66	57	39	2	4	1.1	2	0.4
Sauce, Mornay	0.25	cup	86	57	183	6	6	0.2	15	7
Sauce, pesto	0.25	cup	58	12	311	10	4	0.9	29	7.3
Sauce, soy (wheat & soy)	1	Tbs	18	13	10	1	2	0.1	0	0

MonoF	PolyF	Choles	Calc	Phos	Sod	Pot	Zn	Iron	Magn	VitA	VitE	VitC	Thia	Ribo	Nia	B6	Fola	B12
(g)	(g)	(mg)	(mg)	(mg)	(mg)	(mg)	(mg)	(mg)	(mg)	(µg RE)	(µg α-TE)	(mg)	(mg)	(mg)	(mg)	(mg)	(µg)	(µg)
2.2	0.2	15	2	26	270	52	0.5	0.5	3	0	0.04	0	0.02	0.04	0.7	0.04	0	0.7
3.4	0.6	16	2	28	372	76	0.6	0.3	3	0	0.06	0	0.12	0.06	1	0.1	0	0.38
2.6	2	47	11	60	572	139	1	0.9	9	0	0.32	0	0.04	0.1	2	0.14	2	0.12
—	—	29	76	—	879	—	—	2.6	—	955	—	6	—	—	—	—	—	—
0	0	0	3	6	117	48	0	0.1	3	44	0.08	11	0.01	0.01	0.1	0.02	4	0
0	0	0	32	38	11	191	0.2	0.4	12	0	0.13	3	0.04	0.12	0.3	0.15	10	0
0	0	0	0	0	535	0	0	0	0	0	0	0	0	0	0	0	0	0
6.7	6.6	24	73	145	686	275	1.1	2.4	24	34	2.95	13	0.42	0.23	3.8	0.16	41	0.36
11.1	7.2	30	284	254	512	602	1.9	3	65	137	4.44	11	0.34	0.38	3.8	0.34	78	0.26
6.2	2.5	16	63	79	608	111	0.8	1.9	16	54	0.73	6	0.28	0.21	2.7	0.08	18	0.38
5	2.2	45	83	82	819	76	0.8	2	13	17	0.13	0	0.19	0.15	2.7	0.16	17	0.1
5.8	11.5	32	73	110	478	152	0.8	2.2	19	23	6.27	1	0.28	0.19	3.8	0.24	28	0.12
7	5.9	77	252	257	1311	212	3.4	2.9	26	77	2.44	1	0.18	0.31	2.6	0.16	18	1.63
6.5	11.5	152	84	129	545	128	0.8	2.3	17	73	4.74	0	0.28	0.32	2.2	0.19	40	0.42
8.9	9.4	68	185	311	939	353	1.2	3.5	37	97	1.83	3	0.46	0.42	4.2	0.11	92	1.08
5.2	0.9	58	66	212	608	355	5.3	3.7	31	0	0.15	0	0.3	0.31	5.4	0.24	26	2.11
7.4	2	56	412	488	1174	173	2.1	2.1	26	210	1.52	0	0.28	0.36	2.2	0.06	28	0.4
—	—	20	60	—	420	220	—	1.4	—	0	—	0	—	—	—	—	—	—
1.4	0.4	34	44	117	212	209	2.3	2.2	20	11	0.28	4	0.21	0.25	3.5	0.16	30	0.9
5	5.8	55	249	317	1548	333	2.5	2.2	28	76	2.43	15	0.7	0.35	3.9	0.34	15	1.13
6.6	7.2	28	66	160	901	207	1.3	2.3	32	8	3.55	4	0.5	0.23	3.6	0.2	25	0.48
3.5	4.7	36	56	218	1285	332	1.8	2.1	34	6	2.15	17	0.81	0.28	5.1	0.39	22	0.52
6.8	1.7	44	24	97	670	143	2	2.3	13	0	0.27	0	0.24	0.27	3.6	0.05	48	0.51
8.9	1.2	53	71	142	1341	242	2.7	2.6	24	3	0.21	4	0.29	0.27	4.8	0.13	21	0.99
11.4	8.2	110	215	319	682	380	6.9	4.1	35	119	3.4	0	0.24	0.45	6	0.34	24	2.36
6.7	3.9	2	60	141	293	245	1.1	2.2	56	0	0.12	0	0.27	0.17	5.3	0.13	40	0
9.9	7.6	89	319	321	1308	247	4.2	2.9	36	101	0.7	11	0.18	0.32	3.1	0.22	30	1.45
3.4	6.5	34	56	183	1267	382	3.2	3.4	34	9	2.91	10	0.24	0.25	5.4	0.33	27	1.76
8.2	2.3	36	189	287	1650	394	2.6	2.5	68	80	—	12	1	0.8	5.5	0.14	87	1.09
3.6	7.6	15	74	161	582	174	0.7	2.4	24	22	3	1	0.28	0.2	5.6	0.12	28	0.64
5.1	6.6	62	239	400	1350	345	3.1	3.6	43	88	3.11	0	0.26	0.39	4.2	0.26	29	0.35
2.2	5.4	42	40	166	917	264	2.3	3.1	19	6	2.16	0	0.17	0.26	3.3	0.22	13	0.21
2.8	6.8	35	47	289	1340	336	1.9	2.2	62	9	2.8	0	0.23	0.18	7.9	0.41	32	1.43
0.9	0	0	36	20	20	328	0.2	1.4	20	10	0.42	25	0	0.03	0.3	0.06	24	0
0.5	0	0	66	48	17	585	0.2	1.7	51	70	0.73	34	0.02	0.03	3.1	0.1	41	0
—	—	90	200	200	1100	150	—	0	0	160	—	0	0	0.2	0	—	—	—
—	—	60	300	200	1200	160	—	0	16	160	—	0	0	0.2	0	—	—	—
0	0	0	1	1	31	7	0	0.1	0	22	0.04	0	0	0	0	0.01	0	3.12
7	1	75	300	—	670	—	—	0	—	150	—	0	—	—	—	—	—	—
—	—	11	169	—	372	—	—	1.2	—	279	—	0	—	—	—	—	—	—
0.2	0.2	0	6	6	255	54	0.1	0.3	6	27	0.35	2	0.01	0.01	0.3	0.02	1	0
1.8	0.3	16	7	9	563	14	0	0.2	2	57	0.14	0	0.03	0.03	0.3	0	2	0.02
0.1	0.1	0	1	2	55	8	0	0	1	0	0.03	0	0	0	0	0	1	0
1.9	0.3	16	16	23	261	102	0.1	0.8	9	63	0.19	4	0.04	0.05	0.8	0.03	6	0.06
2.5	1.1	18	134	101	258	63	0.6	0.3	9	84	0.59	0	0.04	0.12	0.2	0.02	5	0.22
1.3	0.4	13	142	110	391	138	0.2	0.1	12	29	0.08	1	0.04	0.14	0.1	0.04	3	0.28
7.5	3.6	44	661	724	1549	397	2.9	1	40	231	2.18	2	0.14	0.56	0.6	0.12	16	1.08
—	—	0	0	1	1	29	—	0	—	3	—	3	0	0	0	—	—	—
0	0	0	1	3	76	21	0	0	1	8	0.02	1	0	0	0.1	0.01	0	0
—	—	0	14	36	14	253	—	0.5	—	96	—	11	0.06	0.05	1.1	—	—	—
1.3	0.9	0	4	19	196	52	0.1	0.3	2	31	0.41	0	0.01	0.03	0.8	0.01	1	0.06
0.9	0.3	10	20	30	92	146	0.2	0.4	11	138	0.26	27	0.03	0.04	0.7	0.05	4	0.03
2.4	0.8	22	16	22	84	98	0.1	0.3	8	195	0.43	5	0.02	0.05	0.3	0.06	6	0.03
0.2	0.3	42	126	157	5440	442	1.4	2.2	7	29	2.63	0	0.02	0.15	4	0.09	12	5.24
—	—	0	0	—	500	—	—	0	—	0	—	0	—	—	—	—	—	—
0.7	0.1	6	16	16	196	16	0.1	0.1	1	28	0.08	0	0.01	0.02	0	0.06	3	0.1
0.3	0	2	5	4	14	7	0	0	1	9	0.03	0	0	0.01	0	0	0	0.01
0	0	0	0	1	1	29	0	0	1	50	0.04	2	0	0	0	0.01	1	0
1.8	2.5	42	11	67	484	114	0.6	0.5	8	12	0.43	1	0.1	0.1	1.2	0.09	13	0.2
2.1	1.2	0	22	44	786	530	0.3	1	30	120	2	16	0.06	0.07	2	0.31	17	0
3.2	1.9	1	16	54	89	216	0.3	1.2	21	254	0.96	0	0.02	0	1.1	0.17	19	0.03
0.6	0.8	0	11	67	235	191	0.4	0.9	25	41	0.22	12	0.03	0.04	1.3	0.06	9	0.04
5	2.6	79	158	127	402	108	0.6	0.4	12	163	1.14	1	0.06	0.16	0.3	0.05	10	0.39
18.1	2.1	18	417	207	422	206	1	2.4	33	86	2.9	5	0.02	0.1	0.4	0.09	16	0.32
0	0	0	3	20	1028	32	0.1	0.4	6	0	0	0	0.01	0.02	0.6	0.03	3	0

Food Item	Qty	Meas	Wgt (g)	Wtr (g)	Cals	Prot	Carb (g)	Fib (g)	Fat (g)	SatF (g)
Sauce, soy, lite, LaChoy	1	Tbs	18	13	15	1	2	0	0	0
Sauce, soy, tamari	1	Tbs	14	10	9	2	1	0.1	0	0
Sauce, spaghetti w/meat, recipe	0.5	cup	124	94	144	8	11	2.1	8	2.3
Sauce, spaghetti w/meatballs, canned	0.5	cup	125	94	128	6	14	0.9	5	1.3
Sauce, spaghetti, Prego	0.5	cup	125	94	135	2	22	1.9	4	1.4
Sauce, spaghetti, canned	0.5	cup	124	94	136	2	20	4.2	6	0.8
Sauce, spaghetti, meat flavor, canned	0.5	cup	125	92	150	4	19	4	7	1.4
Sauce, spaghetti, w/mushrooms, canned	0.5	cup	123	103	108	2	13	1.2	3	0.4
Sauce, spaghetti/marinara	0.5	cup	125	102	94	2	13	2.5	5	0.7
Sauce, stroganoff w/milk & water	0.25	cup	62	48	57	2	7	0.1	2	1.4
Sauce, Szechuan	1	Tbs	16	13	12	0	2	0.2	0	0
Sauce, tartar	2	Tbs	28	10	149	0	1	0.1	16	3.1
Sauce, tartar, nonfat, Kraft	2	Tbs	30	—	23	0	5	0.5	0	0
Sauce, teriyaki	1	Tbs	18	12	15	1	3	0	0	0
Sauce, teriyaki, dry w/water	1	Tbs	18	15	8	0	2	—	0	0
Sauce, tomato, canned, no added salt	0.5	cup	122	109	37	2	9	1.7	0	0
Sauce, white clam	0.25	cup	60	34	149	11	2	0	11	1.4
Sauce, white, dry mix, prep w/milk	0.25	cup	66	54	60	3	5	0.1	3	1.6
Sauce, white, recipe	0.25	cup	62	48	89	2	5	0.1	7	2
Sauce, Worcestershire	1	tsp	6	4	4	0	1	0	0	0
Sauerkraut, canned, low sodium	0.5	cup	71	66	14	1	3	1.8	0	0
Sauerkraut, canned, w/liquid	0.5	cup	118	109	22	1	5	3	0	0
Sausage, Polish, pork	1	oz.	28	15	93	4	0	0	8	2.9
Sausage, braunschweiger	2	piece	57	27	205	8	2	0	18	6.2
Sausage, chorizo, link	1	each	60	19	273	14	1	0	23	8.6
Sausage, kielbasa	1	piece	26	14	81	3	1	0	7	2.6
Sausage, pepperoni, pork/beef	4	piece	22	6	109	5	1	0	10	3.5
Sausage, pork, Chinese	4	oz.	113	44	403	24	7	0	33	—
Sausage, pork, Italian link, cooked	1	each	67	34	216	13	1	0	17	6.1
Sausage, summer, thuringer, beef & pork	1	piece	23	12	77	4	0	0	7	2.8
Sausage, turkey, breakfast type	1	piece	28	17	65	6	0	0	5	1.6
Sausage, turkey, smoked	1	oz.	28	19	55	4	0	0	4	1.3
Scone	1	each	42	12	150	4	18	0.6	7	2.1
Scone, apple kiwi, fat free, Health Valley	1	each	60	35	80	7	15	7	0	0
Scone, whole wheat	1	each	42	11	145	5	18	2.8	7	2.1
Seafood salad	0.5	cup	104	76	166	12	2	0.4	12	1.6
Seafood souffle	0.5	cup	80	57	129	9	4	0.1	8	2.4
Seaweed, kelp, raw	0.5	cup	40	33	17	1	4	0.5	0	0.1
Seaweed, spirulina, dried	0.5	cup	8	0	22	4	2	0.3	1	0.2
Seeds, lupin, cooked, no salt	0.5	cup	83	59	99	13	8	2.3	2	0.3
Sego diet drink	1	cup	256	—	180	9	27	0	4	0.1
Sego lite diet drink	1	cup	256	—	120	9	16	0	2	0.4
Sesame butter, tahini, f/roasted/toasted kernels	1	Tbs	15	0	89	3	3	1.4	8	1.1
Sesame meal, partially defatted	1	oz.	28	1	161	5	7	1.1	14	1.9
Sesame seed kernels, dried	0.25	cup	38	2	221	10	4	4.4	21	2.9
Shallot, freeze dried, chopped	0.25	cup	4	0	12	0	3	0.2	0	0
Shallot, raw, chopped	1	Tbs	10	8	7	0	2	0.1	0	0
Shasta Soda, cherry cola, diet	1	cup	240	239	0	0	0	0	0	0
Shasta Soda, cream soda, diet	1	cup	240	239	0	0	0	0	0	0
Shasta Soda, ginger ale, diet	1	cup	240	239	0	0	0	0	0	0
Sherbet, orange	0.5	cup	96	64	132	1	29	0	2	1.1
Sherry, medium	1	cup	240	206	336	1	19	0	0	0
Shortening, vegetable (Crisco/Fluffo)	1	Tbs	13	0	113	0	0	0	13	3.2
Shrimp jambalaya	0.5	cup	122	88	153	14	13	0.9	5	0.9
Shrimp marinara dinner, Healthy Choice	1	each	298	243	250	10	44	5	4	2
Shrimp patty burger	1	each	120	72	248	18	15	1.3	13	3.4
Shrimp salad	0.5	cup	91	65	141	13	3	0.4	8	1.3
Shrimp w/lobster sauce	0.25	cup	46	32	72	9	2	0.1	3	0.6
Shrimp, curried	0.5	cup	118	88	157	14	7	0.2	8	2.5
Soda, 7-Up, diet	1	cup	240	240	2	0	0	0	0	0
Soda, 7-Up, regular	1	cup	240	233	28	0	7	0	0	0
Soda, Coca Cola, can/bottle	1	cup	240	215	100	0	26	0	0	0
Soda, Coca Cola, classic, can/bottle	1	cup	240	218	94	0	26	0	0	0
Soda, Coca Cola, diet, can/bottle	1	cup	240	240	1	0	0	0	0	0
Soda, Dr. Pepper type	1	cup	245	219	101	0	26	0	0	0.2

MonoF (g)	PolyF (g)	Choles (mg)	Calc (mg)	Phos (mg)	Sod (mg)	Pot (mg)	Zn (mg)	Iron (mg)	Magn (mg)	VitA (μg RE)	VitE (μg α-TE)	VitC (mg)	Thia (mg)	Ribo (mg)	Nia (mg)	B6 (mg)	Fola (μg)	B12 (μg)
—	—	0	3	—	505	—	—	0.1	—	0		0	—	—	—	—	—	—
0	0	0	3	19	810	31	0.1	0.3	6	0	0	0	0.01	0.02	0.6	0.03	3	0
2.8	2.4	23	29	86	565	542	1.7	2	31	229	2.14	18	0.09	0.13	2.9	0.26	12	0.71
2.4	0.8	16	26	56	553	123	1.1	1.6	14	220	2	2	0.08	0.1	1.2	0.16	7	1.18
—	—	0	38	—	587	—	—	1.4	—	96	—	9	—	—	—	—	—	0
3	1.6	0	35	45	618	478	0.3	0.8	30	153	2.49	14	0.07	0.07	1.9	0.44	27	0
3.5	1.6	8	34	57	590	476	0.7	1	30	288	2.96	13	0.07	0.08	2.2	0.44	26	0.25
1.5	0.8	0	15	30	496	333	0.3	1	15	241	1.36	9	0.08	0.08	0.9	0.16	13	0
1.1	2.7	0	32	51	657	565	0.5	1.6	31	138	2.52	21	0.09	0.1	1.7	0.23	12	0
0.6	0.1	8	109	63	381	140	0.2	0.3	8	26	—	0	0.18	0.16	0.2	0.02	2	0.12
0.1	0.1	0	3	3	127	27	0	0.1	3	14	0.17	1	0	0	0.1	0.01	1	0
5.2	8.1	14	5	9	198	22	0	0.3	1	18	4.48	0	0	0.01	0	0.01	1	0
0	0	0	0	—	197	14	—	0	—	0	—	0	—	—	—	—	—	—
0	0	0	4	28	690	40	0	0.3	11	0	0	0	0	0.01	0.2	0.02	4	0
0	0	0	7	13	299	13	0	0.2	5	0	0	0	0	0	0.1	0.01	2	0
0	0.1	0	17	39	741	454	0.3	0.9	23	120	1.72	16	0.08	0.07	1.4	0.19	12	0
7.3	1.1	28	42	141	245	265	1.2	11.7	8	72	1.6	9	0.06	0.18	1.4	0.05	12	40.8
1.2	0.4	9	106	64	199	111	0.1	0.1	66	23	0.4	1	0.02	0.11	0.1	0.02	4	0.26
2.3	2.2	7	65	54	92	86	0.2	0.2	8	78	0.85	1	0.05	0.1	0.2	0.02	4	0.19
0	0	0	6	3	56	45	0	0.3	1	1	0	1	0	0.01	0	0	0	0
0	0	0	21	14	219	121	0.1	1	9	1	0.07	10	0.01	0.01	0.1	0.06	17	0
0	0.1	0	35	24	780	201	0.2	1.7	15	2	0.12	17	0.02	0.03	0.2	0.15	28	0
3.8	0.9	20	3	39	249	67	0.5	0.4	4	0	0.06	0	0.14	0.04	1	0.05	1	0.28
8.5	2.1	89	5	96	652	113	1.6	5.3	6	2405	0.2	0	0.14	0.87	4.8	0.19	25	11.5
11	2.1	53	5	90	741	239	2	1	11	0	0.13	0	0.38	0.18	3.1	0.32	1	1.2
3.4	0.8	17	11	38	280	70	0.5	0.4	4	0	0.06	0	0.06	0.06	0.7	0.05	1	0.42
4.6	1	17	2	26	449	76	0.6	0.3	4	0	0.05	0	0.07	0.06	1.1	0.06	1	0.55
—	—	—	27	245	998	—	—	3.4	—	0	—	0	0.52	0.31	5.3	—	—	—
8	2.2	52	16	114	618	204	1.6	1	12	0	0.17	1	0.42	0.16	2.8	0.22	3	0.87
3	0.3	17	3	26	286	62	0.6	0.6	3	0	0.05	0	0.04	0.08	1	0.06	0	1.27
1.8	1.2	23	5	52	191	76	1	0.5	6	0	0.14	0	0.03	0.08	1.4	0.08	1	0.5
1.6	1	19	5	37	219	59	0.7	0.4	5	0	0.14	0	0.02	0.06	1.2	0.06	1	0.56
2.5	1.4	51	62	61	246	50	0.3	1.2	7	85	0.9	0	0.14	0.16	1.2	0.03	8	0.1
0	0	0	20	—	160	—	—	0.1	—	200	—	12	—	—	—	—	—	—
2.5	1.5	50	55	153	174	189	0.8	1	32	84	1.07	0	0.09	0.11	1.3	0.08	11	0.1
8.3	1.2	64	45	137	274	249	1.6	1	27	27	2.29	7	0.04	0.05	1.2	0.09	16	0.89
3.3	2	112	65	116	303	136	0.8	0.8	14	117	1.49	0	0.05	0.19	1.3	0.08	13	0.53
0	0	0	67	17	93	36	0.5	1.1	48	5	0.35	1	0.02	0.06	0.2	0	72	0
0.1	0.2	0	9	9	79	102	0.2	2.1	15	4	0.38	1	0.18	0.28	1	0.03	7	0
1	0.6	0	42	106	3	203	1.2	1	45	1	0.08	1	0.11	0.04	0.4	0.01	49	0
1.7	1.5	3	200	200	289	481	3	3.6	80	300	—	12	0.3	0.34	4	0.4	80	1.2
0.4	0.9	3	200	200	289	481	3	3.6	80	300	—	12	0.3	0.34	4	0.4	80	1.2
3	3.5	0	64	110	17	62	0.7	1.3	14	1	0.34	0	0.18	0.07	0.8	0.02	15	0
5.1	6	0	43	219	11	115	2.9	4.1	98	2	0.64	0	0.73	0.08	3.6	0.04	8	0
7.8	9	0	49	291	15	153	3.9	2.9	130	3	0.85	0	0.27	0.03	1.8	0.06	36	0
0	0	0	7	11	2	59	0.1	0.2	4	202	0.01	1	0.01	0	0	0.06	4	0
0	0	0	4	6	1	33	0	0.1	2	12	0.01	1	0.01	0	0	0.04	3	0
0	0	0	—	49	37	0	—	—	—	—	—	—	—	—	—	—	—	0
0	0	0	—	—	37	0	—	—	—	—	—	—	—	—	—	—	—	0
0	0	0	—	—	37	0	—	—	—	—	—	—	—	—	—	—	—	0
0.5	0.1	6	52	38	44	92	0.5	0.1	8	13	0.08	3	0.02	0.08	0.1	0.02	5	0.18
0	0	0	19	16	18	200	0.2	0.6	19	0	0	0	0.02	0.06	0.3	0.02	0	0
5.7	3.3	0	0	0	0	0	0	0	0	0	1.06	0	0	0	0	0	0	0
1.8	1.6	93	51	158	327	227	0.9	2.7	31	82	2.12	9	0.09	0.05	2.3	0.12	5	0.6
—	—	55	60	—	260	—	—	1.8	—	60	—	1	—	—	—	—	—	—
5.4	3.5	143	58	197	299	328	1.1	2.3	39	29	2.7	5	0.1	0.1	2.7	0.22	9	0.78
2.2	4.2	103	43	140	195	183	0.8	1.7	26	21	2.56	3	0.02	0.03	1.6	0.14	8	0.65
0.8	1.3	64	21	91	248	105	0.6	0.9	15	10	0.86	1	0.05	0.05	1.2	0.07	6	0.39
2.9	2	91	113	181	316	218	0.9	1.5	30	94	2.04	2	0.06	0.15	1.6	0.08	6	0.67
0	0	0	5	—	7	18	—	0.1	—	0	—	0	0	0	—	0	0	0
0	0	0	1	—	2	5	—	0	—	0	0	0	0	0	0	0	—	0
0	0	0	7	35	5	2	0	0.1	2	0	0	0	0	0	0	0	0	0
0	0	0	9	40	9	0	0	0.1	3	0	0	0	0	0	0	0	0	0
0	0	0	10	18	4	12	0.2	0.1	2	0	0	0	0.02	0.05	0	0	0	0
0	0	0	7	27	24	2	0.1	0.1	1	0	0	0	0	0	0	0	0	0

Food Item	Qty	Meas	Wgt (g)	Wtr (g)	Cals	Prot	Carb (g)	Fib (g)	Fat (g)	SatF (g)
Soda, Dr. Pepper type, decaf, sugar free, 12 oz can	1	each	355	354	4	0	0	0	0	0
Soda, Pepsi, diet	1	cup	240	239	0	0	0	0	0	0
Soda, Pepsi, regular	1	cup	240	212	100	0	27	0	0	0
Soda, Slice, apple, diet	1	cup	237	233	0	0	0	0	0	0
Soda, Slice, mandarin orange, diet	1	cup	237	233	0	0	0	0	0	0
Soda, Sprite, can/bottle	1	cup	240	213	93	0	25	0	0	0
Soda, Sprite, diet, can/bottle	1	cup	240	240	3	0	0	0	0	0
Soda, Tab, can/bottle	1	cup	240	239	1	0	0	0	0	0
Soda, club	1	cup	237	236	0	0	0	0	0	0
Soda, cola, caffeine-free, can/bottle	1	cup	240	212	107	0	27	0	0	0
Soda, cola, diet, w/aspartame+saccharin	1	cup	237	236	2	0	0	0	0	0
Soda, cola-type, regular	1	cup	247	221	101	0	26	0	0	0
Soda, cola/coke, diet, caffeine-free	1	cup	240	239	0	0	0	0	0	0
Soda, cola/coke, diet, w/aspartame, can/bottle	1	cup	237	236	2	0	0	0	0	0
Soda, cola/pepper type, diet, w/saccharin	1	cup	237	236	0	0	0	0	0	0
Soda, cream	1	cup	247	214	126	0	33	0	0	0
Soda, cream, sugar-free, 12 fl oz can	1	each	355	354	0	0	0	0	0	0
Soda, diet, lemon lime, Slice	1	cup	240	234	0	0	1	0	0	0
Soda, ginger ale	1	cup	244	223	83	0	21	0	0	0
Soda, ginger ale, sugar-free, 12 fl oz can	1	each	355	354	0	0	0	0	0	0
Soda, grape, carbonated	1	cup	248	220	107	0	28	0	0	0
Soda, lemon lime	1	cup	245	220	98	0	26	0	0	0
Soda, Mountain Dew	1	cup	240	—	113	0	31	0	0	0
Soda, orange, Minute Maid, can/bottle	1	cup	240	209	113	0	31	0	0	0
Soda, Pepsi, diet, caffeine free	1	cup	240	239	0	0	0	0	0	0
Soda, root beer	1	cup	247	220	101	0	26	0	0	0
Sorbet, fruit, citrus flavor	0.5	cup	100	76	92	0	23	0.1	0	0
Sorbet, fruit, non-citrus flavor	0.5	cup	100	82	70	1	17	0	0	0
Souffle, cheese	0.5	cup	56	40	98	6	3	0	7	2.8
Souffle, spinach	0.5	cup	68	50	109	5	1	1.4	9	3.6
Soup, Home Cookin', hearty lentil, RTS	0.5	cup	122	105	65	4	12	2.5	0	0.2
Soup, Pasta Fagioli, fat free, Health Valley	0.5	cup	120	107	40	3	8	2	0	0
Soup, Scotch broth, w/water	0.5	cup	120	111	40	2	5	0.6	1	0.6
Soup, bean & ham, chunky, RTS	0.5	cup	122	96	115	6	14	5.6	4	1.7
Soup, bean and 'frank', w/water	1	cup	150	125	113	6	13	3.4	4	1.3
Soup, bean with bacon, prep w/water	0.5	cup	126	107	86	4	11	4.3	3	0.8
Soup, beef and mushroom, w/water	0.5	cup	122	113	37	3	3	0.1	2	0.7
Soup, beef broth/bouillon, condensed, prepared	0.5	cup	120	117	8	1	0	0	0	0.1
Soup, beef noodle, prep w/water	0.5	cup	122	112	42	2	4	0.4	2	0.6
Soup, beef stroganoff, chunky style	0.5	cup	120	96	118	6	11	0.7	6	2.5
Soup, beef, chunky, RTS	0.5	cup	120	100	85	6	10	0.7	3	1.3
Soup, bisque, tomato, prepared, w/milk	0.5	cup	126	102	99	3	15	0.3	3	1.6
Soup, bisque, tomato, w/water	0.5	cup	124	108	62	1	12	0.2	1	0.3
Soup, black bean, w/water	0.5	cup	124	108	58	3	10	2.2	1	0.2
Soup, bouillabaisse	0.5	cup	114	88	121	17	2	0.3	4	1
Soup, broth, chicken, dry cube, prepared	0.5	cup	122	118	6	0	1	0	0	0
Soup, broth/bouillon, beef, canned, low sodium	0.5	cup	120	115	19	2	0	0	1	0.2
Soup, broth/bouillon, beef, dry cube, prepared	0.5	cup	120	118	4	0	0	0	0	0
Soup, broth/bouillon, beef, dry, w/water	0.5	cup	122	118	10	1	1	0	0	0.2
Soup, broth/bouillon, chicken, condensed, prepared	0.5	cup	122	117	20	2	0	0	1	0.2
Soup, cauliflower, dry, w/water	0.5	cup	128	119	35	1	5	0.1	1	0.1
Soup, cheese, condensed	1	cup	257	198	311	11	21	2.1	21	13.3
Soup, cheese, prepared w/milk	0.5	cup	126	103	115	5	8	0.5	7	4.6
Soup, cheese, prepared w/water	0.5	cup	124	109	78	3	5	0.5	5	3.3
Soup, chicken & vegetable, chunky, RTS	1	cup	240	200	166	12	19	0.2	5	1.4
Soup, chicken and dumpling, prep w/water	0.5	cup	120	111	48	3	3	0.2	3	0.7
Soup, chicken gumbo, prep w/water	0.5	cup	122	114	28	1	4	1	1	0.2
Soup, chicken mushroom, w/water	0.5	cup	122	110	66	2	5	0.1	5	1.2
Soup, chicken noodle & meatballs, RTS	0.5	cup	124	112	50	4	4	0.3	2	0.5
Soup, chicken noodle, chunky, RTS	0.5	cup	120	101	88	6	9	1.9	3	0.7
Soup, chicken noodle, chunky, RTS	1	cup	240	202	175	13	17	3.8	6	1.4
Soup, chicken noodle, prep w/water	0.5	cup	120	111	37	2	5	0.4	1	0.3
Soup, chicken rice, chunky, RTS	0.5	cup	120	104	64	6	6	0.5	2	0.5
Soup, chicken rice, w/water	0.5	cup	120	113	30	2	4	0.4	1	0.2
Soup, chicken vegetable, prep w/water	0.5	cup	120	112	37	2	4	0.5	1	0.4

MonoF	PolyF	Choles	Calc	Phos	Sod	Pot	Zn	Iron	Magn	VitA	VitE	VitC	Thia	Ribo	Nia	B6	Fola	B12
(g)	(g)	(mg)	(mg)	(mg)	(mg)	(mg)	(mg)	(mg)	(mg)	(µg RE)	(µg α-TE)	(mg)	(mg)	(mg)	(mg)	(mg)	(µg)	(µg)
0	0	0	14	32	21	0	0.3	0.1	4	0	0	0	0.02	0.08	0	0	0	0
0	0	0	0	27	23	5	—	0	—	0	—	0	—	—	—	—	—	0
0	0	0	0	35	23	—	—	0	—	0	—	0	—	—	—	—	—	0
0	0	0	0	0	33	—	—	0	—	0	—	0	—	—	—	—	—	0
0	0	0	0	0	33	—	—	0	—	0	—	0	—	—	—	—	—	0
0	0	0	5	0	22	0	0.1	0.2	2	0	0	0	0	0	0	0	0	0
0	0	0	10	0	0	67	0.1	0.1	—	0	0	0	0	0	0	—	0	0
0	0	0	8	30	4	12	—	0.1	—	0	0	0	0	0	0	0	0	0
0	0	0	12	0	50	5	0.2	0	2	0	0	0	0	0	0	0	0	0
0	0	0	—	33	30	0	—	—	—	—	—	—	—	—	—	—	—	0
0	0	0	9	21	21	0	0.2	0.1	2	0	0	0	0.01	0.05	0	0	0	0
0	0	0	7	30	10	2	0	0.1	2	0	0	0	0	0	0	0	0	0
0	0	0	—	33	37	36	—	—	—	—	—	—	—	—	—	—	—	0
0	0	0	9	21	14	0	0.2	0.1	2	0	0	0	0.01	0.05	0	0	0	0
0	0	0	9	26	38	5	0.1	0.1	2	0	0	0	0	0	0	0	0	0
0	0	0	12	0	30	2	0.2	0.1	2	0	0	0	0	0	0	0	0	0
0	0	0	14	39	57	7	0.2	0.1	4	0	0	0	0	0	0	0	0	0
0	0	0	0	0	23	—	—	0	—	0	—	0	—	—	—	—	—	0
0	0	0	7	0	17	2	0.1	0.4	2	0	0	0	0	0	0	0	0	0
0	0	0	14	39	57	7	0.2	0.1	4	0	0	0	0	0	0	0	0	0
0	0	0	7	0	37	2	0.2	0.2	2	0	0	0	0	0	0	0	0	0
0	0	0	5	0	27	2	0.1	0.2	2	0	0	0	0	0	0	0	0	0
0	0	—	0	0	47	—	—	0	—	0	—	0	—	—	—	—	—	0
0	0	0	5	0	0	13	0.1	0.2	2	0	0	0	0	0	0	0	0	0
0	0	—	0	27	23	—	—	0	—	0	—	0	—	—	—	—	—	0
0	0	0	12	0	32	2	0.2	0.1	2	0	0	0	0	0	0	0	0	0
0	0	0	9	13	8	100	0	0.5	8	27	0.05	26	0.01	0.03	0.2	0.02	22	0
0	0	0	2	0	46	2	0	0	1	0	0	0	0	0	0	0	0	0
2.4	1.4	97	105	100	149	73	0.5	0.4	8	84	0.64	0	0.04	0.18	0.1	0.04	12	0.39
3.4	1.5	92	115	116	381	101	0.6	0.7	19	337	0.61	2	0.05	0.15	0.2	0.06	40	0.68
0	0	0	20	—	430	—	—	1.8	—	200	—	0	—	—	—	—	—	—
0	0	0	20	—	125	—	—	0.1	—	200	—	8	—	—	—	—	—	—
0.4	0.3	2	7	28	506	80	0.8	0.4	2	108	0.04	0	0.01	0.02	0.6	0.04	5	0.13
1.9	0.5	11	39	72	486	213	0.5	1.6	23	198	0.06	2	0.07	0.07	0.9	0.06	15	0.04
1.6	1	8	52	99	656	287	0.7	1.4	28	52	—	1	0.07	0.04	0.6	0.08	18	0.04
1.1	0.9	1	40	66	476	201	0.5	1	23	44	0.04	1	0.04	0.02	0.3	0.02	16	0.02
0.6	0.1	4	2	17	471	77	0.7	0.4	5	0	—	2	0.02	0.03	0.5	0.02	5	0.1
0.1	0	1	7	16	391	65	0	0.2	2	0	0	0	0	0.02	0.9	0.01	2	0.08
0.6	0.2	2	7	23	476	50	0.8	0.5	2	32	0	0	0.03	0.03	0.5	0.02	10	0.1
2.1	1.2	25	24	60	522	168	1.3	1.1	2	98	0.76	0	0.05	0.11	0.1	0.07	7	0.31
1.1	0.1	7	16	60	433	168	1.3	1.2	2	131	0.08	3	0.03	0.08	1.4	0.07	7	0.31
0.9	0.6	11	93	87	555	302	0.3	0.4	13	55	0.5	4	0.06	0.13	0.6	0.07	11	0.21
0.3	0.6	2	20	30	524	209	0.3	0.4	5	36	0.37	3	0.03	0.04	0.6	0.04	7	0
0.3	0.2	0	22	53	599	137	0.7	1.1	21	25	0.04	0	0.04	0.03	0.3	0.05	12	0.01
2	0.7	45	41	170	208	366	0.9	2	37	44	1.15	6	0.12	0.09	2.5	0.19	14	5.21
0.1	0	0	6	6	396	12	0	0.1	1	2	0.02	0	0.01	0.01	0.1	0	1	0.01
0.3	0.1	0	5	36	36	103	0.1	0.3	1	0	0.02	0	0	0.04	1.6	0.01	2	0.12
0	0	0	1	6	578	10	0	0.1	1	0	0	0	0	0.01	0.2	0	0	0
0.1	0	0	5	12	681	18	0	0	4	1	0.01	0	0	0.04	1.7	0.01	2	0.12
0.3	0.1	0	5	37	388	105	0.1	0.3	1	0	0.02	0	0	0.04	1.7	0.01	2	0.12
0.4	0.3	0	5	26	421	52	0.1	0.3	1	0	—	1	0.04	0.04	0.3	0.01	1	0.09
5.9	0.6	59	285	272	1919	308	1.3	1.5	8	218	0.41	0	0.03	0.27	0.8	0.05	8	0
2	0.2	24	144	126	510	171	0.3	0.4	10	74	0.13	1	0.03	0.17	0.3	0.04	5	0.21
1.5	0.1	15	70	68	479	77	0.3	0.4	2	54	—	0	0.01	0.07	0.2	0.01	2	0
2.2	1	17	26	106	1068	367	2.2	1.5	10	600	0.07	6	0.04	0.17	3.3	0.1	12	0.24
1.3	0.7	17	7	30	430	58	0.2	0.3	2	26	0.07	0	0.01	0.04	0.9	0.02	1	0.08
0.3	0.2	2	12	12	477	38	0.2	0.5	2	7	0.02	2	0.01	0.02	0.3	0.03	2	0.01
2	1.2	5	15	13	471	77	0.5	0.4	5	56	0.61	0	0.01	0.06	0.8	0.02	0	0.02
0.8	0.4	5	15	42	520	77	0.2	0.9	5	117	—	4	0.06	0.06	1.2	0.02	11	0.12
1.3	0.8	10	12	36	425	54	0.5	0.7	5	61	0.4	0	0.04	0.08	2.2	0.02	19	0.16
2.7	1.5	19	24	72	850	108	1	1.4	10	122	0.79	0	0.07	0.17	4.3	0.05	38	0.31
0.6	0.3	4	8	18	553	28	0.2	0.4	2	36	0.04	0	0.03	0.03	0.7	0.01	11	0.07
0.7	0.3	6	17	36	444	54	0.5	0.9	5	293	0.04	2	0.01	0.05	2	0.02	2	0.16
0.5	0.2	4	8	11	407	51	0.1	0.4	0	32	0.03	0	0.01	0.01	0.6	0.01	0	0.07
0.6	0.3	5	8	20	472	77	0.2	0.4	4	133	0.04	0	0.02	0.03	0.6	0.02	2	0.06

Food Item	Qty	Meas	Wgt (g)	Wtr (g)	Cals	Prot	Carb (g)	Fib (g)	Fat (g)	SatF (g)
Soup, chicken, chunky, ready to serve	0.5	cup	126	106	89	6	9	0.8	3	1
Soup, chili beef, w/water	0.5	cup	125	106	85	3	11	4.8	3	1.7
Soup, consomme, w/gelatin, prepared mix	0.5	cup	124	118	9	1	1	0	0	0
Soup, crab bisque	0.5	cup	124	100	127	10	6	0.2	7	2.3
Soup, crab, RTS	0.5	cup	122	112	38	3	5	0.4	1	0.2
Soup, cream of asparagus, condensed	1	cup	251	211	173	5	21	1	8	2.1
Soup, cream of asparagus, w/milk	0.5	cup	124	107	81	3	8	0.4	4	1.7
Soup, cream of asparagus, w/water	0.5	cup	122	112	43	1	5	0.2	2	0.5
Soup, cream of bacon, prepared w/water	0.5	cup	122	111	59	2	5	0.1	4	1
Soup, cream of broccoli	0.5	cup	118	96	117	4	8	0.9	8	3
Soup, cream of celery, condensed	1	cup	251	213	181	3	18	1.5	11	2.8
Soup, cream of celery, dry, w/water	0.5	cup	127	119	32	1	5	0.2	1	0.1
Soup, cream of celery, w/milk	0.5	cup	124	107	82	3	7	0.4	5	2
Soup, cream of celery, w/water	0.5	cup	122	113	45	1	4	0.4	3	0.7
Soup, cream of chicken, w/milk	0.5	cup	124	105	96	4	7	0.1	6	2.3
Soup, cream of chicken, w/water	0.5	cup	122	111	59	2	5	0.1	4	1
Soup, cream of mushroom, condensed	1	cup	251	204	259	4	19	0.8	19	5.2
Soup, cream of mushroom, w/milk	0.5	cup	124	105	102	3	8	0.2	7	2.6
Soup, cream of mushroom, w/water	0.5	cup	122	110	65	1	5	0.2	5	1.2
Soup, cream of onion, w/milk	0.5	cup	124	105	93	3	9	0.4	5	2
Soup, cream of onion, w/water	0.5	cup	122	110	54	1	6	0.5	3	0.7
Soup, cream of potato, w/milk	0.5	cup	124	108	74	3	9	0.2	3	1.9
Soup, cream of potato, w/water	0.5	cup	122	113	37	1	6	0.2	1	0.6
Soup, cream of salmon	0.5	cup	124	96	129	14	3	0.1	6	1.7
Soup, cream of shrimp, w/milk	0.5	cup	124	107	82	3	7	0.1	5	2.9
Soup, cream of shrimp, w/water	0.5	cup	122	112	45	1	4	0.1	3	1.6
Soup, cream of vegetable, dry, prep w/water	0.5	cup	130	119	53	1	6	0.3	3	0.7
Soup, egg drop	0.5	cup	122	114	36	4	1	0	2	0.6
Soup, escarole, RTS	0.5	cup	124	120	14	1	1	—	1	0.3
Soup, gazpacho, RTS	0.5	cup	122	114	23	4	2	0.2	0	0
Soup, green pea, canned, w/milk	0.5	cup	127	99	119	6	16	1.4	4	2
Soup, green pea, w/water	0.5	cup	125	104	82	4	13	1.4	1	0.7
Soup, hot & sour/hot & spicy	0.5	cup	122	107	66	6	3	0.2	3	1
Soup, leek, dry, w/water	0.5	cup	127	118	36	1	6	1.5	1	0.5
Soup, lentil & ham, RTS	0.5	cup	124	106	69	5	10	1	1	0.6
Soup, lobster bisque	0.5	cup	124	98	136	10	6	0.1	8	2.9
Soup, lobster gumbo	0.5	cup	122	102	89	5	10	2	4	0.7
Soup, minestrone, Real Italian, Health Valley	4	oz.	113	99	38	4	10	5.2	0	0
Soup, minestrone, chunky, RTS	0.5	cup	120	104	64	3	10	2.9	1	0.7
Soup, minestrone, dry, prepared	0.5	cup	127	116	39	2	6	0.7	1	0.4
Soup, minestrone, w/water	0.5	cup	120	110	41	2	6	0.5	1	0.3
Soup, mushroom & beef stock, w/water	0.5	cup	122	112	43	2	5	0.4	2	0.8
Soup, mushroom barley, w/water	0.5	cup	122	113	37	1	6	0.4	1	0.2
Soup, mushroom, dry, prep w/water	0.5	cup	126	116	48	1	6	0.4	2	0.4
Soup, onion, w/water	0.5	cup	120	112	29	2	4	0.5	1	0.1
Soup, oxtail, dry, w/water	0.5	cup	126	118	35	1	4	0.3	1	0.6
Soup, pea, prepared w/water, low sodium	0.5	cup	125	104	82	4	13	0.4	2	0.7
Soup, pepper pot, prep w/water	0.5	cup	120	109	52	3	5	0.2	2	1
Soup, pork rice and vegetable	0.5	cup	122	109	61	6	4	0.5	2	0.7
Soup, split pea & ham, chunky, RTS	0.5	cup	120	97	92	6	13	2	2	0.8
Soup, split pea and carrot, Health Valley	4	oz.	113	101	52	4	8	1.9	0	0
Soup, split pea and ham, w/water	0.5	cup	126	103	95	5	14	1.1	2	0.9
Soup, stock pot, w/water	0.5	cup	124	112	50	2	6	0.2	2	0.4
Soup, sweet and sour	0.5	cup	122	110	37	2	8	0.9	0	0.1
Soup, tomato beef noodle, w/water	0.5	cup	122	106	70	2	11	0.7	2	0.8
Soup, tomato rice, w/water	0.5	cup	124	109	59	1	11	0.7	1	0.3
Soup, tomato vegetable, dry, prep w/water	0.5	cup	126	118	28	1	5	0.3	0	0.2
Soup, tomato, dry, prep w/water	0.5	cup	132	119	52	1	10	0.3	1	0.5
Soup, tomato, low sodium, RTS	0.5	cup	122	105	70	2	12	0.8	2	1
Soup, tomato, w/milk	0.5	cup	124	105	81	3	11	1.4	3	1.4
Soup, tomato, w/water	0.5	cup	122	110	43	1	8	0.2	1	0.2
Soup, turkey noodle, w/water	0.5	cup	122	113	34	2	4	0.4	1	0.3
Soup, turkey vegetable, w/water	0.5	cup	120	112	36	2	4	0.2	2	0.4
Soup, turkey, chunky, RTS	0.5	cup	118	102	67	5	7	0.5	2	0.6
Soup, turtle and vegetable	0.5	cup	122	110	59	6	2	0.3	2	0.4

MonoF	PolyF	Choles	Calc	Phos	Sod	Pot	Zn	Iron	Magn	VitA	VitE	VitC	Thia	Ribo	Nia	B6	Fola	B12
(g)	(g)	(mg)	(mg)	(mg)	(mg)	(mg)	(mg)	(mg)	(mg)	(µg RE)	(µg α-TE)	(mg)	(mg)	(mg)	(mg)	(mg)	(µg)	(µg)
1.5	0.7	15	13	56	444	88	0.5	0.9	4	65	0.09	1	0.04	0.09	2.2	0.02	2	0.13
1.4	0.1	6	21	74	518	263	0.7	1.1	15	75	0.09	2	0.03	0.04	0.5	0.08	9	0.16
0	0	0	4	20	1649	29	0	0.1	4	0	0	0	0	0.01	0.3	0.01	2	0.06
2.5	1.5	46	125	149	290	242	1.9	0.5	23	74	1.06	2	0.08	0.15	1.5	0.1	23	2.9
0.3	0.2	5	33	44	617	163	0.7	0.6	7	26	0.12	0	0.1	0.04	0.7	0.06	7	0.1
1.9	3.7	10	58	78	1962	346	1.8	1.6	8	90	1.26	6	0.11	0.16	1.6	0.02	48	0.1
1	1.1	11	87	77	521	180	0.5	0.4	10	42	0.42	2	0.05	0.14	0.4	0.03	15	0.25
0.5	0.9	2	15	20	490	87	0.4	0.4	2	22	0.33	1	0.03	0.04	0.4	0.01	11	0.02
1.6	0.7	5	17	18	493	44	0.3	0.3	1	28	0.1	0	0.02	0.03	0.4	0.01	1	0.05
3	1.7	12	123	104	394	214	0.4	0.3	18	104	0.74	22	0.05	0.19	0.3	0.08	19	0.31
2.6	5	28	80	75	1900	246	0.3	1.3	13	60	0.38	1	0.06	0.1	0.7	0.02	5	0.1
0.4	0.3	0	18	16	419	55	0.1	0.3	3	14	0.13	0	0.01	0.02	0.2	0	1	0.02
1.2	1.3	16	93	76	505	155	0.1	0.3	11	34	0.48	1	0.04	0.12	0.2	0.03	4	0.25
0.6	1.3	7	20	18	475	61	0.1	0.3	4	16	0.45	0	0.02	0.02	0.2	0.01	1	0.12
2.2	0.8	14	90	76	523	136	0.3	0.3	9	47	0.12	1	0.04	0.13	0.5	0.03	4	0.27
1.6	0.7	5	17	18	493	44	0.3	0.3	1	28	0.1	0	0.02	0.03	0.4	0.01	1	0.05
3.6	8.9	3	65	85	1736	168	1.2	1	10	0	2.61	2	0.06	0.17	1.6	0.02	8	0.25
1.5	2.3	10	89	78	459	135	0.3	0.3	10	19	0.67	1	0.04	0.14	0.5	0.03	5	0.25
0.9	0.9	1	23	24	24	50	0.3	0.3	2	0	0.62	0	0.02	0.05	0.4	0.01	2	0.02
1.6	0.8	16	89	77	502	155	0.3	0.3	11	35	0.04	1	0.05	0.14	0.3	0.04	11	0.25
1	0.7	7	17	18	464	60	0.1	0.3	2	15	0.37	1	0.03	0.04	0.3	0.01	3	0.02
0.9	0.3	11	83	81	531	161	0.3	0.3	9	34	0.05	1	0.04	0.12	0.3	0.04	5	0.25
0.3	0.2	2	10	23	500	68	0.3	0.2	1	15	0.01	0	0.02	0.02	0.3	0.02	1	0.02
2.2	1.8	37	144	225	767	262	0.8	0.8	22	30	0.89	1	0.03	0.14	4.8	0.2	11	2.77
1.3	0.2	17	82	73	518	124	0.4	0.3	11	27	0.43	0	0.03	0.11	0.3	0.22	5	0.52
0.7	0.1	9	9	16	488	29	0.4	0.3	5	7	0.42	0	0.01	0.01	0.2	0.02	2	0.29
1.3	0.7	0	16	27	585	48	0.1	0.3	5	1	0.62	2	0.61	0.05	0.3	0.01	4	0.06
0.8	0.3	52	10	54	364	110	0.2	0.4	2	20	0.26	0	0.01	0.09	1.5	0.03	8	0.25
0.4	0.2	1	16	40	1931	133	1.1	0.4	2	109	—	2	0.04	0.02	1.2	0.11	17	0.25
0	0	0	12	18	370	112	0.1	0.5	4	131	0.23	4	0.02	0.01	0.5	0.07	5	0
1.1	0.3	9	86	119	485	188	0.9	1	28	29	0.09	1	0.08	0.13	0.7	0.05	4	0.22
0.5	0.2	0	14	62	459	95	0.9	1	20	10	0.05	1	0.05	0.03	0.6	0.03	1	0
1.2	0.5	11	15	80	781	176	0.6	0.9	14	1	0.06	0	0.1	0.11	2.3	0.07	6	0.17
0.4	0	1	15	15	483	44	0.1	0.3	5	0	0.08	1	0.02	0.01	0.1	0.01	4	0.01
0.6	0.2	4	21	92	660	179	0.4	1.3	11	17	0.12	2	0.09	0.06	0.7	0.11	25	0.15
2.9	1.6	36	135	153	429	269	1.3	0.3	25	97	1.14	1	0.05	0.18	0.5	0.07	9	1.29
1.5	1.2	12	54	64	335	305	0.8	0.9	27	103	1.11	14	0.1	0.06	1.1	0.1	34	0.51
0	0	0	19	—	99	—	—	1.7	—	945	—	2	—	—	—	—	—	—
0.5	0.1	2	30	55	432	306	0.7	0.9	7	217	0.36	2	0.03	0.06	0.6	0.12	26	0
0.4	0.1	1	19	30	513	170	0.4	0.5	4	15	0.02	1	0.04	0.02	0.5	0.05	18	0
0.3	0.6	1	17	28	455	157	0.4	0.5	4	117	0.04	1	0.03	0.02	0.5	0.05	18	0
0.7	0.4	4	5	18	484	79	0.7	0.4	5	62	0.28	0	0.02	0.05	0.6	0.02	5	0
0.5	0.4	0	6	30	445	46	0.2	0.3	5	10	0.18	0	0.01	0.04	0.4	0.08	2	0
1.1	0.8	0	33	38	510	100	0	0.3	3	0	0.32	1	0.14	0.06	0.2	0.01	3	0.13
0.4	0.3	0	13	6	527	34	0.3	0.3	1	0	0.14	1	0.02	0.01	0.3	0.02	8	0
0.5	0.1	1	5	30	605	42	0	0.1	5	2	0.04	0	0.01	0.01	0.4	0.01	3	0.13
0.5	0.2	0	14	62	12	95	0.8	1	20	10	0.05	1	0.05	0.04	0.6	0.02	1	0
1	0.2	5	12	20	486	76	0.6	0.4	2	43	0.04	1	0.03	0.02	0.6	0.03	5	0.08
1	0.2	19	9	48	301	110	1	0.5	8	247	0.11	1	0.12	0.07	1.2	0.11	4	0.12
0.8	0.3	4	17	89	482	152	1.6	1.1	19	244	0.07	3	0.06	0.05	1.3	0.11	2	0.12
0	0	0	19	—	109	208	—	2.6	—	945	—	4	0.05	0.08	2.7	0.21	—	—
0.9	0.3	4	11	106	503	200	0.7	1.1	24	23	0.08	1	0.07	0.04	0.7	0.03	1	0.13
0.5	0.9	2	11	27	526	119	0.6	0.4	2	200	—	1	0.02	0.03	0.6	0.04	5	0
0.1	0.1	2	14	24	661	139	0.2	0.3	9	15	0.26	9	0.04	0.03	0.5	0.06	9	0.02
0.9	0.3	2	9	28	459	110	0.4	0.6	4	27	0.39	0	0.04	0.04	0.9	0.04	10	0.1
0.3	0.7	1	11	17	408	165	0.3	0.4	2	38	0.4	7	0.03	0.02	0.5	0.04	7	0
0.2	0	0	4	15	573	52	0.1	0.3	10	10	0.4	3	0.03	0.02	0.4	0.02	5	0
0.5	0.1	0	26	33	472	147	0.1	0.2	7	41	0.42	2	0.03	0.02	0.4	0.05	3	0.04
—	—	4	16	—	25	—	—	0.6	—	51	—	15	—	—	—	—	—	—
0.8	0.6	9	79	74	372	224	0.1	0.9	11	55	1.3	34	0.07	0.12	0.8	0.08	10	0.22
0.2	0.5	0	6	17	348	132	0.1	0.9	4	34	1.24	33	0.04	0.03	0.7	0.06	7	0
0.4	0.2	2	6	24	407	38	0.3	0.5	2	15	0.03	0	0.04	0.03	0.7	0.02	10	0.07
0.7	0.3	1	8	20	453	88	0.3	0.4	2	122	0.07	0	0.01	0.02	0.5	0.02	2	0.08
0.9	0.5	5	25	52	461	181	1.1	1	12	358	0.06	3	0.02	0.05	1.8	0.15	6	1.06
0.6	0.9	30	34	59	236	140	0.3	0.6	9	21	0.33	3	0.04	0.08	0.8	0.05	9	0.28

Food Item	Qty	Meas	Wgt (g)	Wtr (g)	Cals	Prot	Carb (g)	Fib (g)	Fat (g)	SatF (g)
Soup, vegetable & beef broth, w/water	0.5	cup	120	110	41	1	7	0.2	1	0.2
Soup, vegetable beef, dry, prep w/water	0.5	cup	126	119	27	1	4	0.3	1	0.3
Soup, vegetable beef, w/water	0.5	cup	122	112	39	3	5	0.2	1	0.4
Soup, vegetable chicken, low sodium, w/water	0.5	cup	120	100	83	6	10	0.5	2	0.7
Soup, vegetable, canned, low sodium	0.5	cup	120	110	41	1	6	0.4	1	0.2
Soup, vegetable, chunky, RTS	0.5	cup	120	105	61	2	10	0.6	2	0.3
Soup, vegetable, from dry mix, low sodium	0.5	cup	126	118	28	1	5	0.3	0	0.2
Soup, vegetable, vegetarian, w/water	0.5	cup	120	111	36	1	6	0.2	1	0.1
Soup, vichyssoise	0.5	cup	124	108	74	3	9	0.2	3	1.9
Soup, won ton	0.5	cup	120	101	94	7	8	0.5	3	1.1
Sour cream, nonfat	2	Tbs	28	21	31	2	5	0	0	0
Soursop, raw pulp	1	each	225	183	149	2	38	7.4	1	0.1
Soy drink, So Good Lite	1	cup	260	229	114	9	17	2.1	2	0.3
Soy drink, So Good	1	cup	255	222	158	8	13	2	8	0.8
Soy flour, defatted, stirred	1	cup	88	6	290	41	34	15.4	1	0.1
Soy milk	1	cup	240	224	79	7	4	3.1	5	0.5
Soy milk, fat-free, Soy Moo, Health Valley	1	cup	54	48	25	1	5	0.2	0	0
Soybean sprouts, raw	0.5	cup	35	24	43	5	3	0.4	2	0.3
Soybean sprouts, steamed	0.5	cup	47	37	38	4	3	0.4	2	0.3
Soybean, fermented/Natto	0.5	cup	88	48	186	16	13	4.7	10	1.4
Soybeans, dry, cooked	0.5	cup	86	54	149	14	9	5.2	8	1.1
Soybeans, dry, roasted	0.5	cup	86	1	387	34	28	7	19	2.7
Soybeans, green, cooked	0.5	cup	90	62	127	11	10	3.8	6	0.7
Spaghetti, w/meatballs, canned	1	cup	250	195	258	12	28	5.8	10	2.2
Spaghetti, w/sauce & cheese, canned	1	cup	250	200	190	6	38	2.5	2	0
Spaghetti, w/white clam sauce	0.5	cup	124	78	228	13	21	1.1	10	1.3
Spinach, canned, drained, no added salt	0.5	cup	107	98	25	3	4	2.6	1	0.1
Spinach, cooked, drained, no added salt	0.5	cup	90	82	21	3	3	2.2	0	0
Spinach, frozen, cooked, drained, no added salt	0.5	cup	95	86	27	3	5	2.8	0	0
Spinach, frozen, unprepared	0.5	cup	78	71	19	2	3	2.3	0	0
Spinach, raw, chopped	0.5	cup	28	26	6	1	1	0.8	0	0
Spinach, steamed	0.5	cup	14	13	3	0	0	0.4	0	0
Spinach, stir fried	0.5	cup	90	82	20	3	3	2.4	0	0
Sport drink, orange, All Sport	1	cup	240	—	47	0	13	0	0	0
Sports bar, Tiger	1	each	65	11	230	11	40	4	2	—
Spread, Touch of Butter, tub	1	Tbs	14	5	77	0	0	0	9	2
Spring roll w/meat	1	each	64	42	114	5	9	0.7	6	1.5
Squash, acorn, baked cubes	0.5	cup	102	85	57	1	15	4.5	0	0
Squash, acorn, baked, mashed	0.5	cup	122	102	69	1	18	5.4	0	0
Squash, butternut, baked cubes	0.5	cup	102	90	41	1	11	2.9	0	0
Squash, butternut, baked, mashed	0.5	cup	122	108	49	1	13	3.4	0	0
Squash, crookneck, canned slices, drained	0.5	cup	108	104	14	1	3	1.5	0	0
Squash, crookneck, cooked	0.5	cup	90	84	18	1	4	1.3	0	0.1
Squash, hubbard, baked	0.5	cup	120	102	60	3	13	3.2	1	0.2
Squash, scallop, cooked, mashed	0.5	cup	120	102	60	3	13	3.2	1	0.2
Squash, scallop, slices, cooked	0.5	cup	120	114	19	1	4	2.3	0	0
Squash, spaghetti, cooked	0.5	cup	90	86	14	1	3	1.7	0	0
Squash, summer, cooked slices	0.5	cup	78	72	21	1	5	1.1	0	0
Squash, summer, raw slices	0.5	cup	90	84	18	1	4	1.3	0	0.1
Squash, winter, baked cubes	0.5	cup	65	61	13	1	3	1.2	0	0
Squash, winter, cooked w/salt, no sugar, no fat	0.5	cup	102	91	40	1	9	2.9	1	0.1
Squash, zucchini slices, steamed	0.5	cup	120	106	46	1	10	3.3	1	0.2
Squash, zucchini w/peel, frozen, cooked	0.5	cup	90	86	13	1	3	1.1	0	0
Squash, zucchini, baby, raw	1	each	112	106	19	1	4	1.4	0	0
Squash, zucchini, canned, Italian style	1	each	16	15	3	0	0	0.2	0	0
Squash, zucchini, cooked	0.5	cup	114	103	33	1	8	2.3	0	0
Squash, zucchini, raw	0.5	cup	90	85	14	1	4	1.3	0	0
Squash, zucchini, stir fried, no oil	0.5	cup	65	62	9	1	2	0.8	0	0
Stew, beef & vegetable, canned	0.5	cup	90	86	13	1	3	1.1	0	0
Stew, Brunswick	1	cup	245	202	194	14	17	2.4	8	2.4
Stew, lamb, tomato base sauce	1	cup	250	208	174	16	21	3.2	4	1
Stew, oyster, prep w/milk	0.5	cup	126	96	136	9	14	2.9	5	2.2
Stew, oyster, prep w/water	1	cup	245	218	135	6	10	0	8	5
Stew, seafood, tomato base sauce	0.5	cup	120	114	29	1	2	0	2	1.2
Stew, veal, tomato base sauce	0.5	cup	126	104	84	10	8	1.2	1	0.4
	0.5	cup	126	105	95	8	8	1.3	3	1.4

MonoF (g)	PolyF (g)	Choles (mg)	Calc (mg)	Phos (mg)	Sod (mg)	Pot (mg)	Zn (mg)	Iron (mg)	Magn (mg)	VitA (µg RE)	VitE (µg α-TE)	VitC (mg)	Thia (mg)	Ribo (mg)	Nia (mg)	B6 (mg)	Fola (µg)	B12 (µg)
0.3	0.4	1	8	19	405	96	0.4	0.5	4	105	0.16	1	0.02	0.02	0.5	0.03	5	0
0.2	0	0	6	18	501	38	0.1	0.4	11	11	0.02	1	0.02	0.02	0.2	0.03	4	0.13
0.4	0.1	2	9	21	395	87	0.8	0.6	2	95	0.16	1	0.02	0.02	0.5	0.04	5	0.16
1.1	0.5	8	13	53	42	184	1.1	0.7	5	301	0.06	3	0.02	0.08	1.6	0.05	6	0.12
0.5	0.5	0	19	11	21	133	1.1	0.6	3	198	0.27	2	0.02	0.02	0.4	0.06	6	0
0.8	0.7	0	28	36	505	198	1.6	0.8	4	294	0.3	3	0.04	0.03	0.6	0.1	8	0
0.1	0	0	4	15	25	52	0.1	0.3	10	10	0.4	3	0.02	0.02	0.4	0.02	5	0
0.4	0.4	0	11	17	411	105	0.2	0.5	4	151	0.4	1	0.03	0.02	0.5	0.03	5	0
0.9	0.3	11	83	81	531	161	0.3	0.3	9	34	0.05	1	0.04	0.12	0.3	0.04	5	0.25
1.5	0.5	27	16	77	380	157	0.6	0.9	10	48	0.26	2	0.21	0.14	2.3	0.1	10	0.2
0	0	0	36	36	22	62	—	0	—	43	—	0	0	0.06	—	—	—	0.11
0.2	0.2	0	32	61	32	626	0.2	1.4	47	0	0.9	46	0.16	0.11	2	0.13	32	0
0.5	1	0	257	—	94	322	0.5	2.1	—	101	—	5	0.16	0.49	—	0.16	26	0.78
2	4.6	0	252	—	92	316	0.5	2	—	100	—	5	0.15	0.48	—	0.15	26	0.76
0.2	0.5	0	212	593	18	2097	2.2	8.1	255	4	0.17	0	0.61	0.22	2.3	0.5	268	0
0.8	2	0	10	118	29	338	0.6	1.4	46	7	0.02	0	0.39	0.17	0.4	0.1	4	0
0	0	0	90	—	14	4	—	0.3	—	0	—	0	0.02	0.02	0.7	—	—	0
0.5	1.3	0	24	57	5	169	0.4	0.7	25	0	0	5	0.12	0.04	0.4	0.06	60	0
0.5	1.2	0	28	64	5	167	0.5	0.6	28	0	0	4	0.1	0.02	0.5	0.05	38	0
2.1	5.4	0	190	152	6	638	2.6	7.5	101	0	0.01	11	0.14	0.17	0	0.11	7	0
1.7	4.4	0	88	211	1	443	1	4.4	74	1	1.68	1	0.13	0.24	0.3	0.2	46	0
4.1	10.5	0	120	558	2	1173	4.1	3.4	196	2	3.96	4	0.37	0.65	0.9	0.19	176	0
1.1	2.7	0	131	142	13	485	0.8	2.2	54	14	0.01	15	0.23	0.14	1.1	0.05	100	0
3.9	3.9	22	52	113	1220	245	2.4	3.2	20	100	1.5	5	0.15	0.18	2.2	0.12	5	0.82
0.4	0.5	8	40	88	955	303	1.1	2.8	21	120	2.13	10	0.35	0.28	4.5	0.13	6	0
6.6	1.1	24	42	162	218	256	1.4	11.3	20	64	1.46	8	0.19	0.22	2.4	0.07	16	36.2
0	0.2	0	136	47	29	370	0.5	2.5	81	939	1.39	15	0.02	0.15	0.4	0.11	105	0
0	0.1	0	122	50	63	419	0.7	3.2	78	737	0.86	9	0.09	0.21	0.4	0.22	131	0
0	0.1	0	139	46	82	283	0.7	1.4	66	739	0.91	12	0.06	0.16	0.4	0.14	103	0
0	0.1	0	87	32	58	252	0.3	1.6	45	605	0.74	19	0.07	0.12	0.3	0.11	94	0
0	0	0	28	14	22	156	0.1	0.8	22	188	0.53	8	0.02	0.05	0.2	0.06	54	0
0	0	0	13	6	11	73	0.1	0.4	11	89	0.26	2	0.01	0.02	0.1	0.02	18	0
0	0.1	0	89	44	71	502	0.5	2.4	71	545	1.7	22	0.06	0.16	0.6	0.17	149	0
0	0	—	0	23	37	37	—	0	—	0	—	0	—	—	—	—	—	0
—	—	—	350	400	100	280	—	4.5	140	50	20	60	1.5	1.7	20	2	400	6
4.4	1.9	1	3	2	140	4	0	0	0	152	0.43	0	0	0	0	0	0	0.01
2.7	1.6	37	13	58	304	124	0.5	0.8	10	14	0.78	2	0.16	0.13	1.3	0.1	9	0.12
0	0.1	0	45	46	4	448	0.2	1	44	44	0.12	11	0.17	0.01	0.9	0.2	19	0
0	0.1	0	54	55	5	535	0.2	1.1	53	53	0.15	13	0.2	0.02	1.1	0.24	23	0
0	0	0	42	28	4	291	0.1	0.6	30	718	0.17	16	0.07	0.02	1	0.13	20	0
0	0	0	50	33	5	348	0.2	0.7	36	858	0.21	18	0.09	0.02	1.2	0.15	24	0
0	0	0	13	23	5	104	0.3	0.8	14	13	0.13	3	0.02	0.03	0.5	0.04	11	0
0	0.1	0	24	35	1	173	0.4	0.3	22	26	0.11	5	0.04	0.04	0.5	0.08	18	0
0.1	0.3	0	20	28	10	430	0.2	0.6	26	725	0.14	11	0.09	0.06	0.7	0.21	19	0
0	0.1	0	18	34	1	168	0.3	0.4	23	11	0.14	13	0.06	0.03	0.6	0.1	25	0
0	0.1	0	14	25	1	126	0.2	0.3	17	8	0.11	10	0.05	0.02	0.4	0.08	19	0
0	0.1	0	16	11	14	91	0.2	0.3	9	9	0.09	3	0.03	0.02	0.6	0.08	6	0
0	0.1	0	24	35	1	173	0.4	0.3	22	26	0.11	5	0.04	0.04	0.5	0.06	18	0
0	0.1	0	13	23	1	127	0.2	0.3	15	13	0.08	10	0.04	0.02	0.4	0.07	17	0
0	0.3	0	14	20	1	448	0.3	0.3	8	365	0.12	10	0.09	0.02	0.7	0.07	29	0
0.1	0.3	0	17	24	279	521	0.3	0.4	10	425	0.14	12	0.1	0.03	0.8	0.09	33	0
0	0.1	0	14	29	3	223	0.2	0.4	20	29	0.11	7	0.06	0.03	0.3	0.07	17	0
0	0.1	0	19	28	2	216	0.2	0.5	14	48	0.34	4	0.05	0.04	0.4	0.05	9	0
0	0	0	3	15	0	73	0.1	0.1	5	8	0.04	5	0.01	0.01	0.1	0.02	3	0
0	0.1	0	19	33	424	311	0.3	0.8	16	61	0.11	3	0.05	0.04	0.6	0.17	34	0
0	0	0	12	36	3	228	0.2	0.3	20	22	0.11	4	0.04	0.04	0.4	0.07	15	0
0	0	0	10	21	2	161	0.1	0.3	14	22	0.08	6	0.05	0.02	0.3	0.06	14	0
0	0.1	0	14	29	3	223	0.2	0.4	20	28	0.11	7	0.06	0.03	0.3	0.07	16	0
3.1	0.4	34	29	110	1006	426	4.2	2.2	39	262	0.34	7	0.07	0.12	2.4	0.2	31	1.59
1.3	1	34	37	168	451	538	1.4	1.7	46	51	0.57	18	0.12	0.16	5.8	0.37	44	0.18
1.9	0.4	26	18	100	512	361	1.6	1.1	27	157	0.54	7	0.12	0.14	2.7	0.2	17	0.74
2.1	0.3	32	167	162	1041	235	10.3	1	20	44	0.49	4	0.07	0.23	0.3	0.06	10	2.62
0.5	0.1	7	11	24	490	24	5.2	0.5	2	4	0.12	2	0.01	0.02	0.1	0.01	1	1.1
0.5	0.3	48	40	111	493	405	0.9	4.7	22	266	1.27	16	0.09	0.1	1.7	0.17	17	12.2
1.3	0.3	28	18	96	303	273	1	0.7	18	307	0.25	6	0.07	0.12	3.5	0.2	13	0.28

Food Item	Qty	Meas	Wgt (g)	Wtr (g)	Cals	Prot	Carb (g)	Fib (g)	Fat (g)	SatF (g)
Stew, venison, tomato base sauce	0.5	cup	126	105	81	9	9	1.5	1	0.3
Strawberries, cooked, unsweetened	0.5	cup	121	114	24	0	6	2.1	0	0
Strawberries, fresh	0.5	cup	83	76	25	1	6	1.9	0	0
Strawberries, frozen, unsweetened	0.5	cup	74	67	26	0	7	1.6	0	0
Strawberries, sliced, frozen, sweetened, thawed	0.5	cup	128	93	122	1	33	2.4	0	0
Strawberry Julius	1	cup	215	183	170	0	41	0.4	0	0.1
Strudel, berry	1	piece	64	28	159	2	29	1.4	4	0.8
Strudel, cheese	1	piece	64	24	195	6	24	0.4	8	3.9
Strudel, cherry	1	piece	64	25	179	3	29	1.1	6	0.9
Strudel, peach	1	piece	64	36	123	2	23	1.2	3	0.6
Stuffing mix, cornbread, prepared	0.5	cup	100	65	179	3	22	2.9	9	1.8
Subway, Club sandwich on a 6-in. white roll	1	each	246	179	297	21	40	3	5	1
Subway, Cold Cut Trio salad	1	each	330	294	191	13	11	1	11	3
Subway, Spicy Italian sandwich on a 6-in. white roll	1	each	232	148	467	20	38	3	24	9
Subway, Veggie Delite sandwich on a 6-in. white roll	1	each	175	124	222	9	38	3	3	0
Subway, chicken taco salad	1	each	370	322	250	18	15	2	14	5
Subway, meatball sandwich on a 6-in. white roll	1	each	260	181	404	18	44	3	16	6
Subway, pizza salad	1	each	335	288	277	12	13	2	20	8
Subway, seafood & crab salad w/light mayonnaise	1	each	331	298	161	13	11	2	8	1
Subway, tuna salad w/light mayonnaise	1	each	331	294	205	12	11	1	13	2
Subway, tuna sandwich w/light mayonnaise	1	each	178	119	279	11	38	2	9	2
Succotash, cooked from fresh	0.5	cup	96	66	110	5	23	4.3	1	0.1
Succotash, frozen, cooked	0.5	cup	85	63	79	4	17	3.5	1	0.1
Succotash, whole corn & lima beans, canned	0.5	cup	128	105	80	3	18	3.3	1	0.1
Sugar apple (sweetsop), raw	1	each	155	113	146	3	37	6.8	0	0.1
Sugar cane juice	8	oz.	227	198	79	0	21	—	0	—
Sugar, brown, packed	1	tsp	3	0	11	0	3	0	0	0
Sugar, maple, piece	1	each	28	2	100	0	26	0	0	0
Sugar, raw	1	tsp	4	0	15	0	4	0	0	0
Sugar, white, granulated	1	tsp	4	0	16	0	4	0	0	0
Sugar, white, powdered, unsifted	0.25	cup	30	0	117	0	30	0	0	0
Sukiyaki	0.5	cup	81	63	88	10	3	0.6	4	1.5
Sunflower seed butter, salted	1	Tbs	16	0	93	3	4	2	8	0.8
Sunflower seed kernels, dry	0.25	cup	36	2	205	8	7	3.8	18	1.9
Sunflower seed kernels, oil roasted, unsalted	0.25	cup	34	1	208	7	5	2.3	19	2
Sunflower seed, dry roasted	0.25	cup	32	0	186	6	8	3.6	16	1.7
Sunflower seed, oil roasted, salted	0.25	cup	34	1	208	7	5	2.3	19	2
Supplement, Osmolite, prepared, Ross Labs	1	cup	253	199	250	9	36	—	8	—
Sushi, w/egg, rolled in seaweed	0.5	cup	83	62	102	5	12	0.2	4	1
Sushi, w/vegetables & fish	0.5	cup	83	53	119	4	24	0.7	0	0.1
Sushi, w/vegetables, rolled in seaweed	0.5	cup	83	59	97	2	22	0.5	0	0.1
Swamp cabbage, chopped, cooked	0.5	cup	49	46	10	1	2	0.9	0	0
Sweet & sour chicken breast	1	cup	131	103	117	8	15	0.8	3	0.6
Sweet potato, baked, then peeled	0.5	cup	100	73	103	2	24	3	0	0
Sweet potato, candied, cup measure	0.5	cup	98	66	134	1	27	2.4	3	1.3
Sweet potato, canned, w/syrup	0.5	cup	114	88	101	1	24	2.8	0	0
Sweet potato, canned, w/syrup, drained	0.5	cup	98	71	106	1	25	2.9	0	0.1
Sweet potato, flakes prep w/water	0.5	cup	128	96	121	1	29	—	0	0
Sweet potato, peeled, boiled, mashed	0.5	cup	100	73	105	2	24	1.8	0	0.1
Sweetener, NutraSweet, low calorie	5	gram	5	0	19	5	0	0	0	0
Sweetener, saccharin, tablet	1	each	0	0	0	0	0	0	0	0
Sweetener, sugar substitute, saccharin-based, liqui	1	tsp	5	5	0	0	0	0	0	0
Swiss chard, chopped, raw	0.5	cup	18	17	3	0	1	0.3	0	0
Swiss chard, cooked, no added salt	0.5	cup	88	81	18	2	4	1.8	0	0
Syrup, chocolate, thin	2	Tbs	38	14	82	1	22	0.7	0	0.2
Syrup, corn, dark	1	Tbs	20	5	58	0	16	0	0	0
Syrup, corn, light	2	Tbs	41	9	116	0	31	0	0	0
Syrup, maple	2	Tbs	40	13	105	0	27	0	0	0
Syrup, pancake	2	Tbs	39	9	113	0	30	0	0	0
Syrup, pancake, reduced-calorie	2	Tbs	36	20	59	0	16	0	0	0
Syrup, pancake, w/2% maple	2	Tbs	39	12	104	0	27	0	0	0
Tabbouleh/tabbuli	0.5	cup	80	62	93	2	8	2.3	7	0.9
Taco Bell, Pintos & cheese	1	each	128	87	203	10	19	10.7	10	4.3
Taco Bell, burrito, big beef supreme	1	each	298	192	520	24	54	11	23	10
Taco Bell, burrito, chicken	1	each	171	99	345	17	41	—	13	5

MonoF (g)	PolyF (g)	Choles (mg)	Calc (mg)	Phos (mg)	Sod (mg)	Pot (mg)	Zn (mg)	Iron (mg)	Magn (mg)	VitA (µg RE)	VitE (µg α-TE)	VitC (mg)	Thia (mg)	Ribo (mg)	Nia (mg)	B6 (mg)	Fola (µg)	B12 (µg)
0.2	0.2	29	16	104	339	383	1	1.8	22	267	0.43	13	0.11	0.2	2.8	0.2	15	1.61
0	0.2	0	12	15	2	135	0.1	0.3	9	2	0.11	44	0.02	0.05	0.2	0.05	14	0
0	0.2	0	12	16	1	138	0.1	0.3	8	2	0.12	47	0.02	0.06	0.2	0.05	15	0
0	0	0	12	10	1	110	0.1	0.6	8	3	0.2	31	0.02	0.03	0.3	0.02	12	0
0	0.1	0	14	17	4	125	0.1	0.8	9	3	0.18	53	0.02	0.06	0.5	0.04	19	0
0.1	0.1	0	27	—	8	82	—	0.1	—	0	—	6	0.01	0.06	—	0.01	—	0
1.7	1.2	11	15	26	103	55	0.2	0.8	6	53	1.04	5	0.09	0.09	0.8	0.02	6	0.03
2.8	1.1	42	90	87	116	64	0.6	0.8	8	95	0.69	0	0.08	0.16	0.7	0.03	8	0.12
2	2.9	9	19	40	88	100	0.3	0.8	15	79	0.7	3	0.09	0.08	0.8	0.05	8	0.02
1.2	0.9	8	12	22	75	102	0.2	0.6	7	59	0.82	3	0.06	0.07	1	0.02	4	0.02
3.9	2.7	0	26	34	455	62	0.2	0.9	13	85	1.39	1	0.12	0.09	1.2	0.04	97	0.01
—	—	26	29	—	1341	—	—	4	—	120	—	15	—	—	—	—	—	—
—	—	64	46	—	1127	—	—	2	—	282	—	33	—	—	—	—	—	—
—	—	57	40	—	1592	—	—	4	—	169	—	15	—	—	—	—	—	—
—	—	0	25	—	582	—	—	3	—	120	—	15	—	—	—	—	—	—
—	—	52	115	—	990	—	—	3	—	361	—	35	—	—	—	—	—	—
—	—	33	32	—	1035	—	—	4	—	142	—	16	—	—	—	—	—	—
—	—	50	100	—	1336	—	—	2	—	390	—	33	—	—	—	—	—	—
—	—	32	25	—	599	—	—	2	—	284	—	32	—	—	—	—	—	—
—	—	32	29	—	654	—	—	2	—	298	—	32	—	—	—	—	—	—
—	—	16	26	—	583	—	—	3	—	126	—	14	—	—	—	—	—	—
0.1	0.4	0	16	112	16	394	0.6	1.5	51	28	0.32	8	0.16	0.09	1.3	0.11	32	0
0.1	0.4	0	13	60	38	225	0.4	0.8	20	20	0.31	5	0.06	0.06	1.1	0.08	28	0
0.1	0.3	0	14	70	282	208	0.6	0.7	24	19	0.26	6	0.04	0.07	0.8	0.06	40	0
0.2	0.1	0	37	50	14	383	0.2	0.9	33	2	0.92	56	0.17	0.18	1.4	0.31	22	0
—	—	—	30	20	—	—	—	0.2	—	—	—	—	0.02	0.02	0.2	—	—	—
0	0	0	3	1	1	10	0	0.1	1	0	0	0	0	0	0	0	0	0
0	0	0	26	1	3	78	1.7	0.5	5	1	0	0	0	0	0	0	0	0
0	0	0	3	1	2	14	0	0.1	1	0	0	0	0	0	0	0	0	0
0	0	0	0	0	0	0	0	0	0	0	0	0	0	0	0	0	0	0
0	0	0	0	1	0	1	0	0	0	0	0	0	0	0	0	0	0	0
1.6	0.4	77	31	105	381	234	1.8	1.7	24	132	0.55	2	0.06	0.21	1.6	0.18	31	0.78
1.5	5	0	20	118	83	12	0.8	0.8	59	1	7.68	0	0.05	0.04	0.9	0.13	38	0
3.4	11.8	0	42	254	1	248	1.8	2.4	127	2	18.1	1	0.82	0.09	1.6	0.28	82	0
3.7	12.8	0	19	384	1	163	1.8	2.3	43	2	17	0	0.11	0.1	1.4	0.27	79	0
3.7	10.5	0	22	370	1	272	1.7	1.2	41	0	16.1	0	0.03	0.08	2.2	0.26	76	0
3	12.8	0	19	384	204	163	1.8	2.3	43	2	13.5	0	0.11	0.1	1.4	0.27	79	0
—	—	—	125	125	150	240	2.8	2.2	50	125	3.78	38	0.38	0.43	5	0.5	100	1.5
1.6	0.9	98	22	72	274	70	0.6	0.9	12	66	0.8	1	0.07	0.14	0.8	0.07	14	0.21
0.1	0.1	6	13	55	172	108	0.4	1.2	14	86	0.3	2	0.14	0.04	1.5	0.08	8	0.17
0.1	0.1	0	12	34	76	56	0.4	0.8	11	33	0.07	1	0.11	0.02	1	0.07	5	0
0	0	0	26	21	60	139	0.1	0.6	15	255	0.01	8	0.02	0.04	0.2	0.04	17	0
0.8	1.5	23	16	75	732	187	0.7	0.8	21	20	0.39	12	0.06	0.08	3.1	0.18	6	0.08
0	0	0	28	55	10	348	0.3	0.4	20	2182	0.28	25	0.07	0.13	0.6	0.24	23	0
0.6	0.1	8	26	26	69	185	0.1	1.1	11	411	3.72	7	0.02	0.04	0.4	0.04	11	0
0	0.1	0	17	31	50	211	0.2	0.9	15	652	0.26	12	0.03	0.05	0.5	0.06	7	0
0	0.1	0	17	24	38	189	0.2	0.9	12	702	0.27	11	0.02	0.04	0.3	0.06	8	0
0	0.1	0	19	26	57	179	—	0.8	—	1530	—	14	0.03	0.04	0.4	—	—	0
0	0.1	0	21	27	13	184	0.3	0.6	10	1705	0.28	17	0.05	0.14	0.6	0.24	11	0
0	0	0	0	0	2	0	—	0.1	—	0	—	0	0	0	0	—	0	0
0	0	0	0	0	0	1	0	0	0	0	0	0	0	0	0	0	0	0
0	0	0	0	0	1	5	0	0	0	0	0	0	0	0	0	0	0	0
0	0	0	9	8	38	68	0.1	0.3	15	59	0.34	5	0.01	0.02	0.1	0.02	2	0
0	0	0	51	29	157	480	0.3	2	75	275	1.65	16	0.03	0.08	0.3	0.07	8	0
0.1	0	0	5	48	36	84	0.3	0.8	24	1	0.01	0	0	0.02	0.1	0	2	0
0	0	0	4	2	32	9	0	0.1	2	0	0	0	0	0	0	0	0	0
0	0	0	1	1	50	2	0	0	1	0	0	0	0	0	0	0	0	0
0	0	0	27	1	4	82	1.7	0.5	6	0	0	0	0	0	0	0	0	0
0	0	0	0	4	33	1	0	0	1	0	0	0	0	0	0	0	0	0
0	0	0	0	16	72	1	0	0	0	0	0	0	0	0	0	0	0	0
0	0	0	2	4	24	2	0.1	0	1	0	0	0	0	0.01	0	0	0	0
4.7	0.6	0	27	37	321	168	0.3	1.2	23	83	1.08	26	0.04	0.03	0.7	0.06	29	0
—	—	16	160	—	693	384	2.2	1.9	110	267	—	0	0.05	0.15	0.4	0.21	68	0
—	—	55	150	—	1520	—	—	2.7	—	600	—	5	—	—	—	—	—	—
—	—	57	140	—	854	—	—	2.5	—	440	—	1	—	—	—	—	—	—

Food Item	Qty	Meas	Wgt (g)	Wtr (g)	Cals	Prot	Carb (g)	Fib (g)	Fat (g)	SatF (g)
Taco Bell, burrito, seven layer	1	each	234	143	438	13	55	10.7	19	5.8
Taco Bell, cinnamon twist	1	each	35	2	175	1	24	0	8	0
Taco Bell, mexican pizza	1	each	223	119	578	21	43	8.1	36	10.1
Taco Bell, nachos, bellgrande, svg	1	each	287	148	708	19	77	15.6	36	10.1
Taco Bell, nachos, supreme, serving	1	each	145	81	330	10	33	6.6	18	5.9
Taco Bell, taco	1	each	78	46	180	9	12	3	10	4
Taco Bell, taco, soft, chicken	1	each	128	81	212	15	22	2.1	7	2.6
Taco Bell, taco, soft, steak	1	each	100	63	180	12	16	1.6	8	2
Taco Bell, taco, soft, supreme	1	each	124	79	227	10	20	2.6	12	6.1
Taco Bell, taco, supreme	1	each	106	68	206	9	13	2.8	13	6.6
Taco Time, Mexi-fries, svg	1	each	130	75	330	3	31	1	20	7
Taco Time, burrito, bean, crispy	1	each	149	82	354	11	34	4	21	4
Taco Time, burrito, beef, crispy	1	each	149	65	466	22	32	1	28	10
Taco Time, burrito, combo, soft	1	each	255	153	520	27	48	4	25	10
Taco Time, chicken fajita salad	1	each	297	198	541	28	39	2	31	7
Taco Time, taco, natural super	1	each	283	173	575	28	49	4	31	13
Taco shell, Ortega	2	each	30	0	140	2	20	2	7	1
Taco shell, baked	2	each	26	2	122	2	16	2	6	0.8
Taco, chicken	1	each	78	44	174	16	9	1.2	8	3.2
Tahini (sesame butter)	1	Tbs	15	0	91	3	3	1.4	8	1.2
Tamale, w/meat	1	each	70	36	183	7	16	2.9	10	3.7
Tamales, Old El Paso	1	each	69	49	110	2	10	1.7	6	2.3
Tamarind, raw	5	each	10	3	24	0	6	0.5	0	0
Tangelo, fresh	1	each	95	82	45	1	11	2.3	0	0
Tangerine, canned in light syrup	0.5	cup	126	105	77	1	20	0.9	0	0
Tangerine, fresh	1	each	84	74	37	1	9	1.9	0	0
Taro chips	10	each	23	0	115	1	16	1.7	6	1.5
Taro shoots, cooked slices	0.5	cup	70	67	10	1	2	0.4	0	0
Taro slices, cooked	0.5	cup	66	42	94	0	23	3.4	0	0
Taro, raw slices	0.5	cup	52	37	58	1	14	2.1	0	0
Taro, tahitian, cooked slices	0.5	cup	68	59	30	3	5	0.7	0	0.1
Tarragon, ground	0.25	tsp	0	0	1	0	0	0	0	0
Tart, lemon meringue	1	each	117	53	329	4	43	0.6	16	4
Tea, brewed	1	cup	240	239	2	0	1	0	0	0
Tea, camomile	1	cup	240	239	2	0	0	0	0	0
Tea, decaf, low calorie, frozen, prepared	1	cup	245	243	7	0	2	0	0	0
Tea, from instant, sweetened, w/lemon	1	cup	262	239	89	0	22	0	0	0
Tea, from instant, unsweetened	1	cup	237	236	2	0	0	0	0	0
Tea, herbal, brewed	1	cup	237	237	2	0	0	0	0	0
Tea, instant, w/lemon, diet, dry, prepared	1	cup	238	236	5	0	1	0	0	0
Tea, instant, w/lemon, prepared	1	cup	238	237	5	0	1	0	0	0
Tea, presweetened, w/low calorie sweetener	1	cup	245	243	5	0	1	0	0	0
Tempeh	0.5	cup	83	46	165	16	14	4.5	6	0.9
Toaster pastry, Pop Tarts, brown sugar cinnamon	1	each	50	5	220	3	32	1	9	1
Toaster pastry, fruit filled, Pop Tart	1	each	52	6	204	2	37	1.1	5	0.8
Tofu (soybean curd, reg)	0.5	cup	124	108	76	8	2	0.2	5	0.7
Tofu yogurt	1	cup	262	203	254	9	43	0.5	5	0.7
Tofu, fried, w/Nigari	1	oz.	28	14	77	5	3	1.1	6	0.8
Tofu, okara, w/Nigari	0.5	cup	61	50	47	2	8	2.5	1	0.1
Tofu, raw, firm, prepared, w/Nigari	0.5	cup	126	105	97	10	4	0.5	6	0.8
Tomatillo, raw, chopped	0.5	cup	66	60	21	1	4	1.2	1	0.1
Tomatillo, raw, whole	1	each	34	31	11	0	2	0.6	0	0
Tomato juice, canned, low sodium	1	cup	244	229	42	2	10	2	0	0
Tomato juice, canned, w/salt	1	cup	244	229	42	2	10	1	0	0
Tomato paste, canned	0.25	cup	66	48	54	2	13	2.7	0	0.1
Tomato paste, canned, no added salt	0.5	cup	66	48	54	2	13	2.7	0	0.1
Tomato puree, canned, low sodium	0.5	cup	125	109	50	2	12	2.5	0	0
Tomato puree, canned, w/salt	0.5	cup	125	109	50	2	12	2.5	0	0
Tomato sauce w/mushrooms, canned	0.5	cup	122	108	43	2	10	1.8	0	0
Tomato slices, raw	2	piece	40	38	8	0	2	0.4	0	0
Tomato wedge w/tomato juice, canned	0.5	cup	130	120	34	1	8	1.3	0	0
Tomato, Italian/plum, raw, whole	1	each	62	58	13	1	3	0.7	0	0
Tomato, Roma, raw	1	each	62	58	13	1	3	0.7	0	0
Tomato, cherry	10	each	170	159	36	1	8	1.9	1	0.1
Tomato, fresh, stewed w/bread crumbs	0.5	cup	50	41	40	1	7	0.9	1	0.3

MonoF (g)	PolyF (g)	Choles (mg)	Calc (mg)	Phos (mg)	Sod (mg)	Pot (mg)	Zn (mg)	Iron (mg)	Magn (mg)	VitA (µg RE)	VitE (µg α-TE)	VitC (mg)	Thia (mg)	Ribo (mg)	Nia (mg)	B6 (mg)	Fola (µg)	B12 (µg)
—	—	21	165	—	1058	—	—	3	—	248	—	5	—	—	—	—	—	—
—	—	0	0	—	238	28	—	0.4	—	50	—	0	0.1	0.04	0.7	0.04	—	—
—	—	46	253	—	1054	408	5.4	3.6	80	405	—	5	0.32	0.34	3	1.12	60	—
—	—	32	184	—	1205	674	—	3.3	—	138	—	3	0.1	0.34	2.2	—	—	—
—	—	22	110	—	593	—	—	2	—	73	—	3	—	—	—	—	—	—
—	—	25	80	—	330	159	—	1.1	—	100	—	0	0.05	0.14	1.2	0.12	—	—
—	—	37	85	—	571	—	—	0.8	—	64	—	1	—	—	—	—	—	—
—	—	20	62	—	797	—	—	1.1	—	31	—	0	—	—	—	—	—	—
—	—	31	87	—	515	—	—	1.6	—	131	—	3	—	—	—	—	—	—
—	—	33	94	—	328	—	—	1	—	141	—	0	—	—	—	—	—	—
9	4	—	13	46	360	315	—	1	—	0	—	4	0.06	0.01	1	—	—	0
11	6	11	143	216	302	347	2	4	—	12	—	—	0.33	0.2	2	0.35	13	—
12	6	52	180	253	571	463	4	4	—	28	—	2	0.24	0.37	5	0.33	68	—
14	1	54	271	392	826	713	5	7	—	90	—	5	0.45	0.44	5	0.6	70	—
10	11	73	177	267	490	442	2	3	—	127	—	20	0.26	0.36	9	0.44	66	—
17	1	66	300	414	763	749	5	7	—	107	—	5	0.46	0.48	5	0.58	74	—
3	1	0	60	—	200	70	—	0.7	—	20	—	—	—	—	—	—	—	—
2.3	2.2	0	42	64	95	46	0.4	0.6	27	0	0.95	0	0.06	0.01	0.4	0.08	27	0
3.2	1.4	46	95	154	106	167	1.3	1	28	39	0.85	1	0.08	0.13	4.2	0.25	16	0.2
3.2	3.7	0	21	119	0	69	1.6	1	53	1	0.34	0	0.24	0.02	0.8	0.02	15	0
4.3	1.4	24	32	80	229	154	1.1	1.9	29	18	0.43	4	0.24	0.18	2.9	0.12	5	0.18
2.7	0.5	10	13	—	197	—	—	0.6	—	—	—	—	—	—	—	—	—	—
0	0	0	7	11	3	63	0	0.3	9	0	0.07	0	0.04	0.02	0.2	0.01	1	0
0	0	0	38	13	0	172	0.1	0.1	10	20	0.23	50	0.08	0.04	0.3	0.06	29	0
0	0	0	9	13	8	98	0.3	0.5	10	106	0.43	25	0.07	0.06	0.6	0.05	6	0
0	0	0	12	8	1	132	0.2	0.1	10	77	0.2	26	0.09	0.02	0.1	0.06	17	0
1	3	0	14	30	79	174	0.1	0.3	19	0	1.13	1	0.04	0.01	0.1	0.1	5	0
0	0	0	10	18	1	241	0.4	0.3	6	4	0.7	13	0.03	0.04	0.6	0.08	2	0
0	0	0	12	50	10	319	0.2	0.5	20	0	0.29	3	0.07	0.02	0.3	0.22	13	0
0	0	0	22	44	6	307	0.1	0.3	17	0	1.24	2	0.05	0.01	0.3	0.15	12	0
0	0.2	0	102	46	37	427	0.1	1.1	35	121	1.85	26	0.03	0.14	0.3	0.08	5	0
0	0	0	5	1	0	12	0	0.1	1	2	0.01	0	0	0	0	0	1	0
6.8	3.9	74	14	56	272	54	0.4	1.3	8	34	1.56	3	0.15	0.19	1.2	0.04	11	0.14
0	0	0	0	2	7	89	0	0	7	0	0	0	0	0.03	0	0	12	0
0	0	0	5	0	2	22	0.1	0.2	2	5	0.19	0	0.02	0.01	0	0	1	0
0	0	0	0	2	7	90	0	0	7	0	0	0	0	0.03	0	0	13	0
0	0	0	5	3	8	50	0.1	0.1	5	0	0	0	0	0.05	0.1	0	10	0
0	0	0	5	2	7	47	0.1	0	5	0	0	0	0	0	0.1	0	1	0
0	0	0	5	0	2	21	0.1	0.2	2	0	0	0	0.02	0.01	0	0	1	0
0	0	0	5	2	24	40	0.1	0.1	5	0	0	0	0	0.01	0.1	0	5	0
0	0	0	5	2	14	50	0.1	0	5	0	0	0	0	0.02	0.1	0	1	0
0	0	0	5	2	24	42	0.1	0.1	5	0	0	0	0	0.01	0.1	0	5	0
1.4	3.6	0	77	171	5	305	1.5	1.9	58	57	0.02	0	0.11	0.09	3.8	0.25	43	0.83
—	—	0	0	40	210	—	0.6	1.8	—	150	—	0	0.15	0.17	2	0.2	40	—
2.2	2	0	14	58	218	58	0.3	1.8	9	150	1.19	0	0.15	0.19	2	0.2	34	0
1	2.6	0	138	114	10	149	0.8	1.4	34	1	0.01	0	0.06	0.05	0.7	0.06	55	0
1.1	2.7	0	309	100	92	123	0.8	2.8	105	8	0.81	7	0.16	0.05	0.6	0.05	16	0
1.3	3.2	0	105	81	5	41	0.6	1.4	17	0	0.01	0	0.05	0.01	0	0.03	8	0
0.2	0.5	0	49	37	5	130	0.3	0.8	16	0	0	0	0.01	0.01	0.1	0.07	16	0
1.2	3.2	0	204	185	10	222	1.3	1.8	58	1	0.02	0	0.12	0.13	0	0.08	42	0
0.1	0.3	0	5	26	1	177	0.1	0.4	13	7	0.25	8	0.03	0.02	1.2	0.04	5	0
0.1	0.1	0	2	13	0	91	0.1	0.2	7	4	0.13	4	0.02	0.01	0.6	0.02	2	0
0	0.1	0	22	46	24	537	0.3	1.4	27	137	2.22	45	0.12	0.08	1.6	0.27	49	0
0	0.1	0	22	46	881	537	0.3	1.4	27	137	2.22	45	0.12	0.08	1.6	0.27	49	0
0.1	0.1	0	23	52	517	614	0.5	1.3	33	160	2.82	28	0.1	0.12	2.1	0.25	15	0
0.1	0.1	0	23	52	58	614	0.5	1.3	33	160	2.82	28	0.1	0.12	2.1	0.25	15	0
0	0.1	0	21	50	42	533	0.3	1.6	30	160	3.15	13	0.09	0.07	2.2	0.19	14	0
0	0.1	0	21	50	499	533	0.3	1.6	30	160	3.15	13	0.09	0.07	2.2	0.19	14	0
0	0.1	0	16	39	554	466	0.3	1.1	23	116	1.72	15	0.09	0.13	1.6	0.16	12	0
0	0.1	0	2	10	4	89	0	0.2	4	25	0.15	8	0.02	0.02	0.3	0.03	6	0
0	0.1	0	34	30	283	328	0.2	0.6	14	76	0.5	19	0.07	0.04	0.9	0.15	13	0
0	0.1	0	3	15	6	138	0.1	0.3	7	38	0.24	12	0.04	0.03	0.4	0.05	9	0
0	0.1	0	3	15	6	138	0.1	0.3	7	38	0.24	12	0.04	0.03	0.4	0.05	9	0
0.1	0.2	0	8	41	15	377	0.2	0.8	19	105	0.65	32	0.1	0.08	1.1	0.14	26	0
0.5	0.4	0	13	19	230	125	0.1	0.5	8	34	0.64	9	0.06	0.04	0.6	0.04	6	0

Food Item	Qty	Meas	Wgt (g)	Wtr (g)	Cals	Prot	Carb (g)	Fib (g)	Fat (g)	SatF (g)
Tomato, green, fried	1	each	144	104	237	4	16	2	18	4.7
Tomato, green, raw, chopped	0.5	cup	90	84	22	1	5	1	0	0
Tomato, green, raw, whole	1	each	123	114	30	1	6	1.4	0	0
Tomato, raw, chopped	0.5	cup	90	84	19	1	4	1	0	0
Tomato, raw, wedge	1	piece	31	29	7	0	1	0.3	0	0
Tomato, raw, whole, medium size	1	each	123	115	26	1	6	1.4	0	0.1
Tomato, red, fried	1	each	101	74	164	3	11	1.2	13	3.3
Tomato, stewed, canned, low sodium	0.5	cup	128	116	36	1	9	1.3	0	0
Tomato, sun dried pieces	10	piece	20	3	52	3	11	2.5	1	0.1
Tomato, sun dried, oil pack, drained	10	each	30	16	64	2	7	1.7	4	0.6
Tomato, yellow, sun dried	0.5	cup	27	6	79	3	15	3.2	1	0.2
Tomatoes w/green chilies, canned	0.5	cup	120	114	18	1	4	1.2	0	0
Tomatoes, canned, no salt added	0.5	cup	120	112	23	1	5	1.2	0	0
Tomatoes, raw, diced, cooked	0.5	cup	120	111	32	1	7	1.2	0	0.1
Tomatoes, sun dried, whole	0.5	cup	27	4	70	4	15	3.3	1	0.1
Topping, Marshmallow creme	2	Tbs	38	8	122	0	30	0	0	0
Topping, butterscotch	2	Tbs	41	13	103	1	27	0.4	0	0
Topping, caramel	2	Tbs	41	13	103	1	27	0.4	0	0
Topping, chocolate hot fudge	2	Tbs	42	9	149	2	27	1.2	4	1.7
Topping, nuts in syrup	2	Tbs	41	8	167	2	22	0.7	9	0.8
Topping, pineapple	2	Tbs	42	14	108	0	28	0.4	0	0
Topping, strawberry	2	Tbs	42	14	108	0	28	0.4	0	0
Tortellini, spinach	0.5	cup	61	37	116	6	13	0.5	4	1.6
Tortilla chips, Doritos	20	piece	36	1	180	3	23	2.3	9	1.8
Tortilla chips, Doritos, grab bag	1	each	64	1	319	4	40	4.1	17	3.2
Tortilla chips, baked, low fat, Tostitos	1	oz.	28	—	111	3	24	2	1	0
Tortilla chips, baked, low fat, unsalted, Tostitos	1	oz.	28	—	111	3	24	2	1	0
Tortilla chips, nacho flavor (Doritos)	1	cup	26	0	129	2	16	1.4	7	1.3
Tortilla chips, nacho flavor, light	10	each	16	0	71	1	12	0.8	2	0.5
Tortilla chips, ranch flavor, Doritos	10	piece	18	0	88	1	12	0.7	4	0.8
Tortilla chips, taco flavor, Doritos	1	oz.	28	0	136	2	18	1.5	7	1.3
Tortilla, corn, 6 inch	1	each	30	13	67	2	14	1.6	1	0.1
Tortilla, flour, 10.5 inch	1	each	57	15	185	5	32	1.9	4	1
Tortilla, flour, 8 inch	1	each	35	9	115	3	20	1.2	3	0.6
Tortilla, whole wheat	1	each	35	11	73	3	20	1.9	0	0.1
Tostada, bean & chicken	1	each	157	106	250	20	18	3.4	11	5.4
Tostada, beef & cheese	1	each	163	101	315	19	23	—	16	10.4
Tostada, w/guacamole	2	each	261	189	360	12	32	—	23	9.9
Trail mix, regular	0.5	cup	75	7	347	10	34	3.8	22	4.2
Trail mix, regular, unsalted	0.5	cup	75	7	347	10	34	3.8	22	4.2
Trail mix, regular, w/chocolate chips, salted	0.5	cup	73	5	353	10	33	4	23	4.4
Trail mix, regular, w/chocolate chips, unsalted	0.5	cup	73	5	353	10	33	4	23	4.4
Trail mix, tropical	0.5	cup	70	6	285	4	46	4.5	12	5.9
Tuna noodle casserole, recipe	1	cup	202	151	237	17	25	1.4	7	1.9
Tuna salad	0.5	cup	102	65	192	16	10	0	9	1.6
Tuna, bass, freshwater, baked/broiled fillet	1	each	62	43	90	15	0	0	3	0.6
Tuna, light, canned in water, drained	1	cup	154	115	179	39	0	0	1	0.4
Turkey breast, roasted, Healthy Favorites	1	oz.	28	—	22	4	1	0	0	0
Turkey patty, breaded, fried	3	oz.	85	42	241	12	13	0.4	15	4
Turkey pot pie, Banquet	1	each	198	129	370	10	38	3	20	8
Turkey roll, light & dark meat	2	piece	57	40	84	10	1	0	4	1.2
Turkey roll, light meat	2	piece	57	41	83	11	0	0	4	1.2
Turkey, canned in water, Swanson	0.5	cup	124	78	180	32	8	2	4	1
Turkey, dark & light meat, skinless, roasted	4	oz.	113	74	193	33	0	0	6	1.9
Turkey, dark meat, roasted	4	oz.	113	68	251	31	0	0	13	4
Turkey, dark meat, skinless, roasted	4	oz.	113	72	212	32	0	0	8	2.7
Turkey, fryer, breast meat, roasted	3	oz.	85	58	115	26	0	0	1	0.2
Turkey, ground, cooked patty	1	each	82	49	194	23	0	0	11	2.8
Turkey, light meat, roasted	4	oz.	113	71	223	32	0	0	9	2.6
Turkey, roasted	4	oz.	113	70	236	32	0	0	11	3.2
Turkey, tom, breast, roasted	4	oz.	113	72	214	32	0	0	8	2.4
Turkey, tom, leg, roasted	4	oz.	113	69	234	32	0	0	11	3.4
Turkey, tom, roasted	4	oz.	113	70	229	32	0	0	10	3
Turkey, tom, skinless, roasted	4	oz.	113	74	191	33	0	0	5	1.8
Turkey, w/gravy, frozen, heated	1	cup	240	204	161	14	11	0	6	2

MonoF	PolyF	Choles	Calc	Phos	Sod	Pot	Zn	Iron	Magn	VitA	VitE	VitC	Thia	Ribo	Nia	B6	Fola	B12
(g)	(g)	(mg)	(mg)	(mg)	(mg)	(mg)	(mg)	(mg)	(mg)	(µg RE)	(µg α-TE)	(mg)	(mg)	(mg)	(mg)	(mg)	(µg)	(µg)
7.7	4.5	32	85	84	242	269	0.3	1.3	17	81	1.93	24	0.15	0.16	1.2	0.1	12	0.11
0	0.1	0	12	25	12	184	0.1	0.5	9	58	0.34	21	0.05	0.04	0.4	0.07	8	0
0	0.1	0	16	34	16	251	0.1	0.6	12	79	0.47	29	0.07	0.05	0.6	0.1	11	0
0	0.1	0	4	22	8	200	0.1	0.4	10	56	0.34	17	0.05	0.04	0.6	0.07	14	0
0	0	0	2	7	3	69	0	0.1	3	19	0.12	6	0.02	0.02	0.2	0.02	5	0
0.1	0.2	0	6	30	11	273	0.1	0.6	14	76	0.47	24	0.07	0.06	0.8	0.1	18	0
5.4	3.2	23	54	56	167	202	0.2	0.8	12	58	1.35	14	0.1	0.12	0.9	0.07	12	0.08
0	0.1	0	42	26	282	303	0.2	0.9	15	69	0.48	14	0.06	0.04	0.9	0.02	7	0
0.1	0.2	0	22	71	419	685	0.4	1.8	39	17	0	8	0.11	0.1	1.8	0.07	14	0
2.6	0.6	0	14	42	80	470	0.2	0.8	24	39	0.16	31	0.06	0.12	1.1	0.1	7	0
0.4	0	0	32	—	23	—	—	2.3	—	49	—	5	—	—	—	—	—	0
0	0	0	24	17	483	129	0.2	0.3	13	47	0.46	7	0.04	0.02	0.8	0.12	11	0
0	0.1	0	36	23	178	265	0.2	0.7	14	72	0.38	17	0.05	0.04	0.9	0.11	9	0
0.1	0.2	0	7	37	13	335	0.1	0.7	17	89	0.46	27	0.08	0.07	0.9	0.11	16	0
0.1	0.3	0	30	96	566	925	0.5	2.4	52	24	0	11	0.14	0.13	2.4	0.09	18	0
0	0	0	1	3	19	2	0	0.1	1	0	0	0	0	0	0	0	0	0
0	0	0	22	19	143	34	0.1	0.1	3	11	0	0	0	0.04	0	0.01	1	0.04
0	0	0	22	19	143	34	0.1	0.1	3	11	0	0	0	0.04	0	0.01	1	0.04
1.6	0.1	1	34	57	147	154	0.3	0.6	22	2	1.24	0	0.02	0.09	0.1	0.03	2	0.09
2	5.6	0	16	46	17	86	0.4	0.4	26	2	0.36	0	0.07	0.05	0.2	0.08	9	0
0	0	0	9	3	27	135	0.2	0.2	1	1	0	25	0.01	0	0	0.01	1	0
0	0	0	10	6	9	31	0.2	0.4	2	1	0.06	11	0	0.01	0.1	0.01	1	0
1.6	0.7	79	72	84	126	69	0.5	1.2	12	95	0.66	1	0.12	0.19	0.9	0.05	17	0.24
5.6	1.3	0	55	74	190	71	0.6	0.5	32	7	0.49	0	0.03	0.07	0.5	0.1	4	0
9.9	2.3	0	98	131	336	125	1	1	56	13	0.87	0	0.05	0.12	0.8	0.18	6	0
—	—	0	—	—	142	—	—	—	—	—	—	—	—	—	—	—	—	—
—	—	0	—	—	0	—	—	—	—	—	—	—	—	—	—	—	—	—
3.9	0.9	1	38	63	184	56	0.3	0.4	21	11	0.35	0	0.03	0.05	0.4	0.07	4	0.01
1.4	0.3	0	25	51	160	44	—	0.3	16	7	0.13	0	0.04	0.04	0.1	0.04	4	0
2.5	0.6	0	25	43	110	44	0.2	0.3	16	5	0.24	0	0.02	0.04	0.3	0.04	3	0
4.1	1	1	44	68	224	62	0.4	0.6	25	26	0.39	0	0.07	0.06	0.6	0.08	6	0
0.2	0.3	0	52	94	48	46	0.3	0.4	20	0	0.05	0	0.03	0.02	0.4	0.07	34	0
2.1	0.6	0	71	70	272	74	0.4	1.9	15	0	0.52	0	0.3	0.17	2	0.03	70	0
1.3	0.4	0	44	44	169	46	0.3	1.2	9	0	0.32	0	0.19	0.1	1.3	0.02	44	0
0.1	0.2	0	10	82	171	82	0.5	0.7	26	0	0.43	0	0.1	0.02	0.9	0.07	8	0
4	1.6	54	169	239	436	367	2.3	1.8	48	87	1.88	4	0.11	0.2	4.6	0.32	54	0.26
3.3	1	41	217	179	897	572	3.7	2.9	64	96	—	3	0.1	0.55	3.2	0.23	75	1.17
8.5	3	39	423	232	799	650	4.1	1.6	73	217	—	4	0.13	0.57	2	0.26	115	0.99
9.4	7.2	0	58	259	172	514	2.4	2.3	119	2	2.66	1	0.35	0.15	3.5	0.22	53	0
9.4	7.2	0	58	259	8	514	2.4	2.3	119	2	2.66	1	0.35	0.15	3.5	0.22	53	0
9.9	8.2	3	80	283	88	473	2.3	2.5	118	4	7.81	1	0.3	0.16	3.2	0.19	48	0
9.9	8.2	3	80	283	20	473	2.3	2.5	118	4	7.81	1	0.3	0.16	3.2	0.19	48	0
1.7	3.6	0	40	130	7	496	0.8	1.8	67	4	1.55	5	0.32	0.08	1	0.23	29	0
1.5	3.2	41	34	155	772	182	1.2	2.3	30	13	1.18	1	0.18	0.15	7.8	0.2	10	1.52
3	4.2	13	17	182	412	182	0.6	1	20	28	0.97	2	0.03	0.07	6.9	0.08	8	1.23
1.1	0.8	54	64	159	56	283	0.5	1.2	24	22	0.46	1	0.05	0.06	0.9	0.09	10	1.43
0.2	0.5	46	17	251	521	365	1.2	2.4	42	26	0.82	0	0.05	0.11	20.5	0.54	6	4.6
0	0	8	—	—	333	—	—	0.4	—	—	—	—	—	—	—	—	—	—
6.4	4	53	12	230	680	234	1.2	1.9	13	9	2.03	0	0.08	0.16	2	0.17	24	0.19
—	—	45	40	—	850	—	—	1.1	—	150	—	0	—	—	—	—	—	—
1.3	1	31	18	95	332	153	1.1	0.8	10	0	0.19	0	0.05	0.16	2.7	0.15	3	0.13
1.4	1	24	23	104	277	142	0.9	0.7	9	0	0.08	0	0.05	0.13	4	0.18	2	0.14
—	—	70	0	—	440	—	—	0	—	0	—	0	—	—	—	—	—	—
1.2	1.6	86	28	242	79	338	3.5	2	30	0	0.37	0	0.07	0.21	6.2	0.52	8	0.42
4.1	3.5	101	37	222	86	311	4.7	2.6	26	0	0.69	0	0.07	0.27	4	0.36	10	0.41
1.9	2.4	96	36	231	90	329	5.1	2.6	27	0	0.73	0	0.07	0.28	4.1	0.41	10	0.42
0.1	0.2	71	10	190	44	248	1.5	1.3	25	0	0.08	0	0.04	0.11	6.4	0.48	5	0.33
4	2.7	84	21	162	88	222	2.4	1.6	20	0	0.28	0	0.04	0.14	4	0.32	6	0.27
3.2	2.3	86	24	236	71	323	2.3	1.6	30	0	0.15	0	0.06	0.15	7.1	0.53	7	0.4
3.6	2.8	93	30	230	77	318	3.4	2	28	0	0.38	0	0.06	0.2	5.8	0.46	8	0.4
2.8	2	85	24	238	76	328	2.4	1.6	31	0	0.2	0	0.07	0.15	6.9	0.56	7	0.41
3.2	3	102	40	227	91	319	4.9	2.6	26	0	0.92	0	0.07	0.29	3.9	0.39	10	0.42
3.4	2.6	93	31	230	82	320	3.4	2	28	0	0.47	0	0.07	0.21	5.6	0.48	8	0.41
1.1	1.5	87	28	243	84	341	3.6	2	30	0	0.48	0	0.08	0.21	6	0.53	9	0.43
2.3	1.1	43	34	194	1329	146	1.7	2.2	19	31	0.84	0	0.06	0.3	4.3	0.24	10	0.58

Food Item	Qty	Meas	Wgt (g)	Wtr (g)	Cals	Prot	Carb (g)	Fib (g)	Fat (g)	SatF (g)
Turkey, white meat, skinless, roasted	4	oz.	113	78	159	34	0	0	1	0.4
Turnip greens, raw, chopped	0.5	cup	28	25	7	0	2	0.9	0	0
Turnip greens, raw, cooked	0.5	cup	72	67	14	1	3	2.5	0	0
Turnip, raw cubes	0.5	cup	65	60	18	1	4	1.2	0	0
Turnip, raw cubes, cooked, no added salt	0.5	cup	78	73	16	1	4	1.6	0	0
Turtle meat, cooked	4	oz.	113	80	152	27	0	0	4	0.9
Vanilla cookie crust, recipe, chilled	1	piece	29	2	156	1	15	0	11	2.2
Veal patty, breaded, cooked	3	oz.	85	45	225	18	7	0.4	14	4.8
Veal scallopini	1	piece	96	55	257	18	1	0.2	19	5.6
Veal, ground, broiled	4	oz.	113	76	195	28	0	0	9	3.4
Veal, leg, pan fried, lean	3	oz.	85	52	156	28	0	0	4	1.1
Veal, leg, roasted, lean	4	oz.	113	76	170	32	0	0	4	1.4
Veal, leg, roasted, lean & fat	4	oz.	113	75	181	31	0	0	5	2.1
Veal, loin chop, braised, lean	1	each	69	39	156	23	0	0	6	1.8
Veal, loin, cutlet/chop, braised, lean & fat	1	each	80	42	227	24	0	0	14	5.4
Veal, rib, roasted, lean	4	oz.	113	73	201	29	0	0	8	2.4
Veal, rib, roasted, lean & fat	4	oz.	113	68	259	27	0	0	16	6.1
Veal, shoulder, whole, braised, lean	4	oz.	113	67	226	38	0	0	7	1.9
Veal, sirloin, roasted, lean	4	oz.	113	74	191	30	0	0	7	2.7
Veal, sirloin, roasted, lean & fat	4	oz.	113	71	229	28	0	0	12	5.1
Vegetable juice cocktail (V8), low sodium	1	cup	242	226	46	2	11	1.9	0	0
Vegetable tempura	0.5	cup	32	22	50	1	4	0.4	3	0.6
Vegetables, Japanese stir fry, Bird's Eye	0.5	cup	58	53	18	1	4	1.1	0	0
Vegetables, pickled, giardiniera	0.5	cup	82	74	22	1	5	1.7	0	0
Vegetarian, Garden dog, hotdog	1	each	57	30	120	19	4	1	2	—
Vegetarian, Garden(R) burger, meat only	2.5	oz.	71	41	130	8	18	5	3	1
Vegetarian, Garden(R) sausage patty, meat only	1	each	35	21	65	4	9	2	2	1
Vegetarian, Garden(R) steak, meat only, large	1	each	142	115	369	23	51	14.2	8	2.8
Vegetarian, Garden(R) taco/Veg Mexi	0.25	oz.	35	9	107	6	18	4.8	1	0.6
Vegetarian, bacon bits	4	each	57	5	253	18	16	5.8	15	2.3
Vegetarian, bacon strips	3	each	24	12	74	3	2	0.6	7	1.1
Vegetarian, breakfast links	1	each	25	13	64	5	2	0.7	5	0.7
Vegetarian, breakfast sausage patty	1	each	38	19	48	7	4	1.1	7	1.1
Vegetarian, chicken, breaded, fried	1	oz.	28	20	97	3	1	1.2	3	0.5
Vegetarian, chili	0.5	cup	107	69	141	19	15	3.9	2	0.3
Vegetarian, fish sticks	2	each	57	26	165	13	5	3.5	10	1.6
Vegetarian, frankfurter	1	each	51	30	102	10	4	2.4	5	0.8
Vegetarian, luncheon slice	1	piece	67	31	188	17	6	3.4	11	1.7
Vegetarian, meatballs	7	each	70	41	140	15	6	3.2	6	1
Vegetarian, scallops, breaded, fried	0.5	cup	85	36	257	20	8	5.4	16	2.5
Vegetarian, soyburger	1	each	71	41	142	15	6	3.3	6	1
Vegetarian, soyburger, w/cheese, serving	1	each	135	67	316	21	30	4.1	13	4.2
Vermouth, dry	0.5	cup	120	92	144	0	7	0	0	0
Vinegar, balsamic	1	Tbs	15	13	10	0	2	0	0	—
Vinegar, cider	1	Tbs	15	14	2	0	1	0	0	0
Waffle, Special K, Eggo	1	each	30	11	72	3	15	0	0	0
Waffle, blueberry, 7 inch round	1	each	75	32	186	6	30	1.3	5	1.8
Waffle, buttermilk, Eggo	1	each	39	16	110	2	15	0	4	0.8
Waffle, buttermilk, recipe	1	each	75	32	217	6	25	1.1	10	1.9
Waffle, cornmeal, 7 inch round	1	each	75	31	209	6	28	1.3	8	2
Waffle, cornmeal, frozen, 4 inch	1	each	38	16	106	3	14	0.6	4	1
Waffle, frozen toasted	1	each	35	15	92	2	14	0.8	3	0.5
Waffle, mix prepared w/water	1	each	75	32	218	5	26	1	10	1.7
Waffle, mixed grain, frozen, 4 inch	1	each	38	12	116	3	17	2.1	5	1.2
Waffle, oat bran, Eggo	1	each	38	16	107	3	15	2.1	4	0.6
Waffle, plain, recipe	1	each	75	32	218	6	25	1.1	11	2.2
Waffle, whole grain, 4 inch round	1	each	39	17	107	4	13	1	5	1.6
Waffle, whole grain, frozen	1	each	39	17	107	4	13	1	5	1.6
Walnut, English/Persian, dried, chopped	0.25	cup	30	1	193	4	5	1.4	19	1.7
Walnuts, black, dried	0.25	cup	31	1	190	8	4	1.6	18	1.1
Water	1	cup	237	237	0	0	0	0	0	0
Water, Perrier, 6.5 fl oz bottle	1	each	192	192	0	0	0	0	0	0
Water, bottled, Poland Springs	1	cup	237	237	0	0	0	0	0	0
Water, sparkling mineral, sweet, bottled	1	each	488	445	166	0	43	0	0	0
Water, tonic, sugar-free, 12 fl oz can	1	each	355	354	0	0	0	0	0	0

MonoF (g)	PolyF (g)	Choles (mg)	Calc (mg)	Phos (mg)	Sod (mg)	Pot (mg)	Zn (mg)	Iron (mg)	Magn (mg)	VitA (µg RE)	VitE (µg α-TE)	VitC (mg)	Thia (mg)	Ribo (mg)	Nia (mg)	B6 (mg)	Fola (µg)	B12 (µg)
0.2	0.4	98	17	245	64	314	2.4	1.8	32	0	0.12	0	0.05	0.15	7.9	0.65	7	0.44
0	0	0	52	12	11	81	0.1	0.3	9	209	0.8	16	0.02	0.03	0.2	0.07	53	0
0	0.1	0	99	21	21	146	0.1	0.6	16	396	1.24	20	0.03	0.05	0.3	0.13	85	0
0	0	0	20	18	44	124	0.2	0.2	7	0	0.02	14	0.03	0.02	0.3	0.06	9	0
0	0	0	17	15	39	105	0.2	0.2	6	0	0.02	9	0.02	0.02	0.2	0.05	7	0
1.6	1.3	68	163	247	454	316	1.4	1.9	28	83	1.23	0	0.15	0.21	1.4	0.15	18	1.23
4.6	3.1	11	12	23	151	23	0.1	0.5	3	84	1.48	0	0.06	0.07	0.6	0.02	14	0.03
5.5	2	86	27	164	333	237	2.1	1	20	9	0.8	0	0.06	0.23	6.1	0.3	13	0.79
8.3	4.2	62	45	170	381	228	1.9	0.7	19	165	2.2	0	0.05	0.19	3.6	0.22	10	0.95
3.2	0.6	117	19	246	94	382	4.4	1.1	27	0	0.17	0	0.08	0.31	9.1	0.44	12	1.44
1.4	0.3	91	6	247	66	376	2.9	0.7	27	0	0.36	0	0.06	0.32	10.7	0.43	14	1.28
1.4	0.3	117	7	268	77	446	3.5	1	32	0	0.62	0	0.07	0.37	11.5	0.35	18	1.34
2	0.4	117	7	265	77	441	3.4	1	32	0	0.56	0	0.07	0.36	11.3	0.35	18	1.33
2.3	0.6	86	22	164	58	205	2.8	0.8	19	0	0.29	0	0.04	0.24	7	0.19	10	0.91
5.4	0.9	94	22	176	64	224	2.9	0.9	19	0	0.32	0	0.03	0.24	7.2	0.21	11	0.97
3	0.8	130	14	235	110	353	5.1	1.1	27	0	0.41	0	0.07	0.33	8.5	0.31	16	1.79
6.2	1.1	125	12	223	104	335	4.6	1.1	25	0	0.4	0	0.06	0.31	7.9	0.28	15	1.66
2.5	0.6	147	42	295	110	362	7.9	1.6	32	0	0.51	0	0.07	0.4	7.6	0.3	18	2.2
2.6	0.5	118	16	262	96	414	4	1	31	0	0.52	0	0.07	0.42	10.6	0.39	18	1.69
4.6	0.8	116	15	253	94	398	3.8	1	30	0	0.48	0	0.07	0.4	10.1	0.36	17	1.61
0	0.1	0	27	41	653	467	0.5	1	27	283	0.77	67	0.1	0.07	1.8	0.34	51	0
0.9	1.3	20	8	22	10	56	0.1	0.4	4	73	0.32	1	0.04	0.06	0.4	0.02	7	0.04
—	—	0	16	21	219	96	—	0.4	8	37	—	16	0.03	0.06	0.5	0.05	18	0
0	0.1	0	18	23	562	186	0.1	0.3	10	624	0.23	26	0.04	0.03	0.4	0.11	14	0
—	—	0	20	—	310	500	—	1.4	—	0	—	4	—	—	—	—	—	—
1.5	0.5	11	84	132	289	193	0.9	0	30	10	0.2	0	0.11	0.15	1.1	0.08	10	0.11
0.4	0.1	5	40	68	150	71	0.4	0.2	14	12	0.1	0	0.05	0.07	0.5	0.04	5	0.06
4.2	1.2	31	239	375	822	548	2.5	0	86	28	0.61	0	0.3	0.42	3	0.21	29	0.31
0.4	0.2	0	118	—	80	152	—	0.4	—	18	—	1	—	—	—	—	—	0
3.6	7.7	0	58	124	1008	83	1.1	0.4	54	0	3.93	1	0.34	0.04	0.9	0.05	72	0.68
1.7	3.7	0	6	17	352	41	0.1	0.6	5	2	1.66	0	1.06	0.12	1.8	0.12	10	0
1.1	2.3	0	16	56	222	58	0.4	0.9	9	16	0.52	0	0.58	0.1	2.8	0.21	6	0
1.7	3.5	0	24	86	337	88	0.6	1.4	14	24	0.8	0	0.89	0.15	4.3	0.32	10	0
1.5	1.3	0	7	70	113	85	0.2	0.5	3	0	0.55	0	0.2	0.14	1.3	0.14	16	0.6
0.6	0.9	0	53	216	526	362	1.3	4.2	36	78	1.24	16	0.12	0.07	1.2	0.15	82	0
2.5	5.4	0	54	257	279	342	0.8	1.1	13	0	2.25	0	0.63	0.51	6.8	0.86	58	2.39
1.2	2.7	0	17	175	219	76	0.6	0.9	9	0	0.98	0	0.56	0.61	8.2	0.5	40	1.22
2.6	5.6	0	28	296	576	188	1.1	1.5	15	0	2.01	0	0.64	0.37	7.4	0.74	67	1.74
1.5	3.3	0	20	241	385	126	1.3	1.5	13	0	1.21	0	0.63	0.42	7	0.84	55	1.68
3.8	8.3	0	84	398	434	531	1.2	1.8	20	0	3.5	0	0.97	0.8	10.6	1.33	90	3.72
1.5	3.3	0	21	244	391	128	1.3	1.5	13	0	1.23	0	0.64	0.43	7.1	0.85	55	1.7
4	3.7	13	146	372	931	211	2	2.7	26	45	1.43	1	0.77	0.55	8.1	0.86	70	1.71
0	0	0	8	8	20	48	0	0.4	6	0	0	0	0.02	0.02	0	0.01	0	0
—	—	0	5	—	4	12	—	0.1	—	0	—	0	—	—	—	—	—	—
0	0	0	1	1	0	15	0	0.1	3	0	0	0	0	0	0	0	0	0
0	0	0	21	—	129	16	—	1.9	—	155	—	0	0.16	0.18	2.1	0.21	41	0.62
1.6	0.9	34	219	262	523	154	0.5	1.2	16	29	0.89	2	0.15	0.23	1	0.06	7	0.2
—	—	12	20	—	240	32	—	1.8	—	150	—	0	0.15	0.17	2	0.2	40	0.6
2.5	5.1	50	137	124	451	128	0.6	1.6	14	26	1.5	0	0.2	0.27	1.6	0.04	11	0.16
2.2	3	75	110	108	312	124	0.6	1.6	17	50	1.41	0	0.21	0.27	1.6	0.08	16	0.27
1.1	1.5	38	56	55	158	63	0.3	0.8	9	25	0.72	0	0.1	0.14	0.8	0.04	8	0.14
1.1	1	8	81	147	275	45	0.2	1.6	8	127	0.29	0	0.14	0.17	1.6	0.31	16	0.88
2.7	5.2	38	93	252	458	134	0.4	1.2	15	20	1.5	0	0.16	0.19	1.2	0.08	9	0.2
1.2	2	28	83	104	146	123	0.9	1.4	25	60	0.93	3	0.14	0.19	1.4	0.11	23	0.12
1.1	2	0	8	131	214	189	0.7	0.7	38	57	0.57	0	0.06	0.06	0.8	0.03	15	0.23
2.6	5.1	52	191	143	383	119	0.5	1.7	14	49	1.73	0	0.2	0.26	1.6	0.04	34	0.19
1.9	1	39	84	83	150	91	0.4	0.7	16	25	0.53	0	0.08	0.13	0.7	0.04	7	0.15
1.9	1	39	84	83	150	91	0.4	0.7	16	25	0.53	0	0.08	0.13	0.7	0.04	7	0.15
4.3	11.7	0	28	95	3	151	0.8	0.7	51	4	0.79	1	0.12	0.04	0.3	0.17	20	0
4	11.7	0	18	145	0	164	1.1	1	63	9	0.82	1	0.07	0.03	0.2	0.17	20	0
0	0	0	5	0	7	0	0.1	0	2	0	0	0	0	0	0	0	0	0
0	0	0	27	0	2	0	0	0	0	0	0	0	0	0	0	0	0	0
0	0	0	2	0	2	0	0	0	2	0	0	0	0	0	0	0	0	0
0	0	0	5	0	20	0	0.5	0	0	0	0	0	0	0	0	0	0	0
0	0	0	14	39	57	7	0.2	0.1	4	0	0	0	0	0	0	0	0	0

Food Item	Qty	Meas	Wgt (g)	Wtr (g)	Cals	Prot	Carb (g)	Fib (g)	Fat (g)	SatF (g)
Water, tonic/quinine/carbonated	1	cup	244	222	83	0	22	0	0	0
Water chestnut, Chinese, raw slices	0.5	cup	62	46	60	1	15	1.9	0	0
Watercress, fresh	0.5	cup	17	16	2	0	0	0.3	0	0
Watercress, fresh sprigs	10	each	25	24	3	1	0	0.4	0	0
Watermelon, fresh pieces	0.5	cup	80	73	26	0	6	0.4	0	0
Waxgourd, cooked cubes	0.5	cup	87	84	11	0	3	0.9	0	0
Waxgourd, raw, cubes	0.5	cup	66	63	9	0	2	1.9	0	0
Weiner wraps, franks in dough	1	each	85	39	278	7	15	0.4	21	6.8
Wendy's, Frosty dairy dessert, medium	1	each	324	219	478	12	79	0	12	7.6
Wendy's, Jr cheeseburger, deluxe	1	each	179	104	358	18	36	3	17	6
Wendy's, bacon cheeseburger, w/bun	1	each	170	94	389	20	35	2	20	7.2
Wendy's, chicken sandwich, grilled	1	each	177	109	290	25	33	1.9	7	1.4
Wendy's, hamburger, big classic, w/cheese	1	each	287	170	590	35	47	3	30	12.2
Wendy's, hamburger, single, deluxe	1	each	219	136	420	25	37	3	20	7
Wendy's, junior hamburger	1	each	117	56	268	15	34	2	10	3.5
Wheat berries, whole, cooked	0.5	cup	75	65	42	2	10	1.7	0	0
Wheat bran, crude	0.25	cup	15	1	32	2	10	6.4	1	0.1
Wheat germ, defatted, Viobin	0.5	oz.	15	1	45	4	9	3	0	0
Wheat germ, toasted	2	Tbs	14	1	54	4	7	1.8	2	0.3
Wheat germ, w/brown sugar/honey	1	cup	113	4	420	30	66	11.5	9	1.5
Wheat grain, cracked, dry	4	oz.	113	12	384	16	82	13.1	2	0.4
Wheat sprouts	0.5	cup	54	26	107	4	23	0.6	1	0.1
Whiskey sour, canned	2	Tbs	31	24	37	0	4	0	0	0
Wine, dessert, dry	1	cup	236	189	297	0	10	0	0	0
Wine, dessert, sweet	0.5	cup	118	86	181	0	14	0	0	0
Wine, nonalcoholic	1	cup	232	228	14	1	3	0	0	0
Wine, nonalcoholic, light	1	cup	251	246	15	1	3	0	0	0
Wine, red	1	cup	236	209	170	0	4	0	0	0
Wine, rice	4	oz.	113	89	152	1	6	0	0	0
Wine, rosé	1	cup	236	210	168	0	3	0	0	0
Wine, sangria	4	oz.	113	94	93	0	13	0	0	0
Wine, sherry, dry	0.5	cup	117	104	82	0	2	0	0	0
Wine, sweet vermouth	0.5	cup	120	87	184	0	14	0	0	0
Wine, white, dry	1	cup	238	213	158	0	1	0	0	0
Winged bean/goabean tuber, raw	0.5	cup	50	29	74	6	14	2.8	0	0.1
Wonton, fried, meat filled	3	piece	57	25	183	8	12	0.6	11	2.2
Wonton/eggroll wrapper	3	each	24	7	70	2	14	0.4	0	0.1
Yam, orange, canned in syrup	0.5	cup	114	88	101	1	24	2.8	0	0
Yam, white, cooked	0.5	cup	68	48	79	1	19	2.6	0	0
Yams, orange, baked, then peeled, mashed	0.5	cup	100	73	103	2	24	3	0	0
Yams, orange, canned, mashed	0.5	cup	128	95	129	3	30	2.2	0	0.1
Yams, orange, peeled, boiled, mashed	0.5	cup	100	73	105	2	24	1.8	0	0.1
Yeast, baker's, dry active	1	Tbs	8	1	22	3	3	1.6	0	0
Yeast, brewer's	1	Tbs	8	0	23	3	3	2.5	0	0
Yogurt chips	1	oz.	28	1	146	3	16	0.5	8	2.1
Yogurt, custard fruit, lowfat	1	cup	245	183	250	11	47	0	3	1.7
Yogurt, frozen, banana-strawberry, HaagenDaz	0.5	cup	98	—	170	6	27	—	4	2
Yogurt, frozen, peach, HaagenDaz	0.5	cup	98	—	170	6	26	—	4	2
Yogurt, fruit, lowfat	1	cup	245	183	250	11	47	0	3	1.7
Yogurt, fruit, nonfat, low cal sweetener	1	cup	241	208	122	12	19	1.3	0	0.2
Yogurt, lowfat, vanilla/lemon	1	cup	245	194	209	12	34	0	3	2
Yogurt, nonfat, lemon	1	cup	245	187	223	12	43	0	0	0.3
Yogurt, nonfat, vanilla	1	each	227	173	207	12	40	0	0	0.2
Yogurt, peach, nonfat, Knudsen	6	oz.	170	—	170	8	33	0	0	0
Yogurt, plain, lowfat	1	cup	245	208	155	13	17	0	4	2.4
Yogurt, plain, nonfat	1	cup	245	209	137	14	19	0	0	0.3
Yogurt, plain, whole milk	1	cup	245	215	150	8	11	0	8	5.2

MonoF	PolyF	Choles	Calc	Phos	Sod	Pot	Zn	Iron	Magn	VitA	VitE	VitC	Thia	Ribo	Nia	B6	Fola	B12
(g)	(g)	(mg)	(mg)	(mg)	(mg)	(mg)	(mg)	(mg)	(mg)	(µg RE)	(µg α-TE)	(mg)	(mg)	(mg)	(mg)	(mg)	(µg)	(µg)
0	0	0	2	0	10	0	0.2	0	0	0	0	0	0	0	0	0	0	0
0	0	0	7	39	9	362	0.3	0	14	0	0.74	2	0.09	0.12	0.6	0.2	10	0
0	0	0	20	10	7	56	0	0	4	80	0.17	7	0.02	0.02	0	0.02	2	0
0	0	0	30	15	10	82	0	0	5	118	0.25	11	0.02	0.03	0	0.03	2	0
0.1	0.1	0	6	7	2	93	0.1	0.1	9	30	0.12	8	0.06	0.02	0.2	0.12	2	0
0	0.1	0	16	15	93	4	0.5	0.3	9	0	0.34	9	0.03	0	0.3	0.03	3	0
0	0.1	0	12	12	73	4	0.4	0.3	7	0	0.26	9	0.03	0.07	0.3	0.02	3	0
9.6	3.4	22	137	103	818	131	1	1.2	10	14	0.82	10	0.19	0.16	2	0.06	5	0.59
—	—	54	446	356	260	776	1.4	1.6	65	217	—	0	0.15	0.67	0.5	0.17	25	1.2
—	—	50	179	—	885	—	—	3.4	—	99	—	6	—	—	—	—	—	—
10.5	1.4	61	174	342	870	384	6	3.5	39	82	—	6	0.31	0.32	6.6	0.27	29	2.04
—	—	61	94	—	740	—	—	2.5	—	38	—	6	—	—	—	—	—	—
—	—	102	254	—	1485	588	—	5.5	—	153	—	15	0.46	1.55	6.1	—	—	—
—	—	70	130	—	920	468	—	4.7	—	60	—	6	0.43	0.33	5.8	—	—	—
—	—	30	109	—	605	—	—	3	—	20	—	1	—	—	—	—	—	—
0	0.1	0	4	39	0	50	0.4	0.4	17	0	0.15	0	0.06	0.02	0.8	0.04	6	0
0.1	0.3	0	11	152	0	177	1.1	1.6	92	0	0.35	0	0.08	0.09	2	0.2	12	0
0	0.1	0	10	179	1	174	2.1	1.5	52	250	0.01	—	0.15	0.08	1.2	0.22	63	0.08
0.2	0.9	0	6	162	1	134	2.4	1.3	45	0	2.56	1	0.24	0.12	0.8	0.14	50	0
1.2	5.5	0	56	1142	12	1089	15.7	9.1	307	11	24.9	0	1.51	0.78	5.3	0.56	376	0
0.3	0.9	0	39	392	6	459	3.3	4.4	156	0	0.48	0	0.51	0.24	7.2	0.39	50	0
0.1	0.3	0	15	108	9	91	0.9	1.2	44	0	0.03	1	0.12	0.08	1.7	0.14	20	0
0	0	0	0	2	14	3	0	0	0	0	0	0	0	0	0	0	0	0
0	0	0	19	21	21	217	0.2	0.6	21	0	0	0	0.04	0.04	0.5	0	1	0
0	0	0	9	11	11	109	0.1	0.3	11	0	0	0	0.02	0.02	0.3	0	0	0
0	0	0	21	35	16	204	0.2	0.9	23	0	0	0	0	0.02	0.2	0.05	2	0
0	0	0	23	38	18	221	0.2	1	25	0	0	0	0	0.02	0.2	0.05	3	0
0	0	0	19	33	12	264	0.2	1	31	0	0	0	0.01	0.07	0.2	0.08	5	0.02
0	0	0	6	7	2	28	0	0.1	7	0	0	0	0	0	0	0	0	0
0	0	0	19	35	12	234	0.1	0.9	24	0	0	0	0.01	0.04	0.2	0.06	3	0.02
0	0	0	5	6	8	40	0.1	0.1	4	1	0.01	4	0.01	0.01	0	0.01	2	0
0	0	0	9	16	9	104	0.1	0.5	12	0	0	0	0	0.02	0.1	0.03	1	0.01
0	0	0	10	11	11	110	0.1	0.3	11	0	0	0	0.02	0.02	0.3	0	0	0
0	0	0	22	14	10	146	0.2	0.8	22	0	0	0	0	0.01	0.2	0.05	0	0
0.1	0.1	0	15	22	18	293	0.7	1	12	0	—	0	0.19	0.08	0.8	0.04	10	0
4.9	3.6	39	17	72	250	114	0.7	1.2	13	65	1.71	1	0.24	0.17	1.8	0.1	10	0.17
0	0.1	2	11	19	137	20	0.2	0.8	5	1	0.02	0	0.12	0.09	1.3	0.01	21	0
0	0.1	0	17	31	50	211	0.2	0.9	15	652	0.26	12	0.03	0.05	0.5	0.06	7	0
0	0	0	10	33	5	456	0.1	0.4	12	0	0.11	8	0.06	0.02	0.4	0.16	11	0
0	0	0	28	55	10	348	0.3	0.4	20	2182	0.28	25	0.07	0.13	0.6	0.24	23	0
0	0.1	0	38	67	96	269	0.3	1.7	31	1936	0.35	7	0.04	0.12	1.2	0.3	14	0
0	0.1	0	21	27	13	184	0.3	0.6	10	1705	0.28	17	0.05	0.14	0.6	0.24	11	0
0.2	0	0	5	97	4	150	0.5	1.2	7	0	0.01	0	0.18	0.41	3	0.12	176	0
0	0	0	17	140	10	151	0.6	1.4	18	0	—	0	1.25	0.34	3	0.4	313	0
3.5	2.1	1	37	47	13	63	0.3	0.9	7	3	0.69	0	0.12	0.12	1	0.02	5	0.08
0.7	0.1	10	372	292	143	478	1.8	0.2	36	27	0.07	2	0.09	0.44	0.2	0.1	23	1.14
2	0	60	146	195	50	170	—	0.4	—	—	—	4	—	0.17	—	—	—	—
2	0	40	146	146	45	160	—	0.4	—	—	—	—	—	0.17	—	—	—	—
0.7	0.1	10	372	292	143	478	1.8	0.2	36	27	0.07	2	0.09	0.44	0.2	0.1	23	1.14
0.1	0	3	369	291	139	550	1.8	0.6	41	6	0.17	26	0.1	0.45	0.5	0.11	32	1.11
0.8	0.1	12	419	331	161	537	2	0.2	40	32	0.08	2	0.1	0.49	0.3	0.11	26	1.29
0.1	0	4	436	343	168	559	2.1	0.2	42	4	0.01	2	0.1	0.52	0.3	0.12	27	1.34
0.1	0	4	404	318	155	518	2	0.2	39	4	0.01	2	0.1	0.48	0.3	0.11	25	1.24
0	0	5	250	200	105	370	—	—	—	0	—	0	0.03	0.26	—	—	—	0.9
1	0.1	15	448	353	172	573	2.2	0.2	43	39	0.1	2	0.11	0.52	0.3	0.12	27	1.38
0.1	0	4	488	385	187	625	2.4	0.2	47	5	0.01	2	0.12	0.57	0.3	0.13	30	1.5
2.2	0.2	31	296	233	114	380	1.4	0.1	28	74	0.22	1	0.07	0.35	0.2	0.08	18	0.91

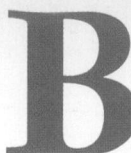
Standards for Body Size

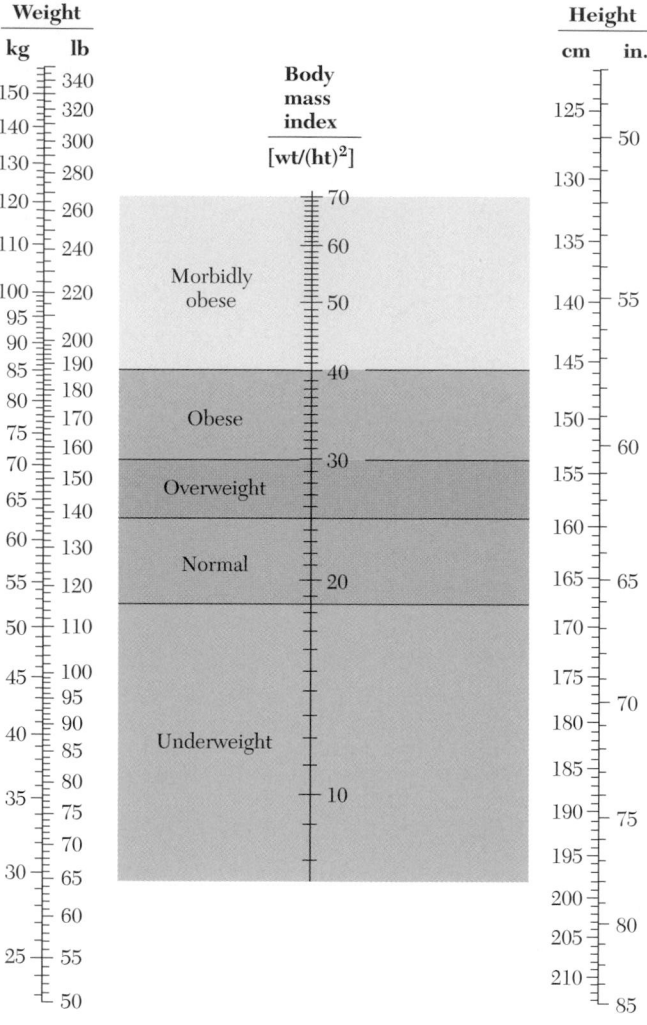

NOMOGRAM FOR DETERMINING BODY MASS INDEX (BMI)

Estimation of Frame Size Using Elbow Breadth*

MEN Height in 1-Inch Heels	Elbow Breadth	WOMEN Height in 1-Inch Heels	Elbow Breadth
5 ft 2 in. to 5 ft 3 in.	$2\frac{1}{2}$ to $2\frac{7}{8}$ in.	4 ft 10 in. to 4 ft 11 in.	$2\frac{1}{4}$ to $2\frac{1}{2}$ in.
5 ft 4 in. to 5 ft 7 in.	$2\frac{5}{8}$ to $2\frac{7}{8}$ in.	5 ft 0 in. to 5 ft 3 in.	$2\frac{1}{4}$ to $2\frac{1}{2}$ in.
5 ft 8 in. to 5 ft 11 in.	$2\frac{3}{4}$ to 3 in.	5 ft 4 in. to 5 ft 7 in.	$2\frac{3}{8}$ to $2\frac{5}{8}$ in.
6 ft 0 in. to 6 ft 3 in.	$2\frac{3}{4}$ to $3\frac{1}{8}$ in.	5 ft 8 in. to 5 ft 11 in.	$2\frac{3}{8}$ to $2\frac{5}{8}$ in.
6 ft 4 in. and over	$2\frac{7}{8}$ to $3\frac{1}{4}$ in.	6 ft 0 in. and over	$2\frac{1}{2}$ to $2\frac{3}{4}$ in.

*If your measurement is within the range indicated, you have a medium frame. Measurements smaller than those listed indicate a small frame, and those larger indicate a large frame. Elbow breadth is measured as the distance between the bony protrusions of the elbow. For this measurement the right arm is raised to the horizontal, and the elbow flexed to 90 degrees, with the back of the hand facing the measurer.

Source: Metropolitan Life Insurance Company.

1983 Metropolitan Life Insurance Co. Height and Weight Tables

Height	Small Frame	Medium Frame	Large Frame
	←——————— lb ———————→		
Men°			
5'2"	128–134	131–141	138–150
5'3"	130–136	133–143	140–153
5'4"	132–138	135–145	142–156
5'5"	134–140	137–148	144–160
5'6"	136–142	139–151	146–164
5'7"	138–145	142–154	149–168
5'8"	140–148	145–157	152–172
5'9"	142–151	148–160	155–176
5'10"	144–154	151–163	158–180
5'11"	146–157	154–166	161–184
6'0"	149–160	157–170	164–188
6'1"	152–164	160–174	168–192
6'2"	155–168	164–178	172–197
6'3"	158–172	167–182	176–202
6'4"	162–176	171–187	181–207
Women†			
4'10"	102–111	109–121	118–131
4'11"	103–113	111–123	120–134
5'0"	104–115	113–126	122–137
5'1"	106–118	115–129	125–140
5'2"	108–121	118–132	128–143
5'3"	111–124	121–135	131–147
5'4"	114–127	124–138	134–151
5'5"	117–130	127–141	137–155
5'6"	120–133	130–144	140–159
5'7"	123–136	133–147	143–163
5'8"	126–139	136–150	146–167
5'9"	129–142	139–153	149–170
5'10"	132–145	142–156	152–173
5'11"	135–148	145–159	155–176
6'0"	138–151	148–162	158–179

°Weights at ages 25 to 59 based on lowest mortality. Weight in pounds according to frame (in indoor clothing weighing 5 lb, shoes with 1" heels).

†Weights at ages 25 to 59 based on lowest mortality. Weight in pounds according to frame (in indoor clothing weighing 3 lb, shoes with 1" heels).

Courtesy of Metropolitan Life Insurance Company.

Birth to 36 months: Boys
Length-for-age and Weight-for-age percentiles

NAME _____

RECORD # _____

Revised November 28, 2000.
SOURCE: Developed by the National Center for Health Statistics in collaboration with
the National Center for Chronic Disease Prevention and Health Promotion (2000).
www.cdc.gov/growthcharts

Birth to 36 months: Girls
Length-for-age and Weight-for-age percentiles

NAME _____

RECORD # _____

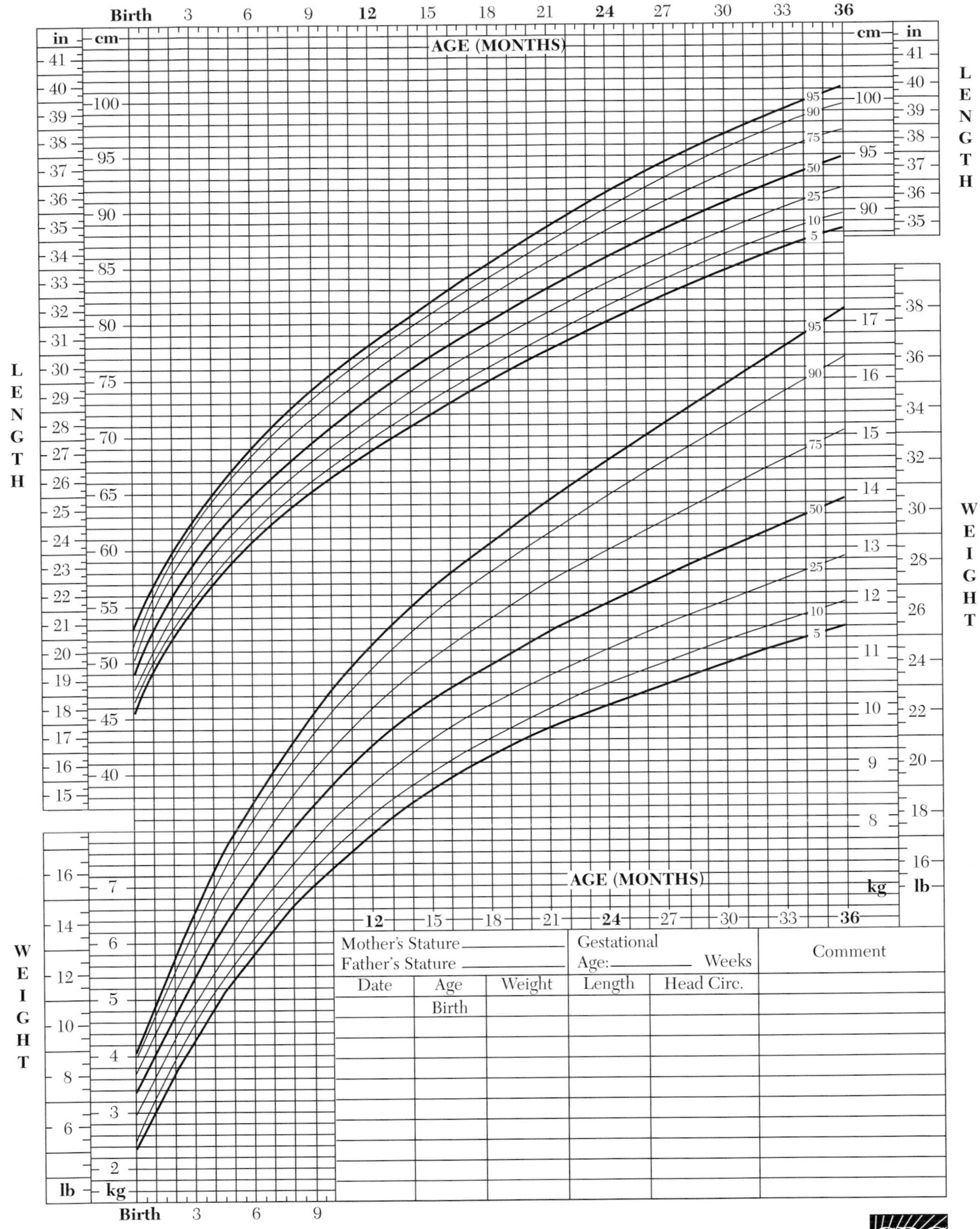

AGE (MONTHS)

Birth 3 6 9 **12** 15 18 21 **24** 27 30 33 **36**

LENGTH

Mother's Stature_____		Gestational		Comment	
Father's Stature_____		Age:_____ Weeks			
Date	Age	Weight	Length	Head Circ.	
	Birth				

AGE (MONTHS)

WEIGHT

Revised November 28, 2000.
SOURCE: Developed by the National Center for Health Statistics in collaboration with
the National Center for Chronic Disease Prevention and Health Promotion (2000).
www.cdc.gov/growthcharts

2 to 20 years: Boys
Body mass index-for-age percentiles

NAME _____

RECORD # _____

Date	Age	Weight	Stature	BMI°	Comments

°To Calculate BMI: Weight (kg) ÷ Stature (cm) ÷ Stature (cm) × 10,000
or Weight (lb) ÷ Stature (in) ÷ Stature (in) × 703

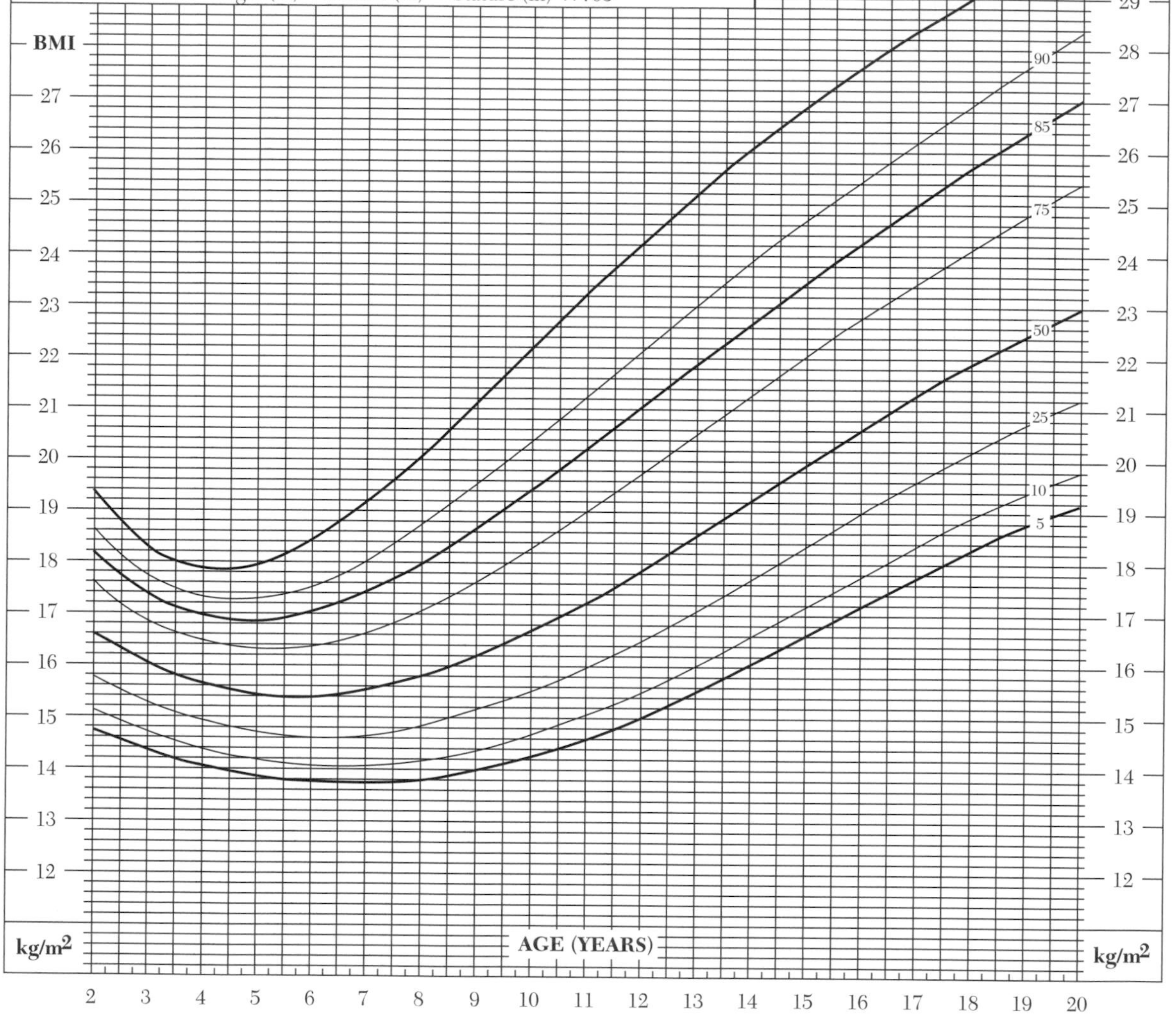

BMI

kg/m²

AGE (YEARS)

kg/m²

95
90
85
75
50
25
10
5

2 3 4 5 6 7 8 9 10 11 12 13 14 15 16 17 18 19 20

SOURCE: Developed by the National Center for Health Statistics in collaboration with
the National Center for Chronic Disease Prevention and Health Promotion (2000).
www.cdc.gov/growthcharts

2 to 20 years: Girls
Body mass index-for-age percentiles

NAME _____

RECORD # _____

Date	Age	Weight	Stature	BMI°	Comments

°To Calculate BMI: Weight (kg) ÷ Stature (cm) ÷ Stature (cm) × 10,000
or Weight (lb) ÷ Stature (in) ÷ Stature (in) × 703

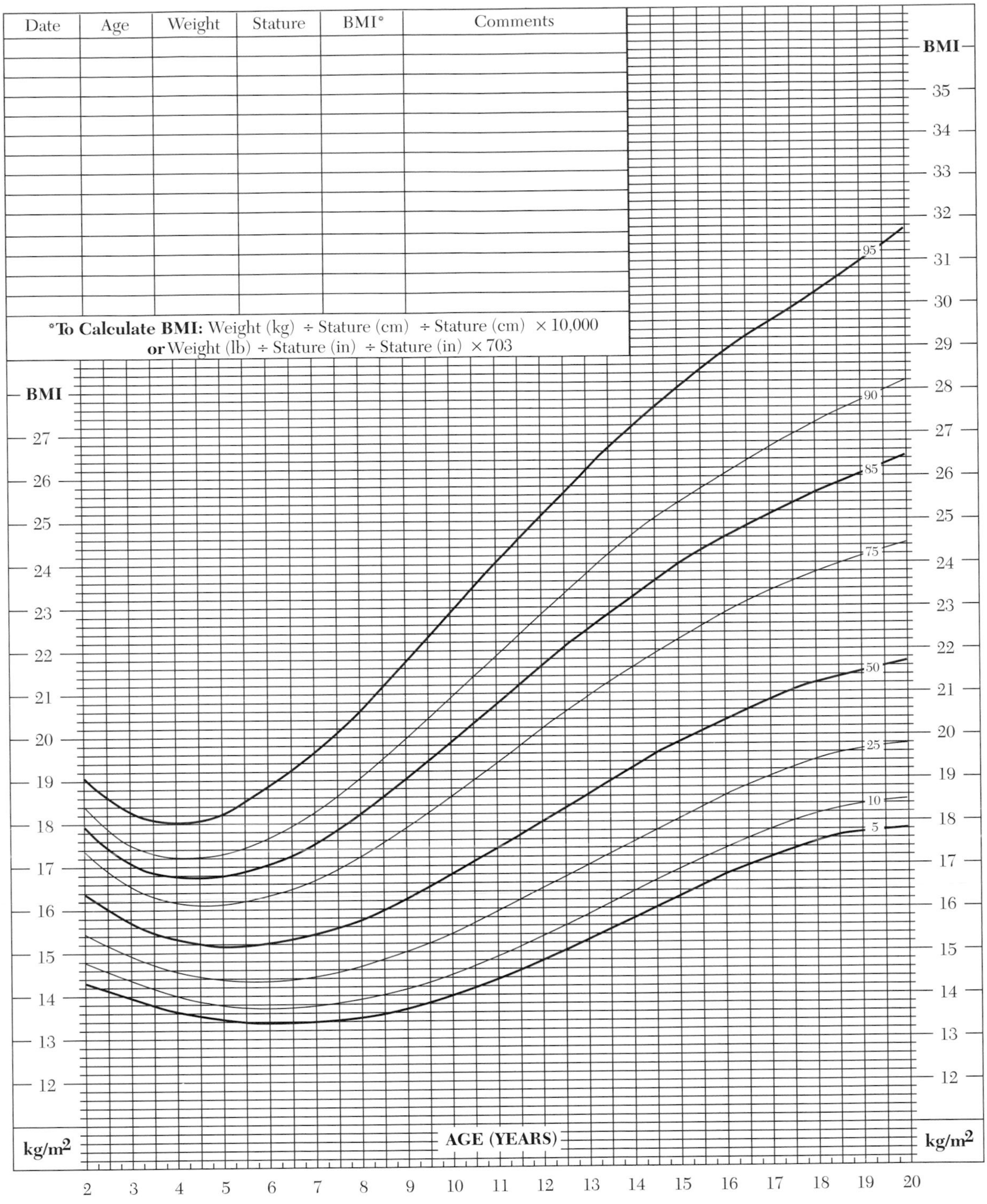

BMI

BMI

35
34
33
32
31
30
29
28
27
26
25
24
23
22
21
20
19
18
17
16
15
14
13
12

95
90
85
75
50
25
10
5

kg/m²

AGE (YEARS)

kg/m²

2 3 4 5 6 7 8 9 10 11 12 13 14 15 16 17 18 19 20

SOURCE: Developed by the National Center for Health Statistics in collaboration with
the National Center for Chronic Disease Prevention and Health Promotion (2000).
www.cdc.gov/growthcharts

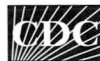

Weight-for-Height Tables for Adults— Gerontology Center Recommendations

Height (ft and in)	Gerontology Research Center* (Age-Specific Weight Range in Pounds for Men and Women)				
	20–29 yr	30–39 yr	40–49 yr	50–59 yr	60–69 yr
4'10"	84–111	92–119	99–127	107–135	115–142
4'11"	87–115	95–123	103–131	111–139	119–147
5'0"	90–119	98–127	106–135	114–143	123–152
5'1"	93–123	101–131	110–140	118–148	127–157
5'2"	96–127	105–136	113–144	122–153	131–163
5'3"	99–131	108–140	117–149	126–158	135–168
5'4"	102–135	112–145	121–154	130–163	140–173
5'5"	106–140	115–149	125–159	134–168	144–179
5'6"	109–144	119–154	129–164	138–174	148–184
5'7"	112–148	122–159	133–169	143–179	153–190
5'8"	116–153	126–163	137–174	147–184	158–196
5'9"	119–157	130–168	141–179	151–190	162–201
5'10"	122–162	134–173	145–184	156–195	167–207
5'11"	126–167	137–178	149–190	160–201	172–213
6'0"	129–171	141–183	153–195	165–207	177–219
6'1"	133–176	145–188	157–200	169–213	182–225
6'2"	137–181	149–194	162–206	174–219	187–232
6'3"	141–186	153–199	166–212	179–225	192–238
6'4"	144–191	157–205	171–218	184–231	197–244

*Values in this table are for height without shoes and weight without clothes.

Normal Blood Values of Nutritional Relevance

 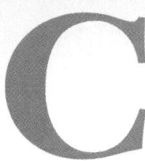

Red blood cells	
Men	4.6–6.2 million/mm^3
Women	4.2–5.2 million/mm^3
White blood cells	5,000–10,000/mm^3
Hematocrit	
Men	40–54 ml/100 ml
Women	36–47 ml/100 ml
Children	35–49 ml/100 ml
Hemoglobin	
Men	14–18 g/100 ml
Women	12–16 g/100 ml
Children	11.2–16.5 g/100 ml
Ferritin	
Men	20–300 ng/ml
Women	20–120 ng/ml
Calcium	9–11 mg/100 ml
Iodine	3.8–8 μg/100 ml
Iron	
Men	75–175 μg/100 ml
Women	65–165 μg/100 ml
Zinc	0.75–1.4 μg/ml
Magnesium	1.8–3.0 mg/100 ml
Potassium	3.5–5.0 mEq/liter
Sodium	136–145 mEq/liter
Chloride	100–108 mEq/liter
Vitamin A	20–80 μg/100 ml
Vitamin B$_{12}$	200–800 pg/100 ml
Vitamin C	0.6–2.0 mg/100 ml
Carotene	48–200 μg/liter
Folate	2–20 ng/ml
pH	7.35–7.45
Total protein	6.6–8.0 g/100 ml
Albumen	3.0–4.0 g/100 ml
Cholesterol	<200 mg/100 ml
LDL Cholesterol	<130 mg/100 ml
HDL Cholesterol	≥40 mg/100 ml
Triglycerides	<150 mg/100 ml
Glucose	60–100 mg/100 ml blood, 70–120 mg/100 ml serum

Source: Handbook of Clinical Dietetics, American Dietetic Association,© 1981 by Yale University Press (New Haven, Conn.); and Committee on Dietetics of the Mayo Clinic, *Mayo Clinic Diet Manual* (Philadelphia: W. B. Saunders Company, 1981), pp. 275–277.

• BLOOD PRESSURE LEVELS

Blood pressure is measured in millimeters of mercury (mm Hg). The classifications in the following table are for persons who are not taking antihypertensive drugs and are not acutely ill. When systolic and diastolic pressures fall into different categories, the physician will select the higher category to classify the person's blood pressure status. Diagnosis of high blood pressure is based on the average of two or more readings taken at each of two or more visits after an initial screening.

Classification of Blood Pressure for Adults Age 18 Years and Older, With Recommended Follow-Up

Category	Systolic (mm Hg)		Diastolic (mm Hg)	Follow-Up Recommended
Optimal°	<120	and	<80	Recheck in 2 years
Normal	<130	and	<85	Recheck in 2 years
High normal	130–139	or	85–89	Recheck in 1 year
Hypertension				
STAGE 1 (Mild)	140–159	or	90–99	Confirm within 2 months
STAGE 2 (Moderate)	160–179	or	100–109	Evaluate within 1 month
STAGE 3 (Severe)	≥180	or	≥110	Evaluate immediately or within 1 week depending on clinical situation

°Unusually low readings should be evaluated for clinical significance.

Source: Sixth Report of the Joint National Committee on Detection, Evaluation, and Treatment of High Blood Pressure, NIH, 1997.

Classification of Blood Lipid Levels (mg/100 ml)

LDL Cholesterol

< 100	Optimal
100–129	Above optimal
130–159	Borderline high
160–189	High
≥ 190	Very high

Total Cholesterol

< 200	Desirable
200–239	Borderline high
≥ 240	High

HDL Cholesterol

< 40	Low
≥ 60	High

Triglycerides

< 150	Normal
150–199	Borderline high
200–499	High
≥ 500	Very high

Source: National Cholesterol Education Program. Adult Treatment Panel III Report, 2001.

Sources of Information on Nutrition

 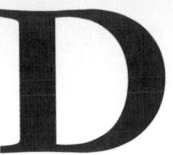

Many publications are available at little or no cost from the government. For individual publications or catalogs, contact:

Superintendent of Documents
U.S. Government Printing Office
Washington, DC 20402
www.access.gpo.gov/su_docs/

National Technical Information Service
5285 Port Royal Road
Springfield, VA 22162

National Research Council
National Academy of Sciences
2102 Constitution Ave. N.W.
Washington, DC 20418
www.nas.edu/

Consumer Information Service
Department 609K
Pueblo, CO 81009
www.pueblo.gsa.gov/

Food Safety and Inspection
  Administration
U.S. Department of Agriculture
Washington, DC 20250
www.usda.gov/fsis/

National Council on Aging
1828 L Street NW
Washington, DC 20036
www.ncoa.org/

Alliance for Food & Fiber
Food Safety Hotline
(800) 266-0200
www.foodsafetyalliance.org/

Center for Food Safety and Applied
  Nutrition
Food and Drug Administration
200 C Street SW
Washington, DC 20204
(800) 332-4010
www.cfsan.fda.gov/

National Lead Information Center
(800) 424-5323
www.epa.gov/opptintr/lead/nlic.htm

Food and Agriculture Organization
North American Regional Office
1325 C St. S.W.
Washington, DC 20025
www.fao.org/

Food and Drug Administration
5600 Fishers Lane
Rockville, MD 20852
www.fda.gov/

The Food and Nutrition Information
  Center
National Agriculture Library
Room 304
10301 Baltimore Blvd.
Beltsville, MD 20705
www.nal.usda.gov/fnic/

National Center for Health Statistics
6265 Belcrest Road
Hyattsville, MD 20782
www.nchs.gov/

National Cancer Institute
Office of Cancer Communications
Building 31, Room 10A18
Bethesda, MD 20205
www.nih.nci.gov/

National Center for Complementary
  and Alternative Medicine
National Institutes of Health
Bethesda, MD 20205
nccam.nih.gov/

Seafood Safety Hotline
(800) 332-4010; (202) 205-4314

U.S. EPA Safe Drinking Water Hotline
(800) 426-4791

Office of Dietary Supplements
  National Institutes of Health
Bethesda, MD 20205
www.odp.od.nih.gov/ods/

Agriculture Research Service
U.S. Department of Agriculture
3700 East West Hwy.
Hyattsville, MD 20782
www.usda.ars.gov/

National Institute on Aging
Information Office
Building 21, Room 5C35
Bethesda, MD 20205
www.nih.gov/nia/

National Heart, Lung, and Blood
  Institute
Information Office
Building 31, Room 4A21
Bethesda, MD 20205
www.nhlbi.nih.gov/

National Institute of Dental Research
Information Office
Building 31, Room 2C34
Bethesda, MD 20205

Health and Welfare Canada
Canadian Government Publishing
  Center
Minister of Supply and Services
Ottawa, Ontario K1A 0S9
www.hc-sc.gc.ca

National Weight Central Information
  Network
National Institutes of Health
Bethesda, MD 20205
www. niddk.nih.gov/WIN

World Health Org.
Geneva, Switzerland
www.who.int/

Many private and international organizations also publish reputable food and nutrition information. Some of these include:

American Dietetic Association
216 W. Jackson Blvd.
Suite 800
Chicago, IL 60606–6995

National Dairy Council
6300 North River Road
Rosemont, IL 60018–4233
www.nationaldairycouncil.org/

American Heart Association
7320 Grenville Ave.
Dallas, TX 75231
www.americanheart.org/

American Anorexia and Bulemia
   Assoc., Inc.
165 W. 46th St., Suite 1108
New York, NY 10036
www.aabainc.org

American College of Sports Medicine
401 W. Michigan Street
Indianapolis, IN 46202-3233
(317) 637-9200; fax: (317) 634-7817
www.acsm.org/

American Council on Exercise
5820 Oberlin Drive, Suite 102
San Diego, CA 92121
(800) 529-8227
www.acefitness.org/

American Diabetes Association
Diabetes Information Service Center
1660 Duke St.
Alexandria, VA 22314
www.diabetes.org/

American Cancer Society
90 Park Ave.
New York, NY 10016
www.cancer.org/

Canadian Dietetic Association
480 University Ave., Suite 601
Toronto, Ontario M5G 1V2 Canada
www.dietitians.ca/

American Academy of Pediatrics
141 Northwest Point Boulevard
Elk Grove Village, IL 60007-1098
(847) 434-4000; fax: (847) 434-8000
www.aap.org/

The Food and Agriculture Organization
North American Regional Office
1325 C St. S.W.
Washington, DC 20025
www.fao.org

ILSI Human Nutrition Institute
1126 Sixteenth Street NW
Washington, DC 20036
(202) 659-0524; fax: (202) 659-3617
www.ilsi.org/hni.html

Institute of Food Technologists
221 N. LaSalle Street, Suite 300
Chicago, IL 60601-1291
(312) 782-8424; fax: (312) 782-8348
www.ift.org/

Canadian Nutritional Recommendations and Guidelines

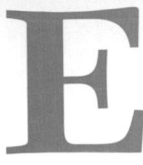

Nutrition Recommendations for Canadians

- The Canadian diet should provide energy consistent with the maintenance of *body weight* within the recommended range.
- The Canadian diet should include *essential nutrients* in amounts recommended.
- The Canadian diet should include no more than 30 percent of energy as fat (33 grams/1000 kcalories or 39 grams/5000 kilojoules) and no more than 10 percent as saturated fat (11 grams/1000 kcalories or 13 grams/5000 kilojoules).
- The Canadian diet should provide 55 percent of energy as *carbohydrate* (138 grams/1000 kcalories or 165 grams/5000 kilojoules) from a variety of sources.
- The *sodium* content of the Canadian diet should be reduced.
- The Canadian diet should include no more than 5 percent of total energy as *alcohol*, or two drinks daily, whichever is less.
- The Canadian diet should contain no more *caffeine* than the equivalent of four regular cups of coffee per day.
- Community water supplies containing less than 1 milligram per liter should be *fluoridated* to that level.

NOTE: Italics added to highlight areas of concern.

Source: Health and Welfare Canada, *Nutrition Recommendations: The Report of the Scientific Review Committee* (Ottawa: Canadian Government Publishing Centre, 1990).

Canada's Guidelines for Healthy Eating

1. Enjoy a VARIETY of foods.
2. Emphasize cereals, breads, other grain products, vegetables, and fruit.
3. Choose lower-fat dairy products, leaner meats, and foods prepared with little or no fat.
4. Achieve and maintain a healthy body weight by enjoying regular physical activity and healthy eating.
5. Limit salt, alcohol, and caffeine.

Source: Minister of Supply and Services, Canada, 1992. Cat. No. 1139–252/1992E.

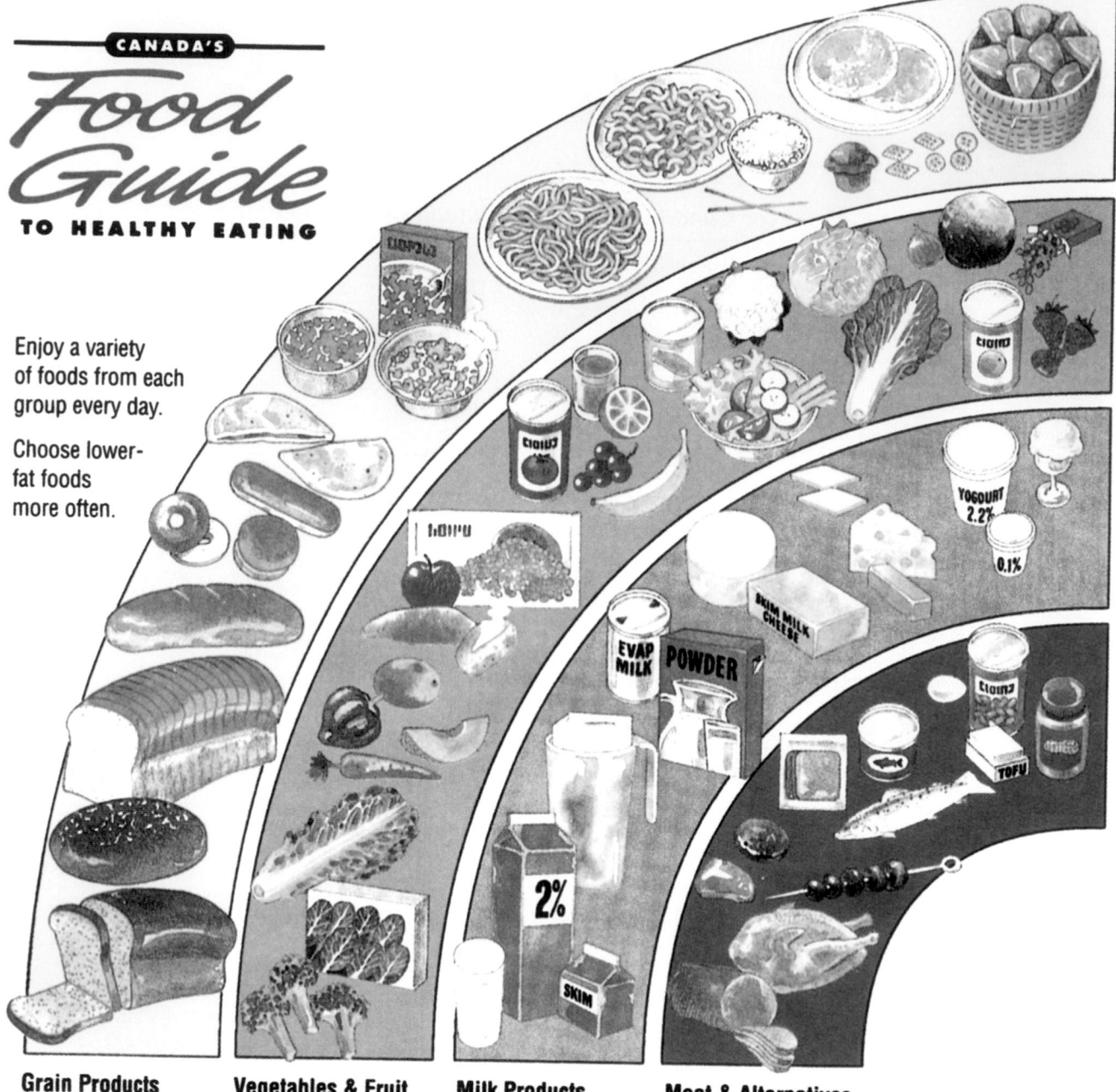

CANADA'S

Food Guide

TO HEALTHY EATING

Enjoy a variety of foods from each group every day.

Choose lower-fat foods more often.

Grain Products
Choose whole grain and enriched products more often.

Vegetables & Fruit
Choose dark green and orange vegetables and orange fruit more often.

Milk Products
Choose lower-fat milk products more often.

Meat & Alternatives
Choose leaner meats, poultry and fish, as well as dried peas, beans and lentils more often.

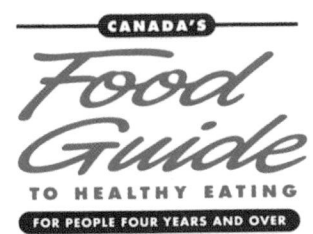

Different People Need Different Amounts of Food

The amount of food you need every day from the 4 food groups and other foods depends on your age, body size, activity level, whether you are male or female and if you are pregnant or breast-feeding. That's why the Food Guide gives a lower and higher number of servings for each food group. For example, young children can choose the lower number of servings, while male teenagers can go to the higher number. Most other people can choose servings somewhere in between.

Grain Products
5-12
SERVINGS PER DAY

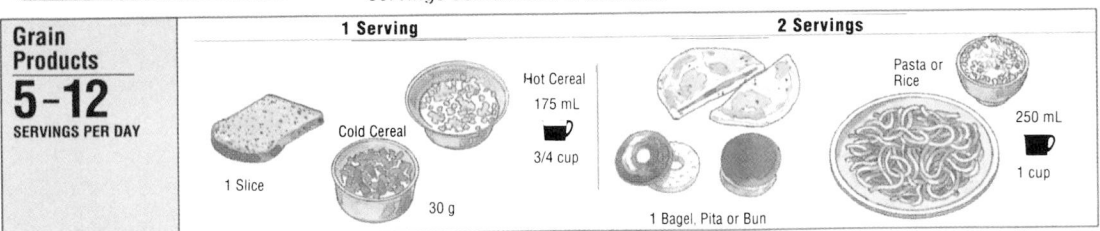

Vegetables & Fruit
5-10
SERVINGS PER DAY

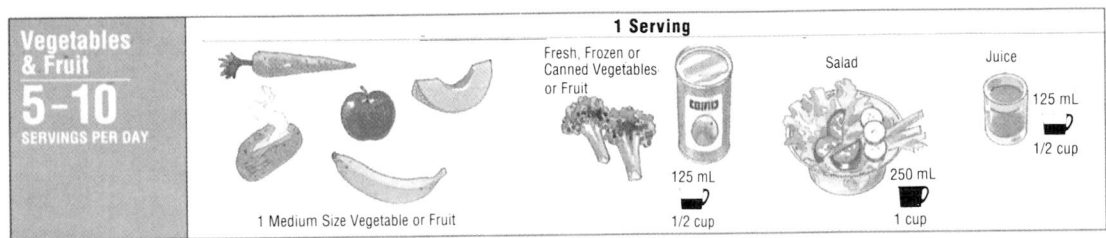

Milk Products
SERVINGS PER DAY
Children 4-9 years: 2-3
Youth 10-16 years: 3-4
Adults: 2-4
Pregnant & Breast-feeding
Women: 3-4

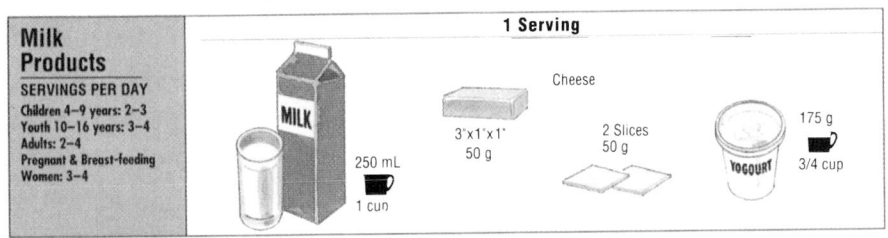

Meat & Alternatives
2-3
SERVINGS PER DAY

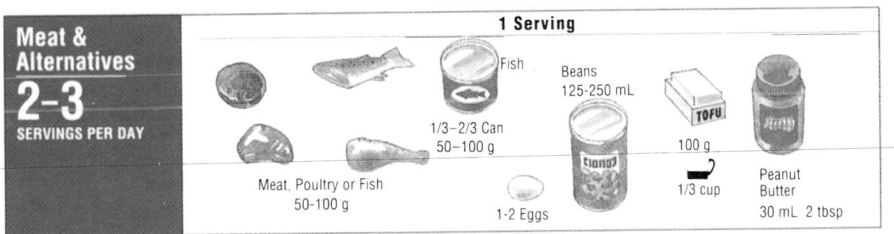

Other Foods

Taste and enjoyment can also come from other foods and beverages that are not part of the 4 food groups. Some of these foods are higher in fat or Calories, so use these foods in moderation.

Key Nutrients in Canada's Food Guide to Healthy Eating

Each food group is essential. That's because it provides its own set of nutrients.

Grain Products	+	Vegetables & Fruits	+	Milk Products	+	Meat & Alternatives	=	The Food Guide
protein				protein		protein		protein
				fat		fat		fat
carbohydrate		carbohydrate						carbohydrate
fibre		fibre						fibre
thiamin		thiamin				thiamin		thiamin
riboflavin				riboflavin		riboflavin		riboflavin
niacin						niacin		niacin
folacin		folacin				folacin		folacin
				vitamin B$_{12}$		vitamin B$_{12}$		vitamin B$_{12}$
		vitamin C						vitamin C
		vitamin A		vitamin A				vitamin A
				vitamin D				vitamin D
				calcium				calcium
iron		iron				iron		iron
zinc				zinc		zinc		zinc
magnesium		magnesium		magnesium		magnesium		magnesium

• GUIDE TO FOOD LABELING AND ADVERTISING, CANADIAN FOOD INSPECTION AGENCY

What Is Nutrition Labeling?

- It is a **standardized presentation** of the nutrient content of a food.

- It is designed to provide useful information that is **not misleading or deceptive.**

- It is **voluntary,** but if applied should comply with the Guidelines on Nutrition Labeling° and with the *Food and Drug Regulations*, which regulate the format, nutrient content information, nomenclature, units of measurement, per-serving basis and declaration of serving size.

- It consists of the **heading,** a statement of the **serving size,** the «core list» (energy, protein, fat, and carbohydrate) plus optional nutrient declarations given equal prominence, in a standardized order.

Nomenclature, Order of Listing, and Units

1. **Heading**

2. **Serving size:** metric units as sold (household measure should be declared in brackets).

3. **Energy** (expressed in both Calories and kilojoules), **protein, fat** and **carbohydrate** constitute the «core list» and must be included when the nutrition labeling format is used. All must be expressed in grams.

4. If one of these **fat components**, excluding linoleic acid, is listed, all four (in addition to fat) must be listed. Linoleic acid may be listed provided the four fat components and fat are also listed.

5. Declaration of one **carbohydrate** component does not require the declaration of any others. All sugar alcohols must be declared by name when used.

6. If either **sodium or potassium** is listed, both must be listed. Both must be expressed in milligrams.

7. **Vitamins and mineral nutrients** must be stated as % of Recommended Daily Intake. If less than 5% of Recommended Daily Intake, they may be listed provided no claims relate to them. Only the names shown may be used in nutrition labeling.

Source: Online at www.cfia-acia.agr.ca/english/ppc/label/5-0-0.html

---

°*Guidelines on Nutrition Labeling*, Guideline No. 2 (Ottawa: Health Canada, Health Protection Branch, May 2, 1996).

Nutrition Information Nutritionnelle

per × g or mL per serving (× cups, item, etc.)
par portion de × g ou mL (× tasses, unités, etc.)

Energy/Énergie	× Cal
	× kJ
Protein/Protéines	× g
Fat/Matières grasses	× g
polyunsaturates/polyinsaturés	× g
linoleic acid/acide linoléique	× g
monounsaturates/monoinsaturés	× g
saturates/saturés	× g
cholesterol/cholestérol	× mg
Carbohydrate/Glucides	× g
sugars/sucres	× g
sugar alcohols (named)	× g
polydextrose	× g
starch/amidon	× g
dietary fibre/fibres alimentaires	× g
Sucralose	× mg
Aspartame	× mg
Acesulfame-potassium/acésulfame-potassium	× mg
Sodium	× mg
Potassium	× mg

Percentage of Recommended Daily Intake
Pourcentage de l'Apport Quotidien Recommandé

Vitamin A/Vitamine A	× %
Vitamin D/Vitamine D	× %
Vitamin E/Vitamine E	× %
Vitamin C/Vitamine C	× %
Thiamine or/ou Vitamin B^1/Vitamine B^1	× %
Riboflavin/Riboflavine or/ou Vitamin B^2/Vitamine B^2	× %
Niacin/Niacine	× %
Vitamin B^6/Vitamine B^6	× %
Folacin/Folacine	× %
Vitamin B^{12}/Vitamine B^{12}	× %
Pantothenic Acid or Pantothenate/	× %
Acide Pantothénique ou Pantothénate	
Calcium	× %
Phosphorus/Phosphore	× %
Magnesium/Magnésium	× %
Iron/Fer	× %
Zinc	× %
Iodine/Iode	× %

F Nutrient Intake Recommendations by the World Health Organization

Recommended Intakes of Nutrients—WHO—1974

Age	Body Weight (kg)	Energy[1] (kcal)	(mJ)	Protein[1,2] (gm)	Vitamin A[3,4] (μg)	Vitamin D[5,6] (μg)
Children						
<1	7.3	820	3.4	14	300	10.00
1–3	13.4	1360	5.7	16	250	10.0
4–6	20.2	1830	7.6	20	300	10.0
7–9	28.1	2190	9.2	25	400	2.5
Male adolescents						
10–12	36.9	2600	10.9	30	575	2.5
13–15	51.3	2900	12.1	37	725	2.5
16–19	62.9	3070	12.8	38	750	2.5
Female adolescents						
10–12	38.0	2350	9.8	29	575	2.5
13–15	49.9	2490	10.4	31	725	2.5
16–19	54.4	2310	9.7	30	750	2.5
Adult man						
(moderately active)	65.0	3000	12.6	37	750	2.5
Adult woman						
(moderately active)	55.0	2200	9.2	29	750	2.5
Pregnancy						
(later half)		+350	+1.5	38	750	10.0
Lactation						
(first 6 months)		+550	+2.3	46	1200	10.0

[1]Energy and Protein Requirements. Report of a Joint FAO/WHO Expert Group, FAO, Rome, 1972.

[2]As egg or milk protein.

[3]Requirements of vitamin A, thiamin, riboflavin and niacin. Report of a Joint FAO/WHO Expert Group, FAO, Rome, 1965.

[4]As retinol.

[5]Requirements of ascorbic acid, vitamin D, vitamin B_{12}, folate and iron. Report of a Joint Applied FAO/WHO Expert Group, FAO, Rome, 1970.

[6]As cholecalciferol.

[7]Calcium requirements. Report of a FAO/WHO Expert Group, FAO, Rome, 1961.

[8]On each line the lower value applies when over 25 % of calories in the diet come from animal foods, and the higher value when animal foods represent less than 10 % of calories.

Thiamin[3] (mg)	Riboflavin[3] (mg)	Niacin[3] (mg)	Folic Acid[5] (μg)	Vitamin B$_{12}$[5] (μg)	Ascorbic Acid[5] (mg)	Calcium[7] (gm)	Iron[5,8,9] (mg)
0.3	0.5	5.4	60	0.3	20	0.5–0.6	5–10
0.5	0.8	9.0	100	0.9	20	0.4–0.5	5–10
0.7	1.1	12.1	100	1.5	20	0.4–0.5	5–10
0.9	1.3	14.5	100	1.5	20	0.4–0.5	5–10
1.0	1.6	17.2	100	2.0	20	0.6–0.7	5–10
1.2	1.7	19.1	200	2.0	30	0.6–0.7	9–18
1.2	1.8	20.3	200	2.0	30	0.5–0.6	5–9
0.9	1.4	15.5	100	2.0	20	0.6–0.7	5–10
1.0	1.5	16.4	200	2.0	30	0.6–0.7	12–24
0.9	1.4	15.2	200	2.0	30	0.5–0.6	14–28
1.2	1.8	19.8	200	2.0	30	0.4–0.5	5–9
0.9	1.3	14.5	200	2.0	30	0.4–0.5	14–28
+0.1	+0.2	+2.3	400	3.0	50	1.0–1.2	(9)
+0.2	+0.4	+3.7	300	2.5	50	1.0–1.2	(9)

[9]For women whose iron intake throughout life has been at the level recommended in this table, the daily intake of iron during pregnancy and lactation should be the same as that recommended for nonpregnant, nonlactating women of childbearing age. For women whose iron status is not satisfactory at the beginning of pregnancy, the requirement is increased, and in the extreme situation of women with no iron stores, the requirement can probably not be met without supplementation.

Source: Passmore, Nicol and Rao. *Handbook on Human Nutritional Requirements*. Geneva, WHO Monogr. Ser. No. 61, 1974, Table 1.

ADDENDUM: Dietary allowances, official or unofficial for many European countries, as of 1976 or earlier, appear in the Proceedings of the Second European Nutrition Conference, Munich, 1976. (Nutr. Metab. 21:210, 1977.)

The Population Nutrient Goals From WHO

	Limits for Population Average Intakes	
	Lower Limit	Upper Limit
Total fat	15% of energy	30% of energy[a]
Saturated fatty acids	0% energy	10% of energy
Polyunsaturated fatty acids	3% of energy	7% of energy
Dietary cholesterol	0 mg/day	300 mg/day
Total carbohydrate	55% of energy	75% of energy
Complex carbohydrates[b]	50% of energy	75% of energy
Dietary fibre[c]		
As non-starch polysaccharides (NSP)	16 g/day	24 g/day
As total dietary fibre	27 g/day	40 g/day
Free sugars[d]	0% of energy	10% of energy
Protein	10% of energy	15% of energy[e]
Salt	—[e]	6 g/day

Total energy

Energy intake needs to be sufficient to allow for normal childhood growth, for the needs of pregnancy and lactation, and for work and desirable physical activities, and to maintain appropriate body reserves of energy in children and adults. Adult populations on average should have a body-mass index (BMI) of 20–22.

(BMI = body mass in kg/[height in metres]^2).

The lower limit defines the minimum intake needed to prevent deficiency diseases, while the upper limit expressed the maximum intake compatible with the prevention of chronic diseases.

[a]An interim goal for nations with high fat intakes; further benefits would be expected by reducing fat intake towards 15% of total energy.

[b]A daily minimum intake of 400 g vegetables and fruits, including at least 30 g of pulses, nuts, and seeds, should contribute to this component.

[c]Dietary fibre includes the non-starch polysaccharides (NSP), the goals for which are based on NSP obtained from mixed food sources. Since the definition and measurement of dietary fibre remain uncertain, the goals for total dietary fibre have been estimated from the NSP values.

[d]These sugars include monosaccharides, disaccharides, and other short-chain sugars extracted from carbohydrates by refining. These refined, or purified, sugars do not include the natural sugars consumed when eating fruits and vegetables or drinking milk.

[e]Not defined.

Source: Diet, nutrition and the prevention of chronic diseases. A report of the WHO Study Group on Diet, Nutrition and Prevention of Noncommunicable Diseases. Nutr. Rev. 49:291–301, 1991.

U.S. Nutrition Recommendations

Estimated Sodium, Chloride, and Potassium Minimum Requirements of Healthy Persons[a]

Age	Weight (kg)[a]	Sodium (mg)[a,b]	Chloride (mg)[a,b]	Potassium (mg)[c]
Months				
0–5	4.5	120	180	500
6–11	8.9	200	300	700
Years				
1	11.0	225	350	1,000
2–5	16.0	300	500	1,400
6–9	25.0	400	600	1,600
10–18	50.0	500	750	2,000
>18[d]	70.0	500	750	2,000

[a]No allowance has been included for large, prolonged losses from the skin through sweat.

[b]There is no evidence that higher intakes confer any health benefit.

[c]Desirable intakes of potassium may considerably exceed these values (~3,500 mg for adults).

[d]No allowance included for growth. Values for those below 18 years assume a growth rate at the 50th percentile reported by the National Center for Health Statistics (Hamill et al., 1979) and averaged for males and females.

Nutrition and Your Health:
DIETARY GUIDELINES FOR AMERICANS

AIM FOR FITNESS...
▲ Aim for a healthy weight.
▲ Be physically active each day.

BUILD A HEALTHY BASE...
■ Let the Pyramid guide your food choices.
■ Choose a variety of grains daily, especially whole grains.
■ Choose a variety of fruits and vegetables daily.
■ Keep food safe to eat.

CHOOSE SENSIBLY...
● Choose a diet that is low in saturated fat and cholesterol and moderate in total fat.
● Choose beverages and foods to moderate your intake of sugars.
● Choose and prepare foods with less salt.
● If you drink alcoholic beverages, do so in moderation.

...for good health

Dietary Guidelines for Americans, 1980 to 2000

1980	1985	1990	1995	2000
7 Guidelines	**7 Guidelines**	**7 Guidelines**	**7 Guidelines**	**10 Guidelines, clustered into 3 groups**
Eat a variety of foods.	Eat a variety of foods.	Eat a variety of foods.	Eat a variety of foods.	**Aim for Fitness** — Aim for a healthy weight.
Maintain ideal weight.	Maintain desirable weight.	Maintain healthy weight.	Balance the food you eat with physical activity—maintain or improve your weight.	Be physically active each day.
				Build a Healthy Base — Let the Pyramid guide your food choices.
Avoid too much fat, saturated fat, and cholesterol.	Avoid too much fat, saturated fat, and cholesterol.	Choose a diet low in fat, saturated fat, and cholesterol.		Choose a variety of grains daily, especially whole grains.
Eat foods with adequate starch and fiber.	Eat foods with adequate starch and fiber.	Choose a diet with plenty of vegetables, fruits, and grain products.	Choose a diet with plenty of grain products, vegetables, and fruits.	Choose a variety of fruits and vegetables daily.
				Keep food safe to eat.
			Choose a diet low in fat, saturated fat, and cholesterol.	**Choose Sensibly** — Choose a diet that is low in saturated fat and cholesterol and moderate in total fat.
Avoid too much sugar.	Avoid too much sugar.	Use sugars only in moderation.	Choose a diet moderate in sugars.	Choose beverages and foods to moderate your intake of sugars.
Avoid too much sodium.	Avoid too much sodium.	Use salt and sodium only in moderation.	Choose a diet moderate in salt and sodium.	Choose and prepare foods with less salt.
If you drink alcohol, do so in moderation.	If you drink alcoholic beverages, do so in moderation.	If you drink alcoholic beverages, do so in moderation.	If you drink alcoholic beverages, do so in moderation.	If you drink alcoholic beverages, do so in moderation.

Shading indicates how the order in which the guidelines are presented has changed over time

Source: Center for Nutrition Policy and Promotion, USDA, May 30, 2000.

Healthy People 2010

Goals

1. Increase quality and years of healthy life.

2. Eliminate health disparities.

Leading Health Indicators

1. Physical activity
2. Overweight and obesity
3. Tobacco use
4. Substance abuse
5. Responsible sexual behavior
6. Mental health
7. Injury and violence
8. Environmental quality
9. Immunization
10. Access to health care

Focus Areas

Access to quality health services

Arthritis, osteoporosis, and chronic back conditions

Cancer

Chronic kidney disease

Diabetes

Disability and secondary conditions

Educational and community-based programs

Environmental health

Family planning

Food safety

Health communication

Heart disease and stroke

HIV

Immunization and infectious diseases

Injury and violence prevention

Maternal, infant, and child health

Medical product safety

Mental health and mental disorders

Nutrition and overweight

Occupational safety and health

Oral health

Physical activity and fitness

Public health infrastructure

Respiratory diseases

Sexually transmitted diseases

Substance abuse

Tobacco use

Vision and hearing

Source: Healthy People 2010. Available online at www.health.gov/healthypeople.

National Cholesterol Education Program Step I and Step II Diets*

Nutrient	Recommended Intake as Percent of Total Kcalories	
	Step I	Step II
Total Fat	30% or less	30% or less
Saturated fatty acids	8–10%	Less than 7%
Polyunsaturated fatty acids	Up to 10%	Up to 10%
Monounsaturated fatty acids	Up to 15%	Up to 15%
Carbohydrate	55% or more	55% or more
Protein	Approximately 15%	Approximately 15%
Cholesterol	Less than 300 mg/day	Less than 300 mg/day
Total kcalories	To achieve and maintain desired weight	To achieve and maintain desired weight

*Recommendations available online at amhrt.org/Heart_and_Stroke_A_Z_Guide/dietg.html

American Institute for Cancer Research Diet & Health Guidelines for Cancer Prevention

1. Choose a diet rich in a variety of plant-based foods.
2. Eat plenty of vegetables and fruits.
3. Maintain a healthy weight and be physically active.
4. Drink alcohol in moderation, if at all.
5. Select foods low in fat and salt.
6. Prepare and store foods safely.
   And, always remember . . .
   Do not smoke or use tobacco in any form.

Source: American Institute of Cancer Research. Available online at www.aicr.org/reduce.htm.

American Cancer Society*

Choose most foods you eat from plant sources.

Limit your intake of high-fat foods, particularly from animal sources.

Be physically active: Achieve and maintain a healthy weight.

Limit consumption of alcoholic beverages, if you drink at all.

°Available online at www.cancer.org/statistics/cff98/nutrition.html

National Cancer Institute Dietary Guidelines*

Reduce fat intake to 30% of kcalories or less.

Increase fiber to 20—30 grams/day, with an upper limit of 35 grams.

Include a variety of fruits and vegetables in the daily diet.

Avoid obesity.

Consume alcoholic beverages in moderation, if at all.

Minimize consumption of salt-cured, salt-pickled, and smoked foods.

°Available online at rex.nci.nih.gov/NCI_Pub_Interface/ActionGd_Web/guidelns.html

Dietary Approaches to Stop Hypertension: DASH Diet

When making changes, start small.

Center your meal around carbohydrates such as pasta, rice, beans, or vegetables.

Treat meat as one part of the whole meal, instead of the focus.

Use fruit and lowfat low-energy foods such as sugar-free gelatin for desserts and snacks.

A 2000-kcalorie diet should include
   7–8 servings of grains and grain products
   4–5 servings of vegetables
   4–5 servings of fruit
   2–3 servings of lowfat and nonfat dairy foods
   2 or fewer servings of meat, poultry, and fish
   one-half serving of nuts, seeds, or legumes

Source: Dietary Approaches to Stop Hypertension. Available online at dash.bwh.harvard.edu

Food Guide Pyramid
A Guide to Daily Food Choices

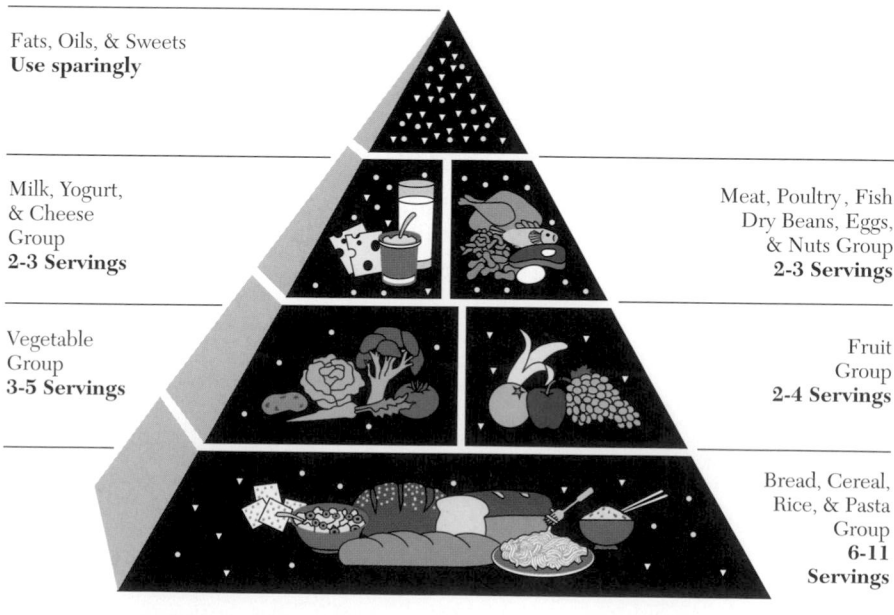

Fats, Oils, & Sweets
Use sparingly

Milk, Yogurt, & Cheese Group
2-3 Servings

Meat, Poultry, Fish, Dry Beans, Eggs, & Nuts Group
2-3 Servings

Vegetable Group
3-5 Servings

Fruit Group
2-4 Servings

Bread, Cereal, Rice, & Pasta Group
6-11 Servings

Key
• Fat (naturally occurring and added)   ▼ Sugars (added)
These symbols show fats, oils, and added sugars in foods.

Number of Food Guide Pyramid Servings for Three Daily Energy Levels*

	1600 kcalories (sedentary women and some older adults)	2200 kcalories (children, teenage girls, active women, and many sedentary men)	2800 kcalories (teenage boys, many active men, and some very active women)
Bread, Cereal, Rice & Pasta Group	6	9	11
Vegetable Group	3	4	5
Fruit Group	2	3	4
Milk, Yogurt, & Cheese Group	2–3†	2–3†	2–3†
Meat, Poultry, Fish, Dry Beans, Eggs, & Nuts Group	2 (5 oz total)	2 (6 oz total)	3 (7 oz total)

*Assumes that food choices are mostly low-fat and low kcalorie.

†Women who are pregnant or breastfeeding, teenagers, and young adults to age 24 need three servings.

U.S. Department of Agriculture. The Food Guide Pyramid. Home and Garden Bulletin 252, 1992, revised 1996.

A Modifed Food Guide Pyramid for Vegetarians

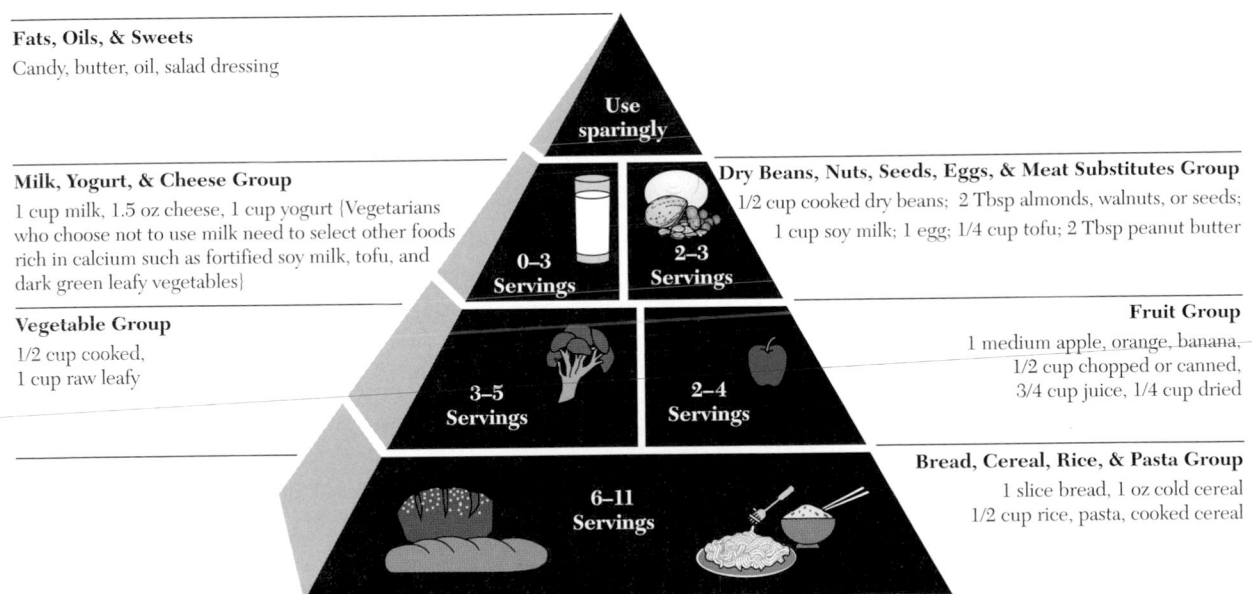

Fats, Oils, & Sweets
Candy, butter, oil, salad dressing

Use sparingly

Milk, Yogurt, & Cheese Group
1 cup milk, 1.5 oz cheese, 1 cup yogurt {Vegetarians who choose not to use milk need to select other foods rich in calcium such as fortified soy milk, tofu, and dark green leafy vegetables}

0–3 Servings

Dry Beans, Nuts, Seeds, Eggs, & Meat Substitutes Group
1/2 cup cooked dry beans; 2 Tbsp almonds, walnuts, or seeds; 1 cup soy milk; 1 egg; 1/4 cup tofu; 2 Tbsp peanut butter

2–3 Servings

Vegetable Group
1/2 cup cooked, 1 cup raw leafy

3–5 Servings

Fruit Group
1 medium apple, orange, banana, 1/2 cup chopped or canned, 3/4 cup juice, 1/4 cup dried

2–4 Servings

Bread, Cereal, Rice, & Pasta Group
1 slice bread, 1 oz cold cereal 1/2 cup rice, pasta, cooked cereal

6–11 Servings

Dietary Reference Intakes (DRIs): Tolerable Upper Intake Levels (UL[a]): Vitamins

Life Stage Group	Vitamin A (μg/d)[b]	Vitamin D (μg/d)	Vitamin E (mg/d)[c,d]	Vitamin K	Vitamin C (mg/d)	Thiamin	Riboflavin	Niacin (mg/d)[d]	Vitamin B6 (mg/d)	Folate (μg/d)[d]	Vitamin B12	Pantothenic Acid	Biotin	Choline (g/d)	Carotenoids[e]
Infants															
0–6 mo	600	25	ND[f]	ND	ND	ND	ND	ND	ND	ND	ND	ND	ND	ND	ND
7–12 mo	600	25	ND	ND	ND	ND	ND	ND	ND	ND	ND	ND	ND	ND	ND
Children															
1–3 y	600	50	200	ND	400	ND	ND	10	30	300	ND	ND	ND	1.0	ND
4–8 y	900	50	300	ND	650	ND	ND	15	40	400	ND	ND	ND	1.0	ND
Males, Females															
9–13 y	1,700	50	600	ND	1,200	ND	ND	20	60	600	ND	ND	ND	2.0	ND
14–18 y	2,800	50	800	ND	1,800	ND	ND	30	80	800	ND	ND	ND	3.0	ND
19–70 y	3,000	50	1,000	ND	2,000	ND	ND	35	100	1,000	ND	ND	ND	3.5	ND
>70 y	3,000	50	1,000	ND	2,000	ND	ND	35	100	1,000	ND	ND	ND	3.5	ND
Pregnancy															
≤18 y	2,800	50	800	ND	1,800	ND	ND	30	80	800	ND	ND	ND	3.0	ND
19–50 y	3,000	50	1,000	ND	2,000	ND	ND	35	100	1,000	ND	ND	ND	3.5	ND
Lactation															
≤18 y	2,800	50	800	ND	1,800	ND	ND	30	80	800	ND	ND	ND	3.0	ND
19–50 y	3,000	50	1,000	ND	2,000	ND	ND	35	100	1,000	ND	ND	ND	3.5	ND

[a]UL=The maximum level of daily nutrient intake that is likely to pose no risk of adverse effects. Unless otherwise specified, the UL represents total intake from food, water, and supplements. Due to lack of suitable data, ULs could not be established for vitamin K, thiamin, riboflavin, vitamin B12, pantothenic acid, biotin, or carotenoids. In the absence of ULs, extra caution may be warranted in consuming levels above recommended intakes.

[b]As preformed vitamin A only.

[c]As α-tocopherol; applies to any form of supplemental α-tocopherol.

[d]The ULs for vitamin E, niacin, and folate apply to synthetic forms obtained from supplements, fortified foods, or a combination of the two.

[e]β-Carotene supplements are advised only to serve as a provitamin A source for individuals at risk of vitamin A deficiency.

[f]ND=Not determinable due to lack of data of adverse effects in this age group and concern with regard to lack of ability to handle excess amounts. Source of intake should be from food only to prevent high levels of intake.

Source: Trumbo, P., Schlicker, S., and Poos, M. Dietary Reference Intakes: vitamin A, vitamin K, arsenic, boron, chromium, copper, iodine, manganese, molybdenum, nickel, silicon, vanadium, and zinc. J. Am. Diet. Assoc. 101:294–301, 2001.

Dietary Reference Intakes (DRIs): Tolerable Upper Intake Levels (UL[a]): Minerals

Life Stage Group	Arsenic[b] (mg/d)	Boron (mg/d)	Calcium (g/d)	Chromium (mg/d)	Copper (μg/d)	Fluoride (mg/d)	Iodine (μg/d)	Iron (mg/d)	Magnesium (mg/d)[c]	Manganese (mg/d)	Molybdenum (μg/d)	Nickel (mg/d)	Phosphorus (g/d)	Selenium (μg/d)	Silicon[d]	Vanadium (mg/d)[e]	Zinc (mg/d)
Infants																	
0–6 mo	ND[f]	ND	ND	ND	ND	0.7	ND	40	ND	ND	ND	ND	ND	45	ND	ND	4
7–12 mo	ND	ND	ND	ND	ND	0.9	ND	40	ND	ND	ND	ND	ND	60	ND	ND	5
Children																	
1–3 y	ND	3	2.5	ND	1,000	1.3	200	40	65	2	300	0.2	3	90	ND	ND	7
4–8 y	ND	6	2.5	ND	3,000	2.2	300	40	110	3	600	0.3	3	150	ND	ND	12
Males, Females																	
9–13 y	ND	11	2.5	ND	5,000	10	600	40	350	6	1,100	0.6	4	280	ND	ND	23
14–18 y	ND	17	2.5	ND	8,000	10	900	45	350	9	1,700	1.0	4	400	ND	ND	34
19–70 y	ND	20	2.5	ND	10,000	10	1,100	45	350	11	2,000	1.0	4	400	ND	1.8	40
>70 y	ND	20	2.5	ND	10,000	10	1,100	45	350	11	2,000	1.0	3	400	ND	1.8	40
Pregnancy																	
≤18 y	ND	17	2.5	ND	8,000	10	900	45	350	9	1,700	1.0	3.5	400	ND	ND	34
19–50 y	ND	20	2.5	ND	10,000	10	1,100	45	350	11	2,000	1.0	3.5	400	ND	ND	40
Lactation																	
≤18 y	ND	17	2.5	ND	8,000	10	900	45	350	9	1,700	1.0	4	400	ND	ND	34
19–50 y	ND	20	2.5	ND	10,000	10	1,100	45	350	11	2,000	1.0	4	400	ND	ND	40

[a]UL=The maximum level of daily nutrient intake that is likely to pose no risk of adverse effects. Unless otherwise specified, the UL represents total intake from food, water, and supplements. Due to lack of suitable data, ULs could not be established for arsenic, chromium, and silicon. In the absence of ULs, extra caution may be warranted in consuming levels above recommended intakes.

[b]Although the UL was not determined for arsenic, there is no justification for adding arsenic to food or supplements.

[c]The ULs for magnesium represent intake from a pharmacological agent only and do not include intake from food and water.

[d]Although silicon has not been shown to cause adverse effects in humans, there is no justification for adding silicon to supplements.

[e]Although vanadium in food has not been shown to cause adverse effects in humans, there is no justification for adding vanadium to food and vanadium supplements should be used with caution. The UL is based on adverse effects in laboratory animals and these data could be used to set a UL for adults but not children and adolescents.

[f]ND=Not determinable due to lack of data of adverse effects in this age group and concern with regard to lack of ability to handle excess amounts. Source of intake should be from food only to prevent high levels of intake.

Source: Trumbo, P., Schlicker, S., and Poos, M. Dietary Reference Intakes: vitamin A, vitamin K, arsenic, boron, chromium, copper, iodine, manganese, molybdenum, nickel, silicon, vanadium, and zinc. J. Am. Diet. Assoc. 101:294–301, 2001.

H Ethnic Diets Planning Tools

The Mediterranean Diet Pyramid

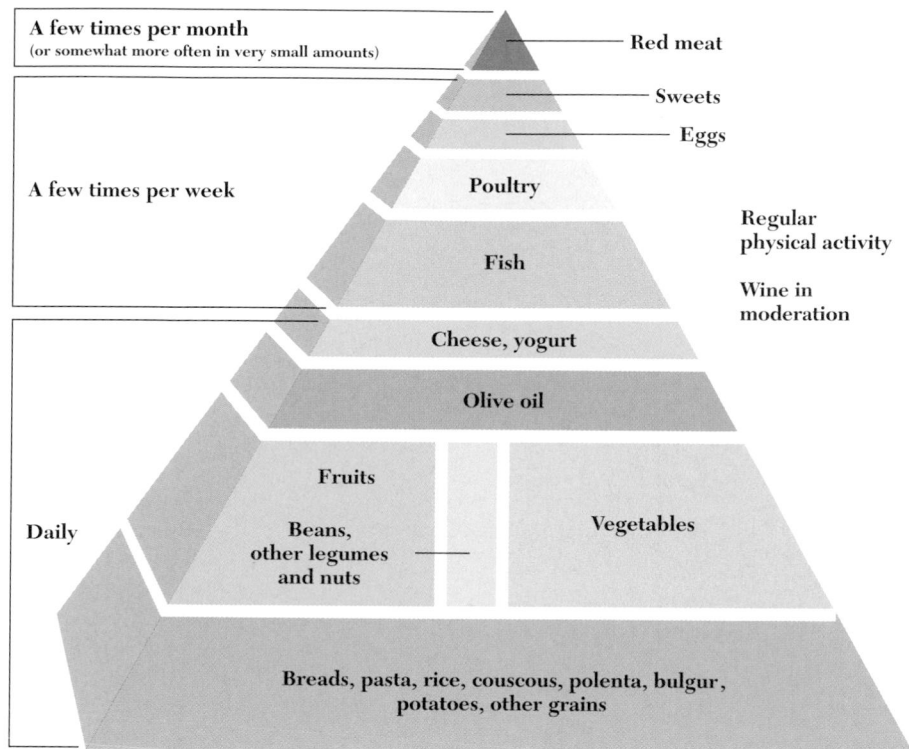

A few times per month
(or somewhat more often in very small amounts)

— Red meat

— Sweets

— Eggs

A few times per week

Poultry

Fish

Regular
physical activity

Wine in
moderation

Cheese, yogurt

Olive oil

Fruits

Daily

Beans,
other legumes
and nuts

Vegetables

Breads, pasta, rice, couscous, polenta, bulgur,
potatoes, other grains

©1994 Oldways Preservation & Exchange Trust.

HEALTH HINTS FROM THE MEDITERRANEAN DIET PYRAMID

• Eat most food from plant sources, including fruits, vegetables, potatoes, breads, beans, nuts, and seeds.

• Use seasonally fresh, locally grown food with a minimum of processing.

• Let olive oil be your principal fat, replacing other fats, oils, butter and margarine.

• Eat red meat only a few times per month and favor the lean cuts.

• If you drink wine, enjoy only 1 or 2 glasses a day, preferably with meals.

• Engage in regular exercise to promote a healthy weight, fitness, and well-being.

Asian Diet Pyramid

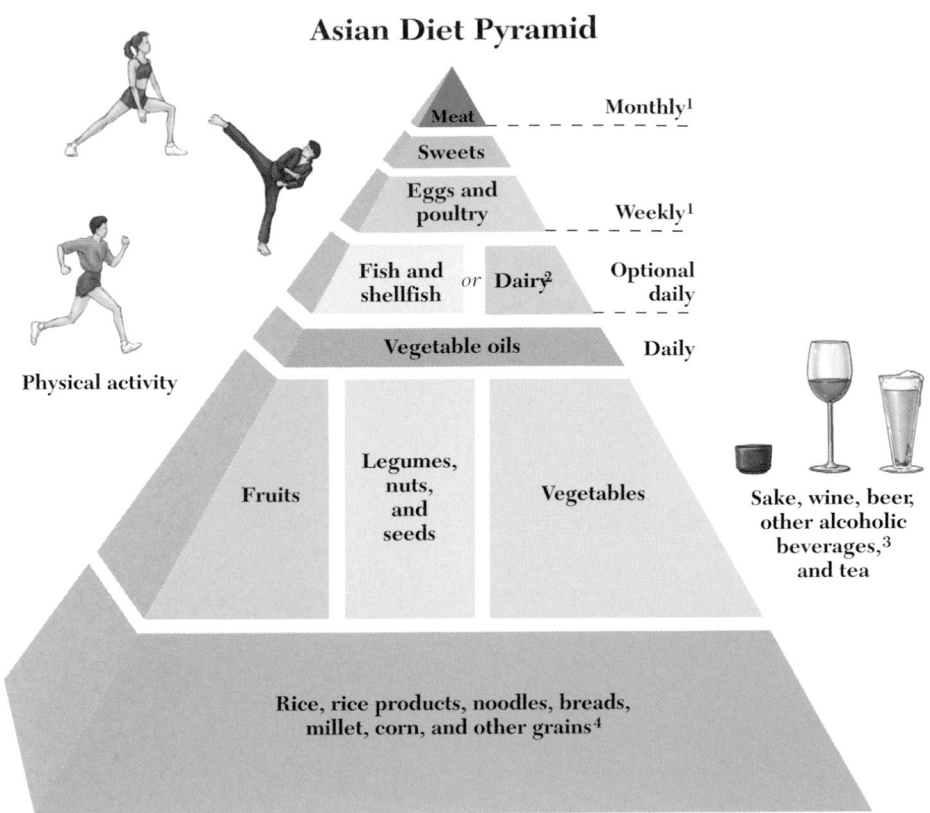

Meat — Monthly[1]

Sweets

Eggs and poultry — Weekly[1]

Fish and shellfish *or* Dairy[2] — Optional daily

Vegetable oils — Daily

Physical activity

Fruits

Legumes, nuts, and seeds

Vegetables

Sake, wine, beer, other alcoholic beverages,[3] and tea

Rice, rice products, noodles, breads, millet, corn, and other grains[4]

©1995 Oldways Preservation & Exchange Trust

[1]Or more often in very small amounts.
[2]Dairy foods are generally not part of the healthy, traditional diets of Asia, with the notable exception of India. In light of current nutrition research, if dairy foods are consumed on a daily basis, they should be used in low to moderate amounts, and preferably be low in fat.
[3]Wine, beer, and other alcoholic beverages should be consumed in moderation and primarily with meals, and avoided whenever consumption would put an individual or others at risk.
[4]Minimally refined whenever possible.

Mexican American Foods and the Food Guide Pyramid

bacon
butter
candy
cream cheese
fried pork rinds
lard
margarine
soft drinks
sour cream
vegetable oil

cheddar cheese
custard
evaporated milk
ice cream
jack cheese
powdered milk
queso blanco,
  fresco,
  or mexicano

beef,
black beans,
chicken, eggs, fish,
garbanzo beans,
kidney beans, lamb,
nuts, peanut butter,
pinto beans, pork,
sausage, tripe

agave
beets
cabbage
carrots
cassava
chilis
corn
elote
iceberg lettuce
jicama

green tomatoes
onion
peas
potato
prickly pear
  cactus leaves
purslane
squash
sweet potatoes
tomato
turnips

apple
avocado
banana
cherimoya
guava
mango

orange
papaya
pineapple
platano
zapote

bolillo
bread
cake
cereal
corn tortilla
crackers

flour tortilla
fried flour tortilla
graham crackers
macaroni
masa
oatmeal

pastry
rice
sopa
spaghetti
sweet bread
taco shell

© 1993 *Pyramid Packet*, Penn State Nutrition Center, 5 Henderson Building, University Park, PA 16802; (814)865-6323

Sources: Algert, Susan J., and Teri Hall Ellison, Contributors. *Ethnic and Regional Food Practices—A Series: Mexican American Food Practices, Customs, and Holidays*; Diabetes Care and Education Practice Group of the American Dietetic Association, 1989; *Comidas Hispana en Dietas Diabetica* (*Spanish Foods in Diabetic Diets*). Visiting Nurse Association of Milwaukee, 1975.

African American Foods and the Food Guide Pyramid

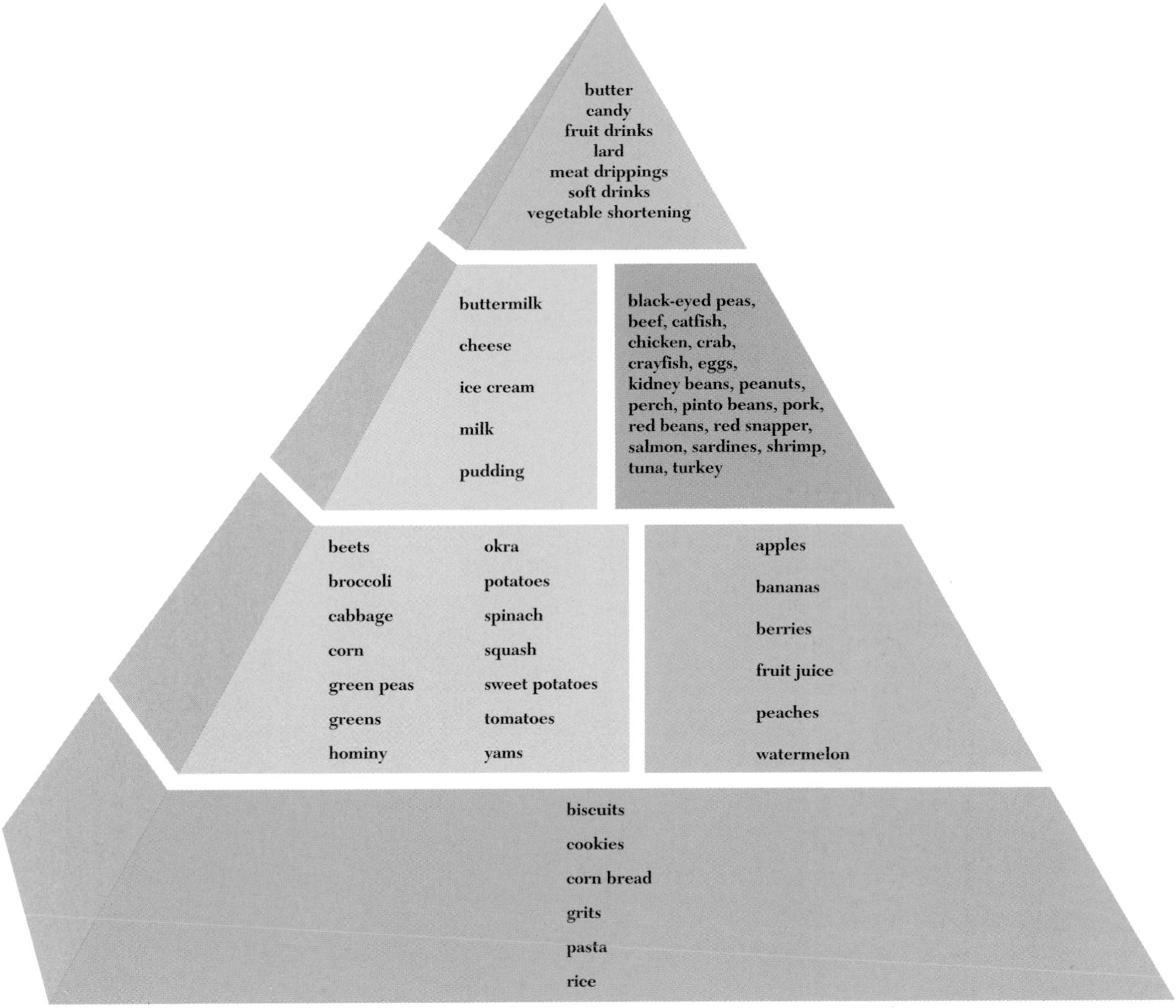

butter
candy
fruit drinks
lard
meat drippings
soft drinks
vegetable shortening

buttermilk

cheese

ice cream

milk

pudding

black-eyed peas,
beef, catfish,
chicken, crab,
crayfish, eggs,
kidney beans, peanuts,
perch, pinto beans, pork,
red beans, red snapper,
salmon, sardines, shrimp,
tuna, turkey

beets	okra	apples
broccoli	potatoes	bananas
cabbage	spinach	berries
corn	squash	
green peas	sweet potatoes	fruit juice
greens	tomatoes	peaches
hominy	yams	watermelon

biscuits

cookies

corn bread

grits

pasta

rice

© 1993 *Pyramid Packet*, Penn State Nutrition Center, 5 Henderson Building, University Park, PA 16802; (814)865-6323
Source: Kittler, Pamela Goyan, and Kathryn Sucher. *Food and Culture in America* (New York: Van Nostrand Reinhold, 1989).

Chinese American Foods
and the Food Guide Pyramid

bacon fat,
butter,
coconut milk,
corn oil,
duck sauce, honey, lard,
maltose syrup, peanut oil,
sesame oil, sesame paste,
soybean oil, suet, sugar

buffalo milk

cow's milk

fish bones

soybean milk

yogurt

bean paste, beef,
chestnuts, chicken,
duck, eggs,
fish (e.g., carp, catfish),
lamb,
legumes (e.g., mung
  beans, soy beans),
pork, quail, rice birds,
shellfish and other seafood
(e.g., shrimp, squid), squab

amaranth, arrowheads, bamboo shoots,
bitter gourd, black mushroom, bok choy,
cabbage, celery, chayote, chilis,
Chinese broccoli, choy sum, dried wood ear,
eggplant, garland chrysanthemum, garlic,
ginger, green beans, hairy cucumber, leek,
lotus root, mustard greens, okra, onions,
Oriental radish, peas, pickled cucumber, potatoes,
scallion, spinach, sprouts, straw mushrooms, taro,
tomatoes, turnip, water chestnut, watercress,
winter melon, yard-long beans

carambola, Chinese banana,

Chinese pear, guava, jujube,

kumquats, litchi, longan, mango,

orange, papaya, persimmon,

pummelo, watermelon

barley	glutinous rice	nin goh	rice flour
bing	hua juan	noodles, including cellophane noodles, rice sticks, rice vermicelli	steamed rice
dumplings	mianbao		sorghum
		rice congee	Wonton wrappers
fried rice	mantou		zong-zi

© 1993 *Pyramid Packet*, Penn State Nutrition Center, 5 Henderson Building, The Pennsylvania State University, University Park, PA 16802; (814)865-6323
Sources : Kee Maggie Ma. *Ethnic and Regional Food Practices—A Series: Chinese American Food Practices, Customs and Holidays*. Diabetes Care and Education
Practice Group of the American Dietetic Association, 1990; Kittler, Pamela Goyan, and Kathryn Sucher. *Food and Culture in America* (New York; Van
Nostrand Reinhold, 1989).

Indian Foods and the Food Guide Pyramid

butter, chocolate, coconut milk, coconut oil, ghee, groundnut oil, honey, jam, jaggery, mustard oil, sesame oil, soft drinks, sugar, sunflower oil, toffees, vanaspati

buffalo's milk, buttermilk (lassi), cow's milk, curds, chhena, ice cream, kheer, khoya, kulfi milk powder, paneer, peda, raita, rasmalai, rossogolla, sondesh, srikhand, sweet curds

almonds, cashew nuts, chana, chicken, coconut chutney, dal, eggs, groundnut, kabob, kheema, mutton, pappad, pulses, rajma, rasam, sambar, soyabean nuggets, sprouted beans

aviyal	capsicum	onions
bitter gourd	carrots	pakora
brinjal	cauliflower	peas
(aubergine)	cucumber	plantain
cabbage	drumsticks	potatoes
	gourds	pumpkin
	green beans	radishes
	green papaya	salad
	lotus stem	sweet potatoes
	lady's finger	tomatoes
	leafy greens	vegetable curry

apples	mango
bananas	melons
cheeku	oranges
custard apple	papaya
fruit chutney	pineapple
goose berries	plums
grapes	pomegranates
guava	raisins
Indian pears	sharbat
jackfruit	sweet lime
lychees	tamarind

bhatura	naan	puris	steamed rice
dhokla	parboiled rice	roti (made from millet, rice flour)	uppma
dosas	pressed rice	rice noodles	vermicelli
idlis	puffed rice		white bread
makai ki roti	pullao	sago	

© 1996 *Multicultural Pyramid Packet*, Penn State Nutrition Center, 5 Henderson Building, University Park, PA 16802, (814)865-6323
Sources: Barer-Stein, Thelma. *You Eat What You Are—A Study of Ethnic Food Traditions* (Toronto: McClelland and Stewart, Ltd., 1979); Dalal, *Tarla Dalal's New Indian Vegatarian Cooking* (Bombay: India Book Distributors, 1986); Kittler, Pamela Goyan, and Kathryn Sucher. *Food and Culture in America* (New York: Van Nostrand Reinhold, 1989); Madhur, Jaffrey. *A Taste of India* (London: Pan Books, Ltd., 1985); Sahni, Julie. *Classic Indian Cooking* (New York: William Morrow and Company, Inc. 1980); Santha, Rama Rau. *The Cooking of India* (New York: Time-Life Books [Foods of the World], 1969). Pyramid prepared by Uma Srinath.

Jewish Foods and the Food Guide Pyramid

cream
cheese,
gribenes,
honey, jelly,
margarine,
marmalade,
mayonnaise,
olive oil, preserves,
schmaltz, sesame seed oil,
sherbert, sour cream, sugar

cottage cheese

edam cheese

farmers' cheese

Gouda cheese

milk

Swiss cheese

yogurt

almonds, beef,
beef tongue, bob,
brisket, chick peas,
chopped liver,
corned beef, dry beans,
eggs, flanken,
gefilte fish, herring,
lentils, lox, pastrami,
poultry salmon, sardines,
smelt, smoked fish, split peas,
tripe, veal

artichokes	green beans	potatoes
asparagus	greens	sorrel
beets/borscht	latke	spinach
broccoli	leeks	squash
brussel sprouts	olives	sweet
cabbage	onion	potatoes
carrot	peas	tomatoes
cauliflower	peppers	turnips
corn	pickles	yams
garlic		

bananas	figs
citrus fruits	grapes
dates	melons
dried apples	prunes
dried apricots	raisins
dried pears	sabra

bagel	bubke	crepe	honey cake	leckach	pita bread
barley	bulgur	dumplings	kasha	matzoh	pumpernickel bread
bialy	bulke	farfel	kichlach	noodle pudding	rye bread
blintz	challah	hard rolls	knaidlach	pastry	teiglach

© 1993 *Pyramid Packet*, Penn State Nutrition Center, 5 Henderson Building, University Park, PA 16802; (814)865-6323

Sources: Higgins, Catherine, and Hope S. Warshaw, contributors. *Ethnic and Regional Food Practices—A Series: Jewish Food Practices, Customs, and Holidays.* Diabetes Care and Education Practice Group of the American Dietetic Association, 1989; Barer-Stein, Thelma. *You Eat What You Are—A Study of Ethnic Food Traditions* (Toronto: McClelland and Stewart Ltd., 1979).

Current Navajo Foods and the Food Guide Pyramid

butter, fruit-flavored ades and punches, lard, margarine, mayonnaise, salad dressing, shortening, soda pop, vegetable oil

cheese

goat's milk

low fat milk

non-fat dry milk

whole milk

beef, blood sausage, chicken, deer, dry beans, eggs, elk, fish, frankfurter, ham, mutton, peanut butter, piñon nuts, pork, prairie dog, processed meats/Spam®

carrots	potato	apple	grapes
celery	red/green chilis	apricots	juniper berries
corn	spinach	avocado	kiwi
green beans	squash	banana	Navajo melon
hominy	squash blossoms	canned friut	orange
lettuce	steamed corn	cantaloupe	raisins
Navajo spinach	tomato	casabas	sumac berries
onion	yellow hot peppers	fruit juice	watermelon

alkaad	macaroni
blue corn bread	pancakes
blue corn mush	spaghetti
blue dumplings	tortillas
cereal	waffles
fry bread	white bread
kneel down bread	whole grain bread

© 1993 *Pyramid Packet*, Penn State Nutrition Center, 5 Henderson Building, University Park, PA 16802; (814)865-6323

Sources: Pelican, Suzanne, and Karen Bachman-Carter. *Ethnic and Regional Food Practices—A Series: Navajo Food Practices, Customs, and Holidays.* Diabetes Care and Education Practice Group of the American Dietetic Association, 1991; Navajo Health and Nutrition Survey (unpublished). Navajo Area Indian Health Service.

Puerto Rican Foods and the Food Guide Pyramid*

bacon,
butter,
cocoa,
fruit drinks,
honey, jelly, lard,
margarine, olive oil,
soft drinks, sugar cane,
vegetable oil

bread pudding, flan, goat's milk, low-fat milk, queso blanco, queso del país, rice pudding, skim milk, tembleque, whole milk, yogurt	achiote, almonds, black beans, cow organ meats, chorizos, egg, gandules, garbonzo beans, maní, pescado, pollo, puerco, habichuelas, res, ternera, turkey, walnuts

batata
berro
berzas
calabaza
carrots
eggplant
garlic
green beans
green pepper
grelos

lettuce
maiz
ñame
onion
okra
pumpkin
tomatoes
viandas
yautía
yuca

apples
acerola
avocado
bananas
breadfruit
cantaloupe
fruit nectars
grapefruit
grapes
guava
kiwi

kumquats
lemons
mammaee apple
mangos
olives
oranges
papaya
parcha
pineapple
plátano
pomegranate

quenepas
strawberries
watermelon

cake   cornmeal   waffles

cereal   farina   white rice

coditos   oatmeal   whole wheat bread

© 1996 *Multicultural Pyramid Packet*, Penn State Nutrition Center, 5 Henderson Building, University Park, PA 16802, (814)865-6323
* May be used with Cuban and Dominican populations.
Sources: Dooley, Eliza B.K. *Puerto Rican Cookbook* (Virginia: Dietz, 1948); Internet: http://www.cu-online.com/~maggy/pr.html;
Internet: http://pubweb.acns.nwu.edu/%7Ecotto/pr.html; Rivera, Jeanie. Personal interview, 1 April 1996; Ruíz, Leondro.
Personal interview, 26 May 1996; "Buen Provecho..." *Bienvenidos* 1994; V asquez, Susana. Personal Interview, 10 April 1996.

Vietnamese American Foods
and the Food Guide Pyramid

coconut milk
peanut oil
sesame oil
sesame paste
vegetable oil

Calcium comes from
the use of fish bones.

beef
chicken
crab
duck
pork
shrimp
squid
white-flesh fish

artichokes	eggplant	sweet potato
asparagus	garlic	tofu
broccoli	gia	tomato
ca tim	green beans	
cabbage	leeks	
carrots	mang	
cauliflower	mung beans	
com choy	onion	
corn	potato	
cucumber	rau muong	
dau hu	squash	

banana	lychee
carambola	mango
grapes	orange
guava	pandeo
jejube	papaya
lemon	pineapple
lit chi	watermelon
logan coconut	

banh trang	cha gio	mung bean vermicelli
bun	French bread	white rice
cellophane noodles	mein	xoi

© 1996 *Multicultural Pyramid Packet*, Penn State Nutrition Center, 5 Henderson Building, University Park, PA 16802; (814)865-6323

Sources: Passimore, Jackie. *Asia, the Beautiful Cookbook* (San Francisco: Collins Publishers, 1990); Routhier, Nicole. *The Foods of Vietnam* (New York: Stewart, Taborr and Chang, 1989); Solomon, Charmaine. *Complete Asian Cookbook* (New York: McGraw-Hill Book Co., 1982); Le, Laura, personal interview April 1996; Le, Tuan, personal interview, April 1996; Waiter at The Pho Express Restaurant. personal interview, April 1996.

I Exchange Lists

Foods are listed with their serving sizes, which are usually measured after cooking. When you begin, you should measure the size of each serving. This may help you learn to «eyeball» correct serving sizes.

The following chart shows the amount of nutrients in one serving from each list.

The exchange lists provide you with a lot of food choices (foods from the basic food groups, foods with added sugars, free foods, combination foods, and fast foods). This gives you variety in your meals. Several foods, such as dried beans and peas, bacon, and peanut butter, are on two lists. This gives you flexibility in putting your meals together. Whenever you choose new foods or vary your meal plan, monitor your blood glucose to see how these different foods affect your blood glucose level.

Groups/Lists	Carbo-hydrate (grams)	Protein (grams)	Fat (grams)	Calories
Carbohydrate Group				
Starch	15	3	1 or less	80
Fruit	15	—	—	60
Milk				
Skim	12	8	0–3	90
Low-fat	12	8	5	120
Whole	12	8	8	150
Other carbohydrates	15	Varies	Varies	Varies
Vegetables	5	2	—	25
Meat and Meat Substitute Group				
Very lean	—	7	0–1	35
Lean	—	7	3	55
Medium-fat	—	7	5	75
High-fat	—	7	8	100
Fat Group	—	—	5	45

© 1995 by the American Diabetes Association, Inc., and the American Dietetic Association.

• STARCH LIST

One starch exchange equals 15 grams carbohydrate, 3 grams protein, 0–1 grams fat, and 80 calories.

Bread
Bagel ....½ (1 oz)
Bread, reduced-calorie.........................2 slices (1½ oz)
Bread, white, whole-wheat, pumpernickel, rye ....1 slice (1 oz)
Bread sticks, crisp, 4 in. long × ½ in.......................2 (⅔ oz)
English muffin ....½
Hot dog or hamburger bun.....................................½ (1 oz)
Pita, 6 in. across ....½
Roll, plain, small ....1 (1 oz)
Raisin bread, unfrosted..1 slice (1 oz)
Tortilla, corn, 6 in. across 1
Tortilla, flour, 7–8 in. across..1
Waffle, 4½ in. square, reduced-fat..................................1

Cereals and Grains
Bran cereals ....½ cup
Bulgur ....½ cup

Cereals ....½ cup
Cereals, unsweetened, ready-to-eat............................¾ cup
Cornmeal (dry) ....3 Tbsp
Couscous ....⅓ cup
Flour (dry) ....3 Tbsp
Granola, low-fat ....¼ cup
Grape-Nuts ....¼ cup
Grits ....½ cup
Kasha ....½ cup
Millet ....¼ cup
Muesli ....¼ cup
Oats ....½ cup
Pasta ....½ cup
Puffed cereal ....1½ cups
Rice milk ....½ cup
Rice, white or brown ....⅓ cup
Shredded Wheat ....½ cup
Sugar-frosted cereal ....½ cup
Wheat germ ....3 Tbsp

Dried Beans, Peas, and Lentils
(Count as 1 starch exchange, plus 1 very lean meat exchange.)
Beans and peas (garbanzo, pinto, kidney, white, split, black-eyed) ...½ cup
Lima beans...⅔ cup
Lentils ....½ cup
Miso 🖝₊ ....3 Tbsp

🖝₊ = 400 mg or more of sodium per serving.

Starchy Vegetables
Baked beans ....⅓ cup
Corn ....½ cup
Corn on cob, medium ....1 (5 oz)
Mixed vegetables with corn, peas, or pasta ....1 cup
Peas, green ....½ cup
Plantain ....½ cup
Potato, baked or boiled..1 small (3 oz)
Potato, mashed ....½ cup
Squash, winter (acorn, butternut)..................................1 cup
Yam, sweet potato, plain ....½ cup

Crackers and Snacks
Animal crackers...8
Graham crackers, 2½ in. square...3
Matzoh ....¾ oz
Melba toast..4 slices
Oyster crackers 24
Popcorn (popped, no fat added or low-fat microwave) ....3 cups
Pretzels ....¾ oz
Rice cakes, 4 in. across 2
Saltine-type crackers...6
Snack chips, fat-free (tortilla, potato) ....15–20 (¾ oz)
Whole-wheat crackers, no fat added ....2–5 (¾ oz)

Starchy Foods Prepared With Fat
(Count as 1 starch exchange, plus 1 fat exchange.)

Biscuit, $2\frac{1}{2}$ in. across 1
Chow mein noodles .... $\frac{1}{2}$ cup
Corn bread, 2 in. cube .... 1 (2 oz)
Crackers, round butter type 6
Croutons .... 1 cup
French-fried potatoes .... 16–25 (3 oz)
Granola .... $\frac{1}{4}$ cup
Muffin, small .... 1 ($1\frac{1}{2}$ oz)
Pancake, 4 in. across 2
Popcorn, microwave .... 3 cups
Sandwich crackers, cheese or peanut butter filling 3
Stuffing, bread (prepared) .... $\frac{1}{3}$ cup
Taco shell, 6 in. across 2
Waffle, $4\frac{1}{2}$ in. square 1
Whole-wheat crackers, fat added .... 4–6 (1 oz)

• Fruit List

One fruit exchange equals 15 grams carbohydrate and 60 calories. The weight includes skin, core, seeds, and rind.

Fruit

Apple, unpeeled, small .... 1 (4 oz)
Applesauce, unsweetened .... $\frac{1}{2}$ cup
Applies, dried .... 4 rings
Apricots, fresh .... 4 whole ($5\frac{1}{2}$ oz)
Apricots, dried .... 8 halves
Apricots, canned .... $\frac{1}{2}$ cup
Banana, small .... 1 (4 oz)
Blackberries .... $\frac{3}{4}$ cup
Blueberries .... $\frac{3}{4}$ cup
Cantaloupe, small .... $\frac{1}{3}$ melon (11 oz) or 1 cup cubes
Cherries, sweet, fresh .... 12 (3 oz)
Cherries, sweet, canned .... $\frac{1}{2}$ cup
Dates 3
Figs, fresh .... $1\frac{1}{2}$ large or 2 medium ($3\frac{1}{2}$ oz)
Figs, dried .... $1\frac{1}{2}$
Fruit cocktail .... $\frac{1}{2}$ cup
Grapefruit, large .... $\frac{1}{2}$ (11 oz)
Grapefruit sections, canned .... $\frac{3}{4}$ cup
Grapes, small .... 17 (3 oz)
Honeydew melon .... 1 slice (10 oz) or 1 cup cubes
Kiwi .... 1 ($3\frac{1}{2}$ oz)
Mandarin oranges, canned .... $\frac{3}{4}$ cup
Mango, small .... $\frac{1}{2}$ fruit ($5\frac{1}{2}$) or $\frac{1}{2}$ cup
Nectarine, small .... 1 (5 oz)
Orange, small .... 1 ($6\frac{1}{2}$ oz)
Papaya .... $\frac{1}{2}$ fruit (8 oz) or 1 cup cubes
Peach, medium, fresh .... 1 (6 oz)
Peaches, canned .... $\frac{1}{2}$ cup
Pear, large, fresh .... $\frac{1}{2}$ (4 oz)
Pears, canned .... $\frac{1}{2}$ cup
Pineapple, fresh .... $\frac{1}{4}$ cup
Pineapple, canned .... $\frac{1}{2}$ cup
Plums, small .... 2 (5 oz)
Plums, canned .... $\frac{1}{2}$ cup
Prunes, dried 3
Raisins .... 2 Tbsp
Raspberries .... 1 cup
Strawberries .... $1\frac{3}{4}$ cup whole berries
Tangerines, small .... 2 (8 oz)
Watermelon .... 1 slice ($13\frac{1}{2}$ oz) or $1\frac{1}{4}$ cup cubes

Fruit Juice

Apple juice/cider .... $\frac{1}{2}$ cup
Cranberry juice cocktail .... $\frac{1}{3}$ cup
Cranberry juice cocktail, reduced-calorie .... 1 cup
Fruit juice blends, 100% juice .... $\frac{1}{3}$ cup
Grape juice .... $\frac{1}{3}$ cup
Grapefruit juice .... $\frac{1}{2}$ cup
Orange juice .... $\frac{1}{2}$ cup
Pineapple juice .... $\frac{1}{2}$ cup
Prune juice .... $\frac{1}{3}$ cup

• Milk List

One milk exchange equals 12 grams carbohydrate and 8 grams protein.

Skim and Very Low-Fat Milk
(0–3 grams fat per serving)

Skim milk .... 1 cup
$\frac{1}{2}$% milk .... 1 cup
1% milk .... 1 cup
Nonfat or lowfat buttermilk .... 1 cup
Evaporated skim milk .... $\frac{1}{2}$ cup
Nonfat dry milk .... $\frac{1}{3}$ cup dry
Plain nonfat yogurt .... $\frac{3}{4}$ cup
Nonfat or lowfat fruit-flavored yogurt sweetened with aspartame or with a non-nutritive sweetener .... 1 cup

Low-Fat
(5 Grams Fat per Serving)

2% milk .... 1 cup
Plain lowfat yogurt .... $\frac{3}{4}$ cup
Sweet acidophilus milk .... 1 cup

Whole Milk
(8 grams fat per serving)

Whole milk .... 1 cup
Evaporated whole milk .... $\frac{1}{2}$ cup
Goat's milk .... 1 cup
Kefir .... 1 cup

• OTHER CARBOHYDRATES LIST

One exchange equals 15 grams carbohydrate, or 1 starch, or 1 fruit, or 1 milk.

Food	Serving Size	Exchanges per Serving
Angel food cake, unfrosted	1/12 cake	2 carbohydrates
Brownie, small, unfrosted	2 in. square	1 carbohydrate, 1 fat
Cake, unfrosted	2 in. square	1 carbohydrate, 1 fat
Cake, frosted	2 in. square	2 carbohydrates, 1 fat
Cookie, fat-free	2 small	1 carbohydrate
Cookie or sandwich cookie with creme filling	2 small	1 carbohydrate, 1 fat
Cupcake, frosted	1 small	2 carbohydrates, 1 fat
Cranberry sauce, jellied	1/4 cup	2 carbohydrates
Doughnut, plain cake	1 medium (1 1/2 oz)	1 1/2 carbohydrates, 2 fats
Doughnut, glazed	3 3/4 in. across (2 oz)	2 carbohydrates, 2 fats
Fruit juice bars, frozen, 100% juice	1 bar (3 oz)	1 carbohydrate
Fruit snacks, chewy (pureed fruit concentrate)	1 roll (3/4 oz)	1 carbohydrate
Fruit spread, 100% fruit	1 Tbsp	1 carbohydrate
Gelatin, regular	1/2 cup	1 carbohydrate
Gingersnaps	3	1 carbohydrate
Granola bar	1 bar	1 carbohydrate, 1 fat
Granola bar, fat-free	1 bar	2 carbohydrates
Hummus	1/3 cup	1 carbohydrate, 1 fat
Ice cream	1/2 cup	1 carbohydrate, 2 fats
Ice cream, light	1/2 cup	1 carbohydrate, 1 fat
Ice cream, fat-free, no sugar added	1/2 cup	1 carbohydrate
Jam or jelly, regular	1 Tbsp	1 carbohydrate
Milk, chocolate, whole	1 cup	2 carbohydrates, 1 fat
Pie, fruit, 2 crusts	1/6 pie	3 carbohydrates, 2 fats
Pie, pumpkin or custard	1/8 pie	1 carbohydrate, 2 fats
Potato chips	12–18 (1 oz)	1 carbohydrate, 2 fats
Pudding, regular (made with lowfat milk)	1/2 cup	2 carbohydrates
Pudding, sugar-free (made with lowfat milk)	1/2 cup	1 carbohydrate
Salad dressing, fat-free 🥄	1/4 cup	1 carbohydrate
Sherbet, sorbet	1/2 cup	2 carbohydrates
Spaghetti or pasta sauce, canned 🥄	1/2 cup	1 carbohydrate, 1 fat
Sweet roll or Danish	1 (2 1/2 oz)	2 1/2 carbohydrates, 2 fats
Syrup, light	2 Tbsp	1 carbohydrate
Syrup, regular	1 Tbsp	1 carbohydrate
Syrup, regular	1/4 cup	4 carbohydrates
Tortilla chips	6–12 (1 oz)	1 carbohydrate, 2 fats
Yogurt, frozen, lowfat, fat-free	1/3 cup	1 carbohydrate, 0–1 fat
Yogurt, frozen, fat-free, no sugar added	1/2 cup	1 carbohydrate
Yogurt, low-fat with fruit	1 cup	3 carbohydrates, 0–1 fat
Vanilla wafers	5	1 carbohydrate, 1 fat

🥄 = 400 mg or more of sodium per serving.

• VEGETABLE LIST

Vegetables that contain small amounts of carbohydrates and calories are on this list. Vegetables contain important nutrients. Try to eat at least 2 or 3 vegetable choices each day. In general, one vegetable exchange is:

1/2 cup of cooked vegetable or vegetable juice, or

1 cup of raw vegetables

If you eat 1 to 2 vegetable choices at a meal or snack, you do not have to count the calories or carbohydrates because they contain small amounts of these nutrients.

One vegetable exchange equals 5 grams carbohydrate, 2 grams protein, 0 grams fat, and 25 calories.

Artichoke
Artichoke hearts
Asparagus
Beans (green, wax, Italian)
Bean sprouts
Beets
Broccoli
Brussels sprouts
Cabbage
Carrots
Cauliflower
Celery
Cucumber
Eggplant
Green onions or scallions
Greens(collard, kale, mustard, turnip)
Kohlrabi
Leeks
Mixed vegetables (without corn, peas, or pasta)
Mushrooms
Okra
Onions
Pea pods
Peppers (all varieties)
Radishes
Salad greens (endive, escarole, lettuce, romaine, spinach)
Sauerkraut 🥄
Spinach

Summer squash

Tomato

Tomatoes, canned

Tomato sauce ✎

Tomato/vegetable juice ✎

Turnips

Water chestnuts

Watercress

Zucchini

✎ = 400 mg or more sodium per exchange.

Cheese:
4.5%-fat cottage cheese...¼ cup
Grated Parmesan...2 Tbsp
Cheeses with 3 grams or less fat per ounce ....1 oz
Other:
Hot dogs with 3 grams or less fat per ounce ✎ ....½ oz
Processed sandwich meat with 3 grams or less fat per ounce, such as
turkey pastrami or kielbasa...1 oz
Liver, heart (high in cholesterol)..1 oz

✎ = 400 mg or more sodium per exchange.

• VERY LEAN MEAT AND SUBSTITUTES LIST

One exchange equals 0 grams carbohydrate, 7 grams protein, 0–1 grams fat, and 35 calories.

One very lean meat exchange is equal to any one of the following items.

Poultry: Chicken or turkey (white meat, no skin),
Cornish hen (no skin)..1 oz
Fish: Fresh or frozen cod, flounder, haddock, halibut, trout; tuna, fresh
or canned in water..1 oz
Shellfish: Clams, crab, lobster, scallops, shrimp, imitation shellfish ....1 oz
Game: Duck or pheasant (no skin), venison, buffalo, ostrich ....1 oz
Cheese with 1 gram or less fat per ounce:
Nonfat or low-fat cottage cheese ....¼ cup
Fat-free cheese...1 oz
Other: Processed sandwich meats with 1 gram or less fat per ounce, such
as deli thin, shaved meats, chipped beef ✎, turkey ham ....1 oz
Egg whites..2
Egg substitutes, plain...¼ cup
Hot dogs with 1 gram or less fat per ounce ✎..................1 oz
Kidney (high in cholesterol) ....1 oz
Sausage with 1 gram or less fat per ounce ....1 oz

Count as one very lean meat and one starch exchange.

Dried beans, peas, lentils (cooked).................................½ cup

✎ = 400 mg or more sodium per exchange.

• LEAN MEAT AND SUBSTITUTES LIST

One exchange equals 0 grams carbohydrate, 7 grams protein, 3 grams fat, and 55 calories.

One lean meat exchange is equal to any one of the following items.

Beef: USDA Select or Choice grades of lean beef trimmed of fat, such as
round, sirloin, and flank steak; tenderloin; roast (rib, chuck, rump);
steak (T-bone, porterhouse, cubed), ground round ....1 oz
Pork: Lean pork, such as fresh ham; canned, cured, or boiled ham;
Canadian bacon ✎; tenderloin, center loin chop ....1 oz
Lamb: Roast, chop, leg ....1 oz
Veal: Lean chop, roast..1 oz
Poultry: Chicken, turkey (dark meat, no skin), chicken white meat (with
skin), domestic duck or goose (well-drained of fat, no skin)..............1 oz
Fish:
Herring (uncreamed or smoked)...1 oz
Oysters..6 medium
Salmon (fresh or canned), catfish ....1 oz
Sardines (canned)..2 medium
Tuna (canned in oil, drained)..1 oz
Game: Goose (no skin), rabbit..1 oz

• MEDIUM-FAT MEAT AND SUBSTITUTES LIST

One exchange equals 0 grams carbohydrate, 7 grams protein, 5 grams fat, and 75 calories.

One medium-fat meat exchange is equal to any one of the following items.

Beef: Most beef products fall into this category (ground beef, meatloaf,
corned beef, short ribs, Prime grades of meat trimmed of fat, such as
prime rib) ....1 oz
Pork: Top loin, chop, Boston butt, cutlet......................1 oz
Lamb: Rib roast, ground...1 oz
Veal: Cutlet (ground or cubed, unbreaded).....................1 oz
Poultry: Chicken dark meat (with skin), ground turkey or ground
chicken, fried chicken (with skin)...................................1 oz
Fish: Any fried fish product ....1 oz
Cheese: With 5 grams or less fat per ounce
Feta...1 oz
Mozzarella ....1 oz
Ricotta ....¼ cup (2 oz)
Other:
Egg (high in cholesterol, limit to 3 per week) 1
Sausage with 5 grams or less fat per ounce.........................1 oz
Soy milk..1 cup
Tempeh...¼ cup
Tofu..4 oz or ½ cup

• HIGH-FAT MEAT AND SUBSTITUTES LIST

One exchange equals 0 grams carbohydrate, 7 grams protein, 8 grams fat, and 100 calories.

Remember, these items are high in saturated fat, cholesterol, and calories and may raise blood cholesterol levels if eaten on a regular basis. One high-fat meat exchange is equal to any one of the following items.

Pork: Spareribs, ground pork, pork sausage ....1 oz
Cheese: All regular cheeses, such as American ✎, cheddar, Monterey
Jack, Swiss ....1 oz
Other: Processed sandwich meats with 8 grams or less fat per ounce,
such as bologna, pimento loaf, salami ....1 oz
Sausage, such as bratwurst, Italian, knockwurst, Polish, smoked ......1 oz
Hot dog (turkey or chicken) ✎ 1 (10/lb)
Bacon ....2 slices (20 slices/lb)
Count as one high-fat meat plus one fat exchange.

Hot dog (beef, pork, or combination) ✎ 1 (10/lb)
Peanut butter (contains unsaturated fat) ....2 Tbsp

✎ = 400 mg or more sodium per exchange.

• FATS LIST

Monounsaturated Fats

One fat exchange equals 5 grams fat and 45 calories.

Avocado, medium..⅛ (1 oz)
Oil (canola, olive, peanut)..1 tsp
continued
Olives: ripe (black) ....8 large
    Green, stuffed 🔸...10 large
Nuts
    Almonds, cashews..6 nuts
    Mixed (50% peanuts)...6 nuts
    Peanuts...10 nuts
    Pecans..4 halves
Peanut butter, smooth or crunchy...2 tsp
Sesame seeds...1 Tbsp
Tahini paste...2 tsp

🔸 = 400 mg or more sodium per exchange.

Polyunsaturated Fats

One fat exchange equals 5 grams fat and 45 calories.

Margarine: stick, tub, or squeeze..1 tsp
    Lower-fat (30% to 50% vegetable oil)..............................1 Tbsp
Mayonnaise: regular..1 tsp
    Reduced-fat..1 Tbsp
Nuts, walnuts, English...4 halves
Oil (corn, safflower, soybean)...1 tsp
Salad dressing: regular 🔸..1 Tbsp
    Reduced-fat..2 Tbsp
Miracle Whip Salad Dressing®: regular.......................................2 tsp
    Reduced-fat..1 Tbsp
Seeds: pumpkin, sunflower...1 Tbsp

🔸 = 400 mg or more sodium per exchange.

Saturated Fats*

One fat exchange equals 5 grams of fat and 45 calories.

Bacon, cooked...1 slice (20 slices/lb)
Bacon, grease..1 tsp
Butter: stick...1 tsp
    Whipped...2 tsp
    Reduced-fat..1 Tbsp
Chitterlings, boiled...2 Tbsp (½ oz)
Coconut, sweetened, shredded..2 Tbsp
Cream, half and half..2 Tbsp
Cream cheese: regular...1 Tbsp (½ oz)
    Reduced-fat..2 Tbsp (1 oz)
Fatback or salt pork, see below†
Shortening or lard..1 tsp
Sour cream: regular...2 Tbsp
    Reduced-fat..3 Tbsp

*Saturated fats can raise blood cholesterol levels.

Use a piece 1 in. × 1 in. × ¼ in. if you plan to eat the fatback cooked with vegetables. Use a piece 2 in. × 1 in. × ½ in. when eating only the vegetables with the fatback removed.

• FREE FOODS LIST

A *free food* is any food or drink that contains less than 20 calories or less than 5 grams of carbohydrate per serving. Foods with a serving size listed should be limited to three servings per day. Be sure to spread them out throughout the day. If you eat all three servings at one time, it could affect your blood glucose level. Foods listed without a serving size can be eaten as often as you like.

Fat-Free or Reduced-Fat Foods

Cream cheese, fat-free...1 Tbsp
Creamers, nondairy, liquid...1 Tbsp
Creamers, nondairy, powdered...2 tsp
Mayonnaise, fat-free...1 Tbsp
Mayonnaise, reduced-fat..1 tsp
Margarine, fat-free...4 Tbsp
Margarine, reduced-fat..1 tsp
Miracle Whip®, nonfat..1 Tbsp
Miracle Whip®, reduced-fat..1 tsp
Nonstick cooking spray
Salad dressing, fat-free..1 Tbsp
Salad dressing, fat-free, Italian..2 Tbsp
Salsa...¼ cup
Sour cream, fat-free, reduced-fat...1 Tbsp
Whipped topping, regular or light...2 Tbsp

Sugar-Free or Low-Sugar Foods

Candy, hard, sugar-free..1 candy
Gelatin dessert, sugar-free
Gelatin, unflavored
Gum, sugar-free
Jam or jelly, low-sugar or light...2 tsp
Sugar substitutes°
Syrup, sugar-free..2 Tbsp

°Sugar substitutes, alternatives, or replacements that are approved by the Food and Drug Administration (FDA) are safe to use. Common brand names include: Equal® (aspartame), Sprinkle Sweet® (saccharin), Sweet One® (acesulfame K), Sweet-10® (saccharin), Sugar Twin® (saccharin), Sweet 'n Low® (saccharin).

Drinks

Bouillon, broth, consommé 🔸
Bouillon or broth, low-sodium
Carbonated or mineral water
Cocoa powder, unsweetened...1 Tbsp
Coffee
Club soda
Diet soft drinks, sugar-free
Drink mixes, sugar-free
Tea
Tonic water, sugar-free

Condiments

Catsup..1 Tbsp
Horseradish
Lemon juice
Lime juice
Mustard
Pickles, dill 🔸...1½ large
Soy sauce, regular or light 🔸
Taco sauce...1 Tbsp
Vinegar

Seasonings

Be careful with seasonings that contain sodium or are salts, such as garlic or celery salt, and lemon pepper.

Flavoring extracts
Garlic
Herbs, fresh or dried
Pimento
Spices
Tabasco® or hot pepper sauce
Wine, used in cooking
Worcestershire sauce

🔸 = 400 mg or more of sodium per choice.

• COMBINATION FOOD LIST

Many of the foods we eat are mixed together in various combinations. These combination foods do not fit into any one exchange list. Often it is hard to tell what is in a casserole dish or prepared food item. This is a list of exchanges for some typical combination foods. This list will help you fit these foods into your meal plan. Ask your dietitian for information about any other combination foods you would like to eat.

Food	Serving Size	Exchanges per Serving
Entrees		
Tuna noodle casserole, lasagna, spaghetti with meatballs, chile with beans, macaroni and cheese 🔖	1 cup (8 oz)	2 carbohydrates, 2 medium-fat meats
Chow mein (without noodles or rice)	2 cups (16 oz)	1 carbohydrate, 2 lean meats
Pizza, cheese, thin crust 🔖	¼ of 10 in. (5 oz)	2 carbohydrates, 2 medium-fat meats, 1 fat
Pizza, meat topping, thin crust 🔖	¼ of 10 in. (5 oz)	2 carbohydrates, 2 medium-fat meats, 2 fats
Pot pie 🔖	1 (7 oz)	2 carbohydrates, 1 medium-fat meat, 4 fats
Frozen entrees		
Salisbury steak with gravy, mashed potato 🔖	1 (11 oz)	2 carbohydrates, 3 medium-fat meats, 3–4 fats
Turkey with gravy, mashed potato, dressing 🔖	1 (11 oz)	2 carbohydrates, 3 lean meats
Entree with less than 300 calories 🔖	1 (8 oz)	2 carbohydrates, 3 lean meats
Soups		
Bean 🔖	1 cup	1 carbohydrate, 1 very lean meat
Cream (made with water) 🔖	1 cup (8 oz)	1 carbohydrate, 1 fat
Split pea (made with water) 🔖	½ cup (4 oz)	1 carbohydrate
Tomato (made with water) 🔖	1 cup (8 oz)	1 carbohydrate
Vegetable beef, chicken noodle, or other broth-type 🔖	1 cup (8 oz)	1 carbohydrate

🔖 = 400 mg or more sodium per exchange.

• FAST FOODS LIST*

Food	Serving Size	Exchanges per Serving
Burritos with beef 🔖	2	4 carbohydrates, 2 medium-fat meats, 2 fats
Chicken nuggets 🔖	6	1 carbohydrate, 2 medium-fat meats, 1 fat
Chicken breast and wing, breaded and fried 🔖	1 each	1 carbohydrate, 4 medium-fat meats, 2 fats
Fish sandwich/tartar sauce 🔖	1	3 carbohydrates, 1 medium-fat meat, 3 fats
French fries, thin	20–25	2 carbohydrates, 2 fats
Hamburger, regular	1	2 carbohydrates, 2 medium-fat meats
Hamburger, large 🔖	1	2 carbohydrates, 3 medium-fat meats, 1 fat
Hot dog with bun 🔖	1	1 carbohydrate, 1 high-fat meat, 1 fat
Individual pan pizza 🔖	1	5 carbohydrates, 3 medium-fat meats, 3 fats
Soft-serve cone	1 medium	2 carbohydrates, 1 fat
Submarine sandwich 🔖	1 sub (6 in.)	3 carbohydrates, 1 vegetable, 2 medium-fat meats, 1 fat
Taco, hard shell 🔖	1 (6 oz)	2 carbohydrates, 2 medium-fat meats, 2 fats
Taco, soft shell 🔖	1 (3 oz)	1 carbohydrate, 1 medium-fat meat, 1 fat

🔖 = 400 mg or more of sodium per serving.

*Ask at your fast-food restaurant for nutrition information about your favorite fast foods.

Food Labeling Information

Sample Label for a Granola Bar

Nutrition Facts

Serving Size 1 bar (24g)
Servings Per Container 12

Amount Per Serving

Calories 120   Calories from Fat 45

	% Daily Value*
Total Fat 5g	**8%**
Saturated Fat 1g	**5%**
Cholesterol 0mg	**0%**
Sodium 65mg	**3%**
Total Carbohydrate 17g	**6%**
Dietary Fiber 1g	**4%**
Sugars 6g	
Protein 2g	

Vitamin A 0%	•	Vitamin C 0%	
Calcium 0%	•	Iron 4%	

* Percent Daily Values are based on a 2,000 calorie diet. Your daily values may be higher or lower depending on your calorie needs:

	Calories:	2,000	2,500
Total Fat	Less than	65g	80g
Sat Fat	Less than	20g	25g
Cholesterol	Less than	300mg	300mg
Sodium	Less than	2,400mg	2,400mg
Total Carbohydrate		300g	375g
Dietary Fiber		25g	30g

Calories per gram:
Fat 9 • Carbohydrate 4 • Protein 4

Ingredients: Rolled oats, sugar, sunflower oil, brown sugar syrup, honey, salt, soy lecithin

Daily Reference Values

Food Component	Daily Reference Value (2000 kcal)
Total fat	Less than 65 g (30% of energy)
Saturated fat	Less than 20 g (10% of energy)
Cholesterol	Less than 300 mg
Total carbohydrate	300 g (60% of energy)
Dietary fiber	25 g (11.5 g/1000 kcal)
Sodium	Less than 2400 mg
Potassium	3500 mg
Protein	50 g (10% of energy)

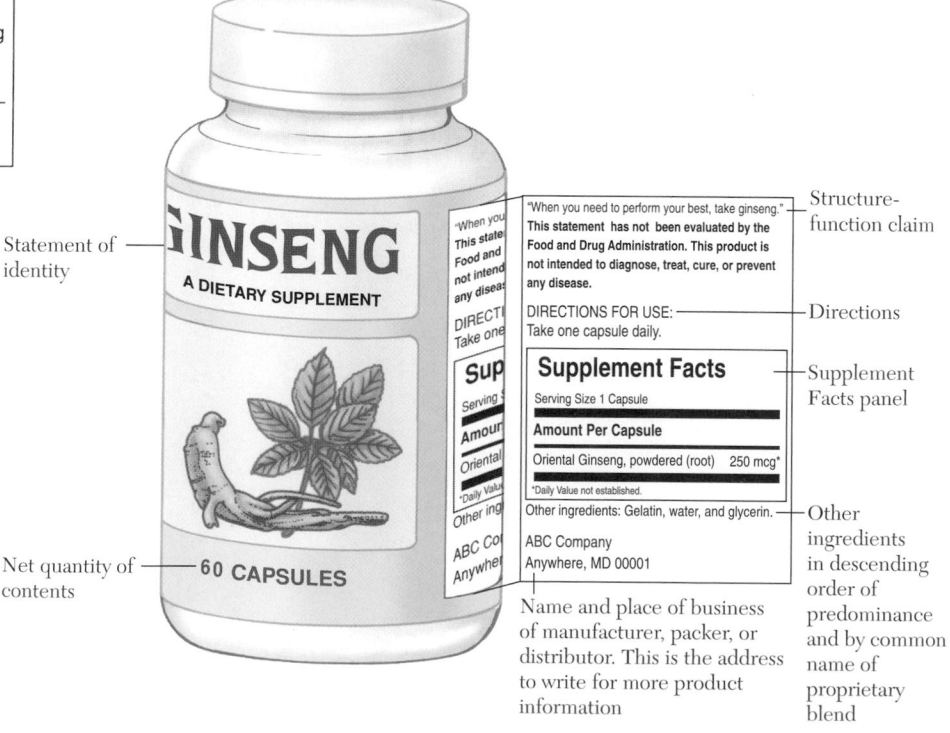

Statement of identity

Net quantity of contents

Structure-function claim

Directions

Supplement Facts panel

Other ingredients in descending order of predominance and by common name of proprietary blend

Name and place of business of manufacturer, packer, or distributor. This is the address to write for more product information

GINSENG
A DIETARY SUPPLEMENT

"When you need to perform your best, take ginseng." This statement has not been evaluated by the Food and Drug Administration. This product is not intended to diagnose, treat, cure, or prevent any disease.

DIRECTIONS FOR USE:
Take one capsule daily.

Supplement Facts
Serving Size 1 Capsule

Amount Per Capsule

Oriental Ginseng, powdered (root)   250 mcg*

*Daily Value not established.

Other ingredients: Gelatin, water, and glycerin.

ABC Company
Anywhere, MD 00001

60 CAPSULES

Recommended Dietary Intakes (RDIs)*

Vitamins and Minerals	Units of Measurement	Adults and Children 4 or More Years of Age	Infants	Children Under 4 Years of Age	Pregnant or Lactating Women
Vitamin A	International Units (micrograms)†	5000 (1000 µg)	1500	2500	8000
Vitamin D	International Units (micrograms)†	400 (10 µg)	400	400	400
Vitamin E	International Units (micrograms)†	30 (10 µg)	5	10	30
Vitamin C	Milligrams	60	35	40	60
Folic acid	Micrograms	400	0.1	0.2	0.8
Thiamin	Milligrams	1.5	0.5	0.7	1.7
Riboflavin	Milligrams	1.7	0.6	0.8	2.0
Niacin	Milligrams	20	8	9	20
Vitamin B_6	Milligrams	2.0	0.4	0.7	2.5
Vitamin B_{12}	Micrograms	6.0	2	3	8
Biotin	Micrograms	300	0.05	0.15	0.30
Pantothenic acid	Milligrams	10	3	5	10
Calcium	Milligrams	1000	0.6	0.8	1.3
Phosphorus	Milligrams	1000	0.5	0.8	1.3
Iodine	Micrograms	150	45	70	150
Iron	Milligrams	18	15	10	18
Magnesium	Milligrams	400	70	200	450
Copper	Milligrams	20	0.6	1.0	2.0
Zinc	Milligrams	15	5	8	15
Vitamin K	Micrograms	80	—‡	—‡	—‡
Chromium	Micrograms	120	—	—	—
Selenium	Micrograms	70	—	—	—
Molybdenum	Micrograms	75	—	—	—
Manganese	Milligrams	2	—	—	—
Chloride	Milligrams	3400	—	—	—

*Based on National Academy of Sciences' 1968 Recommended Dietary Allowances.

†The RDIs for fat-soluble vitamins are expressed in International Units (IU). Values that are approximately equivalent in micrograms are given in parentheses.

‡No values yet established for vitamin K, chromium, selenium, molybdenum, manganese, or chloride for this population.

Nutrient Content Descriptors Commonly Used on Food Labels

Free	Means that a product contains no amount of, or a trivial amount of, fat, saturated fat, cholesterol, sodium, sugars, or kcalories. For example, "sugar free" and "fat free" both mean less than 0.5 g per serving. Synonyms for "free" include "without," "no," and "zero."
Low	Used for foods that can be eaten frequently without exceeding the Daily Value for fat, saturated fat, cholesterol, sodium, or kcalories. Specific definitions have been established for each of these nutrients. For example, "lowfat" means that the food contains 3 g or less per serving, and "low cholesterol" means that the food contains less than 20 mg of cholesterol per serving. Synonyms for "low" include "little," "few," and "low source of."
Lean and extra lean	Used to describe the fat content of meat, poultry, seafood, and game meats. "Lean" means that the food contains less than 10 g fat, less than 4.5 g saturated fat, and less than 95 mg of cholesterol per serving and per 100 g. "Extra lean" means that the food contains less than 5 g fat, less than 2 g saturated fat, and less than 95 mg of cholesterol per serving and per 100 g.
High	Can be used if a food contains 20% or more of the Daily Value for a particular nutrient. Synonyms for "high" include "rich in" and "excellent source of."
Good source	Means that a food contains 10 to 19% of the Daily Value for a particular nutrient per serving.
Reduced	Means that a nutritionally altered product contains 25% less of a nutrient or of energy than the regular or reference product.
Less	Means that a food, whether altered or not, contains 25% less of a nutrient or of energy than the reference food. For example, pretzels may claim to have "less fat" than potato chips. "Fewer" may be used as a synonym for "less."
Light	May be used in different ways. First, it can be used on a nutritionally altered product that contains one-third fewer kcalories or half the fat of a reference food. Second, it can be used when the sodium content of a low-calorie, lowfat food has been reduced by 50%. The term "light" can be used to describe properties such as texture and color as long as the label explains the intent—for example, "light and fluffy."
More	Means that a serving of food, whether altered or not, contains a nutrient that is at least 10% of the Daily Value more than the reference food. This definition also applies to foods using the terms "fortified," "enriched," or "added."
Healthy	May be used to describe foods that are low in fat and saturated fat and contain no more than 360 mg of sodium and no more than 60 mg of cholesterol per serving and provide at least 10% of the Daily Value for vitamins A or C, or iron, calcium, protein, or fiber.
Fresh	May be used on foods that are raw and have never been frozen or heated and contain no preservatives.

Source: Federal Register 58. Washington, D.C.: U.S. Government Printing Office, Superintendent of Documents, Jan. 6, 1993.

FDA-Approved Health Claims*

Calcium and osteoporosis	Adequate calcium intake throughout life helps maintain bone health and reduce the risk of osteoporosis.
Sodium and hypertension (high blood pressure)	Diets low in sodium may reduce the risk of high blood pressure in some people.
Dietary fat and cancer	Diets low in fat may reduce the risk of some types of cancer.
Saturated fat and cholesterol and risk of coronary heart disease	Diets low in saturated fat and cholesterol help reduce blood cholesterol and, thus the risk of heart disease.
Fiber-containing grain products, fruits, and vegetables, and cancer risk	Diets low in fat and rich in fiber-containing grain products, fruits, and vegetables may reduce the risk of some types of cancer.
Fruits, vegetables, and grain products that contain fiber, particularly soluble fiber, and risk of coronary heart disease	Diets low in saturated fat and cholesterol and rich in fruits, vegetables, and grain products that contain fiber, particularly soluble fiber, may reduce the risk of coronary heart disease.
Fruits and vegetables and cancer	Diets low in fat and rich in fruits and vegetables may reduce the risk of some types of cancer.
Folic acid and neural tube birth defects	Adequate folic acid intake by the mother reduces the risk of birth defects of the brain or spinal cord in her baby.
Soluble fiber from certain foods and risk of coronary heart disease.	Diets low in fat, saturated fat, and cholesterol that include soluble fiber from whole oats or psyllium seed husk may reduce the risk of heart disease.
Dietary sugar alcohol and dental caries (cavities)	Sugar-free foods that are sweetened with sugar alcohols do not promote tooth decay and may reduce the risk of dental caries.
Soy protein and risk of coronary heart disease	Soy protein included in a diet that is low in saturated fat and cholesterol may reduce the risk of coronary heart disease by lowering blood cholesterol levels.
Plant sterol/stanol esters and risk of coronary heart disease	Plant sterols and plant stanols included in a diet that is low in saturated fat and cholesterol may reduce the risk of coronary heart disease by lowering blood cholesterol levels.

*A food carrying a health claim must be a naturally good source (10% or more of the Daily Value) for one of six nutrients (vitamin A, vitamin C, protein, calcium, iron, or fiber) and must not contain more than 20% of the Daily Value for fat, saturated fat, cholesterol, or sodium. These claims have been approved for use on food labels. The FDA continues to evaluate new claims, many of which are in various stages of approval.

Energy Expenditure for Various Activities

 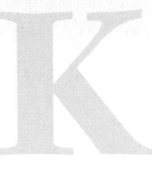

Type of Activity	Kcalories per Hour (by body weight)				
	100 lb	120 lb	150 lb	180 lb	200 lb
Aerobics (heavy)	363	435	544	653	726
Aerobics (medium)	227	272	340	408	454
Aerobics (light)	136	163	204	245	272
Archery	159	190	238	286	317
Backpacking	408	490	612	735	816
Badminton (doubles)	181	218	272	327	363
Badminton (singles)	231	278	347	416	463
Basketball (nonvigorous)	431	517	646	776	862
Basketball (vigorous)	499	599	748	898	998
Bicycling (6 mph)	159	190	238	286	317
Bicycling (10 mph)	249	299	374	449	499
Bicycling (11 mph)	295	354	442	531	590
Bicycling (12 mph)	340	408	510	612	680
Bicycling (13 mph)	385	463	578	694	771
Billiards	91	109	136	163	181
Bowling	177	212	265	318	354
Boxing—competition	603	724	905	1086	1206
Boxing—sparring	376	452	565	678	753
Calisthenics (heavy)	363	435	544	653	726
Calisthenics (light)	181	218	272	327	363
Canoeing (2.5 mph)	150	180	224	269	299
Canoeing (5 mph)	340	408	510	612	680
Carpentry	227	272	340	408	454
Climbing (mountain)	454	544	680	816	907
Disco dancing	272	327	408	490	544
Ditch digging (hand)	263	316	395	473	526
Fencing	340	408	510	612	680
Fishing (bank/boat)	159	190	238	286	317
Fishing (in waders)	249	299	374	449	499
Football (touch)	340	408	510	612	680
Gardening	145	174	218	261	290
Golf (carry clubs)	227	272	340	408	454
Golf (pull cart)	163	196	245	294	327
Golf (ride in cart)	113	136	170	204	227
Handball (vigorous)	454	544	680	816	907
Hiking (X-country)	249	299	374	449	499
Hiking (mountain)	340	408	510	612	680
Horseback trotting	231	278	347	416	463
Housework	181	218	272	327	363

(continued)

Type of Activity	Kcalories per Hour (by body weight)				
	100 lb	120 lb	150 lb	180 lb	200 lb
Hunting (carry load)	272	327	408	490	544
Ice hockey (vigorous)	454	544	680	816	907
Ice skating (10 mph)	263	316	395	473	526
Jazzercize (heavy)	363	435	544	653	726
Jazzercise (medium)	227	272	340	408	454
Jazzercise (light)	136	163	204	245	272
Jog (9 min/mile)	499	599	748	898	998
Jog (10 min/mile)	454	544	680	816	907
Jog (12 min/mile)	385	463	578	694	771
Jog (13 min/mile)	317	381	476	571	635
Jog (14 min/mile)	272	327	408	490	544
Jog (15 min/mile)	227	272	340	408	454
Jog (17 min/mile)	181	218	272	327	363
Lawn mowing (hand)	295	354	442	531	590
Lawn mowing (power)	163	196	245	294	327
Musical instrument playing	113	136	170	204	227
Racquetball (social)	385	463	578	694	771
Racquetball (vigorous)	454	544	680	816	907
Roller skating	231	278	347	416	463
Rowboating (2.5 mph)	200	239	299	359	399
Rowing (11 mph)	590	707	884	1061	1179
Run (5 min/mile)	816	980	1224	1469	1633
Run (6 min/mile)	703	844	1054	1265	1406
Run (7 min/mile)	612	735	918	1102	1224
Run (8 min/mile)	544	653	816	980	1088
Sailing	159	190	238	286	317
Shuffleboard/skeet	136	163	204	245	272
Skiing (X-country)	454	544	680	816	907
Skiing (downhill)	363	435	544	653	726
Square dancing	272	327	407	490	544
Swimming (competitive)	680	816	1020	1224	1361
Swimming (fast)	426	512	639	767	853
Swimming (slow)	349	419	524	629	698
Table tennis	236	283	354	424	472
Tennis (doubles)	227	272	340	408	454
Tennis (singles)	295	354	442	531	590
Tennis (vigorous)	385	463	578	694	771
Volleyball	231	278	347	416	463
Walking (20 min/mile)	159	190	238	286	317
Walking (26 min/mile)	136	163	204	245	272
Water skiing	317	381	476	571	635
Weight lifting (heavy)	408	490	612	735	816
Weight lifting (light)	181	218	272	327	363
Wood chopping (sawing)	295	354	442	531	590

Data reprinted with permission from N-Squared Computing, First Databank Division of the Hearst Corporation.

Calculations and Conversions

Weights and Measures

Measure	Abbreviation	Equivalent
1 gram	g	1000 milligrams
1 milligram	mg	1000 micrograms
1 microgram	μg	1/1000000 of a gram
1 nanogram	ng	1/1000000000 of a gram
1 picogram	pg	1/1000000000000 of a gram
1 kilogram	kg	1000 grams 2.2 lb
1 pound	lb	454 grams 16 ounces
1 teaspoon	tsp	approximately 5 grams
1 tablespoon	Tbsp	3 teaspoons
1 ounce	oz	28.4 grams
1 cup	c	8 fluid ounces 16 tablespoon
1 pint	pt	2 cups 16 fluid ounces
1 quart	qt	2 pints 32 fluid ounces
1 gallon	gal	128 fluid ounces 4 quarts
1 liter	l	1.06 quarts 1000 milliliters
1 milliliter	ml	1000 microliters
1 deciliter	dl	100 milliliters
1 kcalorie	kcal	1000 calories 4.167 kilojoules
1 kilojoule	kJ	1000 joules

Converting Vitamin A Units into μg Vitamin A

Form and source	Amount equal to l μg vitamin A
Preformed vitamin A in food or supplements	1 μg
	1 RAE
	1 μg RE
	3.3 IU
β-carotene in foods°	12 μg
	1 RAE
	2 μg RE
	20 IU
α-carotene or β-cryptoxanthin in food	24 μg
	1 RAE
	2 μg RE
	40 IU

°β-carotene in supplements may be better absorbed than β-carotene in food and so provides more vitamin A activity. It is estimated that 2 μg of β-carotene dissolved in oil provides 1 μg of vitamin A activity.

Calculating Dietary Folate Equivalents in Fortified Foods

The folate listed on labels of fortified foods is primarily folic acid, which is more available than natural forms of folate. In order to compare the folate content of these foods to recommendations, the amount of folic acid must be converted to dietary folate equivalents, espressed as μg DFE. This calculation assumes that all of the folate in these foods is from added folic acid.

Determine the amount of folic acid in the fortified food:

- Multiply the Daily Value for folate by the % Daily Values listed on the label.
- Daily Value is 400 μg.

Convert the μg folic acid into μg DFE:

- Multiply the μg folic acid by 1.7.
- Folic acid added to a food in fortification provides 1.7 times more available folate per μg than folate naturally present in foods.

For example:

- A serving of English muffins provides 6% of the Daily Value for folate:

    To find the μg folic acid: 400 μg × 6% = 24 μg folic acid

    To convert to μg DFE: 24 μg folic acid × 1.7 = 40 μg DFE

Converting Vitamin E Values into mg α-Tocopherol

To estimate the α-tocopherol intake from foods:

- If values are given as mg α-TEs:

$$\text{mg } \alpha\text{-TE} \times 0.8° = \text{mg } \alpha\text{-tocopherol}$$

- If values are given in IUs:

    First, determine if the source of the α-tocopherol is natural or synthetic.

    - For natural α-tocopherol:

        $$\text{IU of natural } \alpha\text{-tocopherol} \times 0.67 = \text{mg } \alpha\text{-tocopherol}$$

    - For synthetic α-tocopherol (dl-α-tocopherol):

        $$\text{IU of synthetic } \alpha\text{-tocopherol} \times 0.45 = \text{mg } \alpha\text{-tocopherol}$$

°Based on dietary data from the NHANES III study, approximately 80% of the α-tocopherol equivalents from food are from α-tocopherol and can thus contribute to the body's requirement for vitamin E.

Answers to Critical Thinking Questions

 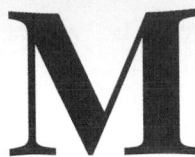

• CHAPTER 1: WHAT IS WRONG WITH THIS EXPERIMENT?

Was the study well controlled? No. Muscle strength was tested before the supplement was given to establish any differences between groups not due to the supplement, but other controls were missing. There was no placebo used to make the control group indistinguishable from the experimental group. The diet was not well controlled. No information was obtained about what the subjects were consuming before or during the study. Subjects were asked not to change their diets, but the study provided no way to assess whether some subjects changed their diets during the experiment. There was also no control of physical activity. If subjects in the experimental group began lifting weights during the study, the differences in muscle strength may have been due to this rather than the supplement.

Was the proper number of experimental subjects used? There is no mention of the statistical methods used to determine the correct number of subjects, but 25 in each group is probably enough to establish reliable results.

Was quantifiable data evaluated? Yes. Muscle strength is quantifiable and can be measured repeatedly.

Is the conclusion valid? No. Since the diets and exercise regimens of the two groups were not evaluated and controlled, these variables could have caused the observed differences in muscle strength. In addition, because no statistics are presented, the 5-pound increase in leg strength may not have represented a true statistical difference between the two groups.

• CHAPTER 2: USING THE FOOD GUIDE PYRAMID

Does Jarad's diet meet the minimum number of servings recommended by the Food Guide Pyramid? He meets the recommendations for all groups except fruits.

Bread, Cereal, Rice, & Pasta	6–11 servings are recommended; he had 7.
Vegetable	3–5 servings are recommended; he had about 3½.
Fruit	2–4 servings are recommended; he had only 1.
Milk, Yogurt, & Cheese	2–3 servings are recommended; he had about 3½.
Meat, Poultry, Fish, Dry Beans, Eggs, & Nuts	2–3 servings are recommended; he had 3.

How many foods did he have during the day that contribute primarily sugar and/or fat? He had 4; it is recommended that fats, oils, and sweets be consumed sparingly.

Suggest a nutrient-dense sandwich order that includes selections from at least 3 Food Guide Pyramid food groups. One sandwich idea is a whole grain roll with turkey, lettuce, tomatoes, peppers, and mustard. Adding a slice of cheese will add a food from the Milk, Yogurt, and Cheese Group.

• CHAPTER 2: NUTRITIONAL ASSESSMENT

Should she be concerned about the nutrients she is consuming in excess of her goal? Use the DRI tables to determine if they are likely to pose a risk. Her vitamin C intake is 146% of goal: this amount has not been shown to cause side effects and is well below the UL of 2000 mg. Her vitamin A intake is 147% of goal. Vitamin A can be toxic but only if it is consumed as preformed vitamin A (retinoids), which is found in animal products. Plant sources of vitamin A provide carotenoids, which are not toxic. For women in Alison's age group, the UL is set at 3000 μg per day of preformed vitamin A from the diet and from supplements. Even if all the vitamin A in Alison's diet were from retinoids, it would be below the UL. The UL for calcium is 2.5 grams per day—her intake is well below this, so it is in a safe range of intake.

• CHAPTER 3: GASTROINTESTINAL PROBLEMS CAN AFFECT NUTRITION

What type of foods should be avoided? Fatty foods should be avoided because fat in the GI tract causes the gallbladder to contract. This contraction causes pain when there are gallstones in the gallbladder.

• CHAPTER 4: LOSING WEIGHT ON A LOW CARBOHYDRATE DIET

Which groups of the Food Guide Pyramid are likely to be low in John's diet? If he follows this diet, he will consume less than the recommended number of servings from the Bread, Cereal, Rice, and Pasta Group and the Fruit

Group. He is also likely to consume less than recommended from the Vegetable Group and the Milk, Yogurt, and Cheese Group.

Why can ketosis develop in type 1 diabetes even when plenty of carbohydrate is consumed? Type 1 diabetics do not produce enough insulin. Without insulin, glucose cannot enter cells. Without adequate glucose in the cells, fat cannot be completely broken down and ketones are formed. Ketosis occurs in a type 1 diabetic even when plenty of carbohydrate is consumed because glucose cannot enter the cells where it is needed.

• CHAPTER 4: BUILDING A HEALTHY BASE

How many grams of fiber are in Katie's modified diet? Does it meet the recommendations? Her modified diet provides approximately 21.5 grams of fiber, which is below the AI of 25 grams per day for young adult women.

Does Katie's modified diet meet the recommendations for 2–4 servings of fruits, 3–5 servings of vegetables, and 6–11 servings of grains? Yes. Her modified diet provides about 7 servings of grains, 4 servings of fruit, and 3½ servings of vegetables.

• CHAPTER 5: DIETARY FAT AND HEART DISEASE RISK

What risk factors does Rafael have for developing cardiovascular disease? He is at risk because he is male and his mother died of a heart attack before the age of 65. His stress level is moderate, but his risk is increased by a total blood cholesterol level that is over 200 mg/dl, by LDL cholesterol in the high risk range, and by HDL cholesterol that is less than 40 mg/dl. His diet exceeds the recommendations for fat, saturated fat, and cholesterol and contains fewer servings of fruits and vegetables and more meat than is recommended.

What dietary and lifestyle changes would you recommend to reduce his risks? He could increase the number of servings of whole grains, fruits, and vegetables he eats each day, use lowfat dairy products, and reduce his intake of high-fat meats. He could increase his exercise and reduce his stress level.

If Rafael were to replace all of the added fat in his diet with olive oil, would he reduce his risk of cardiovascular disease to the level found in Mediterranean countries? No, olive oil is only one component of a total dietary pattern and lifestyle that is associated with a lower risk of cardiovascular disease. He would also need to change other aspects of his diet and lifestyle.

• CHAPTER 5: FITTING FAT INTO YOUR DIET

Does Stella's original diet meet the serving recommendations of the Food Guide Pyramid for grains, vegetables, and fruit? Do her choices from these groups follow the selection tips of the Food Guide Pyramid? No. Stella's diet includes only 4 servings of grains but should have at least 6. It contains 3 servings of vegetables, which meets the recommendations, but only 1 serving of fruit, which is below the suggested 2 to 4 servings. Her choices do not follow the selection tips. All 3 vegetables are potatoes, so there is little variety; they are also fried, which increases fat and kcalories in the diet. Many of her other choices are also high in fat and low in nutrient density.

A computer analysis shows that her total energy intake is 2100 kcalories. What is the percent of kcalories from fat in her original diet? 93.6 grams × 9 kcal/gram = 842 kcal/2100 kcal × 100 = 40%

What is the percentage of energy from fat in her modified diet, assuming it also contains 2100 kcalories? Does this diet meet the serving and selection recommendations of the Food Guide Pyramid for grains, vegetables, and fruits? 50.9 grams × 9 kcal/gram = 458 kcal/2100 kcal × 100 = 22%

Yes. Her modified diet does meet the Food Guide Pyramid recommendations. It includes about 8 servings of grains, 5 servings of vegetables, and 4 servings of fruits. Most of her choices are high in nutrient density.

• CHAPTER 6: WHAT DOES NITROGEN BALANCE TELL US?

What is his nitrogen balance? His balance is 0 grams. Intake is equal to output, so he is in nitrogen balance.

What is her nitrogen balance? She is in positive nitrogen balance by 2.4 grams.

Does her nitrogen balance make sense metabolically? Yes. Subject C is pregnant, so she is retaining nitrogen that is being used to synthesize new tissue.

• CHAPTER 6: CHOOSING A VEGETARIAN DIET

How much protein would this diet provide if he decided to eliminate dairy products? It would provide 46.7 grams.

Does his diet meet the Food Guide Pyramid recommendations for vegetarians? He meets the recommendations for all groups except vegetables, which should be increased to at least 3 servings:

	Recommended	Ajay's Diet
Grains	6–11	9
Vegetables	3–5	2
Fruits	2–4	3
Dairy	0–3	$2\frac{1}{2}$
Meat Substitutes	2–3	2

• CHAPTER 7: BALANCING INTAKE AND EXPENDITURE

What is her EER? April is 23 years old, 64 inches tall, and weighs 140 pounds.

$$64 \text{ inches} \times 0.0254 \text{ meters/inch} = 1.63 \text{ meters}$$

$$140 \text{ pounds}/2.2 \text{ pounds/kg} = 63.6 \text{ kg}$$

The PA value for an adult woman in the "low active" category is 1.12

$$\begin{aligned} EER = 354 &- (6.91 \times \text{Age in years}) \\ &+ PA\,[(9.36 \times \text{weight in kg}) \\ &+ (726 \times \text{height in meters})] \end{aligned}$$

Using April's information:

$$\begin{aligned} EER = 354 &- (6.91 \times 23) + 1.12[(9.36 \times 63.6) \\ &+ (726 \times 1.63)] = 2187 \text{ kcal/day} \end{aligned}$$

How does her EER compare to her intake? April consumes 2450 kcal/day, and her EER is only 2187 kcal/day. She is therefore consuming about 263 kcalories more than she is expending. This will cause a weight gain of approximately $\frac{1}{2}$ pound a week.

What would her EER be with the added 2 hours per day of tennis? Adding 2 hours of tennis a day would put April in the "very active" category so her PA value would be 1.45.

$$\begin{aligned} EER = 354 &- 6.91\,(23) + 1.45\,[(9.36 \times 63.6) \\ &+ (726 \times 1.63)] = 2774 \text{ kcal/day} \end{aligned}$$

Is she destined to become obese? She is not destined to be obese, but to maintain her weight in a healthy range she probably needs to monitor her kcaloric intake more carefully and exercise more than an individual with no genetic tendency to carry excess body fat. If she makes small changes in her diet and exercise patterns that she can stick with, she is more likely to succeed.

• CHAPTER 7: DO YOU THINK THIS DIET WILL WORK?

Does this program include an exercise component? No. The amino acid supplement is supposed to convert fat into energy, but no exercise recommendations are given.

Does the program promote changes in eating habits and lifestyle that will encourage achieving and maintaining a healthy weight? No. It tries for a quick fix rather than promoting small changes that will last a lifetime.

• CHAPTER 8: FOUR HUNDRED OF FORTIFIED FOLATE

List some substitutions that would increase Marcia's intake of naturally occurring folate and folic acid from fortified foods. She could increase her intake of naturally occurring folate by replacing the french fries at lunch with a leafy green vegetable such as a spinach salad. To increase her intake from fortified foods, she could choose a fortified breakfast cereal. The amounts added to cereals are typically greater than the amount added to other grain products.

Would you recommend Marcia take a folate supplement? Yes. Unless Marcia plans her diet more carefully, she would benefit from a folic acid supplement.

• CHAPTER 9: HOW MUCH VITAMIN A IS IN YOUR FAST FOOD MEAL?

Use the Food Guide Pyramid to suggest foods that John could add to improve his diet. Be sure to select foods high in vitamin A or vitamin A precursors. He can improve his diet by increasing the number of servings from the Vegetable Group, the Fruit Group, and the Milk, Yogurt, & Cheese Group. By selecting yellow orange colored foods like carrots, sweet potatoes, cantaloupe, and mangos as well as leafy green vegetables like broccoli and spinach, he will get plenty of vitamin A precursors. The additional servings of milk will add preformed vitamin A as well as calcium to his diet.

John's meals are also low in vitamin C. What foods could he add to his diet to increase his intake of vitamin C? If some of the selections he adds from the Fruit Group are citrus fruits, he will easily meet his need for vitamin C. Other fruits that are good sources of vitamin C include strawberries, kiwis, and cantaloupe. Vegetables that are good sources include broccoli and peppers.

• CHAPTER 10: A DIET FOR HEALTH

How does the modified diet compare to the recommendations of the Food Guide Pyramid? to Rashamel's current diet?

	FGP	Current	Modified
Grains	6–11	8	10
Vegetables	3–5	1	5
Fruit	2–4	3	5
Milk	2–3	1	4
Meat	2–3	2	2

How could this diet be changed to reduce the energy content without reducing the calcium? Yuka could use nonfat milk instead of lowfat milk and reduce the number of servings from other groups as shown in Table 10.2. Someone who needs only 1800 kcals should consume fewer servings of grains, vegetables, and fruits.

• CHAPTER 11: INCREASING IRON INTAKE

What dietary factors could contribute to Odelia's poor iron status?

1. The RDA for a young female vegetarian is 33 mg per day. Her total iron intake is marginal at 12 mg per day.

2. The iron in her diet comes from plant sources. This might contribute to her deficiency because the iron in plants is nonheme iron, which is poorly absorbed.

3. The diet is low in vitamin C-rich foods. This may contribute to her deficiency because vitamin C enhances iron absorption.

4. The switch to stainless steel cookware may have reduced her iron intake because iron leaches from iron cookware, increasing the iron content of the food being prepared.

What modifications could Odelia make to increase the iron content of her dinner? She could cook the meal in an iron pot. She could add tomatoes or lime juice to the meal; the acid would increase the amount of iron leached from the iron cookware into the food. She could have orange juice instead of apple juice with dinner. The vitamin C in the orange juice would enhance the iron absorption of the foods in that meal. She could add beans (a good vegetarian source of iron) to the rice. Tea, which contains tannins that inhibit iron absorption, could be consumed later in the morning.

Does Odelia's diet meet the recommendations of the Food Guide Pyramid for vegetarians? Are there other nutrient deficiencies for which she may be at risk? She needs to add a serving of dairy products and of legumes or nuts to her diet to meet the recommendations. Also, the only fruit she consumes is apple juice; she should add more variety from this group. She is unlikely to be at risk of calcium, vitamin D, or vitamin B_{12} deficiency because she consumes dairy products, but the lack of meat in her diet puts her at risk of zinc deficiency.

• CHAPTER 12: SUPPLEMENTAL CHOICES

What would you recommend to Hazel? She should stop taking these supplements because the amounts of nutrients are so high that she is exceeding the UL for some. She can ensure she meets all her nutrient needs by taking a multivitamin/mineral supplement that contains no more than 100% of the Daily Value for any nutrient. She can also increase her nutrient intake by improving her diet. By increasing her intake of dairy products to the amount recommended by the Food Guide Pyramid, she will meet her needs for calcium; by increasing her intake of fruits, especially citrus fruits, to the recommended level, she can increase her intake of vitamin C. If she decides not to take a supplement, consuming a fortified breakfast cereal will help ensure she gets plenty of B vitamins.

• CHAPTER 13: INCORPORATING EXERCISE SENSIBLY

What is Nicole's EER now that she is in the active physical activity category?

$$EER = 354 - (6.91 \times \text{Age in yrs})$$
$$+ PA\,[(9.36 \times \text{Weight in kg})$$
$$+ (725 \times \text{Height in meters})]$$

Age = 45 yrs, PA = 1.27, Weight = 63.6 kg, Height = 1.63m

$$EER = 354 - (6.91 \times 45) + 1.27\,[(9.36 \times 63.6)$$
$$+ (726 \times 1.63)] = 2302 \text{ kcal/day}$$

• CHAPTER 13: AN ERGOGENIC BOOST?

What would you recommend Andrew do? If Andrew participates in sprint events requiring short bursts of activity, creatine might improve his performance. To have this benefit, he needs to continue to take the supplement and there are no good long-term studies on creatine safety. There is little risk if Andrew wants to try the supplement to see if his performance is improved, but he should be cautious about taking it over the long term. The evidence supporting the benefits of chromium picolinate is questionable so, although the risks of taking it are small, they still outweigh the benefits.

• CHAPTER **14:** NUTRIENT NEEDS FOR A SUCCESSFUL PREGNANCY

Chevron is overweight. Should she still add these foods to her diet? Yes. All pregnant women should gain weight during pregnancy to allow for the healthy growth of the fetus. Even though she is overweight, Chevron needs to slowly gain weight during the last two trimesters of her pregnancy.

How could her original diet be improved to increase nutrient density? Chevron could reduce the number of french fries she has at lunch and replace them with a more nutrient-dense vegetable such as carrot sticks or pepper slices. She could have juice instead of orange soda. She could have two cookies instead of three and replace the third cookie with a glass of lowfat milk. This will keep her energy intake the same but increase the nutrients she obtains.

Does Chevron's diet meet the iron needs of pregnancy without supplements? Her current diet provides 10.5 mg of iron—significantly less than the RDA of 27 mg per day for pregnant women.

• CHAPTER **15:** AT RISK FOR MALNUTRITION

Suggest some dietary changes that would increase Bobby's iron intake and absorption. To increase his iron intake, his food could be cooked in iron cookware, an extra serving of red meat might be included in spaghetti sauce or as a pizza topping, and dried fruit could be used for snacks. To increase iron absorption, Bobby could consume iron-containing foods with foods that are high in vitamin C. For instance, a snack of iron-fortified breakfast cereal consumed with a glass of orange juice would provide iron and enhance its absorption.

Suggest some activities you enjoyed as a child that would help Bobby to increase his activity level. He could try a family walk or a game of catch after dinner, a bike ride, a stroll to the park to play on the swings, or a weekend hike in the woods.

• CHAPTER **15:** LESS FOOD MAY NOT MEAN FEWER KCALORIES

How could she modify her original diet to reduce her energy intake, provide the essential nutrients she needs, and keep up her busy schedule? She could go back to her original breakfast, which is fast and easy. For lunch, she could have a turkey sandwich, apple, and a glass of milk but skip the chips. For a snack, she could have either the burger, the shake, or the fries, but not all three.

For dinner, if she has the ham sandwich from her original diet, she will be consuming less energy and more nutrients than she does with the candy bar and chips.

• CHAPTER **16:** AVERTING MALNUTRITION

How does Shirley's diet compare to the recommendations of the Food Guide Pyramid for people over 70? Her intake of grain products (particularly whole grains) and fruits and vegetables does not meet recommendations. These deficiencies make her fiber intake lower than recommended.

Suggest foods Shirley could add to improve her diet without increasing the time she spends cooking. She could switch to a vitamin B_{12}-fortified whole grain breakfast cereal. She could increase her intake of whole grains by having whole grain toast with breakfast. She could increase her fluid intake by including a glass of water at lunch and some herbal tea after dinner. She could increase her fluid and fruit intake by having a glass of fruit juice with breakfast. She could increase her vegetable intake by adding vegetables to the soup she has for lunch.

• CHAPTER **17:** ARE THESE CHOICES SAFE?

How might raw vegetables and fruit salad become contaminated? Because they are not cooked, bacteria that come in contact with them either directly or via cross-contamination will not be destroyed by cooking. Both fruits and vegetables can become contaminated with pathogens in the field or during transport. Produce may also become contaminated by cutting boards, knives, or other utensils that are used to prepare raw meats and not washed before being used for the fruits and vegetables.

After the party is over, what foods would you consider safe to keep as leftovers and what would you throw out? The fruit salad, raw vegetables, chips, crackers and cheese, and cookies would be the safest to keep. The cooked items that were left at room temperature for hours (lasagna, stuffed mushrooms, cheesecake, and talames) should be discarded, as should the chicken salad and onion dip.

• CHAPTER **17:** INDIVIDUAL RISK-BENEFIT ANALYSIS

What other changes can Rex make to minimize the risks associated with his family's typical diet while including foods that are beneficial? To decrease the risks associated with using raw eggs, he can advise his son that he does not need the protein shakes but that if he wants to drink them, he should use nonfat dry milk rather than raw eggs to increase the protein. He can have his daughter wait for the cookies to bake before tasting them. To decrease the risks associated with eating fish, he can try a wider variety of fresh and saltwater fish to avoid an excess of any one type. Because the risks of eating raw fish are greater, he can limit sushi to a rare treat purchased only from a restaurant that he knows buys the fish fresh daily. The pesticide risks from consuming produce are small compared with the benefits of a diet high in fruits and vegetables. To reduce the amounts of pesticides ingested, fruits and vegetables can be washed thoroughly or consumed without the skins. He can also reduce pesticide consumption by purchasing organic produce, but he must consider that it is more expensive. He can also buy locally grown produce and keep up his summer vegetable garden.

• CHAPTER 18: WHAT CAN YOU DO?

What impact will the following changes Keesha makes have on the environment? Bringing her juice in a thermos reduces the amount of garbage (packaging, disposable cups, etc.) she produces from her meals; composting reduces the amount of garbage sent to the dump; buying organically grown produce supports agricultural techniques that reduce the amount of chemical fertilizers and pesticides used; buying locally grown foods reduces the energy cost of transporting and storing produce grown at distant locations.

Suggest some other changes Keesha could make to decrease her impact on the environment? She could reduce energy use in her home by buying a timer for her household thermostat and water heater so they automatically turn down during the hours when no one is home. Modifying her diet to consume smaller portions of animal products would save energy because animal products cost more energy to produce than plant products. To reduce the amount of packaging, she could buy foods in larger containers and select products with less packaging. She could take her lunch to work in reusable containers rather than in disposable lunch bags.

Glossary

Absorption The process of taking substances from the gastrointestinal tract into the interior of the body.

Accidental contaminants Substances not regulated by the FDA that unexpectedly enter the food supply.

Accutane A drug that is used orally to treat severe acne. It is a derivative of vitamin A.

Acesulfame K (Acesulfame potassium) An artificial sweetener that contains no energy and is 200 times as sweet as sugar.

Acetylcholine A neurotransmitter that functions in the brain and other parts of the nervous system.

Acetyl-CoA A common intermediate consisting of a 2-carbon compound attached to a molecule of CoA that is produced from the metabolism of carbohydrate, fat, and protein.

Acid A substance that releases hydrogen ions (H^+) in solution.

Active transport The transport of substances across a cell membrane with the aid of a carrier molecule and the expenditure of energy. This may occur against a concentration gradient.

Acute Effects that develop rapidly.

Adaptive thermogenesis Adjustments in energy expenditure induced by factors such as changes in ambient temperature and food intake.

Adequate Intake (AI) A DRI value used as a goal for intake when no RDA can be determined. These values are an approximation of the average nutrient intake that appears to sustain a desired indicator of health.

ADI (Acceptable Daily Intake) The amount of a sweetener that can be safely consumed daily over a lifetime without adverse effects.

Adipocytes Fat-storing cells.

Adipose tissue Tissue found under the skin and around body organs that is composed of fat-storing cells.

Adolescent growth spurt An 18- to 24-month period of peak growth velocity that begins at about ages 10 to 13 in girls and 12 to 15 in boys.

Adrenaline A hormone secreted by the adrenal gland in response to stress that causes changes, such as an increase in heart rate, in preparation for "fight or flight"; also called epinephrine.

Aerobic exercise Exercise such as jogging, swimming, or cycling that increases heart rate and requires oxygen in metabolism. This type of exercise improves cardiovascular fitness.

Aerobic metabolism Metabolism requiring oxygen. In aerobic metabolism, glycolysis, the citric acid cycle, and the electron transport chain break down carbohydrates, fatty acids, and amino acids to carbon dioxide and water and produce ATP.

Aflatoxin An extremely potent carcinogen that is produced by a mold that grows on peanuts, corn, and grains.

Agar A polysaccharide extract of seaweed that is used in foods as an emulsifier, stabilizer, and gel.

Age-related bone loss Bone loss that occurs in both men and women as they advance in age.

AIDS (acquired immune deficiency syndrome) The syndrome caused by HIV infection that causes the immune system to fail, resulting in frequent recurrent infections that ultimately result in death.

Alcohol An energy-containing molecule that contains 7 kcalories per gram and is made by the fermentation of carbohydrates from plant products; the type of alcohol that is consumed in the diet is called ethanol.

Alcohol dehydrogenase An enzyme with activity in the stomach and liver that converts ethanol to acetaldehyde.

Alcoholic hepatitis Inflammation of the liver caused by alcohol consumption.

Alcohol-related birth defects *See* Fetal alcohol effects.

Aldosterone A hormone secreted by the adrenal glands that increases sodium reabsorption and therefore enhances water reabsorption by the kidney.

Alginate A polysaccharide extract of brown algae used in the processing of food, primarily dairy products.

Alimentary canal *See* Gastrointestinal tract.

Allergen A foreign substance, usually a protein, that stimulates an immune response.

Allergy An adverse reaction involving the immune system that results from exposure to a specific allergen.

Alpha-carotene A carotenoid, some of which can be converted into vitamin A, that is found in leafy green vegetables, carrots, and squash.

Alpha-linolenic acid An 18-carbon omega-3 polyunsaturated fatty acid known to be essential in humans.

Alpha-tocopherol (α-tocopherol) The only form of tocopherol (vitamin E) active in humans.

Alzheimer's disease A disease that results in the relentless and irreversible loss of mental function.

Amenorrhea Delayed onset of menstruation or the absence of three or more consecutive menstrual cycles.

Amino acid pool All of the amino acids in body tissues and fluids that are available for protein synthesis.

Amino acids The building blocks of proteins. Each contains a carbon atom bound to a hydrogen atom, an amino group, an acid group, and a side chain.

Amniotic fluid The liquid in the amniotic sac that surrounds and protects the fetus during development.

Amniotic sac A membrane surrounding the fetus that contains the amniotic fluid.

Amylopectin A plant starch that is composed of long branched chains of glucose molecules.

Amylose A plant starch that is composed of long unbranched chains of glucose molecules.

Anabolic Energy-requiring processes in which simpler molecules are combined to form more complex substances.

Anabolic steroids Synthetic fat-soluble hormones that mimic testosterone and are used by some athletes to increase muscle strength and mass.

Anaerobic metabolism or **anaerobic glycolysis** Metabolism in the absence of oxygen. In glycolysis, two molecules of ATP are produced from each molecule of glucose. Glucose is metabolized in this way when the blood cannot deliver oxygen to the tissues quickly enough.

Androstenedione A compound (known as Andro) that can be converted into testosterone and estrogen inside the body. It is a dietary supplement used by athletes to increase muscle mass and strength.

Anecdotal Information based on a story of personal experience.

Anemia A condition in which there is a reduced number of red blood cells or a reduced amount of hemoglobin, which reduces the oxygen-carrying capacity of the blood.

Angiotensin II A compound that causes blood vessel walls to constrict and stimulates the release of the hormone aldosterone.

Anisakis disease A disease caused by infection of the gastrointestinal tract with an Anisakis roundworm that contaminates raw fish.

Anorexia nervosa An eating disorder characterized by self-starvation, a distorted body image, and low body weight.

Antacid A drug used to neutralize acidity in the gastrointestinal tract.

Anthropometric measurements External measurements of the body, such as height, weight, limb circumference, and skinfold thickness.

Antibiotic A substance that inhibits the growth of or destroys microorganisms; used to treat or prevent infection.

Antibodies Proteins produced by cells of the immune system that destroy or inactivate foreign substances in the body.

Anticaking agent A substance added to dry food products to prevent clumping.

Anticarcinogen A compound that can counteract the effect of cancer-causing substances.

Anticoagulant A substance that delays or prevents blood coagulation.

Antidiuretic hormone (ADH) A hormone secreted by the pituitary gland that increases the amount of water reabsorbed by the kidney and therefore retained in the body.

Antioxidant A substance that is able to neutralize reactive oxygen molecules and protect the body from oxidative damage.

Antithiamin factors Substances in food that destroy the vitamin thiamin. Some are enzymes and are destroyed by cooking; others are not inactivated by cooking.

Anus The lower opening of the digestive tract through which the feces leave the body.

Apolipoprotein B A protein embedded in the outer shell of low-density lipoprotein (LDL) particles that binds to LDL receptor proteins on body cells.

Appetite The desire to consume specific foods that is independent of hunger.

Arachidonic acid A 20-carbon omega-6 polyunsaturated fatty acid that can be synthesized from linoleic acid.

Arginine A nonessential amino acid found in protein.

Ariboflavinosis The condition resulting from a deficiency of riboflavin.

Arteriole A small artery that carries blood to capillaries.

Artery A blood vessel that carries blood away from the heart.

Arthritis A disease characterized by inflammation of the joints, pain, and sometimes changes in structure.

Artificial sweetener A chemically manufactured sweetener that differs from simple sugars in chemical structure and often provides little or no energy when ingested.

Ascorbic acid The chemical term for vitamin C.

Aseptic processing A method that places sterilized food in a sterilized package using a sterile process.

Asparagine A nonessential amino acid found in protein.

Aspartame An artificial sweetener that is 200 times as sweet as sugar and is composed of the amino acids phenylalanine and aspartic acid.

Aspartic acid A nonessential amino acid found in protein.

Asthma A respiratory disorder characterized by wheezing and difficulty in breathing.

Atherosclerosis A type of cardiovascular disease that involves the buildup of fatty material in the artery walls.

Atoms The smallest units of an element that still retain the properties of that element.

ATP (adenosine triphosphate) The high-energy molecule used by the body to perform energy-requiring activities.

Atrophic gastritis An inflammation of the stomach lining that causes a reduction in stomach acid and allows bacterial overgrowth.

Attention deficit hyperactive disorder A condition that is characterized by a short attention span, a high level of activity, excitability, and distractibility.

Autoimmune disease A disease that results from immune reactions that destroy normal body cells.

Avidin A protein found in raw egg whites that binds biotin, preventing its absorption.

B

Bacteria (singular, **bacterium**) Tiny single-celled organisms found throughout the environment. Most are harmless or beneficial, but a few types can cause disease in humans.

Balance study A study that compares the total amount of a nutrient that enters the body with the total amount that leaves the body.

Basal Energy Expenditure (BEE) The amount of energy needed to keep an awake, resting body alive.

Basal Metabolic Rate (BMR) The rate at which energy is expended to keep an awake, resting body alive. It is measured after 12 hours without food or exercise.

Base A substance that accepts hydrogen ions in solution.

Bee pollen A mixture of pollen, bee saliva, and plant nectar that collects on the legs of bees; sold as an ergogenic aid.

Behavior modification A process used to gradually and permanently change habitual behaviors.

Benzocaine A local anesthetic used in some weight-loss products.

Beriberi A thiamin deficiency disease that is characterized by muscle weakness, loss of appetite, and nerve degeneration.

Beta-carotene (β-carotene) A pigment found in many yellow and red-orange fruits and vegetables that is a precursor of vitamin A.

Beta-cryptoxanthin A carotenoid found in corn, green peppers, and lemons that can provide some vitamin A activity.

Bile A substance made in the liver and stored in the gallbladder. It is released into the small intestine to aid in fat digestion and absorption.

Bile acids Emulsifiers present in bile that are synthesized by the liver from cholesterol.

Binge The consumption of a large amount of food in a discrete period of time associated with a feeling that eating is out of control.

Binge-eating disorder An eating disorder characterized by recurrent episodes of binge-eating in the absence of purging behavior.

Bioavailability A general term that refers to how well a nutrient can be absorbed and used by the body.

Bioelectric impedance analysis A technique for estimating body composition that measures body water by directing electric current through the body and calculating resistance to flow.

Biological value A measure of protein quality determined by comparing the amount of nitrogen retained in the body with the amount absorbed from the diet.

Biotechnology A set of techniques used to manipulate DNA for the purpose of changing the characteristics of an organism or creating a new product; also called genetic engineering.

Blood pressure The amount of force exerted by the blood against the artery walls.

Body mass index (BMI) An index of weight in relation to height that is used to compare body size with a standard; it is equal to body weight (in kilograms) divided by height (in meters squared).

Bolus A ball of chewed food mixed with saliva.

Bomb calorimeter An instrument used to determine the energy content of food. It measures the heat energy released when a food is combusted.

Bone remodeling The process whereby bone is continuously broken down and reformed to allow for growth and maintenance.

Botulism A severe food-borne intoxication that results from consuming the toxin produced by *Colostridium botulinum*.

Bovine somatotropin (bST) A hormone naturally produced by cows that stimulates the production of milk. A synthetic version of this hormone is now being produced by genetic engineering.

Bovine Spongiform Encephalopathy (BSE) A fatal neurological disease that affects cattle (Mad cow disease) and may be transmitted to humans by consuming beef by-products.

Bran The protective outer layers of whole grains. It is a concentrated source of dietary fiber.

Brewer's yeast The type of yeast used in brewing beer; a good source of B vitamins and often used as a nutritional supplement.

Brown adipose tissue A type of fat tissue that has a greater number of mitochondria than the more common white adipose tissue. It can waste energy by producing heat and is believed to be responsible for some of the change in energy expenditure in adaptive thermogenesis in rodents.

Brush border Refers to the microvilli surface of the intestinal mucosa, which contains some digestive enzymes.

Buffer A substance that reacts with an acid or base by picking up or releasing hydrogen ions to prevent changes in pH.

Bulimia nervosa An eating disorder characterized by the consumption of large amounts of food at one time (bingeing), followed by purging behavior such as vomiting and the use of laxatives to eliminate food from the body.

C

Caffeine A bitter white substance found in coffee, tea, chocolate, and other foods; a stimulant and a diuretic.

Calcitonin A hormone produced by the thyroid gland that stimulates bone mineralization and inhibits bone breakdown, thus lowering blood calcium levels.

Calorie The amount of heat required to raise the temperature of 1 g of water 1 degree Celsius; equal to 4.18 joules.

Calorimetry A technique for measuring energy expenditure.

Campylobacter jejuni A bacterium common in raw milk and undercooked meat that causes food-borne illness.

Cancer A disease characterized by cells that grow and divide without restraint and have the ability to grow in different locations in the body.

Capillaries Small, thin-walled blood vessels where the exchange of gases and nutrients between blood and cells occurs.

Caprenin An artificial fat made from a triglyceride containing poorly absorbed fatty acids; provides 5 kcal per gram.

Carbohydrate A compound containing carbon, hydrogen, and oxygen in the same proportions as in water; includes sugars, starches, and most fibers.

Carbohydrate loading See Glycogen supercompensation.

Carbon dioxide A waste product produced by cellular respiration that is eliminated from the body by the lungs.

Carcinogen A substance that causes cells to multiply out of control, eventually resulting in cancer.

Cardiorespiratory system The circulatory and respiratory systems which together deliver oxygen and nutrients to cells.

Cardiovascular Refers to the heart and blood vessels.

Cardiovascular disease Any disease affecting the heart and blood vessels.

Caries or **dental caries** Cavities, or decay of the tooth enamel caused by acid produced when bacteria growing on the teeth metabolize carbohydrate.

Carnitine A molecule that is needed to transport fatty acids and some amino acids into the mitochondria for metabolism. Supplements of carnitine are marketed to athletes to enhance performance.

Carotenoids Natural pigments synthesized by plants and many microorganisms. They give yellow and red-orange fruits and vegetables their color.

Carpal tunnel syndrome Numbness, tingling, weakness, and pain in the hand caused by pressure on the nerves.

Carrageenan A seaweed polysaccharide extracted from the algae Irish moss and used as a thickener mainly in dairy products.

Casein The predominant protein in cow's milk.

Cash crops Crops grown to be sold for monetary return rather than to be used for food locally.

Cassava A starchy root that is the staple of the diet in many parts of Africa.

Catabolic Refers to the processes by which substances are broken down into simpler molecules releasing energy.

Catalase An iron-containing enzyme that destroys peroxides.

Cataracts A disease of the eye that results in cloudy spots on the lens (and sometimes the cornea) which obscure vision.

Cell differentiation Structural and functional changes that cause cells to mature into specialized cells.

Cell membrane The membrane that encloses the cell contents.

Cells The basic structural and functional units of plant and animal life.

Cellular respiration The reactions that break down carbohydrates, fats, and proteins in the presence of oxygen to produce carbon dioxide, water, and energy in the form of ATP.

Cellulite Subcutaneous fat that has a lumpy appearance because strands of connective tissue connect it to underlying structures.

Cellulose An insoluble fiber that is the most prevalent structural material of plant cell walls.

Cephalic phase The phase of gastric secretion that is stimulated by the sight, smell, and taste of food.

Certified food color A food color that has been tested and certified for safety, quality, consistency, and strength of color.

Ceruloplasmin A copper-containing protein that converts iron to the ferric form, which can bind to iron storage and iron transport proteins.

Cesarean section The surgical removal of the fetus from the uterus.

Chemical bonds Forces that hold atoms together.

Chemical score A measure of protein quality determined by comparing the amount of the limiting amino acid in a food with that in a reference protein.

Chinese restaurant syndrome See MSG symptom complex.

Choice grade A USDA-regulated grade of beef with a modest amount of marbled fat.

Cholecalciferol The chemical name for vitamin D_3. It can be formed in the skin of animals by the action of sunlight on a form of cholesterol called 7-dehydrocholesterol.

Cholecystokinin (CCK) A hormone released by the duodenum that signals the pancreas to secrete digestive enzymes and causes the gallbladder to contract and release bile into the duodenum.

Cholesterol A lipid made only by animal cells that consists of multiple chemical rings.

Cholic acid A bile acid.

Choline A compound needed for the synthesis of the phospholipid phosphatidylcholine and the neurotransmitter acetylcholine. It is important for a number of biochemical reactions, and there is evidence that it is essential in the diet during certain stages of life.

Chromium picolinate A form of chromium sold as a supplement promoted to change body composition. Chromium is involved in insulin action, and supplements claim to increase lean body mass, decrease body fat, and delay fatigue. There is little evidence of their effectiveness as an ergogenic aid.

Chronic Effects that develop slowly over a long period.

Chylomicron A lipoprotein that transports lipids from the mucosal cells of the intestine and delivers triglycerides to other body cells.

Chyme A mixture of partially digested food and stomach secretions.

Chymotrypsin A protein-digesting enzyme produced in an inactive form in the pancreas and activated in the small intestine, where it aids digestion.

Circulatory system The organ system consisting of the heart, blood, and blood vessels, which transports material to and from cells.

Cirrhosis Chronic liver disease characterized by the loss of functioning liver cells and the accumulation of fibrous connective tissue.

Citric acid cycle Also known as the Krebs cycle or the tricarboxylic acid cycle, this is the stage of respiration in which 2 carbons of acetyl-CoA are broken down, producing carbon dioxide.

Clones Copies that are identical to the original.

Clostridium botulinum A bacterium that produces a deadly toxin and grows in a low-acid, low-oxygen environment, such as inside certain canned goods.

Clostridium perfringens A bacterium found in meat and poultry that can cause food-borne illness.

Coagulation The process of blood clotting.

Cobalamin The chemical term for vitamin B_{12}.

Coenzymes Small nonprotein organic molecules that act as carriers of electrons or atoms in metabolic reactions and are necessary for the proper functioning of many enzymes.

Cofactor An inorganic ion or coenzyme required for enzyme activity.

Colic A condition in young infants characterized by inconsolable crying. It is believed to be due to pain from gas buildup in the gastrointestinal tract or immaturity of the central nervous system.

Collagen The major protein in connective tissue.

Colon The largest portion of the large intestine.

Colostrum The first milk, which is secreted in late pregnancy and up to a week after birth. It is rich in protein and immune factors.

Complete dietary protein Dietary protein that provides essential amino acids in the proportions needed to support cellular protein synthesis.

Complex carbohydrates Carbohydrates composed of sugar molecules linked together in straight or branching chains. They include oligosaccharides, starches, and fibers.

Compression of morbidity The postponement of the onset of chronic disease so that disability occupies a smaller and smaller proportion of the life span.

Concentration gradient A condition that exists when the amount of a dissolved substance is greater in one area than it is in another.

Conception The union of sperm and egg (ovum) that results in pregnancy.

Condensation reaction A type of chemical reaction in which two molecules are joined to form a larger molecule and water is released.

Conditionally essential amino acid An amino acid that is essential in the diet only under certain conditions or at certain times of life; also called semiessential amino acids.

Connective tissue One of the four human tissue types; includes cartilage, bone, blood, adipose tissue, and the coverings of some organs.

Constipation Infrequent or difficult defecation.

Control group The group of participants in an experiment receiving no experimental treatment; otherwise, members of the control group are identical to the experimental group. A control group is used as a basis of comparison.

Cornea The clear, transparent fibrous outer coat of the eye.

Coronary heart disease A disease of the heart and blood vessels that supply blood to the heart.

Correlation Two or more factors occurring together.

Cortical bone Dense compact bone that forms the sturdy outer surface layer of bone.

Covalent bond A type of chemical bond formed when two atoms share a pair of electrons.

Creatine A compound that can be converted into creatine phosphate, which replenishes muscle ATP during short bursts of activity. Creatine is a dietary supplement used by athletes to increase muscle mass and delay fatigue during short intense exercise.

Creatine phosphate A high-energy compound found in muscle that can be broken down to make ATP.

Cretinism A condition resulting from deficient maternal iodine intake during pregnancy that causes stunted growth and poor mental development in offspring.

Criterion of adequacy A measure or outcome that can be examined to determine the biological effect of a particular level of nutrient intake; established for each nutrient and gender and life-stage group when developing Dietary Reference Intakes.

Critical control points Possible points in food production, manufacturing, and transportation where contamination could occur or be prevented or eliminated.

Critical periods Times in growth and development when an organism is more susceptible to harm from poor nutrition or other environmental factors.

Cross-contamination The transfer of contaminants from one food to another.

Cross-sectional data Information obtained by a single broad sampling of many different individuals in a population.

Crude fiber Fiber that remains after a food has been treated in the laboratory with acid and base. It consists primarily of cellulose and lignin.

Cyclamate An artificial sweetener that was common in the United States in the 1960s; banned after it was found to cause cancer in laboratory animals.

Cycle of malnutrition A cycle in which malnutrition is perpetuated by an inability to meet nutrient needs at all life stages.

Cysteine A conditionally essential sulfur-containing amino acid; when methionine is available in sufficient quantities, cysteine is not essential in the diet.

Cystic acne A chronic inflammatory disease of the skin in which cysts and nodules are common and scarring may occur.

Cytoplasm The cellular material outside the nucleus that is contained by the cell membrane.

D

Daily Reference Values (DRVs) Reference values established for protein and seven nutrients for which no original RDAs were established. The values are based on dietary recommendations for reducing the risk of chronic disease.

Daily Values Nutrient reference values used on food labels to help consumers see how foods fit into their overall diets.

DASH diet A dietary pattern that is plentiful in fruits and vegetables and lowfat dairy products and therefore high in potassium, magnesium, calcium, and fiber, and low in saturated fat and cholesterol.

Deamination The removal of the amino group from an amino acid.

Dehydration A condition that results when the output of water exceeds water input, due to either low water intake or excessive loss.

Delaney Clause A clause added to the 1958 Food Additives Amendment of the Pure Food and Drug Act that prohibits the intentional addition to foods of any compound that has been shown to induce cancer in animals or humans at any dose.

Dementia A deterioration of mental state resulting in impaired memory, thinking, and/or judgment.

Denaturation The alteration of a protein's three-dimensional structure.

Dental caries *See* Caries.

Deoxyribose The 5-carbon sugar that is part of DNA.

Depletion-repletion study A study that feeds subjects a diet devoid of a nutrient until signs of deficiency appear, and then adds the nutrient back to the diet to a level at which symptoms disappear.

Dermatitis An inflammation of the skin.

DHA *See* Docosahexaenoic acid.

DHEA (dehydroepiandosterone) A precursor of the sex hormones testosterone, estrogen, and progesterone; sold as a dietary supplement to slow aging and to increase muscle mass.

Diabetes mellitus A disease of carbohydrate metabolism caused by either insufficient insulin production or decreased sensitivity of cells to insulin. It results in elevated blood glucose levels.

Diacylglycerol or **diglyceride** A molecule of glycerol with two fatty acids attached.

Diaphragm A muscular wall separating the abdomen from the thoracic cavity containing the heart and lungs.

Diarrhea An intestinal disorder characterized by frequent or watery stools.

Dicumarol An anticoagulant that was isolated from moldy clover.

Dietary fiber Nondigestible carbohydrates and lignins that are found intact in plants.

Dietary Folate Equivalent (DFE) The amount of folate equivalent to 1 µg of folate naturally occurring in food, 0.6 µg of synthetic folic acid from fortified food or supplements consumed with food, or 0.5 µg synthetic folic acid consumed on an empty stomach.

Dietary Guidelines for Americans A set of nutrition recommendations designed to promote population-wide dietary changes to reduce the incidence of nutrition-related chronic disease.

Dietary Reference Intakes (DRIs) A set of four reference values for the intake of nutrients and food components that can be used for planning and assessing the diets of healthy people in the United States and Canada.

Dietary supplement A product intended for ingestion in the diet that contains one or more of the following ingredients: vitamins, minerals, herbs, botanicals, or other plant-derived substance; amino acids; concentrates or extracts.

Diet history A dietary intake assessment method that collects information about dietary habits and patterns and combines methods such as 24-hour recall, food frequency, and a food diary in order to determine an individual's typical food intake.

Diet-induced thermogenesis *See* Thermic effect of food (TEF).

Diffusion The movement of molecules from an area of higher concentration to an area of lower concentration without the expenditure of energy.

Digestion The process of breaking food into components small enough to be absorbed into the body.

Digestive system The organ system responsible for the ingestion, digestion, and absorption of food and the elimination of food residues; includes the gastrointestinal tract as well as a number of accessory organs.

Digestive tract *See* Gastrointestinal tract.

Diglyceride *See* Diacylglycerol.

Dipeptide Two amino acids linked by a peptide bond.

Direct calorimetry A method of calculating energy use that measures the amount of energy released as heat.

Direct food additives Substances intentionally added to foods. They are regulated by the FDA.

Disaccharide A sugar formed by linking two monosaccharides.

Dissociate To separate two charged ions.

Diuretic A drug that promotes fluid excretion.

Diverticula Sacs or pouches that protrude from the wall of the large intestine.

Diverticulitis A condition in which diverticula in the large intestine become inflamed.

Diverticulosis A condition in which outpouchings (or sacs) form in the wall of the large intestine.

DNA (deoxyribonucleic acid) The genetic material found in the nucleus that codes for the synthesis of proteins.

Docosahexaenoic acid (DHA) A 22-carbon omega-3 polyunsaturated fatty acid found in fish that may be needed in the diet of newborns. It can be synthesized from alpha-linolenic acid.

Dolomite A calcium supplement composed of ground-up limestone.

Double-blind study An experiment in which neither the study participants nor the researchers know who is in a control or an experimental group.

Down syndrome A disorder caused by extra genetic material that results in distinctive facial characteristics, mental retardation, and other health problems.

Duodenum The upper segment of the small intestine that connects to the stomach.

E

Eating disorder A psychological disorder affecting eating behavior and the regulation of food intake or energy balance.

Eclampsia A life-threatening condition that may occur during pregnancy. It is characterized by high blood pressure, protein in the urine, convulsions, and coma.

Edema Swelling of body tissue due to the buildup of fluid in the intestitial space.

Eicosanoids Regulatory molecules that can be synthesized from omega-3 and omega-6 fatty acids.

Eicosapentaenoic acid (EPA) A 20-carbon omega-3 polyunsaturated fatty acid found in fish that can be synthesized from alpha-linolenic acid but may be essential in humans under some conditions.

Electrolytes Substances that separate in water to form positively and negatively charged ions. In nutrition this term refers to sodium, potassium, and chloride.

Electrons High-energy particles carrying a negative charge that orbit the nucleus of an atom.

Electron transport chain The final stage of cellular respiration in which electrons are passed down a chain of molecules to oxygen, forming water and producing ATP.

Elements Substances that cannot be broken down into products with different properties.

Elimination diet A diet that eliminates potential allergy-causing foods from an individual's diet. Used in conjunction with a food challenge to identify any foods that cause an allergic reaction.

Embryo The developing human from two to eight weeks after fertilization. All organ systems are formed during this time.

Empty kcalories A term that refers to foods that contribute energy but few other nutrients.

Emulsifier A substance with both water-soluble and fat-soluble portions that can break fat into tiny droplets and suspend it in a watery fluid.

Endocrine system Organ system composed of cells, tissues, and organs that secrete hormones to help control body functions.

Endoplasmic reticulum A cellular organelle involved in the synthesis of proteins and lipids and composed of a system of membranous tubules, channels, and sacs in the cytoplasm; rough endoplasmic reticulum has ribosomes on its outside surface.

Endorphin A chemical released by the brain during exercise that acts as a natural tranquilizer; may be the cause of the euphoria known as runner's high.

Endosperm The largest portion of a kernel of grain. It is primarily starch and serves as a food supply for the sprouting seed.

Endurance The length of time one can perform a task.

Energy The capacity to do work.

Energy balance A state in which body weight remains stable because the amount of energy consumed in the diet equals the amount expended.

Enrichment The addition of nutrients to a food to restore those lost in processing to a level equal to or higher than originally present.

Environmental Protection Agency (EPA) U.S. government agency responsible for determining acceptable levels of environmental contaminants in the food supply and for establishing water quality standards.

Enzymes Protein molecules that accelerate the rate of specific chemical reactions without being changed themselves.

Epidemiology The study of the interrelationships between health and disease and other factors in the environment or lifestyle of different populations.

Epiglottis A flap of cartilage that serves as a valve during swallowing to prevent food from passing into the lung passage.

Epinephrine A hormone secreted by the adrenal gland in response to stress that causes changes, such as an increase in heart rate, in preparation for "fight or flight"; also called adrenaline.

Epithelial tissue One of the four human tissue types; includes the cells that cover external body surfaces and line internal cavities and tubes.

Ergogenic aids Anything designed to increase work or improve performance.

Ergot A toxin produced by a mold that grows on grains, particularly rye.

Esophagus A portion of the gastrointestinal tract that extends from the pharynx to the stomach.

Essential amino acid An amino acid that cannot be synthesized by the human body in sufficient amounts to meet needs and therefore must be included in the diet.

Essential fatty acid A fatty acid that must be consumed in the diet because it cannot be made by the body or cannot be made in sufficient quantities to meet needs.

Essential fatty acid deficiency The condition that results when the diet does not supply sufficient amounts of the essential fatty acids.

Essential hypertension High blood pressure that has no obvious external cause.

Essential nutrients Nutrients that must be provided in the diet because the body either cannot make them or cannot make them in sufficient quantities to satisfy its needs.

Essential or **indispensable amino acids** Amino acids that cannot be synthesized by the human body in sufficient amounts to meet needs and therefore must be included in the diet.

Estimated Average Requirements (EARs) Intakes that meet the estimated nutrient needs (as defined by a specific indicator of adequacy) of 50% of individuals in a gender and life-stage group.

Estimated Energy Requirements (EER) The current DRI recommendations for energy needs. They predict the amount of energy needed to maintain energy balance in a healthy person of a defined age, gender, height, weight, and level of physical activity.

Estrogen A steroid hormone secreted by the ovaries and by the placenta that is involved in the maintenance of pregnancy and the maintenance and development of female sex organs and secondary sex characteristics.

Exchange Lists A system of grouping foods based on their carbohydrate, protein, fat, and energy content.

Excretory system Organ system involved in the elimination of metabolic waste products; includes the lungs, skin, and kidneys.

Experimental controls Factors included in an experimental design that limit the number of variables, allowing an investigator to examine the effect of only the parameters of interest.

Experimental groups Groups of participants in an experiment who are subjected to an experimental treatment.

Extracellular fluid The fluid located outside cells. It includes fluid found in the blood, lymph, gastrointestinal tract, spinal column, eyes, and joints, and that found between cells and tissues.

F

Facilitated diffusion The movement of substances across a cell membrane from an area of greater concentration to an area of lower concentration with the aid of a carrier molecule. No energy is required.

Fad bulimia A type of bulimia that is more a trend than a psychological disorder; binge episodes are typically less dramatic and emotional than those of a true bulimic and are common among teenagers and young adults who are concerned about a few extra pounds of body weight.

Failure to thrive The inability of a child's growth to keep up with normal growth curves.

Fallopian tubes (oviducts) Narrow ducts leading from the ovaries to the uterus.

Famine A widespread lack of access to food due to a disaster that causes a collapse in the food production and marketing systems.

Fasting hypoglycemia Low blood sugar that is not related to food intake; often caused by an insulin-secreting tumor.

Fat A lipid that is solid at room temperature; commonly used to refer to all lipids or specifically to triglycerides.

Fat-free mass Body mass composed of all tissue except adipose tissue.

Fatigue The inability to continue an activity at an optimal level.

Fat-soluble vitamin A vitamin that does not dissolve in water; includes vitamins A, D, E, and K.

Fatty acid A lipid made up of a chain of carbons linked to hydrogens with an acid group at one end.

Fatty liver The accumulation of fat in the liver.

Fatty streak A cholesterol deposit in the artery wall.

FDA See Food and Drug Administration.

Feces Body waste, including unabsorbed food residue, bacteria, mucus, and dead cells, which is excreted from the gastrointestinal tract by way of the anus.

Fermentation A process in which microorganisms metabolize components of a food and therefore change the composition, taste, and storage properties of the food.

Ferritin The major iron storage protein.

Fertilization The union of sperm and egg (ovum).

Fetal Alcohol Effects (FAE) Also called alcohol-related birth defects (ARBD) and refers to mild symptoms such as learning disabilities, behavioral abnormalities, and motor impairments seen in an infant whose mother consumed alcohol during pregnancy.

Fetal Alcohol Syndrome (FAS) A characteristic group of severe physical and mental abnormalities in an infant resulting from alcohol consumed by the mother during pregnancy.

Fetus The developing human from the ninth week after conception to birth. Growth and refinement of structures occur during this time.

Fiber Substances in food that are not broken down by the digestive processes in the human stomach and small intestine.

Fitness The ability to perform routine physical activity without undue fatigue.

Flexibility Range of motion.

Fluorhydroxyapatite A fluoride-containing mineral deposit in the tooth enamel that is resistant to acid.

Foam cell A cholesterol-filled white blood cell.

Food additives Substances that can reasonably be expected to become a component of a food during processing. The foods that may contain them and the amounts that may be present are regulated by the FDA.

Food and Drug Administration (FDA) U.S. government agency responsible for the safety and wholesomeness of all food except red meat, poultry, and eggs; also sets standards and enforces regulations for food labeling and for food and color additives.

Food-borne illness An illness that can be transmitted to humans through food or water.

Food-borne infection Illness produced by the ingestion of food containing microorganisms that can multiply inside the body and produce effects that are injurious.

Food-borne intoxication Illness caused by consuming a food containing a toxin.

Food challenge The introduction of foods into the diet one at a time to determine if allergy symptoms occur.

Food Code A set of recommendations published by the FDA for the handling and service of food sold in restaurants and other establishments that serve food.

Food diary Dietary intake assessment method in which the individual is asked to keep a record of all food and beverage consumed for a defined period.

Food disappearance study A method of determining the food use by a population in which the amount of food that leaves the marketplace provides an estimate of the amount of food used by the population.

Food frequency A dietary intake assessment method which obtains information about an individual's typical food consumption patterns.

Food Guide Pyramid A system of food groups developed by the USDA as a guide to the number of servings of different types of foods needed to provide an adequate diet and comply with current nutrition recommendations.

Food insecurity An inability to acquire appropriate foods in a socially acceptable way.

Food intolerance An adverse reaction to a food that does not involve the immune system.

Food processing Any alteration of food from the way it is found in nature.

Food self-sufficiency The ability of an area to produce enough food to feed its population.

Food shortage Insufficient food to feed a population.

Fortification A term used generally to describe the addition of nutrients to foods, such as the addition of vitamin D to milk.

Frame size An estimation of the proportion of body weight due to bone.

Free radical One type of highly reactive molecule that causes oxidative damage to cells.

Fructose A monosaccharide found in fruits and honey that is composed of six carbon atoms arranged in a ring structure; commonly called fruit sugar.

Functional fiber Isolated nondigestible carbohydrates that have been shown to have beneficial physiological effects in humans.

Functional foods Foods that provide health benefits.

G

Galactose A monosaccharide composed of six carbon atoms arranged in a ring structure; when combined with glucose, it forms the disaccharide lactose.

Gallbladder An organ of the digestive system that stores bile, which is produced by the liver.

Gastric juice A substance produced by the gastric glands of the stomach that contains pepsinogen and hydrochloric acid.

Gastric phase The phase of gastric secretion triggered by the entry of food into the stomach; involves the release of gastrin and the secretion of mucus, acid, and enzymes from the gastric glands.

Gastrin A hormone secreted by the mucosa of the stomach that stimulates the secretion of enzymes and acid in the stomach.

Gastrointestinal tract A hollow tube consisting of the mouth, pharynx, esophagus, stomach, small intestine, large intestine, rectum, and anus in which digestion and absorption of nutrients occur; also called the alimentary canal and digestive tract.

Gastroplasty A surgical procedure that staples the lower part of the stomach, decreasing the storage capacity and consequently the amount of food that can be consumed at one time; also called stomach stapling.

Gel A jelly-like suspension of a liquid in a solid system that is semisolid in consistency.

Gelatin A protein derived from collagen that is deficient in the amino acid tryptophan.

Gene A length of DNA that contains the instructions for making a protein.

Gene expression Refers to the events of protein synthesis in which the information coded in a gene is used to synthesize a protein.

Generally Recognized As Safe (GRAS) A group of chemical additives that are generally recognized as safe based on their long-standing presence in the food supply without obvious harmful effects.

Genetic engineering *See* Biotechnology.

Germ The embryo or sprouting portion of a kernel of grain. It contains vegetable oil, vitamins, and minerals.

Gestation The time between conception and birth, which lasts about nine months (or about 40 weeks) in humans.

Gestational diabetes A consistently elevated blood glucose level that develops during pregnancy and returns to normal after delivery.

Ginseng An herb used in traditional Chinese medicine; claims are made that it improves athletic performance and increases sexual potency.

Glucagon A hormone secreted by the pancreas that stimulates the breakdown of liver glycogen and the synthesis of glucose to increase blood sugar.

Gluconeogenesis The synthesis of glucose from simple noncarbohydrate molecules. Amino acids from protein are the primary source of carbons for glucose synthesis.

Glucose A monosaccharide that is the primary form of carbohydrate used to produce energy in the body. It is the sugar referred to as blood sugar.

Glutamic acid A nonessential amino acid that is found in protein and in monosodium glutamate (MSG).

Glutathione peroxidase A selenium-containing enzyme that protects the cell from oxidative damage by degrading reactive chemical species called peroxides.

Glycemic index A ranking of the effect that the consumption of a single carbohydrate-containing food has on blood glucose in relation to a reference carbohydrate such as white bread or glucose.

Glycemic response The rate, magnitude, and duration of the rise in blood glucose that occurs after a meal or food is consumed.

Glyceride The most common type of lipid; consists of one, two, or three fatty acids attached to a molecule of glycerol.

Glycerol A 3-carbon molecule that forms the backbone of triglycerides and phosphoglycerides; also used as a humectant in food.

Glycogen A carbohydrate made of many glucose molecules linked together in a highly branched structure. It is the storage form of carbohydrate in animals.

Glycogen supercompensation or **carbohydrate loading** A regimen of diet and exercise training, followed in preparation for endurance activities, that is designed to maximize muscle glycogen stores.

Glycolysis A metabolic pathway in the cytoplasm of the cell that splits glucose into two 3-carbon pyruvate molecules. The energy released is used to make two ATP molecules.

Goiter An enlargement of the thyroid gland that is caused by a deficiency of iodine.

Goitrogens Substances that interfere with the utilization of iodine or the function of the thyroid gland.

GRAS *See* Generally recognized as safe.

Growth hormone A hormone secreted by the pituitary gland that stimulates growth.

Guar gum A branched polysaccharide from guar plants used as an additive to increase the viscosity of food.

Gum A plant polysaccharide and its derivatives that can dissolve in water and swell to form viscous solutions.

Gum arabic A branched polysaccharide from acacia trees; it is colorless, odorless, and tasteless, and is used as an additive to increase the viscosity of food.

Gum tragacanth A branched polysaccharide from thorny shrubs that grow in the semidesert of the Near East; used as an additive to thicken foods and to stabilize emulsions.

H

Hazard Analysis Critical Control Point (HACCP) A food safety system that focuses on identifying and preventing hazards that could cause food-borne illness.

Health claim A statement made about the relationship between a nutrient or food and a disease or health condition.

Healthy People A set of national health promotion and disease prevention objectives for the U.S. population.

Heart attack A condition in which an artery supplying blood to the heart becomes blocked, cutting off blood flow and hence oxygen and nutrients to a segment of the heart muscle, resulting in tissue death.

Heartburn A burning sensation in the chest caused when acidic stomach contents leak into the esophagus through the gastroesophageal sphincter.

Heat cramp A muscle cramp caused by an imbalance of sodium and potassium as a result of excessive exercise without adequate fluid and electrolyte replacement.

Heat exhaustion Low blood pressure, rapid pulse, fainting, and sweating caused when dehydration decreases blood volume so much that blood can no longer both cool the body and provide oxygen to the muscles.

Heat stroke Elevated body temperature as a result of fluid loss and the failure of the temperature regulatory center of the brain.

Heimlich maneuver A procedure used to dislodge an object blocking an air passage; involves the application of sharp, firm pressure to the abdomen just below the rib cage.

Heme iron A readily absorbed form of iron found in animal products that is chemically associated with proteins such as hemoglobin and myoglobin.

Hemicellulose An insoluble fiber that is a structural component of plant cell walls.

Hemochromatosis An inherited condition that results in increased iron absorption and leads to iron deposits throughout the body and tissue damage.

Hemoglobin An iron-containing protein in red blood cells that binds and transports oxygen through the bloodstream to cells.

Hemolytic anemia A condition in which there is an insufficient number of red blood cells because many have burst open.

Hemorrhoids Swollen veins in the anal or rectal area.

Hemosiderin An insoluble iron-protein compound formed in the liver when the iron storage capacity of ferritin is exceeded.

Hepatic portal circulation The system of blood vessels that collects nutrient-laden blood from the digestive organs and delivers it to the liver.

Hepatic portal vein The vein that transports blood from the gastrointestinal tract to the liver.

Hepatitis Inflammation of the liver.

Herb The leaves, flowers, stems, roots, seeds, or any other part of a nonwoody seed-bearing plant that dies down to the ground after flowering.

Herbicide An agent that kills weeds.

Heterocyclic amines (HAs) A class of mutagenic substances produced when there is incomplete combustion of amino acids during the cooking of meats—for example, when meat is charred.

High-Density Lipoprotein (HDL) A lipoprotein that picks up cholesterol from cells so that it can be eliminated from the body. A low level of HDL increases the risk of cardiovascular disease.

High-fructose corn syrup A sweetener made from corn syrup that is composed of approximately half fructose and half glucose.

Histamine A substance produced by cells of the immune system as part of a nonspecific response that leads to inflammation.

HIV (Human Immunodeficiency Virus) A virus that infects cells of the immune system and eventually leads to AIDS.

Homeostasis A physiological state in which a stable internal body environment is maintained.

Homocysteine A sulfur-containing amino acid that is produced from the metabolism of methionine. Elevated blood levels increase the risk of cardiovascular disease.

Hormone A chemical messenger that is produced in one location, released into the blood, and elicits responses at other locations in the body.

Hormone sensitive lipase An enzyme present in adipose cells that responds to chemical signals by breaking down triglycerides into fatty acids and glycerol for release into the bloodstream.

Humectant A substance added to foods to retain moisture.

Hunger Internal signals that stimulate one to acquire and consume food.

Hydrochloric acid An acid secreted by the gastric glands of the stomach to aid in digestion.

Hydrogenation The process whereby hydrogens are added to the carbon-carbon double bonds of unsaturated fatty acids, making them more saturated.

Hydrogen peroxide A reactive oxygen-containing compound that can form free radicals and cause oxidative damage. It can be eliminated by the selenium-containing enzyme glutathione peroxidase.

Hydrolysis A type of reaction in which a large molecule is broken into two smaller molecules by the addition of water.

Hydrolyzed protein *See* Protein hydrolysate.

Hydroxyapatite A compound composed of calcium and phosphorus that is deposited in the protein matrix of bone to give it strength and rigidity.

Hyperactivity Overactive, excitable, distractible behavior that is characteristic of attention deficit hyperactive disorder.

Hypercarotenemia A condition caused by an accumulation of carotenoids in the adipose tissue, causing the skin to appear yellow-orange.

Hypertension Blood pressure that is consistently elevated to 140/90 mm of mercury or greater.

Hypoglycemia A symptomatic low blood glucose level, usually below 40 to 50 mg of glucose per 100 ml of blood.

Hypothalamus The region of the brain that monitors and regulates conditions and activities in the body, including food intake and energy expenditure.

Hypothermia A condition in which body temperature drops below normal. Hypothermia depresses the central nervous system, resulting in the inability to shiver, sleepiness, and eventually coma.

Hypothesis An educated guess made to explain an observation or to answer a question.

I

Ileocecal valve The structure that separates the ileum of the small intestine from the large intestine.

Ileum The 11-foot segment of the small intestine that connects the jejunum with the large intestine.

Immunization An injection of a killed or inactivated organism into the body to stimulate the immune system to develop antibodies against the active disease-causing organism.

Impaired glucose tolerance A fasting blood sugar level above the normal range but not high enough to be classified as diabetes (110–126 mg/dl).

Implantation The process that begins about a week after fertilization by which the developing ball of cells embeds in the uterine lining.

Incomplete protein A protein that is deficient in one or more of the amino acids required for protein synthesis in humans.

Indirect calorimetry A method of estimating energy use that compares the amount of oxygen consumed with the carbon dioxide expired.

Indirect food additives Substances that are expected to unintentionally enter foods during manufacturing or from packaging. They are regulated by the FDA.

Infant mortality rate The number of deaths during the first year of life per 1000 live births.

Inorganic Substances that contain no carbon atoms.

Inositol A compound that is often included in B vitamin supplements; functions as part of a phospholipid in the human brain but is not a dietary essential; also called myo-inositol.

Insensible losses Fluid losses that are not perceived by the senses, such as evaporation of water through the skin and lungs.

Insoluble fiber Fiber that, for the most part, does not dissolve in water. It includes cellulose, hemicelluloses, and lignin.

Insulin A hormone made in the pancreas that allows the uptake of glucose by body cells and has other metabolic effects such as stimulating the synthesis of glycogen in liver and muscle.

Insulin-dependent diabetes *See* Type 1 diabetes.

Integrated Pest Management (IPM) A method of agricultural pest control that reduces pesticide usage by integrating nonchemical and chemical techniques.

Intermediate-Density Lipoprotein (IDL) A lipoprotein produced by the removal of triglycerides from VLDLs, most of which are then transformed to LDLs.

International Unit (IU) A unit of measure used to express requirements of some vitamins.

Interstitial fluid The portion of the extracellular fluid located in the spaces between cells.

Interstitial space The fluid-filled spaces between cells.

Intervention study A study of a population in which there is an experimental manipulation of some members of the population and observations and measurements are made to determine the effects of this manipulation.

Intestinal microflora Microorganisms that inhabit the large intestine.

Intestinal phase The phase of gastric secretion that is begun by the entry of food into the small intestine.

Intracellular fluid The fluid located inside cells.

Intrinsic factor A protein produced in the stomach that is needed for the absorption of adequate amounts of vitamin B_{12}.

Ion An atom or group of atoms that carries a negative or a positive electrical charge.

Iron deficiency anemia A condition that occurs when the oxygen-carrying capacity of the blood is decreased because there is insufficient iron to make hemoglobin. It is diagnosed clinically when red blood cells are small and pale and hemoglobin is less than normal.

Irradiation A process of exposing foods to radiation to kill contaminating organisms and retard ripening and spoilage of fruits and vegetables.

Isoleucine An essential amino acid found in protein.

Isotope An alternative form of an element that has a different atomic mass, which may or may not be radioactive.

J

Jejunum The 8-foot-long section of the small intestine lying between the duodenum and the ileum.

Juvenile-onset diabetes *See* Type 1 diabetes.

K

Keratin A hard protein that makes up hair and nails.

Keratomalacia Advanced xerophthalmia, characterized by softening of the cornea and irreversible blindness.

Keshan disease A heart disease that occurs in an area of China where the soil is very low in selenium.

Ketones or **ketone bodies** Molecules formed when there is not sufficient carbohydrate to completely metabolize the acetyl-CoA produced from fat breakdown.

Ketosis High levels of ketones in the blood.

Kilocalorie (kcal) A unit of heat that is used to express the amount of energy provided by foods. It is the amount of heat required to raise the temperature of 1 kilogram of water 1 degree Celsius (1 kcalorie = 4.18 kjoules).

Kilojoule (kjoule or kJ) A measure of work that can be used to express energy intake and energy output. It is the amount of work required to move an object weighing 1 kilogram a distance of 1 meter under the force of gravity (4.18 kjoules = 1 kcalorie).

Kwashiorkor A form of protein-energy malnutrition in which only protein is deficient. It is most common in young children who are unable to meet their high protein needs with the available diet.

L

Lactase An enzyme located in the brush border of the small intestine that breaks the disaccharide lactose into glucose and galactose.

Lactation The production and secretion of milk by the mammary gland.

Lacteal A lymph vessel in the intestine that can accept large particles such as the products of fat digestion.

Lactic acid An end product of anaerobic metabolism and an additive used in food to maintain acidity or form curds.

Lactitol The sugar alcohol formed from lactose.

Lacto-ovo vegetarian One who eats no animal flesh but eats eggs and dairy products such as milk and cheese.

Lactose A disaccharide made of glucose linked to galactose that is found in milk.

Lactose intolerance The inability to digest lactose because of a deficiency of the enzyme lactase. It causes symptoms such as intestinal gas and bloating after dairy products are consumed.

Lacto-vegetarian One who eats no animal flesh or eggs but eats dairy products.

Large-for-gestational-age An infant weighing greater than 4 kg (8.8 lb) at birth.

Large intestine The portion of the gastrointestinal tract that includes the colon and rectum; some water and vitamins are absorbed, and bacteria act on food residues here.

Laxative A substance that eases the excretion of feces.

LDL receptor See Low-density lipoprotein receptor.

Lean body mass Body mass attributed to nonfat body components such as bone, muscle, and internal organs. It is also called fat-free mass.

Leavening agent A substance added to food that causes the production of gas, resulting in an increase in volume.

Lecithin A phosphoglyceride composed of a glycerol backbone, two fatty acids, a phosphate group, and a molecule of choline; often used as an emulsifier in foods.

Legume The starchy seed of plants that produce bean pods; includes peas, peanuts, beans, soybeans, and lentils.

Leptin A protein hormone produced by adipocytes that signals information about the amount of body fat.

Leptin receptors Proteins that bind the hormone leptin. In response to this binding, they trigger events that cause changes in food intake and energy expenditure.

Let-down A hormonal reflex triggered by the infant's suckling that causes milk to be released from the milk ducts and flow to the nipple.

Leucine An essential amino acid found in protein.

Life expectancy The average length of life for a population of individuals.

Life span The maximum age to which a member of a species can live.

Lignin An insoluble fiber responsible for the hard woody nature of plant stems.

Limiting amino acid The essential amino acid that is available in the lowest concentration in relation to the body's needs.

Linoleic acid An omega-6 essential fatty acid with 18 carbons and 2 double bonds.

Lipases Fat-digesting enzymes.

Lipid bilayer Two layers of phosphoglyceride molecules oriented so that the fat-soluble fatty acid tails are sandwiched between the water-soluble phosphate-containing heads.

Lipids Organic molecules, most of which do not dissolve in water, that provide energy and insulation and serve as precursors in the synthesis of certain hormones; include fatty acids, glycerides, phospholipids, and sterols.

Lipoic acid A coenzyme needed in the reaction that forms acetyl-CoA; not a dietary essential.

Lipoprotein lipase An enzyme that breaks down triglycerides into free fatty acids and glycerol; attached to the outside of the cells that line the blood vessels.

Lipoproteins Particles containing a core of lipids surrounded by a shell of protein and phospholipid.

Liposuction A procedure that suctions out adipose tissue from under the skin; used to decrease the size of local fat deposits such as on the abdomen or hips.

Locust bean gum A branched polysaccharide that is produced from the endosperm of the seed of the carob plant; used as an additive to increase viscosity in cheese products and sausages.

Longevity The duration of an individual's life.

Longitudinal data Information obtained by repeatedly sampling the same individuals in a population over time.

Low birth weight infant An infant born weighing less than 2.5 kg (5.5 lb).

Low-Density Lipoprotein (LDL) A lipoprotein that transports cholesterol to cells. Elevated LDL cholesterol increases the risk of cardiovascular disease.

Low-density lipoprotein receptor A protein on the surface of cells that binds to LDL particles and allows their contents to be taken up for use by the cell.

Low-input agriculture or **sustainable agriculture** Methods of producing food that leave the environment able to restore itself and continue to produce food for future generations.

Lumen The inside cavity of a tube, such as the gastrointestinal tract.

Lutein A carotenoid found in corn and green peppers that provides some protection against macular degeneration.

Lycopene A carotenoid that gives the red color to tomatoes. It cannot be converted to vitamin A.

Lymphatic system The system of lymph vessels and other lymph organs and tissues that drains excess fluid from the space between cells and provides immune function.

Lymph vessel or **lacteal** A tubular component of the lymphatic system that carries fluid away from body tissues. Lymph vessels in the intestine are known as lacteals and can transport large particles such as the products of fat digestion.

Lysosome A cellular organelle containing degradative enzymes.

M

Macrocytes Larger-than-normal mature red blood cells that have a shortened life span.

Macronutrients Nutrients needed by the body in large amounts. These include water and the energy-yielding nutrients carbohydrates, lipids, and proteins.

Macular degeneration Degeneration of a portion of the retina that results in a loss of visual detail and blindness.

Major minerals Minerals needed in the diet in amounts greater than 100 mg per day or present in the body in amounts greater than 0.01% of body weight.

Malnutrition Poor nutritional status resulting from a dietary intake either above or below that which is optimal.

Maltase An enzyme found in the brush border of the small intestine that breaks maltose into two molecules of glucose.

Maltose A disaccharide made of two glucose molecules linked together.

Mannitol The sugar alcohol formed from the sugar mannose.

Marasmus A form of protein-energy malnutrition in which a deficiency of energy in the diet causes severe body wasting.

Maturity-onset diabetes *See* Type 2 diabetes.

Maximal oxygen consumption or *VO_2 max* The maximum amount of oxygen that can be consumed by the tissues during exercise.

Maximum heart rate The maximum number of beats per minute that the heart can attain. It declines with age and can be estimated by subtracting age in years from 220.

Megaloblastic or *macrocytic anemia* A condition in which there are abnormally large immature and mature red blood cells and a reduction in the total number of red blood cells.

Megaloblasts Large immature red blood cells that are formed when developing red blood cells are unable to divide normally.

Melatonin A hormone involved in regulating the body's cycles of sleep and wakefulness. Levels decline with age. Supplements are claimed to boost antioxidant defenses, improve immune function, and slow aging.

Menaquinones The forms of vitamin K synthesized by bacteria and found in animals.

Menarche The onset of menstruation. It occurs normally in girls between the ages of 10 and 15.

Menopause Physiological changes that mark the end of a woman's capacity to bear children.

Menstruation The cyclic discharge of the uterine lining that, in the absence of pregnancy, occurs about every four weeks during the reproductive years of female humans.

Metabolism The sum of all the chemical reactions that take place in a living organism.

Metallothionein A protein that binds zinc and copper in intestinal cells and limits their absorption.

Methionine An essential sulfur-containing amino acid found in protein.

Methyl group A chemical group consisting of a carbon atom bound to three hydrogen atoms.

Micelles Particles formed in the small intestine when droplets of lipid are emulsified by bile acids.

Microbe An organism too small to be seen without a microscope; also called microorganism.

Microflora *See* Intestinal microflora.

Micronutrients Nutrients needed by the body in small amounts. These include vitamins and minerals.

Microorganism An organism such as a bacterium, too small to be seen without a microscope.

Microvilli Minute projections on the mucosal cell membrane that increase the absorptive surface area in the small intestine.

Mineral An element needed by the body in small amounts for structure and to regulate chemical reactions and body processes.

Miscarriage or *spontaneous abortion* Interruption of pregnancy prior to the seventh month.

Mitochondrion (*mitochondria*) The cellular organelle that is responsible for generating energy in the form of ATP via aerobic metabolism; the citric acid cycle and electron transport chain are located here.

Modified Atmosphere Packaging (MAP) A type of food packaging in which the gases inside the package are changed to control or retard chemical, physical, and microbiological changes.

Modified starch or *modified food starch* Starch that has been treated to enhance its ability to thicken or form a gel.

Molds Multicellular fungi that form a filamentous branching growth.

Molecular biology The study of cellular function at the molecular level.

Molecules Units of two or more atoms of the same or different elements bonded together.

Monoacylglycerol or *monoglyceride* A molecule of glycerol with one fatty acid attached.

Monosaccharide A single sugar molecule, such as glucose.

Monosodium glutamate (MSG) An additive used as a flavor enhancer, commonly used in Chinese food; made up of the amino acid glutamate bound to sodium.

Monounsaturated fatty acid A fatty acid containing one carbon-carbon double bond.

Morbidity The incidence or state of disease or disability.

Morbid obesity A condition in which an individual's body weight is 100 pounds (45.5 kg) above desirable body weight, or the body mass index is greater than 40.

Morning sickness Nausea and vomiting that affects many women during the first few months of pregnancy and that in some women can continue throughout the pregnancy.

mRNA (messenger RNA) A molecule that carries the information in a gene to ribosomes in the cytoplasm so proteins can be synthesized.

MSG symptom complex Symptoms of headache, flushing, tingling, burning sensations, and chest pain reported by some individuals after consuming monosodium glutamate (MSG); commonly referred to as Chinese restaurant syndrome.

Mucosa The layer of tissue lining the gastrointestinal tract and other body cavities.

Mucus A viscous fluid secreted by glands in the gastrointestinal tract and other parts of the body. It acts to lubricate, moisten, and protect cells from harsh environments.

Mutagen Any agent that causes a change in a cell's genetic material.

Mutations Changes in DNA caused by chemical or physical agents.

Myelin A soft, white fatty substance that covers nerve fibers and aids in nerve transmission.

Myocardial infarction Heart attack.

Myoglobin An iron-containing protein in muscle cells that binds oxygen.

Myo-inositol *See* Inositol.

N

National Health and Nutrition Examination Survey (NHANES) An ongoing set of surveys designed to monitor the overall nutritional status of the U.S. population; combines food consumption information with medical histories, physical examinations, and laboratory measurements.

National Organic Program A USDA program that provides guidelines and certification for organic food production.

Nervous system A system of nerve cells organized in message sending, message receiving, and information processing pathways.

Net protein utilization A measure of protein quality determined by comparing the amount of nitrogen retained in the body with the amount eaten in the diet.

Neural tube A portion of the embryo that develops into the brain and spinal cord.

Neural tube closure A developmental event in which neural tissue forms a groove and the sides fold together to form a tube; is completed about 28 days after fertilization.

Neural tube defect A defect in the formation of the neural tube that occurs early in development and results in defects of the brain and spinal cord such as anencephaly and spina bifida.

Neurotransmitter   A chemical substance produced by a nerve cell that can stimulate or inhibit another cell.

Niacin equivalent (NEs)   A unit used to express the amount of niacin present in food including that which can be made from its precursor, tryptophan. One NE is equal to 1 mg of niacin or 60 mg of tryptophan.

Nicotinamide   A form of niacin.

Nicotinamide adenine dinucleotide (NAD)   A coenzyme made from niacin that transports electrons.

Nicotinamide adenine dinucleotide phosphate (NADP)   A coenzyme made from niacin that is needed as an electron carrier in synthetic reactions.

Nicotinic acid   A form of niacin.

Nitrogen balance   A state in which nitrogen intake is equal to nitrogen excretion.

Nitrosamines   Carcinogenic compounds produced by reactions between nitrites and amino acids.

Nonessential or **dispensable amino acids**   Amino acids that can be synthesized by the human body in sufficient amounts to meet needs.

Nonheme iron   A poorly absorbed form of iron found in both plant and animal products that is not part of the iron complex found in hemoglobin and myoglobin.

Noninsulin-dependent diabetes   See Type 2 diabetes.

Nucleus   The central core of an atom, consisting of positively charged protons and electrically neutral neutrons. In cells, it is an organelle containing DNA.

Nursing bottle syndrome   Extreme tooth decay in the upper teeth resulting from putting a child to bed with a bottle containing milk or other sweetened liquid.

Nutrient density   A measure of the nutrients provided by a food relative to the energy it contains.

Nutrients   Chemical substances in foods that provide energy, structure, and regulation of body processes.

Nutrification   The process of adding one or more nutrients to commonly consumed foods with the goal of adding to the nutrient intake of a group of people.

Nutrition   A science that studies the interactions that occur between living organisms and food.

Nutritional assessment   The process of determining the nutritional status of individuals or groups for the purpose of identifying nutritional needs and planning personal health care or community programs to meet these needs.

Nutritional status   State of health as it is influenced by the intake and utilization of nutrients.

Nutrition support claims   Claims often included on the labels of dietary supplements that describe the relationship between a nutrient and a deficiency disease that could result if the nutrient were lacking in the diet.

Nutrition transition   The shift in dietary pattern from a diet high in complex carbohydrates and fiber to a more varied diet higher in fats, saturated fat, and sugar that occurs as incomes increase.

O

Obese   A condition characterized by excess body fat. It is defined as a body mass index of 30 kg/m^2 or greater, or a body weight that is 20% or more above the desirable body weight standard.

Obesity genes   Genes that code for proteins involved in the regulation of body fat. When they are abnormal, the result is abnormal amounts of body fat.

Oil   A lipid that is liquid at room temperature.

Oleic acid   A monounsaturated fatty acid with 18 carbons.

Olestra (sucrose polyester)   An artificial fat made of sucrose with fatty acids linked to it that cannot be digested or absorbed. It has been approved by the FDA for use in certain snack foods.

Oligosaccharides   Short chain carbohydrates containing 3 to 10 sugar units.

Omega-3 (ω-3) fatty acid   A fatty acid containing a carbon-carbon double bond between the third and fourth carbons from the omega end; includes alpha-linolenic acid found in vegetable oils and eicosapentaenoic acid (EPA) and docosahexaenoic acid found in fish oils.

Omega-6 (ω-6) fatty acid   A fatty acid containing a carbon-carbon double bond between the sixth and seventh carbons from the omega end; includes linoleic and arachidonic acid.

Opsin   A protein in the retina of the eye involved in the visual cycle.

Organ   A discrete structure composed of more than one tissue that performs a specialized function.

Organelles   Cellular organs that carry out specific metabolic functions.

Organic food   A food produced according to the production and handling standards established by the National Organic Program of the USDA.

Organic molecules   Substances that contain carbon atoms.

Osmosis   The passive movement of water across a membrane to equalize the concentration of dissolved solutes on both sides.

Osteoarthritis   The form of arthritis common in the elderly that is characterized by a wearing down of the joint surfaces and pain when the joint is moved.

Osteoblasts   Cells responsible for the deposition of bone.

Osteoclasts   Large cells responsible for bone breakdown.

Osteomalacia   A vitamin D deficiency disease in adults that causes weak bones and an increase in bone fractures.

Osteoporosis   A bone disorder characterized by a reduction in bone mass, an increase in bone fragility, and an increased risk of fractures.

Overnutrition   Poor nutritional status resulting from a dietary intake in excess of that which is optimal for health.

Overweight   A body mass index of 25 to 29.9 kg/m^2, or a body weight 10% to 19% above the desirable body weight standard.

Oviduct   See Fallopian tubes.

Ovum   The female reproductive cell.

Oxalates   Organic acids found in spinach, rhubarb, and other leafy green vegetables that can bind certain minerals and decrease their absorption.

Oxaloacetate   A 4-carbon compound derived from carbohydrate that combines with acetyl-CoA in the first step of the citric acid cycle.

Oxidation   The loss of electrons.

Oxidative damage   Damage caused by highly reactive oxygen molecules that steal electrons from other compounds, causing changes in structure and function.

Oxidative stress   A condition that occurs when there are more reactive oxygen molecules than can be neutralized by available antioxidant defenses. It occurs either because excessive amounts of reactive oxygen molecules are generated or because antioxidant defenses are deficient.

Oxidized LDL cholesterol   A substance formed when the cholesterol in LDL particles is oxidized by reactive oxygen molecules. It is key in the development of atherosclerosis because it is taken up by scavenger receptors on white blood cells.

Oxytocin   A hormone released by the posterior pituitary that stimulates the ejection or let-down of milk during lactation.

P

Palmitic acid   A saturated fatty acid containing 16 carbons.

Pancreas   An organ that secretes digestive enzymes and bicarbonate ions into the small intestine during digestion. It also secretes the hormones insulin and glucagon into the blood.

Pancreatic amylase A starch-digesting enzyme found in pancreatic juice.

Pancreatic juice The secretion of the pancreas containing bicarbonate to neutralize acid and enzymes for the digestion of carbohydrates, fats, and proteins.

Papain A protein-digesting enzyme found in papaya.

Para-aminobenzoic acid (PABA) A chemical that is part of the folic acid molecule but that alone has no vitamin activity and cannot be used by the body to synthesize folic acid; effective at blocking ultraviolet (UV) light and thus is used in topical sunscreens.

Parasites Organisms that live at the expense of others without contributing to the survival of the host.

Parathyroid hormone (PTH) A hormone secreted by the parathyroid gland that acts to increase blood calcium levels.

Parietal cells Large cells in the stomach lining that produce and secrete intrinsic factor and hydrochloric acid.

Partially hydrogenated vegetable oil Vegetable oil that has been modified by hydrogenation to decrease the number of unsaturated bonds, therefore raising the melting point and improving the storage characteristics.

Pasteurization The process of heating food products to kill disease-causing organisms.

Pathogen An organism capable of causing disease.

Peak bone mass The maximum bone density attained at any time in life, usually occurring in young adulthood.

Pectin A soluble fiber found in plant cell walls that forms a gel when mixed with acid and sugar.

Peer review Review of the design and validity of a research experiment by experts in the field of study who did not participate in the research.

Pellagra A niacin deficiency disease that is characterized by dermatitis, dementia, diarrhea, and, ultimately, death.

Pepsin A protein-digesting enzyme produced by the stomach. It is secreted in the gastric juice in an inactive form (pepsinogen) and activated by acid in the stomach.

Pepsinogen An inactive protein-digesting enzyme produced by gastric glands and activated to pepsin by acid in the stomach.

Peptic ulcer An open sore in the lining of the stomach, esophagus, or small intestine.

Peptide Two or more amino acids joined by peptide bonds.

Peptide bond A chemical linkage between the amino group of one amino acid and the acid group of another.

Periodontal disease A degeneration of the area surrounding the teeth, specifically the gum and supporting bone.

Peristalsis Coordinated muscular contractions that move food through the gastrointestinal tract.

Pernicious anemia An anemia resulting from vitamin B_{12} deficiency that occurs because dietary vitamin B_{12} cannot be absorbed due to a lack of intrinsic factor. If not treated with vitamin B_{12} injections, nerve damage will result.

Peroxide A reactive chemical that can form free radicals and cause cellular damage.

Pesticide A substance used to prevent or decrease damage to plants from insects and microorganisms.

pH A measure of the level of acidity or alkalinity of a solution compared to neutrality.

Pharynx A funnel-shaped opening that connects the nasal passages and mouth to the respiratory passages and esophagus. It is a common passageway for food and air and is responsible for swallowing.

Phenylalanine An essential amino acid found in protein that cannot be metabolized by individuals with phenylketonuria (PKU).

Phenylketone The product of phenylalanine breakdown produced when phenylalanine cannot be converted to tyrosine; when blood levels get too high, brain damage results.

Phenylketonuria (PKU) An inherited disease in which the body cannot metabolize the amino acid phenylalanine. If the disease is untreated, toxic by-products accumulate in the blood and cause mental retardation.

Phenylpropanolamine A stimulant used in some weight-loss aids to blunt appetite.

Phosphoglyceride A phospholipid composed of a glycerol backbone with two fatty acids and a phosphate group attached; mixes well with both watery and oily substances and is an important component of cell membranes.

Phospholipid A lipid containing a phosphate group.

Photosynthesis The metabolic process by which plants trap energy from the sun and use it to make sugars from carbon dioxide and water.

Phylloquinones The forms of vitamin K found in plants.

Phytic acid or **phytate** An inorganic phosphorus-containing compound found in seeds and grains that can bind minerals and decrease their absorption.

Phytochemical A substance found in plant foods that is not an essential nutrient but has health-promoting properties.

Phytoestrogen An estrogen-like molecule produced by plants.

Phytosterol Compound produced by plants that has a structure similar to cholesterol.

Pica An abnormal craving for and ingestion of unusual food and nonfood substances such as clay, laundry starch, and paint chips.

Placebo A fake medicine or supplement that is indistinguishable in appearance from the real thing. It is used to disguise the control and experimental groups in an experiment.

Placenta An organ produced from both maternal and embryonic tissues. It secretes hormones, transfers nutrients and oxygen from the mother's blood to the fetus, and removes wastes.

Plaque The cholesterol-rich material that is deposited in the blood vessels of individuals with atherosclerosis. It consists of cholesterol, smooth muscle cells, fibrous tissue and, eventually, calcium.

Platelet A cell fragment found in blood that is involved in blood clotting.

Polar A term used to describe a molecule that has a positive charge at one end and a negative charge at the other.

Polychlorinated biphenyls (PCBs) Carcinogenic industrial compounds that have found their way into the environment and, subsequently, the food supply. Repeated exposure causes them to accumulate in biological tissues over time.

Polycyclic aromatic hydrocarbons (PAHs) A class of mutagenic substances produced during cooking when there is incomplete combustion of organic materials—for example, when fat drips on a grill.

Polypeptide A chain of three or more amino acids joined together by peptide bonds.

Polysaccharides Complex carbohydrates containing many sugar units linked together.

Polyunsaturated fatty acid A fatty acid that contains two or more double bonds.

Postmenopausal bone loss The accelerated bone loss that occurs in women for about five years after estrogen production decreases.

Postmenopausal osteoporosis *See* Type I osteoporosis.

Precursor Inactive form of a substance that can be converted into the active form.

Preeclampsia A form of pregnancy-induced hypertension that causes an increase in blood pressure, edema, and protein in the urine.

Pregnancy-induced hypertension A spectrum of conditions involving a rise in blood pressure during pregnancy.

Premature or *preterm infant* An infant born before 37 weeks of gestation.

Premenstrual syndrome (PMS) A syndrome of mood swings, food cravings, bloating, tension and depression, headaches, acne, and anxiety, among other symptoms, that results from the hormonal changes during the days prior to menstruation.

Preservative A compound that prevents spoilage and extends the shelf life of a product by retarding chemical, physical, or microbiological changes.

Preterm infant *See* Premature infant.

Prime grade A USDA-regulated grade of beef with the largest amount of marbled fat.

Progesterone A female sex hormone needed for development and function of the uterus and mammary glands.

Programmed cell death The death of cells at specific predictable times.

Prolactin A hormone released from the anterior pituitary that stimulates the breasts to produce milk.

Pro-oxidant A substance that promotes oxidative damage.

Protein An organic molecule made up of one or more intertwining chains of amino acids.

Protein complementation The process of combining proteins from different sources so that they collectively provide the proportions of amino acids required to meet needs.

Protein digestibility-corrected amino acid score A measure of protein quality that is calculated by adjusting the amino acid score with a correction for digestibility.

Protein efficiency ratio A measure of protein quality determined by comparing the weight gain of a laboratory animal fed a test protein with the weight gain of an animal fed a reference protein.

Protein-Energy Malnutrition (PEM) A condition characterized by wasting and an increased susceptibility to infection that results from the long-term consumption of insufficient energy and protein to meet needs.

Protein hydrolysate or *hydrolyzed protein* A mixture of amino acids or amino acids and polypeptides that results when a protein is completely or partially broken down by treatment with acid or enzymes.

Protein quality A measure of how efficiently a protein in the diet can be used to make body proteins.

Protein-sparing modified fast A very-low-kcalorie diet of high protein content designed to maximize the loss of fat and minimize the loss of protein from the body.

Prothrombin A blood protein required for blood clotting.

Provitamin or *vitamin precursor* A compound that can be converted into the active form of a vitamin in the body.

Psyllium A plant product high in soluble fiber that is used in over-the-counter bulk-forming laxatives.

Puberty A period in life characterized by rapid growth and physical changes that ends in the attainment of sexual maturity.

Purging Behaviors such as self-induced vomiting and misuse of laxatives and diuretics used to rid the body of energy.

Pyloric sphincter A muscular valve that helps regulate the rate at which food leaves the stomach and enters the small intestine.

Pyridoxal phosphate The active coenzyme form of vitamin B_6.

Pyridoxamine A form of vitamin B_6.

Pyridoxine A form of vitamin B_6; a general name used to refer to vitamin B_6, including pyridoxal, pyridoxine, and pyridoxamine.

Pyruvate A 3-carbon molecule produced when glucose is broken down by glycolysis.

R

Raffinose An oligosaccharide found in beans and other legumes that cannot be digested by human enzymes in the stomach and small intestine.

Reactive hypoglycemia Low blood sugar that occurs an hour or so after the consumption of high-carbohydrate foods; results from an overproduction of insulin.

Recommended Dietary Allowances (RDAs) Intakes that are sufficient to meet the nutrient needs of almost all healthy people in a specific life-stage and gender group.

Rectum The portion of the large intestine that connects the colon and anus.

Reference Daily Intakes (RDIs) Reference values established for vitamins and minerals that are based on the highest amount of each nutrient recommended for any adult age group by the 1968 RDAs.

Refined Refers to the process whereby the coarse parts of foods are removed, leaving behind a product of more uniform composition.

Renewable resources Resources that are restored and replaced by natural processes and can therefore be used forever.

Renin An enzyme produced by the kidney that aids in the conversion of angiotensin to its active form, angiotensin II.

Rennin An enzyme produced by the stomach of infants and young children that acts on the milk protein casein to convert it to a curdy substance.

Reserve capacity The amount of functional capacity that an organ has above and beyond what is needed to sustain life.

Respiratory system Organ system that includes the lungs and air passageways involved in the exchange of oxygen from the environment with carbon dioxide waste from cells by way of the bloodstream.

Resting Energy Expenditure (REE) Energy expenditure at rest. It is measured after 5 or 6 hours without food or exercise.

Resting heart rate The number of times that the heart beats per minute while a person is at rest.

Resting Metabolic Rate (RMR) The rate of energy expenditure at rest. It is measured after 5 to 6 hours without food or exercise.

Retin-A A drug that is a vitamin A derivative used topically to treat acne.

Retinal The aldehyde form of vitamin A, which is needed for the visual cycle.

Retinoic acid The acid form of vitamin A, which is needed for cell differentiation, growth, and reproduction.

Retinoids The chemical forms of preformed vitamin A: retinol, retinal, and retinoic acid.

Retinol The alcohol form of vitamin A, which can be interconverted with retinal.

Retinol-binding protein A protein that is necessary to transport vitamin A from the liver to tissues in need.

Retinol Activity Equivalent (RAE) The amount of retinol, β-carotene, α-carotene, or β-crytoxanthin that must be consumed to equal the vitamin A activity of 1 μg of retinol.

Rhodopsin A light-sensitive compound found in the retina of the eye that is composed of the protein opsin loosely bound to retinal.

Ribose The 5-carbon sugar that is part of RNA.

Ribosome The cell organelle where protein synthesis occurs.

Rickets A vitamin D deficiency disease in children that is characterized by poor bone development due to inadequate calcium deposition.

Risk-benefit analysis The process of weighing the risk of ingesting a substance against the benefits it provides; if the risk is small and the benefits great, small amounts of this substance may be acceptable.

Risk factor A characteristic or circumstance that is associated with the occurrence of a particular disease.

RNA (ribonucleic acid) A single-stranded nucleic acid. It carries information in DNA from the nucleus to the cytoplasm, is a component of ribosomes, and delivers amino acids for protein synthesis.

Royal jelly The substance that is produced by worker bees to feed the queen; marketed as an ergogenic aid.

S

Saccharin An artificial sweetener used in diet products that contains no energy and is about 300 times sweeter than sugar.

Saliva A watery fluid produced and secreted into the mouth by the salivary glands. It contains lubricants, enzymes, and other substances.

Salivary amylase An enzyme secreted by the salivary glands that breaks down starch into smaller units.

Salivary glands The internal structures that secrete saliva at the sides of and below the face and in front of the ears.

Salmonella A bacterium that commonly causes food-borne illness.

Satiety The feeling of fullness and satisfaction caused by food consumption that eliminates the desire to eat.

Saturated fatty acid A fatty acid in which the carbon atoms are bound to as many hydrogens as possible and which therefore contains no carbon-carbon double bonds.

Scavenger receptor A protein on white blood cells that binds to oxidized LDL cholesterol, allowing it to enter the cell.

Scientific method The general approach of science that is used to explain observations about the world around us.

Scurvy A vitamin C deficiency disease.

Seasonal affective disorder A disorder characterized by depression and carbohydrate cravings during the fall and winter months.

Secondary lactase deficiency Lactase deficiency that occurs as a result of disease and may resolve after the disease has ended.

Secretin A hormone released by the duodenum that signals the pancreas to secrete bicarbonate ions and stimulates the liver to secrete bile into the gallbladder.

Select grade A USDA-regulated grade of beef with a medium amount of marbled fat.

Selectively permeable Describes a membrane or barrier that will allow some substances to pass freely but will restrict the passage of others.

Semiessential amino acid See Conditionally essential amino acid.

Semivegetarian One who avoids only certain types of meat, fish, or poultry; e.g., an individual who avoids all red meat but continues to consume poultry and fish.

Serotonin A neurotransmitter that functions in the sleep center of the brain.

Set point A level at which body fat or body weight seems to resist change despite changes in energy intake or output.

Sickle cell anemia An inherited disease in which hemoglobin structure is altered. Red blood cells containing the altered hemoglobin are sickle-shaped; rupture easily, causing anemia; and block small blood vessels, causing inflammation and pain.

Simple carbohydrates Carbohydrates known as sugars that include monosaccharides and disaccharides.

Simple diffusion The movement of substances from an area of greater concentration to an area of lower concentration. No energy is required.

Simplesse An artificial fat made from egg and milk proteins that contains about 1.3 kcalories per gram.

Simple sugar See Simple carbohydrates.

Single-blind study An experiment in which either the study participants or the researchers (but not both) are unaware of who is in a control or an experimental group.

Skinfold thickness A measurement of subcutaneous fat used to estimate total body fat.

Small-for-gestational-age An infant born at term weighing less than 2.5 kg (5.5 lb).

Small intestine A tube-shaped organ of the digestive tract where digestion of ingested food is completed and most of the absorption occurs.

Smooth muscle Involuntary muscles that cause constriction of the gastrointestinal tract, blood vessels, and glands.

Sodium bicarbonate A compound that is part of an important buffer system in pancreatic juice and in the bloodstream.

Sodium caseinate A form of the milk protein casein that is frequently used as a food additive.

Sodium-potassium ATPase An energy-requiring protein pump in the cell membrane that pumps sodium out of the cell and potassium into the cell.

Solanine A toxic substance naturally occurring in potatoes; inhibits the action of neurotransmitters.

Soluble fiber Fiber that either dissolves when placed in water or absorbs water. It includes pectins, gums, and some hemicelluloses.

Solutes Dissolved substances.

Solution A solvent containing a dissolved substance.

Solvent A fluid in which one or more substances dissolve.

Sorbitol A sugar alcohol formed from the sugar sorbose; used as a sweetener or humectant in food.

Sperm The male reproductive cell.

Sphincter A muscular valve that helps control the flow of materials in the gastrointestinal tract.

Spina bifida A neural tube defect in which part of the spinal cord is exposed through a gap in the backbone, causing varying degrees of disability.

Spontaneous abortion See Miscarriage.

Spores A dormant state of some bacteria that is resistant to heat but can germinate and produce a new organism when environmental conditions are favorable.

Sports anemia A temporary decrease in hemoglobin concentration that occurs during exercise training. It occurs as an adaptation to training and does not impair delivery of oxygen to tissues.

Stabilizer A substance added to food to stabilize its consistency.

Standards of identity Regulations that define the allowable ingredients, composition, and other characteristics of foods.

Staphylococcus A bacterium, commonly found in the nasal passages, that can contaminate food and cause food-borne illness.

Starch A carbohydrate made of many glucose molecules linked in straight or branching chains. The bonds that hold the glucose molecules together can be broken by the human digestive enzymes.

Starchyose An oligosaccharide found in beans and other legumes that cannot be digested by human enzymes in the stomach and small intestine.

Starvation The condition that occurs when insufficient food is ingested to maintain health.

Stearic acid An 18-carbon saturated fatty acid that, unlike other saturated fats, does not raise blood cholesterol levels.

Steroid hormone A hormone that is made from cholesterol; includes the male and female sex hormones.

Sterol A lipid that contains multiple ring structures.

Stomach A muscular pouchlike organ of the digestive tract that mixes food and secretes gastric juice into the lumen and the hormone gastrin into the blood.

Stroke A blood clot or bleeding in the brain that causes brain tissue death.

Stroke volume The volume of blood pumped by each beat of the heart.

Stunting A decrease in linear growth rate which is an indicator of the nutritional well-being in populations of children.

Subcutaneous fat Adipose tissue located under the skin which is not associated with a great increase in the risk of chronic diseases.

Subscapular The region just below the shoulder blade that is a common location for measuring skinfold thickness.

Subsistence crops Crops grown as food for the local population.

Sucralose An artificial sweetener that is about 600 times sweeter than sucrose; trichlorogalactosucrose. It is heat stable, and so can be used in baked products.

Sucrase An enzyme in the brush border of the small intestine that breaks sucrose into glucose and fructose.

Sucrose A disaccharide commonly known as table sugar that is made of glucose linked to fructose.

Sudden Infant Death Syndrome (SIDS or crib death) The unexplained death of infants, usually during sleep.

Sugar alcohol A sweetener that is structurally related to sugars but provides less energy than monosaccharides and disaccharides because it is not as well absorbed.

Sulfites Sulfur-containing compounds used as preservatives to prevent oxidation in dried fruits and vegetables and to prevent bacterial growth in wine.

Superoxide dismutase (SOD) An enzyme that protects the cell from oxidative damage by neutralizing superoxide radicals. One form of the enzyme requires zinc and copper for activity, and another form requires manganese.

Superoxide radical A type of reactive oxygen molecule that can form free radicals leading to oxidative damage. They can be neutralized by the enzyme superoxide dismutase.

Sustainable Refers to methods of using resources that prevents overuse of natural systems and allows the environment to be maintained indefinitely without a decline.

Sustainable agriculture *See* Low-input agriculture.

T

Tannins Substances found in tea and some grains that can bind certain minerals and decrease their absorption.

Taurine An amino acid found only in animal foods that is not used in protein synthesis but is necessary for nerve function and vision and the synthesis of bile acids;

made in the adult human in sufficient quantities but may be essential in premature infants.

Teratogen A chemical, biological, or physical agent that causes birth defects.

Testosterone A steroid hormone secreted by the testes that is involved in the maintenance and development of male sex organs and secondary sex characteristics.

Texturizer A substance added to food to change its texture.

Theory An explanation based on scientific study and reasoning.

Thermal distress A condition resulting from the inability of the body to dissipate heat as fast as it is produced.

Thermic effect of food (TEF) or diet-induced thermogenesis The energy required for the digestion, absorption, metabolism, and storage of food. It is equal to approximately 10% of daily energy intake.

Thiamin pyrophosphate The active coenzyme form of thiamin.

Threshold effect A reaction that occurs at a certain level of ingestion and increases as the dose increases. Below that level there is no reaction.

Thyroid gland A gland located in the neck that produces thyroid hormones and calcitonin.

Thyroid hormones Hormones produced by the thyroid gland that regulate metabolic rate.

Thyroid-stimulating hormone A hormone that stimulates the synthesis and secretion of thyroid hormones from the thyroid gland.

Tocopherol The chemical name for vitamin E.

Tolerable Upper Intake Level (UL) The maximum daily intake by an individual that is unlikely to pose risks of adverse health effects to almost all individuals in the specified life-stage and gender group.

Tolerances Allowable levels of pesticide residues in foods, set by the EPA.

Total Energy Expenditure (TEE) The sum of basal energy expenditure, TEF and the energy used in physical activity, regulation of body temperature, deposition of new tissue, and production of milk.

Total fiber The sum of dietary fiber and functional fiber.

Total parenteral nutrition (TPN) A method of providing complete nutrition without use of the gastrointestinal tract by infusing a nutrient-rich solution directly into the bloodstream.

Toxic The capacity to produce injury at some level of intake.

Toxin A substance with the ability to cause harm at some level of exposure; also called toxicant.

Trabecular bone The spongy bone that forms the inner bone lattice that supports the cortical shell.

Trace elements or trace minerals Minerals required in the diet in amounts less than 100 mg per day or present in the body in amounts less than 0.01% of body weight.

Transamination The process by which an amino group from one amino acid is transferred to a carbon compound to form a new amino acid.

Transcription The process of copying the information in DNA to a molecule of mRNA.

Trans fatty acid An unsaturated fatty acid in which the hydrogens are on opposite sides of the double bond.

Transferrin An iron transport protein in the blood.

Transit time The time between the ingestion of food and the elimination of the solid waste from that food.

Translation The process of translating the mRNA code into the amino acid sequence of a protein.

Treatment groups *See* Experimental groups.

Triacylglycerol or triglyceride The major form of lipid in food and the major storage form of lipid in the body. It consists of three fatty acids attached to a glycerol molecule.

Triceps Region at the back of the upper arm that is a common site for measuring skin-fold thickness.

Trichinosis The disease caused by infection with the roundworm *Trichinella spiralis* after eating undercooked contaminated pork or game meats; the juvenile form of this roundworm migrates to the muscles and causes flu-like symptoms and muscle pain and weakness.

Triglyceride *See* Triacylglycerol.

Trimester A term used to describe each third or three-month period of a pregnancy.

Tripeptide Three amino acids linked together by peptide bonds.

Tropical oils A term used in the popular press to refer to the saturated oils—coconut, palm, and palm kernel oil—that are derived from plants grown in tropical regions.

Trypsin A protein-digesting enzyme that is secreted from the pancreas in inactive form and activated in the small intestine.

Tuber The starchy underground storage organ of plants.

Tumor A growth of tissue that forms an abnormal mass that serves no physiological function.

Tumor initiator A substance that causes mutations and therefore may predispose a cell to becoming cancerous.

Tumor promoter A substance that stimulates a mutated cell to begin dividing.

Twenty-four-hour recall A dietary intake assessment method in which an interviewer asks an individual to recall all food and drink consumed for the past 24 hours.

Type 1 diabetes A disease that most commonly develops during childhood and is characterized by elevated blood glucose that results when insufficient insulin is produced by the pancreas; also called insulin-dependent diabetes and juvenile-onset diabetes.

Type 2 diabetes A disease that most commonly occurs in overweight adults and is characterized by elevated blood glucose resulting from an insensitivity of the cells to the action of insulin; also called noninsulin-dependent and maturity-onset diabetes.

Type I osteoporosis or **postmenopausal osteoporosis** A loss of bone serious enough to cause fractures; a disproportionate loss of trabecular bone related to the drop in estrogen that occurs with menopause.

Type II osteoporosis or **age-related osteoporosis** The loss of bone mass serious enough to cause fractures; occurs in both cortical and trabecular bone and is related to advanced age.

Tyrosine A conditionally essential amino acid; when phenylalanine is available in sufficient quantities, tyrosine is not essential in the diet.

U

Ubiquinone A compound that transports electrons in the electron transport chain but that is not essential in the diet; also called coenzyme Q.

UL *See* Tolerable Upper Intake Level (UL).

Ulcer An open sore.

Undernutrition Poor nutritional status resulting from a dietary intake below that which meets nutritional needs.

Underwater weighing A method that calculates body composition by comparing an individual's body weight while on land with his or her weight while submerged in water.

Underweight A body mass index of less than 18.5 kg/m², or a body weight 10% or more below the desirable body weight standard.

Unsaturated fatty acid A fatty acid that contains one or more carbon-carbon double bonds.

Urea A nitrogen-containing waste product from the breakdown of proteins that is excreted in the urine.

Urine A fluid produced by the kidneys consisting of metabolic wastes, excess water, and dissolved substances.

U.S. Department of Agriculture (USDA) U.S. government agency responsible for monitoring the safety and wholesomeness of meat, poultry, and eggs.

U.S. Recommended Daily Allowances (U.S. RDAs) Standard reference values for nutrients designed to be used on food labels; generally equal to the highest nutrient recommendations in any age or sex category from the published 1968 RDAs. Replaced by the RDIs.

Uterus A female organ for containing and nourishing the embryo and fetus from the time of implantation to the time of birth.

V

Variable A factor or condition that is changed in an experimental setting.

Vegan A pattern of food intake that eliminates all animal products.

Vegetarian One who eats either no animal products or limited categories of animal products.

Vegetarianism A pattern of food intake that eliminates some or all animal products.

Veins Vessels that carry blood toward the heart.

Venule A small vein that drains blood from capillaries and passes it to larger veins for return to the heart.

Very low birth weight infant An infant born weighing less than 1.5 kg (3.3 lb).

Very-Low-Density Lipoproteins (VLDLs) A lipoprotein assembled by the liver that carries lipid from the liver and delivers triglycerides to body cells.

Very-low-kcalorie diet A weight-loss diet that provides fewer than 800 kcalories per day.

Villi (villus) Fingerlike protrusions of the lining of the small intestine that participate in the digestion and absorption of foodstuffs.

Viruses Minute particles not visible under an ordinary microscope that depend on body cells for their metabolic and reproductive needs.

Visceral fat Adipose tissue deposited in the abdominal cavity around the internal organs. High levels are associated with an increased risk of heart disease, high blood pressure, stroke, diabetes, and breast cancer.

Vitamins Organic compounds needed in the diet in small amounts to promote and regulate the chemical reactions and processes needed for growth, reproduction, and the maintenance of health.

W

Warfarin An anticoagulant drug that acts by inhibiting the action of vitamin K. It is a derivative of dicumarol; also used as rat poison.

Water A molecule composed of two hydrogen atoms and one oxygen atom; essential nutrient needed by the human body in large amounts.

Water-soluble vitamin A vitamin that dissolves in water; includes the B vitamins and vitamin C.

Wear and tear hypothesis A hypothesis that proposes that the changes that occur with age result from the accumulation of cellular damage over time.

Weight cycling or **yo-yo dieting** The cycle of repeatedly losing and regaining weight.

Wheat germ oil An oil pressed from the germ of wheat that is sold as an ergogenic aid.

Whole wheat flour A flour that contains all components of the wheat kernel: the bran, the germ, and the endosperm.

X

Xanthan gum A plant extract used as a stabilizer in processed foods.

Xerophthalmia A spectrum of eye conditions resulting from vitamin A deficiency. It is characterized by a lack of mucus, which leaves the eye dry and vulnerable to cracking and infection; may lead to blindness.

Xylitol The sugar alcohol formed from the sugar xylose; used in sugarless gum.

Y

Yo-yo diet syndrome *See* Weight cycling.

Z

Zeaxanthin A carotenoid found in corn and green peppers that provides some protection against macular degeneration.

Zygote The cell produced by the union of sperm and ovum during fertilization.

Zoochemical A substance found in animals foods (*zoo* means animal) that are not essential nutrients but may have health-promoting properties.

Index

Dietary Reference Intakes: Recommended Intakes for Individuals: Carbohydrates, Fiber, Fat, Fatty Acids, and Protein

Life Stage Group	Carbohydrate (g/day)	Fiber (g/day)	Fat (g/day)	Linoleic Acid (g/day)	α-Linolenic Acid (g/day)	Protein (g/kg/day)	Protein (g/day)
Infants							
0–6 mo	60°	ND	31°	4.4°[†]	0.5°[‡]	1.52°	9.1°
7–12 mo	95°	ND	30°	4.6°[†]	0.5°[‡]	1.5	13.5
Children							
1–3 y	130	19°	ND	7°	0.7°	1.10	13
4–8 y	130	25°	ND	10°	0.9°	0.95	19
Males							
9–13 y	130	31°	ND	12°	1.2°	0.95	34
14–18 y	130	38°	ND	16°	1.6°	0.85	52
19–30 y	130	38°	ND	17°	1.6°	0.80	56
31–50 y	130	38°	ND	17°	1.6°	0.80	56
51–70 y	130	30°	ND	14°	1.6°	0.80	56
> 70 y	130	30°	ND	14°	1.6°	0.80	56
Females							
9–13 y	130	26°	ND	10°	1.0°	0.95	34
14–18 y	130	26°	ND	11°	1.1°	0.85	46
19–30 y	130	25°	ND	12°	1.1°	0.80	46
31–50 y	130	25°	ND	12°	1.1°	0.80	46
51–70 y	130	21°	ND	11°	1.1°	0.80	46
> 70 y	130	21°	ND	11°	1.1°	0.80	46
Pregnancy	175	28°	ND	13°	1.4°	1.1	RDA+25g
Lactation	210	29°	ND	13°	1.3°	1.1	RDA+25g

ND = not determined

°Values are AI (Adequate Intakes)

[†]Refers to all n-6 polyunsaturated fatty acids

[‡]Refers to all n-3 polyunsaturated fatty acids

Acceptable Macronutrient Distribution Ranges (AMDR) for Healthy Diets as a Percent of Energy

Age	Carbohydrate	Added Sugars	Total Fat	Linoleic Acid	α-Linolenic Acid	Protein
1–3 y	45–65	≤25	30–40	5–10	0.6–1.2	5–20
4–18 y	45–65	≤25	25–35	5–10	0.6–1.2	10–30
≥ 19 y	45–65	≤25	20–35	5–10	0.6–1.2	10–35

PA Values for Different Physical Activity Levels (Used to Calculate EER)

Age/Gender	Sedentary	Low Active	Active	Very Active
3–18 y				
Boys	1.00	1.13	1.26	1.42
Girls	1.00	1.16	1.31	1.56
≥ 19 y				
Men	1.00	1.11	1.25	1.48
Women	1.00	1.12	1.27	1.45